SUCCESS!
in
Dental Hygiene

[COMPLETE REVIEW]

Demetra Daskalos Logothetis, RDH, MS
Director and Professor, Dental Hygiene Program
University of New Mexico
Albuquerque, New Mexico

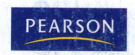

PEARSON

Upper Saddle River, New Jersey 07458

Library of Congress Cataloging-in-Publication Data

Logothetis, Demetra Daskalos
    Success! in dental hygiene / Demetra Logothetis.—1st ed.
    p.; cm.
    Includes bibliographical references and index.
    ISBN-13: 978-0-13-171751-0
    ISBN-10: 0-13-171751-0
    1. Dental hygiene—Examinations, questions, etc. I. Title.
    [DNLM: 1. Dental Care—United States—Examination
Questions. 2. Dental Care—United States—Outlines. 3. Dental
Hygienists—United States—Examination Questions. 4. Dental
Hygienists—United States—Outlines. WU 18.2 L832s 2009]
    RK60.5.L637 2009
    617.6′01076—dc22
                                                    2008027395

Notice: Care has been taken to confirm the accuracy of the information presented in this book. The author, editors, and the publisher, however, cannot accept any responsibility for errors or omissions or for the consequences of the application of the information in this book and make no warranty, express or implied, with respect to its contents.

The author and the publisher have exerted every effort to ensure that drug elections and dosages set forth in this text are in accord with current recommendations and practice at time of publication. However, in view of ongoing research, changes in government regulations, and the constant flow of information relating to drug therapy and drug reactions, the reader is urged to check the package inserts of all drugs for any change in indications of dosage and for added warnings and precautions. This is particularly important when the recommended agent is a new and/or infrequently employed drug.

The author and publisher disclaim all responsibility for any liability, loss, injury or damage incurred as a consequence, directly or indirectly, of the use and application of any of the contents of this volume.

Publisher: Julie Levin Alexander
Assistant to Publisher: Regina Bruno
Executive Editor: Mark Cohen
Associate Editor: Melissa Kerian
Assistant Editor: Nicole Ragonese
Media Editor: Amy Peltier
Development Editor: Alexis Breen Ferraro
Managing Production Editor: Patrick Walsh
Production Liaison: Christina Zingone
Production Editor: Jessica Balch, Pine Tree Composition
Manufacturing Manager: Ilene Sanford
Manufacturing Buyer: Pat Brown
Creative Design Director: Christy Mahon

Senior Art Director: Maria Guglielmo
Interior Design: Wanda España
Director of Marketing: Karen Allman
Executive Marketing Manager: Katrin Beacom
Media Project Manager: Stephen Hartner
Media Production: Red Frog
Director, Image Resource Center: Melinda Patelli
Manager, Rights and Permissions: Zina Arabia
Manager, Visual Research: Beth Brenzel
Image Permission Coordinator: Silvana Attanasio
Composition: Pine Tree Composition, Inc.
Printer/Binder: CJK
Cover Printer: Phoenix Color Corp.

Pearson® is a registered trademark of Pearson plc.

Pearson Education Ltd., London
Pearson Education Singapore, Pte. Ltd
Pearson Education Canada, Inc.
Pearson Education–Japan
Pearson Education Australia PTY, Limited

Pearson Education North Asia, Ltd., Hong Kong
Pearson Educación de Mexico, S.A. de C.V.
Pearson Education Malaysia, Pte. Ltd.
Pearson Education Upper Saddle River, New Jersey

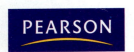

10 9 8 7 6 5 4 3 2 1
ISBN-13: 978-0-13-171751-0
ISBN-10:   0-13-171751-0

To my husband Nick, for his inspiration, encouragement, patience, and love. Forever thanks for being such an incredible person in my life.

To my beautiful children, Stacey and Costa, for the joy and happiness they bring.

Contents

Preface

SUCCESS! in Dental Hygiene is a review textbook designed to assist the dental hygiene student in preparing for the National Dental Hygiene Board Examination by offering an easy outline content format to study. This book is also an excellent tool for preparing students to take state or regional board examinations. It offers a comprehensive section on local anesthesia and pain control for students who must take a local anesthesia examination to become licensed to administer local anesthesia. Key topics that may be covered on the board examination are included in this book. With the easy-to-use outline format you can quickly indentify the important ideas, concepts, and facts that are presented. Important terms are defined where necessary, and illustrations are included where they will help illuminate and clarify information. The concept of the review book is to make it easier to understand information you have learned elsewhere in courses, from textbooks, and in the field. The purpose of the outline format is to help you focus your review on the most important information and use your study time effectively.

The textbook is designed to provide the most important information needed to take any dental hygiene board examination, and is organized based on the National Dental Hygiene Board Specifications with the intent to help students prepare for the exam, and understand the breakdown of the exam's contents. This is an important feature in the book, and different from any other dental hygiene review textbook. The textbook is divided into three sections according to the examination format. Secion I, Scientific Basis for Dental Hygiene Practice, encompasses all the basic science coursework. This is an important section for students to review since most students have taken some of these courses as prerequisites and will need to refresh or relearn some information. Section II, Provision of Clinical Dental Hygiene Services, includes information on assessing patient characteristics through comprehensive material on medical history review; head and neck examination; periodontal, oral, and occlusal evaluation; and clinical testing. It includes a complete radiology section along with x-rays to complement the text. Information on infection control, dental emergencies, patient education, pain control, and management of the medically compromised patient can be found in this section under planning and managing dental hygiene care. Section II also includes material on performing periodontal procedures, reassessment and maintenance, preventive agents, ethical and legal issues, and dental materials. Section III, Community Health and Research Principles, includes coursework related to community dental health and research methods.

SUCCESS! in Dental Hygiene is in outline format for easy reading and memorization. Key concepts (⚷) are provided throughout the text to assist the student in retaining important information necessary to be successful at passing the examination.

This textbook is excellent for refreshing the student's memory prior to board examinations on information they have already learned in an easy-to-use, "dental hygiene in a nutshell" format. However, I also encourage students to use this textbook at the beginning of their dental hygiene education to help study for exams and provide a continuous review of essential material leading up to the national, regional, or state board examinations.

Fifty multiple-choice study questions at the end of each chapter follow the format of questions that appear on the examination. Working through these questions after reviewing each chapter outline will help you assess your strengths and weaknesses in each topic of study. Correct answers and comprehensive rationales are included.

SUCCESS! in Dental Hygiene includes three simulated national board dental Hygiene Examinations, with rationales for the correct answers. Two simulated board examinations are included at the end of the text and the companion CD-ROM, and an additional, interactive examination is included on the CD-ROM only. These exams parallel the National Board Dental Hygiene Examination in test question content and length. This allows the student to work through each examination to determine their strengths and weaknesses.

Acknowledgments

I would like to express my sincere thanks to the many individuals who helped with this textbook. I would like to thank the contributors to this textbook for their hard work, perseverance, and attention to detail. A special thank you to Christine Nathe who always went above and beyond to assist me on this text, as well as with any of the Division's work, and to Gloria Lopez who works so hard for me granting me time to devote myself to projects such as this. Thank you to all the individuals who allowed me to use their pathology slides and x-rays in this text. A special thank you to Sandra Johnston who took many of the photos for the case studies, and to the junior dental hygiene students who allowed me to use photos from their patient cases. I would also like to thank all the reviewers for offering wonderful feedback and advice.

A sincere thank you to Mark Cohen, Executive Editor for Pearson Health Science, for his support and encouragement. Also to Melissa Kerian, Associate Editor, for all her help, and to Alexis Breen Ferraro, Developmental Editor Triple SSS Press Media Development, for keeping me on track with this project.

Demetra Daskalos Logothetis

About the Author

Demetra Daskalos Logothetis, RDH, MS, is the Director and Professor of the Dental Hygiene Program at the University of New Mexico (UNM). She has been a faculty member at UNM since 1986, and has served as Program Director since 1996. She received her Master of Science degree in Dental Hygiene Education and Administration from the University of Missouri–Kansas City. She co-developed the Master of Science in Dental Hygiene Degree Program at UNM, and has been on several committees for the development of the Collaborative Dental Hygiene Practitionier. She has served on several national dental hygiene committees, including Chair of the American Dental Education Association Council of Allied Program Directors and a member of the Western Regional Clinical Exam Subcommittee. She is an editor for *Contact International* (the official newsletter of the International Federation of Dental Hygienists), and on the review board for *Access* (a national magazine by the American Dental Hygienist's Association). She has received several faculty teaching excellence awards from the University of New Mexico, and was awarded the Outstanding Alumni Achievement Award from the University of Missouri–Kansas City, the Roy J. Reinhart Professional Excellence and Service Award from the University of Missouri–Kansas City School of Dentistry, and the University of New Mexico Distinguished Alumnus Award.

Introduction to the National Board Examination

PREPARATION, FORMAT, AND STRATEGIES

Three of the most stressful times for students pursuing a career in dental hygiene are waiting for confirmation that they have been accepted into a dental hygiene program, preparing to take the National Board Examination, and then waiting for confirmation that they have "passed" the examination.

This introduction is intended for dental hygiene students who are preparing to take the National Board Examination, as well as licensed hygienists who are faced with the formidable task of retaking the examination. Reasons for the latter include dental hygienists who have not practiced for a period of time or have moved to an area that requires passing scores from a current National Board Examination.

A major component of success for passing any examination is familiarity with the test itself. This introduction presents the reader with practical information about the examination, as well as helpful study hints, methods to develop a positive attitude, and strategies for overcoming test anxiety. All of these elements are essential to successfully passing the National Board Examination.

ADMINISTRATION OF THE EXAMINATION

The National Board Dental Hygiene Examination is administered by the Joint Commission on National Dental Examinations. This Commission is composed of 15 members who include representatives from dental schools, dental practices, state dental examining boards, dental hygienists, and the public. The examination is given to determine qualifications of dental hygienists who seek licensure for the practice of dental hygiene by assessing their ability to recall information from biomedical, dental, and dental hygiene sciences, as well as their ability to apply critical thinking skills in a problem-solving context.

ELIGIBILITY REQUIREMENTS

To take the National Board Dental Hygiene Examination, a candidate must qualify as a dental hygiene student or graduate of an accredited dental hygiene program. A dental hygiene student is eligible for examination when the dental hygiene program director certifies the student is within four months of anticipated graduation. Further information on eligibility requirements can be obtained in the *National Board Dental Hygiene Examination Candidate's Guide,* which is available by writing the Joint Commission on National Dental Examinations, 211 E. Chicago Avenue, Suite 1846, Chicago, IL 60611-2678 or by phone at (312)440-2678.

TESTING CANDIDATES WITH A DISABILITY

At the discretion of the Joint Commission, special arrangements may be made to enable a candidate with a disabling condition to be examined. To request special arrangements, the candidate must submit a request by the application deadline for the testing date the applicant has chosen. It is advised to make the request at least 90 days before the testing date, which will provide time to make special arrangements or provide additional information.

The applicant must provide with the request documentation of the disability and its effect on the candidate's ability to participate in National Board Examination under normal conditions. If the candidate is a student in an accredited dental hygiene program, a letter from a school official fulfills this requirement. Otherwise, a letter from a physician or other appropriate professional is required. The candidate should propose in the request the type of special arrangement needed. Special arrangements are approved to give the candidate an opportunity equivalent to other candidates, but not to provide an advantage over other candidates.

TESTING SCHEDULE

The testing schedule for the Dental Hygiene National Board Examination is listed in the *Candidate's Guide.* The examination is given three times a year. A deadline for application precedes each examination by five weeks. Seven and one half hours are allocated for the test. Candidates are to report to the testing center at 8:00 A.M., at which time instructions are given and the test materials distributed. The morning session begins at 8:30 A.M. and ends at noon. One hour is allocated for lunch. The afternoon session begins at 1:00 P.M. and the examination concludes at 5:00 P.M.

EXAMINATION FORMAT

The morning session of the examination, Component A, is composed of 200 stand-alone multiple-choice items. The afternoon session, Component B, consists of 150 multiple-choice items that refer to case-based studies. All of the questions consist of a stem, which poses the problem, and a set of possible answers. There can be as few as three possible answers or as many as eight options. There is only one *best* answer, although there may be several options that might also be correct. It is the candidate's responsibility to determine which choice answers the question in most cases, under most circumstances. Often detractors are given as choices, but are not the *best* selections. The topics are interspersed throughout the examination, with the exceptions of items pertaining to Community Dental Health. Those questions are included at the end of the morning session and are based on community dental scenerios, which the Commission refers to as testlets.

DISTRIBUTION OF ITEMS

Component A contains 200 items that include the Scientific Basis for Dental Hygiene Practice, Provision of Clinical Dental Hygiene Services, and Community Health. Five percent of the test items simultaneously address behavioral science; another 5% addresses professional responsibility, including ethics and risk management. The distribution of items is approximately as outlined below:

I. Scientific Basis for Dental Hygiene Practice (60)

    A. Anatomic sciences (15)

        1. Anatomy (11)

          a. Head and neck anatomy (6)

          b. Dental anatomy—Includes tooth morphology, eruption sequence, and occlusion (5)

            (1) General anatomy (2)

            (2) Root anatomy (3)

        2. Histology and embryology (4)

    B. Physiology—This content area can contain information on *anything* related to human physiology (4)

    C. Biochemistry and nutrition (7)

    D. Microbiology and immunology (11)

    E. Pharmacology (10)

    F. Pathology (13) (1*)

        1. General (5)

        2. Oral (7)

*Item is designated under the general topic

II. Provision of Clinical Dental Hygiene Services (120)

A. Assessing patient characteristics (16) (3*)

  1. Medical and dental history (3)

  2. Head and neck examination (1)

  3. Periodontal evaluation, including stains and deposits (6)

  4. Oral evaluation (2)

  5. Occlusal evaluation (1)

B. Obtaining and interpreting radiographs (14) (7*)

  1. Principles of radiophysics and biology (1)

  2. Principles of radiologic health (3)

  3. Technique (1)

  4. Recognition of normal and abnormal (2)

C. Planning and managing dental hygiene care (34)

  1. Infection control (4)

  2. Recognition of emergency situations and provision of appropriate care (5)

  3. Individualized patient education (11) (1*)

    a. Planning individualized instruction (3)

    b. Provision of instruction for prevention and management of oral diseases (7)

      (1) Dental caries (2)

      (2) Periodontal diseases (3)

      (3) Oral conditions (2)

  4. Anxiety and pain control (4)

  5. Recognition and management of compromised patients (3)

  6. Dental hygiene treatment strategies (4)

    a. Diagnosis (1)

    b. Treatment plan (2)

    c. Case presentation (1)

D. Performing periodontal procedures (19)

  1. Etiology and pathogenesis of periodontal disease (4)

  2. Prescribed therapy (10) (3)

    a. Periodontal debridement (5)

    b. Surgical support services (1)

    c. Chemotherapeutic agents (1)

  3. Reassessment and maintenance (i.e., implant care) (5)

E. Using preventive agents (9)

    1. Fluoride—systemic and topical (5)

      a. Mechanisms of action (1)

      b. Toxicology (2)

      c. Methods of administration (2)

        (1) Water fluoridation (1)

        (2) Self-administered (1)

    2. Sealants (3)

      a. Mechanisms of action (1)

      b. Techniques for application (2)

      c. Other preventive agents (1)

F. Providing supportive treatment services (7) (1*)

    1. Properties and manipulation of materials (3)

    2. Polishing natural and restored teeth (1)

    3. Making of impressions and preparation of study casts (1)

    4. Other supportive services (e.g., tooth desensitization) (1)

G. Professional responsibility (17) (1*)

    1. Ethical principles, including informed consent (8)

    2. Regulatory compliance (3)

    3. Patient and professional communication (5)

III. Community Health/Research Principles (24)

A. Promoting health and preventing disease in groups (5)

B. Participating in community programs (11)

    1. Assessing populations and defining objectives (5)

    2. Designing, implementing, and evaluating programs (6)

C. Analyzing scientific literature, understanding statistical concepts, and applying research results (8)

Each testlet presents a short scenario. The body includes two to three paragraphs. There are at least five multiple-choice questions based on each scenario, which are dependent on the main body. Each question has four to five responses, with one correct *best* response. The testlet topics may include, but are not limited to, a wide range of populations such as:

1. Geriatric

2. Medically compromised

3. Special needs

4. Preschoolers
5. Grade schoolers
6. Adolescents
7. Veterans and the military
8. Ethnic populations
9. Immigrant populations

Component B is composed of 150 items based on dental hygiene cases. There are between 10 and 15 items per case. The examination may include a case study of one of the following types of patients:

1. Geriatric
2. Adult-periodontal
3. Pediatric
4. Special needs
5. Medically compromised

The case studies address knowledge and skills required in assessing patient characteristics, obtaining and interpreting radiographs, planning and managing dental hygiene care, performing periodontal procedures, preventive agents, and supportive treatment.

TYPES OF QUESTIONS

Nine question formats are used in the National Board Examination. These question types are interspersed throughout the examination and vary in difficulty. The question formats include:

1. **Completion.** These questions pose a problem in the stem and the correct answer will complete the statement.

   Example: Carbohydrates may be stored in the body as

   a. fiber.   d. adipose tissue.
   b. glucose.   e. polysaccharides.
   c. glycogen.

2. **Question type.** This is composed of a question as the stem, followed by possible answers.

   Example: Which of the following are thick-walled vessels that are predominately elastic in nature?

   a. veins   d. arterioles
   b. venules   e. capillaries
   c. arteries

3. **Negative items.** These questions will be given in a negative format. They will contain such words as EXCEPT, NOT, or LEAST in the stem. These words will be listed in bold capital letters in the test booklet.

   Example: Each of the following is affected by saliva EXCEPT one. Which one is the EXCEPTION?

a. swallowing	d. protein digestion
b. dental caries	e. carbohydrate breakdown
c. oral microflora	

4. **Paired true/false.** These questions contain two sentences relating to the same topic. The candidate must decide whether each statement is true or false.

   Example: Protection from excessive exposure to radiation is aided by use of aluminum filters and a lead diaphragm. The filters reduce the soft radiation reaching the patient's face, and the diaphragm controls the area exposed.

   a. Both statements are TRUE.

   b. Both statements are FALSE.

   c. The first statement is TRUE, the second is FALSE.

   d. The first statement is FALSE, the second is TRUE.

5. **Cause and effect.** The stem contains a statement and a reason, which are written as a single sentence and connected by the word "because." The candidate must decide if the statement and reason are correct, and whether there is a causal relationship between them.

   Example: A tooth whose sealant has worn away requires an immediate restoration because this tooth is more susceptible to decay than a tooth that has never been sealed.

   a. Both statement and reason are correct and related.

   b. Both statement and reason are correct but not related.

   c. The statement is correct but the reason is not.

   d. The statement is NOT correct but the reason is an accurate statement.

   e. Neither the statement nor the reason is correct.

6. **Combination answers.**   These questions present a dual-part answer in a table or column form. Your answer is based on the combination of the items presented.

Example: Which of the following combinations is MOST likely to cause moderate fluorosis (without systemic toxicity)?

Concentration of Fluoride in Water (in ppm)	Age of Individuals (in years)
a. 0.5	2
b. 2	4
c. 3	6
d. 8	7
e. 10	8

7. **Sequencing questions.**   These items ask you to place steps in a procedure or chronology in the proper sequence.

Example: What are the stages of learning (from lower to higher) as depicted in the "Learning Ladder"?

(1) self-interest

(2) habit

(3) awareness

(4) unawareness

(5) involvement

(6) action

    a. 4, 3, 1, 5, 6, 2

    b. 4, 3, 5, 1, 6, 2

    c. 1, 3, 4, 5, 6, 2

    d. 1, 3, 5, 4, 6, 2

8. **Testlet** (Community Dental Health). These test items give a brief case study, or scenario, and base the question on the information presented.

Example: As she examines four classrooms of children, a dental hygienist uses an index designed to assess past and present dental caries. She notices that many of the children either presently have caries, or have had them in the past. These findings far exceed those reported by other researchers—both for the population being examined and for similar groups. Which of the following types of epidemiological investigations is the hygienist conducting?

    a. Analytical   d. Experimental

    b. Descriptive   e. Cross-sectional

    c. Prospective

Key to sample questions 1–8:

(1) c	(5) e
(2) c	(6) c
(3) d	(7) a
(4) a	(8) b

9. **Case-based items.** A case study of a patient is given with a synopsis of the patient's history, a clinical examination chart, radiographs, and clinical photographs. The patient's history will include the following information:

   - Synopsis of patient's history including age, gender, height, weight, and vital signs
   - Medical history: Under care of physician, hospitalizations, medical conditions, current medications, and pregnancy status
   - Dental history: Gingival bleeding, oral hygiene care, dental care, and dental concerns
   - Social history: Tobacco and alcohol use, unusual weight loss or gain, occupational and recreational information
   - Patient's chief complaint

   The clinical examination chart represents the patient's clinical findings. Restorations are not charted, but carious lesions may be charted. Periodontal probing depths and furcations are listed. Supplemental oral examination findings may include attrition, recession, plaque, and calculus deposits.

   Radiographs presented may be a complete mouth series, bitewings, or a panoramic film. The radiographs are labeled Right and Left and are of good quality. In addition to radiographs, photographs of study models may be given. Color photographs are utilized when needed.

PREPARING FOR THE EXAM

Simulate the Required Behavior

When studying for an examination, the most effective approach is to closely simulate the behavior you'll ultimately be required to perform. For example, if you're studying for the difficult National Dental Hygiene Board Examination, it's important that you practice answering difficult dental hygiene questions without access to your notes or textbook. Equally important, you need to practice answering questions that someone else has chosen. After all, you're not the one picking items for the exam, so asking yourself questions that you have made up on your own is usually a poor way to simulate the behavior called for on an exam. That is one of the reasons why the mock board examinations at the end of this textbook are so essential when preparing for the National Dental Hygiene Board Examination—they provide you with difficult practice items that someone else has written.

To prepare for this examination, one of the best study strategies is a two-tiered approach in which you study alone at first and study with others afterward. During the first phase, carefully review your notes and the textbook, perhaps creating flashcards to help you remember definitions, theories, and other important material. Then, once you feel confident of the material, study with one or more classmates. During this second phase, trade off asking each other questions without allowing the person who is answering to look at the textbook or any notes. If you are studying with more than one partner, just form a circle and rotate the role of question-asker.

This kind of studying is highly efficient because it allows others to pick the material, thereby exposing gaps in your knowledge (just as an exam does). Moreover, if the questions people ask are comparable in difficulty to exam questions, you'll be able to estimate your performance on the upcoming exam (e.g., if you can answer 80% of the study questions, you'll probably get about 80% correct on the exam). The only serious drawback to this method is that it can be a waste of time if you or your partners haven't finished studying all the material in advance. Group time should be reserved mainly for *practice*—not for review and discussion.

Spaced Practice Is Better than Massed Practice

Quite a bit of research suggests that spaced practice is generally superior to massed practice. For example, all things being equal, you'll get more mileage out of three 2-hour blocks than one 6-hour block, even though the total amount of time studying is identical in both cases. So if you have a particularly busy schedule and can only spend a few hours studying, be sure to use them well. Late-night cramming is usually a recipe for poor retention, mental and physical fatigue, and careless mistakes on the exam.

Don't Psych Yourself Out

It's been demonstrated that when you carry extra emotional baggage—"I've got to ace this exam" or "If I mess up, I'll never get to practice dental hygiene"—performance suffers, so don't lose the big picture. The most constructive approach is to focus on the task at hand, put in as much time studying as you can afford, and just do your best.

A certain amount of anxiety is normal (or even useful) when studying for an exam, but if you feel overwhelmed or feel that uncontrollable emotions are interfering with your exam performance, you may be suffering from test anxiety. If you think this is a possibility, you should take a course on text anxiety. The course may be able to recommend techniques to reduce your anxiety (e.g., relaxation training).

TAKING THE TEST

Look Over the Test and Pace Yourself

When you first get the exam, don't just plunge into answering test items. Instead, thumb through the pages and get the lay of the land. Once you've looked through the entire test, try to estimate what pace you should maintain in order to finish approximately 10 minutes before the period is over. That way, you'll have a little time at the end to check for careless mistakes like skipped questions or misread items.

Some of the worst problems occur when students enter a time warp and forget to check the clock, or when they spend too much time on one or two difficult items. To prevent this from happening, one trick you can use is to scribble the desired "finish time" time for each section right on the test booklet. That way, you'll be prompted to check the clock after completing each part of the exam.

Take Short Breaks

Try taking a few breaks during the exam by stopping for a moment, shutting your eyes, and taking some deep breaths. Periodically clearing your head in this way can help you stay fresh during the exam session. Remember, you get no points for being the first person to finish the exam, so don't feel like you have to race through all the items—even two or three 30-second breaks can be very helpful.

Don't Skip Around

Skipping around the exam can waste valuable time, because at some point you will have to spend time searching for the skipped questions and rereading them. A better approach is to answer each question in order. If you are truly baffled by a question, mark the answer you believe to be right, place a question mark next to the question, and come back to it later if you have time. Try to keep these flagged questions to a bare minimum (e.g., fewer than 10% of all items).

Don't Be Afraid to Change Your First Answer

Research has shown that changing answers on a multiple-choice or true–false exam is neither good nor bad: If you have a good reason for changing your answer, change it. The origin of the myth that people always change from "right" to "wrong" is that those (i.e., the wrong ones) are the only ones you will see when you review your exam—you won't notice the ones you changed from "wrong" to "right."

What to Do if More than One Answer Seems Correct

If you're utterly stumped by a question, here are some strategies to help you narrow the field and select the correct answer:

1. Ask how the two answers differ (just the answers, ignore the question); maybe jot down how the two answers differ. Then look at the question again and ask yourself, How is this difference important for this question? If you really think there's absolutely no difference between the two answers (e.g., just two words that mean the same thing), then look again at the answers you've eliminated—maybe one of them is actually the correct one. Read the question over separately with each separate answer. Cover up all the other answers as you read the question over separately with each specific answer. This reduces the

distracting effects of the wrong answers and can make it easier for you to see intuitively which answer makes better sense.

2. Ask yourself whether the answer you're considering completely addresses the question. If the test answer is only partly true or is true only under certain narrow conditions, then it's probably not the right answer. If you have to make a significant assumption in order for the answer to be true, ask yourself whether this assumption is obvious enough that the test constructor would expect everyone to make it. If not, it is most likely not correct.

3. If you think an item is a trick question, think again. Very few test constructors would ever write a question intended to be deceptive. If you suspect that a question is a trick item, make sure you're not reading too much into the question, and try to avoid imagining detailed scenarios in which the answer *could* be true. In most cases, "trick questions" are only tricky because they're not taken at face value.

Tips on Answering Multiple-Choice Questions

Tip #1: Read the question carefully before you begin eliminating answers. Make sure you understand what you are being asked and specifically look out for the word NOT in the question.

Tip #2: Make sure you read through every answer even if you are sure the first or second is correct.

Tip #3: As you go through each answer, cross through the ones that you know are incorrect. If you have four possible answers and you can eliminate two you've increased your odds for a correct answer to 50%.

Tip #4: One method for "guessing" as long as you are not penalized is to choose the longest answer choice.

Tip #5: A second method for "guessing" is to always choose the same answer for each question you're unsure of *unless* you are sure that answer is not correct.

Tip #6: Pay close attention to the grammar of the question so that it matches the answer you've chosen.

Tip #7: If opposite answers are given as choices, one of them is often the right answer.

Tip #8: Be careful of "all of the above" and "none of the above" questions. These are sometimes the correct choice but are also often used as a distractor to confuse students. Be sure the choices available pertain to the question. Sometimes correct statements are included that have nothing to do with the question you're working on. In a question with an "all of the above" choice, if you see at least two correct statements, then "all of the above" is probably the answer.

Tip #9: Beware of negatives. If a negative such as "none," "not," "never," or "neither" occurs in the question, then you're looking for a "catch". Read these carefully and be positive you understand the question. There will be an answer that matches even if your thinking is backwards.

Tip #10: Words such as "every," "all," "none," "always," and "only" are superlatives that indicate the correct answer must be an undisputed fact, and are less likely to be correct than ones that use conditional words like "usually" or "probably."

Tip #11: "Usually," "often," "generally," "may," and "seldom" are qualifiers that could indicate a true statement.

Tip #12: Answer the questions without assuming too much. Don't be led astray by overanalyzing. Read the question and assume all the information is there for a reason. Ask for clarification if needed.

Tip #13: Look for grammatical clues. If the stem ends with the indefinite article "an," for example, then the correct response probably begins with a vowel.

Tip #14: The longest response is often the correct one, because the instructor tends to load it with qualifying adjectives or phrases.

Tip #15: Look for verbal associations. A response that repeats key words that are in the stem is likely to be correct.

Tip #16: Use the test booklet to write helpful learning aids such as key phrases, tooth numbering systems, and mnemonics. Refer to them when needed.

Tip #17: Avoid making any stray marks on the answer sheet. It may be read as an answer.

Tip #18: Keep your answer sheet on a hard surface when recording your answers. Do not place it on top of the test booklet, as it may prevent your marks from being dark enough to be recorded.

Tip #19: NEVER leave a question blank. There are no penalties for incorrect answers. By leaving a question blank, you may also increase your chances of marking the wrong space.

Tip #20: Utilize all *positive* resources—1996 Pilot examination, instructors, mock Boards, study groups, and/or past graduates.

TEST ANXIETY

It is impossible not to experience some anxiety when preparing to take the National Board Examination. Knowing the format of the Board will help reduce some of that anxiety. One method of reducing stress is to take practice tests to determine your individual strengths and weaknesses.

Practice Tests

Many dental hygiene programs administer a "mock Board" to help students prepare for taking the National Board. It is important to remember that when taking a mock examination, the test needs to be realistic and comparable to the "real thing." This means that the mock Board should be taken within the same time parameters, have the same number of questions, follow the same format, and be given in a similar setting that the actual examination will be given (i.e., classroom or auditorium). It is ideal to take the mock examination in the same room that the Board will be given. There are two mock Board examinations at the end of this text, and one on the accompanying CD-ROM. Take these exams under the same time constraints as the actual Board exam, and grade your exam at the end. Review all missed questions to understand why you got the question wrong. For the questions you got correct, make sure you understand why the distractors are incorrect.

Recently the Joint Commission on Dental Examinations released an examination in the new format. It includes multiple-choice questions as well as case-based questions. The American Dental Association has released copies of the 1996 Pilot National Board Examination. This test is available to dental hygiene programs. The pilot examination was given to senior dental hygiene students nationwide to determine the validity and reliability of the examination. It is an abbreviated version of the actual examination, and is composed of 100 stand-alone multiple-choice items and 75 multiple-choice questions on the case-based studies. The pilot examination, therefore, is exactly half the length of the National Board. To make a mock Board examination totally realistic, it is necessary to add 100 stand-alone items and 75 more items for the case-based portion of the test. Representative-type questions to add might include those from previous course examinations that have been replaced. Case-based items can be found in some textbooks and are also available on CD and online (i.e., the Proctor and Gamble [P&G] case studies ae available on the Internet or provided by P&G at no charge to dental hygiene programs). These additional questions can be added to the pilot examination to complete the requisite number of items that appear on the National Board. It is important to review both of these released examinations prior to the examination. Contact the Commission on Dental Accreditation or ask your dental hygiene program director to assist you on obtaining copies of these examinations.

When taking a practice test or mock examination, it is imperative that the student have a complete 8 1/2-hour day without interruptions to complete the test. This will enable the student to experience not only the questions presented on the examination, but also the physical aspect of an examination of this caliber.

After the practice test has been taken, it should be graded with a key to determine the student's performance. It can then be determined which subjects are the student's strong or weak areas, and hence additional study time can be allocated based on the student's needs. It is also important to understand how the examination will be graded, using a conversion scale for final test scores.

Before the Examination

The day before the examination should be spent doing something enjoyable and calming. *This is not the time to cram for the examination.* Studying at the last minute may only confuse and panic the candidate. If possible, try to keep physically and mentally occupied. Try to get a good night's rest before the examination. On the morning of the examination, plan to eat a light, healthy breakfast. Surround yourself with *positive* thoughts and people before the test. Avoid being around any negative people. You need to be positive and enthusiastic as you take the test. Arriving at the test site in a relaxed, calm mood will help tremendously when taking the test as well. Your attitude, positive or negative, will be reflected in your test scores!

SCORING THE EXAMINATION

Two factors affect a candidate's scores: the number of items answered correctly and the conversion scale for the examination. In addition, if a test item is found to be defective, the Joint Commission will exclude the test item from scoring. Also, up to 15% of the items included in the test determine the standards of quality for the examination. These pretest items are not included in the scoring process and do not contribute to the candidate's scores. The conversion scale is based on the performance of a reference group. This group consists of all students enrolled in accredited dental hygiene programs who are examined for the first time.

A score of 75 is used as a passing score for the National Board Examination. This is not a raw score. This means that a candidate does not need to correctly answer 75% of all of the questions to pass the examination. The number of correct answers required is determined by the conversion scale. An average *raw score* of approximately 65% converts to a *standard score* of 80–85. Typically, less than 10% of all first-time candidates score below a 75. Over 90% pass!

Adequately preparing for the National Board Examination will enable the candidate to think positively, reduce anxiety, and become confident in test-taking. Remember, positive expectations bring positive results. All things come to those who go after them. If you can dream it, you can do it! Good luck!

EXAMINATION TIPS

The following are examination tips that will help you during the exam.

- Underline or circle the negative words in the test booklet when you come to them.
- Write T or F above each sentence in the test booklet. THEN select your answer. Avoid trying to answer the entire question before you determine the validity of each sentence.
- Underline or circle the word "because" in the test booklet. Determine if the statement (the first part of the question) is correct or incorrect; then determine if the reason (the part of the question that follows "because") is correct or incorrect. Write a T or F over each part of the question in the test booklet. THEN determine if the statements are related to each other and choose the correct answer.
- Determine what the question is asking (i.e., What concentration of fluoride will cause moderate fluorosis without systemic toxicity?) Use only the information you need. Avoid extraneous material; it can be confusing.

- Write the number of each step, starting with #1, and continue to the end. THEN select the answer by matching your order with the choices given.
- Determine WHAT the question is asking (What type of study is the hygienist using?). Use only material presented that is needed to answer the question. Avoid being confused by the other information given.

SUGGESTED READINGS, WEBSITES, AND PROFESSIONAL ORGANIZATIONS OF INTEREST TO DENTAL HYGIENISTS

Suggested Reading

Palmer, *Diet and Nutrition in Oral Health.* Prentice Hall, Upper Saddle River, New Jersey, 2007.

Weinberg; Westphal; Froum; Palat, *Comprehensive Periodontics for the Dental Hygienists.* Prentice Hall, Upper Saddle River, New Jersey, 2006.

Kimbrough; Henderson. *Oral Health Education.* Prentice Hall, Upper Saddle River, New Jersey, 2006.

Cooper; Wiechmann. *Essentials of Dental Hygiene: Preclinical Skills.* Prentice Hall, Upper Saddle River, New Jersey, 2005.

Cooper; Wiechmann. *Essentials of Dental Hygiene: Clinical Skills.* Prentice Hall, Upper Saddle River, New Jersey, 2005.

Madigan; Martinko; Parker, *Brock Biology of Microorganisms.* Prentice Hall, Upper Saddle River, New Jersey, 2003.

Johnson; Thompson, *Essentials of Dental Radiography.* Prentice Hall, Upper Saddle River, New Jersey, 2007.

Adams; Holland; Bostwick, *Pharmacology for Nurses: A Pathophysiologic Approach.* Prentice Hall, Upper Saddle River, New Jersey, 2005.

Rice, *Medical Terminology with Human Anatomy.* Prentice Hall, Upper Saddle River, New Jersey, 2008.

Nathe, Dental Public Health, *Contemporary Practice for the Dental Hygienist.* Prentice Hall, Upper Saddle River, New Jersey, 2005.

Websites

Academy of General Dentistry—http://www.agd.org

American Academy of Pediatric Dentistry—http://www.aapd.org

American Association of Dental Research—http://www.dentalresearch.org

American Association of Public Health Dentistry-—http://www.aaphd.org

American Dental Association—http://www.ada.org

American Dental Education Association—http://www.adea.org

American Dental Hygienists' Association—http://www.adha.org

American Public Health Association—http://www.apha.org

Anxiety Center (test anxiety)—http://www.healthyplace.com/communities/anxiety/treatment/test_strategies.asp

Association of Schools of Allied Health Professionals—http://www.www.asahp.org

Canadian Dental Association—http://www.cda-adc.ca

Canadian Dental Hygienists Association—http://www.cdha.ca

Canadian Public Health Association—http://www.cpha.ca

Centers for Disease Control and Prevention—http://www.cdc.gov

FDI World Dental Federation—http://www.fdiworlddental.org

Hispanic Dental Association—http://www.hdassoc.org

International Association for Dental Research—http://www.iadr.com

International Association for Disability and Oral Health—http://www.iadh.org

International Federation of Dental Hygienists—http://www.ifdh.org

National Center for Dental Hygiene Research—http://www.usc.edu/hsc/dental/dhnet

National Dental Hygienists' Association/National Dental Association—http://www.ndaonline.org

Oral Pathology (a reference site for oral pathology topics, people, places, and links)—http://www.oralpath.com

Oral Pathology Image Database—http://www.uiowa.edu/~oprm/AtlasHome.html

Special Care Dentistry—http://www.foscod.org

Study guides and strategies—http://www.studygs.net/tsttak1.htm

University of Illinois at Chicago, The Academic Center for Excellence (test anxiety)—http://www.uic.edudepts/conselctr/ace/testanxiety.htm

University of North Carolina, Counseling and Psychological Services (testing skills)—http://www.caps.unc.edu/testtake.html

University of Southern California (Oral Pathology)—www.usc.edu/hsc/dental/opath

World Health Organization—http://www.who.org

Contributors

Caren M. Barnes, RDH, MS
Coordinator of Clinical Research and Professor,
  Surgical Specialties
College of Dentistry
University of Nebraska Medical Center
Lincoln, Nebraska

Marsha L. Baltes, PhD
Adjunct Associate Professor
Indiana University School of Medicine
Instructor, Dental Hygiene
Indiana University–Purdue University
Fort Wayne, Indiana

Joseph E. Baughman, DDS
Supervising Dentist, Dental Hygiene
West Central College
Douglasville, Georgia

Barbara L. Bennett, CDA, RDH, MS
Division Director, Allied Health Programs
Program Chair, Dental Hygiene
Texas State Technical College
Harlingen, Texas

Linda D. Boyd, RDH, MS, RD
Associate Professor, Dental Hygiene
Idaho State University
Boise, Idaho

Jacqueline N. Brian, LDH, MS
Division of Dental Education
Indiana University–Purdue University
Fort Wayne, Indiana

Mary Danusis Cooper, LDH, MSEd
Division of Dental Education
Indiana University–Purdue University
Fort Wayne, Indiana

Charlene C. Goodwin, RDH, MSEd, MS
Assistant Professor, Dental Hygiene
Macon State College
Macon, Georgia

Emma Henderson, RDH, BS
Associate Faculty, Dental Hygiene
Indiana University–Purdue University
Fort Wayne, Indiana

Heather O. Mapp, RDH, MEd
Program Director, Dental Hygiene
Lanier Technical Institute/Gainesville College
Gainesville, Georgia

Christine Nathe, RDH, MS
Professor, Dental Hygiene
University of New Mexico
Albuquerque, New Mexico

Patricia J. Nunn, RDH, MS
Dean and Dental Hygiene Program Director
Utah College of Dental Hygiene
Orem, Utah

Phillip E. O'Shaughnessy, DDS, MSD
Assistant Professor, Emeritus
Indiana University School of Dentistry
Adjunct Associate Professor, Emeritus
Indiana University School of Medicine
Indiana University–Purdue University
Coroner, Allen County
Fort Wayne, Indiana

Carole A. Palmer, EdD, RD
Professor and Co-head, Nutrition
  and Preventive Dentistry
Tufts University School of Dental Medicine
Boston, Massachusetts

Frieda Atherton Pickett, RDH, MS
Adjunct Associate Professor, Dental Hygiene
East Tennessee State University
Johnson City, Tennessee

Jeffrey A. Platt, DDS, MS
Assistant Professor, Restorative Dentistry
Indiana University School of Dentistry
Indianapolis, Indiana

Betsy Reynolds, RDH, MS
Associate Clinical Professor
University of Colorado
Denver, Colorado

Michelle L. Sensat, RDH, MS
Assistant Professor, Dental Hygiene
College of Dentistry
University of Nebraska Medical Center
Lincoln, Nebraska

Marilyn J. Stolberg, DDS
Director, Dental Hygiene and Clinical
  Education
Ferris State University
Big Rapids, Michigan

Barbara J. Stubbs, RDH, MS
Assistant Professor, Dental Hygiene
Armstrong Atlantic State University
Savannah, Georgia

Ruth Fearing Tornwall, RDH, MS
Instructor IV, Dental Hygiene
Lamar Institute of Technology
Beaumont, Texas

Lauri Weichmann, RDH, MPA
Coordinator, Dental Hygiene
Carl Sandburg College
Galesburg, Illinois

Gail F. Williamson, RDH, MS
Professor, Dental Diagnostic Sciences
Oral and Maxillofacial Imaging
Department of Oral Surgery, Medicine
  and Pathology
Indiana University School of Dentistry
Indianapolis, Indiana

Reviewers

Susan Callahan Barnard, DHSc, RDH
Dental Hygiene Program Coordinator and
    Assistant Professor
Bergen Community College
Paramus, New Jersey

Kimberly S. Beistle, BA, RDH, MSA, CDA,
    PhD(c)
Program Coordinator, Dental Hygiene
Ferris State University
Big Rapids, MI

Barbara L. Bennett, CDA, RDH, MS
Division Director, Allied Health Programs
Program Chair, Dental Hygiene
Texas State Technical College
Harlingen, Texas

Linda D. Boyd, RDH, RD, EdD
Associate Professor, Dental Hygiene
Idaho State University
Boise, Idaho

Roderic Caron, DMD
Supervising Dentist
New Hampshire Technical Institute
Concord, New Hampshire

Alice S. Derouen, RDH, MEd
Director, Dental Hygiene Program
Horry-Georgetown Technical College
Conway, South Carolina

Mary Galagan, RDH, MHA
Instructor, Dental Hygiene
Pierce College
Lakewood, Washington

Marie Varley Gillis, RDH, MS
Associate Professor and Director,
    Dental Hygiene Program
Howard University
Washington, D.C.

Connie Grossman, MEd, RDH
Assistant Professor and Program Coordinator
Columbus State Community College
Columbus, Ohio

Kristyn Hawkins, LDH, BGS
Clinical Lecturer, Dental Hygiene
Indiana University South Bend
South Bend, Indiana

Pamela Karns, RDH, BSDH
Coordinator, Dental Hygiene Program
John A. Logan College
Carterville, Illinois

Nancy T. Keselyak, RDH, MA
Associate Professor, Dental Hygiene
University of Missouri–Kansas City
Kansas City, Missouri

Laura Mueller-Joseph, RDH, MS EdD
Chair, Dental Hygiene
Farmingdale State University of New York
Farmingdale, New York

Renee G. Prajer, RDH MS
Assistant Professor, Dental Hygiene
University of New Haven
West Haven, Connecticut

Judith E. Romano, RDH, MA
Department Chair, Dental Hygiene
Hudson Valley Community College
Troy, New York

Cindy Schroeder-Drucks, RDH, BS
Assistant Professor, Dental Hygiene
University of Medicine and Dentistry
    of New Jersey
Scotch Plain, New Jersey

Nancy Shearer, RDH, BS, MEd
Coordinator, Dental Hygiene Program
Cape Cod Community College
West Barnstable, Massachusetts

Barbara M. Sidel, RDH, MA
Instructor, Dental Hygiene
Delaware Technical and Community College
Dover, Delaware

Mea Weinberg, DMD, MSD, RPh
Clinical Associate Professor
New York University College of Dentistry
New York, New York

Andrea K. Westmoreland, RDH, MEd
Director, Dental Hygiene
Coastal Bend College
Beeville, Texas

Scientific Basis for Dental Hygiene Practice

1 Anatomical Science

Anatomical sciences encompasses the study of the morphology of the body at macroscopic and microscopic levels and illustrates how structure relates to function. Anatomical sciences are concerned with understanding the structural and functional relationships of the body's organ systems. A knowledge of anatomy provides the foundation for careers and research in dental and dental hygiene professions. An understanding of the complex relationships between structure and function is fundamental for research in the areas of neuroanatomy, reproductive and developmental biology, cell biology, biological anthropology, and comparative anatomy.

chapter objectives

After completion of this chapter, the learner should be able to:

➤ Identify normal bony anatomy of the head and neck region

➤ Identify the joints of the skull

➤ Identify paranasal sinuses

➤ Describe muscles of the head and neck region and muscles of mastication

➤ Describe blood supply to the head and neck

➤ Identify veins of the head and neck

➤ Describe the nervous system

➤ Describe the lymphatic system

➤ Identify salivary glands

➤ Discuss tooth morphology

➤ Describe eruption patterns

➤ Identify tissues of the oral cavity

➤ Discuss tooth development

➤ Describe dental anatomy and tooth morphology

➤ HEAD AND NECK ANATOMY

I. Anatomic Terminology

   A. Dorsal side—Backbone side (also called posterior)

   B. Ventral side—Belly side (also called anterior)

   C. Superior—Describes something that is on top, area that faces toward the head of the body

   D. Inferior—Describes something that is below, area that faces away from the head

   E. Midline—Vertical line dividing the center of the body

   F. Medial—Toward the midline

   G. Lateral—Away from the midline

   H. Frontal section—Slices through the frontal view of the head and neck (Figure 1-1■)

   I. Sagittal section—Slices through the sagittal view of the head and neck (Figure 1-2■), parallel with the median plane

   J. Transverse or cross section—Through the head (Figure 1-3■), horizontal plane

   K. Cranial—Pertaining to the head

   L. Cervical—Pertaining to the neck

   M. Superficial—Structures located toward the surface of the body

   N. Deep—Structures located inward, away from the body surface

   O. Internal—Inner side of the wall of a hollow structure

   P. External—Outer side of the wall of a hollow structure

   Q. Joint—Joining of two bones

   R. Ligaments—Strong connective tissue; hold bones together

II. Skull

   A. Cranium—Primarily involved in housing and protecting the brain

   B. Visceral structures—Related to the face

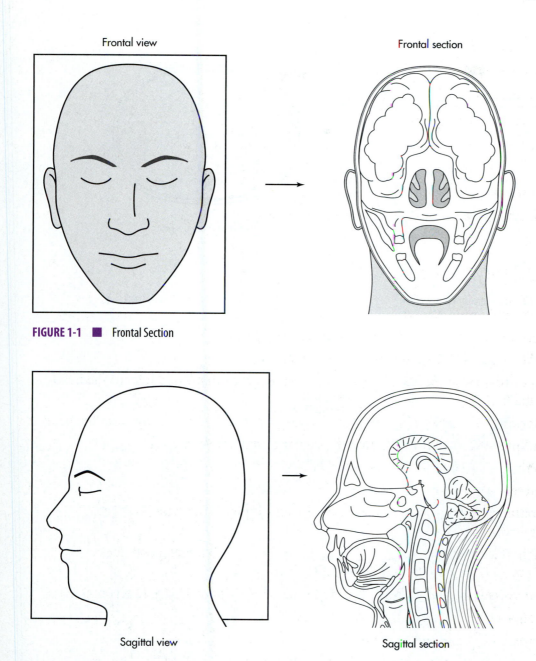

Frontal view

Frontal section

FIGURE 1-1 ■ Frontal Section

Sagittal view

Sagittal section

FIGURE 1-2 ■ Sagittal Section

III. Bones of the Neck

  A. Cervical vertebrae—Provide strong support for the neck and protective tunnel for important nerves and blood vessels; there are seven cervical vertebrae named by number (Figure 1-4■)

    1. c-1 "atlas"; holds up the cranium

    2. c-2 "axis"; medial protuberance allows rotation around it

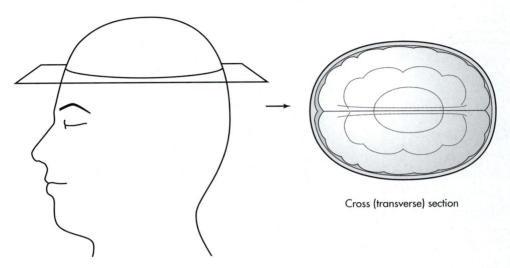

Cross (transverse) section

FIGURE 1-3 ■ Transverse or Cross Section

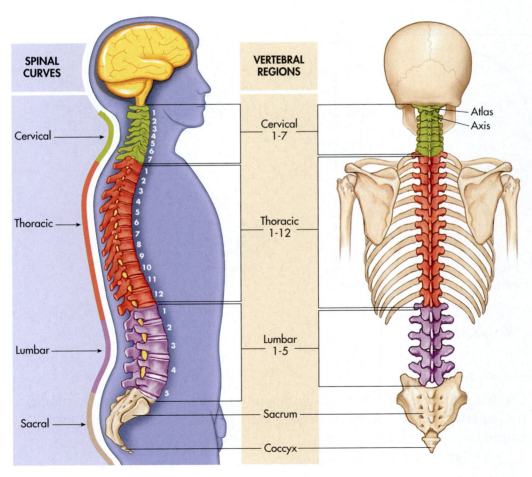

FIGURE 1-4 ■ Vertebral Column

    3. c-3

    4. c-4

    5. c-5

    6. c-6

    7. c-7

B. Hyoid bone—Bone of the neck; attached to several muscles but to no other bone (Figure 1-5■)

    1. Located in the anterior midline, superior to the thyroid cartilage

    2. Forms the base of the tongue and larynx

    3. U-shaped bone, free-floating bone

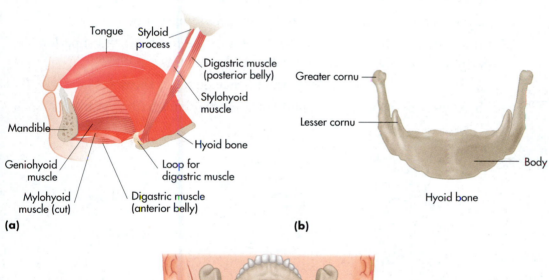

(a)

(b)

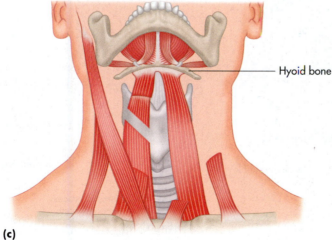

(c)

FIGURE 1-5 ■ Hyoid Bone

4. The mobility of the hyoid bone is necessary for mastication, swallowing, and speech

C. Skull (bones of cranium)

    1. Occipital bone—Single, large bone that forms the posterior, inferior portion of cranium; along its superior margin the occipital bone contacts the two pariental bones at the lambdoidal suture (Figure 1-6■); Figures 1-7b■ and 1-8■ present an inferior view of the skull showing the orientation of the occipital bone and its relationships with other bones in the floor of the cranium; the occipital bone contains:

        a. Foramen magnum—Provides passage for the large spinal cord as it exits the brain; hypoglossal canals transmit cranial nerve (CN) XII

        b. Occipital condyles (paired)—Located lateral to foramen magnum; forms a joint with the first cervical vertebra (atlas)

        c. Hypoglossal canals—Transmits cranial nerve (CN) XII

        d. Portion of jugular foramen—Forms with temporal bone

    2. Frontal bone—Single, large bone that forms the forehead and superior portion of the orbits (Figures 1-6 and 1-7); contains

        a. Supraorbital ridges—Bony prominence under eyebrows

        b. Zygomatic process of frontal bone—Articulates with zygoma

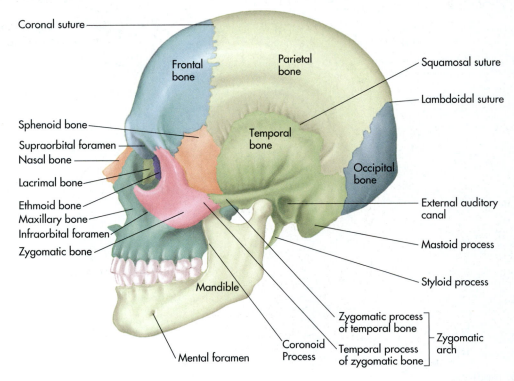

FIGURE 1-6 ■ Adult Skull Part I

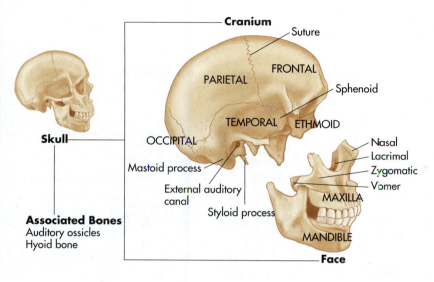

Cranium

Suture

FRONTAL

PARIETAL

Sphenoid

TEMPORAL ETHMOID

OCCIPITAL

Nasal
Lacrimal
Zygomatic
Vomer

Skull

Mastoid process

External auditory canal

Styloid process

MAXILLA

MANDIBLE

Associated Bones
Auditory ossicles
Hyoid bone

Face

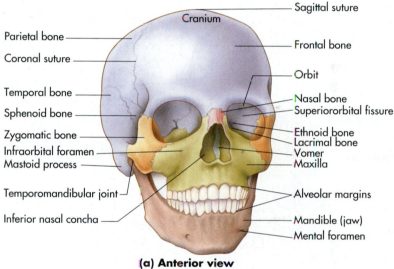

Sagittal suture

Cranium

Parietal bone

Frontal bone

Coronal suture

Orbit

Temporal bone

Nasal bone
Superiororbital fissure

Sphenoid bone

Zygomatic bone

Ethnoid bone
Lacrimal bone

Infraorbital foramen

Vomer

Mastoid process

Maxilla

Temporomandibular joint

Alveolar margins

Inferior nasal concha

Mandible (jaw)
Mental foramen

(a) Anterior view

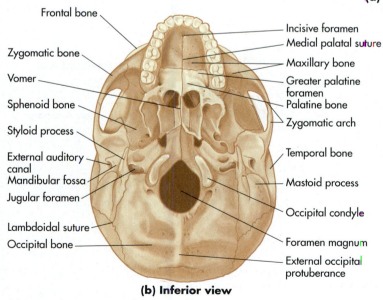

Frontal bone

Incisive foramen
Medial palatal suture

Zygomatic bone

Vomer

Maxillary bone

Sphenoid bone

Greater palatine foramen
Palatine bone

Styloid process

Zygomatic arch

External auditory canal
Mandibular fossa

Temporal bone

Jugular foramen

Mastoid process

Lambdoidal suture

Occipital condyle

Occipital bone

Foramen magnum

External occipital protuberance

(b) Inferior view

FIGURE 1-7 ■ Adult Skull Part II

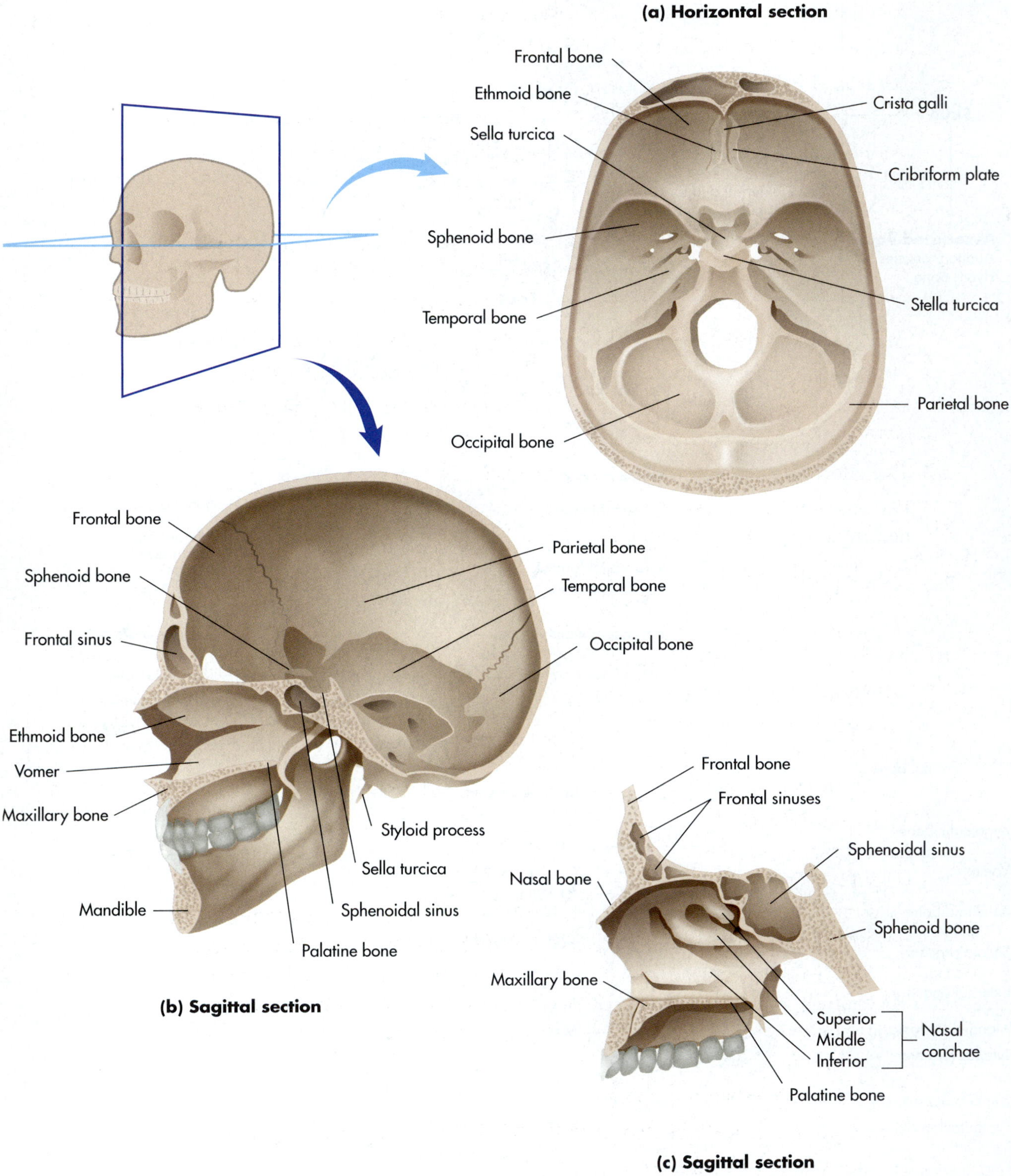

(a) Horizontal section

Frontal bone

Ethmoid bone

Sella turcica

Sphenoid bone

Temporal bone

Occipital bone

Crista galli

Cribriform plate

Stella turcica

Parietal bone

Frontal bone

Sphenoid bone

Frontal sinus

Ethmoid bone

Vomer

Maxillary bone

Mandible

Palatine bone

Sphenoidal sinus

Sella turcica

Styloid process

Parietal bone

Temporal bone

Occipital bone

(b) Sagittal section

Frontal bone

Frontal sinuses

Nasal bone

Maxillary bone

Sphenoidal sinus

Sphenoid bone

Superior
Middle
Inferior
} Nasal conchae

Palatine bone

(c) Sagittal section

FIGURE 1-8 ■ Adult Skull Part III

c. Glabella—Smooth elevation between eyebrows

d. Lacrimal fossa—Contains lacrimal gland

e. Paired frontal paranasal sinuses

3. Pariental bones—superior, paired, flat bones that articulate with the frontal, occipital, temporal, and sphenoid bones (Figures 1-7 and 1-8); together the pariental bones form the roof and the superior walls of the cranium, they interlock along the sagittal suture

D. Temporal bones—Paired bones that form the lateral wall of cranium. Contact the pariental bones along the squamosal suture (Figure 1-6); contain three portions

1. Squamous portion—Large, flat area of bone that forms cranial wall

a. Articular fossa—Portion that articulates with mandibular condyle

b. Articular eminence—Elevation located anterior to articular fossa

c. Postglenoid process—Prevents mandibular condyle from displacing posteriorly

2. Tympanic portion—Forms external acoustic meatus

3. Petrous portion—Inferior and medial portion that contains organs of hearing and balance; contains

a. Mastoid process and air cells—Process located posterior to external acoustic meatus; composed of air spaces that communicate with the middle ear; provides a site for the attachment of muscles that rotate or extend the head

b. Styloid process—Pointed projection that serves for attachment of muscles and ligaments; anchors muscles and ligaments associated with the tongue and hyoid bone

c. Stylomastoid foramen—Opening through which CN VII exits cranium

4. Mandibular fossa—Anterior to the external auditory canal and is a transverse depression; marks the point of articulation with the mandible (Figure 1-7b)

E. Sphenoid bone—"Keystone," single butterfly-shaped bone of the cranium that is centrally located and supports the base of the brain; the wings can be seen most clearly on the superior surface (Figure 1-8a) from the front (Figure 1-7a) or side (Figure 1-6); it is covered by other bones; like the frontal bone, the sphenoid bone also contains a pair of sinuses called sphenoidal sinuses (Figure 1-8b); the sphenoid bone contains:

1. Two paranasal sinuses in the body

2. Sella turcica—Located superior to the body; contains pituitary gland

3. Greater wings—Form lateral wall of skull

4. Foramen ovale (Figure 1-9■)—Where mandibular division of V_3 leaves cranium

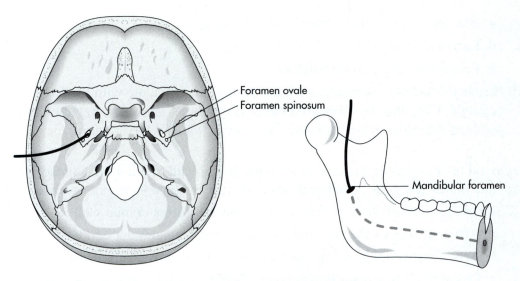

Foramen ovale
Foramen spinosum

Mandibular foramen

FIGURE 1-9 ■ Formen Ovale, where the Mandibular Nerve (V₃) Exits onto the Mandible

5. Foramen spinosum—Where middle meningeal artery (branch of maxillary artery) gains access to interior portion of skull

6. Foramen rotundum (Figure 1-10■)—Where maxillary nerve (V₂) exits

7. Lesser wings—Form part of anterior cranial fossa

8. Medial and lateral pterygoid plates (paired)—Extend inferiorly; where some muscles attach

9. Superior orbital fissure (Figure 1-11■)—Connects the orbit with the cranial cavity; CNs III, IV, VI, and ophthalmic division (V₁) travel through it

10. Carotid foramen—Also includes part of temporal bone; where carotid arteries enter cranium

11. Pterygoid hamuli (Figure 1-12■)—Two tiny hooks important to muscles that pass around them, pterygomandibular raphe

12. Sella turcica (Figure 1-8)—Located in middle of sphenoid bone; pituitary fossa; pituitary gland rests in the fossa and is attached to the base of the brain

F. Ethmoid—Single walnut-shaped bone in frontal bone, midline bone that forms posterior portion of nasal cavity and inferior, medial part of anterior cranial fossa (Figure 1-7a)

1. Numerous sinuses or air cells

2. Cribriform plate—Perforated bone through which sensory nerves from nose ascend to olfactory bulbs of CN I

3. Crista galli—Prominent ridge projects above the superior surface of the ethmoid (Figure 1-8)

4. Perpendicular plate—Posterior, superior portion of nasal septum

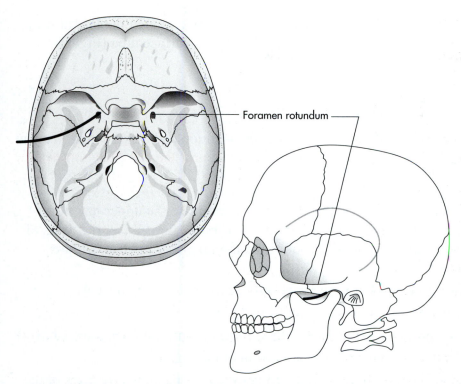

FIGURE 1-10 ■ Foramen Rotundum, where the Maxillary Nerve (V$_2$) Exits

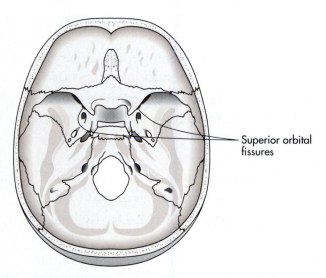

FIGURE 1-11 ■ Superior Orbital Foramen, where Ophthalmic Division (V$_1$) Exits

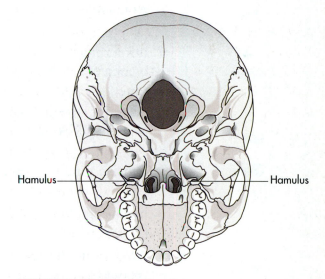

FIGURE 1-12 ■ Pterygoid Hamuli

5. Superior and middle nasal conchae—Bony projections in the lateral wall of the nasal cavity; increase mucous membrane surface area (Figures 1-7a, 1-8b,c)

➤ FACE

Bones of the face support facial features and provide dentition and movement of the jaw for speaking, swallowing, and eating. Of the 14 facial bones, only the mandible is moveable.

I. Facial Bones

A. Maxillae—Paired, fused, complex bones that comprise the upper jaw; form the floor and medial portion of the rim of the orbit (Figure 1-7a), the walls of the nasal cavity, and the anterior roof of the mouth or hard palate (Figure 1-8b); contain

    1. Maxillary sinuses—Large space in body of each bone (Figure 1-9)

    2. Frontal process—Articulates with frontal bone

    3. Zygomatic process—Articulates with zygoma to form cheek (Figures 1-6, 1-7)

    4. Palatine process—Forms anterior portion of hard palate

       a. Median palatine suture—Located between the palatine processes of the maxillae (Figures 1-7, 1-8b)

    5. Orbital process—Forms floor of orbit and infraorbital rim

    6. Alveolar process—Bone that surrounds and supports maxillary teeth; bone is more porous than mandible, can use infiltration anesthesia

    7. Infraorbital foramen—Located inferior to orbit; opening for maxillary branch of CN V (V_2) (Figure 1-7a); landmark for infraorbital injection

    8. Maxillary tuberosity—Located posterior to last molar; perforated by posterior superior alveolar foramina through which the posterior superior alveolar (PSA) nerves and blood vessels pass and is injection site for PSA nerves

    9. Incisive foramen—Behind the central incisors; nasopalatine nerve exits and is injection site for the nasopalatine injection (Figures 1-7, 1-8b)

    10. Nasal septum—Vertical midline structure divides the nasal cavity in half (Figure 1-7a)

    11. Anterior nasal spine—Small projection of bone at the beginning of nasal septum; may appear in periapical films of maxillary anterior teeth

    12. Canine eminence—Prominence of canine root; landmark for ASA injection

B. Mandible—Single, only freely moveable bone of the skull; symphysis is midline fusion of the right and left embryological processes, largest and strongest facial bone (Figures 1-7, 1-8b)

    1. Mental protuberance—Midline bony prominence of chin, also called symphysis

2. Mental foramen—Opening on exterior body where mental nerve enters to join inferior alveolar nerve, mental nerve exits and is landmark for the mental nerve block (Figure 1-7a)

3. Body of the mandible—Horizontal portion of heavy bone that bears the teeth

4. Alveolar process—Bone that surrounds and supports mandibular teeth; alveolar process of posterior teeth is more dense than the mandibular incisors

5. Ramus—Vertical shaft that extends from body to condyle and coronoid process, masseter muscle, temporalis muscle, internal pterygoid muscle, stylomandibular ligament (Figure 1-13■)

6. Angle—Corner where ramus and body meet, masseter muscle, internal pterygoid muscle (Figure 1-13)

7. Coronoid process—Sharp termination of anterior ramus; attachment for temporalis and masseter muscle (Figure 1-13)

8. Condyle—Egg-shaped process connected to ramus by the neck; articulates with temporal bone as part of temporomandibular joint (Figure 1-13)

9. Coronoid notch—Concave area between coronoid process and mandibular condyle; landmark for inferior alveolar block (Figure 1-13)

10. External oblique line—Anterior border of coronoid process that extends as a bony ridge on the body; attachment site for muscle of the cheek the buccinator; landmark for inferior alveolar, lingual injections; visible on posterior radiographs (Figure 1-13)

11. Internal oblique ridge—Interior of mandible parallel to external oblique line; attachment for portion of constrictor muscle; visible on posterior radiographs; landmark for inferior alveolar block (Figure 1-13)

12. Genial tubercles—Small, raised, roughened area on inner medial surface of mandible; muscle attachment area for geniohyoid and genioglossus muscle; also called mental spines (Figure 1-13)

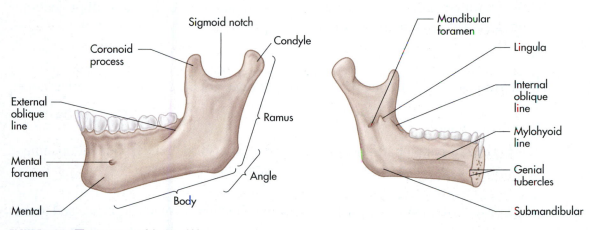

FIGURE 1-13 ■ Structures of the Mandible

13. Mylohyoid line—Ridge on inner surface that separates sublingual from submandibular fossae; attachment of mylohyoid muscle that forms floor of mouth (Figure 1-13)

14. Sublingual fossa—Shallow depression for sublingual salivary gland

15. Submandibular fossa—Deeper depression for submandibular salivary gland (Figure 1-13)

16. Mandibular canal—Inferior alveolar nerve travels along canal after exiting mandibular foramen

17. Mandibular foramen—Opening of the mandibular canal on inner surface of ramus for the inferior alveolar artery, nerve, and vein (Figure 1-13)

18. Lingula—Spicule of bone that guards mandibular foramen (Figure 1-13) protecting inferior alveolar, nerve and vein

19. Pterygoid fovea—Triangular depression below condyle; where lateral pterygoid muscle attaches

20. Mental fossa—Near chin depression, where mentalis muscle attaches (Figure 1-13)

C. Zygomatic bones (zygoma) (Figures 1-6, 1-7a)

1. Paired facial bones that form cheeks

2. Articulates with frontal, maxillary, and temporal bones

D. Vomer—Single, midline bone that forms inferior, posterior part of nasal septum (Figures 1-7a, 1-8b). Supports a prominent partition that forms part of the nasal septum, along with the ethmoid bone.

E. Lacrimal bones—Small, paired bones located in medial wall of orbit adjacent to nasolacrimal duct; smallest bones of cranium (Figures 1-6, 1-7a). They articulate with the frontal, ethmoid, and maxillary bones.

F. Nasal bones—Paired facial bones that form bridge of nose. Articulate with the superior frontal bone and the maxillary bones (Figures 1-6, 1-7a).

G. Inferior nasal conchae—Paired bones; third and inferior lateral wall projection in the nose; separate bone (Figure 1-7a). Their shape helps slow airflow and deflects arriving air toward the olfactory (smell) receptors located near the upper portions of the nasal cavity.

H. Hyoid bone—Only bone of the body that does not articulate with another bone; muscle attachment for hyoid muscles used in swallowing

I. Palatine bone

1. Greater palatine foramen—Also called anterior palatine foramen; opening of pterygopalatine canal; greater palatine nerve (Figure 1-7); location of greater palatine injection

2. Middle and posterior palatine foramen—Palatine nerve to soft palate and tonsils

3. Midpalatine suture—Suture dividing the palate in half (Figure 1-7b)

II. Joints of the Skull

A. Sutures—Immoveable joints; bones are joined by fibrous tissue

   1. Coronal suture—Joins frontal bone anteriorly and parietal bones posteriorly (Figure 1-6)

   2. Sagittal suture—Joins right and left parietal bones (Figure 1-7a)

   3. Lambdoidal suture—Joins occipital with parietal bones (Figure 1-6)

   4. Squamosal—Temporal and parietal bones

   5. Temporozygomatic—Zygomatic and temporal bones

   6. Median palatine—Palatine bones (Figure 1-7b)

   7. Tranverse palatine—Maxilla and palatine bones (Figure 1-7b)

B. Temporomandibular joint (TMJ)—Movable joint allowing hinge-type movement and gliding-type movement between temporal bone and mandible (Figure 1-14■)

   1. Contains a fibrous meniscus or disc

   2. Articulations

      a. Condyle of mandible—Egg-shaped bone that articulates against the articular eminence

      b. Mandibular fossa

      c. Articular eminence of temporal bone

      d. Condyle and the eminence are covered with fibrous connective tissue and no blood vessels, which makes the TMJ different from all other joints

      e. Most frequently used joint in the body

   3. Meniscus

      a. Biconcave disk between the condyle and the eminence

      b. Acts as a cushion

      c. Composed of fibrous connective tissue

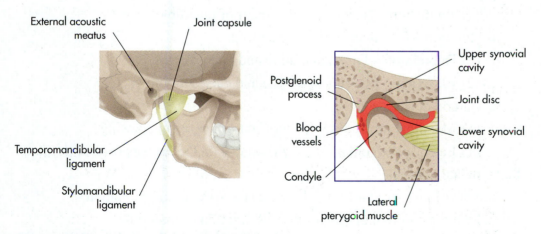

External acoustic meatus

Joint capsule

Temporomandibular ligament

Stylomandibular ligament

Postglenoid process

Blood vessels

Condyle

Lateral pterygoid muscle

Upper synovial cavity

Joint disc

Lower synovial cavity

FIGURE 1-14 ■ Lateral View of the Joint Capsule of the Temporomandibular Joint

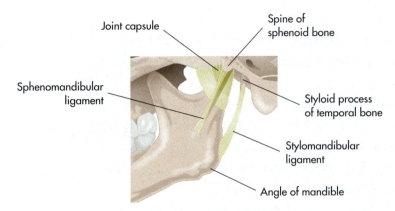

Joint capsule

Spine of
sphenoid bone

Sphenomandibular
ligament

Styloid process
of temporal bone

Stylomandibular
ligament

Angle of mandible

FIGURE 1-15 ■ Internal View of the Temporomandibular Joint

4. Temporomandibular capsule—Attaches the condyle to the temporal bone by a connective tissue band encircling the joint

5. Reinforced by external ligaments (Figure 1-15■)

    a. Stylomandibular ligament—Connects styloid process of temporal bone to posterior border of ramus of the mandible

    b. Sphenomandibular ligament—Connects angular spine of sphenoid bone with lingula of mandible; not an actual part of joint, but helps stabilize it

    c. Temporomandibular joint ligament—Prevents excessive retraction of joint

6. Synovial membrane

    a. Innermost aspect of the joint capsule lined with thin epithelial membrane

    b. Produces lubricating synovial fluid used to protect and cushion the joint

7. Movements of TMJ

    a. Gliding—Condyles move forward or backward on articular eminence

        (1) Protrusion—Forward movement of mandible

        (2) Retraction—Backward movement of mandible

    b. Rotation—Condyles rotate on meniscus

        (1) Depression—Drops mandible and opens mouth

        (2) Elevation—Elevates mandible and closes mouth

    c. Lateral deviation

        (1) Mandible protrudes to either right or left, as in chewing

        (2) Lateral pterygoid muscle will contract on the side opposite of deviation

8. Associate muscles

    a. Lateral pterygoid—Protrusion and lateral deviation of mandible

    b. Posterior portion of temporalis—Retraction of mandible

        c. Suprahyoids—Opening jaw

        d. Masseter, temporalis, and medial pterygoid—Closing jaw

    9. Temporomandibular myofacial pain-dysfunction syndrome

        a. Conditions that may lead to syndrome

            (1) Malocclusions

            (2) Lack of coordination between meniscus and condylar movement, allowing head of condyle to slip off disc

            (3) Meniscus tears

            (4) Arthritis

            (5) Malformations

            (6) Tumors

III. Cranial Fossae

  A. Anterior cranial fossa

    1. Formed by cribriform plate of ethmoid bone, lesser wing of sphenoid bone, and frontal bone

    2. Contains frontal lobe of cerebrum

  B. Middle cranial fossa

    1. Formed by greater wing of the sphenoid, temporal, and anterior portion of the occipital bones

    2. Contains temporal lobe of cerebrum

  C. Posterior cranial fossa

    1. Formed by temporal and occipital bones

    2. Contains cerebellum, pons, and medulla

IV. Paranasal sinuses (Figure 1-16■)

  A. Paired air-filled cavities in bone, which make head lighter and easier to hold erect

  B. Lined with mucous membrane

  C. All communicate with nasal cavity and found in the following bones

    1. Frontal

    2. Sphenoid

    3. Ethmoid

    4. Maxillae

V. Orbit

  A. Composed of seven bones

  B. Contains the eyeball and muscles that control its movements

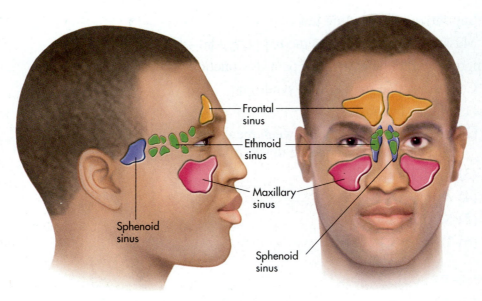

FIGURE 1-16 ■ Lateral View of the Skull and Paranasal Sinuses

    C. Superior orbital fissure—Transmits CN III, IV, and VI and ophthalmic branch of V (V₁)

    D. Optic foramen—Transmits optic nerve from eye to brain (CN II)

    E. Inferior orbital fissure—Contains mandibular branch V (V₃)

➤ MUSCLES

Muscles are divided into groups—muscles of mastication, muscles of facial expression, cervical muscles, suprahyoid muscles, infrahyoid muscles, muscles of the pharynx, pharyngeal muscles, palatine muscles, and tongue muscles. The innervation of each group of muscles reflects embryologic development from different branchial arches.

I. Definitions

    A. Tendons—Connective tissue that attaches muscles to bones

    B. Origin—Stationary attachment of muscle

    C. Insertion—Attachment that moves

    D. Ligament—Dense regular connective that attaches bone to bone

    E. Joint—Where two bones come together

II. Muscles of Mastication (Table 1-1■)

    A. Insertion—Mandible, hence a common function—movement of mandible

    B. Innervation—Motor branch of trigeminal nerve, which follows mandibular division, V₃

    C. Action—Assist with speaking, swallowing, and mastication

TABLE 1-1 Muscles of Mastication			
Muscle	**Origin**	**Insertion**	**Function**
Temporalis	Floor of temporal fossa	Coronoid process of the mandible	Elevates and retracts mandible
Masseter	Zygomatic arch	Angle and ramus of mandible	Elevates mandible
Medial pterygoid	Pterygoid fossa of sphenoid	Medial surface of the angle of mandible	Elevates mandible
Lateral pterygoid	Lateral surface of the lateral pterygoid plate; greater wing of the sphenoid bone	Pterygoid fovea of mandible	Depresses, protrudes, and laterally deviates mandible

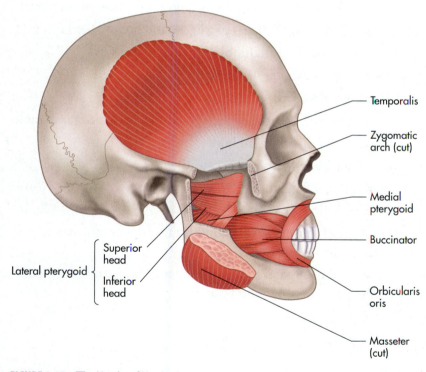

FIGURE 1-17 ■ Muscles of Mastication

   D. Muscles include (Figure 1-17■)
       1. Temporalis muscle—Fan-shaped
          a. Origin—Temporal fossa
          b. Insertion—Coronoid process of mandible

Chewing

Chewing is a complex process in the mastication of food. If a point is placed on the chin while chewing, it revolves in a small circle. In addition to the superior/inferior movement of the mandible, there is a great deal of lateral movement brought about by the muscles of mastication. When the mandible is drawn to the right, for example, the right temporalis and masseter muscles contract along with the left medial pterygoid muscle. The remaining muscles of mastication must be relaxed. Moving to the left, the opposite muscles must contract and relax. While this is occurring, the mandible is moving up and down.

      c. Innervation—Mandibular branch of CN V

      d. Action—Elevates and retracts mandible; called closing the mandible

  2. Masseter muscle—Band-like muscle that forms a great portion of the cheek

      a. Origin—Anterior and medial surfaces of zygomatic arch

      b. Insertion—Angle and ramus of mandible

      c. Innervation—Mandibular branch of CN V

      d. Action—Elevates mandible; called clenching muscle

  3. Medial (internal) pterygoid muscle—Deeper, yet similar to masseter muscle

      a. Origin—Pterygoid fossa of sphenoid bone

      b. Insertion—Medial surface of angle of mandible

      c. Innervation—Mandibular branch of CN V

      d. Action—Elevates mandible

  4. Lateral (external) pterygoid muscle—Horizontal muscle that attaches to medial surface of mandible

      a. Origin—Superior head of greater wing of sphenoid bone; inferior head of lateral pterygoid plate of sphenoid bone

      b. Insertion—Pterygoid fovea of mandible

      c. Innervation—Mandibular branch of CN V

      d. Action

        (1) Both right and left sides protrude mandible

        (2) Use of one side allows lateral deviation of mandible

        (3) Inferior heads allows slight depression of mandible

III. Muscles of Facial Expression (Figure 1-18■)

  A. Origins—Usually from bone, yet muscles insert into facial tissues; this allows for movement resulting in facial expression

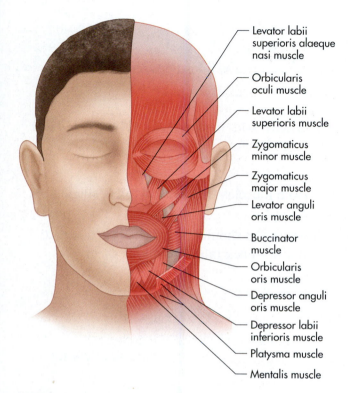

Levator labii
superioris alaeque
nasi muscle

Orbicularis
oculi muscle

Levator labii
superioris muscle

Zygomaticus
minor muscle

Zygomaticus
major muscle

Levator anguli
oris muscle

Buccinator
muscle

Orbicularis
oris muscle

Depressor anguli
oris muscle

Depressor labii
inferioris muscle

Platysma muscle

Mentalis muscle

FIGURE 1-18 ■ Muscles of Facial Expression

B. Innervation—Facial nerve, CN VII

C. Facial muscles that move mouth include

   1. Orbicularis oris muscle—Circular muscle around mouth; purses lips

   2. Depressor anguli oris muscle—Depresses corner of mouth

   3. Depressor labii inferioris muscle—Depresses lower lip

   4. Mentalis muscle—Draws chin to pucker

   5. Buccinator muscle—Draws corner of lip laterally and helps form cheek;
also keeps food pushed back on occlusal surface of teeth; assists in
mastication

   6. Risorius muscle—Widens mouth

   7. Levator labii superioris muscle—Elevates upper lip

   8. Levator labii superioris alaeque nasi muscle—Elevates upper lip and ala of nose

   9. Zygomaticus major muscle—Elevates angle of mouth, as in smiling

  10. Zygomaticus minor muscle—Elevates upper lip

  11. Levator anguli oris muscle—Elevates angle of mouth, as in smiling

  12. Platysma muscle—Raises skin of neck and pulls down corners of mouth

D. Other muscles of facial expression (Figure 1-18)

    1. Orbicularis oculi muscle—Closes eyelid

    2. Corrugator supercilii muscle—Causes frown lines between eyebrows

    3. Frontal belly of epicranius muscle—Raises eyebrows

IV. Cervical Muscles—Important as landmarks in the neck (Figure 1-19■)

A. Innervation—Accessory nerve, CN XI

B. Muscles include

    1. Sternocleidomastoid muscle—Both muscles flex head, while a single muscle will turn head

    2. Trapezius muscle—Allows shrugging of shoulders and holds head erect; runs from head to shoulders and down back in a continuous sheet

V. Suprahyoid Muscles

A. Location—Superior to hyoid bone

B. Insertion—Hyoid bone

C. Action—Assist in chewing (contract to depress mandible) and swallowing (contract to lift hyoid and larynx, closing the glottis)

D. Muscles include

    1. Digastric muscle—Has two bellies; act as pulley opening or depressing the mandible (Figure 1-20■)

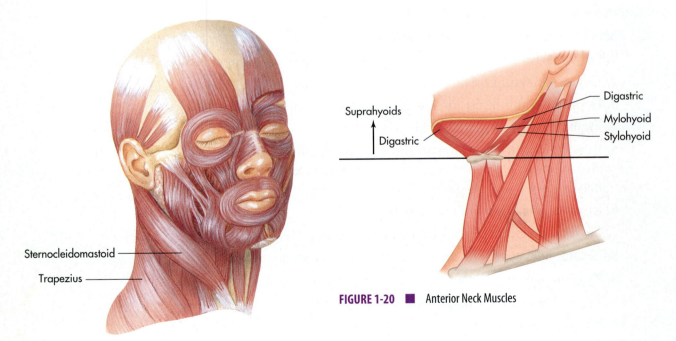

Suprahyoids

Digastric

Digastric

Mylohyoid

Stylohyoid

FIGURE 1-20 ■ Anterior Neck Muscles

Sternocleidomastoid

Trapezius

FIGURE 1-19 ■ Posterior Neck Muscles

    a. Posterior belly—Innervated by facial nerve, CN VII

    b. Anterior belly—Innervated by mylohyoid nerve, branch of V_3

  2. Stylohyoid muscle—Innervated by facial nerve, CN VII; act to tighten or stabilize the hyoid bone during actions of other muscles (Figure 1-20)

  3. Mylohoid muscle—Forms floor of mouth; provides firm base for tongue and helps depress mandible; innervated by mylohyoid nerve, branch of V_3 (Figure 1-20)

  4. Geniohyoid muscle—Innervated by branches of first cervical nerve; insertion at hyoid bone; acts to stabilize hyoid (Figure 1-21■)

VI. Infrahyoid Muscles (Figure 1-22■)

  A. Location—Inferior to hyoid bone

  B. Innervation—Second and third cervical nerves

  C. Action—Depresses and stabilizes hyoid bone

  D. Four pairs of hyoid muscles—Include sternothyroid, sternohyoid, omohyoid, and thyrohyoid muscles

VII. Muscles of the Pharynx (Figure 1-23■)

  A. Action—Involved in speaking, swallowing, and middle ear function

  B. Innervation—Glossopharyngeal and pharyngeal plexus (IX, X)

  C. Includes the stylopharyngeus and pharyngeal constrictor muscles

VIIII. Muscles of the Palate

  A. Innervation—Pharyngeal plexus (glossopharyngeal and vagus nerves) except for tensor veli palatini muscle, which is supplied by trigeminal nerve

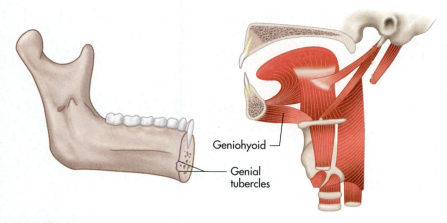

Geniohyoid

Genial tubercles

FIGURE 1-21 ■ Geniohyoid Muscle

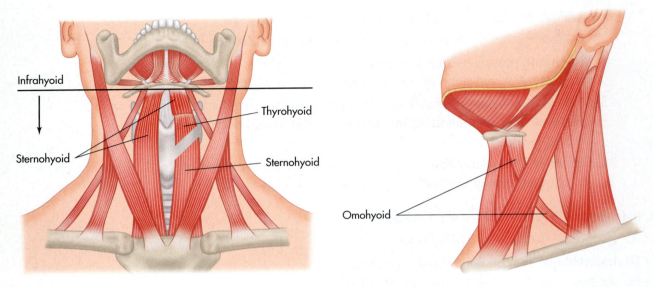

FIGURE 1-22 ■ Infrahyoid Muscles

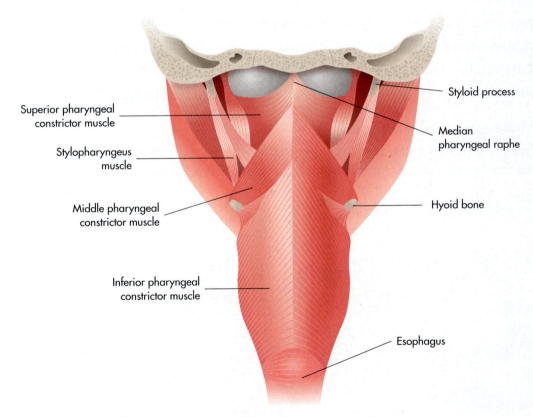

FIGURE 1-23 ■ Posterior View of the Muscles of the Pharynx

B. Action

  1. During swallowing, movement of soft palate separates nasopharynx from oropharynx, preventing food from entering nasal cavity

  2. Movement of soft palate is also used in speaking

C. Muscles of palate include

  1. Palatoglossus muscle—Forms anterior tonsillar pillar (Figure 1-24■)

  2. Palatopharyngeus muscle—Forms posterior tonsillar pillar (Figure 1-25■)

  3. Levator veli palatini muscle—Elevates soft palate (Figure 1-25)

  4. Tensor veli palatini muscle—Stiffens soft palate (Figure 1-25)

  5. Muscle of the uvula—Allows uvula to adapt in closing off nasopharynx (Figure 1-25)

IX. Muscles of the Tongue (Figure 1-24)

A. Innervation—Hypoglossal nerve, CN XII

B. Muscles include

  1. Intrinsic—Located within the tongue

  2. Extrinsic—Have different origins, but all insert into tongue

    a. Genioglossus muscle

      (1) Origin—Genial tubercles

      (2) Action—Protrudes tongue and prevents it from falling back and obstructing the airway

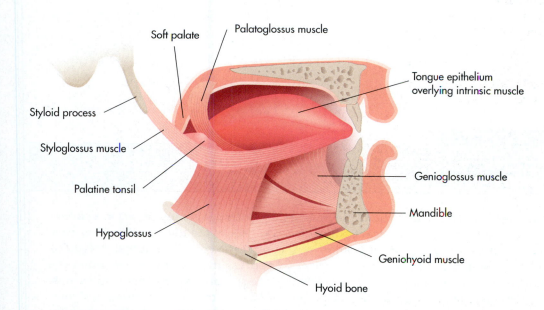

FIGURE 1-24 ■ Intrinsic and Extrinsic Muscles of the Tongue

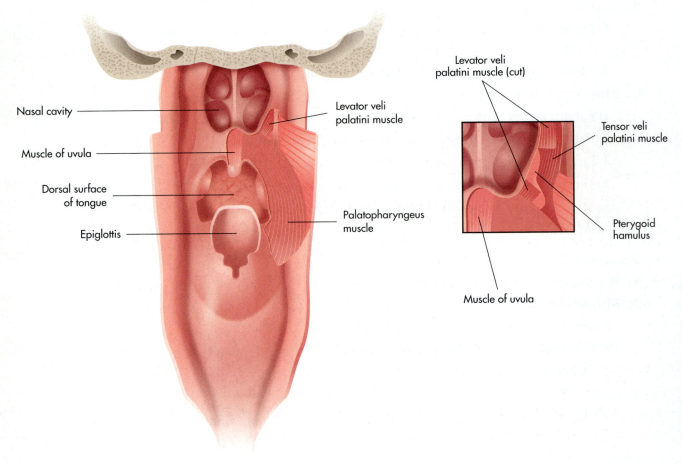

Nasal cavity

Muscle of uvula

Dorsal surface of tongue

Epiglottis

Levator veli palatini muscle

Palatopharyngeus muscle

Levator veli palatini muscle (cut)

Tensor veli palatini muscle

Pterygoid hamulus

Muscle of uvula

FIGURE 1-25 ■ Posterior View of the Muscles of the Soft Palate

Integrated Function of Muscles of Mastication

The muscles of mastication, suprahyoid muscles, and infrahyoid muscles act in a coordinated manner to perform mastication and chewing. To elevate the mandible (i.e., closing the mouth), the muscles of mastication must contract (except the external pterygoid). The suprahyoids and infrahyoid must relax. To depress the mandible (i.e., open the mouth), the muscles of mastication must relax, and the suprahyoids and infrahyoids must contract. In swallowing, the mandible must be fixed by contracting the muscles of mastication, the suprahyoids must be contracted to lift the hyoid and larynx to close the glottis, and the infrahyoids must be relaxed.

b. Styloglossus muscle

    (1) Origin—Styloid process

    (2) Action—Retracts tongue

c. Hyoglossus muscle

    (1) Origin—Hyoid bone

    (2) Action—Depresses tongue

➤ CIRCULATORY SYSTEM

I. Blood Supply to the Head and Neck (Figures 1-26■, 1-27■, 1-28a■)— Provided through the three branches of the aorta

  A. Left subclavian artery—Carries blood to left arm; a branch, the left vertebral artery, delivers blood to brain

  B. Left common carotid artery—Splits into two branches; carries blood to most of head, neck, and brain by its two branches (Figure 1-29■)

    1. Left internal carotid artery—To brain

    2. Left external carotid artery—To head and neck

  C. Right brachiocephalic artery—Short branch of arch that immediately divides into two arteries

    1. Right subclavian artery—Gives rise to right vertebral artery to brain

    2. Right common carotid artery—Splits into

      a. Right internal carotid artery to brain

      b. Right external carotid artery to head and neck

II. Blood Supply to the Brain (Figure 1-28b)—Rich blood supply to the brain is provided by

  A. Two anterior right and left internal carotid arteries that enter skull through carotid canals

  B. Two posterior vertebral arteries that enter skull through foramen magnum

  C. These four arteries join and connect around the base of the brain to form circle of Willis

  D. Middle meningeal arteries—Branches of maxillary arteries that enter cranium through foramen spinosum to supply blood to the meninges of the brain

III. Blood Supply to the Face (structures external to the skull)—Comes from branches of external carotid arteries

  A. Anterior branches of external carotid artery

    1. Superior thyroid artery—To superior portion of thyroid gland

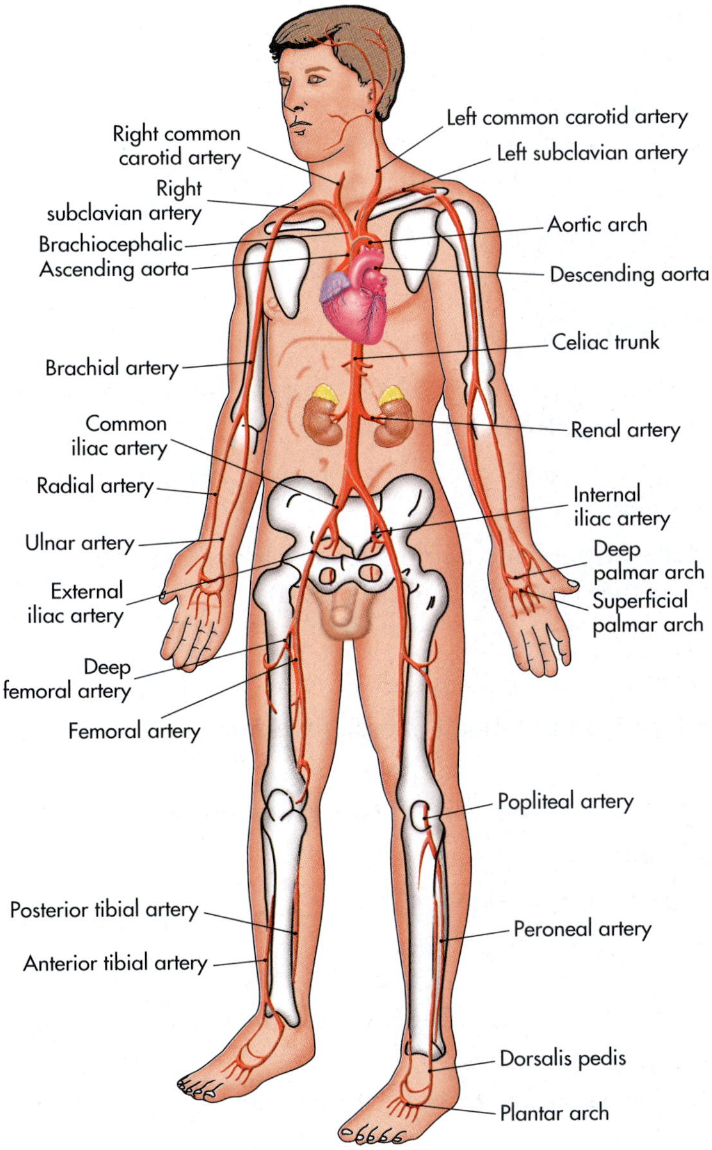

FIGURE 1-26 ■ Arterial System

2. Lingual artery—Branches at level of hyoid bone; runs deep to suprahyoid muscles, supplying adjacent muscles, including floor of mouth through its branch—sublingual artery—and terminates by supplying the tongue

3. Facial artery—Extends medial to mandible, then crosses mandible's lower border and travels to medial corner of eye, giving off numerous branches along the way

  a. Submental artery—To chin

  b. Inferior labial artery—To lower lip

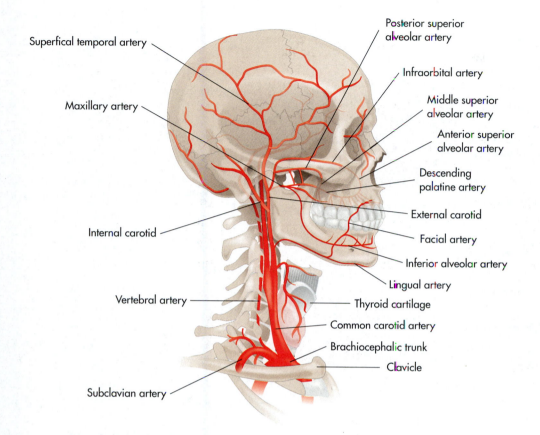

Superfical temporal artery

Maxillary artery

Internal carotid

Vertebral artery

Subclavian artery

Posterior superior alveolar artery

Infraorbital artery

Middle superior alveolar artery

Anterior superior alveolar artery

Descending palatine artery

External carotid

Facial artery

Inferior alveolar artery

Lingual artery

Thyroid cartilage

Common carotid artery

Brachiocephalic trunk

Clavicle

FIGURE 1-27 ■ Anterior Supply of the Head and Neck

    c. Superior labial artery—To upper lip

    d. Lateral nasal artery—To side of nose

    e. Angular artery—To medial corner of eye

    f. Ascending palatine artery—To nasopharyngeal area, especially the palatine tonsils

Blood Supply to the Brain

The brain and its coverings receive arterial blood from three main sources: the internal carotid, the vertebral arteries, and the meningeal arteries. The internal carotid enters the skull through the internal carotid canal, which is adjacent to the body of the sphenoid in the middle cranial fossa. The vertebral arteries arise off the subclavian arteries and enter the posterior cranial cavity through the foramen magnum. The branches of the vertebral and internal carotid join together at the circle of Willis. The middle meningeal arteries arise from the maxillary artery and reenter the middle cranial fossa via the foramen spinosum, carrying blood to the dura.

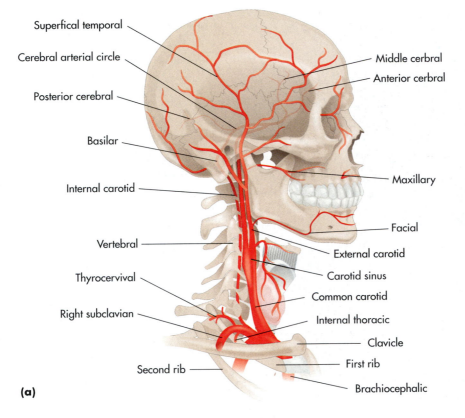

(a)

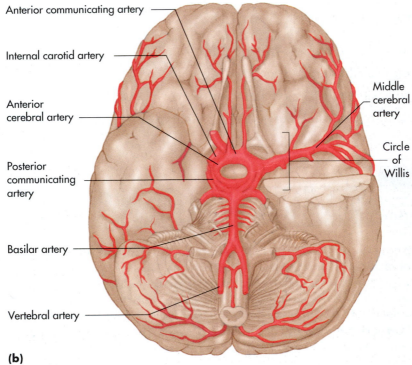

(b)

FIGURE 1-28 ■ Arteries of the Neck, Head, and Brain

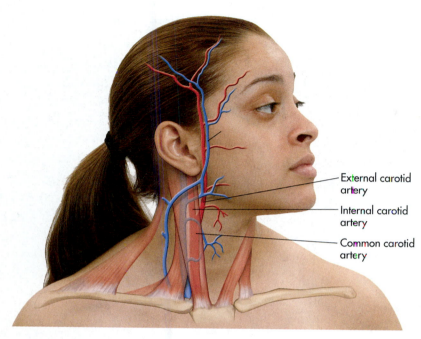

FIGURE 1-29 ■ Common Carotid Artery

B. Medial branch of external carotid artery—Ascending pharyngeal artery supplies pharyngeal walls and soft palate

C. Posterior branches of external carotid artery include

   1. Occipital artery—Supplies occipital region as well as sternocleidomastoid muscle

   2. Posterior auricular artery—To posterior surface of ear, tympanic cavity, and adjacent scalp

D. Terminal branches of external carotid artery include

   1. Superficial temporal artery—Courses through parotid gland, supplying it and area around ear and temporal region

   2. Maxillary artery (Figure 1-30■)—Originates at level of neck of mandible and gives rise to following branches

     a. Middle meningeal artery—Enters skull through foramen spinosum to supply the meninges of brain and bones of skull

     b. Inferior alveolar artery—Enters mandibular canal through mandibular foramen and supplies mandible and mandibular teeth, floor of mouth, and mental region

       (1) Mylohyoid artery—Supplies mylohyoid muscle and floor of mouth

       (2) Mental artery—Exits mental foramen to supply chin region

       (3) Incisive artery—Branches off inferior alveolar artery and divides into dental and alveolar branches to anterior teeth

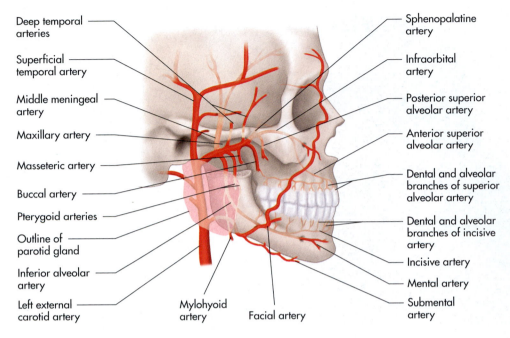

Deep temporal arteries

Superficial temporal artery

Middle meningeal artery

Maxillary artery

Masseteric artery

Buccal artery

Pterygoid arteries

Outline of parotid gland

Inferior alveolar artery

Left external carotid artery

Mylohyoid artery

Facial artery

Sphenopalatine artery

Infraorbital artery

Posterior superior alveolar artery

Anterior superior alveolar artery

Dental and alveolar branches of superior alveolar artery

Dental and alveolar branches of incisive artery

Incisive artery

Mental artery

Submental artery

FIGURE 1-30 ■ Branches of the Maxillary Artery

c. Muscular branches

(1) Deep temporal arteries supply temporalis muscle

(2) Pterygoid arteries supply medial and lateral pterygoid muscles

(3) Masseteric artery supplies masseter muscle

(4) Buccal artery supplies buccinator muscle and buccal region

d. Posterior superior alveolar artery—Supplies posterior teeth and maxillary sinus

e. Infraorbital artery—Travels in infraorbital canal

(1) Anterior superior alveolar artery—Arises from infraorbital artery and gives off to dental and alveolar branches to maxillary teeth; anastomoses with posterior superior alveolar artery

f. Greater palatine artery and lesser palatine arteries—Descend in pterygopalatine canal to supply hard and soft palates, respectively

g. Sphenopalatine artery—Termination point of maxillary artery; supplies nasal cavity; gives rise to the nasopalatine artery that accompanies nasopalatine nerve through incisive foramen of the maxilla

IV. Veins of the Head and Neck (Figure 1-31■)

A. Unlike veins in the rest of the body; valveless, which may contribute to spread of infection

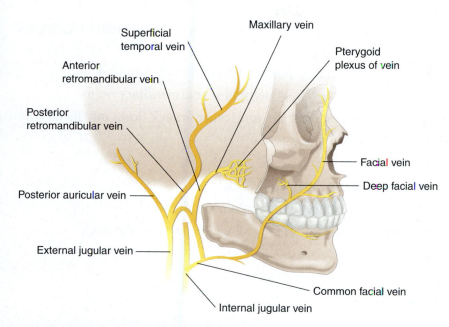

Superficial
temporal vein

Maxillary vein

Anterior
retromandibular vein

Pterygoid
plexus of vein

Posterior
retromandibular vein

Facial vein

Deep facial vein

Posterior auricular vein

External jugular vein

Common facial vein

Internal jugular vein

FIGURE 1-31 ■ Venous Drainage of the Head and Neck

B. Generally follow same path as arteries and share a common name, except for
the following

  1. Venous dural sinuses—Intracranial structures formed by dura into which
the brain, meninges, and skull drain

    a. Several external veins drain into this system, creating potential for
spread of infection

    b. System drains into internal jugular vein; some of named sinuses include

      (1) Superior sagittal sinus

      (2) Inferior sagittal sinus

      (3) Cavernous sinus

      (4) Transverse sinus

  2. Pterygoid plexus—Collection of anastomosing veins surrounding maxillary
artery in infratemporal fossa; area that PSA injection is given and can cause
hematoma or intravenous injection; clinician must be careful when
performing local anesthesia in this area

    a. Connects with facial and retromandibular veins

    b. Protects maxillary artery from compression during mastication

     c. Drained by maxillary vein

     d. Close proximity to maxillary tuberosity makes it vulnerable to accidents during dental procedures

3. Retromandibular vein—Located posterior to ramus of mandible

     a. Formed by merger of superficial temporal and maxillary veins

     b. One branch forms external jugular vein; other branch flows into facial vein

     c. Travels through parotid gland

4. Internal jugular vein

     a. Drains most of tissues of head and neck

     b. Originates in cranial cavity; exits jugular foramen

     c. Found with internal carotid artery and vagus nerve in the neck

5. External jugular vein

     a. Usually smaller than internal jugular

     b. Located more laterally in the neck

     c. Receives much of outflow from the retromandibular vein

     d. Drains only extracranial tissues

➤ NERVOUS SYSTEM

The nervous system causes muscles to contract, stimulates glands to secrete, regulates the blood system, and allows for sensation to be felt. It is made up of the central, peripheral, and autonomic nervous systems (Figure 1-32■).

  I. Central Nervous System (CNS)—includes brain and spinal column

    A. Brain

      1. Divided into three areas (Figure 1-33■)

        a. Pair of cerebral hemispheres, which are divided into five lobes

          (1) Frontal—Controls abstract thought and voluntary muscle control

          (2) Parietal—Integrates incoming stimuli, contains center for speech and conscious sensations

          (3) Temporal—Receives auditory perception

          (4) Occipital—Contains vision center

          (5) Insula—Function unknown

        b. Cerebellum is made up of two cerebellar hemispheres and controls muscle coordination (Figure 1-34■)

        c. Brainstem is divided into four areas (Figure 1-34)

          (1) Diencephalon—Contains thalamus and hypothalamus

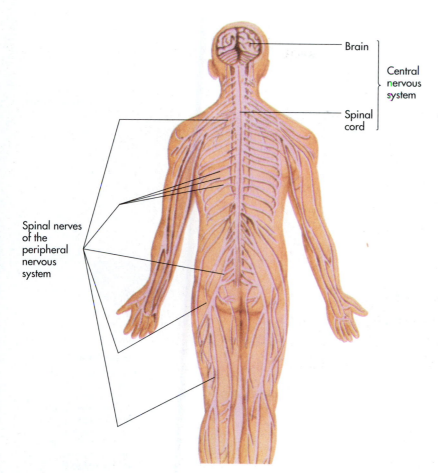

FIGURE 1-32 ■ Nervous System

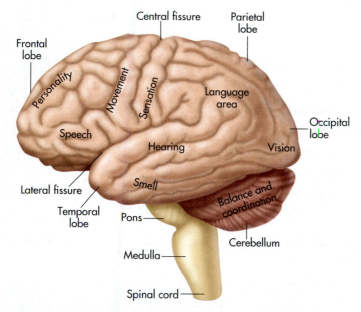

FIGURE 1-33 ■ Cerebral Hemispheres

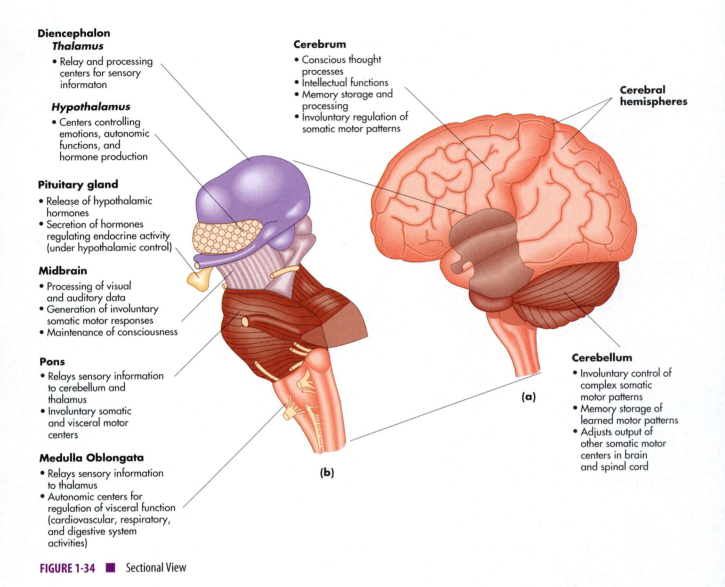

Diencephalon
Thalamus
• Relay and processing centers for sensory informaton

Hypothalamus
• Centers controlling emotions, autonomic functions, and hormone production

Pituitary gland
• Release of hypothalamic hormones
• Secretion of hormones regulating endocrine activity (under hypothalamic control)

Midbrain
• Processing of visual and auditory data
• Generation of involuntary somatic motor responses
• Maintenance of consciousness

Pons
• Relays sensory information to cerebellum and thalamus
• Involuntary somatic and visceral motor centers

Medulla Oblongata
• Relays sensory information to thalamus
• Autonomic centers for regulation of visceral function (cardiovascular, respiratory, and digestive system activities)

Cerebrum
• Conscious thought processes
• Intellectual functions
• Memory storage and processing
• Involuntary regulation of somatic motor patterns

Cerebral hemispheres

(a)

Cerebellum
• Involuntary control of complex somatic motor patterns
• Memory storage of learned motor patterns
• Adjusts output of other somatic motor centers in brain and spinal cord

(b)

FIGURE 1-34 ■ Sectional View

    (2) Midbrain—Function unknown; may be involved with basic instinctual reflexes

    (3) Pons—Contains nuclei of various nerves including the facial and trigeminal

    (4) Medulla oblongata—Contains center for certain vital functions such as breathing, vascular control, and heart rate

II. Peripheral Nervous System

  A. Spinal nerves

    1. Contain 31 pairs of nerves designated by spinal foramen from which they exit; C1 to C8, T1 to T12, L1 to L5, S1 to S5, and the coccygeal nerve

B. Cranial nerves

    1. Afferent component (general somatic afferent)

        a. Sensory perception

        b. Proprioception

        c. Pain, touch, temperature, and pressure

        d. Sense of movement

        e. Skeletal muscle, skin, oral mucosa, alveolar bone, teeth, and TMJ

    2. Efferent component (special visceral efferent)

        a. provides function of the muscles of mastication

    3. 12 pairs of nerves designated by names and Roman numerals (Figure 1-35■ and Table 1-2■)

        a. Olfactory cranial nerve (I)—Receives sense of smell

        b. Optic cranial nerve (II)—Receives sight

        c. Oculomotor cranial nerve (III)—Moves eyeballs and contains autonomic fibers for lens curvature and pupil size

        d. Trochlear cranial nerve (IV)—Eyeball movement

        e. Trigeminal cranial nerve (V)—Includes three divisions

            (1) Ophthalmic division (V_1)—Sensory for upper one-third of face

            (2) Maxillary division (V_2)—Sensory for middle one-third of face, including maxillary teeth, palate, and upper lip

            (3) Mandibular division (V_3)—Sensory of lower one-third of face, including mandibular teeth, tongue, and lower lip; as a motor nerve, it serves the muscles of mastication and mylohyoid muscle

        f. Abducens cranial nerve (VI)—Eyeball movement

        g. Facial cranial nerve (VII)—Muscles of facial expression and carries back taste sensation from anterior two-thirds of tongue

            (1) Contains fibers of the autonomic nervous system to submandibular and sublingual salivary glands via the chorda tympani nerve

Perception

Generally, there are three main types of perception—exteroception, intraception, and proprioception. Exteroception receives stimuli from outside the body (e.g., pain, sight, hearing). Intraception receives stimuli from inside the body (e.g., thirst, hunger). Proprioception is muscle sense (e.g., knowing how many fingers are raised on one's hand without looking or touching). It is very important in coordination of movement.

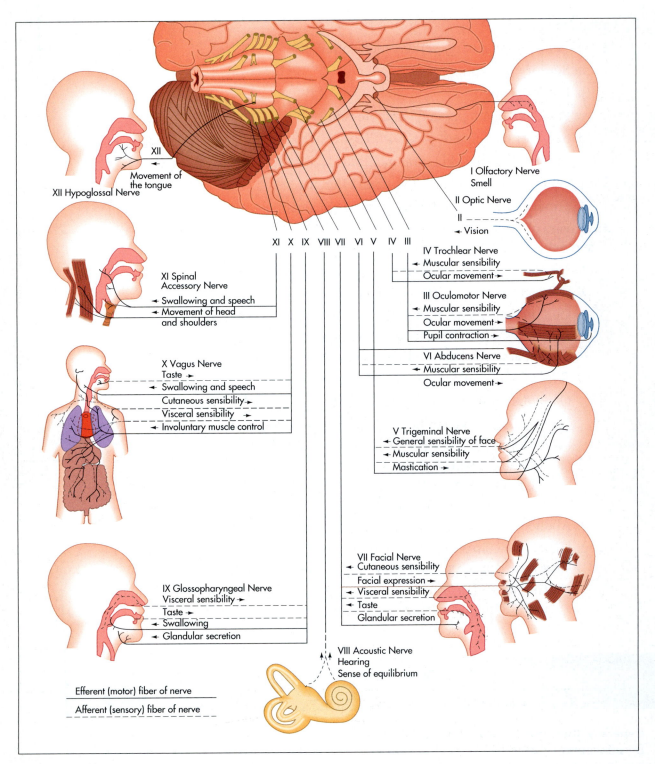

FIGURE 1-35 ■ Twelve Cranial Nerves

TABLE 1-2 SUMMARY OF CRANIAL NERVES

Nerve	Area	Pathology	Sensory/Motor	Mnemonic
Olfactory (I)	Sense of smell	Anosmia	Sensory	Some
Optic (II)	Sight	Blindness	Sensory	Say
Oculomotor (III)	Muscle-eye; proprioception	Deviation of eyeball	Motor	Marry
Trochlear (IV)	Muscle-eye; proprioception	Deviation of eyeball	Motor	Money
Trigeminal (V₁)	Skin of face and scalp	Loss of general sensation	Both Sensory	But
(V₂)	Mucosa of mouth, nose, and maxillary teeth	Loss of general sensation	Sensory	
(V₃)	Muscles of mastication and myohyoid muscle	Paralysis of these muscles	Motor	
(V₃)	Proprioception, mandibular teeth, mucosa of floor of mouth, tongue	Loss of muscle coordination and sensation	Sensory	
Abducens (VI)	Muscle-eye; proprioception	Deviation of eyeball	Motor	My
Facial (VII)	Taste-tongue; proprioception	Loss of taste, affects anterior 2/3 of the tongue	Both Sensory	Brother
	Muscles of facial expression; submandibular, sublingual, and salivary glands	Bell's palsy	Motor; autonomic fibers	
Vestibulocochlear (VIII)	Hearing, balance	Deafness, dizziness	Sensory	Says
Glossopharyngeal (IX)	Posterior 1/3 of tongue, soft palate, pharynx; proprioception	Loss of taste, posterior 1/3 of tongue	Both Sensory	Big

(continued)

TABLE 1-2 SUMMARY OF CRANIAL NERVES (*continued*)

Nerve	Area	Pathology	Sensory/Motor	Mnemonic
	Pharyngeal muscles, parotid salivary gland	Paralysis of pharyngeal muscles; difficulty in swallowing	Motor; autonomic fibers	

Vagus (X)	Pharynx; proprioception
	
	Pharynx and larynx
		Loss of some reflex (swallow)
		
		Loss of speech; difficulty in swallowing
			Both
			  Sensory
			
			  Motor
				Brains

Accessory (XI)	Trapezius and sternocleido-mastoid muscles	Difficulty turning head and lifting shoulders	Motor	Matter
Hypoglossal (XII)	Intrinsic and extrinsic muscles of tongue	Paralysis of tongue	Motor	Most

(2) Innervates lacrimal gland and mucus glands in the nasal cavity (travels with branches of V)

h. Vestibulocochlear (auditory) cranial nerve (VIII)—Receives sound stimuli via cochlear division and equilibrium via vestibular branch

i. Glossopharyngeal cranial nerve (IX)—Receives taste sensation from posterior one-third of tongue and motor control to a throat muscle; supplies autonomic fibers to parotid salivary gland

j. Vagus cranial nerve (X)—Provides motor nerve to several laryngeal muscles, taste sensation from base of tongue, and autonomic control of many visceral organs (e.g., heart, lungs, and gastrointestinal tract)

k. Accessory cranial nerve (XI)—Provides motor innervation to several neck and laryngeal muscles

l. Hypoglossal cranial nerve (XII)—Provides motor nerve to several extrinsic and all intrinsic tongue muscles

4. Pathology associated with cranial nerves

a. Olfactory—Damage may result in anosmia, which is total or partial loss of ability to smell

(1) Total loss—Relatively uncommon; partial loss is quite common in aging process, with men generally losing more olfactory ability than women

Chorda Tympani

The chorda tympani is a branch of the facial nerve that exits the skull via the petrotympanic fissure in the mandibular fossa. It passes inferiorly and joins the lingual nerve from which it branches to the salivary glands. It carries autonomic motor nerves to the submandibular and sublingual salivary glands and receives taste fibers from the anterior two-thirds of the tongue.

    (2) Temporary anosmia—Quite common in people suffering from colds when mucus covers nerve endings

b. Optic—Damage may result in partial or total loss of sight in one or both eyes, depending on where the injury or affliction occurs

c. Oculomotor—Damage may result in loss of certain eye movements

    (1) Carries autonomic nerve fibers controlling pupil size and lens curvature

    (2) Contains motor fibers to levator palpebrae superioris muscle, which raises upper eyelid

    (3) Injury to this nerve may result in eye droop (ptosis)

d. Trochlear—Injury results in loss of function of superior oblique muscle; lateral and downward movement of eyeball is lost

e. Trigeminal—Damage is rare, but may occur when mandibular third molar is removed and inferior alveolar nerve (located in the inferior alveolar canal) may be damaged; results in temporary or permanent loss of sensation to lower lip; trigeminal neuralgia occurs when patient expresses excruciating pain in the distribution of maxillary or mandibular nerves

f. Abducens—Damage results in loss of ability to move eyeball laterally; instead, eyeball turns inward due to overreaction of medial rectus muscle

g. Facial—Damage to the nerve in the skull, middle ear, stylomastoid foramen, or as it passes through parotid gland may result in Bell's palsy or facial paralysis (drooping of the lower eyelid, sagging of the mouth, and lack of expression on the affected side), loss of taste in anterior portion of tongue, and decreased production of tears

h. Vestibulocochlear—Damage to the

    (1) Vestibular division results in loss of balance and dizziness (Ménière's disease); usually temporary

    (2) Cochlear division results in loss of hearing; associated with aging

i. Glossopharyngeal—Damage to this nerve may result in loss of taste to posterior one-third of tongue and secretion from parotid gland (parasympathetic fibers)

    j. Vagus—Damage of recurrent branch may result in partial loss of speech; hoarseness

    k. Accessory—Damage is rare; congenital spasticity of one sternocleidomastoid muscle results in the condition of wryneck, with permanent contracture and torsion of the neck

    l. Hypoglossal—Damage results in partial loss of tongue movement or deviation to one side

III. Specific Innervation of Dental and Oral Structures for Local Anesthesia

A. Maxillary nerve—Branches used in dental anesthesia include

  1. Posterior superior alveolar—Nerves enter maxilla through the posterior superior alveolar foramina from

    a. Third molar and facial gingiva

    b. Second molar and facial gingiva

    c. First molar (except mesiobuccal root) and facial gingiva

  2. Middle superior alveolar—Sensation received from

    a. Mesiobuccal root of first molar

    b. Second premolar

    c. First premolar

  3. Anterior superior alveolar—Sensation received from

    a. Canine

    b. Central and lateral incisors

  4. Posterior palatine (greater palatine)—Sensation received from

    a. Greater palatine—Sensation received from

      (1) Lingual gingiva of molars and premolars

      (2) Posterior four-fifths of hard palate

    b. Lesser palatine—Soft palate

  5. Anterior palatine (nasopalatine)—Sensation received from lingual gingiva of anterior teeth

B. Mandibular nerve—Branches include

  1. Inferior alveolar nerve—Receives general sensation from all mandibular teeth

    a. Mental nerve—Receives general sensation from facial gingiva of mandibular anterior teeth, chin, lower lip, and labial mucosa

    b. Incisive nerve—Branches from anterior mandibular teeth and surrounding periodontium

  2. Long buccal nerve—Receives general sensation from facial gingiva of molars and premolars

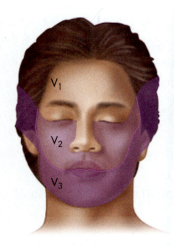

FIGURE 1-36 ■ Divisions of the Trigeminal Nerve

3. Lingual nerve—Receives general sensation from all mandibular lingual gingiva, body of tongue, and floor of mouth

IV. Trigeminal Nerve (Figure 1-36■)

Predominantly sensory; largest cranial nerve of the superficial and deep face; mainly sensory but has a motor and autonomic component.

A. Ophthalmic division (Figure 1-37■)—Purely sensory

- Smallest of the three major divisions of the trigeminal nerve
- Exits from the middle cranial fossa by way of the superior orbital fissure

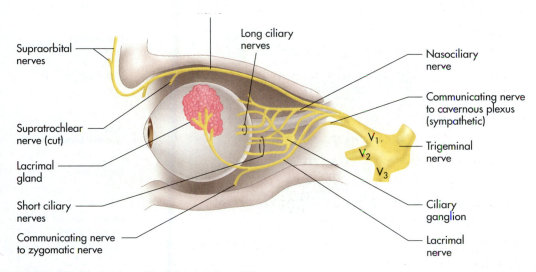

FIGURE 1-37 ■ Divisions of the Ophthalmic Nerve (V₁)

- Three branches: lacrimal, frontal, and nasociliary
- Enters orbit by passing through superior fissure as sensory-only nerves
  1. Nasociliary—Sensory from nasal cavity and orbit
     a. Long cilary—Supplies eyeball
     b. Posterior ethmoidal—Supplies mucous membrane of posterior ethmoidal air cells and sphenoid sinus
     c. Infratrochlear—Supplies skin of eyelids, lacrimal caruncle, lacrimal sac, adjacent conjunctiva, side of nose
     d. Anterior ethmoidal—Supplies anterior ethmoidal air cells, mucosa of anterior portion of septum, lateral nasal
  2. Frontal—Sensory from forehead
     a. Supraorbital—Supplies skin of upper eyelid and scalp
     b. Supratrochelar—Supplies skin of medial portion of upper eyelid and adjacent forehead
  3. Lacrimal—Sensory from area adjacent to lacrimal gland; supplies lacrimal gland, adjacent conjunctiva, skin of the lateral angle of the upper eyelid

B. Maxillary division (V_2) (Figure 1-38■)—Purely sensory; passes into foramen rotundum via pterygopalatine fossa, receiving numerous sensory branches thoughout maxillary region

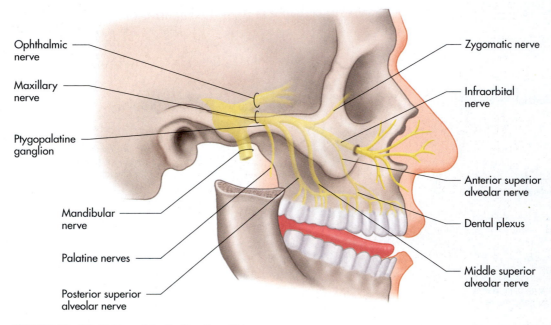

FIGURE 1-38 ■ Divisions of the Maxillary Nerve (V_2)

1. Meningeal nerve
   a. Passes back into middle cranial fossa via foramen spinosum
   b. Carries sensory fibers from dura mater
2. Posterior superior alveolar nerve—Branches off in the pterygopalatine fossa and passes through pterygomaxillary fissure; then enters the PSA foramina on posterior wall of maxillary tuberosity carrying sensation from molars and maxillary sinus, except for mesiobuccal root of maxillary first molar
3. Zygomatic nerve—Branches carry sensation from molar (cheek) portion of face
4. Greater and lesser palatine nerves (Figure 1-39■)
   a. Pass through pterygopalatine fossa inferiorly entering oral cavity through greater and lesser palatine foramina
   b. Carry sensory fibers from the posterior four-fifths (to canine) of hard palate, soft palate, tonsillar area
5. Nasopalatine (anterior palatine) nerve (Figure 1-39)
   a. Leaves pterygopalatine fossa via sphenopalatine foramen into nasal cavity, then passes anteriorly and inferiorly to nasopalatine foramen (incisive), supplies septum, anterior palate where it communicates with greater palatine nerve at the canine palatal tissue
   b. Carries fibers from maxillary anterior teeth and tissues and nasal septum
6. Infraorbital nerve—Forward continuation of maxillary nerve
   a. Enters orbit via inferior orbital fissure, passing through infraorbital canal, and exits through infraorbital canal and foramen
   b. Carries sensory fibers from lower eyelid and adjacent tissue
7. Middle superior alveolar nerve—Branch of infraorbital nerve and maxillary division; when present, carries sensory fibers from maxillary premolar teeth

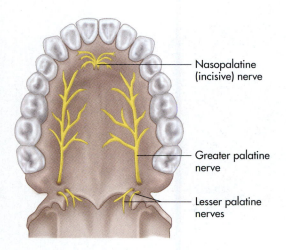

Nasopalatine (incisive) nerve

Greater palatine nerve

Lesser palatine nerves

FIGURE 1-39 ■ Pterygoid Palatine Nerves

and mesiobuccal root of maxillary first molar and surrounding tissues, including buccal gingiva

8. Anterior superior alveolar nerve—Branch of infraorbital nerve and maxillary division; carries sensory fibers from maxillary central and lateral incisors, canines, and associated tissues

C. Mandibular division (V₃) (Figure 1-40■)

1. Only division that carries both sensory and motor fibers; the largest of the three divisions of the trigeminal nerve; exits via oval foramen (foramen ovale)

2. Exits middle cranial fossa via foramen ovale

3. Main branches include

a. Motor fibers—Control muscles of mastication, and mylohyoid and anterior belly of digastric muscles

b. Auriculotemporal nerve—Carries sensation from area anterior to external ear

c. Inferior alveolar nerve—Gives off the mylohyoid nerve (efferent nerve to the mylohyoid muscle and anterior belly of the digastric muscle) before entering mandibular foramen

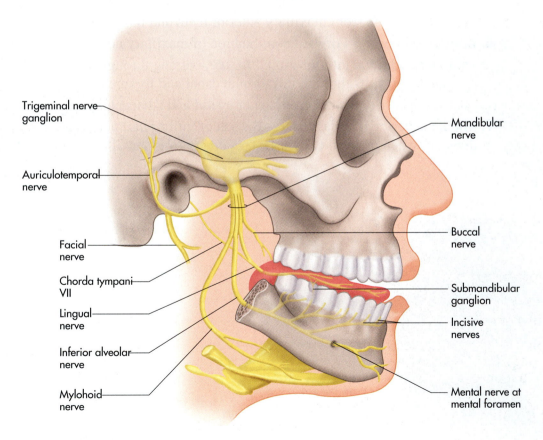

FIGURE 1-40 ■ Branches of the Mandibular Nerve (V₃)

(1) Enters inferior alveolar canal via mandibular foramen and carries sensory fibers from all mandibular teeth

(2) Once in the canal, it divides into the mental nerve leaving the mandible via

    (a) Mental foramen, which carries sensation from lower lip and adjacent mucous membranes

    (b) Incisive nerve, which continues in the canal to anterior teeth

d. Lingual nerve—Travels under tongue receiving general sensation from anterior two-thirds of tongue, floor of mouth, lingual gingiva of mandibular teeth, and taste sensation from the same area via the chorda tympani (VII)

(1) May be visible as it lies subcutaneously posterior to the third molar where it may be damaged by dental procedures in this area

(2) Lies close to inferior alveolar nerve near mandibular foramen where it is also anesthestized during an inferior alveolar block

e. Buccal nerve—Carries sensation from a portion of the cheek and mucous membrane adjacent to molars and premolars

V. Facial Nerve (VII)

A. Carries both sensory and motor fibers

B. Arises from pons and takes a circuitous route through middle ear

C. Exits through stylomastoid foramen of the temporal bone and gives off two branches, the posterior auricular nerve and a branch to the posterior belly of the digastric and stylogyoid muscles (Figure 1-41■); the facial nerve then passes

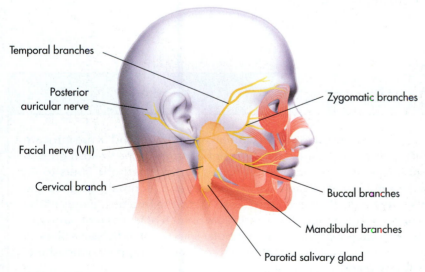

FIGURE 1-41 ■ Pathway of the Branches of the Facial Nerve to the Muscles of Facial Expression

into the parotid salivary gland and divides into numerous branches to supply the muscles of facial expression, but not the parotid gland; bone must be hit during the inferior alveolar injection to prevent anesthetic being deposited in parotid gland and causing temporary facial paralysis

D. Chorda tympani nerve—Branches off facial nerve as it transverses middle ear

1. Passes through petrotympanic fissure in mandibular fossa where it joins lingual nerve
2. Carries autonomic motor fibers to sublingual and submandibular salivary glands
3. Receives taste fibers from anterior two-thirds of tongue
4. Some of its fibers join branches of V_1 and V_2 and carry autonomic motor fibers to the lacrimal gland and mucous glands of maxillary sinus and nasal cavity

VI. Glossopharyngeal Nerve

A. Arises from medulla and primarily supplies tongue and pharynx

B. Carries autonomic motor nerve fibers to parotid salivary gland via the auriculotemporal nerve and receives general sensory and taste fibers from posterior one-third of tongue

C. Carries general motor fibers to a throat muscle and sensation from pharynx

D. Carries afferent fibers from carotid sinus that help control blood pressure

VII. Autonomic Nerve Fibers

A. Two neurons long

B. Fiber before synapse area (ganglion) is termed preganglionic and fibers after the synapse are termed postganglionic

Parasympathetic Fibers and the Trigeminal Nerve

Pathways of the parasympathetic nerve fibers of cranial nerves III, VII, and IX are intricate and somewhat confusing. After the nerve leaves its point of origin in the brain, it goes to various branches of the trigeminal nerve. Nerve III gives parasympathetic fibers to V_1, which carries the autonomic fibers to the ciliary ganglion and lacrimal gland via the nasociliary branch of V_1. Nerve VII gives off branches to V_2, to the mucous glands of the nasal cavity, and a branch (chorda tympani) to the lingual branch of V_3, to carry parasympathetic stimulation to the sublingual and submandibular salivary glands. Nerve IX gives parasympathetic fiber to the auriculotemporal branch of V_3 carrying parasympathetic fibers to the parotid salivary gland

The Autonomic Nervous System

The autonomic nervous system controls many organs at a subconscious level, such as heart rate, breathing rate, and salivary flow. The fibers of the system are found in various nerves of the peripheral nervous system. It is made up of two divisions, the craniosacral (parasympathetic) found in fibers of the III, VII, IX, and X cranial nerves and the thoracolumber found in spinal nerves thoracic 1 to lumbar 3 or 4. The sympathetic division produces effects that occur when one is fearful, fighting, or fleeing. The craniosacral division has the opposite effect.

C. Synapse area for all the sympathetic fibers is superior sympathetic ganglion, which is found in the neck

D. Parasympathetic ganglia—Always found near organ they are controlling

1. Pterygopalatine ganglion—Found in pterygopalatine fossa; serves nerve VII, lacrimal gland, and mucus glands

2. Otic ganglion—Found just inferior to foramen ovale; serves nerve IX to parotid gland

3. Submandibular ganglion—Serves chorda tympani branch of nerve VII to submandibular, sublingual, and minor salivary glands

➤ LYMPHATIC SYSTEM

The lymphatic system is a network of thin-walled vessels and lymph nodes returning fluid from the tissue spaces into the venous system. The presence of one-way valves ensures lymph flow back to general circulation.

I. Lymph Nodes

A. Characteristics

1. Lymph nodes filter toxic products from tissue fluid (lymph) to prevent them from entering general circulation

2. Lymph nodes and vessels are variable in location, and there is a great deal of overlapping coverage

3. Lymph nodes are not normally palpable but, when infected, swell and become palpable, indicating the possible area of infection

4. Lymph fluid from the head and neck ultimately drains into the right or left jugular lymphatic trunk, which empties into the venous system at the junction of the internal jugular and subclavian veins

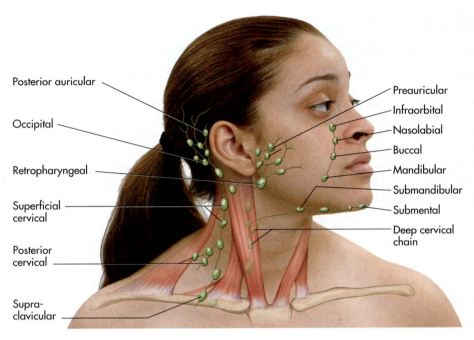

Posterior auricular

Occipital

Retropharyngeal

Superficial cervical

Posterior cervical

Supra-clavicular

Preauricular

Infraorbital

Nasolabial

Buccal

Mandibular

Submandibular

Submental

Deep cervical chain

FIGURE 1-42 ■ Lymph Nodes

5. Lymph vessels have valves, similar to many veins in the body (but not in the head), that allow only a one-way flow of lymph through the vessels and nodes

B. Lymph nodes of the head and neck (Figure 1-42■)

1. Occipital lymph nodes—Superficial nodes that drain lymph fluid from base of skull

2. Retroauricular (posterior auricular) lymph nodes—Superficial nodes that drain lymph fluid from posterior scalp and external ear

3. Anterior auricular lymph nodes—Superficial nodes that drain lymph fluid from area anterior to external ear

4. Superficial parotid lymph nodes—Superficial nodes that drain lymph from parotid gland and adjacent tissue

5. Facial lymph nodes—Superficial nodes that follow path of facial vein and drain into submandibular lymph nodes

   a. Infraorbital (malar)—Drains infraorbital area

   b. Nasolabial—Drains area near nose and upper lip

   c. Buccal—Drains area at corner of mouth

   d. Mandibular—Drains mandibular area

6. Submental lymph nodes—Located on the mylohyoid muscle and drain lymph fluid from chin, lower lip, cheeks, tip of tongue, and incisor teeth

7. Submandibular lymph nodes—Located along inferior border of mandible and drain lymph fluid from chin, lips, nose, cheeks, anterior hard palate,

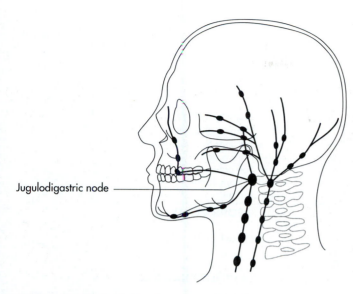

Jugulodigastric node

FIGURE 1-43 ■ Jugulodigastric

sublingual and submandibular salivary glands, and all teeth except mandibular incisors and maxillary third molars

8. External and anterior jugular lymph nodes—Follow path of external jugular vein and drain lymph fluid from lower portion of ear and parotid gland

9. Superior deep cervical lymph nodes—Located under sternocleidomastoid muscle superior to where omohyoid muscle crosses internal jugular vein

   a. Primary nodes for posterior nasal cavity, soft palate, posterior hard palate, base of tongue, and maxillary third molars

   b. Jugulodigastric lymph node (tonsillar node) is palpable when the pharynx or palatine tonsils are inflamed (Figure 1-43■)

10. Inferior deep cervical lymph nodes—Located under sternocleidomastoid muscle, inferior to where omohyoid muscle crosses internal jugular vein

    a. Primary nodes for posterior scalp and neck and structures inferior to neck

    b. Jugulo-omohyoid lymph nodes occur at crossing of omohyoid muscle and internal jugular vein; drains tongue and submental region

➤ TONSILS

The tonsils are large masses of lymphoid tissue found around the opening to the pharynx. Their function is to protect the airway and help fight infection. The tonsils are quite large in youth, but tend to regress with age. When enlarged, pharyngeal tonsils may block the nasopharynx opening of the auditory tube, resulting in a nasal quality of speech and drainage from the middle ear. Palatine tonsils may block the oropharynx.

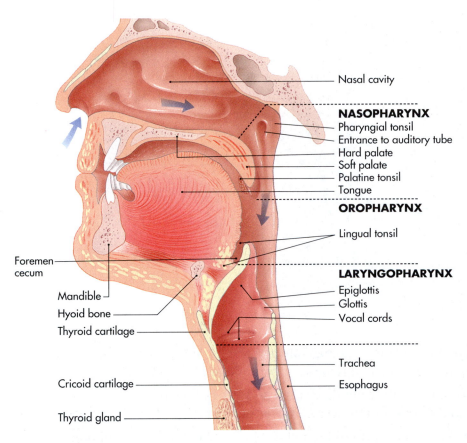

Nasal cavity

NASOPHARYNX
Pharyngial tonsil
Entrance to auditory tube
Hard palate
Soft palate
Palatine tonsil
Tongue

OROPHARYNX

Lingual tonsil

Foremen
cecum

LARYNGOPHARYNX

Mandible
Hyoid bone
Thyroid cartilage

Epiglottis
Glottis
Vocal cords

Trachea
Esophagus

Cricoid cartilage

Thyroid gland

FIGURE 1-44 ■ Nose, Nasal Cavity, and Pharynx

I. Types (Figure 1-44■)

A. Palatine tonsil—Located at posterior lateral border of mouth at the border of the pharynx in a depression between palatopharyngeal fold and glossopharyngeal fold

    1. Palatopharyngeal fold (posterior tonsillar pillar)—Consists of a layer of mucous membrane covering palatopharyngeal muscle

    2. Palatoglossal fold (anterior tonsillar pillar)—Consists of a layer of mucous membrane covering palatoglossus muscle

B. Pharyngeal tonsil (adenoids)—Located on posterior wall of the nasopharynx; may block the auditory (eustachian) tube, which runs from the middle ear to the nasopharynx, thus decreasing drainage and complicating middle ear infections

C. Lingual tonsil—Located at base of the dorsal surface of tongue; consists of a mass of lymphoid tissue

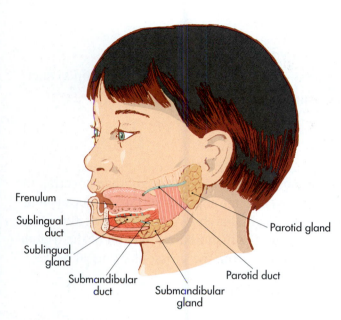

FIGURE 1-45 ■ Salivary Glands

➤ SALIVARY GLANDS

Numerous accessory salivary and mucous glands, as well as the parotid, sublingual, and submandibular salivary glands, are controlled parasympathetically by cranial nerves VII and IX. All glands are controlled sympathetically by branches arising from the superior sympathetic ganglion in the neck (Figure 1-45■).

I. Parotid Gland

    A. Largest gland directly under skin of each cheek

    B. Located in front and below ear

    C. Empties through parotid (Stensen's) duct

    D. Secretes mostly serous fluid

    E. Involved with mumps

II. Submandibular Gland

    A. Pair of encapsulated glands below the angle of mandible directly below the surface skin and on top of the suprahyoid muscle; located on lingual surface of mandible beneath posterior part of tongue

    B. Empties through submandibular (Wharton's) duct that travels in floor of the mouth toward the anterior midline where it empties through a mucosal papilla, a sublingual caruncle located on either side of the lingual frenum

    C. Secretes both serous and mucous fluid

III. Sublingual Gland

   A. Paired glands located anterior to submandibular gland

   B. Ducts may open individually or unite to form the sublingual (Bartholin's) duct

   C. Secretes both serous and mucous fluid

➤ TONGUE

The tongue is composed almost entirely of muscle, with mucous membrane covering the inferior surface and a specialized epithelium covering the superior surface (Figure 1-46■).

Because the tongue forms from different branchial arches, it has different nerve supplies—the anterior two-thirds of the tongue from the mandibular division of the trigeminal and facial nerves and the posterior one-third is from the glossopharyngeal nerve.

I. Markings on the Superior Surface (Dorsum)

   A. Sulcus terminalis

      1. Inverted V-shape, which points toward the throat

      2. Marks division line between anterior and posterior portion of tongue

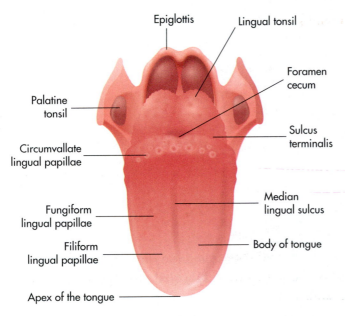

FIGURE 1-46 ■ Papilla of the Tongue

B. Foramen cecum

   1. Pit located at posterior point of the sulcus terminalis

   2. Marks site of origin for the thyroid gland before its migration to the neck

C. Median lingual sulcus—Longitudinal depression down midline of tongue

D. Papillae—Protrusions located on superior surface of tongue

   1. Circumvallate papillae—Flattened protrusions surrounded by a sulcus

     a. 8–12 in number

     b. Located just anterior to the sulcus terminalis in a V-shape

     c. Serous glands (Ebner's salivary gland lies inferior to circumvallate papillae)

     d. Contain taste buds

   2. Fungiform papillae

     a. Mushroom-shaped papillae, red protrusions primarily located on the apex and sides of tongue

     b. Contain taste buds

   3. Filiform papillae—Flame-shaped papillae

     a. Most numerous

     b. Conical shape

     c. Covers anterior two-thirds of surface

     d. Only papillae not containing taste buds

   4. Foliate papillae

     a. Located at lateral sides of base of tongue

     b. Few are present, if any

     c. Contain some taste buds

E. Lingual tonsil

II. Inferior Surface (ventral)—Covered by a thin and translucent mucous membrane, making the lingual vein very visible

A. Fimbriated fold

   1. Plica fimbriatae run laterally to each deep lingual vein

   2. Marks location of the deeper lingual artery, which runs anteriorly under it

B. Lingual frenum—Fold of mucous membrane that attaches inferior surface of the tongue to genial tubercle area

III. Muscles of the Tongue—Divided into two groups (Figure 1-24)

A. Intrinsic—Determines shape; organized into vertical, horizontal, and longitudinal groups allowing tongue to make many intricate movements

B. Extrinsic—Controls position; inserted on the body of tongue from outside locations

1. Styloglossus muscle—Arises from the styloid process, inserts on the lateral side of the body of tongue, and is innervated by hypoglossal nerve (XII)

2. Hyoglossus muscle—Arises from hyoid bone, inserts on the lateral side of the tongue, and is innervated by hypoglossal nerve (XII)

3. Genioglossus muscle—Arises from genial tubercles of mandible, inserts on the posterior surface of tongue, and is innervated by hypoglossal nerve (XII)

4. Palatoglossus muscle—Arises from the soft palate, inserts on the posterior portion of tongue, and is innervated by nerves of the pharyngeal plexus (IX and X)

IV. Blood Supplied by Lingual Artery—Anterior branch of the external carotid artery

V. Innervation—Mixed

A. General sensation

1. V_3—Conveys sensory information from anterior two-thirds of tongue

2. IX—Conveys sensory information from posterior one-third of tongue

B. Taste

1. Supplied by facial (VII) nerve—Conveys taste from anterior one-third of tongue

2. Glossopharyngeal (IX) nerve—Conveys taste on posterior one-third of tongue

3. Vagus (X) nerve—Conveys taste on base of tongue

C. Motor control—Supplied by hypoglossal (XII) nerve; motor fibers to the intrinsic and extrinsic muscles with exception of palatoglossus (IX and X)

VI. Types of Taste Buds (Figure 1-47■)—Differ in their perception to taste quality

A. Sour—Located primarily along posterior border of tongue

B. Sweet—Located primarily at apex of tongue

C. Salty—Located primarily along anterior border of tongue

D. Bitter—Located at base of tongue

Innervation of the Tongue

- General sensation—lingual branch of V_3 and IX
- Taste—includes VII, IX, and X
- Motor control—includes XII

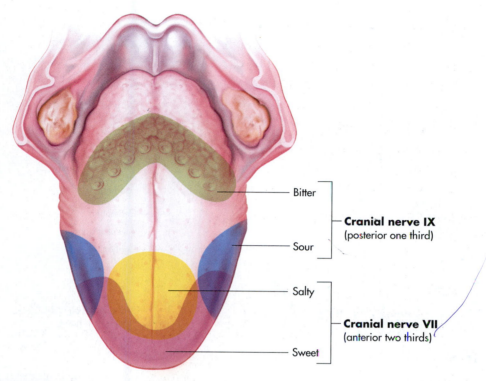

Bitter

Sour

Cranial nerve IX
(posterior one third)

Salty

Cranial nerve VII
(anterior two thirds)

Sweet

FIGURE 1-47 ■ Taste Cells

➤ DENTAL ANATOMY

Morphology

Morphology is the study of form and structure.

I. Definitions (Figure 1-48■)

A. Anatomic crown—Part of tooth covered by enamel (above the cementoenamel juntion [CEJ])

B. Anatomic root—Part of tooth covered by cementum (below the CEJ)

C. Clinical crown—Part of tooth visible above gingival margin

D. Clinical root—Part of tooth attached to alveolar bone by periodontal ligament (begins at gingival line and ends at apex)

E. Cementoenamel junction—Point where enamel of crown meets cementum of root (separates anatomic crown from anatomic root)

F. Longitudinal groove—Groove (concavity) running longitudinally down root surface

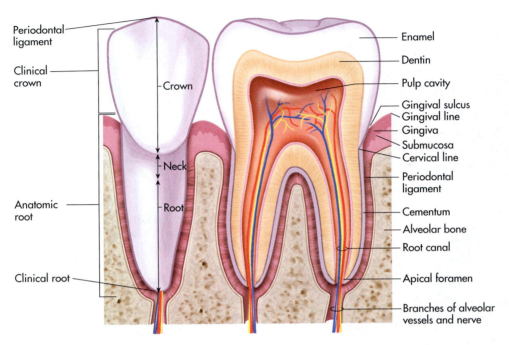

FIGURE 1-48 ■ Longitudinal Section

II. Three Periods of Dentition

A. Primary (Deciduous) (Table 1-3■)

1. Consists of 20 teeth: 8 incisors, 4 canines, and 8 molars
2. Eruption of individual mandibular teeth usually precede the maxillary teeth
3. Teeth in both jaws erupt in pairs, one on the right and one on the left
4. Usually ends with the eruption of the permanent mandibular first molar

B. Mixed (Figure 1-49■)

1. Begins at approximately 6 years of age and ends at approximately 12 years of age

TABLE 1-3 DECIDUOUS TEETH AND APPROXIMATE ERUPTION TIMES	
Central incisors	6.5–8 months
Lateral incisors	7–9 months
First molars	12–16 months
Canines	6–21 months
Second molars	21–30 months

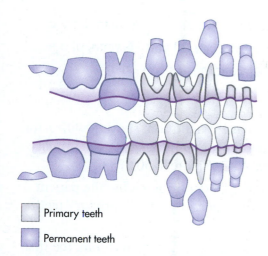

☐ Primary teeth

☐ Permanent teeth

FIGURE 1-49 ■ Mixed Dentition at Approximately 6 Years of Age

2. This period exists while both primary and secondary teeth are simultaneously present

3. Usually ends with the exfoliation of the primary maxillary canine

C. Permanent (Table 1-4■)

1. Succedaneous—Teeth that have primary predecessors; incisors, canines, and premolars

2. First teeth to emerge into the oral cavity are usually the mandibular first molars

TABLE 1-4 PERMANENT TEETH AND APPROXIMATE ERUPTION TIMES		
	Mandibular Teeth	**Maxillary Teeth**
Central incisor	6–7 years	7–8 years
Lateral incisor	7–8 years	8–9 years
Canine	9–10 years	11–12 years
First premolar	10–12 years	10–11 years
Second premolar	11–12 years	10–12 years
First molar	6–7 years	6–7 years
Second molar	11–13 years	12–13 years
Third molar	17–21 years	17–21 years

3. Crowns of permanent teeth are completed between 4 and 8 years of age

4. Roots of permanent teeth are completed between 10 and 16 years of age

5. Completed at approximately 12 years through rest of life

III. Numbering Systems

A. Universal—Uses numbers 1–32 for the permanent dentition, starting with 1 for maxillary right third molar clockwise around lower arch to 32; for the primary dentition the alphabet is used, starting with A–T (Figure 1-50■)

B. Palmer—Brackets represent the four quadrants of dentition facing the patient and permanent teeth are numbered 1–8 on each side of midline; primary teeth use same bracket, but alphabet letters A–E

C. International—Uses two digits for each permanent and deciduous tooth; the first digit denotes the dentition, arch, and side while the second digit denotes the tooth

IV. Generalizations Related to Permanent Teeth

A. Facial surface, mesiodistally, is wider than lingual surface

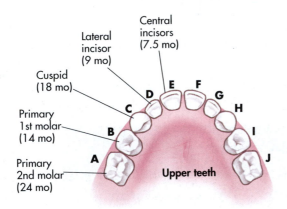

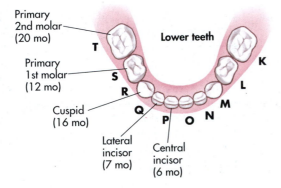

FIGURE 1-50 ■ Universal System of Deciduous Teeth

B. Longitudinal grooves

    1. Anterior teeth—May or may not be present; if present, they most likely will occur on distal surface

        a. Maxillary central incisor—LEAST likely to have longitudinal grooves on the mesial and distal surfaces than any other maxillary or mandibular tooth

    2. Posterior teeth—More prominent and developed on mesial surface

C. Roots

    1. Multirooted teeth—Named for position they occupy in relation to crown surfaces and to each other

        a. Maxillary—Trifurcated; include lingual (longest), mesiofacial, and distofacial roots

        b. Mandibular—Bifurcated; mesial and distal roots

    2. Deviate from norm more frequently than crowns

    3. Apices diverge distally except for mandibular canine, which deviates mesially

    4. All premolars exhibit single roots except for maxillary first, which usually is bifurcated

V. Characteristics of Specific Teeth

A. Maxillary central incisor

    1. Exhibits longest crown in permanent dentition; greatest width is mesiodistally

    2. Mesial and distal surfaces—Converge lingually on a well-developed cingulum

    3. Lingual surface is smaller than facial surface

    4. Incisal edge—Located in center of crown labiolingually

    5. Root—Cone-shaped with blunt apex; one root canal, and proximal surface has a prominent CEJ at incisal curvature

B. Maxillary lateral incisor

    1. Resembles central incisor, but narrower mesiodistally and faciolingually

    2. Displays greatest variance in size and shape of all anterior teeth

    3. Cingulum is narrow

    4. Lingual fossa (pit)—More pronounced than central incisor

    5. Root—Longer and more rounded than central incisor; blunt apex that bends distally; has one root canal

C. Mandibular central incisor

    1. Smallest and simplest tooth in permanent dentition

    2. Crown is bilaterally symmetrical

       3. Lingual crown surface has no distinct anatomy

       4. One root canal

       5. Centered cingulum

       6. Root is longer than crown

D. Mandibular lateral incisor

       1. Less symmetrical, yet slightly larger in all dimensions than mandibular central incisor

       2. Incisal edge has a distinct distolingual twist, and the cingulum is displaced toward the distal

       3. One root canal

       4. Proximal root concavities give double-rooted appearance

E. Maxillary canine

       1. Longest tooth in permanent dentition

       2. Labial surface has distinct labial ridge

       3. Lingual surface has large cingulum

       4. Wide labiolingual dimension

       5. Incisal has single cusp, which is centered over root

       6. Distinct longitudinal depression located on distal root surface; one root canal

       7. Apex may deviate distally

       8. Abrupt tapering of the lingual root surface

       9. Distal coronal concavity and root surface concavity

F. Mandibular canine

       1. Crown is long and narrow compared with maxillary canine

       2. Labial ridge is not as pronounced as maxillary canine

       3. Cingulum is relatively small and off-centered toward distal

       4. Incisal outline is more symmetrical than maxillary canine

       5. Longitudinal depressions are on mesial and distal surfaces of root; one root canal

       6. Root generally has mesial and distal grooves

       7. Proximal root concavities are present

       8. Root is occasionally bifurcated into a facial and lingual root (most common anterior tooth to have bifurcated root)

G. Maxillary first premolar

       1. Crown is wide buccolingually with two cusps—one buccal and one lingual

       2. Mesial and distal pits on occlusal surface

       3. Mesial surface has a longitudinal depression on cervical part of crown and root

4. Long central groove ends with mesial marginal groove, which crosses over mesial marginal ridge

5. Bifurcated root in apical one-third; two root canals

6. Prominent mesial root concavity begins on the crown cervical to the mesial contact and extends apically to the furcation

H. Maxillary second premolar

1. Smaller than first premolar, buccal and lingual cusps are similar in size

2. Occlusal surface more rounded; has a short central groove with a pit at each end

3. No mesial crown concavity or groove

4. Single root, which is longer than the maxillary first premolar; one or two root canals

5. Prominent mesial and distal grooved root surface concavity; mesial root concavity not as pronounced as first premolar

I. Mandibular first premolar

1. Cusps

    a. Buccal cusp—long and sharp, centered over root axis

    b. Lingual cusp is small and nonfunctional

2. Lingual surface has mesiolingual groove that crosses mesial marginal ridge

3. Mesial marginal ridge more cervically located than distal marginal ridge, which is distinct to this tooth

4. Single rooted; one root canal

5. May have deep proximal root concavity on the distal root surface

J. Mandibular second premolar

1. Two common types include

    a. Two-cusps—one buccal cusp and one lingual cusp; H-shaped occlusal pattern

    b. Three-cusps—one buccal cusp and two lingual cusps; Y-shaped occlusal pattern

2. Root is longer than mandibular first premolar; one root canal

K. Maxillary first molar

1. Largest tooth in maxillary arch with its greatest dimension buccolingually

2. Cusps—include five: four major and one minor (cusp of Carabelli), which is located on mesiolingual cusp

3. Rhomboidal occlusal view outline

4. Exhibits oblique ridge on occlusal surface, which crosses from distobuccal cusp to mesiolingual cusp

     5. Roots include

        a. Mesiobuccal (two canals)

        b. Distobuccal (one canal)

        c. Lingual root, longest (one canal)

        d. Furcations on mesial, facial, and distal surfaces

L. Maxillary second molar

    1. Overall size is smaller than maxillary first molar

    2. Crown is similar to maxillary first molar except that cusp of Carabelli is absent

    3. Exhibits three roots—mesiofacial, distofacial, and lingual—that are nearly parallel to one another; three root canals

M. Maxillary third molar

    1. Size is generally smaller and poorly developed

    2. Number of cusps can vary from one to eight

    3. Often impacted

    4. Roots are frequently fused; three root canals

N. Mandibular first molar

    1. First permanent tooth to erupt into oral cavity (all primary teeth may still be present)

    2. Largest tooth in mandibular arch with its greatest dimension mesiodistally

    3. Cusps include five—two buccal, two lingual, and one distal cusp

    4. Two buccal grooves—Y-shaped occlusal groove pattern; mesiobuccal, which frequently ends in a pit; and distobuccal

    5. Occlusal surface has two transverse ridges

    6. Bifurcated roots—mesial and distal; three root canals—mesial has two canals and distal has one canal

O. Mandibular second molar

    1. Crown's greatest dimension is mesiobuccal with only one buccal groove

    2. Distal cusp is absent

    3. Roots are more parallel than mandibular first premolar; three root canals—mesial root has two canals and distal root has one canal

P. Mandibular third molar

    1. Small and poorly developed

    2. Most frequently impacted tooth

    3. Roots are generally fused; three root canals—mesial root has two canals and distal root has one canal

VI. Morphological Differences between Primary and Permanent Dentition

A. Primary teeth are smaller, whiter in color, and less mineralized than permanent teeth

B. Primary teeth have constricted cervical area; cervical ridges are pronounced, especially on buccal aspect of first primary molar

C. Occlusal tables of primary teeth are faciolingually narrower, and the anatomy of the cusps are not as pronounced as permanent teeth

D. Enamel and dentin are thin throughout entire crown

E. Pulp chambers are large; pulp horns extend close to occlusal surface

F. Developmental and supplemental grooves are less pronounced

G. Roots—slender and longer than permanent teeth

    1. Anterior teeth—long compared with the crown size; bend labially

    2. Posterior teeth—widely spread; second molar roots are more widely spread than first molar roots, just opposite of permanent molars

H. Fewer anomalies and variations than permanent teeth

VII. Clinical Consideration and Developmental Disturbances of Permanent Maxillary Teeth

A. Maxillary central incisor

    1. Dwarfed root—Tooth with very short roots in comparison to crown

    2. Hutchinson's incisor—Notched central incisor that develops as a result of congenital syphilis

    3. Supernumerary teeth—Extra teeth in the jaw; most commonly located in the midline and molar regions of the maxilla, followed by the premolar region in the mandible

    4. Diastema—Any spacing between teeth in the same arch

    5. Mesiodens—Supernumerary teeth in the midline of the maxilla, most common supernumerary teeth

B. Maxillary lateral incisor

    1. Dens in Dente—An invagination of the enamel organ within the crown of the tooth; splitting of a single forming tooth germ; crown appears doubled in width; "tooth within a tooth"

    2. Microdontia—Very small, normally shaped teeth

    3. Peg lateral—Conical in shape and tapers toward the incisal to a blunt point

    4. Congenitally missing—The condition of the teeth never having been developed; second most commonly missing tooth

    5. Germination—splitting of a single forming tooth germ; crown appears doubled in width

   C. Maxillary canine

       1. Tubercles—Overcalcification of enamel resulting in small cusp-like elevations on the crown

       2. Dilaceration—A severe bend or distortion of a tooth root and crown; 45-degree to more than 90-degree distortion

       3. Dentigerous cyst—Odontogenic cyst that forms from reduced enamel epithelium; forms around the crown of an impacted or unerupted tooth

       4. Impacted—Describing teeth not completely erupted that are fully or partially covered by bone and/or soft tissue

       5. Germination—Splitting of a single forming tooth germ; crown appears doubled in width

   D. Maxillary first premolar—Roots can occasionally penetrate the maxillary sinus

   E. Maxillary first molar

       1. Concrescence—A fusion or growing together of two adjacent teeth at the root through the cementum

       2. Mulberry molars—Molars with multiple cusps that develop as a result of congenital syphilis

       3. Tubercles—Overcalcification of enamel resulting in small cusp-like elevations on the crown

   F. Maxillary third molar

       1. Impacted—Teeth not completely erupted that are fully or partially covered by bone and/or soft tissue

       2. Congenitally missing—The condition of never having been developed; most commonly missing teeth

       3. Microdontia—Very small, normally shaped teeth

       4. Peg third molars—Conical in shape and tapers toward the incisal to a blunt point

       5. Dentigerous cyst—Odontogenic cyst that forms from the reduced enamel epithelium, forms around the crown of an impacted or unerupted tooth

       6. Accessory roots—Extra root or roots on a tooth, probably caused by trauma, metabolic dysfunction, or pressure

       7. Supernumerary teeth—Extra teeth in the jaw; more common in maxillay arch but does occur in the mandible; commonly called distomolars, paramolars, or fourth molars

VIII. Clinical Consideration and Developmental Disturbances of Permanent Mandibular Teeth

   A. Mandibular central incisor

       1. Accessory roots—Extra root or roots on a tooth, probably caused by trauma, metabolic dysfunction, or pressure

B. Mandibular lateral incisor

    1. Accessory roots—Extra root or roots on a tooth

C. Mandibular Canine

    1. Accessory roots—Bifurcated root

    2. Dilacerations—A severe bend or distortion of a tooth root and crown

D. Mandibular second premolar—Premature loss of primary mandibular second molar can result in impacted second premolar; on occasion congenitally missing

E. Mandibular third molar

    1. Impacted—Teeth not completely erupted that are fully or partially covered by bone and/or soft tissue

    2. Anodontia—No teeth are present in the jay

    3. Accessory roots—Extra root or roots on a tooth

    4. Dentigerous cyst—Cyst around the crown of an unerupted or developing tooth

➤ HISTOLOGY AND EMBRYOLOGY

Histology deals with the structure, function, and composition of tissue.

  I. Tissue—Group of cells that work together to perform special functions

    A. Types—Epithelium, connective, nervous, and muscle

      1. Epithelial—Tissue that covers outer body (skin) or lines mucous membranes (mouth, stomach, and intestine); gives rise to the enamel organ

        a. Surface tissue

          (1) Simple—Single layer of epithelial cells; delicate tissue; lines blood vessels

          (2) Columnar—Single layer of cells, but appear to be in layers; lines upper respiratory tract and intestines

          (3) Stratified—Consists of several layers of epithelial cells; sturdier tissue; lines oral cavity, salivary glands, and most surfaces of the body

        b. Glandular tissue—Consists of surface epithelium that invaginates into underlying connective tissue (CT) to produce secretions

          (1) Exocrine or ducted glands—Retains surface connection (i.e., salivary and sweat glands)

          (2) Endocrine or ductless glands—Loses surface connection (i.e., thyroid and pituitary glands)

      2. Connective—Contains fewer cells and more intercellular substance (ICS); holds body parts together

        a. Types

          (1) Fibrous—Underlies epithelium of skin and oral mucosa; makes up tendons and ligaments

(2) Bone—Supports body

(3) Cartilage—Gives support and allows for skeletal growth

3. Nerve—Made up of nerve cells and tissue; classified as motor or sensory; react to stimuli and transmit impulses

   a. Central nervous system (somatic)—Includes brain and spinal cord

   b. Peripheral nervous system (visceral)—Involves nerves to and from brain and spinal cord; includes smooth muscle nerves (e.g., heart, liver, glands)

   c. Neurons—Basic functioning units of the nervous system that transmit messages throughout the body (Figure 1-51■)

4. Muscle—Responsible for contractions, movements

   a. Skeletal muscles—Limbs, trunk, jaw, face; striated, needs many nuclei to operate

   b. Smooth muscles—Digestive tract, eyes, blood vessels; not striated

   c. Cardiac muscles—Heart; striated

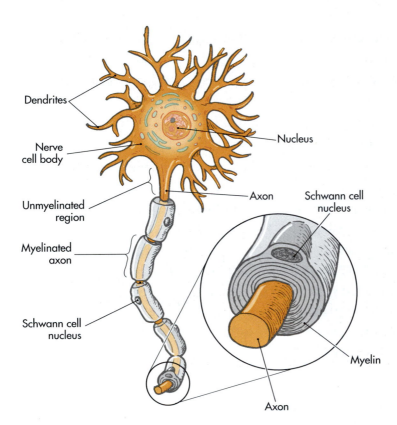

FIGURE 1-51 ■ Neuron

II. Tissues of the Tooth and Surrounding Periodontium (Dental Histology)

A. Enamel—Consists of 96% inorganic and 4% organic material; covers anatomic crown; forms from enamel organ; hardest biological tissue in the body

  1. Amelogenesis—Formation of enamel

    a. Ameloblasts—Enamel-forming cells; originate from ectodermal tissue

    b. Enamel matrix—Organic matrix; consists of rods, rod sheath, and interrod substance

    c. Hydroxyapatite crystals—Consists of calcium phosphate; found in enamel rods

  2. Formations in enamel

    a. Hunter-Schreger bands—Display curvature of enamel rods that run perpendicular to dentinoenamel junction (DEJ); viewed in cross section

    b. Lines (Striae) of Retzius—Depressions that run from DEJ toward occlusal/incisal; viewed in cross section and lines appear brown

    c. Enamel tufts—Undercalcified part of enamel rods; extend from DEJ outward into enamel; appear like "brushes"

    d. Enamel spindles—Originate from odontoblasts; extend from dentinal fibers and cross over DEJ into enamel

    e. Enamel lamellae—Defects in enamel that appear as fine lines on the facial surface

    f. Perikymata—Horizontal ridges that appear on surface formed by lines of Retzius

    g. Nasmyth's membrane—Consists of

      (1) Primary enamel cuticle—Last product of ameloblasts

      (2) Secondary enamel cuticle—Product of reduced enamel epithelium

  3. Effects on enamel

    a. Erosion—Chemical damage to enamel (Figure 1-52■)

    b. Abrasion—Abnormal wear on enamel (Figure 1-53■)

    c. Attrition—Normal wear and tear on enamel (Figure 1-54■)

    d. Abfraction—Wedge-shaped notches of teeth caused by malocclusion or biomechanical forces; located at the cervical areas of teeth (Figure 1-55■)

B. Dentin

  1. Consists of 70% inorganic and 30% organic material

  2. Located in crown and root

  3. Makes up bulk of tooth

  4. First tissue to mineralize during tooth development

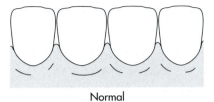

Normal

Eroded

FIGURE 1-52 ■ Erosion

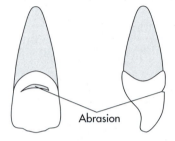

Abrasion

FIGURE 1-53 ■ Abrasion

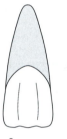 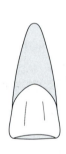

8 years   80 years

FIGURE 1-54 ■ Attrition

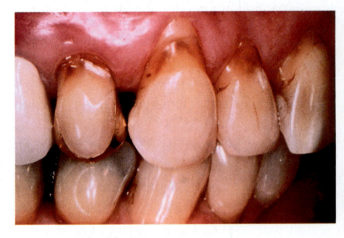

FIGURE 1-55 ■ Abfraction

5. Forms from dental papilla

    a. Odontogenesis—Formation of dentin

        (1) Odontoblast—Cells that form organic matrix of dentin

            (a) Collagen fibers and ground substance—Make up the 30% organic material

            (b) Hydroxyapatite crystals—Make up the 70% inorganic material, which form mineralized matrix

        (2) Dentinal tubules—Tubules that extend from dentinoenamel junction to pulp; contain cytoplasm of pulp cell

        (3) Dentinal fibers—Nerve fibers located in tubules; transmit nerve impulses

(4) Predentin—located next to pulp; consists of organic matrix that has not mineralized

(5) Tomes granular layer—located in root portion just under cementum; an unmineralized area of dentin

(6) Interglobular dentin—usually located in crown portion just under DEJ; an unmineralized area of dentin that occurs during tooth formation

(7) Reactive dentin—Forms immediately in localized areas where dental tubules have been traumatized due to caries, attrition or bruxism, or thermal conditions

(8) Secondary dentin—produced throughout life of tooth, in response to stimuli such as caries or trauma; located next to pulp; modified type of dentin, usually found in older teeth

(9) Sclerotic dentin—dentin tubules filled with calcuim salt because of degeneration of odontoblast

(10) Dead tract—odontoblasts have degenerated, but tract is not filled with calcium salt

(11) Lines of Von Ebner—incremental lines of dentin

C. Cementum

1. Consists of 50% inorganic and 50% organic matters

2. Covers root dentin

3. Primary function is to provide medium for attachment of periodontal ligament

4. Histologically similar to bone

5. Forms from dental sac

a. Cementogenesis—Formation of cementum

(1) Cementoblast—Produces organic matrix of cementum; located in periodontal ligament

(a) Collagen fibers—Make up matrix

(b) Hydroxyapatite crystals—Consist of calcium phosphate; form mineralized matrix

(2) Cementocytes—Cementoblasts that become surrounded by organic matrix

(a) Lacuna—"Little space" occupied by cementocytes

(b) Canaliculi—"Little canal" area occupied by threadlike projections of cementocytes

(3) Types

(a) Acellular—Without cells; located in apical half

(b) Cellular—Contains cells; located in cervical half

(4) Cementoid—Located on outer surface and is hypocalcified

(5) Sharpey's fibers—Bundles of fibers of periodontal ligament that embed into cementoid

(6) Hypercementosis—Excessive amount of cementum growth, forming ball-shaped growths on the apices (Figure 1-56■)

D. Pulp—Innermost soft tissue occupying the hollowed-out inner portion of the dentin; space is called the pulp chamber and root canal; comprised of soft connective tissue with lots of matrix and few cells (Figure 1-57■)

1. Noncalcified tissue that develops from dental papilla

2. Makes up vascular and nerve portion of tooth

    a. Formation of pulp—Calcification does not occur

        (1) Fibroblasts—Form and maintain pulp tissue; primary cell

        (2) Histocytes and undifferentiated mesenchymal cells—Act as defense mechanism

        (3) Odontoblast—Used in repair

        (4) Korff's fibers—Important in formation of dentin matrix

        (5) Pulp stones (denticles)—Mineralized bodies of irregular shape (Figure 1-58■)

    b. Functions

        (1) Formative—Odontoblast produce dentin throughout life of tooth

        (2) Sensory—Nerves bring sense of pain, heat, and cold

        (3) Nutritive—Blood brings nutrients to pulp

        (4) Defensive—Odontoblasts respond to injury or decay

E. Periodontal ligament (PDL)(Figure 1-59■; see Figure 1-60■ for periodontal ligament bundles)

1. Specialized connective tissue derived from fibers of the dental sac

2. Attaches tooth cementum to alveolus

3. Produces cementum and lamina dura

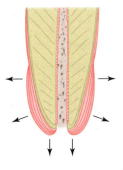

FIGURE 1-56 ■ Hypercementosis

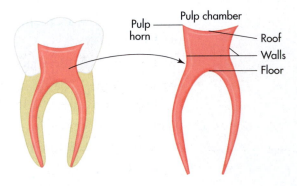

FIGURE 1-57 ■ Pulp

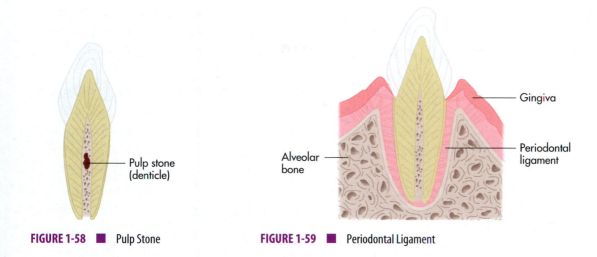

FIGURE 1-58 ■ Pulp Stone

FIGURE 1-59 ■ Periodontal Ligament

a. Formation—Does not calcify

  (1) Fibroblasts—Form fibrils of ligament

  (2) Collagen—Make up fibrils

  (3) Made up of groups of fiber bundles called principal fiber bundles and gingival fibers

    (a) Principal fiber group (Figure 1-61■)

      i) Alveolar crest fibers—Extend from cementum to alveolar crest; help resist horizontal movement; resist tilting, intrusive, extrusive, and rotation forces

      ii) Horizontal fibers—Extend from cementum to bone; resist horizontal pressure, and tilting forces

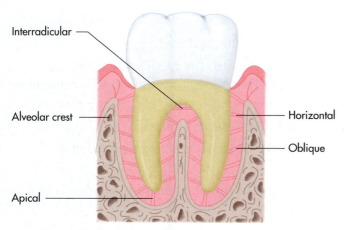

FIGURE 1-60 ■ Periodontal Ligament Bundles

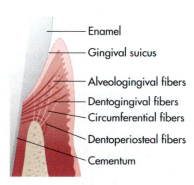

FIGURE 1-61 ■ Cross Section Showing Gingival Fiber Groups

iii) Oblique fibers—Most numerous; extend from cementum obliquely to bone in a coronal direction; prevent apex from being "jammed" against base of socket; resists retrusive and rotational forces, most numerous of fibers

iv) Apical fibers—Extend from cementum at apex to bone; radiate around apex; resists extrusive forces

v) Interradicular fibers—Located between roots of multirooted teeth; help stabilize tooth; resists intrusive, extrusive, and tilting and rotational forces

(b) Gingival fiber groups (Figure 1-61)—Hold gingiva to tooth surface; extend from cementum to lamina propria of free gingiva

i) Dentogingival fibers (free gingiva)—Fibers attach from the cementum in the cervical region into the free gingiva to give support to the gingiva

ii) Alveologingival fibers (attached gingiva)—Fibers attach from the alveolar crest into the free and attached gingiva to provide support

iii) Circumferential fibers (circular)—Extend horizontally around the neck of the tooth to help to maintain the tooth in position

iv) Dentoperiosteal (alveolar crest)—Extend from the cervical cementum over the alveolar crest to the periosteum of the bone

v) Transseptal fibers—Extend from cementum of one tooth to cementum of an adjacent tooth; mesial and distal only

(4) Sharpey's fibers—Terminal end of periodontal ligament that is embedded in cementum on one side and alveolar bone on the other

F. Alveolar bone

1. Part of the mandible and the maxilla that surrounds and supports teeth

2. Consists of 50% organic and 50% inorganic material

3. Consists of the lamina dura, which surrounds the tooth socket, and supporting bone; it is dependent upon the presence of dental roots and when teeth are lost the alveolar bone is resorbed

4. Provides attachment for the periodontal ligament fibers

5. Alveolar bone proper—Faces the root of the tooth, also referred to as lamina dura

a. Cribriform plate—Allows communication between blood vessels and nerves in the periodontal ligament

        (1) Compact bone (cortical plate)—Makes up outside wall of mandible/maxilla

        (2) Trabecular bone (spongy)—Makes up the inside wall of mandible/maxilla

        (3) Bone marrow—Projects into spaces around trabeculae

            (a) Red—Forms function of hemopoiesis (forms blood)

            (b) Yellow—Consists of adipose; contains no blood-producing function

        (4) Bone that allows Sharpey's fibers to insert

    b. Lamina dura—Radiographically appears as radiopaque caused by the two-dimensional view of the compact bone

    c. Periosteum—Consists of connective tissue that covers outside of bone

    d. Endosteum—Consists of connective tissue that covers inside of bone

    e. Tissue

        (1) Osteoblasts—Cells that form bone

        (2) Osteocytes—Osteoblasts that are trapped in lacunae; osteocytic cell processes extend into canaliculi and maintain contact with adjacent osteocytes

        (3) Osteoclasts—Cells that resorb bone

        (4) Lacunae—Space in bone matrix that is occupied by osteocyte; "little space"

        (5) Canaliculi—Connect lacunae

        (6) Lamellae—Thin layers of mature bone

            (a) Lamellar—Lamellae that follow circumference of bone Circumferential bone—Makes up outer perimeter of adult bone Subendosteal—Makes up surface of trabecular bone

            (b) Haversian system—Lamellae arranged in concentric circles around a central canal

            (c) Haversian canal—Central canal that carries capillary-like blood vessels

            (d) Volkmann's canal—Canal through which blood vessels pass in and out of bone

G. Gingiva—Specialized mucous membrane that firmly attaches to underlying bone

    1. Composed of connective (fibrous) and epithelial tissues (stratified squamous)

    2. Structure (Figure 1-62■)

        a. Gingival sulcus—Space between gingiva and tooth; encircles all around tooth; also called periodontal pocket if it were diseased

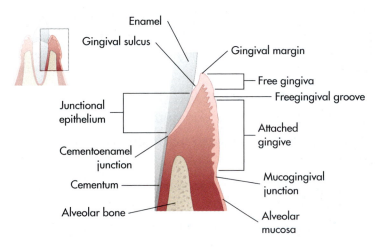

FIGURE 1-62 ■ Cross Section Showing the Parts of the Gingiva

   b. Free gingiva (marginal)—Consists of gingiva not attached to tooth surface

   c. Epithelial attachment (junctional)—Point where epithelium attaches to tooth; located at base of sulcus; made up of nonkeratinized stratified squamous epithelium causing it to be vulnerable to disease

   d. Free gingival groove—Depression located opposite alveolar crest and denotes sulcus depth

   e. Attached gingiva—Located beneath free gingival groove and attaches to bone

   f. Mucogingival junction—Point where attached gingiva ends; layer between gingiva and underlying bone

   g. Rete ridges (pegs)—Fingerlike extensions of epithelium into the lamina propria found in the free gingival; help to strengthen gingiva (Figure 1-63■)

III. Embryology

   A. Primary germ layers

      1. Ectoderm—Forms epithelial tissue (lining or protective tissue); outer covering of body and lining of oral cavity

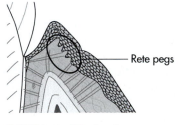

Rete pegs

FIGURE 1-63 ■ Rete Pegs

2. Mesoderm—Forms mesenchyme, which becomes connective tissue for all tooth components, skeletal and muscular systems, cementum, dentin, and pulp; EXCEPT enamel

3. Endoderm—Forms epithelial tissue lining of internal organs

B. Stomodeum

1. Future mouth of embryo

2. Formed from the fusion of the frontal process and branchial arch I (the other branchial arches will become the posterior part of the tongue, larynx, pharynx, hyoid, inner and middle ear)

3. Surrounded by coalescing pharyngeal arches

C. Tongue—Develops during the fourth week of embryonic life and will develop from six processes

1. Circumvallate papillae—Form the border between the ectoderm and endoderm coverings of the tongue; mark the division between the anterior two-thirds or body of the tongue and the posterior one-third or root

IV. Facial Development (Figures 1-64■, 1-65■, 1-66■)

A. Frontonasal process—Contains future brain (begins in fourth week of gestation)

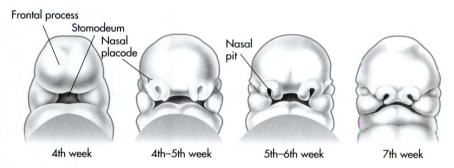

FIGURE 1-64   ■   Developing Face

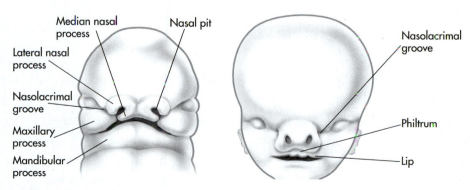

FIGURE 1-65   ■   Face Formation

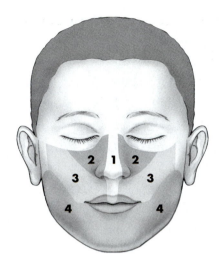

FIGURE 1-66 ■ Development of the Face:
1) Medial Nasal Process; 2) Lateral Nasal Process;
3) Maxillary Process; 4) Mandibular Process

    B. Lateral and median nasal processes—On both right and left sides
        1. Lateral—Forms sides of nose
        2. Median—Forms middle of nose
        3. Globular process develops the premaxilla, maxillary incisors, nasal septum, philtrum of lip
    C. Branchial arch I
        1. Maxillary process—Forms maxilla, all maxillary teeth EXCEPT incisors, cheeks, most of upper lip, and lateral palatine processes, which become palatal shelves that fuse at midline
        2. Mandibular process—Forms mandible and all mandibular teeth; Meckel's cartilage acts as a temporary "jawbone" until the bone of the mandible envelops it and most of it disappears
        3. Palate—Formed by three processes coalescing: two maxillary processes, lateral palatine processes, and one globular process (primary palatine); cleft lip or cleft palate results if processes do not come together properly

V. Tooth Development

    A. Dental lamina—Thickened oral epithelium (ectoderm) that will become occlusal border of mandible and maxilla
    B. Tooth germ—Invagination of dental lamina into the underlying connective tissue (mesoderm)
        1. Enamel organ (dental organ)—Formed from oral epithelium of dental lamina, forms enamel; first part of tooth germ to form; develops from dental lamina

   2. Dental papilla—Formed from connective tissue; becomes dentin and pulp; forms dentin and pulp

   3. Dental sac or follicle—Formed from connective tissue; becomes PDL, cementum, lamina dura

C. Layers of enamel organ (Figure 1-67■)

   1. Outer enamel epithelium—Consists of low cuboidal cells

   2. Stellate reticulum—Consists of star-shaped epithelial cells

   3. Stratum intermedium—Consists of flat epithelial cells

   4. Inner enamel epithelium—Consists of cuboidal cells, and will become the ameloblasts

D. Basement membrane

   1. Separates enamel organ from underlying dental papilla

   2. DEJ is located in this area as it develops

E. Reduced enamel epithelium

   1. Results as the four cell layers of the enamel organ become compressed

   2. Protects tooth until it erupts

   3. Enamel cuticle

      a. Primary enamel cuticle—Last product of ameloblast; mineralized

      b. Secondary enamel cuticle—Product of reduced enamel epithelium; nonmineralized

   4. Hertwig epithelial root sheath

      a. Strands of cells of the reduced enamel epithelium that bring about dentin formation

      b. Determines outline of root dentin and number of roots

   5. Epithelial rests (rests of Malassez)—Remnants of Hertwig's epithelial root sheath in periodontal ligament

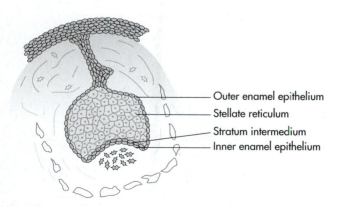

FIGURE 1-67 ■ Layers of Enamel Organ

VI. Oral Cavity

A. Oral mucous membrane

1. Categories

a. Masticatory mucosa—Keratinized; includes gingiva and hard palate

b. Lining mucosa—Nonkeratinized; includes nonmasticatory areas, such as cheeks, soft palate, and underside of tongue

c. Specialized mucosa—Applied to mucous membrane located on dorsum (top) of tongue; includes papillae

2. Functions

a. Protect

b. Secrete (e.g., nasal passages, salivary glands)

c. Absorb—Has ability to take in solution; nutritive

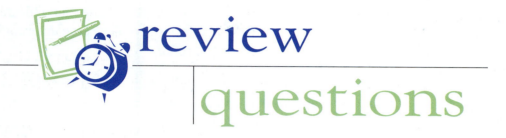

review questions

DIRECTIONS Each of the questions or incomplete statements below is followed by suggested answers or completions. Select the **one** answer that is best in each case.

1. The inferior alveolar artery is a branch of which of the following arteries?
   A. Maxillary
   B. Temporal
   C. Occipital
   D. Facial

2. The left common carotid artery branches off the:
   A. Brachiocephalic artery
   B. Arch of the aorta
   C. Left subclavian artery
   D. Superior sagittal sinus

3. The external auditory meatus is found in which of the following bones?
   A. Sphenoid
   B. Temporal
   C. Occipital
   D. Parietal

4. Within the mandibular canal, near the mental foramen, the inferior alveolar nerve is formed by the mental nerve and which other branch?
   A. Incisive
   B. Lingual
   C. Mylohyoid
   D. Buccal

5. The cribriform plate is a portion of which of the following bones?
   A. Frontal
   B. Sphenoid
   C. Temporal
   D. Ethmoid

6. Cleft lip results from lack of fusion of the:
   A. Mandibular process with the maxillary process
   B. Right mandibular process with the left mandibular process
   C. Maxillary process with the medial nasal elevations
   D. Right and left palatine processes

7. The internal jugular vein empties into the:
   A. Subclavian artery
   B. Subclavian vein
   C. Arch of the aorta
   D. Thoracic duct

8. Which of the following bones contains a paranasal sinus?
   A. Sphenoid
   B. Mandible
   C. Occipital
   D. Zygomatic

review questions

9. Which of the following muscles forms the anterior tonsillar pillar?
   A. Palatopharyngeus
   B. Mylohyoid
   C. Stylohyoid
   D. Palatoglossus

10. Which of the following muscles is NOT a suprahyoid muscle?
    A. Geniohyoid
    B. Stylohyoid
    C. Omohyoid
    D. Mylohyoid

11. Which of the following nerves innervates the buccinator muscle?
    A. Trigeminal
    B. Facial
    C. Glossopharyngeal
    D. Hypoglossal

12. Which of the following branches of the trigeminal nerve consists of motor and sensory fibers?
    A. V_1
    B. Ophthalmic
    C. V_2
    D. Mandibular

13. Which of the following muscles inserts on the coronoid process of the mandible?
    A. Masseter
    B. Lateral pterygoid
    C. Medial pterygoid
    D. Temporalis

14. Which of the following arteries exits the foramen apical to the mandibular premolars?
    A. Posterior superior alveolar
    B. Mental
    C. Lingual
    D. Incisive

15. Which of the following foramen is located on the medial aspect of the mandible and has the inferior alveolar nerve entering it?
    A. Infraorbital
    B. Ovale
    C. Supraorbital
    D. Mandibular

16. Which of the following bones is completely surrounded by soft tissue and does NOT articulate with any other bone?
    A. Vomer
    B. Hyoid
    C. Mandible
    D. Styloid

17. Which of the following sutures separates the occipital bone from the paired parietal bones?
    A. Coronal
    B. Sagittal
    C. Zygomaxillary
    D. Lambdoidal

18. Which of the following salivary glands is predominately serous in its secretory product?
    A. Submandibular
    B. Sublingual
    C. Parotid
    D. Minor salivary glands

19. Which of the following cranial nerves provides sensory taste innervation to the posterior one-third of the tongue?
    A. Abducens
    B. Trigeminal
    C. Trochlear
    D. Glossopharyngeal

20. After a mandibular injection, a patient experiences paralysis of the muscles of facial expression on that side of the face. Which of the following nerves was MOST likely anesthetized?
    A. V_1
    B. V_3
    C. IV
    D. VII

21. Which of the following groups of lymph nodes provides primary lymphatic drainage for the mandibular incisors?
    A. Superficial parotid
    B. Submandibular
    C. Facial
    D. Submental

22. Which of the following processes in the skull is located immediately anterior to the mandibular fossa?
    A. Articular eminence
    B. Styloid
    C. Mental
    D. Mastoid

23. What is the movement of the mandible when the mandibular condyle moves forward on the articular eminence of the temporal bone?
    A. Rotation
    B. Protrusion
    C. Depression
    D. Elevation

24. Which of the following glands lies immediately inferior to the circumvallate papillae?
    A. Parathyroid
    B. Ebner's
    C. Thyroid
    D. Parotid

25. Which of the following alveolar nerves innervates the mesiobuccal root of the maxillary first molar?
    A. Anterior superior
    B. Middle superior
    C. Posterior superior
    D. Inferior

26. Which of the following divisions of the trigeminal nerve enters through the superior orbital fissure?
    A. V_1
    B. V_2
    C. V_3
    D. All divisions

27. Which of the following factors ensures the flow of lymph in one direction?
    A. Sphincters
    B. Valves
    C. Blood pressure
    D. Hydrostatic pressure of lymph

28. Which of the following bones is a small projection located on the medial surface of the ramus anterior to the mandibular foramen?
    A. Lingula
    B. Epiglottis
    C. Vomer
    D. Articular eminence

29. Which of the following organs is associated with the circle of Willis?
    A. Heart
    B. Liver
    C. Brain
    D. Spleen

30. Which lingual papillae are located just anterior to the sulcus terminalis?
    A. Fungiform
    B. Foliate
    C. Filiform
    D. Circumvallate

31. Compared with the permanent teeth, all of the following are characteristics of primary teeth EXCEPT one. Which one is the EXCEPTION?
    A. Smaller pulp size
    B. Whiter in color
    C. Smaller in overall size
    D. Less mineralized enamel

32. Which of the following tissues makes up the bulk of the tooth?
    A. Enamel
    B. Cementum
    C. Dentin
    D. Pulp

33. The number of roots a tooth will develop is determined by the:
    A. Dental sac
    B. Hertwig's root sheath
    C. Periodontal ligament
    D. Cementum

34. Which of the following components is the primary crystalline material of bone?
    A. Magnesium
    B. Carbonate
    C. Potassium
    D. Hydroxyapatite

35. Which of the following is the first mineralized tissue to appear in any developing tooth?
    A. Enamel
    B. Cementum
    C. Dentin
    D. Pulp

36. Rests of Malassez represent remnants of which of the following?
    A. Outer enamel epithelium
    B. Hertwig's root sheath
    C. Stratum intermedium
    D. Stellate reticulum

37. Which of the following compositions represents normal enamel?
    A. 25% hydroxyapatite, 75% organic compounds
    B. 55% hydroxyapatite, 45% organic compounds
    C. 70% hydroxyapatite, 30% organic compounds
    D. 96% hydroxyapatite, 4% organic compounds

38. The attachment apparatus (cementum, PDL, and bone) originates from the:
    A. Inner enamel epithelium
    B. Outer enamel epithelium
    C. Stellate reticulum
    D. Dental sac

39. Which of the following is a derivative of ectoderm?
    A. Dentin
    B. Enamel
    C. Cementum
    D. Alveolar bone

40. Which of the following BEST defines the lines of Retzius?
    A. Cracks in newly formed enamel
    B. Defective enamel rods
    C. Trapped odontoblastic processes
    D. Incremental lines of enamel formation

41. The last layer of enamel produced by ameloblasts, before tooth eruption, is the:
    A. Perikymata
    B. Imbrication line
    C. Primary cuticle
    D. Secondary cuticle

42. Of the following permanent teeth, which is MOST likely to exhibit the cusp of Carabelli?
    A. Mandibular right second premolar
    B. Mandibular right first molar
    C. Maxillary right canine
    D. Maxillary right first molar

43. Which permanent premolar usually exhibits a bifurcated root?
    A. Maxillary first
    B. Maxillary second
    C. Mandibular first
    D. Mandibular second

44. Which permanent premolar has a functional buccal cusp and a nonfunctional lingual cusp?
    A. Mandibular first
    B. Maxillary first
    C. Mandibular second
    D. Maxillary second

45. A lingual groove is commonly found on the permanent premolar crown surface of the:
    A. Mandibular first
    B. Y-type mandibular second
    C. H-type mandibular second
    D. Maxillary first

46. Maxillary permanent molars are the only group of teeth that normally exhibit:
    A. A transverse ridge
    B. Two roots
    C. An oblique ridge
    D. A masticatory function of grinding

47. A permanent molar, which exhibits four cusps and two roots, is MOST likely the:
    A. Maxillary first
    B. Maxillary second
    C. Mandibular first
    D. Mandibular second

48. Which of the following roots is the longest on the permanent maxillary second molar?
    A. Mesial
    B. Mesiobuccal
    C. Lingual
    D. Distobuccal
    E. Distal

49. A cingulum is normally located:
    A. Between two cusp ridges
    B. On the same surface as the transverse ridge
    C. On the lingual surface of anterior teeth
    D. On the buccal surface of posterior teeth

50. The periodontal ligament is located between the:
    A. Enamel and dentin
    B. Dentin and cementum
    C. Cementum and bone
    D. Bone and enamel

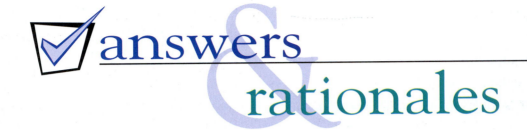

answers & rationales

1.

A. The inferior alveolar artery is a branch of the maxillary artery. The temporal, occipital, and facial arteries are branches of the external carotid artery.

2.

B. The left common carotid artery is a branch off the arch of the aorta. The brachiocephalic artery goes to the right arm and right side of the head, the left subclavian artery goes to the left arm, and the superior sagittal sinus is a dural venous sinus within the skull.

3.

B. The external auditory meatus is found in the temporal bone with the postglenoid process and articular fossa of the temporomandibular joint located anteriorly and the mastoid process located posteriorly. The sphenoid, occipital, and parietal bones are not associated with the hearing organ.

4.

A. The inferior alveolar nerve is formed by the merger of the incisive nerve, composed of dental branches from anterior mandibular teeth, and the mental nerve from the chin and lower lip. The lingual nerve arises from the body of the tongue to join the maxillary division of the trigeminal nerve. The mylohyoid nerve is efferent to the mylohyoid muscle and anterior belly of the digastric muscle and joins the inferior alveolar nerve posterior to the mandibular canal. The buccal nerve carries sensation from the cheek and buccal region of the oral cavity.

5.

D. The cribriform plate is the portion of the horizontal plate of the ethmoid that lies in the anterior cranial fossa and is the opening for the olfactory nerve to enter the superior aspects of the nasal cavity.

6.

C. Cleft lips usually develop slightly lateral to the midline due to a failure of the maxillary process to fuse with the medial nasal process. The mandibular and maxillary processes only meet at the angle of the mouth. The right and left mandibular processes fuse to form the single mandible. Failure of fusion of the palatine processes results in a cleft palate.

7.

B. The arch of the aorta and the subclavian artery are part of the arterial system and do not receive venous blood. The thoracic duct is a collection vessel of the lymphatic system.

8.

A. The sphenoid, frontal, maxilla, and ethmoid bones contain paranasal sinuses.

9.

D. The palatoglossus muscle forms the anterior tonsillar pillar and the palatopharyngeal muscle forms the posterior tonsillar pillar—both structures found where the oral cavity opens into the oropharynx. The mylohyoid and stylohyoid muscles are suprahyoid muscles.

10.

C. The omohyoid muscle is an infrahyoid muscle that has an origin on the superior border of the scapula and inserts on the lateral border of the hyoid. The other three muscles are suprahyoid muscles inserting on the hyoid bone.

11.

B. The buccinator muscle is innervated by the facial nerve (VII) and is therefore not considered a muscle of mastication (innervated by V). The glossopharyngeal nerve innervates the pharynx and the hypoglossal muscles of the tongue.

12.

D. The mandibular branch carries sensory fibers from the teeth and supporting structures and motor fibers to muscles of mastication. V_1 is the ophthalmic division of the trigeminal. V_2 is the maxillary division of the trigeminal, both of which are only sensory.

13.

D. The masseter, temporalis, and lateral and medial pterygoid muscles are muscles of mastication. The temporalis muscle inserts on the coronoid process of the mandible, while the remaining three insert at the temporomandibular joint, ramus, angle, and body of the mandible.

14.

B. The mental artery exits the mental foramen on the anterior surface of the mandible. The posterior superior alveolar artery is located in the maxilla. The lingual artery is a branch from the maxillary artery providing the blood supply to the tongue and the floor of the mouth. The incisive artery is a continuation of the inferior alveolar artery distally and anteriorly within the mandible.

15.

D. The infraorbital foramen is in the maxilla, inferior to the orbit where the infraorbital nerve exits. The foramen ovale is in the base of the skull through which a portion of the trigeminal nerve exits the skull. The supraorbital foramen is superior to the orbital rim.

16.

B. The hyoid bone is a U-shaped bone in the upper neck that does not articulate with any other bone. The vomer bone forms a portion of the nasal septum, the mandible articulates with the temporal bone, and the styloid is a process projecting from the temporal bone at the base of the skull.

17.

D. The coronal suture separates the frontal bone from the paired parietal bones. The sagittal suture separates the paired parietal bones, and the zygomaxillary suture separates the maxilla from the zygomatic bone.

18.

C. The parotid is composed of mostly serous fluid. The submandibular gland is almost an even mixture of serous and mucinous secretory fluid. The sublingual gland is predominately mucous fluid and the minor salivary glands are mostly mucinous secretions.

19.

D. The glossopharyngeal nerve supplies taste to the posterior one-third of the tongue and the facial nerve supplies taste to the anterior two-third of the tongue via the chorda tympani. This is because developmentally the anterior and posterior parts of the tongue arose from two different branchial arches. The abducens (VI) provides motor fibers to a muscle of the eye. The trigeminal (V) provides motor and sensory to the teeth, sinus, gingiva, and muscles of mastication. The trochlear (IV), the smallest of the cranial nerves, provides motor to a muscle of the eye.

20.

D. The facial nerve (VII) courses through the capsule of the parotid gland where it divides into branches innervating the muscles of facial expression. It may become anesthetized with deep mandibular block injections. The ophthalmic division (V_1) of the trigeminal is sensory only. The mandibular division (V_3) of the trigeminal provides both sensory and motor fibers. The trochlear nerve (IV) innervates a muscle of the eyeball.

21.

D. The superficial parotid nodes are too far superior for lymphatic drainage of the mandibular incisors, which drain into the submental nodes located just inferior to the mandibular incisors. The submandibular and facial nodes are the secondary group of nodes, which drain the submental nodes.

22.

A. The articular eminence is a protrusion of bone anterior to the mandibular fossa. The styloid process is a projection that is immediately inferior to the auditory canal. The mental process forms the anterior chin, and the mastoid process is a projection posterior to the mandibular auditory canal.

23.

B. Gliding movement involves protrusion, where the condyle moves forward on the articular eminence and retraction, where the condyle moves backward. Elevation and depression are both forms of rotation, where the condyle rotates on the meniscus.

24.

B. Ebner's glands give serous secretions and aid in cleansing chemical stimulants from the taste buds. The parathyroids lie in the neck on the posterior surface of the thyroid. The thyroid lies in the neck inferior to the thyroid cartilage, and the parotids are major salivary glands that lie anterior to the ear.

25.

B. The middle superior alveolar nerve innervates the maxillary premolars and the mesiobuccal root of the maxillary first molar. The anterior superior alveolar nerve primarily innervates the maxillary anteriors. The posterior superior alveolar nerve primarily innervates the maxillary sinus and maxillary molars, except the mesiobuccal root of the maxillary first molar. The inferior alveolar nerve innervates the mandibular teeth, becoming the incisive nerve beyond the mental foramen.

26.

A. Cranial nerves V_1, along with III, IV, VI, and blood vessels travel within the superior orbital fissure. The foramen rotundum is the opening for the V_2 division, which later enters the infraorbital canal. The foramen ovale is the opening for the V_3 division.

27.

B. The lymphatic vessels contain valves to reduce backflow of lymph. Sphincters are absent in the lymphatic vessels. The blood pressure has no effect on lymphatic flow. There is little or no hydrostatic pressure present in lymphatic vessels.

28.

A. The lingula is anterior to the mandibular foramen and projects posteriorly to partially cover the foramen. The epiglottis is a flap of dense soft tissue that covers the trachea during swallowing. The vomer is a vertical plate of bone that forms a portion of the nasal septum. The articular eminence is a projection of bone anterior to the mandibular fossa.

29.

C. The circle of Willis is an anastomoses of basilar and internal carotid arteries at the base of the brain. The heart, liver, and spleen do not contain intracerebral arteries.

30.

D. Circumvallate are 8–12 large papillae located just anterior to the sulcus terminalis. Fungiform papillae are mushroom-shaped and are located on the apex and sides of the tongue. The numerous filiform papillae are found throughout the anterior portion of the tongue, while the foliate papillae are found at the lateral margins of the tongue.

31.

A. The pulp chamber of deciduous teeth is proportionately larger than permanent teeth. Deciduous teeth are whiter in color, smaller in size, and have less mineralized enamel than permanent teeth.

32.

C. Dentin makes up the bulk of the tooth because it is located in both the crown and root portions. Enamel covers the outer covering of the anatomic crown and the cementum covers the anatomic root. The pulp decreases in size as the tooth ages.

33.

B. Hertwig's root sheath determines the number of roots a tooth will develop. The dental sac forms the periodontal ligament, cementum, and lamina dura.

34.

D. The primary crystalline mineral of bone, enamel, dentin, and cementum is hydroxyapatite.

35.

C. Dentin is the first mineralized tissue to develop. The production of enamel is stimulated by the presence of predentin and shortly follows dentin formation. Cementum and pulp develop later in the tooth development process.

36.

B. Rests of Malassez form Hertwig's root sheath.

37.

D. Enamel is made up of 96% hydroxyapatite and 4% organic material.

38.

D. The dental sac forms the attachment apparatus. The inner enamel epithelium leads to the development of preameloblasts. The outer enamel epithelium forms the outer layer of the enamel organ. The stellate reticulum is a layer of the enamel organ.

39.

B. The enamel organ develops from the basal layer of the oral epithelium—a derivative of ectoderm. Dentin, cementum, and alveolar bone are derivatives of mesoderm.

40.

D. The lines of Retzius represent enamel formed in increments.

41.

C. Perikymata (imbrication line) is a surface manifestation of the lines of Retzius. The secondary cuticle is Nasmyth's membrane.

42.

D. The permanent maxillary first molars exhibit the cusp of Carabelli on the mesiolingual cusp.

43.

A. The remaining premolars all have single roots.

44.

A. The remaining teeth have functional cusps.

45.

B. The Y-type mandibular second molar has three cusps—one buccal and two lingual, which are separated by the lingual groove.

46.

C. Maxillary permanent molars have an oblique ridge—characteristic of only these teeth. Transverse ridges are common on permanent premolars and mandibular molars. Maxillary molars have three roots, not two. The remaining permanent posterior teeth share the common masticatory function of grinding.

47.

D. The mandibular second molar displays two roots and four cusps. The maxillary first molar has three roots and may have five cusps. The maxillary second molar has four cusps and three roots. The mandibular first molar has five cusps and two roots.

48.

C. The lingual root is the longest of the permanent maxillary molars.

49.

C. Cingulums are routinely located on the lingual surface of anterior teeth.

50.

C. The periodontal ligament is located between the cementum and bone. The dentinoenamel junction separates the enamel from the dentin. The Tomes' granular layer is located under the cementum. The bone and enamel do not connect.

2 Physiology

P hysiology is the study of how living organisms perform their vital functions, and human physiology is the study of the functions of the human body. Physiology examines the function of anatomical structures; it considers the physical and chemical processes responsible for the characteristics of life, or vital functions. An understanding of these vital functions allows the dental hygienist the ability to locate oral infections.

chapter objectives

After completion of this chapter, the learner should be able to:

➤ Identify the components of cells

➤ Discuss nonmembranous and membranous organelles

➤ Describe membrane transport

➤ Discuss the integumentary, muscular, nervous, endocrine, circulatory, respiratory, digestive, urinary, and reproductive systems

➤ Discuss the components and functions of blood and the lymphatic system

I. Levels of Organization

A. Chemical level—Atoms form molecules

B. Cellular level—Molecules form organelles that perform a specific function (Example: cell)

C. Tissue level—Similar cells work together to perform a specific function (Example: cardiac muscle tissue)

D. Organ level—Consists of two or more different tissues that work together (Example: heart)

E. Organ system level—Organ and elements that work as a system (Example: circulatory system)

II. Directional Terms

A. Anterior—Front: before (Eye is anterior to ear)

B. Ventral—Belly side; on the front (Lingual frenum is on the ventral side of the tongue)

C. Posterior—Back; behind (Ear is posterior to the nose)

D. Dorsal—On the back (Papillae are on the dorsal surface of the tongue)

E. Lateral—Toward the outside of the body (Eyes are lateral to the nose)

F. Cranial or cephalic—Toward the head

G. Caudal—Toward the tail

H. Inferior—Below; at a lower level (Lips are inferior to the nose)

I. Superior—above or higher (Eyes are superior to the mouth)

J. Proximal—Toward an attached base (Thigh is proximal to the foot)

K. Distal—Away from an attached base (Fingers are distal to the wrist)

L. Superficial—At or near the body surface (Alveolar mucosa is superficial to underlying alveolar bone)

M. Deep—Farther from body surface (Bone is deep to surrounding muscle tissue)

III. Body Cavities—Areas in the Body Where Vital Organs Are Suspended in Chambers

A. Dorsal—Fluid-filled space that includes the cranial cavity and the spinal cavity

B. Ventral—Contains three main parts: thoracic cavity, abdominal cavity, and pelvic cavity, which contain organs that maintain basic life processes

IV. Components of Cells (Figure 2-1■)

A. Cell membrane—Lipid bilayer that provides isolation, protection, and support (controls the entrance/exit)

B. Cytosol—Fluid component of cytoplasm (distributes materials by diffusion)

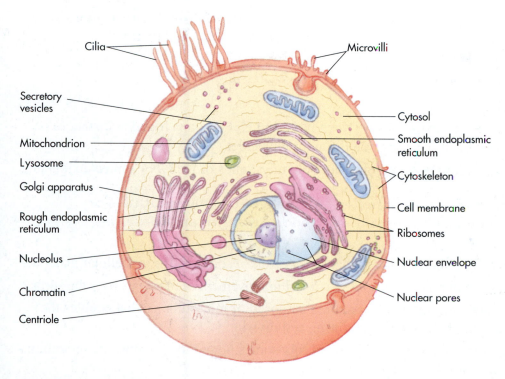

Cilia

Microvilli

Secretory
vesicles

Cytosol

Mitochondrion

Smooth endoplasmic
reticulum

Lysosome

Cytoskeleton

Golgi apparatus

Cell membrane

Rough endoplasmic
reticulum

Ribosomes

Nucleolus

Nuclear envelope

Chromatin

Nuclear pores

Centriole

FIGURE 2-1 ■ Components of a Representive Cell

V. Chemical Bonds

A. Ionic—Result from gain or loss of electrons between atoms (Ionic bonds are broken when the substance dissolves in water)

B. Covalent—Produced when electrons are shared between atoms

C. Polar covalent

    1. Result when sharing of electrons between atoms is unequal

    2. Have charged portions that attract opposite charges and other polar molecules (Examples: water, functional groups of most organic molecules); tend to be hydrophilic (attract water)

D. Ionic—Result from gain or loss of electrons between atoms (Ionic bonds are broken when the substance dissolves in water)

E. Covalent—Produced when electrons are shared between atoms

F. Polar covalent

    1. Result when sharing of electrons between atoms is unequal

    2. Have charged portions that attract opposite charges and other polar molecules

    3. Examples: water, functional groups of most organic molecules

    4. Tend to be hydrophilic (attract water)

    G. Nonpolar covalent—Result when the sharing of electrons between atoms is equal or the molecule is symmetrical, thus canceling the polarity

        1. Examples: carbon dioxide, long-chain hydrocarbons

        2. Tend to be gydrophobic (repel water)

    H. Hydrogen

        1. Electrical attractions between NH+ and C=O groups found at distances on the same molecule or on different molecules

        2. Cause coiling of proteins and hold the strands of the DNA molecule together

VI. Nonmembranous Organelles—Cytoskeleton (Microtubules or Microfilaments) Proteins that Provide Strength and Materials (Figure 2-2■)

    A. Microvilli—Microfilaments that facilitate the absorption of extracellular materials

    B. Cilia—Membrane extensions that assist in movement of materials over the surface

    C. Centrioles—Cylindrical structure composed of microtubules that enables the movement of chromosomes during cell division

    D. Ribosomes—Protein + RNA fixed robosomes bound to endoplasmic reticulum, free ribosomes scattered in cytoplasm; performs protein synthesis

VII. Membranous Organelles (Figure 2-3■)

    A. Endoplasmic reticulum (ER)—Membranous channels in cytoplasm; synthesizes secretory products and intercellular transport and storage

    B. Rough ER—Has ribosomes attached; synthesizes secretory proteins

    C. Smooth ER—Lacks ribosomes; synthesizes lipids and carbohydrates

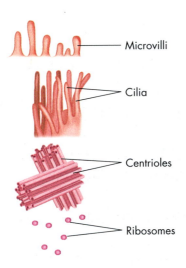

Microvilli

Cilia

Centrioles

Ribosomes

FIGURE 2-2 ■ Nonmembranous Organelles

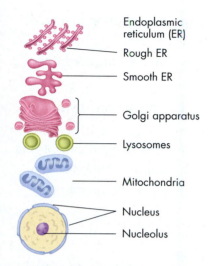

Endoplasmic
reticulum (ER)
— Rough ER

— Smooth ER

— Golgi apparatus

— Lysosomes

— Mitochondria

— Nucleus
— Nucleolus

FIGURE 2-3 ■ Membranous Organelles

D. Golgi apparatus—Flattened chamber that stores and packages secretory products, forms lysosomes

E. Lysosomes—Vesicles containing powerful digestive enzymes, removes damaged organelles or pathogens in cells

F. Mitochondria—Organelles containing enzymes that regulate the reactions that provide energy for the cell; contain the enzymes and cytochromes for the Krebs cycle; produces ATP

G. Nucleus—Nucleoplasm surrounded by double membrane and connects to the endoplasmic reticulum; control center of the cell; stores and processes DNA

H. Nucleolus—Contains the DNA and RNA, located in the nucleoplasm; synthesizes rRNA (ribosomal ribonucleic acid) and assembles ribosomal subunits

VIII.   Membrane Transport

A. Key terms

1. Permeability—Determines which substances enter or leave the cytoplasm

2. Impermeable—No substance can cross the cell membrane

3. Freely permeable—Any substance can cross the cell membrane without difficulty

4. Selectively permeable—Free passage of some substances and restricting passage of others. Based on size, electrical charge, molecular shape, lipid solubility

5. Passive processes—Ions or molecules move across cell membrane without needing energy; includes diffusion, osmosis, facilitated diffusion

6. Active processes—Require energy from the cell to move ions or molecules across the cell membrane; usually in the form of ATP

B. Diffusion—Movement of molecules from area of high concentration to area of low concentration

    1. Concentration gradient—Difference between high and low concentrations

    2. Diffusion across cell membrane (Figure 2-4■)

        a. Molecules can independently diffuse across a cell membrane by lipid solubility and size of molecule

        b. Alcohol, fatty acids, steroids, dissolved gases such as oxygen and carbon dioxide enter and leave the cell by diffusion through lipid bilayers

        c. Water-soluble compounds diffuse through channels in the membrane because they are small

    3. Osmosis (Figure 2-5■)

        a. Diffusion of water molecules across a membrane

        b. Occurs across a selectively permeable membrane that is freely permeable to water but not to solutes (dissolved materials)

        c. Will flow toward the solution with the highest concentration of solutes

C. Filtration

    1. Water and small solute molecules are forced across a membrane due to hydrostatic pressure gradient; example: heart pushes blood through the circulatory system, generating blood pressure; kidney filtration is an essential step in the production of urine

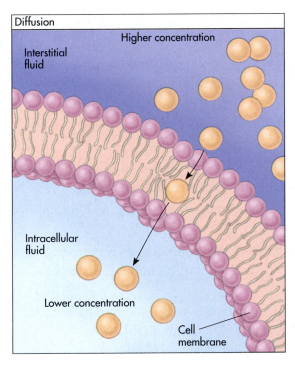

FIGURE 2-4 ■ Diffusion across Cell Membranes

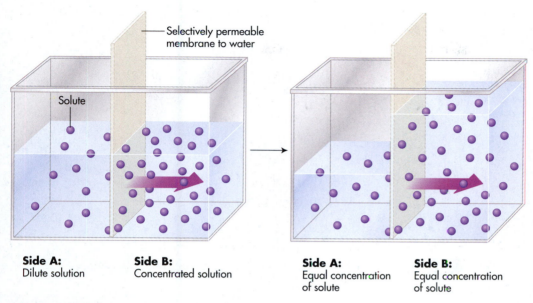

Side A:
Dilute solution

Side B:
Concentrated solution

Side A:
Equal concentration
of solute

Side B:
Equal concentration
of solute

FIGURE 2-5 ■ Osmosis

D. Carrier-mediated transport—Process by which membrane proteins bind specific
ions or organic material and move them across the cell membrane; can be
passive (not ATP required) or active (ATP required)

   1. Facilitated diffusion—Molecules that are too large to fit through membrane
channels, and insoluble lipids are transported by binding to receptor sites on
the protein that moves it into the cell (Figure 2-6■)

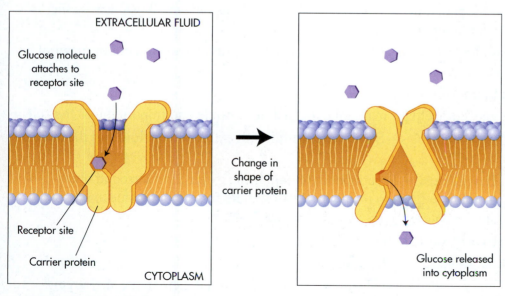

FIGURE 2-6 ■ Facilitated Diffusion

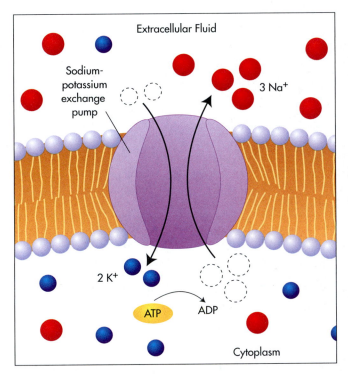

FIGURE 2-7 ■ Sodium–Potassium Exchange Pump

2. Active transport (Figure 2-7■)

   a. Utilizing ATP, the molecules or ions move across the membrane regardless of their intracellular or extracellular concentrations

   b. Carrier proteins called ion pumps actively transport sodium (Na+), potassium (K+), calcium (Ca+), and magnesium (Mg+) across the membrane

E. Vesicular transport—Formation of a vesicle provides movement of material in or out of the cell

   1. Endocytosis

   a. Extracellular material collected in a vesicle and imported into the cell

   b. Pinocytosis—Small vesicles fill with extracellular fluid and then pinch off; "cell drinking"

   2. Phagocytosis—Pseudopodia (cytoplasmic extensions surround object) → membrane fuses to form vesicle → vesicle fuses to a lysome and breaks down contents; "cell eating" (Figure 2-8■)

   3. Exocytosis (outside)

   a. Reverse of endocytosis

   b. Vesicle is created within cell and fuses to cell membrane, discharging contents to extracellular fluid; examples: hormones, mucus, waste products

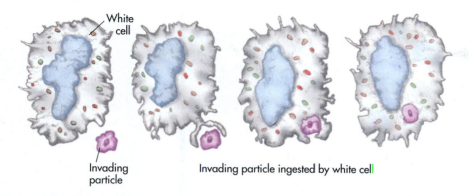

White cell

Invading particle

Invading particle ingested by white cell

FIGURE 2-8 ■ Phagocytosis

F. Cell division

    1. Meiosis—Division of reproductive cells; produces sperm or ova

    2. Mitosis—Division of somatic cells; vast majority of cell division; includes three stages: prophase, metaphase, and telophase

    3. Interphase—Interval of time between cell division when DNA replication occurs

➤ INTEGUMENTARY SYSTEM

- Provides mechanical protection against environmental hazards
- Contains skin, hair, sweat glands, nails, and sensory receptors

I. Skeletal System

Provides mechanical support, stores energy reserves, stores calcium and phosphate reserves; 206 bones

A. Characteristics of skeletal system

    1. Axial skeleton (Figure 2-9■)

        a. Bones of the skull, spinal column, ribs, sternum; framework of the head and trunk of the body

    2. Appendicular skeleton (Figure 2-10■)

        a. Bones of the upper and lower extremities and supporting bones; provides internal support of arms and legs, moves the axial skeleton

    3. Bone marrow

        a. Red marrow—Filled with blood vessels and connective tissue, manufactures RBC, WBC, and platelets

        b. Yellow marrow—Contains mainly fat

    4. Shapes of bone

        a. Long, short, flat, irregular

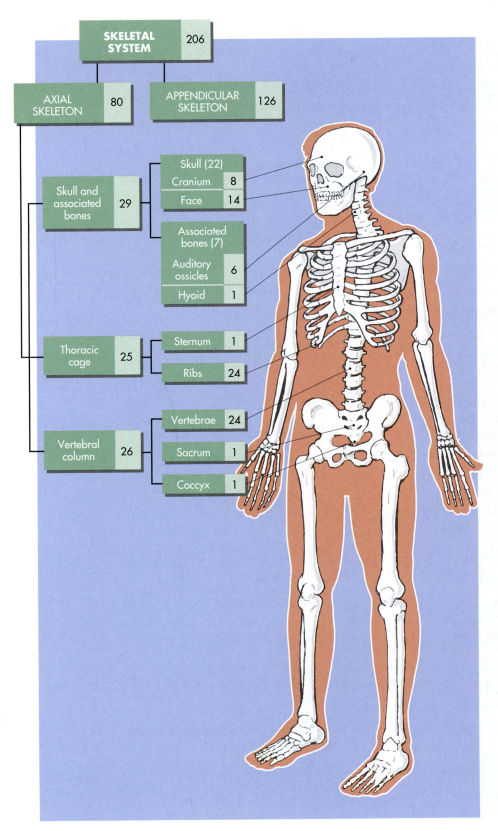

FIGURE 2-9 ■ Axial Skeleton

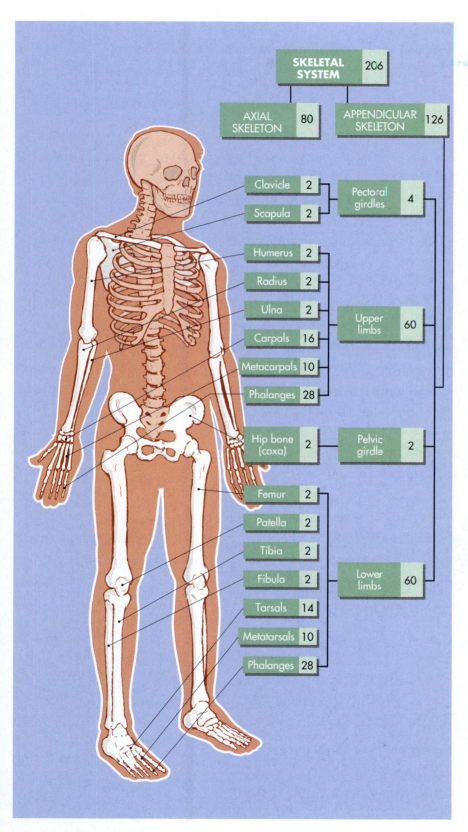

FIGURE 2-10 ■ Appendicular Skeleton

5. Types of bone

    a. Compact—Dense, solid; example: main shaft of femur

    b. Cancellous—Spongy, bony rods covered by marrow; example: found at the end of femur (epiphysis)

6. Cells of the bone

    a. Osteocytes—Mature bone cells

    b. Osteoclasts—Dissolve bony matrix, which regulates the calcium and phosphate concentrations in body fluids

    c. Osteoblasts—Produce new bone

7. Periosteum

    a. Fibrous covering that isolates the bone, provides a route for blood and nerves

8. Diseases or conditions

    a. Osteomyelitis—Infection of bone-forming tissue

    b. Osteoporosis—Loss of bone mass; brittle, soft bones result

    c. Cleft palate—Failure of palate to form and join correctly

    d. Fractures—Breaks of the bone or cartilage

    e. Temporomandibular joint—Degeneration of the joint where the mandible articulates with the temporal bone

9. Cartilage

    a. Nonvascular connective tissue; found where two bones join and areas such as nose and ear

B. Functions

    1. Supports the body against the pull of gravity

    2. Protects soft parts of the body (thoracic cage protects the lungs and heart)

    3. Produces blood cells (hematopoesis) in the marrow of certain bones

    4. Stores mineral salts, such as calcium

    5. Provides a site for muscle attachments

II. Anatomy

A. Bones

    1. Types

        a. Long bones—Covered on the outside by periosteum

        (1) Parts

            (a) Epiphyses—Growing ends

            (b) Diaphysis—Shaft

            (c) Bone marrow—Inside cavity

            (d) Articular cartilage—Covers ends that articulate with other bones

    (2) Composition

       (a) Compact bone is dense with osteocytes (bone cells)

       (b) Cancellous bone (spongy bone) is less dense, but very strong

       (c) Osteoblasts—Develop new bone

       (d) Osteoclasts—Resorb bone

       (e) Bone is living and constantly being resorbed and reformed

b. Skull—Cranium (protects brain) and facial bones

    (1) Cranial bones include frontal, parietal, occipital, temporal, sphenoid, and ethmoid

    (2) Facial bones

       (a) Consist of maxillae, palatine, zygomatic, lacrimal, nasal, vomer, inferior nasal conchae, and mandible

       (b) Hyoid bone—Only bone that does not articulate with another bone

    (3) Sutures—Separate bones (fuse with age)

    (4) Some bones contain paranasal sinuses; they are lined with mucous membrane and make bones of skull lighter; sinuses drain into nasal cavity

c. Vertebral column—Consists of 7 cervical, 12 thoracic, 5 lumbar, 5 (fused) sacral vertebrae, and 1 coccyx

    (1) Intervertebral discs—Fibrocartilaginous material that separates vertebrae

    (2) Atlas—First cervical vertebrae; articulates with occipital bone of cranium

    (3) Axis—Second cervical vertebrae

    (4) Exhibits four curvatures

d. Thoracic cage

    (1) 12 pairs of ribs

    (2) Sternum—Anterior bone for attachment for upper ribs

    (3) Thoracic vertebrae—Where all ribs articulate

    (4) Function—Protects heart and lungs

e. Pectoral girdle—Connects upper limb to axial skeleton

    (1) Clavicles (collarbones)

    (2) Scapulae (shoulder blades)

f. Upper limbs

    (1) Humerus—Upper arm

    (2) Ulna and radius—Located in forearm

    (3) Carpals—Located in wrist

    (4) Metacarpals and phalanges—Located in hand

g. Pelvic girdle—Forms attachment for lower limb with axial skeleton; female pelvis is shallower and wider than male pelvis

(1) Coxal bone—Consists of 2 ilium, 2 ischium, and 1 pubis

(2) Sacrum

(3) Coccyx

h. Lower limbs

(1) Femur—Located in thigh; top is defined by a greater trochanter and articulating head and neck

(2) Tibia and fibula—Comprise lower leg

(3) Patella—Kneecap

(4) Tarsal bones—Make up ankles; calcaneus—bone of heel

(5) Metatarsals and phalanges—Make up foot

B. Joints

1. Types

a. Synarthroses—Found in the cranium; immovable

b. Amphiarthroses—Connected by hyaline cartilage or fibrocartilage; slightly moveable

(1) Vertebrae—Separated by intervertebral discs

(2) Pubic symphysis—Located between pubic bones

c. Diarthroses

(1) Contain synovial joints—Articular cartilage with synovial membrane that produces synovial fluid. (Figure 2-11■)

(2) Types of diarthroses

(a) Saddle joint—Located in thumb

(b) Ball-and-socket joint—Located in hip and shoulder

(c) Pivot joint—Located between radius and ulna, and atlas and axis

(d) Hinge joint—Located in elbow and knee

(e) Gliding joint—Located in wrist and ankle

(f) Condyloid joint—Located between metacarpals and phalanges

C. Connective tissue

1. Types

a. Ligament—Binds two bones together; made up of fibrous connective tissue

b. Tendon—Connects muscles to bones; made up of fibrous connective tissue; helps stabilize joints

c. Bursae—Consists of fluid-filled sac; eases friction between moving tendons and ligaments over fixed structures

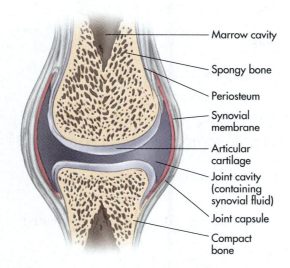

- Marrow cavity
- Spongy bone
- Periosteum
- Synovial membrane
- Articular cartilage
- Joint cavity (containing synovial fluid)
- Joint capsule
- Compact bone

FIGURE 2-11 ■ Freely Movable Synovial Joint

III. Physiology

A. Bones are living structures that are constantly being remodeled

B. Marrow is very active tissue, constantly producing blood cells

C. Movements by synovial joints

    1. Flexion

      a. Decreases joint angle

      b. Example—Bending the knee

      c. Dorsiflexion—Flexes foot upward

      d. Plantar flexion—Flexes foot downward

    2. Extension

      a. Increases joint angle

      b. Example—Straightening the knee

    3. Abduction

      a. Moves body part laterally, away from the midline

      b. Example—Swinging arm out to the side

    4. Adduction

      a. Moves body part toward midline

      b. Example—pulling arm in to the side

    5. Rotation

      a. Moves body part around its own axis

      b. Example—Turning head back and forth

    6. Supination—Rotates lower arm so palm faces upward

    7. Pronation—Rotates lower arm so palm faces downward

    8. Circumduction—Moving body part in wide circles; example: moving arms in large circles

    9. Inversion—Turns foot so the sole is facing midline

    10. Eversion—Turns foot so the sole is facing outward

    11. Elevation—Lifts body part, such as shrugging the shoulders

    12. Depression—Drops body part such as dropping shoulders or opening jaw

IV. Hormones Important to Bone Growth and Homeostasis

A. Growth hormone (GH)

    1. Necessary for normal growth and development of the skeleton, secreated from the anterior pituitary

    2. Hyposecretion of GH during childhood produces a dwarf

    3. Hypersecretion of GH produces a giant; in adulthood produces acromegaly (shape of bones, especially those in the face, become exaggerated)

B. Thyroid hormones

    1. Normal production of thyroid hormones establishes the background rates of cellular metabolism

    2. Overproduction or underproduction of thyroid hormones cause very serious metabolic problems

C. Estrogen

    1. Important for growth in length of bone and for bone maintenance

    2. Maintains female secondary sex characteristics, such as body hair distribution and the location of adipose tissue deposits

    3. Affects central nervous system activity, including sexual behaviors and drives

    4. Maintains functional accessory reproductive glands and organs

    5. Initiates the repair and growth of the endometrium

    6. Present in varying amounts in both sexes

D. Testosterone

    1. Important for growth in mass and density of bone

    2. Affects metabolic operations throughout the body, notably stimulating protein synthesis and muscle growth

    3. Promotes the production of functional sperm

    4. Maintains the secretory glands of the male reproductive tract

    5. Determines secondary sex characteristics such as the distribution of facial hair and body fat

    6. Present in varying amounts in both sexes

E. Parathyroid hormone

    1. Exerts the primary control in calcium homeostasis; when calcium level falls, parathyroid hormone is secreted

    2. Raises calcium by increasing vitamin D production, increased reabsorption of calcium in the kidney

    3. Increases osteoclastic activity to release calcium into the blood

F. Calcitonin

    1. Normally important only in children and is secreted by special cells in the thyroid

    2. Functions to stimulate the uptake of calcium into growing bone and the deposition of bone matrix; can be used to aid uptake of calcium in osteoporosis patients

V. Diseases Related to Bone

A. Osteoporosis

    1. Disorder involving demineralization of bone usually associated with older individuals and is related to several factors:

        a. Deficiency of dietary calcium

        b. Reduced estrogen levels common in postmenopausal women

        c. Reduced activity and exercise

        d. Reduced weightbearing stress on the bones (this is important in stimulating bone growth and replacement at any age)

B. Rickets

    1. Vitamin D deficiency in children (vitamin D is necessary for absorption of calcium)

    2. Results from improper mineralization that results in stunted growth and weakened bones

C. Osteoarthritis

    1. Noninflammatory type of arthritis resulting in degeneration of the bones and joints; especially weight bearing

D. Osteomalacia

    1. Vitamin D deficiency in adults

    2. Causes demineralization of the bones (softening of the bones)

    3. Periodontal disease, delayed tooth eruption

E. Osteomyelitis

    1. Inflammation of the bone and bone marrow due to infection

    F. Paget's disease

        1. Metabolic disorder of unknown cause that involves the destruction of normal bone tissue and replaces it with tissue of irregular and unorganized structure

        2. Enlargement of bone; when in maxilla and mandible, increased spacing of teeth

        3. Radiographic manifestations: "cotton wool" appearance, hypercementosis, loss of lamina dura

    G. Rheumatoid Arthritis

        1. Chronic form of arthritis

        2. Autoimmune disease

VI. Disease of Joints

    A. Arthritis—Inflammation of a joint

    B. Gout—Inflammation of a joint caused by excessive uric acid

VII. Homeostasis—Produces elements of the blood that carry oxygen and helps to maintain pH

➤ MUSCULAR SYSTEM

I. Functions

    A. Stabilization—Tendons of muscles cross joints and give them stability

    B. Oppose force of gravity—Solid structure of bones allows us to remain upright; muscle contraction opposes force of gravity

    C. Movement—Contraction of muscle produces movement (Figure 2-12■)

        1. Skeletal muscle—Produces movement of skeletal system, eyeball, soft tissue of the face, and breathing

        2. Smooth muscle—Produces movement of digestive tract and blood vessels

        3. Cardiac muscle—Produces movement of heart (contraction)

    D. Heat—Biochemical process of muscle contraction gives off heat as a by-product, which maintains body temperature

II. Characteristics of Muscles

    A. Fiber—Groups of muscle cells

    B. Fascia—Sheet of connective tissue that covers, supports, and separates fibers

    C. Excitability or irritability—Muscle response to stimuli

    D. Extensibility—Ability to stretch or spread

    E. Tone—Tension of muscular system

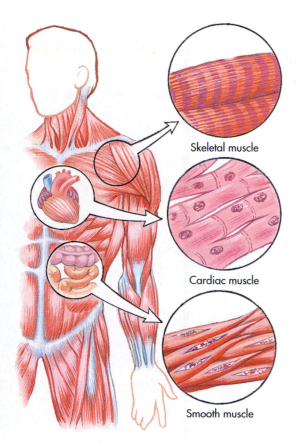

Skeletal muscle

Cardiac muscle

Smooth muscle

FIGURE 2-12 ■ Types of Muscles

F. Contraction—Become shorter and thicker

   1. Isometric—No change in length of muscle but tension is increased

   2. Isotonic—Muscle tension remains the same but muscle shortens

G. Relaxation—Release and return to normal form

H. Tendon—Cord that attaches muscle to bone

I. Aponeurosis—Broad, flat extension that attaches muscle to bone or muscle to muscle

J. Ligaments—Sheets of connective tissue that act to connect or support two or more bones

K. Antagonistic pairs—When one set of muscles contracts, the other relaxes; provide movement

L. ATP—Energy required for muscle contraction, requires oxygen or lactic acid will result; energy transfer molecule

M. Glycogen—Stored in muscle for reserve energy, broken down by glycolysis

III. Anatomy

A. Skeletal muscle (striated muscle)

1. Microscopic anatomy

    a. Myofibrils—Contractile elements made up of smaller myofilaments, which are made up of actin and myosin

        (1) Actin and myosin

            (a) Give skeletal muscle its striated appearance

            (b) Slide past each other, causing myofibrils to shorten (contract)

        (2) Run length of muscle

2. Innervation of skeletal muscle

    a. Motor unit—Consists of motor neuron, which goes to several muscle fibers

    b. Neuromuscular junction—Point where motor neuron innervates muscle fiber

    c. Contraction—Requires energy (adenosine triphosphate, ATP) and calcium

3. Muscle contraction

    a. Origin of muscle—Attaches to end of stationary bone

    b. Insertion of muscle—Attaches to end of moving bone

    c. Functions

        (1) Can only shorten during contraction

        (2) For every movement, there is usually an opposite movement; therefore muscles work in pairs as antagonist muscles

            (a) Example: flexors and extensors (biceps and triceps brachii acting at the elbow)

        (3) Several muscles may be involved in one movement

            (a) Prime mover muscle—Does most of the work of a movement

            (b) Synergist muscle—Assists in movement

            (c) Types of contractions

                (1) Isotonic contraction—Muscle shortens and movement occurs

                (2) Isometric contraction—Muscle contracts, but does not shorten or produce movement

                (3) Muscle tone—Even at rest, some fibers are always contracting to keep muscle from being flaccid

4. Specific skeletal muscles (Figures 2-13a■ and 2-13b■)

    a. Muscles of facial expression—Supplied by cranial nerve VII

    b. Muscles of mastication—Supplied by cranial nerve V

    c. Muscles of head, neck, and trunk—Include antagonists sternocleidomastoid and trapezius

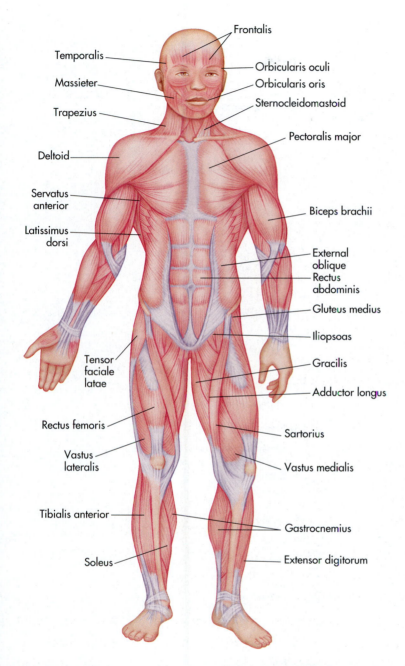

Frontalis
Temporalis
Orbicularis oculi
Massieter
Orbicularis oris
Trapezius
Sternocleidomastoid
Deltoid
Pectoralis major
Servatus anterior
Latissimus dorsi
Biceps brachii
External oblique
Rectus abdominis
Gluteus medius
Iliopsoas
Tensor faciale latae
Gracilis
Adductor longus
Rectus femoris
Sartorius
Vastus lateralis
Vastus medialis
Tibialis anterior
Gastrocnemius
Soleus
Extensor digitorum

FIGURE 2-13a ■ Overview of the Major Skeletal Muscles: Anterior View

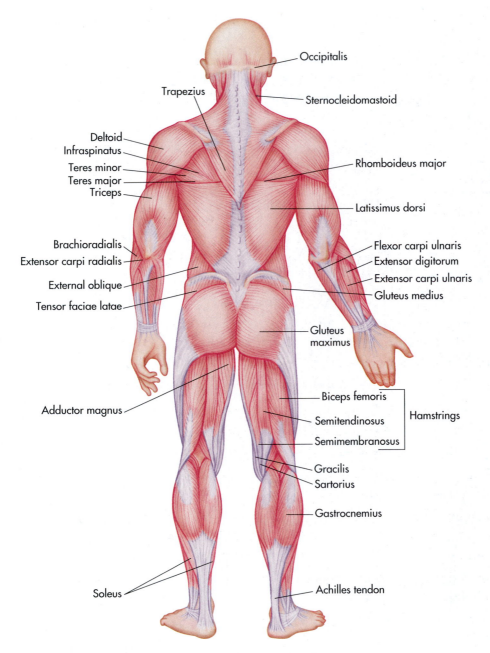

FIGURE 2-13b ■ Overview of the Major Skeletal Muscles: Posterior View

   d. Abdominal muscles—Contain contents of abdominal cavity; assist in maintaining upright posture; include external and internal obliques, transversus abdominus, and rectus abdominus

   e. Muscles of pectoral girdle—Help hold upper arm in socket; provide movement at shoulder; include deltoids, pectoralis majors and minors, lastissimus dorsi, and serratus anterior

   f. Muscles of forearm—Include antagonists triceps brachii, brachialis, and biceps brachii

   g. Muscles of wrist (also move the hand)—Include flexor carpi ulnaris, extensor carpi ulnaris, flexor carpi radialis, and extensor carpi radialis

   h. Muscles of hand—Include flexor digitorum and extensor digitorum

   i. Muscles of hip and thigh

      (1) Iliopsoas—Flexes thigh

      (2) Gluteus maximus—Extends thigh

      (3) Gluteus medius—Abducts thigh

      (4) Adductor group—Adducts thigh

   j. Muscles of leg

      (1) Quadriceps femoris group—Extends lower leg

      (2) Hamstring group—Flexes lower leg and extends hip

   k. Muscles of ankle

      (1) Gastrocnemius and soleus—Form Achilles tendon, which attaches to calcaneus of the heel; plantar flexion

      (2) Tibialis anterior—Dorsiflexion and inversion

      (3) Peroneus (fibularis) muscles—Eversion and plantar flexion

   l. Muscles of foot

      (1) Flexor digitorum longus—Flexes toes

      (2) Extensor digitorum longus—Extends toes

   m. Extraocular (eyeball) muscles—Movement of the eyes; origin is in bony orbit, insertion is on eye

   n. Diaphragm—Separates thoracic from abdominal cavity; contracts during inspiration, relaxes during expiration

B. Smooth muscle

   1. Located in walls of hollow internal organs (gastrointestinal tract and blood vessels)

   2. Involuntary—Controlled by autonomic nervous system

   3. Contains no striations

   4. Slower to contract than striated muscle

   5. Maintains contraction longer than striated muscle

   6. Does not fatigue easily

C. Cardiac muscle

   1. Involuntary muscle found only in heart

   2. Striated

   3. Relaxes completely between contractions

IV. Physiology

A. All-or-none law

1. Only applies to muscle fiber, not to entire muscle

2. Stimulation of muscle fiber either causes it to or not to contract—Strength of muscle contraction is dependent on total number of fibers contracting

B. Muscle twitch—Single stimulus causes muscle to contract and then relax

C. Summation—Muscle fibers contract in rapid succession

D. Tetanus—Sustained maximum contraction

E. Fatigued muscle—Can no longer contract because of lack of ATP

F. Oxygen debt—Continued need for oxygen after vigorous exercise; lactic acid accumulates during exercise because oxygen is necessary for its metabolism

V. Muscle Metabolism

A. Anaerobic glycolysis

1. Initial way of utilizing glucose in all cells to provide ATP when insufficient oxygen is available for aerobic metabolism

2. Does not require oxygen

3. Occurs in cytoplasm, not mitochondria, allowing for quick bursts of speed or strength

4. Slows down as pyruvic acid (product of glycolysis) builds up

5. Pyruvic acid is converted to lactic acid by fermentation, allowing an extension of glycolysis

6. Lactic buildup slows metabolism and causes muscle fatigue; lactic acid must be reconverted to pyruvic acid and metabolized aerobically in the muscle or liver

B. Aerobic metabolism

1. Performed exclusively in the mitochondria

2. Pyruvic acid (product of glycolysis) must be metabolized aerobically

3. Pyruvic acid is converted to an acetyl group and put into the Krebs cycle; energy is released in the form of ATP as high energy electrons; waste products of aerobic metabolism are CO_2 and H_2O

4. Aerobic metabolism is used for endurance activities

VI. Muscular Conditions or Diseases

A. Spasm—Sudden involuntary muscle contraction

B. Fibromyalgia—Chronic pain in the muscle and soft tissue surrounding the joints

C. Muscular dystrophy—Congenital disorder characterized by progressive degeneration of skeletal muscle

    D. Polymyositis—Disease causing muscle inflammation and weakness from an unknown cause

    E. Myasthenia gravis—Autoimmune disorder causing loss of muscle strength and paralysis

VII. Homeostasis—Muscular Activity Helps to Maintain Body Temperature (98.6°C/37°C)

➤ NERVOUS SYSTEM

I. Function

    A. Regulates systems of the body

    B. Coordinates systems of the body

    C. Maintains homeostasis

    D. Responds to stimuli, both internal and external

        1. Permits sensory input

        2. Integrates input into central nervous system (CNS)

        3. Stimulates motor output

II. Components of Nervous System

    A. Neuron—Basic structural unit of the nervous system

    B. Dendrites—Nerve fibers that conduct impulses toward the cell body

    C. Axon—Nerve fibers that conduct impulses away from the cell body

    D. Synapse—Junction where chemicals are released from the ends of axons to allow the stimuli to jump to the next dendrite

    E. Myelin sheath—Layer of Schwann cells that insulate and protect the nerve

    F. Afferent division of the PNS—Brings sensory information to the CNS

    G. Efferent division—Carries motor commands to muscles and glands

    H. Somatic nervous system—Part of PNS that provides voluntary control over skeletal muscles

    I. Neurotransmitters—Chemicals that transfer information from one neuron to another neuron or effector cell; examples: acetylcholine (ACH), norepinephrine (NE), dopamine

    J. Reflex—Automatic motor responses that help the body maintain homeostasis; examples: heart rate, sneezing, and swallowing

    K. Ganglia—Groups of neuron cell bodies

    L. Nerves—Bundles of axons

    M. Centers—Collections of neuron cell bodies that share a particular function

N. Tracts—bundles of axons inside the CNS that share common origins, destinations, and functions

O. Pathways—Link the centers of the brain with the rest of the body

P. Meninges—Specialized membranes that protect and support the brain; three layers: dura mater, arachnoid, and pia mater

Q. Blood–brain barrier—Isolates the neural tissue in the CNS from general circulation

R. Spinal cord—Serves as major highway for the passage of sensory impulses to the brain and motor impulses from the brain

S. Epidural space—Separates the spinal dura mater from the walls of the vertebral canal

III. Anatomy

A. Divisions

1. Central nervous system

a. Brain (Figure 2-14■)

(1) Contains unmyelinated gray matter and myelinated white matter

(2) Contains four ventricles that are filled with cerebrospinal fluid (CSF)

(3) Brainstem

(a) Medulla oblongata—Controls and regulates heartbeat, breathing, and blood pressure

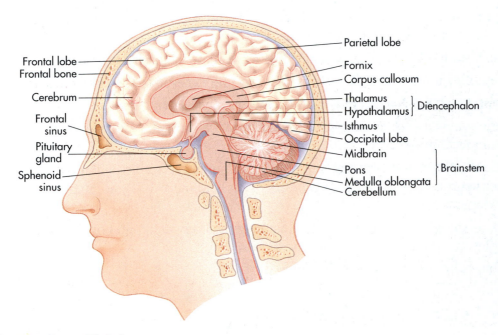

FIGURE 2-14 ■ Brain

(b) Pons—Also regulates breathing; connects cerebellum with CNS

(c) Midbrain—Tracts to and from other parts of the CNS

(4) Diencephalon

(a) Hypothalamus

i) Maintains homeostasis

ii) Regulates hunger, thirst, body temperature, sleep, blood pressure, and water balance

iii) Works with pituitary gland

iv) Functions in conjunction with endocrine system

(b) Thalamus—Central relay station for afferent impulses into brain

(5) Cerebellum

(a) Functions in muscle coordination to produce smooth motion

(b) Maintains muscle tone

(c) Maintains and restores balance

(6) Cerebrum—Site of consciousness and reasoning

(a) Functions

i) Controls interpretation of sensory imput

ii) Initiates muscular movement

(b) Parts

i) Right and left cerebral hemispheres—Lobes include frontal, parietal, occipital, and temporal

ii) Corpus callosum—Bridge of fibers that joins right and left hemispheres

iii) Basal ganglia—Clusters of gray matter involved in movement; dysfunction associated with Parkinson's disease

iv) Limbic system—Involved in learning and memory; site of generation of emotions

b. Spinal cord—Center for reflex activity

(1) Contains unmyelinated gray matter and myelinated white matter

(2) Ascending tracts carry sensory input to brain

(3) Descending tracts carry motor output from brain and cord to muscles

c. Meninges—Three membranes that cover brain and spinal cord

(1) Dura mater—Tough, outermost cover

(2) Arachnoid mater—Consists of middle layer; CSF circulates in subarachoid space

(3) Pia mater—Involves innermost layer

d. CSF—Made up of clear fluid, which is produced inside brain

(1) Supplies CNS with nutrients

(2) Acts as cushion for the CNS

(3) Circulates around brain and cord

(4) Blockage in system leads to hydrocephalus

2. Peripheral nervous system (PNS)

a. Cranial nerves—All 12 pairs are concerned with head and neck, except for vagus (X), which also innervates viscera in thorax and abdomen

b. Spinal nerves—Consists of 31 pairs, innervate segmentally, carry impulses to and from spinal cord

c. Autonomic nervous system (motor division of PNS) (Table 2-1■)

(1) Function—Innervates smooth and cardiac muscles and glands

(2) Consists of a two-neuron system: preganglionic and postganglionic

(3) Is not under conscious control

(4) Two divisions

(a) Sympathetic nervous system (Figure 2-15■)

i) Arises from thoracic and lumbar parts of spinal cord

ii) Uses neurotransmitter norepinephrine

iii) Involved in "fight-or-flight" response

iv) Inhibits digestion

v) Dilates pupils

vi) Increases heart and respiratory rates

(b) Parasympathetic nervous system (Figure 2-16■)

i) Arises from cranial (some cranial nerves have parasympathetic components) and sacral parts of cord

ii) Uses the neurotransmitter acetylcholine

iii) Promotes functions of body during a relaxed state

iv) Constricts pupils

v) Digestion of food takes place

vi) Normal, resting heart rate; heartbeat is not fast or forceful

d. Nervous tissue

(1) Neurons—Conduct nerve impulses (Figure 2-17■)

(a) Dendrites—Receive information from other neurons and send impulses toward cell body

(b) Axons—Send impulses away from cell body

(c) Cell body—Contains cell nucleus

TABLE 2-1 THE EFFECTS OF THE SYMPATHETIC AND PARASYMPATHETIC DIVISIONS OF THE ANS ON VARIOUS ORGANS

Structure	Sympathetic Innervation Effect	Parasympathetic Innervation Effect
Eye	Dilation of pupil Focusing for distance vision	Constriction of pupil Focusing for near vision
Skin Sweat glands Arrector pili muscles	 Increases secretion Contraction, erection of hairs	 None (not innervated) None (not innervated)
Tear Glands	None (not innervated)	Secretion
Cardiovascular System Blood vessels Heart	 Vasoconstriction and vasodilation Increases heart rate, force of contraction, and blood pressure	 None (not innervated) Decreases heart rate, force of contraction, and blood pressure
Adrenal Glands	Secretion of epinephrine and norepinephrine by adrenal medullae	None (not innervated)
Respiratory System Airways Respiratory rate	 Increases diameter Increases rate	 Decreases diameter Decreases rate
Digestive System General level of activity Liver	 Decreases activity Glycogen breakdown, glucose synthesis and release	 Increases activity Glycogen synthesis
Skeletal Muscles	Increases force of contraction, glycogen breakdown	None (not innervated)
Urinary System Kidneys Urinary bladder	 Decreases urine production Constricts sphincter, relaxes urinary bladder	 Increases urine production Tenses urinary bladder, relaxes sphincter to eliminate urine
Reproductive System	Increased glandular secretions; ejaculation in males	Erection of penis (males) or clitoris (females)

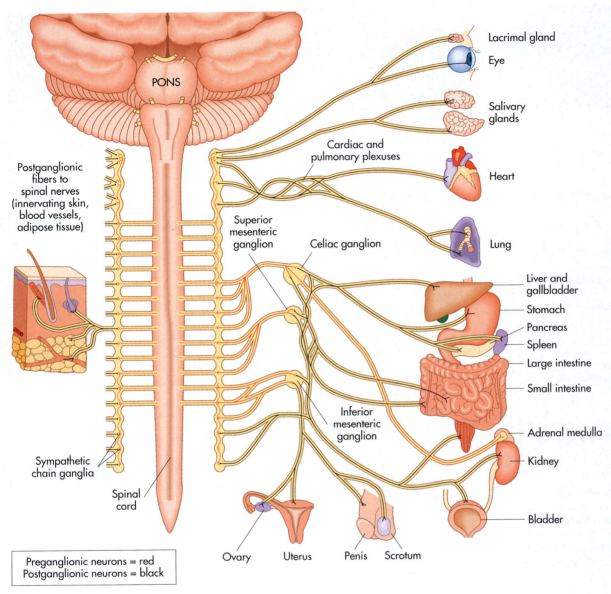

Lacrimal gland

Eye

Salivary glands

Cardiac and pulmonary plexuses

Heart

Lung

Liver and gallbladder

Stomach

Pancreas

Spleen

Large intestine

Small intestine

Adrenal medulla

Kidney

Bladder

PONS

Postganglionic fibers to spinal nerves (innervating skin, blood vessels, adipose tissue)

Superior mesenteric ganglion

Celiac ganglion

Inferior mesenteric ganglion

Sympathetic chain ganglia

Spinal cord

Ovary   Uterus   Penis   Scrotum

Preganglionic neurons = red
Postganglionic neurons = black

FIGURE 2-15 ■ Sympathetic Division

(d) Myelin (Figure 2-18■)

    (1) Formed by Schwann cells

    (2) Wraps around some fibers, giving a white appearance ("white matter")

    (3) Acts as insulation and increases transmission speed

    (4) Nodes of Ranvier—Constrictions located at regular intervals along myelinated nerve fiber where nerve membrane is exposed directly to the extracellular medium

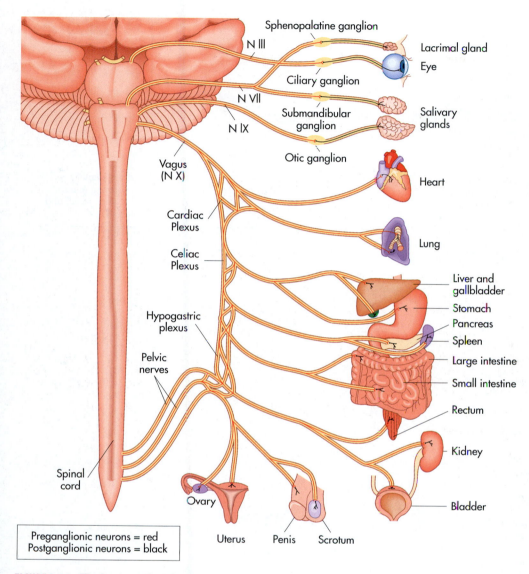

FIGURE 2-16 ■ Parasympathetic Division

(e) Types

    (1) Motor (efferent)—Long axon; conducts impulses from CNS to muscles

    (2) Sensory (afferent)—Conducts impulses from body to CNS

    (3) Interneurons—Connects neurons within CNS

(2) Neuroglial cells—Located within CNS to nourish, support, and protect neurons

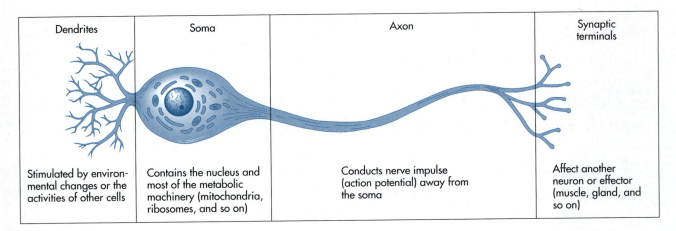

Dendrites	Soma	Axon	Synaptic terminals
Stimulated by environmental changes or the activities of other cells	Contains the nucleus and most of the metabolic machinery (mitochondria, ribosomes, and so on)	Conducts nerve impulse (action potential) away from the soma	Affect another neuron or effector (muscle, gland, and so on)

FIGURE 2-17 ■ Neural Tissue

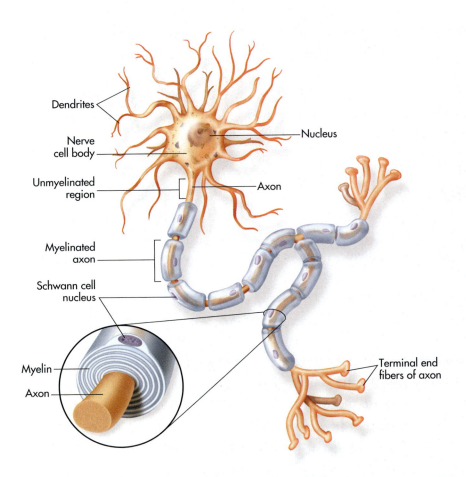

FIGURE 2-18 ■ Structure of a Myelinated Nerve Fiber

IV. Physiology

A. Nerve impulse

   1. Involves change in polarity in axonal membrane

   2. Utilizes sodium and potassium

B. Synapse

   1. Location where an axon of one neuron meets dendrites on another neuron

   2. Axon and dendrites do not touch

   3. Chemical messengers, neurotransmitters, relay nerve impulse across synapse

   4. Some neurotransmitters are acetylcholine, norepinephrine, dopamine, and serotonin

   5. Diseases associated with imbalance of neurotransmitters are Parkinson's disease (dopamine) and depression (norepinephrine and/or serotonin)

C. Reflexes and reflex arc

   1. Reflex—Involuntary, automatic response to an external or internal stimulus

   2. Examples: changes in heart rate, sneezing, gagging, vomiting, swallowing, and urination

   3. Reflex arc—Sensory neuron synapses with an interneuron in spinal cord; the interneuron synapses with motor neuron to muscle, which will cause reaction to the stimulus (e.g., knee-jerk)

V. Diseases or Conditions Affecting the Nervous System

A. Neuritis—Inflammation of the nerves

B. Multiple sclerosis (MS)—Disease that destroys the myelin sheath of neurons in the CNS

C. Parkinson's disease—Nerve disease characterized by tumors, muscle weakness, unsteady gait

D. Bell's palsy—Facial paralysis

E. Alzheimer's—Chronic, organic mental disorder consisting of dementia; more prevalent in adults between 40 and 60 years of age

F. Encephalitis—Inflammation of the brain due to disease factors such as rabies, influenza, measles, or smallpox

G. Epilepsy—Recurrent disorder of the brain in which convulsive seizures and loss of consciousness occur

H. Meningitis—Inflammation of the membranes of the spinal cord and brain that is caused by a microorganism

I. Tic douloureux—Painful condition in which the trigeminal nerve is affected by pressure or degeneration

VI. Homeostasis—Whole nervous system, especially neurotransmitters and reflexes; works with the endocrine system to maintain homeostasis of the body

    A. Blood glucose at 0.1%

    B. pH of the blood at 7.4

    C. Blood pressure at 120/80

    D. Blood temperature at 37°C (98.6°F)

➤ ENDOCRINE SYSTEM

I. Functions

    A. Composed of glands that release hormones

    B. Works with nervous system, which is fast-acting, to coordinate functioning of all parts of body

    C. Slow-acting endocrine glands release hormones into blood that have a specific function on target tissue

II. Anatomy (Figure 2-19■)

    A. Hypothalamus—Part of brain that controls heart rate, body temperature, and water balance; contains the pituitary gland

        1. Pituitary gland—Connected to hypothalamus by a stalk

        2. Produces releasing factors and hormones that travel down stalk to pituitary gland

    B. Posterior pituitary gland—Releases two hormones that are produced in hypothalmus

        1. Antidiuretic hormone (ADH)—Also called vasopressin

            a. Induces reabsorption of water from the kidneys, preventing dehydration

            b. Deficiency causes diabetes insipidus

        2. Oxytocin—Target organs are breast and smooth muscle in uterus; causes uterus to contract during labor and milk to be released when baby nurses

    C. Anterior pituitary gland—Production of hormones is regulated by factors from hypothalamus (Figure 2-20■)

        1. Growth hormone (GH)—Affects overall growth of individual, especially epiphyseal plates of long bones

            a. Pituitary dwarf—Results from deficiency in GH during childhood

            b. Giant—Results from having too much GH during childhood

            c. Acromegaly—Results from too much GH in adulthood

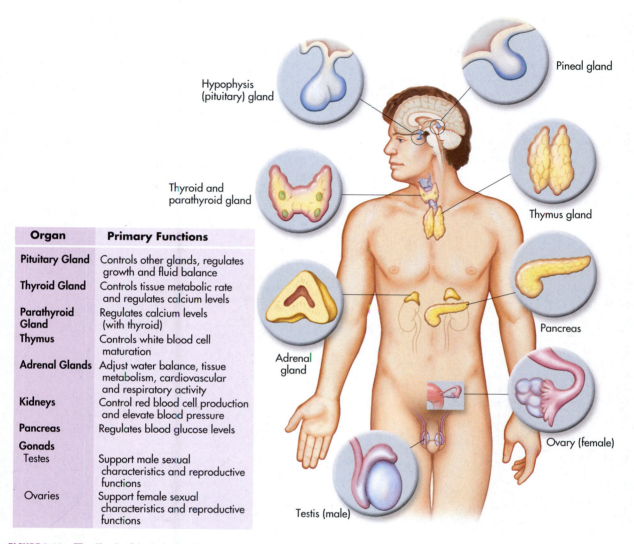

Organ	Primary Functions
Pituitary Gland	Controls other glands, regulates growth and fluid balance
Thyroid Gland	Controls tissue metabolic rate and regulates calcium levels
Parathyroid Gland	Regulates calcium levels (with thyroid)
Thymus	Controls white blood cell maturation
Adrenal Glands	Adjust water balance, tissue metabolism, cardiovascular and respiratory activity
Kidneys	Control red blood cell production and elevate blood pressure
Pancreas	Regulates blood glucose levels
Gonads	
Testes	Support male sexual characteristics and reproductive functions
Ovaries	Support female sexual characteristics and reproductive functions

FIGURE 2-19 ■ Glands of the Endocrine System

2. Prolactin (PRL)—Produced after childbirth; causes mammary glands to produce milk

3. Melanocyte-stimulating hormone (MSH)—Active in frogs; human concentration very low

4. Thyroid-stimulating hormone (TSH)—Stimulates thyroid to produce thyroid hormones; release is determined by blood concentration of thyroid hormones; when thyroid hormones are low, TSH is released (negative feedback)

5. Adrenocorticotropic hormone (ACTH)—Stimulates adrenal cortex to secrete cortisol and aldosterone

6. Gonadotropic hormone—Stimulates ovaries in females and testes in males to secrete sex hormones

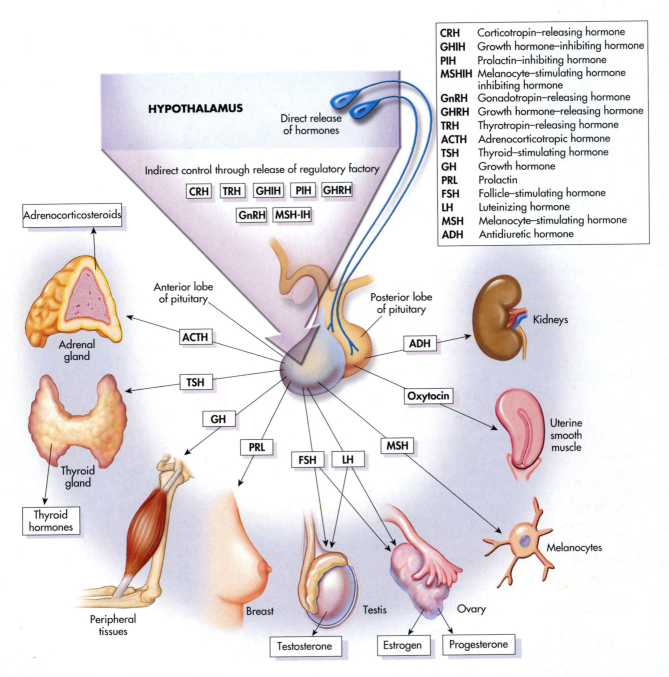

CRH	Corticotropin–releasing hormone
GHIH	Growth hormone–inhibiting hormone
PIH	Prolactin–inhibiting hormone
MSHIH	Melanocyte–stimulating hormone inhibiting hormone
GnRH	Gonadotropin–releasing hormone
GHRH	Growth hormone–releasing hormone
TRH	Thyrotropin–releasing hormone
ACTH	Adrenocorticotropic hormone
TSH	Thyroid–stimulating hormone
GH	Growth hormone
PRL	Prolactin
FSH	Follicle–stimulating hormone
LH	Luteinizing hormone
MSH	Melanocyte–stimulating hormone
ADH	Antidiuretic hormone

FIGURE 2-20 ■ Hormones of the Anterior Pituitary

D. Thyroid gland—Secretes calcitonin, which helps regulate body calcium level; TSH causes thyroid gland to secrete thyroid hormones, which controls metabolic rate

  1. Iodine

    a. Required for production of thyroid hormones

    b. Goiter (an enlargement of the gland)—Caused by lack of iodine

  2. Cretinism—In children, caused by insufficient production of thyroid hormones

  3. Myxedema—In adults, caused by insufficient production of thyroid hormones

  4. Graves' disease—Caused by too much thyroid hormones

E. Parathyroid glands—Located behind the thyroid glands

  1. Produce parathyroid hormone (PTH), which also regulates calcium level in the body

  2. Tetany occurs when blood calcium level becomes too low

F. Adrenal medulla—Controlled by sympathetic division of autonomic nervous system; produces epinephrine and norepinephrine, which causes the following results:

  1. Increases blood glucose level, breathing, and metabolic and heart rates

  2. Dilates bronchioles and increases breathing rate

  3. Dilates blood vessels to skeletal muscle

  4. Constricts blood flow to gastrointestinal tract

  5. Increases heart rate and force of contraction

G. Adrenal cortex

  1. Produces mineralocorticoid, aldosterone, which controls levels of sodium and potassium and regulates blood pressure

  2. Produces glucocorticoid, cortisol, which depresses immune responses and is a potent anti-inflammatory agent; also increases glucose formation and facilitates the breakdown of fat and protein

H. Pancreas

  1. Parts

    a. Exocrine—Produces digestive juices that flow into duodenum

    b. Endocrine—Islets of Langerhans (islands of tissue within the pancreas) produce insulin and glucagon

      (1) Insulin

        (a) Secreted when blood glucose level is high

        (b) Promotes storage of excess glucose as glycogen in liver and buildup of fats and proteins

        (c) Lowers blood glucose level

(d) Disorders associated with insulin

    i) Diabetes mellitus—Due to insufficient insulin production or cell response

        • Symptoms—Polyphagia (excessive eating), polyuria (excessive urination), polydipsia (excessive thirst), weakness, itching, and hyperglycemia (high blood glucose level)

        • Type 1 diabetes—Islet cells do not produce enough insulin

        • Type 2 diabetes—Cell receptors do not respond to insulin

(2) Glucagon

    (a) Secretes when blood glucose level is low

    (b) Promotes breakdown of glycogen into glucose

    (c) Raises blood glucose levels

I. Pineal gland—Produces melatonin, which regulates the sleep—wake cycle

J. Thymus gland (sometimes still called a gland, but primarily a lymphatic organ)—Produces hormones called thymosins, which are used in development of immunity; important in maturation of T lymphocytes; active in childhood

K. Testes

    1. Produce testosterone and secondary sex characteristics

    2. Promote development of sperm and are responsible for male aggression

L. Ovaries—Produce secondary sex characteristics, estrogen, and progesterone; necessary for egg maturation

III. Physiology—Most hormones are regulated by a system of negative feedback with the pituitary gland; blood level of the hormone turns off the releasing factor of the pituitary, thereby slowing or shutting off the production of the hormone (see Figure 2-19)

IV. Conditions of Endocrine System

    A. Acromegaly—Chronic disease of adults resulting in an elongation and enlargement of the bones

    B. Addison's disease—Known as primary adrenal cortical insufficiency; insufficient production of adrenal steroids causes pituitary gland to increase its production of adrenocorticotropic hormones (ACTH) clinical manifestations; oral melonotic macules, or brown pigmentation of skin

    C. Hypothyroidism—Decreased output of thyroid hormone; clinical manifestations:

        1. Children—Thickened lips, enlarged tongue, delayed eruption pattern

2. Adults—Enlarged tongue, reduced salivary flow can occur

    a. Cretinism—during childhood

    b. Myxedema—during adulthood

D. Cretinism—Congenital condition in which a lack of thyroid (hypothyroidism) may result in arrested physical and mental development

E. Myxedema—Condition resulting from a hypofunction of the thyroid gland; symptoms include anemia, enlarged tongue, mental apathy

F. Hyperthyroidism

    1. Excessive production of thyroid hormone; also known as Graves' disease

    2. Children—Premature exfoliation of deciduous teeth, premature eruption of permanent teeth

    3. Adults—Osteoporosis, progressive periodontal disease, burning discomfort of tongue

G. Hyperpituitarism—Excess hormone (growth hormone) production by the pituitary gland, usually caused by benign tumor known as pituitary adenoma; produces gigantism in bones during development, and acromegaly in adult life

H. Cushing's syndrome—Hypersecretion of the adrenal cortex; symptoms include weakness, edema, excess hair growth, skin discoloration, and osteoporosis

I. Myasthenia gravis—Condition with great muscular weakness and progressive fatigue difficulty in chewing and swallowing

J. Diabetes insipidus—Caused by inadequate secretion of a hormone by the posterior lobe of the pituitary gland most common in children

V. Homeostasis—Endocrine system works with nervous system to regulate blood glucose, blood pressure, blood pH, and temperature

➤ CIRCULATORY SYSTEM

I. Function

A. Blood carries everything needed for cellular metabolism to cells and unwanted by-products away from the cells, to lungs and kidneys

B. Blood vessels—Means by which blood gains proximity to cells

C. Heart—Maintains constant movement of blood in blood vessels

II. Anatomic Structures

A. Vascular system (blood vessels)

1. Arteries

   a. Characteristics

   (1) Made up of thick walls with elastic fibers; needed because arterial blood has high pressure

   b. Functions

   (1) Transport (oxygenated) blood away from heart

   (2) Lead to smaller arterioles

2. Capillaries

   a. Characteristics

   (1) Made up of thin walls so oxygen and nutrients can diffuse through to cells

   (2) Arterioles—Branch into capillaries

   (3) Venules—Lead away from capillaries

3. Veins

   a. Characteristics

   (1) thin-walled; some contain valves to prevent blood from flowing backward since venous blood has low pressure

   b. Functions

   (1) Venules—Drain capillary beds that flow into veins

   (2) Most carry unoxygenated blood (carbon dioxide) and wastes away from cells

   (3) Once back to the right side of the heart, venous blood is pumped to lungs

B. Heart—Muscular organ in thorax

1. Characteristics

   a. Contains specialized cardiac muscle tissue

   b. Enclosed in a pericardial sac

   c. Consists of myocardium (muscular layer) and endocardium (internal lining)

   d. Has its own internal electrical conduction system

   (1) Sinoatrial node (pacemaker of the heart)—Sends out impulses for atria to contract approximately 72 beats/minute and sends signals to atrioventricular node

   (2) Atrioventricular node—Receives signals from sinoatrial node and causes ventricles to contract

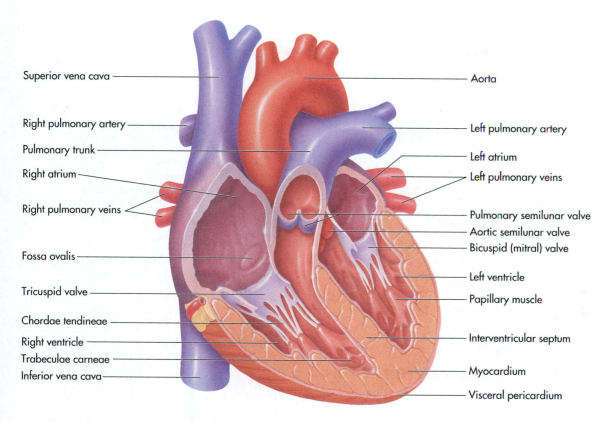

Superior vena cava

Right pulmonary artery

Pulmonary trunk

Right atrium

Right pulmonary veins

Fossa ovalis

Tricuspid valve

Chordae tendineae

Right ventricle

Trabeculae carneae

Inferior vena cava

Aorta

Left pulmonary artery

Left atrium

Left pulmonary veins

Pulmonary semilunar valve

Aortic semilunar valve

Bicuspid (mitral) valve

Left ventricle

Papillary muscle

Interventricular septum

Myocardium

Visceral pericardium

FIGURE 2-21 ■ Structural components of the heart

2. Parts—Composed of four pumping chambers (Figure 2-21■)

a. Right atrium—receives venous blood from body (superior and inferior vena cavae); opens into right ventricle through tricuspid valve; thin-walled

b. Right ventricle—Pumps venous blood through pulmonary valve into pulmonary artery, which leads to lungs; thick-walled

c. Left atrium—Receives arterial (oxygenated) blood from lungs through four pulmonary veins; opens into left ventricle though mitral valve; thin-walled

d. Left ventricle—Pumps arterial blood to entire body; blood flows from left ventricle through aortic valve and into aorta; contains thickest walls of all the chambers

III. Physiology

A. Blood flow (Figure 2-22■)

1. Venous blood—Flows through right side of heart to lungs

2. Arterial blood—Flows through left side of heart to body

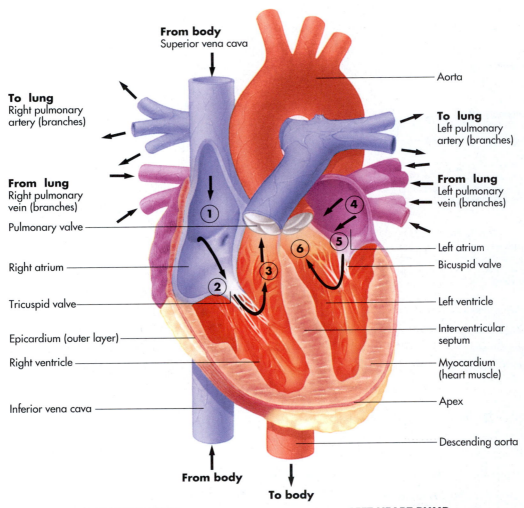

From body
Superior vena cava

Aorta

To lung
Right pulmonary
artery (branches)

To lung
Left pulmonary
artery (branches)

From lung
Right pulmonary
vein (branches)

From lung
Left pulmonary
vein (branches)

Pulmonary valve

Left atrium

Right atrium

Bicuspid valve

Tricuspid valve

Left ventricle

Epicardium (outer layer)

Interventricular
septum

Right ventricle

Myocardium
(heart muscle)

Inferior vena cava

Apex

Descending aorta

From body

To body

RIGHT HEART PUMP

1. Deoxygenated blood returns from the upper and lower body to fill the right atrium of the heart creating a pressure against the atrioventricular (AV) or tricuspid valve.

2. This pressure of the returning blood forces the AV valve open and begins filling the ventricle. The final filling of the ventricle is achieved by the contracting of the right atrium.

3. The right ventricle contracts increasing the internal pressure. This pressure closes the tricuspid valve and forces open the pulmonary valve thus sending blood toward the lung via the pulmonary artery. This blood will become oxygenated as it travels through the capillary beds of the lung and then return to the left side of the heart.

LEFT HEART PUMP

4. Oxygenated blood returns from the lung via the pulmonary vein and fills the left atrium creating a pressure against the bicuspid valve.

5. This pressure of returning blood forces the bicuspid valve open and begins filling the left ventricle. The final filling of the left ventricle is achieved by the contracting of the left atrium.

6. The left ventricle contracts increasing internal pressure. This pressure closes the bicuspid valve and forces open the aortic valve causing oxygenated blood to flow through the aorta to deliver oxygen throughout the body.

FIGURE 2-22 ■ Cardiac Cycle—Systemic Circulation

    3. Structural order of blood flow (into and out of heart)

        a. Inferior and superior vena cavae

        b. Right atrium

        c. Tricuspid valve

        d. Right ventricle

        e. Pulmonary valve

        f. Pulmonary trunk and arteries

        g. Lungs

        h. Pulmonary veins

        i. Left atrium

        j. Mitral valve

        k. Left ventricle

        l. Aortic valve

        m. Aorta

B. Heartbeat (pulse—approximately 72 beats/minute at rest)

    1. Stroke volume—Amount of blood pumped by ventricle during one heartbeat

    2. Cardiac output—Amount of blood pumped by ventricle during 1 minute

C. Cardiac cycle—Contains three

    1. Both atria contract

    2. Both ventricles contract

    3. Heart rests

D. Blood pressure (average normal is 120/80)

    1. Systole—Measured during ventricular contraction

    2. Diastole—Measured during heart relaxation

    3. Hypertension (high blood pressure)

        a. Increased cardiac output (heart rate and/or blood volume increases)

        b. Increased peripheral resistance (arterial constriction)

        c. Hormones epinephrine, norepinephrine, aldosterone, and ADH (an antidiuretic hormone)

        d. Arteries—Elevated blood pressure due to blood leaving the forceful contracting left ventricle

        e. Veins—Blood pressure is lower; muscular contraction assists in moving the venous blood

E. Blood supply of the heart

    1. Coronary arteries—Early branches off the aorta; provides a rich supply of blood to the continual muscular contraction of the myocardium

2. Myocardial infarction (heart attack)—Caused by occlusion of coronary arteries from atherosclerotic plaque or clots

F. Blood supply to the brain—Brain requires constant supply of glucose and oxygen; supplied by 4 arteries: 2 carotids and 2 vertebrals

IV. Homeostasis—Heart and blood vessels are responsible for the blood pressure of 120/80; glucose concentration 0.1%, pH 7.4, and temperature 98.6°F are possible because of the circulation of the blood through vessels and organs; this circulation is propelled by contractions of the heart

➤ BLOOD

I. Functions

A. Transports

1. Oxygen to and carbon dioxide away from cells
2. Nutrients to and wastes away from cells
3. White blood cells to fight infectious invaders
4. Hormones to target organs
5. Clotting elements to break in the vascular system
6. Heat away from areas of high cellular metabolism (contracting muscles)

II. Anatomical Structures (Figure 2-23■)

A. Form elements (45% hematocrit)

1. Red blood cells (RBCs)—Erythrocytes

   a. Contain hemoglobin—Protein carrier for oxygen

   b. Formed in red bone marrow

   c. 4–6 million per cubic mm of blood

2. White blood cells (WBCs)—Leukocytes

   a. Fight infections

   b. Formed in red bone marrow

   c. 5,000–11,000 per cubic mm of blood

   d. Types

   (1) Granular leukocytes

   (a) Neutrophils—Engage in phagocytosis (engulf bacteria); most numerous; release cytotoxic enzymes and chemicals

   (b) Eosinophils—Attack antibody-labeled materials through release of cytotoxic enzmes and/or phagocytosis

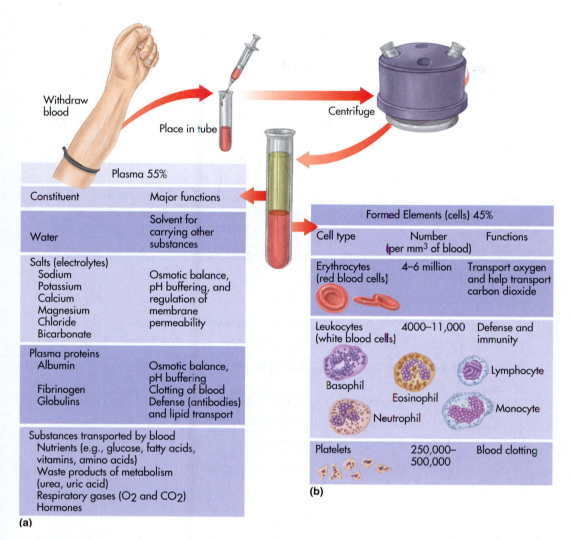

FIGURE 2-23 ■ Composition of Whole Blood: (a) Plasma, the Liquid Portion of Blood; (b) Formed Elements: Red Blood Cells, White Blood Cells, and Platelets

(c) Basophils—Enter damaged tissues and release histamine and other chemicals that reduce inflammation

(2) Agranular leukocytes

(a) Monocytes—Engage in phagocytosis; largest of the WBCs

(b) Lymphocytes—Cells of the lymphatic system responsible for immunity

i) B cells—Mature in bone marrow and produce antibodies

ii) T cells—Mature in thymus; some regulate the immune response, while others attack antigen-bearing cells

(3) Platelets—Used in clotting; amount is 150,000–300,000 per cubic mm of blood

B. Plasma

    1. Consists of liquid part of blood

    2. Accounts for about 55% of whole blood

    3. Composed mostly of water

    4. Includes substances such as hormones, gasses, plasma proteins, salts, and nutrients

III. Physiology

A. Clotting—Includes many factors in addition to platelets, prothrombin, and fibrinogen; creates tangle of threadlike structures that incorporate red blood cells to form clot

B. Types of blood groups—A, B, AB, and O; type O is universal donor because it contains neither A nor B antigens

C. Exchange between blood and tissue fluid

    1. Occurs in capillaries and is dependent on osmotic pressure

    2. Moves water, glucose, oxygen, and amino acids out of blood

    3. Moves water, carbon dioxide, and waste molecules into blood

IV. Homeostasis—Vital in regulating blood pressure

A. Regulates body temperature by shunting blood to skin or internal organs

B. Transports oxygen and carbon dioxide, which assists in maintaining pH

C. Transports nutrients to and wastes away from cells

➤ LYMPHATIC SYSTEM

I. Functions

A. Returns extracellular tissue fluid (lymph) to bloodstream

B. Lymphatic capillaries in gastrointestinal tract absorb fat molecules and transport them to bloodstream

C. Helps defend body against disease

II. Anatomy

A. Lymph vessels (Figure 2-24■)

    1. One-way system of vessels, which carry lymph back to bloodstream

    2. Vessels come from all parts of body

    3. Contain lymph nodes (LN) through which lymph passes; LNs contain many white blood cells that destroy infectious agents

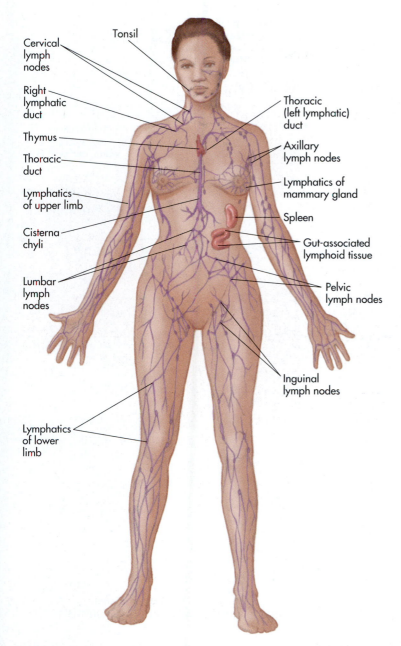

Cervical lymph nodes

Tonsil

Right lymphatic duct

Thymus

Thoracic duct

Lymphatics of upper limb

Cisterna chyli

Lumbar lymph nodes

Lymphatics of lower limb

Thoracic (left lymphatic) duct

Axillary lymph nodes

Lymphatics of mammary gland

Spleen

Gut-associated lymphoid tissue

Pelvic lymph nodes

Inguinal lymph nodes

FIGURE 2-24 ■ Components of the Lymphatic System

B. Spleen—Abdominal organ

    1. Acts as a filter of the blood, much as a lymph node

    2. Filters out broken red blood cells

C. Thymus—Thoracic organ; produces thymosins (hormones); active during childhood; decreases in size in adults; site of maturation of T lymphocytes

D. Red bone marrow—Site where all blood cells (red and white) are produced

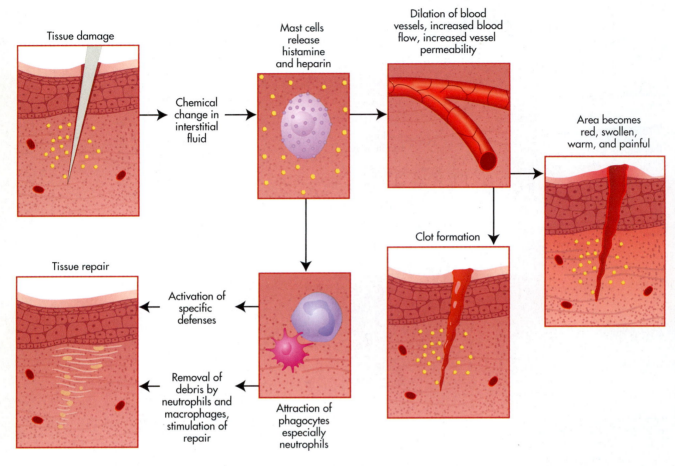

FIGURE 2-25 ■ Inflammation Process

III. Physiology

A. Inflammatory response (Figure 2-25■)

1. Reaction to an injury

2. Releases histamine, which causes capillary dilatation and permeability

3. Swelling occurs

4. White blood cells migrate to site

5. Pus forms as a result of dead WBCs and bacteria

6. Releases bradykinin, which initiates pain

B. Immune response (Figure 2-26■)

1. Antigen—Any substance (microbe, food, pollen, cell) that immune system recognizes as foreign

2. Non-self-recognition of antigen by body

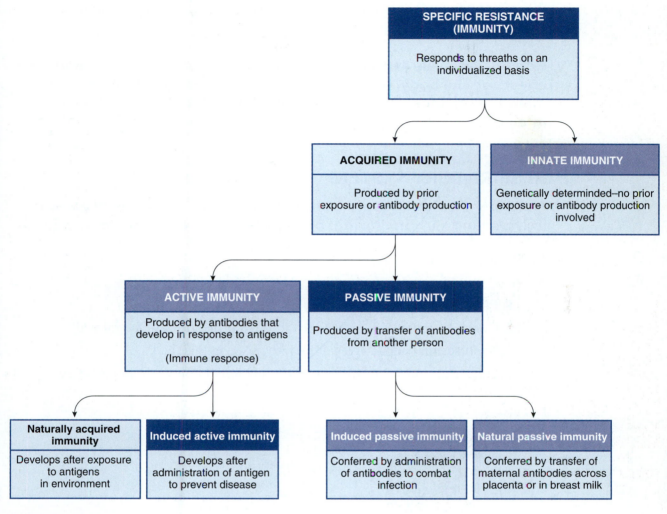

FIGURE 2-26 ■ Types of Immunity

3. Body response—Activates B and T (lymphocytes); B cells produce antibodies, which are proteins that can inactivate antigens; some cells attach to antigen-bearing cells, while others regulate the immune response

4. System is responsible for developing immunity to diseases and immunity rendered by vaccination; results in *active immunity* (can last a lifetime; *passive immunity* occurs when immunoglobulins are received from another individual [short-lived])

IV. Diseases of Lymphatic System

A. Hodgkin's disease—Cancer of the lymphatic cells concentrated in lymph nodes; also called Hodgkin's lymphoma

    B. Non-Hodgkin's lymphoma—Cancer of the lymphatic tissues other than Hodgkin's lymphoma

V. Homeostasis—By keeping the body free of infectious agents and their effects on the body, the lymphatic system plays a vital role in maintaining homeostasis (i.e., body temperature is often elevated in infections)

➤ RESPIRATORY SYSTEM

I. Function—External respiration, which involves exchange of gasses (oxygen and carbon dioxide) between air in alveoli and blood in lungs

II. Anatomy (Figure 2-27■)

    A. Nose

        1. Filters, warms, and humidifies the air

        2. Concha—Increases surface area through projections in lateral wall

        3. Nasolacrimal duct—Eyes drain into nose via this duct

        4. Paranasal sinuses (air-filled cavities in cranial bones) drain into nose

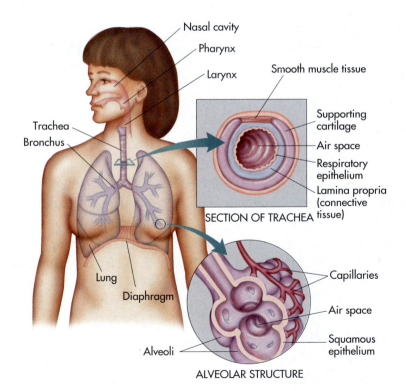

FIGURE 2-27 ■ Respiratory Organs

B. Pharynx (throat)

    1. Opening for nose and mouth

    2. Divided into three parts: nasopharynx, oropharynx, and laryngopharynx

C. Larynx (voice box)—Consists of

    1. Glottis—Top opening of larynx

    2. Epiglottis—Flap protects larynx when food is swallowed

    3. Vocal cords—Contain folds of tissue for speech

D. Trachea

    1. Extends from larynx to thoracic cavity where it splits into bronchi

    2. Aperture is held open with C-shaped rings of cartilage

E. Bronchi

    1. Bronchus (right and left)—One main stem goes to each lung

    2. Contains cartilage to hold lumen open

    3. Continue dividing until there is a tertiary bronchus to each bronchopulmonary segment of lung

F. Bronchioles

    1. Result from branching of tertiary bronchi; lead to alveoli

    2. Contain smooth muscle that can contract and constrict airways (i.e., asthma)

G. Alveoli

    1. Consist of terminal structures of bronchial tree; elastic epithelial sacs

    2. Where external respiration takes place

H. Lungs

    1. Organs that contain bronchial tree, bronchioles, and alveoli

    2. Surrounded by pleural sac

    3. Rich in blood supply for gas exchange

I. Diaphragm—Separates thoracic and abdominal cavities

    1. During inspiration—Contracts and moves downward, creating negative pressure in thoracic cavity and causing air to rush in

    2. During expiration—Relaxes, and elastic tissue of lungs contracts, allowing air to be exhaled

    3. Supplied by phrenic nerve, which comes down from neck

III. Physiology

A. Oxygen—Passes from air in an alveolus across respiratory membrane to enter capillaries surrounding alveolus, where it is picked up by hemoglobin in an RBC and carried to tissue capillaries in body

    B. Ventilation—Involves movement of air in and out of lungs (Figure 2-13)

        1. Diaphragm—Most important muscle involved in ventilation

        2. Rib cage—Also involved in moving air; during inspiration, the ribs move up and increase size of thoracic cavity

    C. Function—Can be determined by tests that measure lung capacity

        1. Tidal volume (TV)—Measures amount of air moving in and out with each breath

        2. Vital capacity (VC)—Measures total amount of air that can be moved in and out of lungs with a single breath

        3. Inspiratory reserve (IRV)—Measures increase inspired beyond tidal volume

        4. Expiratory reserve (ERV)—Measures amount forcefully expired beyond tidal volume

        5. Vital capacity = tidal volume + IRV + ERV

        6. Residual volume—Amount of air that remains in lungs, even after forceful expiration

IV. Diseases of the Respiratory System

    A. Emphysema—Pulmonary condition characterized by shortness of breath and an inability to tolerate physical exertion that occurs as a result of long-term heavy smoking

    B. Pleurisy—Inflammation of the pleura

    C. Pneumonia—Inflammatory condition of the lung resulting from a bacterial and viral infection

    D. Tuberculosis—Infectious disease caused by tubercle bacillus, *Mycobacterium turberculosis*

V. Homeostasis—Respiratory system maintains oxygen content of blood; helps maintain temperature by releasing excess heat and regulates pH of blood by exhaling carbon dioxide

➤ DIGESTIVE SYSTEM

I. Functions

    A. Ingests food

    B. Breaks down food into molecules that can be absorbed across plasma membrane

        1. Proteins—Break down into amino acids

        2. Carbohydrates—Break down into glucose

        3. Fats—Break down into glycerol and fatty acids

    C. Absorbs amino acids, glucose, glycerol, and fatty acids

    D. Eliminates nondigestible foods

Organ	Primary Functions
Salivary Glands	Provide lubrication, produce buffers and the enzymes that begin digestion
Pharynx	Passageway connected to esophagus
Esophagus	Delivers food to stomach
Stomach	Secretes acids and enzymes
Small Intestine	Secretes digestive enzymes, absorbs nutrients
Liver	Secretes bile, regulates blood chemistry
Gallbladder	Stores bile for release into small intestine
Pancreas	Secretes digestive enzymes and buffers; contains endocrine cells
Large Intestine	Removes water from fecal material, stores waste

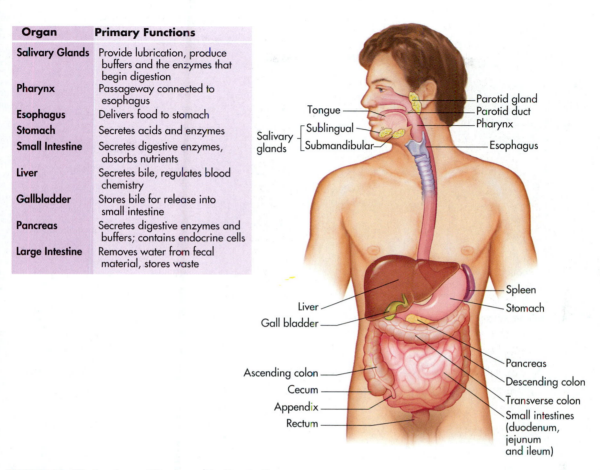

FIGURE 2-28 ■ Functions and Structures of the Digestive Tract

II. Anatomic Structures (Figure 2-28■)

A. Mouth—Food is chewed (masticated) in oral cavity (Figure 2-29■)

  1. Teeth

  2. Tongue

  3. Hard and soft palates

  4. Salivary glands (Figure 2-30■)—Secrete saliva that moisten bolus of food and contain salivary amylase (enzyme that begins breakdown of starch)

B. Tongue—Propels bolus to back of throat, the pharynx, where it moves down into esophagus

C. Esophagus—Muscular tube that passes through diaphragm to reach stomach

D. Stomach—Stores food and starts digestion of proteins

  1. Lined with glands that secrete hydrochloric acid and the enzyme pepsin

  2. Gastroesophageal sphincter—Prevents food from refluxing into esophagus

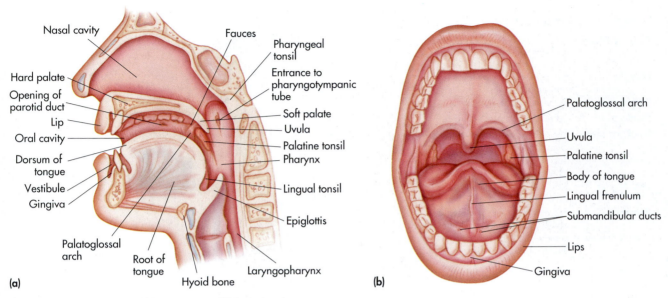

FIGURE 2-29 ■ Oral Cavity: (a) Anterior view; (b) Sagittal section

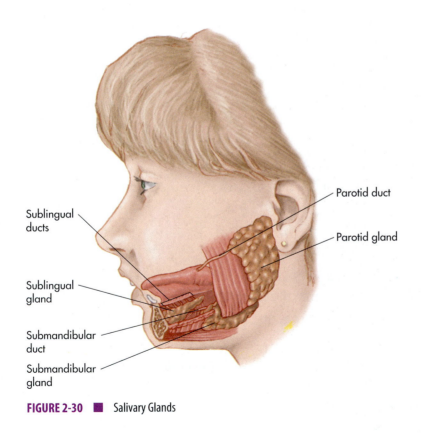

FIGURE 2-30 ■ Salivary Glands

3. Food leaves stomach as chyme and passes through pyloric sphincter into duodenum of small intestine

E. Small intestine—Approximately 10 feet long

    1. Functions

        a. Mechanically and chemically breaks down chyme so nutrients can be absorbed through finger-like projections called villi

           (1) Glucose and amino acids—Absorbed into capillaries and then enter liver via portal vein

           (2) Fats—Enter a lacteal, small vessel of lymphatic system

    2. Parts

        a. Duodenum—Makes up first 10 inches of small intestine

           (1) Receives bile from liver to emulsify fats

           (2) Receives pancreatic juice from pancreas

           (3) Produces intestinal juice that contains enzymes to chemically break down chyme

        b. Jejunum—Makes up next 3 feet of small intestine

        c. Ileum—Makes up last 6–7 feet of small intestine

F. Large intestine—Approximately 5 feet long

    1. Functions

        a. Absorbs water and electrolytes

        b. Stores feces and nondigestible food until they can be eliminated

    2. Parts

        a. Cecum (through the ileocecal valve)—Ileum of small intestine opens into this part of large intestine

        b. Vermiform appendix—Projects off cecum

        c. Ascending colon—Located on right side of abdomen into which cecum opens

        d. Transverse colon—Extends from right to left side of abdomen

        e. Descending colon—Opens into sigmoid colon; located on left side of abdomen

        f. Sigmoid colon (S-shaped segment)—Opens into rectum, which ends in the anus, an external opening

G. Pancreas—An abdominal organ that produces exocrine digestive enzymes and bicarbonate and endocrine hormones, insulin and glucagon

H. Liver

    1. Produces bile that flows via bile duct into duodenum; extra bile is stored in gall bladder, a pouch hanging down from liver

2. Receives nutrients absorbed through portal vein

3. Removes and stores iron

4. Stores fat-soluble vitamins A, D, E, and K

5. Removes and detoxifies poisons

6. Stores glucose as glycogen

7. Destroys old red blood cells

8. Produces plasma proteins

III. Physiology

A. Peristalsis—Rhythmic movements that begin in esophagus and propel food through digestive system

B. Chemical digestion—Breaks down carbohydrates into glucose, proteins into amino acids, and fats into fatty acids and glycerol; all these molecules are small enough to pass through plasma membrane of digestive system

C. Provide nutrition

1. Glucose—Used for immediate energy or stored as glycogen in liver

2. Amino acids—Used for protein synthesis

3. Fats—Reserved as a long-term energy source

4. Vitamins—Essential for cellular metabolism

5. Minerals—Inorganic elements necessary for some metabolism

IV. Homeostasis

A. Water is absorbed in stomach and large intestine to maintain blood volume that helps to regulate normal blood pressure

B. Liver—Assists in controlling glucose concentration (0.1%)

C. Pancreas—Produces bicarbonate, which assists in proper pH (7.4) of the blood and produces insulin and glucagon, which regulate glucose concentration

D. Absorption of nutrients to nourish cells and maintain function

➤ URINARY SYSTEM

I. Functions

A. Remove nitrogenous wastes (by-products of protein metabolism) from blood and excretes them; nitrogenous wastes are in the form of urea, uric acid, creatinine, and ammonium

B. Maintain blood volume—Regulates amount of water excreted and/or reabsorbed

C. Regulate electrolyte balance in blood (i.e., sodium [Na+], potassium [K+], bicarbonate [HCO_3-], and calcium [Ca+])

D. Regulate blood pH by excreting hydrogen (H+) ions

E. Secrete erythropoietin—Stimulates production of RBCs

F. Secrete renin—Helps maintain blood pressure

II. Anatomical Structures (Figure 2-31■)

A. Kidneys—Paired organs in retroperitoneal space

B. Nephrons—Functional unit of kidneys; over 1 million per kidney; each nephron contains

    1. Glomerulus—Capillary cluster through which fluid part of blood flows

    2. Glomerular capsule—Leads to tubular system

    3. Tubular system—Secretes electrolytes and reabsorbs water

    4. Collecting ducts—Urine leaves nephron system and flows into these ducts, which all empty into renal pelvis

C. Ureters—Paired tubes leading from kidneys to urinary bladder

D. Urinary bladder—Pelvic organ used for storage of urine

E. Urethra—Tube leading from urinary bladder to outside; short in females, long in males

F. Urination (micturition)—Emptying of bladder through urethra

G. Renal arteries—Since kidneys regulate blood volume and composition, they have a rich supply of blood from large renal arteries that come directly off descending aorta

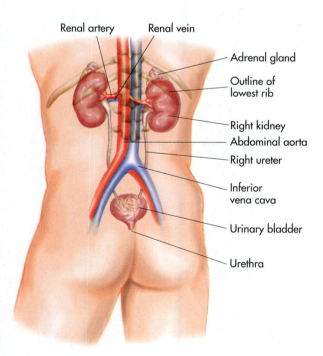

Renal artery   Renal vein

Adrenal gland

Outline of lowest rib

Right kidney

Abdominal aorta

Right ureter

Inferior vena cava

Urinary bladder

Urethra

FIGURE 2-31 ■ Urinary System

III. Physiology

A. Kidney—Function is regulated by the following hormones

1. Aldosterone

a. Secreted by adrenal cortex and regulates sodium (Na+) and potassium (K+)

b. Regulates blood pressure and blood volume with help of enzyme, renin, secreted by kidney

2. ADH (antidiuretic hormone)

a. Secreted by posterior lobe of pituitary gland when body is dehydrated to conserve water

b. Regulates blood pressure and blood volume, which are elevated by actions of aldosterone and ADH

B. Electrolytes—Dissolved in the plasma of blood and regulated by kidneys

1. Sodium and potassium—Used in muscle contraction and nerve impulse conduction

2. Bicarbonate ion (HCO_3)—Maintains pH of blood

IV. Disorders of the Urinary Tract

A. Pyelonephritis—Inflammation of the renal pelvis and the kidney

B. Glomerulonephritis—Inflammation of the kidney

C. Urinary retention—An inability to fully empty the bladder; blockage in the urethra

V. Homeostasis—Maintained by regulating blood volume and pH

➤ REPRODUCTIVE SYSTEM

I. Function

A. Males

1. Produce sperm within the testes—Nurture and transport sperm until they exit the penis

2. Produce sex hormones

B. Females

1. Release eggs from ovary—Nurture and transport egg in uterine tube until it reaches uterus

2. Nurture and house fetus in uterus during pregnancy

3. Produce sex hormones

II. Anatomy

  A. Male

    1. Testes—Contained in scrotum, outside of abdominal cavity

      a. Produce sperm and sex hormones

      b. Must be kept cooler than body temperature for viable sperm

      c. Seminiferous tubules—Where spermatogenesis occurs

      d. Interstitial cells—Produce male sex hormones, androgens

    2. Epididymis—Stores maturing sperm

    3. Vas deferens—Connects epididymis with urethra; portion cut during a vasectomy (for birth control)

    4. Seminal fluid

      a. Secretion that contains sperm during ejaculation

      b. Produced by three glands: seminal vesicles, prostate gland, and bulbourethral glands

    5. Penis—Tip is covered by flap of skin, foreskin, which may be removed (circumcision)

      a. Penetrates vagina during sexual intercourse

      b. Contains erectile tissue that fills with blood to cause an erection

    6. Testosterone

      a. Production is regulated by pituitary gland and is necessary for production and maturation of sperm

      b. Responsible for secondary sex characteristics

  B. Female

    1. Ovaries

      a. Release eggs and produce sex hormones

      b. Graafian follicle—Maturing egg in follicle tissue

      c. Ovulation—Time at which egg is released from follicle

      d. Corpus luteum—Formed by an empty follicle

        (1) If pregnancy does not occur, corpus luteum degenerates 10 days after ovulation

        (2) If pregnancy occurs, corpus luteum persists up to 6 months to produce hormones that maintain pregnancy

    2. Uterine tube (fallopian tube)—Where fertilization usually occurs; transports egg to uterus; egg begins dividing while in uterine tube (several days)

    3. Uterus—Thick-walled, muscular organ

      a. Enlarges to accommodate growing fetus

b. Myometrium—Composes muscular layer

c. Endometrium—Composes lining; rich in blood vessels to supply the placenta

4. Vagina—Fibromuscular organ; also functions as birth canal during parturition (childbirth)

5. External genitalia (vulva)

a. Labia majora and labia minora—Folds of skin around vaginal opening

b. Clitoris—Female counterpart of the penis, but much smaller; contains erectile tissue for sexual excitation and climax

III. Physiology

A. Orgasm

1. Physiological and psychological climax of sexual stimulation

a. In males, results in ejaculation, release of semen, and relaxation of muscular tension

b. In females, is preceded by lubrication of vagina and followed by relaxation of muscular tension

B. Regulation of female hormones

1. Controlled by the hypothalamus, which secretes gonadotropic-releasing factor to pituitary gland

2. Anterior pituitary gland—Secretes follicle-stimulating hormone (FSH) and luteinizing hormone (LH), which target ovaries

3. Ovaries secrete estrogen and progesterone

4. Estrogen

a. Necessary for egg maturation

b. Responsible for secondary sex characteristics

c. Predominates during first half of menstrual cycle

5. Progesterone

a. Secreted by corpus luteum

b. Prepares endometrium to receive a fertilized egg

c. Predominates during second half of menstrual cycle

6. Menstruation

a. Occurs if egg is not fertilized and does not implant in uterus

b. Endometrium is sloughed off

c. Menstrual cycle is usually 28 days

(1) Menstruation occurs during first 5 days

(2) Ovulation occurs about day 14

(3) Period of fertility is approximately from day 10 to day 18

C. Pregnancy

    1. Occurs when sperm and egg (gametes) unite to form an embryo

    2. Placenta transfers nutrients from maternal bloodstream to fetus

    3. Embryonic membranes produce hormone human chorionic gonadotropic hormone (HCG)

    4. Full-term pregnancy lasts 40 weeks

IV. Homeostasis—Sex hormones help to maintain a robust and youthful body, capable of adjusting to stimuli and maintaining homeostasis

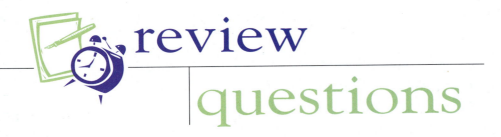

review questions

DIRECTIONS Each of the questions or incomplete statements below is followed by suggested answers or completions. Select the **one** answer that is best in each case.

1. Which of the following blood components is necessary for clotting?
   A. Plasma
   B. Platelets
   C. Neutrophils
   D. Hemoglobin

2. Which of the following heart chambers pumps with the greatest force?
   A. right atrium
   B. right ventricle
   C. left atrium
   D. left ventricle

3. Diastole occurs when the:
   A. Ventricles contract
   B. Ventricles fill
   C. Heart rests
   D. Atria contract

4. All of the following nutrients can be absorbed by the gastrointestinal system EXCEPT one. Which one is the EXCEPTION?
   A. Fatty acids
   B. Glucose
   C. Proteins
   D. Glycerol

5. Which of the following BEST describes the large intestine?
   A. Possesses villi for absorption
   B. Secretes acid and digestive juice
   C. Receives bile from the liver and pancreatic juice from the pancreas
   D. Absorbs water and electrolytes

6. All of the following are functions of the liver EXCEPT one. Which one is the EXCEPTION?
   A. Secretes glucagon
   B. Stores vitamins A, D, E, and K
   C. Removes and detoxifies poisons
   D. Produces bile

7. Which of the following glands BEST regulates blood glucose level?
   A. Thyroid
   B. Pituitary
   C. Pancreas
   D. Adrenal medulla

8. During inflammation, histamine is released and causes:
   A. Swelling
   B. Clotting
   C. Bleeding
   D. Pus formation

9. Which of the following systems produces heat, which helps maintain body temperature at 37°C?
   A. Skeletal
   B. Lymphatic
   C. Digestive
   D. Muscular

10. Which of the following BEST describes a striated (skeletal) muscle?
    A. Contracts slower than smooth muscle
    B. Fatigues more quickly than smooth muscle
    C. Controlled by the autonomic nervous system
    D. Found in hollow organs, such as the intestine

11. Which part of the brain controls respiration?
    A. Medulla
    B. Thalamus
    C. Cerebellum
    D. Cerebrum

12. A synapse is:
    A. The place where an axon of one neuron meets the dendrites of another neuron
    B. Where the nucleus and organelles of a neuron are located
    C. The insulation surrounding the axon
    D. A sensory receptor

13. Sperm are produced in the:
    A. Testes
    B. Epididymis
    C. Vas deferens
    D. Prostate gland

14. Fertilization of the egg MOST commonly occurs in the:
    A. Ovary
    B. Fallopian tube
    C. Uterus
    D. Vagina

15. During a normal human menstrual cycle of 28 days, the period of human fertility occurs in day(s):
    A. 1–5 of the menstrual cycle
    B. 14 only
    C. 10–18
    D. 18–28

16. During respiration, gas exchange occurs in the:
    A. Trachae
    B. Bronchi
    C. Bronchioles
    D. Alveoli

17. The diaphragm:
    A. Contracts during inspiration
    B. Contracts during expiration
    C. Is an abdominal structure
    D. Is located superior to the lungs

18. All of the following are functions of the skeletal system EXCEPT one. Which one is the EXCEPTION?
    A. Protects the soft parts of the body
    B. Produces blood cells
    C. Holds joints together
    D. Stores mineral salts, such as calcium

19. Ribs attach to which of the following vertebrae?
    A. Cervical
    B. Thoracic
    C. Lumbar
    D. Sacral

20. The action of flexion:
    A. Increases the joint angle (straightens it)
    B. Moves the body part laterally away from the midline
    C. Moves the body part toward the midline
    D. Decreases the joint angle (bends it)

21. All of the following are functions of the urinary system EXCEPT one. Which one is the EXCEPTION?
    A. Absorbs glucose
    B. Removes nitrogenous wastes
    C. Maintains blood volume
    D. Regulates electrolytes

22. Which of the following structures provides the opening to the outside for the urinary system?
    A. Nephron
    B. Ureter
    C. Urinary bladder
    D. Urethra

23. Which of the following heart valves separates the right atrium from the right ventricle?
    A. Bicuspid
    B. Tricuspid
    C. Mitral
    D. Semilunar

24. Which of the following tissues lines the inner surface of the heart?
    A. Pericardium
    B. Pleura
    C. Peritoneum
    D. Endocardium

25. Which of the following valves separates the small intestines from the ascending colon?
    A. Pyloric
    B. Mitral
    C. Semilunar
    D. Ileocecal

26. Which of the following veins carry oxygenated blood?
    A. Jugular
    B. Facial
    C. Pulmonary
    D. Maxillary

27. The autonomic nervous system exerts its influence on:
    A. Smooth muscle
    B. Glandular secretion
    C. Cardiac muscle
    D. All of the above

28. Sodium ions are reabsorbed, and potassium and hydrogen ions are secreted, under the control of:
    A. Antidiuretic hormone
    B. Thyroxin
    C. Epinephrine
    D. Aldosterone
    E. Cortisol

29. Functions of the kidney include all of the following EXCEPT:
    A. Regulation of hydrogen ion concentration
    B. Regulation of body fluid volumes
    C. Regulation of serum calcium levels
    D. Regulation of serum sodium levels
    E. Removal of urea, creatinine, and other metabolic end products

30. Filtration in the kidney occurs at the:
    A. Glomerulus
    B. Proximal convoluted tubule and loop of Henle
    C. Distal convoluted tubule
    D. Collecting tubule

31. Functions of the adult liver include all of the following EXCEPT:
    A. Bile formation
    B. Reticuloendothelial activity
    C. Glycogenesis, glycogenolysis, and gluconeogenesis
    D. Erythropoiesis
    E. Detoxication

32. The swallowing mechanism involves which of the following cranial nerves?
    A. Trigeminal
    B. Facial
    C. Glossopharyngeal
    D. Vagus and hypoglossal
    E. All of the above

33. Oxygenated blood flows through which of the following structures?
    A. Pulmonary valve
    B. Right atrioventricular valve
    C. Pulmonary artery
    D. Coronary arteries

34. Digestion means:
    A. Splitting large chemical compounds in foods into simpler substances that can be absorbed
    B. Absorption of small molecular weight end products into body fluids
    C. Hydrolysis
    D. A and C only
    E. B and C only

35. Which hormone promotes glucose transport from blood into cells?
    A. Insulin
    B. Glucagon
    C. Epinephrine
    D. Pancreatin

36. Which hormone is LESS involved in a stress reaction?
    A. Epinephrine
    B. Norepinephrine
    C. Cortisone
    D. Thyroxin
    E. Adrenocorticotropin

37. Cortisol:
    A. Increases the flux of amino acids in the body
    B. Mobilizes stored fat
    C. Promotes gluconeogenesis
    D. All of the above
    E. A and C only

38. Calcitonin:
    A. Potentiates the effect of parathyroid hormone
    B. Is secreted by the thyroid gland
    C. Is released in response to excess serum calcium
    D. All of the above
    E. B and C only

39. Which of the following describe(s) the functions of the hypothalamus?
    A. Temperature control centers
    B. Regulation of visceral activity
    C. Synthesis of hormonal releasing factors
    D. Influencing basic drives like sex, thirst, hunger
    E. All of the above

40. Inability to coordinate muscular activity can be due to a lesion in the:
    A. Cerebellum
    B. Somesthetic cortex
    C. Broca's area
    D. Occipital lobe

41. The primary motor area of the brain is the:
    A. Precentral gyrus
    B. Postcentral gyrus
    C. Temporal lobe
    D. Occipital lobe
    E. Hypothalamus

42. Conduction occurs when a stimulus reduces the membrane potential to a critical level. This level is called:
    A. Summation
    B. Threshold
    C. Facilitation
    D. Action potential
    E. Refractory period

43. The physiological concept that refers to the maintenance of a constant internal environment is:
    A. Hemostasis
    B. Dynamic equilibrium
    C. Homeostasis
    D. Interdependence
    E. Induction

44. The organelles that contain enzymes capable of digesting and destroying cellular debris are called:
    A. Endoplasmic reticulum
    B. Golgi apparatus
    C. Mitochondria
    D. Lysosomes
    E. Ribosomes

45. Transport of water across a cell membrane takes place by:
    A. Osmosis
    B. Facilitated diffusion
    C. Active transport
    D. Diffusion

46. The direction and rate of diffusion of an ion are influenced by the:
    A. Concentration gradient
    B. Gydrostatic pressure gradient
    C. Electrical gradient
    D. All of the above

47. All of the following are derived from endoderm EXCEPT:
    A. Epithelial parts of the respiratory system
    B. Epithelial parts of the gastrointestinal system
    C. Epithelium in the mouth
    D. Epithelium of the pharynx

48. A single motor neuron and the muscle cells supplied by its axon branches is termed a(n):
    A. Efferent neuron
    B. Motor unit
    C. Motor end plate
    D. Sarcoplasmic reticulum
    E. Annulospiral ending

49. Conduction occurs when a stimulus reduces the membrane potential to a critical level. The level is called:
    A. Summation
    B. Threshold
    C. Facilitation
    D. Action potential
    E. Refractory period

50. Which of the following is NOT a leukocyte?
    A. Neutrophil
    B. Thrombocyte
    C. Eosinophil
    D. Basophile
    E. Monocyte

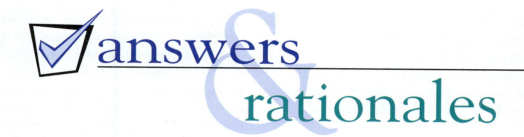

answers & rationales

1.

B. Platelets are part of a complex cascade of reactions that causes clotting. Plasma is the fluid part of blood. Neutrophils are white blood cells used for fighting infection, and hemoglobin is the carrier for oxygen found in red blood cells.

2.

D. The left ventricle is the chamber that pumps blood to the entire body. This is why the left ventricular myocardium is the thickest. The right atrium is the chamber that pumps blood down into the right ventricle. The right ventricle is the chamber that pumps blood to the lungs and the left atrium only needs to pump blood down to the left ventricle.

3.

C. Diastole is the heart at rest. Systole is the highest reading in a blood pressure measurement and represents the force of the contraction of the ventricles. The ventricles are filling when the atria are contracting.

4.

C. Proteins must be broken down into amino acids before absorption can occur. Fatty acids, glycerol, and glucose are in the simplest state for absorption to occur.

5.

D. Fecal matter entering the cecum is watery; therefore it is the job of the large intestine to absorb water and electrolytes to give feces a solid consistency. The small intestine, which has villi for absorption, receives bile from the liver and pancreatic juice from the pancreas. The stomach is responsible for secreting acid and digestive juice.

6.

A. The pancreas secretes glucagon, not the liver. However, the liver stores fat-soluble vitamins A, D, E, and K; removes and detoxifies poisons; and produces bile.

7.

C. The pancreas secretes insulin and glucagon to maintain a fairly constant blood glucose level. The thyroid gland is involved in metabolic rate. Although the pituitary gland controls many glands, it does not control the pancreas. The adrenal medulla is part of the autonomic nervous system and produces epinephrine and norepinephrine.

8.

A. Histamine causes capillary dilation and permeability, which leads to swelling. Histamine plays no part in the clotting mechanism. The fluids that leak out of the capillaries do not contain red blood cells. Pus formation is a late reaction to inflammation, formed by dead white blood cells and infectious agents.

9.

D. Heat is a by-product of the biochemical process of muscle contraction and helps to maintain body temperature. When muscles are very active, as in strenuous exercise, the body may become overheated. In the skeletal system, the metabolic activity is not great enough to produce enough heat to maintain temperature. The lymphatic system is involved in fighting disease and transports fat from the gastrointestinal tract. When blood is diverted to the digestive system during digestion, the body may actually experience a drop in temperature.

10.

B. Striated muscle is used for quick response, as in a reflex, but it cannot maintain contraction for a long time. Smooth muscle is controlled by the autonomic nervous system. Organs are controlled by the autonomic nervous system (we do not consciously think about it) and, therefore, contain smooth muscle.

11.

A. The medulla, or brainstem, controls functions such as breathing, heartbeat, and blood pressure, all of which maintain life. The thalamus is a relay station for afferent information. The cerebellum coordinates skeletal movement. The cerebrum is for higher cortical functioning, such as reasoning and thought processing. A person may live with a nonfunctional cerebrum and an intact medulla. This state is known as brain-dead.

12.

A. Neurotransmitters conduct an impulse across a synapse from the axon of one neuron to the dendrites of another. The cell body of a neuron contains the nucleus and organelles. Some axons are wrapped in myelin that acts as an insulator, thus increasing conduction speed. A receptor is specialized to receive information from the environment (sight, touch, hearing) and generate nerve impulses from it.

13.

A. Sperm are produced in the testes. The epididymis is a highly convoluted tube in which sperm are stored. The vas deferens is a tube that connects the epididymis with the urethra. The prostate gland produces fluid that contributes to semen.

14.

B. While the egg is moving down the fallopian tube, sperm swim up the tube to fertilize it. The egg is released from the ovary unfertilized. The egg must be fertilized and ready to implant by the time it arrives in the uterus in order for pregnancy to occur. The vagina cannot support a placenta, and the egg cannot move back up into the uterus.

15.

C. Sperm can live for several days in the female reproductive tract. Likewise, the egg is viable for several days after ovulation, and may be fertilized for several days after ovulation. The lining is shed during days 1 to 5 of the menstrual cycle. Day 14 is the time of ovulation, but the period of fertility extends before and after this day. If the egg is not fertilized by day 18, it is no longer viable.

16.

D. The alveoli are thin-walled sacs through which oxygen diffuses into, and carbon dioxide out of, the surrounding capillaries. The trachea is a tube that leads to the bronchi of the lungs. Bronchi are too thick-walled (with cartilage) to allow gas exchange to occur. Bronchioles are small tubes, lined with smooth muscle that lead to the alveoli.

17.

A. When the diaphragm contracts it moves down, increasing the capacity of the thoracic cavity, which creates negative pressure and draws in air (inspiration). The diaphragm, which separates the abdomen from the thorax (inferior to the lungs), relaxes during expiration.

18.

C. The function of the muscles, and tendons of muscles and ligaments, is to hold the joints together. The skeletal system protects body parts, produces blood cells, and stores minerals.

19.

B. There are 12 thoracic vertebrae and one rib pair that attach to each vertebrae to form the thoracic cage. Cervical vertebrae are located in the neck and lumbar vertebrae are in the lower back, posterior to the abdomen. The sacrum articulates with the coxal bones to form the pelvic girdle.

20.

D. An example of flexion is bending (at the elbow). Straightening the joint angle is extension. Moving a body part laterally, away, is abduction. Moving a body part toward the midline is adduction.

21.

A. Absorption of glucose is the function of the digestive system. However, the urinary system removes ni-trogenous wastes, maintains blood volume, and regulates electrolytes.

22.

D. The urethra is the tube that leads from the urinary bladder to the urethral opening for emptying the urinary bladder. Nephron is the functional unit of the kidneys. The ureter leads from the kidney to the urinary bladder. The urinary bladder stores the urine.

23.

B. The tricuspid is a three-leaf valve that separates the right atrium from the right ventricle. The bicuspid or mitral valve separates the left atrium from the left ventricle. The semilunar valves are three-cusped valves in the aorta and the pulmonary artery.

24.

D. The endocardium lines the inner surface of the heart. It may become inflamed, which occurs in bacterial endocarditis. The pericardium is the outside lining of the heart. The pleura is the lining around the lung cavity, and the peritoneum lines the abdominal cavity.

25.

D. The ileocecal valve separates the ileum from the cecum, the ascending colon. The pyloric valve is located at the junction of the stomach and duodenum. The mitral valve is located between the left atrium and left ventricle. The semilunar valve is a three-cusped valve located within the pulmonary artery.

26.

C. The pulmonary vein is the only vein to carry freshly oxygenated blood from the lungs to the heart. The jugular, facial, and maxillary veins carry unoxygenated blood.

27.

D. Smooth muscle, glandular secretions, and cardiac muscle are all controlled by the autonomic nervous system (ANS). By acting directly on cardiac muscle, smooth muscle, and glands, the ANS regulates visceral activity. It also helps to control arterial pressure, gastrointestinal mobility, secretion, urinary output, sweating, and body temperature.

28.

D. Sodium ions are reabsorbed and potassium and hydrogen ions are secreted under the control of aldosterone. As each sodium ion is reabsorbed from glomerular filtrate into blood, either a potassium or a hydrogen ion is secreted from blood into glomerular filtrate. The specific ion that is secreted appears to be a matter of numerical chance.

29.

C. Serum calcium levels are regulated principally by increasing or decreasing reabsorption by the intestines. The kidney functions to regulate hydrogen ion concentrations, body fluid volumes, and serum sodium levels. It also helps in the removal of urea, creatinine, and other metabolic end products.

30.

A. Filtration in the kidney occurs in the glomerulus. The glomerulus is the tuft of capillaries in Bowman's capsule where water, electrolytes, amino acids, glucose, urea, and other small molecular-size constituents are filtered from blood. The capillaries of the glomerulus unite to form the outgoing efferent arteriole.

31.

D. Erythropoiesis, or red blood cell formation, takes place in the bone marrow, liver, and spleen of the fetus. Liver and spleen are not involved in the adult. The liver forms bile and is involved in reticuloendothelial activity, glucogenesis, glycogenesis, and gluconeogenesis.

32.

E. The trigeminal nerve is the fifth cranial nerve. It innervates the muscles of mastication; the facila nerve innervates muscles of facial expression; the glossopharyngeal muscle innervates the muscles of the pharynx; and the hypoglossal innervates the muscle of the tongue. Coordination of all of these muscle groups is necessary for swallowing.

33.

D. Oxygenated blood flows through the coronary arteries of the heart. The remaining vessels listed contain deoxygenated blood—the pulmonary valve, the right atrioventricular valve, and the pulmonary artery.

34.

D. Digestion involves splitting the large chemical compounds in foods into simpler substances that can be absorbed. It also involves hydrolysis. By the process of hydrolysis, or breaking down with the addition of water as H+ and OH–, large molecules are split into particles small enough to be absorbed across the intestinal mucosa.

35.

A Insulin, secreted by the beta cells of the pancreas, promotes uptake of glucose by cells. In the liver, insulin increases oxidation of glucose and its conversion to fatty acids. Insulin activity is inadequate in patients with diabetes mellitus.

36.

D. Thyroxin regulates basal metabolic rate. Thyroxin is a hormone secreted by the thyroid gland. It increases the rate of replacement of cartilage by bone at the growth plate.

37.

D. Cortisol increases the flux of amino acids in the body and mobilizes stored fat. It also promotes gluconeogenesis. Cortisol and other related corticosteroids are produced by the adrenal cortex.

38.

E. Calcitonin is secreted by the thyroid gland. It is released in response to excess serum calcium. The effect of calcitonin, or thyrocalcitonin as it is sometimes called, is opposite that of parathyroid hormone.

39.

E. The hypothalamus regulates visceral activity and controls temperature centers and synthesis of hormonal releasing factors. It has an important role in maintaining sexual behavior and function. The hypothalamus is located centrally in the brain, lateral and inferior to the third ventricle.

40.

A. Inability to coordinate muscular activity can be due to a lesion in the cerebellum. The cerebellum is located in the posterior cranial fossa, posterior and inferior to the cerebrum. The cerebellum is connected by afferent and efferent pathways with all other parts of the central nervous system.

41.

A. Each bulge in the brain is called a gyrus. The motor area of the brain is the precentral gyrus, located in the posterior part of the temporal lobe. The postcentral gyrus is the sensory area of the brain.

42.

B. Conduction occurs when a stimulus reduces the membrane potential to a coritical level. This level is called threshold. When the transfer of sodium reduces the cell membrane potential to threshold, impulse conduction is initiated.

43.

C. The physiological concept that refers to the maintenance of a constant internal environment is homeostasis. Among the homeostatic control mechanisms now understood are those maintaining normal concentration of blood constituents, body temperature, volume and pH of the body fluids, blood pressure, and heart rate. While the concept describes a constant state, the constancy is one of dynamic equilibrium in that substances are continually being added to and taken from the internal environment.

44.

D. The organelles that contain enzymes capable of digesting and destroying cellular debris are called lysosomes. Lysosomes are specifically membranous structures containing lytic enzymes capable of breaking down cellular components. Fortunately, they are able to discriminate cellular debris and bacteria from the host.

45.

A. Transport of water across a cell membrane takes place by osmosis. In the process of osmosis, water moves from an area of high water concentration into an area of low water concentration. The force with which a solution draws water into it is called osmotic pressure.

46.

D. The direction and rate of diffusion of an ion are influenced by the concentration gradient, hydrostatic gradients, and electrical gradients. Ions diffuse through a semipermeable membrane from an area of high concentration to an area of low concentration. Ions diffuse faster down a pressure gradient and in a direction that tries to equalize electric charges.

47.

C. Epithelium of the mouth is derived from ectoderm. Specifically, the mouth is lined with stratified squamous epithelium. Epithelial parts of the respiratory system, gastrointestinal system, and pharynx are derived from endoderm.

48.

C. A single motor neuron and the muscle cells supplied by its axon branches are termed a motor end plate. Neurons have two types of processes: axons and dendrites. The axon of the motor nerve divides into several branches, which distribute to different muscle fibers.

49.

B. Conduction occurs when a stimulus reduces the membrane potential to a critical level. This level is called threshold. When the transfer of sodium reduces the cell membrane potential to threshold, impulse conduction is initiated.

50.

B. Thrombocytes are not leukocytes. Granulocytic leukocytes include neutrophils, eosinophils, and basophils. Lymphocytic leukocytes include lymphocytes and monocytes.

3 Biochemistry and Nutrition

The relationship between nutrition and oral health is critical to the overall health of an individual. Nutrition provides the foundation for oral and general health. It is crucial that the dental hygienist has the current knowledge of nutritional recommendations as they relate to general and oral health and disease. The dental hygienist must understand how diet and nutrition can be implicated in oral conditions; must recognize relevant dietary and nutritional conditions; and must manage nutritional issues.

chapter objectives

After completion of this chapter, the learner should be able to:

➤ Discuss nutrients such as carbohydrates, proteins, lipids, and fiber
➤ Discuss vegetarian diets
➤ Understand digestion
➤ Describe micronutrients
➤ Discuss water
➤ Discuss macrominerals and microminerals
➤ Understand nutrition in oral health
➤ Describe nutritional screening
➤ Understand dietary guidelines for Americans
➤ Discuss nutritional assessment and counseling
➤ Describe oral conditions affecting nutrient intake

I. Population Guidelines

A. Dietary Reference Intakes (DRIs)—Represent a set of four standards used to provide a comprehensive measure of nutrition and long-term guidelines that are utilized to both assess and plan diets for healthy individuals in both the United States and Canada; include updated RDAs, upper limits for safe intake (tolerable upper limits, or UL), estimated average requirements (EARs), and adequate intake (AI); outlined by age and gender

1. Estimated average requirement (EAR)—The estimated amount of nutrient needed to meet the requirements of half of the healthy people in a group based on gender, age, and life-stage groups; based on bioavailability, reducing risk of disease, and prevention of nutrient deficiency

2. Recommended Dietary Allowance (RDAs)—Represent calculated nutrient needs for healthy individuals based on gender, age, and life-stage groups; calculated using the EAR as a baseline and then increasing the amounts to satisfy requirements of the majority of healthy individuals (Figure 3-1■)

3. Adequate intake (AI)—Represents an estimate guideline for intake of a nutrient in an individual when an RDA cannot be determined due to lack of scientific data on requirements

4. Tolerable upper limits (UL)—Represent the highest (maximum) level of a daily nutrient that is likely to result in no adverse effects in an individual

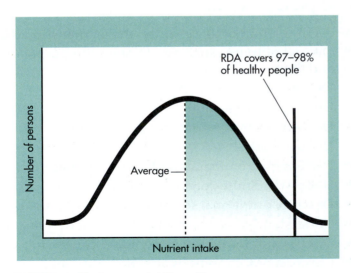

FIGURE 3-1 ■ Recommended Dietary Allowance

B. Healthy People 2010 Initiative—Developed by U.S. Department of Health and Human Services, the initiative focuses on health promotion and disease prevention through healthy choices in diet, weight control, and prevention of other nutritional risk factors (visit the Healthy People 2010 Website at http://www.health.gov/healthypeople/).

II. Nutrients

Nutrients are used by the body to promote growth, maintenance, and repair. The six classes of nutrients obtained from food include carbohydrates, proteins, lipids, vitamins, minerals, and water.

A. Definitions of nutrients

   1. Nutrient—Biochemical substance used by the body for growth, maintenance, and repair

   2. Essential nutrient—Substance that the body cannot make or cannot make in sufficient quantities and must be obtained from an outside source; nutrients required for human life

   3. Nonessential nutrient—Nutrients that the body utilizes but are not required for life

   4. Macronutrients—Essential nutrients that provide energy and are classified as proteins, fats, and carbohydrates

   5. Micronutrients—Essential nutrients that the body needs in small amounts; they serve to regulate and control the functions of the body; all micronutrients are either vitamins or minerals

B. Carbohydrates—Carbohydrates are made up of carbon, hydrogen, and oxygen. They are abundant in nature and provide a cheap source of energy (4 kcal/g). The three major classifications include monosaccharides, disaccharides, and complex polysaccharides.

   1. Functions of carbohydrates

     a. Primary—Available carbohydrates serve as the primary energy for all of the cells in the body by being converted to glucose; the brain and central nervous system utilize only glucose for energy (other tissues may use fat)

     b. Secondary—Spare protein from being used for energy and glucose production; fiber benefits the body by providing bulk in the intestines; helps the elimination and prevention of some dietary lipids from being absorbed; in excess, can be made into triglycerides and stored as fat

     c. Provide an energy source for all body tissues—Source of energy for the brain and red blood cells (RBCs); yields 4 kcal/g

     d. Spares proteins so they can be used for tissue maintenance and repair instead of energy

e. Needed for *oxidation* of fats—If diet is devoid of carbohydrates, body uses fat as energy, but not as efficiently as carbohydrates; ketone bodies are produced

f. Regulates body processes (effect of bulk and fiber aids in *peristalsis*)

g. Aids in palatability of diet (taste)

2. Classifications

a. Monosaccharides

(1) Chemical structure—Consists as a single ring that is one sugar in size; three are important in human nutrition; all contain six carbon atoms (hexoses); structure varies; saccharide = sugar, mono = one, ose = sugar

(2) Galactose—Also known as milk sugar

(a) Component of lactose; never found by itself in nature, always with glucose

(b) Produced from glucose during lactation

(3) Fructose—Also known as fruit sugar or levulose

(a) Sweetest of all sugars

(b) Sources include honey, fruits, corn syrup, and vegetables

(c) Because fructose, like other sugars, is converted to glucose in the liver, there is a delay in the rise of blood glucose when this sugar is eaten by people with true hypoglycemia and diabetes

(4) *Glucose*—Also known as dextrose/blood sugar (Figure 3-2■)

(a) Most important sugar; the final breakdown product of other carbohydrates; also the final form that circulates through the blood and is used by the tissues

(b) Body uses this form best (major energy source for the body)

(c) Sources include honey, fruits, and corn syrup

(d) Glucose can be stored in the liver and muscle tissue as glycogen, a polymer of glucose; the liver converts all other sugars to glucose

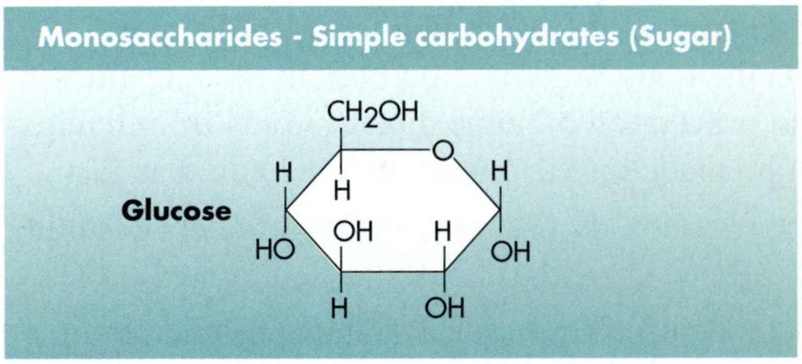

Monosaccharides - Simple carbohydrates (Sugar)

Glucose

FIGURE 3-2 ■ Chemical Structure of Glucose

(e) Normal fasting blood glucose levels are <100 mg/dL, and impaired fasting glucose is 100–125 mg/dL

(5) *Sugar alcohols*—Include sorbitol, mannitol, and xylitol; used as sweeteners

(a) Poorly digested and inhibit rapid rises in blood sugar; often used by people limiting sugar intakes, such as diabetics

(b) Poor absorption causes diarrhea

(c) Xylitol cannot be metabolized by oral bacteria and is considered anticariogenic

i) Chewing xylitol gum for 20 minutes after a meal causes a rise in salivary pH to > 5.5

ii) Recommended dose is 10 g/day or two pieces of xylitol gum after each meal/snack containing fermentable carbohydrates

b. Disaccharides—Double sugars; vary in sweetness; digested to monosaccharides

(1) Chemical structure—Two monosaccharides joined together by a bond; di = two (Figure 3-3■)

(2) Sucrose—Table sugar

(a) Made up of glucose and fructose

(b) Sources include cane, beet, maple, brown, and table sugars, maple syrup, and fruits

(c) The most predominant food preservative used in the world today

(3) Lactose—Milk sugar

(a) Made up of glucose and galactose

(b) Unique to mammals; primary carbohydrate for infants consuming breast milk and milk-based formula

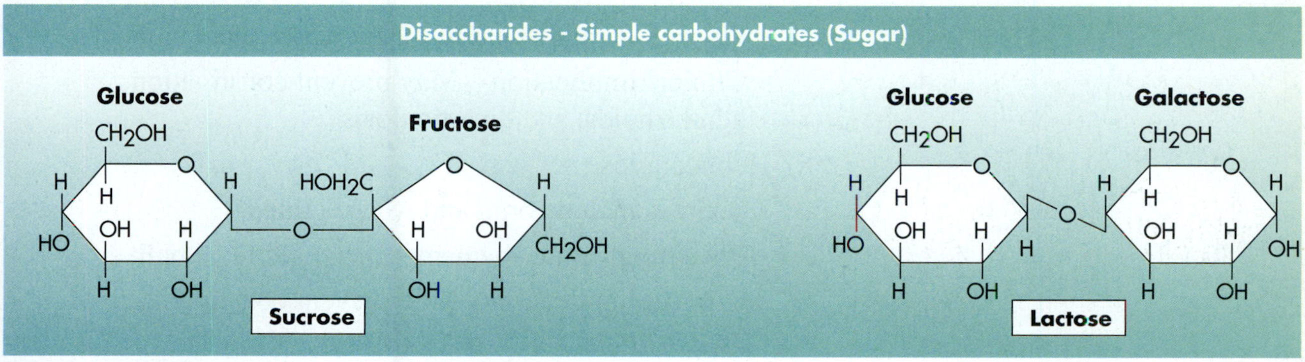

FIGURE 3-3 ■ Chemical Structure of Sucrose and Lactose

(c) Least sweet of all simple sugars

(d) Lactose intolerance is the inability to digest all of the lactose because of a decline in the enzyme lactase that often occurs in adulthood; symptoms include bloating, gas, abdominal discomfort, and diarrhea

  i) Lact = milk; ase = enzyme

  ii) Intestinal bacteria feed off the undigested lactose, which causes these symptoms

  iii) Intolerance is not the same as an allergy

  iv) An allergy to milk is a reaction to one or more of the proteins in milk; can be life threatening; foods with casein and/or whey need to be avoided

  v) Because milk and milk products are the primary dietary source of calcium, eliminating these foods from the diet due to lactose intolerance can result in a calcium deficiency; eating foods with a lower lactose content than milk, such as yogurt and cheese, may reduce symptoms

(4) Maltose—Malt sugar

  (a) Made up of two glucose molecules

  (b) Exists in malt products (e.g., cereal and beer)

  (c) Not usually consumed in foods directly

  (d) Produced when starch is broken down during digestion and during the fermentation process that yields alcohol

c. Polysaccharides (complex)—Poly = many

  (1) Nondigestible (fiber)—Resists digestion in gastrointestinal tract

  (a) Insoluble

    i) Cellulose—Provides bulk/fiber for intestinal mobility

      • Sources include whole wheat flour, bran, and cabbage family

      • Physiological mechanism—Increases fecal bulk

      • Clinical implication—May prevent constipation, hemorrhoids, and diverticulosis

    ii) Hemicellulose

      • Sources include bran and whole grains

      • Physiological mechanism—Increases fecal bulk

      • Clinical implication—May prevent constipation, hemorrhoids, and diverticulosis

        iii) Lignin

- Sources include fruits, mature vegetables, and whole grains
- Physiological mechanism—Decreases free radicals in gastrointestinal (GI) tract
- Clinical implication—Possibly anticariogenic

  (b) Soluble—Lowers blood cholesterol levels; slows glucose absorption

      i) Pectins

- Sources include apples and citrus fruits
- Physiological mechanism—Forms a gel with water

      ii) Gums

- Sources include oats, legumes, barley, and guar
- Used as additives, especially in dairy products (ice cream)

(2) Digestible

  (a) Starch

      i) Sources include legumes, rice, corn, potatoes, and other root vegetables

      ii) Most important carbohydrate

  (b) Glycogen

      i) Animal equivalent to starch

      ii) Made in the liver from glucose after the ingestion of starch and/or sugar that is not immediately needed by the body

      iii) Storage sites—In muscle, it can supply glucose for muscle use; in liver, it helps regulate blood sugar

d. Non-nutritive sweeteners—Provide negligible calories and are noncariogenic

(1) Saccharin—Found primarily in some soft drinks and tabletop sweeteners (Sweet'N Low)

(2) Aspartame—Made from two amino acids, phenylalanine and aspartic acid (NutraSweet/Equal)

  (a) Unstable in prolonged high heat

  (b) Sources include soft drinks, puddings, frozen desserts, and candies

  (c) Must be used in limited amounts by persons with PKU (phenylketonuria), which is the inability to metabolize phenylalanine, and is not recommended for use by individuals with epilepsy

  (d) Does not promote decay or raise blood glucose levels

(3) Acesulfame K

    (a) Sunette/Sweet One; a derivative of acetoacetic acid; also contains potassium

    (b) Not digested; no calories

    (c) Heat stable; uses include gum, nondairy creamers, sodas, puddings, gelatin desserts, dry mixes, and baked goods

(4) Sugar alcohols—Sorbitol, mannitol, and xylitol

    (a) Occur naturally in foods; provide 4 calories per gram

    (b) Essentially noncariogenic: not fermented by oral bacteria (exception in persons with xerostomia; can metabolize *Mutans Streptococcus* at a slow rate; consequently cause dental caries in patients with xerostomia)

    (c) Have a laxative effect on the intestines if greater than 50g/day of sorbitol or greater than 20g/day of mannitol are consumed, causing gas, bloating, and diarrhea

    (d) Xylitol—Clinical studies confirm that xylitol is effective in reducing dental decay and bacterial growth. Xylitol prevents adhesion of *M. Strep* to the tooth surfaces, and it also affects the metabolism of the bacteria so it is less effective at producing organic/lactic acid.

3. Cariogenic potential

  a. Cellulose and other fibrous carbohydrates are considered noncariogenic

  b. Starches can be hydrolyzed to fermentable carbohydrates by the enzyme salivary amylase; breakdown begins in the mouth

    (1) Starch/sugar combinations are highly cariogenic

    (2) All monosaccharides and disaccharides are cariogenic under the right circumstances

    (3) Sucrose is the only carbohydrate used by *Mutans Streptococcus* to form glucans, which permit bacterial colonies to adhere to tooth

  c. Many factors determine ultimate cariogenic potential—Those specific to food include oral retention time, physical form, frequency of intake, and composition

4. Recommended intake: 55–60% of total calories primarily from complex carbohydrates and natural sugars

  a. Recommended fiber intake is 20–35 g/day

  b. Sources include

    (1) Complex carbohydrates—Whole and enriched grains, cereals, pasta, rice, potatoes, legumes, and other root vegetables

(2) Simple carbohydrates—Fruits, dairy products, some vegetables (e.g., sweet corn and carrots), sweets, and soda

5. Disorders of carbohydrate metabolism

a. Diabetes mellitus is characterized by high levels of blood glucose (hyperglycemia) resulting from insulin resistance by the body cells, impaired insulin secretion by the pancreas, and/or increased hepatic glucose production

(1) Classifications

(a) Insulin-dependent (Type 1; IDDM)—Usually begins in childhood

(b) Non-insulin-dependent (Type 2; NIDDM)—Associated with older age, obesity, genetic component, environmental determinants, impaired glucose tolerance, physical inactivity, and race/ethnicity

(2) Symptoms

(a) Type 1—Acetone breath (fruity odor), *polyphagia, polydipsia, polyuria,* dehydration, fatigue, weight loss, and ketoacidosis

(b) Type 2—May or may not exhibit the classic symptoms (polyphagia, polydipsia, and polyuria)

(3) Complications

(a) Chronic complications—Poor circulation, increased infections, blindness, kidney and heart disease, *neuropathy*

(b) Oral complications—Increase in periodontal disease and xerostomia

(4) Treatment goals—Aimed at maintaining blood glucose levels (80–110 mg/dl) and glycocylated hemoglobin or hemoglobin A_1C (< 7%) as near normal as possible

(a) Dietary control (for both Types 1 and 2)—Self-monitor blood glucose 1–2x/week

i) Eat a healthy, low-fat diet (20% protein, 50% carbohydrate, 30% fat)

ii) Divide carbohydrate intake evenly throughout the day

iii) Participate in regular physical activity

iv) Restrict calorie intake if weight loss is needed

v) Limit alcohol intake

(b) Insulin—Self-monitor blood glucose at least 2x/day

i) Recommend frequent small meals to maintain blood glucose levels

ii) Coordinate mealtimes and exercise with insulin

iii) Schedule morning dental appointments to prevent hypoglycemic (blood glucose < 70 mg/dl) episodes

(c) Oral medications—Self-monitor blood glucose at least 1x/day

b. Hypoglycemia—Low levels of blood glucose

(1) Symptoms include mental confusion, blurred vision, weakness, agitation, shakiness, and anger

(2) Treatment—Administer treatment quickly to prevent *insulin shock*

(a) Give 15 grams of rapidly absorbed sugar—such as orange juice or regular soda—3 glucose tablets or 1 tablespoon sugar

(b) Wait 15 minutes and recheck blood glucose; if still not within the normal range, give another 15 grams of carbohydrate until levels are normal

c. Lactose intolerance

(1) Results from a deficiency of the enzyme lactase, which breaks down lactose in dairy products

(2) Prevalent in Asians, North American blacks, and North American whites

(3) Symptoms include abdominal cramping, flatulence, and diarrhea

(4) Diagnosis

(a) Use the "gold standard"—Hydrogen breath test (the patient drinks a lactose load and then exhales into a machine, which will measure the hydrogen production; this indicates if the patient is digesting lactose)

(b) Most people self-diagnose the condition and avoid milk, results in an average calcium intake of 320 mg/day (25% of RDA); places patient at high risk of failing to achieve adequate levels of peak bone mass (risk of osteoporosis)

(5) Dietary recommendations—Patient can consume

(a) Up to 1 cup of milk daily, in a divided dose with meals (as tolerated)

(b) Aged cheese (e.g., Swiss, colby, longhorn) and soft cheese (cream and cottage chesses and ricotta) because they are low in lactose

(c) Reduced lactose products

(d) Calcium-fortified products such as orange juice and cereals

(e) Nondairy sources such as broccoli, spinach, and legumes; however, they are relatively poor sources

C. Proteins—Organic compounds synthesized from amino acids found in food and recirculated amino acids in the body. They are composed of carbon, hydrogen, oxygen, and nitrogen and provide 4 kcal/g.

  1. Classification—All proteins are synthesized from 20 amino acids in two categories

   a. Essential amino acids—There are 9 essential amino acids: histidine, isoleucine, leucine, lysine, methionine, phenylalanine, threonine, tryptophan, and valine

   (1) Needed for protein synthesis

   (2) Amino acids that cannot be made by the body or that cannot be made in sufficient quantities and therefore must be obtained from foods

   (3) Cannot be synthesized from other amino acids

   b. Nonessential amino acids—There are 11 nonessential amino acids: alanine, arginine, asparagine, aspartic acid, cysteine, glutamic acid, glutamine, glycine, proline, serine, and tyrosine

   (1) Needed for protein synthesis

   (2) Can be synthesized in the liver from other amino acids

  2. Types of proteins

   a. Complete proteins have all the essential amino acids present in the body

   (1) Can support tissue synthesis

   (2) Sources include animal and some plants, such as soy

   b. Incomplete proteins have one or more essential amino acids missing or have all amino acids, but in insufficient quantity to support tissue synthesis

   (1) *Deaminated* in liver; carbon fraction used for energy

   (2) Sources include plants, except soy

   c. Complementary proteins

   (1) Combine incomplete proteins with complementary amino acids to make complete protein (e.g., beans and rice)

   (2) Combine complete with incomplete proteins (e.g., cheeses and tortillas)

  3. Functions

   a. Assist with synthesis of all body tissues

   b. Contribute to growth and maintenance

   c. Provide a source of energy if intake of fats and carbohydrates is insufficient

   d. Fluid and electrolyte balance

   e. Constituents of antibodies, enzymes, and hormones

   f. DNA and RNA (genetic material)

   g. Neurotransmitters

   h. Regulation of pH (acid-base balance)

   i. Blood clotting (fibrin)

   j. Vision (opsin)

   k. Pigments (melanin)

4. RDA—Adults 0.8 g/kg

5. Food sources

   a. Complete—Protein from foods that contains all of the essential amino acids in the amounts that the body requires; they may also contain some or all of the nonessential amino acids; include dairy products, meat, fish, and poultry

   b. Incomplete—Protein from foods that does not contain all of the essential acid or does not contain them in sufficient quantity; include whole grains, starchy vegetables, legumes, seeds, and nuts

6. Deficiency—Results in abnormal growth, development, and synthesis of all tissues

   a. Protein-energy (calorie) malnutrition (PEM)

   (1) Kwashiorkor—A condition that results from an infection superimposed on malnutrition; now thought to be a form of food poisoning caused by aflatoxin from moldy grain; severe protein deficiency; symptoms include delayed healing, decreased resistance to infection, skin lesions, loss of hair (alopecia) or change in hair color

   (2) Marasmus—A condition resulting from severe food deprivation or impaired absorption over a long time period; chronic form of PEM in which the deficiency is primarily to protein energy; in advanced stages, it is characterized by muscle wasting, absence of subcutaneous fat, severe growth retardation, and impaired brain development

   b. Phenylketonuria (PKU)—Inability to metabolize phenylalanine (essential amino acid); avoid aspartame found in products such as Nutrasweet™ and Equal™

7. Excess protein intake: Often described as protein intake greater than two times the RDA

   a. Health effects

   (1) Heart disease can result because foods high in protein are also often high in fat, saturated fat, and cholesterol

(2) High-protein diets may result in low intakes of other nutrients from fruits, vegetables, and grains; weight gain may also occur when high-fat, protein-rich foods are eaten often

(3) A diet high in animal proteins has been correlated to an increased risk of some types of cancer

(4) Calcium excretion increases with high-protein diet, possibly increasing the risk of developing osteoporosis

D. Lipids—Insoluble in water, soluble in lipid solvents and composed of carbon, hydrogen, and oxygen; provide 9 kcal/g of energy

1. Biochemistry—Lipids contain the same three elements as carbohydrates: carbon (C)—hydrogen (H), and oxygen (O)—but they contain less oxygen in proportion to hydrogen and carbon

2. Classification

a. Sterols—Cholesterol is synthesized in the liver and available from the diet; needed for cell membranes and production of hormones

(1) Chemical structure—C, H, and O molecules arranged in a multiring structure

(2) Cholesterol—A fat-like waxy substance that is made in the body by the liver and obtained from foods of animal origin; the majority of cholesterol is made by the body from fragments of carbohydrate, lipid, and protein; only a small percent is obtained from the diet

(3) Functions of cholesterol in the body—The major function is to form bile acid, which is needed to digest lipids; cholesterol is also a structural component of cell membranes, myelin, steroid hormones, and vitamin D

(4) Recommended intake of cholesterol—300 mg or less per day; this is not the same as blood cholesterol levels

(5) Food sources—Animal tissues: meats, fish, poultry and organ meats; animal byproducts: egg yolk and dairy products

b. Triglycerides are the primary form of lipids in food—In storage and blood; degree of saturation and length of carbon chain determine characteristics; made up of 1 glycerol and 3 fatty acids

(1) Saturated fatty acids—Contain only single bonds; each carbon atom has 2 hydrogen atoms attached

(a) Usually solid at room temperature

(b) Sources include animal fat and tropical oils

(c) Examples: palmitic and stearic acids

(d) High intake is associated with risk of cardiac disease, recommended intake is 10% or less of total calories per day;

saturated fats raise total cholesterol levels and raise low-density lipoprotein (LDL) or "bad cholesterol" levels

(e) Food sources include animal fats, butter, egg yolks, cocoa butter, whole milk, cheese, chocolate, stick margarine, hydrogenated and tropical oils

(2) Monounsaturated fatty acids—Contain one double bond

    (a) Associated with lowering serum cholesterol by lowering low-density lipoprotein (LDL) and raising high-density lipoprotein (HDL) or "good cholesterol"

    (b) Sources include olive and canola oils, nuts, avocados, peanut butter

    (c) Example: oleic acid

(3) Polyunsaturated fatty acids (PUFA)—Contain more than one double bond

    (a) Polyunsaturated fats lower total cholesterol levels and they may also lower both LDL and HDL cholesterol levels

    (b) Characteristics

        i) Usually liquid at room temperature

        ii) Sources include primarily vegetable oils including corn, soybean, cottonseed, safflower, sesame, and sunflower oils, almonds, filberts, pecans, walnuts, liquid margarine, and fish

(4) Trans-fatty acids are from the *hydrogenation* of polyunsaturated oils

    (a) Can raise serum LDL levels, as do saturated fats, but may cause small lowering of HDL levels

    (b) Sources include stick margarine, shortening, commercial-frying fats, high-fat baked goods, and salty snack chips

(5) Essential fatty acids (EFA)—Fatty acids the body needs, but cannot synthesize; two main EFAs are linoleic (omega-6) and linolenic (omega-3)

    (a) Precursors of eicosanoids (prostaglandins, thromboxanes, leukotrienes) and play a major role in retinal function and brain development

    (b) Sources include vegetable oils, walnuts, and wheat germ

c. Artificial fats or fat replacers—Items that mimic fat in foods, but have different characteristics

(1) Olestra®—Approved by FDA in 1996

    (a) Made of sucrose with 6–8 fatty acids attached

    (b) Cannot be digested or absorbed; may cause excretion of fat-soluble vitamins, so products are fortified

(c) Excess intake can cause diarrhea and gastrointestinal symptoms

(2) Simplesse®—First fat substitute approved by the FDA

(a) Formulated from egg white or milk protein

(b) Provides 1–2 kcal/g

(c) Cannot be used in cooking foods, because it coagulates and becomes rubbery when heated

3. Functions

a. Provide a source of energy—9 kcal/g

b. Act as a carrier of fat-soluble vitamins

c. Provide a source of essential fatty acids

d. Provide food with flavor, texture, palatability, and satiety

e. Provide insulation and protection to body organs

4. Dietary recommendations—Should not consume more than 30% of total calories; 10% of total calories should come from saturated fat

5. Food sources—Animal fats, fish, poultry, vegetable oils, nuts, seeds, and dairy products

6. Diseases—Overconsumption contributes to obesity, which is a major risk factor for many chronic diseases, including diabetes mellitus and cardiovascular disease

E. Fiber

1. Unavailable CHO

a. Polysaccharides that cannot be digested by human digestive enzymes

b. Includes cellulose, hemicelluloses, pectins, gums, mucilages, and nonpolysaccharides such as lignins

c. Intestinal bacteria can digest some fibers and ferment them to form short-chain fatty acids that are absorbed by intestinal cells

2. Recommended intake

a. Adults—20–35 grams of fiber per day

b. Children—Age of the child plus 5 grams per day is recommended by the American Health Foundation for children over the age of 2 years old; example: a 7-year-old child needs 7 + 5 or 12 grams per day

3. Excessive intake of fiber—More than 40 grams per day for adults

a. Effects of excess

(1) Fiber binds up minerals; intake above the recommended amount can negatively affect mineral status

(2) A sudden intake of a lot of fiber, even to the recommended levels; can cause diarrhea or constipation and may even cause an obstruction of the GI tract

(3) May displace energy-dense and nutrient-dense foods

(4) Requires an increase in fluid intake

    4. Water-soluble fiber—Forms a gel in water; used to make jams and jellies

        a. Slows down the transit time of the GI tract; provides satiety; delays hunger

        b. Delays the absorption of glucose, which can help keep blood glucose levels from rising rapidly; helpful in glucose control for people with diabetes

        c. Lowers blood cholesterol by binding up some dietary lipids so that they are not absorbed in the small intestine and prevents bile from being reabsorbed in the large intestine; the liver takes cholesterol from the blood to make more bile; may reduce the risk of heart disease

        d. Food sources—Fruits (apple, citrus), oats, oat bran, barley, and legumes

    5. Water-insoluble fiber—Does not dissolve in water but attracts and holds water

        a. Functions

            (1) Provides bulk and promotes regularity; helps prevent and treat constipation, hemorrhoids, and diverticulosis

            (2) Speeds up the transit time of the GI tract, increases the muscle tone of the intestines, and may protect against colon cancer

III. Vegetarian Diets

  A. Vegan—Also called strict vegetarian or pure vegetarian

    1. A dietary pattern that excludes animal tissues (meat, fish, poultry) and animal by-products (eggs, dairy products)

    2. Includes vegetables, fruits, grains, nuts, and seeds only

    3. Complementary protein combining is necessary to get adequate amounts of the essential amino acids

    4. May be low in high-quality protein, vitamin B_{12}, vitamin D, calcium, iron, and zinc

  B. Lactovegetarian

    1. A dietary pattern that excludes animal tissues (meat, fish, poultry) and eggs

    2. Includes dairy products, vegetables, fruits, grains, nuts, and seeds

    3. If sufficient amounts of dairy products are consumed, along with complementary protein combinations, calcium, vitamin B_{12}, and high-quality protein intake are usually adequate

  C. Ovovegetarian

    1. A dietary pattern that excludes animal tissues (meat, fish, poultry) and dairy products

    2. Includes eggs, vegetables, fruits, grains, nuts, and seeds

3. If egg yolks are consumed often along with complimentary protein combinations, iron, zinc, high-quality protein, and vitamin B_{12} intake are usually adequate

D. Lacto-ovovegetarian

1. A dietary pattern that only excludes animal tissues (meat, fish, poultry)

2. Includes dairy products and eggs in addition to vegetables, fruits, grains, nuts, and seeds

3. Calcium, iron, zinc, and high-quality protein are usually adequate if sufficient amounts of dairy products and egg yolks are consumed

IV. Digestion (Figure 3-4■)

A. Gastrointestinal (GI) tract

1. The GI tract is about 30 feet in length

2. Includes the mouth (oral cavity), esophagus, stomach, small intestine, and large intestine (colon)

3. Accessory organs involved in digestion are the liver, gallbladder, and pancreas

B. Hydrolysis

1. Chemical reaction that splits molecules apart with the addition of water; occurs during the digestion of carbohydrates, lipids, proteins; hydro = water, lysis = breaking

C. Mouth—Mastication occurs

1. Starch digestion begins—Salivary amylase breaks starch, which is composed of chains of glucose molecules, into dextrin and maltose

2. Esophagus

   a. Food pipe

   b. Allows food to pass from the mouth to the stomach

   c. Goes through the diaphram

D. Stomach

1. Holding tank

2. Muscular, elastic, saclike organ

3. Holds each bolus of food swallowed; secretes hydrochloric acid (HCl), some enzymes, and fluids

4. Churns, mixes, and grinds food to form chyme

5. Stretches to give the message of fullness after eating

6. The carbohydrate, lipid, and protein content of the chyme determines the emptying time of the stomach

7. Protein digestion begins—HCl causes protein strands to uncoil and pepsin breaks the strands into smaller fragments of protein

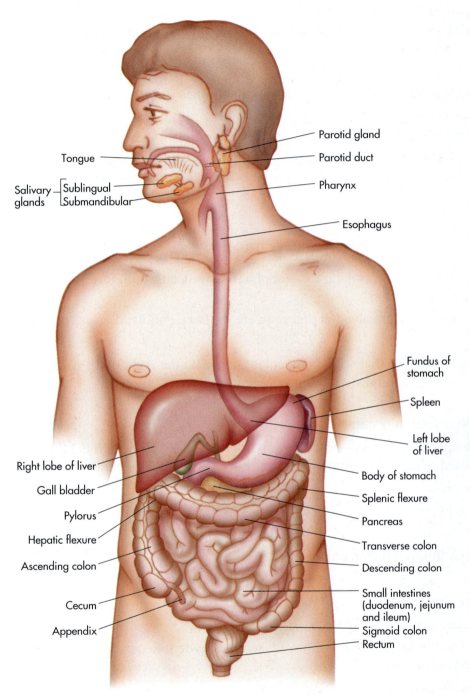

Parotid gland

Parotid duct

Tongue

Salivary glands {Sublingual / Submandibular}

Pharynx

Esophagus

Fundus of stomach

Spleen

Left lobe of liver

Right lobe of liver

Gall bladder

Pylorus

Hepatic flexure

Ascending colon

Cecum

Appendix

Body of stomach

Splenic flexure

Pancreas

Transverse colon

Descending colon

Small intestines (duodenum, jejunum and ileum)

Sigmoid colon

Rectum

FIGURE 3-4 ■ Digestive Process

8. Intrinsic factor—The glycoprotein "intrinsic factor" is secreted by the stomach and attaches to vitamin B_{12}, which facilitates the absorption of B_{12} in the small intestine

E. Small intestine—Bile is secreted only if chyme contains lipid

   1. Size and function

      a. The small intestine is about 10 feet in length with an absorptive surface area equal to a quarter of a football field

      b. "Small" because its diameter is small compared to the large intestine

      c. Villi and microvilli line the small intestine

   2. Three segments

      a. Duodenum—The top portion, about 10 inches long, where sodium bicarbonate and bile are secreted into the small intestine via the common bile duct; where the majority of food digestion occurs, from which nutrients are absorbed

      b. Jejunum—The first two-fifths of the small intestine beyond the duodenum

      c. Ileum—The remaining segment of the small intestine

F. Large intestine (colon)—Most bile is recirculated in the body

   1. Size and function

      a. The remaining portion of the GI tract; about 5 feet in length

      b. Water, some minerals, and undigested residues such as fiber pass into the large intestine where most of the water, electrolytes, and bile salts are absorbed

   2. Three segments

      a. Ascending colon—Goes up the right side of the abdomen

      b. Transverse colon—Passes across the front to the left side

      c. Descending colon—Down the left side of the abdomen and includes the sigmoid colon and rectum where waste products, fiber, bacteria, and any unabsorbed nutrients are stored until they are excreted

G. Mechanical digestion

   1. Mastication—The actions of the teeth, tongue, and muscles of mastication that tear and grind food into small pieces and blend it with saliva; xerostomia affects taste and the ability to swallow foods easily

   2. Saliva—Lubricates food to facilitate taste and swallowing

   3. Epiglottis—Cartilage in the throat that closes off the airway when food or liquids are swallowed

   4. Bolus—Each portion of food that is swallowed and enters the esophagus

5. Peristalsis

    a. Involuntary wavelike muscular contractions of the esophagus, stomach, small intestine, colon, and rectum

    b. It involves circular and longitudinal muscles that rhythmically contract and relax, mixing and churning food as it digests

6. Cardiac sphincter—The circular muscle at the junction between the esophagus and the stomach that closes after a bolus is swallowed to prevent the reflux of stomach contents

7. Chyme—The semiliquid mass of partly digested food, mixed with HCl and expelled from the stomach to the small intestine

8. Pyloric sphincter—The circular muscle at the junction between the stomach and small intestine that regulates the flow of chyme into the small intestine

9. Segmentation—Periodic squeezing by the circular muscles of the intestines that momentarily forces the chyme back a few inches to maximize contact with digestive juices and the absorptive surface of the intestinal walls

10. Ileocecal valve—The circular muscle at the junction of the small intestine and the colon; a sphincter muscle

11. Anus—The last circular muscle of the GI tract that controls the release of waste products (feces); a sphincter muscle

H. Chemical digestion

    1. Saliva—Salivary amylase initiates the chemical digestion of starch

    2. Hydrochloric acid (HCl)

        a. Gastric glands secrete HCl into the stomach, which causes the pH of the stomach to be very acidic; HCl is needed to prepare minerals to be absorbed in the small intestine

        b. Most enzymes, including salivary amylase, are denatured in the stomach but pepsinogen is activated to pepsin, which initiates the chemical digestion of protein

        c. Mucin protects the stomach mucosa from HCl

        d. No significant chemical digestion of carbohydrate or lipid occurs in the stomach

    3. Sodium bicarbonate—Secreted by the pancreas to neutralize the acidic chyme as it enters the small intestine

    4. Bile

        a. Made in the liver, stored in the gallbladder, and secreted into the small intestine (duodenum) when dietary lipids are mixed in the chyme

        b. Made from the cholesterol that the liver produces

      c. An emulsifier that has both water-soluble and fat-soluble portions; allows lipids to mix with a watery solution where lipases can break them down into smaller particles

    5. Pancreatic enzymes—Secreted into the small intestine to digest carbohydrate (carbohydrases), lipid (lipases), and protein (proteases)

V. Micronutrients (trace minerals)—Inorganic substances required by humans in amounts less than 100 mg/day

  A. Water-soluble vitamins (includes the B-complex and C vitamins)

    1. Common characteristics

      a. Easily destroyed or lost during storage and cooking

      b. Absorbed through the portal system

      c. Stored in the body in very limited amounts, therefore required from the diet on a daily basis

      d. Excess is excreted in the urine and feces

      e. Not usually stored in large amounts; short-term storage in the body fluid "pool"

      f. Required in frequent doses every 1–3 days

      g. Toxicity is uncommon from food intake; may occur from supplement overuse

    2. B Vitamins

      a. Many B vitamins are coenzymes; without them certain enzymes are inactive

      b. Some are needed to release the energy in foods for use by the body; others are needed in cellular metabolism

Vitamins

- Substances that the body cannot make at all or that it cannot make in sufficient quantities to sustain life
- The first vitamins discovered contained nitrogen; however, not all vitamins contain nitrogen
- The amounts needed are measured in milligrams (mg) or micrograms (mcg)
- Vitamins do not contain energy/calories but are needed for the body to metabolize carbohydrates, lipids, and proteins, which do contain calories
- vita = life
- amine = contains nitrogen
- 28 grams (g) = about 1 ounce
- 1 g = 1000 mg; 1 mg = 1,000 mcg

c. Deficiencies of single B vitamins rarely occur; if a person shows signs of a deficiency they are often deficient in more than one B vitamin; one exception is vitamin B_{12}

d. Enzymes = various types of proteins needed to cause chemical reactions to occur or to occur at a faster rate

3. Types of water-soluble vitamins

a. Thiamin (vitamin B_1)—Stable to dry heat; destroyed by moist heat and in the presence of alkali, such as baking soda, and by sulfur dioxide used in drying fruits

   (1) Functions as thiamin pyrophosphate (TPP)

      (a) Converts carbohydrates to fat

      (b) Converts two carbon units (transketolase reaction)

      (c) Converts amino acids, carbohydrates, and fats to energy (oxidative decarboxylation)

      (d) Converts glyoxylate to carbon dioxide

   (2) RDA—0.5 mg/1,000 calories of energy intake, with a minimum intake of 1 mg/day for adults

   (3) Food sources include whole/enriched grain products, legumes, and lean pork

   (4) Deficiency is no longer common in the United States

      (a) Types of thiamin deficiency diseases

         i) Beriberi—Symptoms include mental confusion, muscular wasting and chronic polyneuropathy, edema, anorexia, and foot and wrist drop

         ii) Wernicke-Korsakoff syndrome—Symptoms include disorientation, jerky movements of eyes, and a staggering gait

      (b) High-risk groups include alcoholics

      (c) Management is best accomplished with assistance from a professional and includes oral thiamin administration

b. Riboflavin (vitamin B_2) is found in milk and is easily destroyed by light

   (1) Function—Assists with metabolism of carbohydrates, protein, and fat as part of coenzymes flavin mononucleotide (FMN) and flavin adenine dinucleotide (FAD)

   (2) RDA is associated with protein consumption, energy intake, and body size (0.6 mg/1,000 calories for all ages) with a minimum of 1.2 mg/day for adults

(3) Food sources—Present in most plant and animal tissue such as eggs, lean meat, milk, broccoli, enriched breads, and cereals

(4) Deficiency (ariboflavinosis) is rare and usually occurs concurrently with other B-complex vitamin deficiencies

    (a) Oral manifestations include edema of the pharyngeal and oral mucous membranes, *angular cheilosis, stomatitis,* and *glossitis*

    (b) High-risk groups include people with malabsorption syndromes

c. Niacin is found in cells such as nicotinamide; can be converted from amino acid tryptophan; stable in heat

  (1) Functions

    (a) Coenzymes function as cofactors in tissue respiration, glycolysis, and other redox systems

    (b) Assists with structural repair of cells via DNA synthesis

  (2) RDA is expressed as niacin equivalents because excess tryptophan (amino acid) can be broken down to produce niacin (1 niacin equivalent = 60 mg tryptophan); need is related to energy expenditure: 6.6 niacin equivalents/1,000 calories

  (3) Food sources include lean meats, poultry, fish, mushrooms, and peanuts

  (4) Management of deficiency and/or diseases

    (a) Pellegra—Characterized by the 4 Ds (diarrhea, dementia, dermatitis, and death)

    (b) Oral symptoms include glossitis, stomatitis, and burning mouth

    (c) High-risk groups include alcoholics

    (d) Treatment—Provided by a physician with oral administration of 150–600 mg of nicotinic acid or nicotinamide

d. Pyroxidine (vitamin B_6) is found in 3 pyridine forms: pyridoxine, pyridoxal, and pyridoxamine; relatively heat stable in acid, but labile in alkaline

  (1) Functions

    (a) Assists with coenzymes involved in carbohydrate, fat, and protein metabolism

    (b) Converts tryptophan to niacin

    (c) Involved in heme biosynthesis

    (d) Needed for neurotransmitter synthesis

    (e) Helps clear blood of homocysteine

  (2) RDA is 1.3 mg for adults

(3) Food sources include yeast, wheat germ, pork, glandular meats, whole-grain cereals, legumes, potatoes, bananas, and oatmeal

(4) Management of deficiency and/or disease

(a) High-risk groups include alcoholics and drug interactions (e.g., isoniazid, l-Dopa)

(b) Symptoms include hypochromic, microcytic anemia, neurologic disorders in infants and animals, stomatitis, cheilosis, glossitis, irritability, depression, and confusion

(c) Treatment involves 10–15 mg/day; prescribed and monitored by a medical professional

(5) Current issues

(a) Homocysteine—Low intake of B_6 and folic acid are associated with high serum homocysteine, which, in turn, is associated with increased risk of heart attack

(b) Deficiency is associated with decreased immunity in the elderly, probably related to its function in protein synthesis

e. Folate/folic acid (pteroylglutamic acid) is readily soluble in water and destroyed when heated (50–90%) in neutral or alkaline media

(1) Functions

(a) Acts as a coenzyme for synthesis of purines and pyrimidines for DNA synthesis; needed for all cells that are replaced rapidly and need continuous DNA

(b) Involved in the interconversions of amino acids such as the conversion of homocysteine to methionine

(c) Interrelated with vitamin B_{12} (cobalamin); if either one is deficient, hematological changes occur

(d) Used in DNA synthesis and new cell formation; includes cells of the fetus, especially for closure of the neural tube, which develops into the brain and spinal cord; also for cells with a high turnover rate such as those of the oral tissues, GI tract, and RBC maturation

(e) Forms both red and white blood cells in the bone marrow

(f) Important in the prevention of heart disease by breaking down homocysteine, a compound that promotes fatty plaques to form on the walls of blood vessels

(2) RDA is 400 mcg/day for adults

(3) Food sources include enriched breads and cereals, yeast, liver, organ meats, fresh green leafy vegetables, and legumes; the name suggests the word "foliage"

(4) Management of deficiency and/or diseases

    (a) Increased risk of neural tube defects (NTDs); risk can be reduced 60% with intakes of 400 micrograms for all women of childbearing age

        i) Defect occurs in the first couple of weeks of pregnancy and may include cleft palate as well as spinal bifida

        ii) Occurs in approximately 4,000 pregnancies/year

    (b) Megaloblastic anemia

        i) High-risk groups include drug/nutrient interactions (e.g., methotrexate and dilantin), elderly, and alcoholics

        ii) Clinical symptoms include poor growth and fainting

        iii) Oral manifestations include burning tongue and oral mucosa, red and swollen tongue, and angular cheilosis

        iv) Treatment should be provided and monitored by a physician

f. Vitamin B_{12} (cobalamin)

  (1) Functions

    (a) Needed to activate one of the folate coenzymes, DNA and RNA synthesis, maintenance of the myelin sheath, bone cell activity, fatty acid and amino acid metabolism

    (b) Involved in the conversion of homocysteine to methionine

  (2) Absorption

    (a) Hydrochloric acid is necessary to release cobalamin from its peptide bonds

    (b) Gastric secretions contain intrinsic factor, which is a protein carrier for vitamin B_{12}

    (c) Vitamin B_{12} is released from food proteins by pepsin and hydrochloric acid in the stomach; then the intrinsic factor, a glycoprotein secreted by parietal cells in the stomach, attaches to B_{12}, allowing it to be absorbed in the intestine

  (3) RDA is 2.4 mcg/day for adults

  (4) Food sources are found *only* in animal products such as meat, poultry, fish, and dairy products

  (5) Management of deficiency and/or disease

    (a) Pernicious anemia results from deficiency and causes megaloblastic anemia along with a red, beefy tongue; condition can progress to neurological damage with *paresthesia*, numbness and tingling in hands and feet, unsteadiness, *ataxia*, psychological disorders, and overt psychosis if left untreated

(b) High-risk groups include the elderly (secondary to *achlorhydria* or lack of intrinsic factor), vegetarians (lack extrinsic factor); those with resectioned stomachs or ileum

(c) Treatment is vitamin B_{12} given orally or intramuscularly (IM)

g. Pantothenic acid—Deficiency is extremely rare

   (1) Functions as part of coenzyme A (CoA), which is involved in fatty acid metabolism and the TCA cycle

   (2) RDA/AI is 5 mg/day for adults

   (3) Widespread in foods; easily destroyed by heat

h. Biotin—Synthesized by GI bacteria

   (1) Functions

      (a) Part of a coenzyme used in energy metabolism, fat and glycogen synthesis, and amino acid metabolism; involved in oxidation of fatty acids, degradation of amino acids, and purine synthesis

   (2) RDA/AI is 30 mcg for adults

   (3) Food sources: widespread in foods; also some is synthesized by bacteria in the intestines; liver, egg yolk, soybean, and yeast

   (4) Deficiency is rare—Can occur when greater than two dozen egg whites are consumed daily for several months (often seen in people who do body building) because avidin, a protein in raw egg whites, binds biotin; cooking denatures avidin

      (a) High-risk groups include malabsorptions (biotinidase deficiency), long-term anticonvulsant therapy as in epilepsy, or diets high in raw egg whites (avidin binds biotin)

      (b) Symptoms include anorexia, nausea, mental changes, *myalgia*, localized paresthesia, squamous dermatitis of extremities, scaly seborrheic dermatitis, and sometimes alopecia (hair loss)

i. Vitamin C (ascorbic acid)—Readily destroyed by heat, oxidation, and alkali

   (1) Functions—Collagen synthesis necessary for wound healing, scar tissue formation, ligaments, tendons, and the foundation for bones and teeth; an antioxidant to prevent cell damage; synthesis of the thyroid hormone thyroxin; amino acid metabolism; and enhances the absorption of iron

      (a) Acts as a powerful antioxidant-reducing agent

      (b) Involved as a cofactor in hydroxylation of proline and lysine in collagen formation

(c) Participates in synthesis of tyrosine and adrenal hormones

(d) Needed for folate metabolism and leukocyte function

(e) Enhances iron absorption from nonanimal food sources

(2) RDA is 75–90 mg/day for adults

(3) Food sources: green peppers, broccoli, strawberries, citrus fruits, tomatoes, melons, cabbage, and leafy greens

(4) Deficiency—Scurvy, which is characterized by pinpoint hemorrhages, bleeding gums, failure of wounds to heal, rough skin, muscle degeneration and pain, depression, atherosclerotic plaques in blood vessels, joint pain, suppression of the immune system, and microcytic anemia. Severe scurvy can lead to tooth loss, hysteria, heart attack, and massive internal bleeding

(5) Management of deficiency and/or disease

(a) Subclinical deficiency—Symptoms include reduced enzyme activity and leukocyte function, and increased susceptibility to infection

(b) Clinical deficiency results in scurvy, a defect in collagen synthesis

 i) Clinical symptoms include healing impairment, anemia, corkscrew hair, perifollicular petechiae (capillary hemorrhages surrounding hair follicles), bleeding in joints, joint pain, and defective skeletal calcification

 ii) Oral manifestations include hemorrhagic gingivitis with enlarged blue/red gingiva, spontaneous gingival bleeding on provocation, enlarged marginal gingiva, interdental infarcts, loose teeth, and secondary gingival infections (Figure 3-5■)

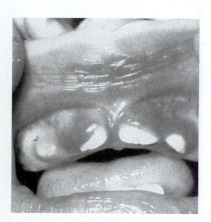

FIGURE 3-5 ■ Scorbutic Gingivae

(c) High-risk groups for marginal deficiency include people who consume no fruits or vegetables or discontinue massive doses of vitamin C, alcoholics, elderly people on limited diets, severely ill people under chronic stress, and infants consuming exclusively cow's milk

(d) Treatment—Ingest 1 gm/day of ascorbic acid by mouth

(6) Toxicity

(a) Severe scurvy can lead to tooth loss, hysteria, heart attack, and massive internal bleeding

(b) May interfere with some medical tests and the action of anticoagulants

B. Fat-soluble vitamins

- Vitamins A, D, E, and K
- Digested and absorbed like lipids; require bile and are first absorbed into the lymph and then enter the blood
- Many require protein carriers to transport them in the body
- Stored in fatty tissues of the body and in the liver
- Needed in periodic doses; average intake over several days
- Toxicity can easily occur from supplement use
- Not readily excreted

1. Characteristics

a. Soluble in organic solvents

b. Absorbed and transported with lipids; require bile and are first absorbed into the lymph and then enter the blood

c. Require protein carriers to transport them in the body

d. Can be stored in the body tissues at toxic levels not readily excreated

2. Types

a. Vitamin A (retinol, retinal, and the precursor forms: carotenes)

(1) Functions

(a) Required for rhodospin (for dark adaptation) and other photosensitive pigments

(b) Cell differentiation; maintenance of epithelial cells, mucous membranes, the cornea, and skin; bone and tooth growth; vision; reproduction; immunity

(c) Prevents infectious disease via role in epithelial tissue maintenance

(d) Provides growth and modeling of bones and teeth

(e) Betacarotene is a precursor to vitamin A

(2) RDA

    (a) Male—900 mcg/day

    (b) Female—700 mcg/day

(3) Food sources

    (a) Retinol (preformed vitamin A)—Liver, butter, fish oil, egg yolk, whole milk, and fortified margarine

    (b) Carotene (provitamin A)—Dark green, yellow, and orange fruits and vegetables

(4) Management of deficiency and/or disease

    (a) Affects 1–5 million infants and preschool children in developing countries

    (b) High-risk groups include those with malabsorption and fat absorption disorders

    (c) Symptoms

        i) Clinical—Includes follicular hyperkeratosis (keratin around hair follicles), night blindness, xerophthalmia (leads to blindness), Bitot's spots (dry patches on the conjunctiva)

        ii) Oral manifestations—*Xerostomia,* impaired growth including teeth and bone, and reduced resistance to infection

        iii) Treatment should be monitored by a physician and involves massive intermittent doses of vitamin A

(5) Prevention of toxicity

    (a) Vitamin A is stored in the tissues and can reach toxic levels

        i) Acute hypervitaminosis A can be induced by single doses of retinol $\geq$ 15,000 mcg/day IU in adults

        ii) Chronic hypervitaminosis A occurs with repeated intake of vitamin A in amounts at least 10 times the RDA (30,000 mcg/day)

    (b) High-risk groups include those with compromised liver function from drugs, hepatitis, or protein-energy malnutrition; pregnant women and children are also especially vulnerable

    (c) Clinical symptoms include nausea, vomiting, fatigue, weakness, headache, bone pain, fragility, anorexia, and may cause birth defects if taken in high doses during pregnancy

    (d) Oral manifestations include cheilosis and gingivitis

    (e) Treatment involves discontinuing supplements; symptoms will usually disappear in weeks or months

b. Vitamin D is both a vitamin and a hormone (hormone = compound made by one organ of the body that affects another part of the body)

(1) Cholecalciferol is synthesized in the skin with exposure to sunlight and also found in animal food sources

(2) Ergocalciferol is found in plant food sources

(3) Functions

(a) Facilitates calcium absorption from intestines; remove and deposits bone mineral (remodeling)

(b) Maintains the blood homeostasis of calcium

(4) RDA for adults

(a) 0–50 years—5 mcg

(b) 50–70 years—10 mcg

(c) 70+ years—15 mcg; this group has increased needs

i) Aging results in a fourfold decrease in capacity of the skin to produce vitamin D_3

ii) Many elderly have limited sun exposure

(5) Food sources include fish liver oils, *fortified* milk, margarine, and butter

(6) Management of deficiency and/or disease

(a) Rickets is a childhood disease associated with malformation of bones due to deficient mineralization of the organic matrix

i) High-risk groups include underprivileged children in northern latitudes; in the United States, black children are at higher risk because skin melanin shields conversion of 7-dehydrocholesterol to active vitamin D

ii) Symptoms include bowlegs, knock-knees, pigeon breast, and frontal *bossing* of skull

iii) Treatment

• Prevent by providing vitamin D supplementation to newborns until the child begins drinking fortified cow's milk at age 1

• Rickets is rarely completely cured so prevention is essential

(b) Osteomalacia is a vitamin D deficiency in adulthood

i) High-risk groups include the elderly living alone, eating an inadequate diet, receiving little sunlight, and women of childbearing age who have been depleted of calcium after multiple pregnancies with inadequate diets

ii) Symptoms include softening of the bones of the extremities, spine, thorax, and pelvis, which leads to deformities, rheumatic-type pain, and general weakness

iii) Prevention

- Supply adequate dietary amounts of vitamin D, calcium, and phosphorus
- Increase exposure to ultraviolet light

iv) Treatment—Provide 25–125 mcg (1,000–5,000 IU)/day of vitamin D along with calcium supplements under medical supervision

(7) Toxicity

(a) Nausea, vomiting, increased blood levels of calcium and phosphorus, calcification of soft tissues (blood vessels, kidneys, heart, lungs), kidney stones and kidney damage, headache, joint pain, fatigue, excessive thirst, muscle weakness (Figure 3-6■)

(8) Self-synthesis

(a) Manufactured by the body from skin exposure to ultraviolet light; light on the face, neck, and hands daily for 10–15 minutes is usually adequate; where sun exposure is limited due to weather, sunscreen, or being homebound, dietary sources must supply total need or a supplement may be recommended

(b) Dark skin pigments block vitamin D synthesis and requires longer exposure times to ultraviolet light

c. Vitamin E (tocopherol)

(1) Functions—An antioxidant; stabilizes cell membranes and protects PUFA and vitamin A in foods and in the body; acts as an antioxidant scavenging free radicals

(2) RDA is measured in milligrams of α-tocopherol equivalents (α-TE)

(a) Adult males—10 mg α-TE

(b) Adult females—8 mg α-TE

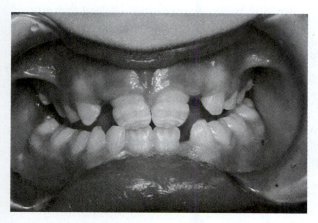

FIGURE 3-6 ■ Vitamin D Toxicity—Oral Effects

Source: © John L. Giunta, DMD, MS

(3) Food sources include seed oils, wheat germ, fruits, vegetables, and animal fats; easily destroyed by heat and exposure to air

(4) Management of deficiency and/or disease

(a) Vitamin E deficiency is uncommon

(b) High-risk groups include those with malabsorption (e.g., cystic fibrosis and AIDS patients) or lipid transport abnormalities, and premature infants

(c) Symptoms include erythrocyte hemolysis (breaking of RBC), hemolytic anemia, impaired vision, speech, and muscular functioning

(d) Treatment is provided under medical supervision and may include water-soluble forms of the vitamin

(5) Toxicity—rare; can interfere with blood clotting; can enhance the effects of anticoagulant medications

d. Vitamin K—Named for *koagulation,* a Danish word

(1) Functions

(a) Synthesis of blood-clotting proteins; essential as a cofactor in blood clotting

(b) Involved in bone crystalline formation; a bone protein that is involved in the regulation of blood calcium

(2) RDA for men is 80 mcg and for women, 65 mcg

(3) Sources—Microflora in the gut produces some vitamin K, the rest is obtained primarily from foods such as green leafy vegetables

(4) Management of deficiency and/or disease

(a) Deficiencies are rare

(b) High-risk groups include those with fat malabsorption problems (e.g., cystic fibrosis and celiac disease), destroyed intestinal flora through long-term antibiotic therapy, on anticoagulant therapy, and newborns

(c) Symptoms include abnormal bleeding

(d) Treatment needs vary:

i) Newborns receive vitamin K intramuscularly (IM) after delivery

ii) Those with fat malabsorption problems may require water-soluble forms

VI. Water

- Water is part of the fluid of every cell; it constitutes about 60% of the adult body (higher for infants, children)
- Water is associated with lean tissue, which is the weight of the body minus the weight of body fat
- Intercellular fluid—Inside of the cells; about two-thirds of the water in the body
- Extracellular fluid—Fluid that is outside of the cells and includes interstitial fluid that is between the cells

A. Functions

1. The major component of the blood and lymph that carries nutrients throughout the body and helps the body get rid of waste products via the urine and feces

2. A solvent for amino acids, glucose, minerals, and vitamins

3. Involved in chemical reactions including hydrolysis and condensation

4. Maintains the structure of large molecules including proteins and glycogen

5. Helps in the regulation of body temperature

6. Involved in maintaining blood volume and blood pressure

7. Acts as a lubricant between cells and around joints

8. Helps to cushion the joints and the eye; during pregnancy, amniotic fluid protects the fetus

B. Water balance—Controlled mainly by the hypothalamus in the brain and the kidneys by the hormones ADH, angiotensin, and aldosterone; ADH = antidiuretic hormone

C. Dehydration—When water output exceeds intake; causes thirst, dry skin and dry mouth, low blood pressure, rapid heart rate, fatigue, headache, impaired physical performance, low urine output, dizziness, and exhaustion

D. Water Intoxication—Rare; can be caused by kidney disease or severe food restriction, as seen in the eating disorder anorexia nervosa when large amounts of water are consumed in the place of food; causes a dilution of electrolytes affecting nerve conduction

E. Minimum intake—In adults, the body must excrete about 2 cups (480 mL) of urine each day to get rid of waste products; therefore, the minimum intake is 2 cups (16 ounces)

F. Optimal intake—Depends on activity level, environmental temperatures, composition of the diet, etc.; approximately one half cup per 100 calories expended or roughly 2½ quarts

G. Sources of water

1. Water itself, other beverages, fruits, vegetables, meats, cheeses, and the water produced during metabolism in the chemical reaction condensation; caffeine and alcohol act as diuretics

VII. Macrominerals—Inorganic substances required by humans in amounts ≥ 100 mg/day

A. Calcium—Most abundant mineral in the body

1. Functions

a. Found primarily in the bones and teeth along with phosphorus-forming hydroxyapatite crystals; provides strength and rigidity; structural component of teeth and bones (99%)

b. A small amount (1%) of calcium is in the blood and other fluids where it participates as an electrolyte in nerve transmission and muscle contraction; also involved in blood clotting, hormone secretion, and calmodulin, which is needed for normal blood pressure

c. Assists with nerve transmission and regulation of heartbeat

d. Assists with blood clotting

2. Goals of DRI/AI

a. Build peak mass

b. Reduce bone loss and prevent osteoporosis

(1) 9–18 years—1,300 mg/day

(2) 19–50 years—1,000 mg/day

(3) 50+ years—1,200 mg/day

3. Sources

a. Dairy products are best absorbed due to the presence of vitamin D and lactose; 1 cup milk = 300 mg calcium

b. Vegetable sources contain *phytates*, *oxalic acid*, and fiber, which *interfere* with absorption

(1) 10 oz. tofu

(2) 4 cups broccoli

(3) 6 cups cooked red beans

c. Fortified juices and cereals

d. Dietary supplements

(1) Calcium carbonate and malate are absorbed best; recommend sugar-free chewable tablets to reduce cariogencity

(2) Avoid oyster shell supplements due to possible lead contamination

4. Types of calcium deficiency diseases—Stunted growth in children, osteoporosis in adults

  a. Osteomalacia is associated with a vitamin D deficiency, resulting in a reduction in the mineral content of bone

  b. Osteoporosis is loss of bone density without a change in composition; fractures occur with minimal stress due to risk factors such as inadequate calcium and vitamin D intake, lack of weight-bearing exercise, estrogen depletion, family history, race (white or Asian), female gender, slight body build, alcohol and tobacco use, medications, and certain disease states

  c. Osteopenia is a decrease in bone mineral density that can be a precursor condition to osteoporosis; however, not every person diagnosed with osteopenia will develop osteoporosis

  d. Management of deficiency and/or disease

    (1) Encourage intake of 1,000–1,300 mg/day of calcium and 10–15 mcg of vitamin D for those under 30 years of age to build adequate peak bone mass and to maintain bone mass in older adults

    (2) Provide tobacco intervention and referral to an addiction medicine specialist for alcohol dependency/abuse

    (3) Suggest to postmenopausal women not taking hormone replacement therapy to discuss the benefits and risks with their physician

    (4) Encourage regular weight-bearing exercise (with a physician's approval)

B. Phosphorus—Second most abundant mineral in the body

  1. Functions

    a. Transfer and release of energy stored as adenosine triphosphate (ATP)

    b. Part of composition of phospholipids, DNA, and RNA

    c. Assists with metabolism of fats, carbohydrates, and proteins

    d. Acts as a buffering system

  2. RDA

    a. 8–18 years—1,250 mg/day

    b. 19–70+ years—700 mg/day

  3. Food sources—Widespread in foods, especially

    a. Proteins, such as meat, poultry, fish, eggs

    b. Milk and milk products

  4. Management of deficiency and/or disease

    a. Hypophosphatemia rarely occurs in a healthy population

(1) High-risk groups include those who excessively use phosphate-binding antacids, have *hyperparathyroidism*, alcoholism, renal insufficiency, and eating disorders

(2) Symptoms include increased calcium excretion, resulting in a negative calcium balance and bone loss

(3) Treatment requires medical supervision

C. Magnesium—Bones contain two-thirds of the body's magnesium

1. Functions

a. Bone mineralization, as a component of many enzymes, energy metabolism, blood clotting, nerve transmission, muscle relaxation, maintenance of enamel, and immunity maintains calcium homeostasis and prevents skeletal abnormalities

(1) Third most prevalent mineral found in teeth

(2) Dentin contains two times the amount present in enamel

b. Receives energy production from ATP

c. Acts as a cofactor for more than 300 enzymes involved in metabolism

d. Assists with calcium in neuromuscular transmission

2. RDA

a. Women—320 mg/day

b. Men—420 mg/day

3. Food sources—Abundant in foods; general diet usually provides adequate amounts found in

a. Whole-grain products

b. Nuts and seeds

c. Legumes

d. Green leafy vegetables—Magnesium is part of the chlorophyll molecule

4. Management of deficiency and/or disease

a. Hypomagnesemia

(1) High-risk groups include those undergoing renal disease, diuretic therapy, hyperthyroidism, diabetes, parathyroid gland disorders, and alcoholics

(2) Symptoms include neuromuscular dysfunction, muscle spasm convulsions, tremors, anorexia, nausea, apathy, and cardiac arrhythmias

(3) Treatment requires medical supervision

VIII. Microminerals (trace elements)—Inorganic substances required by humans in amounts < 100 mg/day

A. Fluoride does not fit the strict definition of an essential nutrient because it has no known metabolic function

    1. Functions

        a. Considered essential because of its beneficial effect on tooth enamel; replaces the hydroxyl ion in *hydroxyapatite,* forming fluorapatite; less soluble and more resistant to acid demineralization

        b. Incorporated into the matrix of bone, improving strength and decreasing bone resorption

        c. Results in a systemic effect primarily when the teeth are forming; results in a topical effect after eruption

    2. DRI/AI

        a. 6 mo. to 1 year—0.5 mg

        b. 1–3 years—0.7 mg

        c. 4–8 years—1.1 mg

        d. Adults—3.1 to 3.8 mg

    3. Sources

        a. Fluoridated drinking water—62% of U.S. water supplies are fluoridated; 1 cup of fluoridated water (1 ppm) provides approximately 0.2 mg of fluoride

        b. Fluoridated dental products—Toothpaste, mouth rinses, and supplements; an average of 0.30 mg fluoride is ingested with each brushing by young children

        c. Food sources include tea, seafood, mechanically deboned poultry, and food cooked in Teflon pans

            (1) Dietary intake of fluoride ranges from 0.3 to 1.0 mg/day for adults

            (2) Ready-to-feed infant formulas contain 0.1–0.2 mg/L of fluoride; fluoride content of powdered or liquid-concentrate formulas depends primarily on the fluoride concentration of the water used to reconstitute them and may range from 0.1 to 1.0 mg/day

    4. Management of deficiency and/or disease

        a. Lack of fluoride results in an increased incidence of caries

        b. Treatment

            (1) Determine the total intake of fluoride from all sources

            (2) If below the AI, prescribe the appropriate level of supplementation

5. Tolerable upper intake levels (UL)

a. Fluorosis—Mottling of the enamel that results from excess fluoride intake during the preeruptive development of teeth

(1) UL is 0.10 mg/kg/day for children 8 years old and younger

(2) Fluorosis ranges from mild with whitish opaque flecks to severe with extrinsic, brownish discoloration, and varying degrees of enamel pitting depending on dose

b. Skeletal fluorosis is characterized by dose-related calcification of ligaments, osteosclerosis, *exostosis*, osteoporosis of long bones, muscle wasting, and neurological defects due to hypercalcification of the vertebrae; UL for people 7–70+ years is 10 mg/day

B. Iron

1. Functions

a. Acts as a component of hemoglobin, which transports oxygen

b. Acts as a catalyst for oxidative reactions in cells including ATP production

c. Essential for normal immune function

d. Critical for normal brain function

2. RDA—18 mg/day for adults

3. Food sources include meats, egg yolk, dark green vegetables, and enriched cereals

a. Heme sources of iron found in animal products are absorbed with about 25% efficiency compared with nonheme sources absorbed at 5%

b. Factors that enhance absorption include vitamin C, animal proteins, increased gastric acidity

c. Factors that decrease absorption include the presence of phytates and oxalates, as well as coffee and tea consumption

4. Management of deficiency and/or disease

a. Most common nutritional deficiency among children and women of childbearing age

b. Iron deficiency anemia results in hypochromic, microcytic anemia

(1) High-risk groups include infants less than 2 years of age, teenage girls, pregnant women, and elderly people

(2) Clinical symptoms include fatigue, pale conjunctiva of eye, tachycardia, anorexia, pica (especially ice eating), koilonychia (spoon-shaped fingernails), and gastritis

(3) Oral manifestations include atrophy of the lingual papillae, burning and redness of the tongue, angular stomatitis, and dysphagia

(4) Treat with ferrous sulfate or ferrous gluconate supplements

5. Toxicity—Iron overload results in oxidative damage to body cells/organs

a. Hemochromatosis—Genetic disease found in 1% of population

(1) High-risk groups include men who have no mechanism for losing iron

(2) Symptoms include fatigue, weakness, chronic abdominal pain, aching joints, *hepatomegaly*, skin pigmentation, diabetes mellitus, arthritis, cancer, and heart disease

(3) Treatment includes drawing blood 2–3 times/week to remove excess iron and limiting heme sources of iron in the diet

C. Zinc

1. Functions

a. Act as a cofactor in more than 120 enzymes involved in cell growth and reproduction

b. Involved in fat, carbohydrate, and protein metabolism

c. Stabilizes DNA and RNA in the cell nucleus

d. Essential for bone growth including osteoblastic activity, formation of bone enzymes, and calcification

e. Involved in collagen synthesis

f. Supports immune function

g. Enhances taste and appetite

2. RDA

a. Women—8 mg/day

b. Men—11 mg/day

3. Food sources include protein-rich foods

a. Glucose, lactose, red wine, and soy protein enhance absorption

b. High intakes of calcium, iron, copper, fiber, phytates, and phosphate salts interfere with absorption

4. Management of deficiency and/or disease

a. High-risk groups include pregnant women, the elderly, vegans, and alcoholics

b. Symptoms include loss of taste acuity, poor appetite, impaired wound healing and growth, mild anemia, skin lesions, and hypogonadism

c. Oral manifestations include changes to the epithelium of the tongue (such as thickening of the epithelium), an increase in cell numbers, and flattened filiform papillae

d. Treatment should be monitored by a physician and registered dietitian

5. Toxicity

a. Chronic ingestion of 100–300 mg/day may result in toxicity

b. Symptoms include vomiting, diarrhea, epigastric pain, lethargy, fatigue, renal damage, and pancreatitis

D. Copper

1. Functions

a. Forms red blood cells

b. Acts as a catalyst in the formation of collagen; involved in the cross-linking of collagen necessary for tensile strength

c. Acts as a cofactor in oxidative reactions and production of neurotransmitters

2. RDA—900 mcg/day

3. Food sources include shellfish, liver, nuts, sesame and sunflower seeds, legumes, and cocoa

4. Deficiency occurs rarely in genetic syndromes, such as *Menkes' syndrome* and malabsorption syndromes; symptoms include neutropenia, bone demineralization, hair and skin depigmentation; causes failure of iron absorption leading to anemia

E. Other trace minerals—Iodine, chromium, cobalt, and selenium

1. Functions

a. Iodine and selenium—Involved in thyroid hormone activity

b. Selenium—Acts with antioxidants to reduce cell damage from free radicals

c. Chromium—Potentiate insulin action

d. Cobalt—Constituent of vitamin B_{12}

2. Food sources include seafood, liver, poultry, milk, grains, and iodized salt

3. Deficiencies are rare, except for iodine

a. 1 billion people worldwide are at risk for iodine deficiency

b. Symptoms include goiter, cretinism, shortened stature, and hypothyroidism

F. Electrolytes—Compounds or ions that dissociate in solution

1. Sodium—Major cation of extracellular fluid

a. Functions

(1) Regulates extracellular fluids

(2) Aids in conduction of nerve impulses

(3) Involved in control of muscle contraction

b. Estimate of requirements for adults is 500 mg/day

c. Food sources include table salt and protein-rich foods

d. Deficiency—Hyponatremia occurs when sodium losses exceed water losses

(1) High-risk groups include those who use excessive diuretics, hyperglycemia in diabetics, and heat exhaustion

(2) Symptoms include nausea, abdominal cramps, headache, confusion, lethargy, and coma

2. Chloride—Principal anion in extracellular fluids

a. Functions

(1) Maintains water balance and osmotic pressure

(2) Maintains acid-base balance in body fluids

b. Estimate of requirements for adults is 750 mg/day

c. Food source is primarily table salt

d. Deficiency results in a loss of appetite, failure to thrive, muscle lethargy, and severe metabolic alkalosis

3. Potassium—Major cation of intracellular fluid

a. Functions

(1) Maintains intracellular fluid levels

(2) Regulates muscle contraction

(3) Facilitates transmission of nerve impulses

(4) Regulates acid-base balance

b. Estimate of requirements of adults is 2,000 mg/day

c. Food sources include fruits, vegetables, and fresh meats

d. Deficiency is rare

IX. Nutrition in Oral Health

A. Systemic effects of nutrients

1. Hard tissues of the oral cavity (Figure 3-7■)

a. Teeth and alveolar bone are made up of collagen fibers in which hydroxyapatite crystals are deposited

(1) Collagen is a protein matrix synthesized by fibroblasts and is a component of the connective tissues of the gingiva and periodontal ligament, as well as the ground substance for the deposition of minerals to form teeth and bone

(a) Vitamin C is required for hydroxylation of the amino acids proline and lysine, to form hydroxyproline and hydroxylysin, which are essential precursors of collagen biosynthesis

(b) Copper is essential for the cross-linking of collagen fibers and provides tensile strength

(c) Other nutrients necessary for collagen synthesis and maintenance include zinc, vitamin A, silicon, and manganese

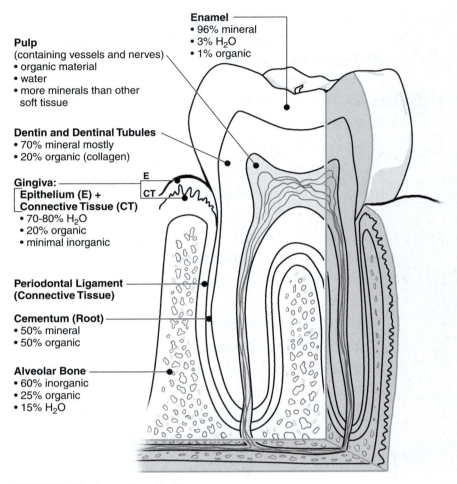

Enamel
• 96% mineral
• 3% H$_2$O
• 1% organic

Pulp
(containing vessels and nerves)
• organic material
• water
• more minerals than other
  soft tissue

Dentin and Dentinal Tubules
• 70% mineral mostly
• 20% organic (collagen)

Gingiva:
Epithelium (E) +
Connective Tissue (CT)
• 70-80% H$_2$O
• 20% organic
• minimal inorganic

E
CT

Periodontal Ligament
(Connective Tissue)

Cementum (Root)
• 50% mineral
• 50% organic

Alveolar Bone
• 60% inorganic
• 25% organic
• 15% H$_2$O

FIGURE 3-7 ■ Composition of Oral Tissues

(2) Odontoblasts and ameloblasts require the same nutrients involved in collagen biosynthesis to synthesize the protein matrix of the dentin and enamel; deficiency during the preeruptive stage may result in hypoplasia

(3) Hydroxyapatite forms the calcified structure of the tooth/bone and requires calcium, phosphorus, magnesium, boron, manganese, vitamin K, and vitamin D; bone is constantly being remodeled by osteoblastic and osteoclastic activity and a constant supply of necessary nutrients is required to maintain bone and prevent bone loss

(4) Fluoride added to the hydroxyapatite crystal reduces solubility of substance to acids, making it more caries-resistant

2. Soft tissues of the oral cavity

a. Oral mucosa is made up of nonkeratinized tissues that line the oral cavity, except for the keratinized tissues found on the hard palate, gingiva, and dorsum of the tongue

(1) Nutrients required for maintenance of tissues include the B-complex vitamins, iron, vitamins A and C, zinc, and protein

(2) Oral cavity may be first site to exhibit signs and symptoms of systemic disease or nutritional deficiencies for several reasons

(a) Rapid rate of cell turnover, every 3–7 days

(b) Tissues are under constant attack by microorganisms

(c) High risk of trauma to oral tissues

b. Salivary glands

(1) Functions of saliva

(a) Lubricates the oral mucosa

(b) Buffers to maintain a neutral pH

(c) Contains minerals that aid in remineralization

(d) Increases oral clearance of bacterial substrates

(e) Possesses antimicrobial properties

(2) Deficient intakes of protein, vitamin A, and iron may result in reduced salivary flow due to salivary gland dysfunction

B. Local effects of nutrients on dental caries

1. Dietary carbohydrates

a. Caries process involves the hydrolyzing of mono- and disaccharides by enzyme salivary amylase to form sucrose, glucose, and fructose

(1) These sugars are substrates for bacterial plaque, primarily *Streptococcus* and *Lactobacillus*, which produce acids (e.g., acetic, formic, lactic, carboxylic, propionic)

(2) The critical pH for demineralization of enamel is 5.5 or less; pH remains low for 20–30 minutes after ingestion of fermentable carbohydrates

b. Caries prevention must focus on modifying the causative factors

(1) Remove plaque

(2) Increase resistance of tooth by demineralization with topical fluorides

(3) Modify cariogenic dietary factors

(a) Evaluate oral retentiveness or length of time teeth are exposed to a lowered pH

i) High sucrose foods deliver high sugar levels, but only for a short time and generally are not retained on tooth

        ii) Highly retentive, starchy foods (cookies, crackers, dry cereals, pretzels, and potato chips) are more cariogenic because they deliver a progressively increasing concentration of sugars over a prolonged period as the starch particles, entrapped on the tooth, are hydrolyzed by the bacteria

(b) Frequency of eating meals and snacks; linear relationship between caries incidence and the number of snacks

(c) Physical form of the carbohydrate

        i) Liquid forms are often found in acidic mediums such as soft and sports drinks and fruit drinks/juices that enhance demineralization

        ii) Sticky carbohydrates, such as raisins and fruit leathers, are highly retentive and cariogenic

(d) Length of interval between meals/snacks

(e) Sequence of food consumption

        i) *Anticariogenic* or cariostatic foods eaten at the end of a meal prevent the lowering of the pH

        ii) Cariostatic foods such as meat are high in protein and fat

        iii) Cheese is anticariogenic; when eaten after sucrose intake, it shortens the length of time the pH remains in the critical area from 15 to 20 minutes to 5 minutes

(f) Amount of fermentable carbohydrate consumed

        i) In one study, the elderly (65–74 years of age) consumed 47–53% more sugar-containing foods than did 19- to 24-year-olds

        ii) Patients with root caries were found to consume twice the sugary liquids and 50% more cakes and cookies than a healthy control group

        iii) A study group with root caries consumed 40% more sugar and 32% more starch than those without root caries

(g) Sugar concentration of the food or beverage

(h) Proximity of eating to bedtime—Primarily a problem if thorough plaque removal does not occur; salivary secretions decrease during sleep

2. Topical fluoride—Enhances the rate of remineralization of the enamel and dentin and reduces the acid production in dental plaque

C. Maintenance of periodontal health

    1. Lack of nutrients does not cause periodontal disease, but it may be a modifying factor once the disease process has been initiated

    2. Effects of nutrition in periodontal health and disease

        a. Healthy epithelial tissue prevents the penetration of bacterial endotoxins into the subgingival tissue; increased permeability of the gingival barrier at the gingival sulcus occurs with deficiencies of vitamin C, folate, and zinc

        b. Maintenance of the integrity of the host's immune response— Important nutrients in the body's immune response include protein, iron, zinc, and vitamin E

        c. Calcification of the alveolar bone and cementum—For maintenance of the calcified tissues, good supplies of protein, calcium, phosphorus, vitamin D, magnesium, vitamin K, and zinc are required

        d. Stimulation of salivary flow to aid in oral clearance—May be enhanced by chewing firm, coarse, and fibrous foods

        e. Repair and healing process—Include protein, vitamins A and C, folate, calcium, iron, and zinc in diet

        f. Amount and type of supragingival plaque—Avoid sugar-rich foods, which enhance undesirable bacteria and use preventive measures to remove plaque from the teeth

X. Nutrition Screening

A. Purpose—To identify patients at nutritional risk

B. Methods

    1. Nutrition Screening Initiative—Developed to screen older adults for nutritional risk

        a. Forms are simple and can be completed by the patient

        b. Screening questions address a number of issues (medical, dental, psychosocial) that may affect a patient's food intake, resulting in nutritional inadequacies

    2. Screening for caries risk

        a. Determine the frequency of meals and snacks

        b. Identify habits, such as frequent use of gum, breath mints, cough drops, or antacids, that may contribute to caries risk

        c. Identify sources of simple and retentive carbohydrates in the diet

XI. Assessment of Nutritional Status

A. Standards for dietary intake

1. Dietary Reference Intake (DRI) will replace the periodic revisions of the Recommended Dietary Allowances (RDA)

    a. Purpose—Will encompass not only prevention of deficiency disease, but also the following

    (1) Role of nutrients in decreasing the risk of chronic and other diseases and conditions

    (2) Upper limits beyond which toxicity may occur

    b. Components

    (1) Estimated Average Requirement (EAR)—Meets estimated needs of 50% of individuals in a given age and gender group

    (2) Adequate Intake (AI)—Experimentally observed estimates of nutrient intake that appear to reduce the risk of chronic and other diseases and conditions; uncertainty in data prevents specific RDA

    (3) Recommended Dietary Allowance (RDA)—Meets nutrient needs of 97% of healthy people

    (4) Tolerable Upper Intake Level (UL)—Maximum intake that is unlikely to pose risk of adverse health effects in 97% of the population

2. Dietary guidelines

    a. Goals

    (1) Provide an adequate and balanced diet that meets the nutritional needs of an individual for maintenance, repair, growth or development, and to maintain the living processes

    (2) Help reduce the risks of developing chronic degenerative diseases

    b. Federal dietary guidelines

    (1) USDA Guide to MyPyramid, Steps to a Healthier You 2005 (Figure 3-8■)

    (a) *One size doesn't fit all.* MyPyramid plan offers you a personal eating plan with the foods and amounts that are right for you. MyPyramid food patterns are designed for the general public ages 2 and over. Places a stronger emphasis than the past editions on calorie control and increasing physical activity (Figure 3-9■).

    (b) The U.S. Department of Agriculture (USDA) and the U.S. Department of Health and Human Services (USDHHS) issue Dietary Guidelines for Americans to advance and promote dietary guidance for all Americans.

Anatomy of MyPyramid

One size doesn't fit all

USDA's new MyPyramid symbolizes a personalized approach to healthy eating and physical activity. The symbol has been designed to be simple. It has been developed to remind consumers to make healthy food choices and to be active every day. The different parts of the symbol are described below.

Activity

Activity is represented by the steps and the person climbing them, as a reminder of the importance of daily physical activity.

Moderation

Moderation is represented by the narrowing of each food group from bottom to top. The wider base stands for foods with little or no solid fats or added sugars. These should be selected more often. The narrower top area stands for foods containing more added sugars and solid fats. The more active you are, the more of these foods you can fit into your diet.

Personalization

Personalization is shown by the person on the steps, the slogan, and the URL. Find the kinds and amounts of food to eat each day at MyPyramid.gov.

Proportionality

Proportionality is shown by the different widths of the food group bands. The widths suggest how much food a person should choose from each group. The widths are just a general guide, not exact proportions. Check the website for how much is right for you.

Variety

Variety is symbolized by the 6 color bands representing the 5 food groups of the Pyramid and oils. This illustrates that foods from all groups are needed each day for good health.

Gradual Improvement

Gradual improvement is encouraged by the slogan. It suggests that individuals can benefit from taking small steps to improve their diet and lifestyle each day.

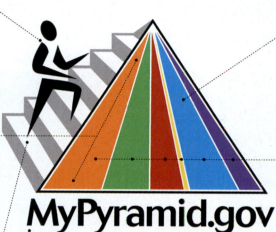

USDA U.S. Department of Agriculture Center for Nutrition Policy and Promotion April 2005 CNPP-16

USDA is an equal opportunity provider and employer.

GRAINS VEGETABLES FRUITS OILS MILK MEAT& BEANS

FIGURE 3-8 ■ MyPyramid

Source: USDA website, http://www.mypyramid.gov

(c) Recommendations for general public (Table 3-1■; see pp. 222–232)

    i) Adequate nutrients within calorie needs

    ii) Physical activity

    iii) Weight management

    iv) Food groups

    v) Fats

    vi) Carbohydrates

    vii) Sodium and potassium

   viii) Alcoholic beverages

    ix) Food safety

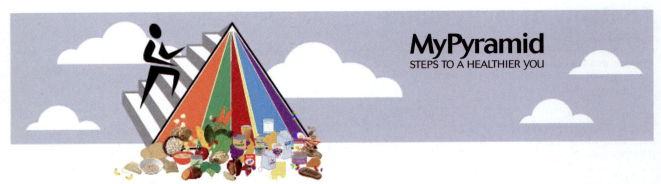

MyPyramid
STEPS TO A HEALTHIER YOU

Based on the information you provided, this is your daily recommended amount from each food group.

GRAINS	VEGETABLES	FRUITS	MILK	MEAT & BEANS
6 ounces	2 1/2 cups	1 1/2 cups	3 cups	5 ounces
Make half your grains whole	**Vary your veggies** Aim for these amounts each week:	**Focus on fruits**	**Get your calcium-rich foods**	**Go lean with protein**
Aim for at least **3 ounces** of whole grains a day	**Dark green veggies** = 3 cups	Eat a variety of fruit	Go low-fat or fat-free when you choose milk, yogurt, or cheese	Choose low-fat or lean meats and poultry
	Orange veggies = 2 cups	Go easy on fruit juices		Vary your protein routine— choose more fish, beans, peas, nuts, and seeds
	Dry beans & peas = 3 cups			
	Starchy veggies = 3 cups			
	Other veggies = 6 1/2 cups			

Find your balance between food and physical activity

Be physically active for at least **30 minutes** most days of the week.

Know your limits on fats, sugars, and sodium

Your allowance for oils is **5 teaspoons a day.**

Limit extras–solid fats and sugars–to **195 calories a day.**

Your results are based on a 1800 calorie pattern.

Name: _____

This calorie level is only an estimate of your needs. Monitor your body weight to see if you need to adjust your calorie intake.

FIGURE 3-9 ■ Sample MyPyramid Recommendations for Adults
Source: USDA website, http://www.mypyramid.gov

B. Methods of evaluating dietary data

1. Use of dietary guidelines to determine overall dietary adequacy is most efficient in the dental office due to limited time and nutritional knowledge

2. Determine cariogenicity of dietary habits—Evaluate frequency and type of retentive starches and sugars consumed

3. Computer analysis—Enter all foods into a database

   a. Evaluate overall nutrient intakes compared to RDAs—An intake below the RDA does not necessarily mean the patient is deficient

      (1) Advantage—Accurate and detailed information on nutrient intake

   (2) Disadvantage—Difficult to translate individual nutrients into the types of foods the patient needs to include in the diet to obtain the desired nutrients

   b. Percentage of simple sugars

   (1) Advantage—Helpful in identifying sources of sugars

   (2) Disadvantage—Does not identify retentive starches and it is difficult to assess frequency of sugar exposure

XII. Nutrition Assessment and Counseling

A. Methods of data gathering for nutrient assessment

1. Food Frequency Questionnaire (FFQ)

   a. Consists of a multiple page survey listing a variety of foods and asking the patient how often the foods are consumed over a period of time, usually from 6 months to a year

   b. Advantages

   (1) Requires little "in office" time

   (2) Allows analysis of food group/general nutrient intakes over time

   c. Disadvantages

   (1) Provides general dietary information

   (2) Cannot evaluate daily frequency of sugar and snacking

   (3) Relies on patient memory for frequency of intake over a long period

2. 24-hour dietary recall

   a. Patient is asked to remember everything consumed during the past 24 hours; interviewer writes everything down and asks probing questions in order to gather more detail

   b. Advantages

   (1) Allows analysis of food group and nutrient consumption

   (2) Can be done quickly

   (3) Gathers data to evaluate sugar/fat intake

   c. Disadvantages

   (1) Patient may not accurately remember the kinds and amounts of food and beverage intake

   (2) Interviewer needs experience asking open-ended questions

   (3) Represents only 1 day of food intake, which may not be typical of the patient's usual diet

   (4) There is a tendency to overreport low intakes and to underreport high intakes

3. 3- to 7-day food record

    a. Requires patient to record the type and amount of food and beverages consumed

    b. Advantages

        (1) Allows evaluation of an average intake over a number of days

        (2) Saves "in office" time

        (3) Allows analysis of food group/nutrient consumption and eating patterns

    c. Disadvantages

        (1) Time-consuming for the patient and compliance is low

        (2) Requires a highly trained person to evaluate the results obtained and develop individual recommendations

B. Nutrition counseling

    1. Components of nutrition counseling

        a. Interviewing—Obtaining information from the patient

        b. Teaching—Nonpersonal, transfer of information

        c. Counseling—Personalized working relationship with the patient to help him or her solve a problem or issue

        d. Follow-up and monitor progress

    2. Requirements for successful counseling

        a. Provide conducive environment

        (1) Physical environment—Provide a private place with no interruptions or threatening surroundings (e.g., dental drill) and work with patient at eye level

        (2) Patient readiness—Work with patient who is not too tired or scared, in a hurry, or has past negative experiences, and is interested in self-help

        (3) Counselor readiness—Shares good attitude; not overstressed or in a hurry; provides unbiased acceptance of all patients in word and body language

C. Interviewing skills

    1. Encourage patient to talk about his or her lifestyle and daily habits

    2. Use open-ended questions to determine values, concepts, and attitudes

    3. Use closed-ended questions to establish facts

    4. Provide active listening—Listen to what is being said and probe further; ask for clarification and acknowledge listening to patient

    5. Be nonjudgmental—Provide neither negative nor positive verbal or nonverbal judgments on patient's statements or habits

   6. Provide attending skills—Maintain eye contact, nod head, or use other means of confirmation to indicate listening without judgment

D. Teaching skills

   1. Determine patient's knowledge first

   2. Clarify confusion; fill in knowledge gaps

   3. Educate patient about the link between nutrition and oral and general health

   4. Elicit continuous feedback to ensure patient comprehension

   5. Provide appropriate amount of information to meet patient's needs; avoid being too simple or too complex

   6. Use appropriate visuals, including patient's own mouth and radiographs

E. Counseling skills

   1. Help patient assess his or her own diet

   2. Have patient summarize results and findings

   3. Have patient determine suggestions for changes

      a. Basic dietary adequacy

      b. Cariogenic dietary habits

   4. Suggest basic diet adequacy

   5. Suggest cariogenic risk factors

   6. Have patient set goals for improvement

   7. Provide suggestions and strategies when needed

   8. Summarize with "reality check" and obtain verbal commitment for course of action

   9. Monitor patient's progress from visit to visit

XIII. Nutrition Considerations in the Life Cycle

A. Infancy

   1. Early childhood caries—A pattern of rampant caries beginning prior to 36 months of age affecting the primary maxillary anterior teeth

      a. 20% of children are at high risk, including Native Americans, Hispanics, and Native Alaskans

      b. Etiology—Due to prolonged and frequent exposure to a bottle or breastfeeding, particularly at night and nap time

      c. Prevention—Educate pregnant women about appropriate infant feeding practices and oral care before delivery

         (1) NEVER put an infant or child to bed with a bottle containing anything other than water

         (2) Avoid having infants sleep with mother and nurse at-will all night

(3) Avoid using sweetened pacifiers

(4) Begin weaning infants to a cup at 6 months; children should be completely weaned to a cup by age 1

B. Childhood

  1. Should eat foods high in nutrient and energy density to meet needs for growth and development; portion sizes are adjusted based on child's size and physiological needs

  2. Children over age 2 years should eat a reduced-fat diet to decrease the risk of diet-related chronic diseases later in life

  3. Excessive juice consumption (> 12 oz/day) may lead to

    a. Obesity due to excessive calories

    b. Short stature (results from juice replacing more nutrient-dense foods)

    c. Caries due to frequent exposure to fermentable carbohydrates

    d. Low-income children are at high risk to develop rampant caries

    e. 90% of children with early childhood caries will develop decay on primary first molars

C. Adolescents—80% of an individual's average caries incidence occurs during adolescence

  1. Dietary habits—Adolescents exert newfound independence in food choices

    a. Generally choose foods low in vitamin A, thiamin, iron, and calcium

    b. Eat fast foods and ready-to-eat snacks high in fat, sugar, protein, and sodium

  2. Eating disorders—Affect 5–11% of adolescents

    a. Anorexia nervosa—50% also practice bulimia

      (1) Diagnostic criteria

        (a) Fail to maintain minimal weight and height for age group

        (b) Fear of being overweight

        (c) Distorted body image

        (d) Amenorrhea in females

      (2) Oral manifestations may include

        (a) Angular cheilitis due to multiple nutrient deficiencies

        (b) Xerostomia resulting from parotid gland dysfunction

        (c) Dental erosion due to self-induced vomiting

    b. Bulimia

      (1) Diagnostic criteria

        (a) Practice a minimum of two binges per week for 3 months; consume large quantities of high-calorie, carbohydrate-rich foods (average intake of food during a binge is 3,400 calories over an hour, with some patients ingesting as much as 50,000 calories in 24 hours)

(b) Feel a lack of control

(c) Compensatory actions to negate the binge's effects

  i) Use laxatives

  ii) Practice self-induced vomiting

  iii) Perform excessive exercise

  iv) Practice strict dieting or fasting

(d) Overly concerned about body weight and shape

(2) Oral manifestations

(a) Perimolysis—Enamel erosion on the lingual surfaces of the maxillary anterior teeth

(b) Evidence of calluses or scars on the first knuckle of the index finger from induced vomiting

(c) Traumatic palatal injuries or bruising from object used to induce vomiting

(d) Possible xerostomia, due to dehydration from vomiting and laxatives

(e) Caries—An increase of 20% due to

  i) Large amounts of fermentable and retentive carbohydrates eaten during a binge

  ii) Exposure to acid during vomiting episodes

  iii) Increase in xerostomia, which reduces the oral clearance of carbohydrates

c. Binge-eating disorder (BED)

(1) Diagnostic criteria—Same binge-eating behaviors as the bulimic patient, but with no purging

(2) Oral manifestation includes increased caries rate due to the frequency of exposure to fermentable carbohydrates

D. Aging

1. Chronic disease—Incidence and prevalence increases as the population ages

a. Cardiovascular disease (CVD) results from atherosclerosis that narrows the arteries and restricts blood flow, which can result in ischemia of the heart, brain, or extremities

(1) Risk factors include increasing age, gender, heredity, tobacco use, *hyperlipidemia*, hypertension, physical inactivity, diets high in saturated fats, diabetes mellitus, and obesity

(2) Prevention includes lowering blood pressure, normalizing lipid levels, maintaining glycemic control, reducing excess body fat, ceasing tobacco use, increasing physical activity, and consuming a healthy, low-fat diet

2. Polypharmacy—Use of multiple drugs at any one time

a. Xerostomia (dry mouth)—Side effect of more than 400 medications including antihistamines, antihypertensives, antidepressants, and antipsychotics

(1) Signs and symptoms associated with xerostomia include

(a) Dysgeusia (changes in taste) due to low levels of saliva that aid in the dissolution of foods and allow the sensation of sweet, sour, salty, and bitter tastes

(b) Difficulty in speaking, swallowing (dysphagia), and chewing due to the lack of saliva to provide lubrication to the oral tissues

(c) Burning or soreness of the oral mucosa

(d) Increased susceptibility to oral *candidiasis*; saliva is needed to

i) Maintain the integrity of the mucous membranes, the first line of defense in innate immunity

ii) Limit growth of bacteria and prevent oral infections via antimicrobial agents, such as immunoglobulins and lysozymes

(e) Difficulty in wearing dentures

(f) Increase in the incidence of severe caries due to loss of saliva, which:

i) Provides substantial buffering capacity to maintain the oral pH near neutrality

ii) Provides some physical cleansing and diluting of toxic bacterial products

iii) Maintains mineral content of the teeth by aiding in ongoing remineralization

(2) Dietary recommendations to prevent caries should focus on

(a) Minimizing the frequency of meals and snacks

(b) Limiting sugary and retentive between-meal snacks such as candy, raisins, crackers, potato chips, pretzels, cookies, and dry cereal

(c) Encouraging consumption of fresh fruits, vegetables, and dairy products as snacks

(d) Encouraging frequent sips of water for hydration and lubrication of the oral mucosa

   (e) Using sialogogues, such as xylitol in sugarless gum, to stimulate saliva

   (f) Ending a meal or snack with cheese (anticariogenic) or rinsing with water when the patient cannot perform an oral hygiene regimen

(3) Tooth loss

   (a) Denture wearers have 75–85% reduced masticatory efficiency

   (b) Effects on dietary intake—Patient alters food intake to reduce chewing or because of fear of choking, therefore patient

   i) Consumes fewer meats, fresh fruits, and vegetables

   ii) Relies on soft foods, which tend to be more retentive, increasing the risk of root caries for those with remaining teeth

   iii) Consumes more refined carbohydrates and sucrose

   iv) Loses teeth because of decrease in nutrient intakes of vitamin A, crude fiber, and calcium

XIV. Oral Conditions Affecting Nutrient Intake

A. Oral cancer

1. Accounts for about 3% of all cancers; long-term prognosis is generally poor

2. Effects on nutrient intake depend on the

   a. Patient's nutritional status before diagnosis

   b. Stage and site of the cancer

   c. Aggressiveness of therapy required in treating the cancer

3. Complications associated with oral cancer include

   a. Chronic pain

   b. Impaired swallowing and chewing, resulting in weight loss

   c. Speech difficulties

   d. Mucositis

   e. Xerostomia

   f. Physical disfigurement

   g. Oral infections, such as candidiasis

4. Nutrition recommendations

   a. Consume small, frequent high-calorie/high-protein meals and snacks primarily consisting of liquid or soft, moist foods

   (1) Add whole milk or cream to puddings, cream soups, and milkshakes

   (2) Add extra cheese to foods

   (3) Add butter or margarine to mashed potatoes and scrambled eggs

   (4) Use pasteurized egg nog in milkshakes

(5) Use commercial supplements or instant breakfast drinks in whole milk for snacks

b. Attempt to eat all solid foods before consuming liquids at meals to prevent early satiety

B. Oral and periodontal surgery

1. Effects on nutrient intake—Usually minimal due to the short duration of inadequate nutrient intakes

   a. High-risk groups include those with poor nutritional status before surgery (e.g., alcoholics, medically compromised patients, and those unable to consume adequate nutrition within 3–5 days postoperatively—this is of particular concern for diabetics)

2. Dietary recommendations for soft/liquid diet

   a. For the medically compromised patient, consult with physician and registered dietitian before surgery for recommendations to replete any nutrient deficiencies

      (1) Recommend a multivitamin supplement at 100% of RDA levels

      (2) Provide a list of nutrient-dense foods and beverages to have during postoperative recovery

   b. Postoperative care—Nutrient requirements increase because of blood loss, increased catabolism, tissue regeneration, and host defense activities

      (1) A liquid diet may be required for the first 1–3 days

         (a) Milkshakes, ice cream, pudding, custards, instant breakfast drinks, and commercial liquid supplements provide calories, protein, and many of the essential nutrients needed for wound healing

         (b) Diabetic patients need to spread their carbohydrate intake evenly throughout the day to keep blood glucose under control and may want to choose sugar-free or no-sugar-added products

         (c) Continue the multivitamin supplement until eating returns to normal

      (2) From days 3–7 postoperatively, the diet may progress from liquid to soft to normal as the patient tolerates

         (a) Add fruit nectars and soft fruits such as applesauce and bananas to the liquid diet

         (b) Additional soft foods include cottage cheese, yogurt, mashed potatoes, macaroni and cheese, scrambled eggs, and oatmeal

C. Oral lesions

1. May complicate nutrient intakes for a few days to months

2. Apthous ulcers, mucositis, stomatitis, and esophagitis are inflammations of the mucous membranes lining the GI tract starting in the mouth

   a. Causes

      (1) Chemotherapy drugs including methotrexate, hydroxyurea, and 5-fluorouracil

      (2) Radiation to the head and neck

      (3) Immune suppression, as in AIDS

   b. Concerns

      (1) Ability to ingest enough food to provide adequate nutrition and prevent weight loss

      (2) Ability to perform home care procedures, which may prevent or reduce the severity of stomatitis

   c. Nutrition recommendations include a liquid or soft diet as discussed under oral cancer

   d. Poorly tolerated foods

      (1) Citrus fruit or juices, such as orange and grapefruit

      (2) Rough, coarse, or dry foods such as raw vegetables, granola, toast, and crackers

      (3) Spicy or salty foods

      (4) Textured or granular foods

      (5) Extremely hot or cold foods

TABLE 3-1 OVERVIEW OF NUTRIENTS

Macronutrients

Nutrient	Major Functions	Deficiency Symptoms	Oral Manifestations of Deficiency	Symptoms of Nutrient Excesses	Dietary Sources	Recommendations	Upper Tolerable Intake Levels
Carbohydrate (CHO)	Energy source (4 kcal/g) Spares protein Needed for oxidation of fats			Dental caries	Complex CHOs: whole and enriched grains, cereals, pasta, and rice Simple CHOs: fruits, dairy, soda, baked goods	CHO: 55–60% of total calories Simple CHOs: ≤10% of total calories Fiber: 20–35 g/day	
(Fibers)	Facilitates normal peristalsis						
Protein	Synthesis of body tissues Growth and maintenance Source of energy w/↓ fat and ↓ CHO intake	Kwashiorkor Marasmus Abnormal growth, development, and synthesis of tissues	Lag period in initiation of wound healing Compromised antibacterial properties of saliva		Complete: dairy, meat, fish, eggs, soy, and poultry Incomplete: whole grains, legumes, nuts, and vegetables	Adults: 0.8 g/kg of body wt/day; 10–15% of total calories	

Nutrient	Functions	Deficiency Symptoms	Effects of Excess	Sources	Recommended Intake	Toxicity
Fat	Source of energy (9 kcal/g); Carries fat-soluble vitamins; Source of essential fatty acids; Provides insulation and protection to body organs; Satiety	Essential fatty acid deficiency symptoms: scaly skin, hair loss, impaired wound healing	Obesity ↑ Incidence of cardiovascular disease; Type 2 diabetes mellitus; Hypertension; Some forms of cancer	Meats, fish, and poultry; Vegetable oils, nuts, and seeds; Dairy products	Fat ≤ 30% of total calories; Saturated fat < 10% of total calories; Essential fatty acids: Linoleic acid: 1–2% of total calories; 3–6 g/day	

Micronutrients

Water-Soluble Vitamins

Nutrient	Functions	Deficiency Symptoms		Sources	Recommended Intake	Toxicity
Thiamin (B_1)	Coenzyme in CHO metabolism	Beriberi; Mental confusion; Muscular wasting; Chronic polyneuropathy		Lean pork; Wheat germ; Enriched breads and cereals; Egg yolks; Legumes	Males 14–70+ yr: 1.2 mg/day; Females 19–70+ yr: 1.1 mg/day	None
Thiamin (B_1)		Anorexia; Wernicke-Korsakoff; Disorientation; Jerky movements of eyes; Staggering gait		Whole grains		

(continued)

TABLE 3-1 OVERVIEW OF NUTRIENTS (*continued*)

Nutrient	Major Functions	Deficiency Symptoms	Oral Manifestations of Deficiency	Symptoms of Nutrient Excesses	Dietary Sources	Recommen-dations	Upper Tolerable Intake Levels
Riboflavin (B_2)	Part of coenzyme CHO, fat, and protein metabolism	Photophobia Loss of visual acuity Burning and itching of the eyes Ariboflavinosis Oral symptoms Greasy erup-tion of the skin in the nasolabial fold	Soreness and burning of lips, mouth, and tongue Edema of pharyngeal and oral mucous membranes Angular cheilosis Stomatitis Glossitis: purple, swollen tongue		Milk products Organ meats Lean meats Eggs Green leafy vegetables	Males 14–70+ yr: 1.3 mg/day Females 19–70+ yr: 1.1 mg/day	None
Niacin (B_3)	Part of coenzyme in release of energy from CHO, fat, and protein Structural repair of cells via DNA synthesis	Muscular weakness Anorexia Indigestion Skin eruptions Pellegra—the Ds Dermatitis Dementia Diarrhea	Irritation and inflamma-tion of mucous membranes of the mouth Sore tongue (beefy tongue)	Liver toxicity "Flushing"	Lean meats, fish, and poultry Peanuts Enriched breads and cereals	Males 14–70+ yr: 16 mg/day Females 14–70+ yr: 14 mg/day	Adults: 30 mg/day
Pyroxidine (B_6)	Coenzyme in protein metabolism Conversion of tryptophan to niacin Neurotransmit-ter synthesis	Hypochromic, microcytic anemia Neurological disorders Confusion Irritability Depression	Stomatitis Cheilosis Glossitis	Severe sensory neuropathy	Yeast Wheat germ Pork Whole-grain cereals Legumes Bananas	Males 14–50 yr: 1.7 mg/day Females 19–50 yr: 1.5 mg/day	Adults: 100 mg/day

	Function	Deficiency		Food Sources	Recommended Intake	Upper Limit
Folate/Folic Acid	Coenzyme in DNA synthesis Interconversion of amino acids Formation of WBCs and RBCs	Alteration of DNA synthesis Megaloblastic anemia Poor growth GI disturbances Neural tube defects	Burning tongue and oral mucosa Red and swollen tongue Angular cheilosis	Liver Legumes Dark green leafy vegetables Lean beef Potatoes	Adults 14–70+ yr: 400 mcg/day	Adults: 1,000 g/day
Folate/Folic Acid	Interrelationship with vitamin B_{12}			Enriched breads and cereals		
Cobalamin (B_{12})	Required for DNA synthesis	Pernicious anemia Megaloblastic anemia Neurological damage with paresthesia Numbness and tingling in hands and feet Unsteadiness Psychological disorders	Red, beefy tongue	Animal products only Meat, poultry, and fish Dairy products Eggs	Adults 14–70+ yr: 2.4 mcg/day	None

(continued)

TABLE 3-1 OVERVIEW OF NUTRIENTS (*continued*)

Nutrient	Major Functions	Deficiency Symptoms	Oral Manifestations of Deficiency	Symptoms of Nutrient Excesses	Dietary Sources	Recommen-dations	Upper Tolerable Intake Levels
Vitamin C (Ascorbic acid)	Antioxidant Cofactor in hy-droxylation of proline and lysine in collagen formation Needed in folate metabolism Enhances iron absorption	Scurvy Healing im-pairment Defective skeletal cal-cification Joint pain Bruise easily Follicular hyper-keratosis	Swollen, hemorrhagic gingivitis Enlarged marginal gingivae Loose teeth Dryness of the mouth	Diarrhea "Rebound scurvy" after sudden dis-continuation of massive doses of vitamin C	Citrus fruits Leafy green vegetables Green pep-pers Broccoli Tomatoes Potatoes Melons	Males: 90 mg/day Females: 75 mg/day	2,000 mg/day

Fat-Soluble Vitamins

Nutrient	Major Functions	Deficiency Symptoms	Oral Manifestations of Deficiency	Symptoms of Nutrient Excesses	Dietary Sources	Recommen-dations	Upper Tolerable Intake Levels
Vitamin A (preformed: retinal and retinol) (precursor: carotenes)	Required for rhodopsin and other photo-sensitive pigments Cellular differ-entiation and prolifer-ation Integrity of the immune system	Ocular changes from night blindness to xeroph-thalmia Increased susceptibility to infection Loss of appetite Hyper-keratosis	Xerostomia Impaired growth of teeth and bone Poor wound healing	Nausea and vomiting Fatigue Weakness Birth defects if taken in excess during pregnancy Bone pain and fragility	Retinol: liver fish oil fortified milk and margarine Carotene: dark green, yellow, and orange fruits and vegeta-bles	Males: 900 mcg/day Females: 700 mcg/day	3,000 mcg/day

| Vitamin D (cholecalciferol) | Facilitates calcium absorption Maintains blood homeostasis of calcium | Rickets (in children): inadequate mineralization of the skeleton, resulting in bowlegs, pigeon breast, and frontal bossing of the skull Osteomalacia (in adults) softening of bones in the extremeties, spine, thorax, and pelvis General weakness | Hypercalcemia Hypercalciuria Deposition of calcium in soft tissues and irreversible renal and cardiovascular damage Death | Fish liver oils Fortified milk, margarine, and butter | 0–50 yr: 5 mcg/day 50–70 yr: 10 mcg/day 70+ yr: 15 mcg/day | Adults: 50 mcg/day |
| Vitamin E (tocopherols) | Antioxidant-scavenging free radicals | Peripheral neuropathy | Relatively nontoxic when taken by mouth High doses may interfere with blood clotting | Vegetable oils Wheat germ Nuts | Adults: 15 mg/day | Adults: 1,000 mg/day |

(continued)

TABLE 3-1 OVERVIEW OF NUTRIENTS (*continued*)

Nutrient	Major Functions	Deficiency Symptoms	Oral Manifestations of Deficiency	Symptoms of Nutrient Excesses	Dietary Sources	Recommen-dations	Upper Tolerable Intake Levels
Vitamin K	Cofactor in blood clotting Involved in bone crystalline formation	Abnormal bleeding		Hemolytic anemia	Green leafy vegetables	Adults: Males: 80 mcg/day Females: 65 mcg/day	
Macrominerals							
Calcium	Component of teeth and bones (99%) Transport function in cell membranes Nerve transmission and regulation of heartbeat Blood clotting	Osteoporosis Amount of bone ↓ and bone fractures with minimal stress	Possible association with alveolar bone loss	Constipation Possible ↑ risk of urinary stone formation Inhibition of absorption of iron and zinc	Dairy products Fortified juices and cereals Legumes Green, leafy vegetables	9–18 yr: 1,300 mg/day 19–50 yr: 1,000 mg/day 50+ yr: 1,200 mg/day	Adults: 2,500 mg/day
Phosphorus	Component of bone mineral Transfer of energy as ATP Component of phospholipids, DNA, and RNA Involved in metabolism of fats, CHOs, and proteins	Bone loss Weakness Anorexia Malaise Pain		↓ blood calcium level	Meat, poultry, and fish Eggs Dairy products	8–18 yr: 1,250 mg/day 19–70+ yr: 700 mg/day	Adults: 4 g/day

	Function	Deficiency	Toxicity	Sources	RDA/DRI	UL
Magnesium	Maintain calcium homeostasis Energy production from ATP Cofactor for over 300 enzymes involved in metabolism	Neuro-muscular dysfunction Muscle spasms Convulsions Tremors Anorexia Cardiac arrhythmias	Nausea and vomiting Hypotension Bradycardia	Whole grains Nuts and seeds Legumes Green, leafy vegetables	Males 30–70+ yr: 420 mg/day Females 30–70+ yr: 320 mg/day	> 9 yr: 350 mg/day (nonfood Mg)

Trace Minerals

	Function	Deficiency	Toxicity	Sources	RDA/DRI	UL
Fluoride	Anticaries effect on tooth enamel Incorporated in bone matrix ↑ strength and ↓ bone resorption	↑ incidence of caries	Dental fluorosis Skeletal fluorosis	Flouridated water Flouridated dental products Tea Seafood Mechanically deboned poultry Food cooked in Teflon pans	6–12 mo: 0.5 mg/day 1–3 yr: 0.7 mg/day 4–8 yr: 1.1 mg/day	0–6 mo: 0.7 mg/day 6–12 mo: 0.9 mg/day 1–3 yr: 1.3 mg/day 4–8 yr: 2.2 mg/day 9–70 yr: 10 mg/day

(continued)

TABLE 3-1 OVERVIEW OF NUTRIENTS (*continued*)

Nutrient	Major Functions	Deficiency Symptoms	Oral Manifestations of Deficiency	Symptoms of Nutrient Excesses	Dietary Sources	Recommendations	Upper Tolerable Intake Levels
Iron	Component of hemoglobin Catalyst cellular reactions Essential for immune function Critical for brain function	Microcytic, hypochromic anemia Fatigue Pale conjunctivae of eyes Anorexia Gastritis Koilonychia (spoon-shaped fingernails)	Atrophy of lingual papillae Burning, red tongue Angular stomatitis Dysphagia	Hemochromatosis Fatigue Weakness Chronic abdominal pain Skin pigmentation Aching joints ↑ risk of heart disease, diabetes mellitus, and cancer	Heme iron Meats, fish, and poultry Eggs Nonheme iron Enriched breads and cereals Dark green leafy vegetables	Adults: Males 8 mg/day Females 15 mg/day 19–50 yr: 18 mg/day 50+ yr: 8 mg/day	45 mg/day
Zinc	Cofactor > 100 enzymes in cell growth Coenzyme energy metabolism Stabilizes DNA and RNA Involved in collagen synthesis Formation of bone enzymes and calcification Taste and appetite Immune function	Poor appetite Skin lesions Impaired growth and wound healing	Loss of taste acuity Flattened filiform papillae of the tongue Thickening of the epithelium of the tongue	Vomiting Diarrhea Epigastric pain Lethargy Fatigue Renal damage	Protein-rich foods	Adults: Males 11 mg/day Females 8 mg/day	40 mg/day

	Function	Deficiency	Toxicity	Sources	RDA	UL
Copper	Formation of red blood cells Cross-linking of collagen	Neutropenia Bone demineralization Hair and skin depigmentation		Shellfish Liver Nuts and seeds Legumes Cocoa	Adults: 900 mcg/day	10 mg/day
Electrolytes						
Sodium	Regulates extracellular fluids Aids in conduction of nerve impulses Control of muscle contraction	Hypo-natremia Nausea Abdominal cramps Headache Confusion Lethargy Coma	Edema Hypertension	Table salt Protein-rich foods (meats and dairy)	Adults: 500 mg/day	
Chloride	Maintains water balance and osmotic pressure Maintains acid-base balance	Loss of appetite Failure to thrive Muscle lethargy Severe metabolic alkalosis		Table salt	Adults: 750 mg/day	

(continued)

TABLE 3-1 OVERVIEW OF NUTRIENTS (*continued*)

Nutrient	Major Functions	Deficiency Symptoms	Oral Manifestations of Deficiency	Symptoms of Nutrient Excesses	Dietary Sources	Recommen-dations	Upper Tolerable Intake Levels
Potassium	Maintains intracellular fluid Regulation of muscle contraction Regulates acid-base balance Facilitates nerve trans-mission	Hypokalemia Weakness Nausea Listlessness Anorexia		Cardiac effects Death	Fruits Vegetables Meats	Adults: 2,000 mg/day	
Water	Universal solvent Medium for metabolic reactions Structural component of cells Transport medium for nutrients Involved in electrolyte balance and homeostasis	Dehydration Weight loss Hypotension Orthostatic hypotension Dry skin ↓ skin turgor ↓ urinary output	Xerostomia Shrinkage of mucous membranes	Water intoxi-cation Headache Nausea and vomiting Muscle twitching Convulsion Blurring of vision	Drinking water Soft drinks Liquid milk Fruits and vegetables	1 ml/kcal or about 2–3 L	

CHO, carbohydrate; WBC, white blood cell; RBC, red blood cell; RE, retinol equivalent; ATP, adenosine triphosphate.

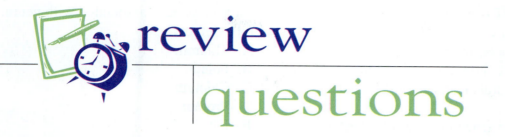

review questions

DIRECTIONS Each of the questions or incomplete statements below is followed by suggested answers or completions. Select the **one** answer that is best in each case.

---

1. An adequate amount of nutrient intake is needed by the oral tissues for all of the following EXCEPT one. Which one is the EXCEPTION?
   A. Growth
   B. Development
   C. Catabolism
   D. Maintenance

2. Essential amino acids must be obtained from the diet. They cannot be synthesized from other amino acids.
   A. The first statement is TRUE, the second is FALSE.
   B. Both statements are TRUE.
   C. The first statement is FALSE, the second is TRUE.
   D. Both statements are FALSE.

3. Which of the following is an example of an essential fatty acid?
   A. Linoleic
   B. Tropical oils
   C. Lecithin
   D. Oleic

4. Which of the following vitamins is NOT fat-soluble?
   A. A
   B. D
   C. C
   D. E

5. Modifiable risk factors for oral disease include all of the following EXCEPT one. Which one is the EXCEPTION?
   A. Dietary factors
   B. Oral hygiene habits
   C. Health status of the hard and soft tissues
   D. Genetics
   E. Immunological response

6. The critical pH at which demineralization of the enamel occurs is
   A. 0
   B. 2.0
   C. 5.5
   D. 7.0
   E. 8.0

7. Functions of saliva include all of the following EXCEPT one. Which one is the EXCEPTION?
   A. Provides buffering capacity
   B. Provides antimicrobial capacity
   C. Speeds oral clearance of bacterial substrates
   D. Provides growth medium for bacteria
   E. Aids in remineralization of the tooth

8. Examples of retentive carbohydrates include all of the following EXCEPT one. Which one is the EXCEPTION?
   A. Crackers
   B. Cheese
   C. Potato chips
   D. Cookies
   E. Pretzels

9. All of the following are common characteristics of water-soluble vitamins EXCEPT one. Which one is the EXCEPTION?
   A. Required from the diet on a daily basis
   B. Absorbed in the small intestine
   C. Stored in the body for long periods
   D. Easily destroyed

10. Good sources of calcium include all the following EXCEPT one. Which one is the EXCEPTION?
    A. Fortified orange juice
    B. Bread
    C. Legumes
    D. Milk
    E. Yogurt

11. A high intake of dietary components that exert negative effects on bone mass include:
    A. Fat
    B. Sugar
    C. Calcium
    D. Alcohol

12. A deficiency in which of the following nutrients has been associated with neural tube defects?
    A. Thiamin
    B. Folate
    C. Calcium
    D. Protein
    E. Fat

13. Severe decay in early childhood is usually evident in:
    A. Primary first molars
    B. Mandibular central and lateral incisors
    C. Maxillary canines
    D. Maxillary central and lateral incisors

14. A deficiency in vitamin A may result in:
    A. Rickets
    B. Abnormal bleeding
    C. Peripheral neuropathy
    D. Night blindness

15. A bulimic patient may use all of the following methods to purge after binge eating EXCEPT one. Which one is the EXCEPTION?
    A. Laxatives
    B. Diuretics
    C. Antidepressants
    D. Excessive exercise
    E. Vomiting

16. One of the MOST common drug–nutrient interactions that can increase the risk of dental caries is:
    A. Dysgeusia
    B. Dysphagia
    C. Xerostomia
    D. Dysphasia

17. The calcium RDA standard for elderly individuals is below the standard set for the general population. This is because elderly people have decreased calcium absorption.
    A. The first statement is TRUE, the second is FALSE.
    B. Both statements are TRUE.
    C. The first statement is FALSE, the second statement is TRUE.
    D. Both statements are FALSE.

18. Diabetic patients may experience all of the following symptoms EXCEPT one. Which one is the EXCEPTION?
    A. Frequent urination
    B. Blurred vision
    C. Decreased hunger
    D. Increased infections

19. A normal fasting blood glucose level, in mg/dL, is:
    A. 40–60
    B. 80–120
    C. 150–200
    D. > 200

20. One of the risk factors for osteoporosis is:
    A. Increased physical activity
    B. Tobacco use
    C. Estrogen therapy
    D. Toxic levels of vitamin D

21. The MOST common nutritional deficiency among women of child-bearing age and children in the United States is:
    A. Zinc
    B. Vitamin C
    C. Iron
    D. Sodium

22. Dairy products are good sources of all of the following nutrients, vitamins, and minerals EXCEPT one. Which one is the EXCEPTION?
    A. Calcium
    B. Zinc
    C. Vitamin D
    D. Protein
    E. Riboflavin

23. Which of the following factors decreases absorption of dietary iron?
    A. Vitamin C
    B. Lactose
    C. Hydrochloric acid
    D. Phytates
    E. Animal proteins

24. According to the USDA Guide to My Pyramid, Steps to a Healthier You 2005, what is the main emphasis of the plan?
    A. Places a stronger emphasis on calorie control and physical activity
    B. Places a stronger emphasis on receiving the recommended food group servings
    C. Places a stronger emphasis on portion control
    D. Places a stronger emphasis on nutritional supplements

25. The form of carbohydrate BEST used by tissues is:
    A. Lactose
    B. Maltose
    C. Sucrose
    D. Glucose
    E. Fructose

26. Carbohydrates provide 4 kcal/g and fats provide 7 kcal/g.
    A. The first statement is FALSE, the second statement is TRUE.
    B. The first statement is TRUE, and the second statement is FALSE.
    C. Both statements are FALSE.
    D. Both statements are TRUE.

27. Glucose is the sole source of energy for the:
    A. Brain
    B. Pancreas
    C. Heart
    D. Liver
    E. Kidney

28. Food sources of vitamin B_{12} include all of the following EXCEPT one. Which one is the EXCEPTION?
    A. Chicken
    B. Milk
    C. Pork
    D. Legumes
    E. Beef

29. Groups at high risk for many nutritional deficiencies include all of the following EXCEPT one. Which one is the EXCEPTION?
    A. Alcoholics
    B. Children
    C. Young adult males
    D. Elderly

30. The elderly have an increased need for vitamin D because of:
    A. Decreased synthesis by the skin
    B. Increased intake of dairy products
    C. Increased absorption in the small intestine
    D. Decreased intake of vitamin C

31. Green leafy vegetables are sources of all of the following nutrients, vitamins, and minerals EXCEPT one. Which one is the EXCEPTION?
    A. Folate
    B. Vitamin B_{12}
    C. Carbohydrates
    D. Magnesium
    E. Iron

32. All of the following nutrients, vitamins, and minerals are involved in collagen synthesis EXCEPT one. Which one is the EXCEPTION?
    A. Vitamin C
    B. Copper
    C. Protein
    D. Iodine
    E. Zinc

33. Individuals with dentures have reduced masticatory efficacy, which results in increased intakes of:
    A. Fiber
    B. Protein
    C. Sucrose
    D. Calcium
    E. Vitamin A

34. Sucrose is made up of the monosaccharides:
    A. Fructose and galactose
    B. Glucose and galactose
    C. Glucose and glucose
    D. Glucose and fructose

35. The intrinsic factor is necessary for the absorption of:
    A. Amino acids
    B. Essential fatty acids
    C. Sucrose
    D. Vitamin B_{12}

36. Formation of glucose from noncarbohydrate substances is called.
    A. Gluconeogenesis
    B. Glycogenesis
    C. Glucogenesis
    D. Glycolysis

37. Pernicious anemia is associated with:
    A. Iron deficiency
    B. Aminopyrine therapy
    C. Vitamin K deficiency
    D. Vitamin B_{12} deficiency

38. An adequate intake of vitamin C is necessary for good repair of a wound because it promotes:
    A. Growth of epithelium
    B. Production of collagens
    C. Budding of capillaries
    D. Phagocytosis of cell fragments

39. The effect of vitamin C deficiency is primarily on:
    A. Epithelial tissues
    B. Connective tissues
    C. Nervous tissues
    D. Muscular tissues
    E. Hematopoietic tissues

40. The bulk of iron stored in the intestinal wall is:
    A. Ferritin
    B. Apoferritin
    C. $FeSO_4$
    D. Hemoglobin
    E. Cytochrome C

41. The prime food factor responsible for dental caries is:
    A. The sugar content of a particular food
    B. Frequent between-meal eating of sweets
    C. Firm, detersive foods
    D. Drinking fluoridated water
    E. Ingestion of a balanced, adequate diet

42. Which of the following is formed in the animal from dietary tryptophan?
    A. Niacin
    B. Thiamin
    C. Folic acid
    D. Riboflavin
    E. Pyridoxine

43. Amino acids are building blocks for:
    A. Vitamins
    B. Minerals
    C. Proteins
    D. All of the above

44. Fat is primarily considered as:
    A. A concentrated source of energy
    B. The cheapest source of energy
    C. A tissue-building substance
    D. A food substance to be avoided

45. The most important carbohydrate available to the body, whether it be by absorption from the diet or by synthesis within the body, is:
    A. Galactose
    B. Starch
    C. Sucrose
    D. Glucose

46. An essential macromineral closely associated with calcium and phosphorus in the structure of bones and teeth is:
    A. Copper
    B. Fluoride
    C. Magnesium
    D. Selenium
    E. Zinc

47. Normal production of sound dentin and enamel requires adequate amounts of which of the following vitamins?
    A. Vitamin A
    B. Vitamin C
    C. Vitamin D
    D. All of the above

48. Which of the following ingredients listed on a product label indicates that it contains sugar?
    A. High fructose corn syrup
    B. Dextrose
    C. Levulose
    D. Glucose
    E. All of the above

49. Perifollicular hemorrhages are associated with a dietary deficiency of:
    A. Ascorbic acid
    B. Choline
    C. Vitamin B complex
    D. Vitamin K
    E. Vitamin E

50. Which mineral is essential for bone formation because it aids in the creation of a protein structure into which calcium is deposited?
    √A. Manganese
    B. Magnesium
    C. Vanadium
    D. Selenium
    E. Chrominum
    F. K

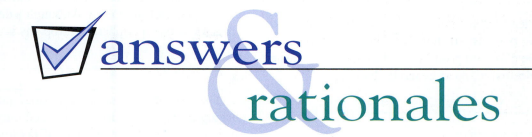

answers & rationales

1.

C. Catabolism is the destructive phase of metabolism in which complex substances are broken down to release nutrients and energy when the body has insufficient nutrients. The oral tissues, like the body, need nutrients for growth, maintenance, repair, and development.

2.

B. Essential amino acids must be obtained from the diet, because the body cannot synthesize them.

3.

A. Linoleic (omega-6) and linolenic (omega-3) are essential fatty acids that must be obtained from the diet. Tropical oils are saturated fats. Lecithin is a phospholipid that acts as an emulsifier for mixing water with oil, as in salad dressings. Oleic acid is a monounsaturated fatty acid found in olive and canola oils.

4.

C. Vitamin C is water-soluble. Vitamins A, D, E, and K are fat-soluble.

5.

D. Genetics is a risk factor that is not modifiable at this time. However, dietary factors, oral hygiene habits, immunological responses, and health status of oral tissues are modifiable factors.

6.

C. The pH at which the oral environment becomes acidic enough to cause minerals to be leached from the tooth surface is 5.5, and on cementum it is 6.7. This is the initial process in caries development. A pH of 7.0 and 8.0 is basic.

7.

D. Because saliva does not contain sucrose and functions as a pH buffer, it does not provide a growth medium for bacteria. Saliva also aids in the remineralization of teeth and the oral clearance of food, as well as provides antimicrobial properties.

8.

B. Cheese is composed of protein and fat. Its anticariogenic effect, due to its high calcium and phosphorus content, assists in raising the pH of saliva and buffers the acids produced by bacteria. Crackers, potato chips, pretzels, and cookies are all capable of producing energy for cariogenic bacteria.

9.

C. Water-soluble vitamins are not stored in the body for long periods, so they must be consumed daily. They are absorbed primarily in the small intestine and easily destroyed, most generally by heat.

10.

B. Bread has little calcium content, but is enriched with B vitamins. Legumes, milk, fortified juice, and yogurt are good sources of calcium.

11.

D. Excessive alcohol consumption has a negative effect on bone mass, a risk factor for osteoporosis, possibly because of its toxic effects on osteoblasts. Ninety-nine percent of calcium is found in the bones and teeth. Fat and sugar do not affect bone mass.

12.

B. The RDA for folate has been increased as a result of studies suggesting an association between low intakes and neural tube defects, such as spinal bifida. A deficiency in thiamin causes beriberi, which can damage the nervous and cardiovascular systems. A calcium deficiency is associated with rickets, osteoporosis, osteomalacia, and tetany. In the United States, there is rarely a deficiency associated with fat and protein.

13.

D. Maxillary central and lateral incisors are the first teeth affected in early childhood caries. The position of the tongue against the nipple causes pooling of the liquid around these teeth when there is extended contact with fermentable carbohydrates. The remaining teeth are protected by the position of the tongue.

14.

D. A deficiency in vitamin A causes night blindness. Rickets is caused by a deficiency in vitamin D and calcium. Vitamin K aids in the formation of prothrombin, a blood-clotting factor. Although a deficiency in vitamin E is rare, peripheral neuropathy is a symptom.

15.

C. The use of antidepressants does not assist in purging of excess calories consumed during a binging episode. However, the use of laxatives and diuretics, vomiting, and excessive exercise are all examples of purging.

16.

C. Xerostomia or dry mouth is a side effect of more than 400 different medications. Decreased saliva flow results in a loss of its buffering effects, thereby causing an increase in the incidence of caries. Dysgeusia is a change of taste a patient may experience. Dysphagia involves difficulty in swallowing and dysplasia describes abnormal growth or development.

17.

C. Because elderly people experience decreased calcium absorption, their need for calcium is higher than the RDA standards.

18.

C. Diabetics usually experience an increase in appetite. They may experience symptoms of frequent urination, blurred vision, and increased infections.

19.

B. The normal range for fasting blood glucose is between 80 and 120 mg/dL. Numbers below the normal range indicate hypoglycemia and numbers above this range indicate hyperglycemia.

20.

B. Individuals who smoke are at a higher risk for developing osteoporosis. Increased physical activity and estrogen therapy are advised as preventive and treatment measures, respectively. Toxic levels of vitamin D lead to calcium being deposited in soft tissues and irreversible cardiovascular and kidney damage.

21.

C. The most common nutritional deficiency of children and women of childbearing age in the United States is iron deficiency. Vitamin C (sources include citrus fruits, broccoli, potatoes, and tomatoes) and zinc (found in protein-rich foods) are easily attained from the diet. A deficiency in sodium is rare because sodium is so readily available.

22.

B. Dairy products are good sources of protein, phosphorus, riboflavin, and vitamins A and D. Zinc is found primarily in protein-rich foods such as oysters, beef, eggs, and peanuts.

23.

D. Iron absorption, like that of calcium and other minerals, can also be affected by food factors such as Phytates (a salt of a phosphoric acid ester) that bind to iron and reduce its absorption. Vitamin C and hydrochloric acid favor iron absorption. Animal proteins are good sources of iron. Lactose is the sugar found in milk.

24.

A. The USDA Guide to MyPyramid, Steps to a Healthier You 2005, stresses the importance of a personal eating plan with the foods and amounts that are right for you. It places a stronger emphasis on calorie control and increasing physical activity.

25.

D. Glucose is the form of carbohydrate used best by body tissues for energy. Maltose, lactose, and sucrose are disaccharides, which must be broken down into monosaccharides before entering the bloodstream. Fructose (levulose) is the sweetest of all the monosaccharides and is a product of the breakdown of sucrose.

26.

B. Carbohydrates provide 4 kcal/g and fats provide 9 kcal/g.

27.

A. Glucose is the sole source of energy for brain and red blood cells. Glucose is used by the pancreas, heart, liver, or kidney—but not as the sole source of energy as with the brain and red blood cells.

28.

D. Vitamin B_{12} is found only in animal sources, not in plant foods. Legumes are pods, such as peas and lentils. They are a plant source.

29.

C. Young adult males tend to have high intakes of nutrients and are not among the groups at risk for deficiencies. Elderly people, alcoholics, and children are all at risk for nutritional deficiencies. The elderly suffer from absorption problems. Children usually consume less calories per day than recommended by the RDA standards. Alcohol interferes with the storage of nearly all nutrients.

30.

A. There is a fourfold decrease in the synthesis of vitamin D by the skin in elderly people. Dairy products assist in the absorption of vitamin D; however, elderly people may experience absorption problems. Vitamin C does not affect the absorption of vitamin D, but diets high in fiber can affect vitamin D absorption.

31.

B. Vitamin B_{12} is obtained from animal sources only. However, folate, carbohydrates, magnesium, and iron can be found in green leafy vegetables.

32.

D. Iodine helps regulate the basal metabolic rate. Protein, copper, zinc, and vitamin C are all involved in collagen synthesis and maintenance.

33.

C. Because denture wearers have reduced masticatory efficacy—75–85% less than natural teeth—an increase in the intake of sucrose and refined carbohydrates, foods easier to chew, is common. Foods rich in fiber, protein, calcium, and vitamin A require more biting and chewing.

34.

D. The disaccharide sucrose is made up of two monosaccharides: glucose and fructose. Glucose and galactose make up the disaccharide lactose. Two molecules of glucose make up maltose. The combination of fructose and galactose do not make up a disaccharide.

35.

D. The intrinsic factor is a protein made in the stomach. If this factor is absent, absorption of vitamin B_{12} is affected. Amino acids travel to the liver through the portal vein. The primary site for fat absorption is the small intestine. Sucrose is broken down into monosaccharides and then transported to the liver through the portal vein.

36.

A. When body metabolism requires glucose, which is not available from recently digested carbohydrates, it calls on the liver to convert its stored glycogen into glucose through the process of glycolysis. When the store is depleted, the liver begins to make new glycogen from amino acids. This partial conversion of protein to glycogen in the liver is known a gluconeogenesis.

37.

D. Pernicious anemia is usually due to a lack of intrinsic factor, which prevents the absorption of the physiologic amount of vitamin B_{12}.

38.

B. Ascorbic acid is absolutely essential for the fibroblast to produce its fibrous protein, collagen. An ascorbic acid deficiency will bring about a reversal of the differentiated cells to the more immature cell types. However, if ascorbic acid is administered, the defect is promptly corrected.

39.

B. Without ascorbic acid for collagen biosynthesis, connective tissue formation would be impaired, and so would healing and scar tissue formation and maintenance. This means that ascorbic acid is essential for the formation and maintenance of intercellular substances in connective tissue.

40.

A. Iron is stored as soluble ferritin within most body tissues, but especially within the reticuloendothelial system and the liver parenchyma. Some iron is held in less mobile masses of aggregate ferritin, call hemosiderin.

41.

B. The Vipeholm study proved several points regarding the dental caries–refined carbohydrate relationship. One point is that the frequency of using sugar is the prime factor in caries activity.

42.

A. Foods that are a good source of tryptophan, such as animal protein (with the exception of gelatin) and vegetable protein, are good sources of niacin because the body has the capacity to convert typtophan into niacin.

43.

C. Amino acids are ordinarily required for synthesis of tissue proteins, and the absence of any one of them could prevent the formation of proteins in the body.

44.

A. Fats are an excellent source of energy. They provide 9 calories per gram of substance compared to 4 calories per gram provided by carbohydrate and protein. In short, they are twice as efficient as a source of energy.

45.

D. Glucose is the form of carbohydrate that the body tissues can best use.

46.

C. Magnesium is present both in enamel and dentin, but its concentration in dentin is about twice that in enamel. A deficiency will produce a reduction in the rate of alveolar bone formation, widening of the periodontal ligament, and gingival hyperplasia.

47.

D. Enamel begins developing prenatally and continues postnatally. Enamel originates from oral epithelial cells that differentiate into ameloblasts, while dentin originates from the odontoblasts. Differentiation of these two important cells, necessary for enamel and dentin formation, is aided by both vitamins A and C. Prenatally, calcium and phosphorus are essential for calcification of the enamel and dentin. However, this process cannot occur in the absence of vitamin D. Deficiency of this vitamin also causes poor growth of enamel cells (ameloblasts) and dentin cells (odontoblasts).

48.

E. Corn syrup, dextrose, levulose, and glucose are all sugars. Corn syrup is a viscous liquid and is the product of incomplete hydrolysis of starch. High fructose corn syrup is derived from sucrose or dextrose. Dextrose is another name for glucose and is produced commercially by the hydrolysis of starch. Levulose is an alternate name for fructose or fruit sugar and it is the sweetest tasting of all the sugars. Glucose is the carbohydrate that body tissues use most efficiently.

49.

A. The hemorrhagic tendency, resulting in abnormal gingival bleeding, may be due to vascular abnormalities associated with vitamin C (ascorbic acid) deficiency. Even though there is no universally accepted agreement as to the mechanism for the weakness of connective tissue, there is evidence of blood vessel fragility with consequent diffuse tissue bleeding. This results in easy bruising, friable bleeding gums, and pinpoint skin and joint hemorrhage. Infection is a consequence of capillary fragility and permeability.

50.

A. Even though the clinical signs and symptoms of a manganese deficiency have not been clearly defined, manganese is an essential nutrient for humans. It is needed for normal bone structure because manganese creates a protein structure into which calcium is deposited.

4 Microbiology, Infectious Diseases, and Infection Control

The study of microbiology is important for dental professionals to prevent the transmission of disease to themselves and their patients. Infection control is the mechanism by which the health professional controls disease transmission.

chapter objectives

After completion of this chapter, the learner should be able to:

➤ Discuss the classification of microorganisms

➤ Discuss the bacterial cell structure and function of microorganisms

➤ Describe eukaryotic cell structure and function

➤ Describe the growth and cultivation of microorganisms

➤ Discuss antimicrobial agents

➤ Describe infection control during dental treatment

➤ Discuss the infectious disease process

➤ Describe the immune system

➤ Discuss viral infections

➤ Discuss bacterial infections

➤ Discuss fungal infections

➤ Describe respiratory tract infections

➤ Describe infection of the gastrointestinal tract

➤ MICROORGANISMS

I. Basic Concepts

A. Most numerous species on earth—Part of normal environment

B. Same characteristics as more complex cells: metabolism, growth, reproduction

C. Microorganisms capable of producing disease—Pathogens

D. Nomenclature—Binomial system

    1. Two-word name

    2. Genus (capitalized) and species (lowercase), with both italicized (e.g., *Streptococcus mutans*)

II. Classifications

A. *Prokaryotes*—Lack nucleus, unicellular, may be anaerobic or aerobic, smallest living organism with ability to survive independently of other organisms (Figure 4-1■)

    1. Shape—(Figure 4-2■)

        a. *Cocci* (singular, *coccus*)—Spherical bacteria

        b. *Bacilli* (singular, *bacillus*) or rods—Cylindrical-shaped bacteria

        c. *Spirilla* (singular, *spirillum*)—Helical-shaped bacteria

        d. *Vibrio* is a genus of Gram-negative bacteria possessing a curved rod shape.

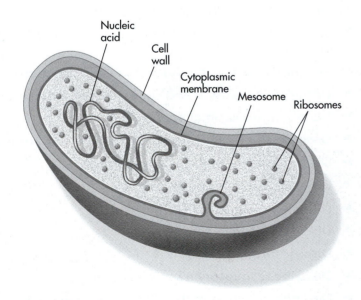

FIGURE 4-1 ■ Components of a Prokaryotic Cell

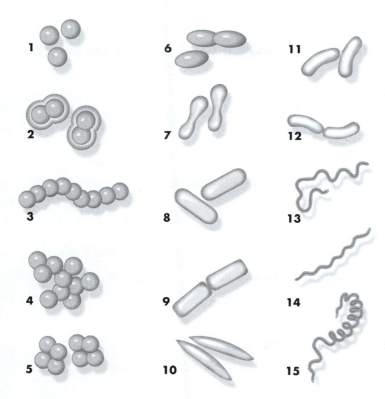

FIGURE 4-2 ■ Variations in Basic Bacterial Morphology: 1. Single Cocci; 2. Pairs of Cocci; 3. Chains of Cocci; 4. Clusters of Cocci; 5. Cocci in Tetrads. 6. Coccobacilli; 7. Club-Shaped Bacilli; 8. Bacilli with Rounded Ends; 9. Bacilli with Square Ends; 10. Bacilli with Tapered Ends (fusiforms); 11. Vibrios; 12. Spirillum; 13. Borrelia; 14. Treponema; 15. Leptospira

2. Cell wall structure

   a. Cytoplasmic membrane—Innermost structure; same in all cells; functional barrier between inside and outside of the cell; energy-producing system for prokaryotic cells

   b. Cell wall—Differs from Gram-positive and Gram-negative cells

   (1) Gram-positive—peptidoglycan; thick (multilayered)

   (2) Gram-negative—more complex; lipopoly saccharide outer membrane and very thin peptidoglycan layer between outer and inner cell membrane

   c. Glycocalyx—External to cell wall; varies from species to species; bacteria secrete polysaccharides to produce slimy gel-type matter; have ability to exclude ink during staining procedures

3. Components of prokaryotic cells—Most species are divided into two different categories based on their reaction to gram stain

    a. Gram stain—Cell staining procedures that differentiates between gram-positive and gram-negative cell walls

        (1) Gram-positive = purple

        (2) Gram-negative = pink

4. Bacteria—*Bacterium* means rod or staff

    a. Most play positive roles—Necessary for many life processes

    b. Extremely adaptable to variable living conditions

    c. All have cell walls

    d. Cause many diseases (pathogenic)

5. *Rickettsiae*—Tiny bacteria transmitted by arthropods (ticks and lice)

6. *Chlamydiae*—Half the size of rickettsiae, cannot be seen with light microscope

7. *Mycoplasms*—Smaller than chlamydiae, only prokaryote without cell wall

8. *Cynobacteria*

    a. Formerly called blue-green algae

    b. Use photosynthesis

    c. Many "fix" nitrogen

B. *Eukaryotes*—Possess a well-defined nucleus, organelles; more advanced life form (Figure 4-3■)

1. Algae (contain chlorophyll)—May have one or many cells

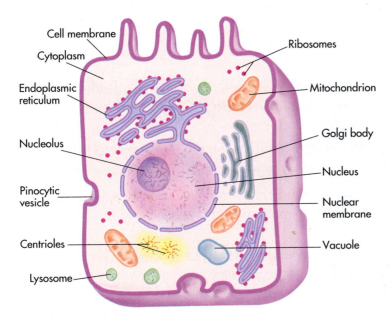

FIGURE 4-3 ■ Main Structural Components of a Eukaryotic Cell

2. Protozoa—Unicellular, nonphotosynthetic

3. Fungi (yeasts and molds)—Nonphotosynthetic; classified by type of spores; mechanism of sexual and asexual spore formation; presence of mycelia

4. Slime molds—Plasmodium

C. *Viruses*—Classified according to type of nucleic acid, morphology; presence of envelope

D. *Helminths*—Multicellular, usually parasites of human gastrointestinal (GI) tract or circulatory system

E. *Prions*—New classification, proteinacious infectious particles; defy many forms of sterilization

III. Metabolic Functions

A. Energy metabolism—Any chemical change or reaction that occurs within the cell

1. Photosynthesis—Process by which autotrophic organisms convert radiant energy from the sun into a form of chemical energy that they use or can be used by living organisms that require organic matter as their energy source (heterotrophic organisms); green plants on land and algae growing in water are responsible for most of the photosynthetic activity on earth

2. Catabolism—Carbohydrates, proteins, and lipids store energy in their chemical bonds that are available for biosynthesis through catabolic reactions; glucose or a polymer of glucose such as starch is the main source of energy for most cells

3. Metabolic energy—Energy obtained by metabolic processes is stored in adenosine triphosphate (ATP) molecules that contain three phosphate groups; two are connected to high-energy bonds readily available for cellular functions; energy released $\rightarrow$ ATP loses phosphate group $\rightarrow$ adenosine diphosphate (ADP) $\rightarrow$ energy and phosphate available; ATP regenerated through the cell respiration process (Figure 4-4■)

4. Glycolysis—Splitting of glucose; series of reactions involving the catabolism of glucose, causing the production of pyruvic acid (Figure 4-5■)

5. Fermentation—The conversion of pyruvic acid into alcohol and organic acids

6. Cell respiration—Krebs cycle and electron transport chain: regenerate ATP *(ADP=P$\rightarrow$ ATP)*

IV. Measurement and Observation of Microorganisms

A. Measurement units

1. Micrometer (mcm = 10^{-6} m)

2. Nanometer (nm = 10^{-9} m)

3. Angstrom unit (Å = 10^{-10} m)

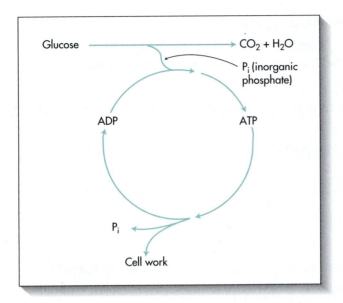

FIGURE 4-4 ■ ATP-ADP Cycle

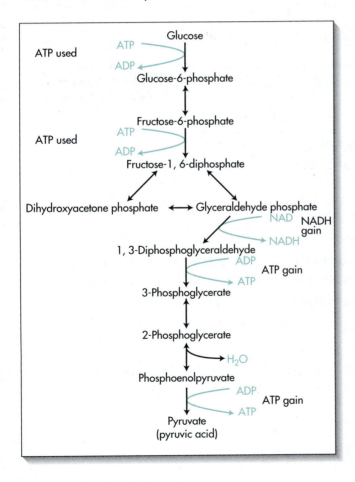

FIGURE 4-5 ■ Simplified Schematic of the Glycolytic pathway

4. Millimeter (mm = 10^{-3} m)

5. Centimeter (cm = 10^{-2} m)

B. Specimen preparation

    1. Living specimens—Hanging drop and temporary wet mount are preparations used

    2. Staining

        a. Improves visualization of dead cells

        b. Some species differentiation

        c. Types

            (1) Acid/base—Shows different cell components

            (2) Single dye (crystal violet, methylene blue, saffranin)

            (3) Differential staining—More than one dye used to group bacteria

                (a) Gram stain—Cell wall thickness, shows penicillin sensitivity

                    i) Gram-positive—Thick cell wall, stains purple or blue, penicillin sensitive

                    ii) Gram-negative—Thin cell wall, stains red, resistant to penicillin

                    iii) Acid fast—Differentiates mycobacteria (*Mycobacterium tuberculosis*) by indicating presence of special cell wall lipids that resist depolarization

                    iv) Dark field microscopy—Necessary to visualize spirochetes

V. Bacterial Cell Structure and Function (Figure 4-1)

A. Morphology

    1. Cocci (single—coccus)

        a. Round or ovoid shape

        b. Occur in pairs (diplococci), chains (streptococci), four-square (tetrad), eight-cube (sarcinae), and clusters (staphylococci)

        c. Predominates in oral health

    2. Bacilli (single—bacillus)

        a. Rodlike or cylindric

        b. Occurs in pairs (diplobacilli), chains (streptobacilli), rounded rods (coccobacilli), and with tapered ends (fusiform bacilli)

    3. Spirilla (single—spirillum)

        a. Spiral or curved

        b. Vibrios—may be portion of a spiral

B. External cell structures

  1. Surface coating (glycocalyx)

   a. Capsules—Thick, organized polysaccharide and/or polypeptides attached to cell wall, protection from pathogens, drugs, phagocytosis, increases virulence (e.g., *Mutans Streptococcus*)

   b. Slime layer—A soluble mass of polysaccharides and/or polypeptides that are unorganized and loosely attached to the cell wall; protects and aids adherence

  2. Appendages

   a. *Flagella*

    (1) Long, rigid protein strands

    (2) Aid in mobility

   b. Axial filaments

    (1) Form of locomotion used by spirochetes

    (2) Aid in mobility

   c. *Pili*

    (1) Join bacteria in preparation for DNA transfer (also allows drug resistance if plasmids)

    (2) Most common in gram-negative bacteria

    (3) Provide attachment

   d. *Fimbriae*

    (1) Shorter, more numerous than pili

    (2) Enables attachment of cell to surfaces (increases virulence)

C. Cell wall—Peptidoglycan macromolecule that maintains shape, prevents cell rupture, supports flagella

  1. Gram-positive

   a. Multilayers of peptidoglycan and teichoic acids

   b. Disrupted by penicillins and lysozymes

  2. Gram-negative

   a. Lipoprotein–lipopolysaccharide–phospholipid outer membrane surrounding thin peptidoglycan layer

   b. Protects cell from phagocytosis, penicillin, lysozyme

   c. Disrupted by antibody lysis, mechanical forces (e.g., scaling), and complement

D. Plasma membrane

  1. Phosopholipid bilayer with fluid mosaic protein layer interspersed

  2. Functions in active transport, as cell barrier

  3. Contains enzymes and protein receptors

E. Cell envelope

1. All external structures and appendages
2. Helps cell adhesion and maintenance
3. Responsible for staining characteristics

F. Internal cell structure

1. Cytoplasm—Fluid space inside plasma membrane; site of biochemical activities; contains ribosomes, granules, chromatin body
2. Genome (nucleoid)—Single chromosome of one molecule of DNA; closed loop without nuclear membrane in nucleoplasm of cell
   a. Plasmids—Extrachromosomal DNA molecules that carry drug resistance information
   b. Transposons—DNA segments that can move without the benefit of homology
3. Ribosomes—Composed of ribosomal ribonucleic acid (RNA) and ribosomal protein, function in protein synthesis
4. Mesosomes—Folds in cytoplasmic membrane caused by drying (artifact)
5. Endospores—Gram-positive cells form these dormant structures
   a. May remain in spore state for years, extremely resistant to heat, drying, chemical disinfection, and radiation
   b. "Live spore test" considered benchmark for sterilization
      (1) Steam and chemical vapor uses spores of *Geobacillus stearothermophilus*
      (2) Dry heat and ethylene oxide sterilizers use spores of *Bacillus atrophaeus*
   c. Produced by genera *Bacillus* and *Clostridium*
6. Inclusions—Storage material, may include polysaccharide granules, granular sulfur, lipids, and vacuoles
7. Photosynthetic apparatus

VI. Eukaryotic Cell Structure and Function

A. Distinct nucleus bound by nuclear membrane; cell has nucleolus and membrane-bound organelles

B. Animal cells

1. Cell membrane surrounds cell and connects with internal membrane system
   a. Functions through active and passive transport in regulation of cell substances
   b. Important in drug sensitivity, phagocytosis, tumor formation, and immune response

2. Nucleus

    a. Controls physiology and reproduction of cell

    b. Composed of nuclear membrane, nucleoli (RNA synthesis), chromosomes (DNA), and nucleoprotein (chromatin)

3. Internal structures

    a. Mitochondria—Energy production through adenosine triphosphate (ATP)

    b. Golgi complex—Protein packaging

    c. Endoplasmic reticulum (ER)—Protein synthesis; rough (has ribosomes attached) and smooth

    d. Lysosomes—Digestive enzymes

    e. Cytoplasm—Intracellular fluid, ions, nutrients, particles for cell function

➤ GROWTH AND CULTIVATION OF MICROORGANISMS

I. Bacterial Growth

A. Binary fission—One parent cell produces two new cells

B. Bacterial growth curve—Phases

    1. Lag phase—During *lag phase*, bacteria adapt themselves to growth conditions. It is the period where the individual bacteria are maturing and not yet able to divide

    2. Log phase—Cell numbers increase in exponential manner (logarithmic) most susceptible to antimicrobials at this phase

    3. Stationary phase—The growth rate slows as a result of nutrient depletion and accumulation of toxic products; this phase is reached as the bacteria begin to exhaust the resources that are available to them

    4. Decline (death) phase—Number of viable cells decrease; bacteria run out of nutrients and die

C. Generation time—Time needed for cell to divide varies widely between species, usually around 20 minutes

D. Growth measurements

    1. Increase in mass, numbers, weight, turbidity

    2. Viable counts of microorganisms

        a. Bacteria—Colony-forming units (CFU)

        b. Viruses—Plaque-forming units (PFU)

II. Conditions that Affect Bacterial Growth

A. Physical conditions

    1. Thermal—May grow within a range, many around 86°F/30°C

2. Acid/alkaline (pH)—Most organisms grow best around neutral pH, between 6 and 8

3. Osmotic pressure

B. Chemical conditions

  1. Atmospheric requirements

    a. Aerobes—Require oxygen

    b. Microaerophilic—Low concentrations of oxygen

    c. Anaerobes—Do not require oxygen

    d. Obligate anaerobes—Cannot tolerate free oxygen

    e. Facultative anaerobes—Aerobic organisms that can grow in the absence of oxygen

  2. Nutrition requirements

    a. Heterotrophic—Organic compounds needed for growth

    b. Autotrophic—Use inorganic compounds

    c. Hypotrophic—Obligate intracellular parasite

III. Antimicrobial Agents

A. Mechanisms of antimicrobial agents

  1. Inhibition of cell wall synthesis (e.g., penicillins)

  2. Disruption of cell membrane (e.g., polymycin)

  3. Inhibition of cell wall synthesis (e.g., tetracyclines)

  4. Inhibition of DNA synthesis (e.g., rifampin)

  5. Competitive inhibition (e.g., sulfa drugs)

B. Antibody assays—Tests to determine exposure to antigen of a specific pathogen; also known as serological reactions

  1. Titer—Most dilute concentration of serum antibody that reacts with antigen

  2. Enzyme-linked immunosuppressant assay (ELISA)—Inexpensive enzyme test for HIV, other pathogens

  3. Neutralization, precipitation, agglutination, flocculation—All common tests

  4. Others: complement fixation, fluorescent antibody technique, radioimmunoassay, monoclonal antibodies, Western blot test

C. Antibiotic resistance and abuse

  1. Many organisms resistant to common antibiotics

  2. Multidrug resistant tuberculosis, *Escherichia coli, Psuedomonoas aeruginosa,* Methicillin-resistant *Staphylococcus aureus*

  3. Exchange of plasmids through pili, transfer of genetic material

TABLE 4-1 COMPARISON OF STERILIZATION METHODS

Method	Methodology	Advantages	Disadvantages
Steam under pressure	15–20 minutes 250–270°F 15–20 lb. pressure Coagulation of protein	Short cycle Good penetration Wide range of materials Packs may be used	Corrosion of instruments Dulls cutting edges Improper loading/poor penetration
Dry heat	1 hr, 320–350°F No pressure Oxidation of cell parts	Safe for metal instruments Does not dull cutting edge No rust, corrosion	Long cycle Poor penetration May destroy some materials
Unsaturated chemical vapor	20–30 minutes 270°F Automatic pressure Gas is toxic	Short cycle No rust, corrosion Does not dull edges Useful for orthodontic wire	Dry instruments before processing Destroys some plastics Ventilation needed
Ethylene oxide (ETO)	Room temp/8–10 hr 120°F 2–3 hours Gas is toxic	Safe for many materials Low temperature Reliable	Long cycle Expensive equipment Ventilation needed Aeration/24 hr.
Glutaraldehyde chloride dioxide	Immersion for 6–10 hours	Used for heat-sensitive items	Irritating to skin, lungs Unable to monitor

IV. Microbial Destruction (Table 4-1■)

A. Definitions of procedures

    1. *Sterilization*—Destruction of all life forms, including spores

    2. *Disinfectant*—Chemical used to kill pathogenic microorganisms on a inanimate object, such as a tabletop

    3. *Antiseptic*—Chemical used to kill pathogenic microorganisms on a living organism, such as the surface of the human body

    4. *Aseptic*—Free of microorganisms

    5. *Sanitize*—To reduce microbial populations to a safe level as determined by public health standards

B. Sterilization monitoring—Critical for infection control effectiveness

    1. Most reliable test of sterilization—Killing of live bacterial endospores

        a. Steam and chemical vapor—*Bacillus stearothermophilus* spores

        b. Dry heat and ethylene oxide—*Bacillus subtilis* var. niger spores

        c. Should be monitored weekly

        d. Accurate documentation must be kept

        e. Control (unexposed, unsterilized) incubated at same time

   2. Internal chemical indicators—"Slow change indicators"

     a. Dyes change color when heat, steam, or gas reaches *inside* of load

     b. Gives warning of gross sterilizer malfunction, *not* proof of sterility

   3. Chemical process indicators

     a. Dyes change color on short exposure to sterilizing conditions

     b. Not proof of sterilization, simply proof of instrument processing

   4. Item classification for sterilization, disinfection, and cleaning

     a. *Critical*—Items that penetrate oral soft tissue or bone; must be sterilized (e.g., surgical bur)

     b. *Semicritical* items—Items that come in contact with mucous membranes; must be sterilized (e.g., dental mirror)

     c. *Noncritical* items—Items that normally do not penetrate or contact mucous membranes, but that may be contaminated; require intermediate-level disinfection (e.g., dental chair)

   5. Sterilization failures

     a. Overloading—Steam, chemical, vapor cannot penetrate

     b. Improper packaging or timing

     c. Unit malfunction

     d. Improper unit operation or maintenance

C. Categories of chemical disinfectants (Table 4-2■)

   1. *High level*—Inactivates all forms of bacteria and spores, fungi, and viruses; high-level chemicals may also be classified as a sterilant, depending on length of contact with item

   2. *Intermediate level*—Inactivates many forms of microorganism spores

   3. *Low level*—Inactivates vegetative bacteria and some lipid-type viruses, does not destroy spores, tubercle bacilli, or nonlipid viruses such as polio

   4. Criteria that products should have

     a. EPA approval

     b. tuberculocidal, bacteriocidal, virucidal, and fungicidal effects

     c. acceptable shelf life, use life, reuse life, and adequate instructions for use

D. Other disinfectants

   1. Heavy metals—Mercury, copper, silver

   2. Alcohols—Skin antiseptics

     a. Ethyl alcohol—Reacts with organic matter, preclean

     b. Isoprophyl alcohol—"Rubbing alcohol," skin cleaner

   3. Hydrogen peroxide—Rinse to debride wounds; effective against anaerobic organisms

TABLE 4-2 COMPARISON OF DISINFECTANTS*

Disinfectant	Example	Scope	Advantages	Limitations
Halogens or chlorines	Sodium hypochlorite (bleach 1:10) EPA-registered surface	Broad spectrum: Bacteriocidal Viricidal Tuberculocidal	Inexpensive Rapid action Broad spectrum	Unstable, mix daily Must preclean Corrosive to metals Irritating to skin
	Chlorine dioxide Not EPA registered	Same as above	Same as above	Same as above Unable to monitor biologically
Synthetic phenols	Omni II EPA-registered surface	Broad spectrum: Tuberculocidal	Broad spectrum Compatible with most materials Residual action	Not sporicidal Mix daily May degrade some plastics Irritating to skin
	Chlorhexidine			Film accumulation Hard to rinse
Iodophors	Biocide EPA registered, Intermediate surface	Broad spectrum: Tuberculocidal Bactericidal Virucidal	Residual action Rapid actions Few reactions Broad spectrum	Stains surfaces Mix daily Inactivated by hard water Reacts with starch wipes
Glutaraldehyde	Cidex EPA registered immersion only— not surface	Chemical sterilant After 6–10 hours Most potent	Effective when immersed for long periods Active with organic matter	Prolonged time Rinse items Not for surfaces Severe tissue and lung irritation

*Disinfectants cannot be biologically monitored.

4. Soaps and detergents—Wetting agents, ionic (e.g., quaternary ammonium compounds); NOT acceptable as surface disinfectants

V. Infection Control during Dental Treatment

A. Equipment should be selected according to the ease of disinfection and degree of contamination

1. Minimal surfaces requiring contact with contaminated hands

a. Foot controls

b. Recessed waste containers with opening in countertop

2. Smooth construction—Minimal seams, buttons, exposed controls

3. Plastics, vinyls, laminates preferred

4. Carpet not recommended in treatment or laboratory areas

B. Surfaces should be compatible with disinfectants

C. Dental unit water lines (DUWL)—Reduce colony-forming units (CFU) or "biofilms" of microorganisms

    1. Water may be contaminated with pathogenic bacteria

        a. Gram-negative bacteria such as *Legionella pneumophila* (implicated in outbreaks of Legionnaire's disease)

        b. *Psuedomonas* dangerous to immunocompromised client

    2. Check antiretraction valves for effectiveness

    3. Self-contained water reservoir with sterile water

    4. Bacterial filtration unit in water line

    5. Flush lines at beginning of day for 3–5 minutes, 20–30 seconds between clients, and with disinfecting agent followed by rinse at end of day

D. General housekeeping—Clean surfaces not associated with client treatment routinely with soap and water, minimize surface clutter

E. Preparation for client care

    1. Surface-disinfect noncritical items (those that do not penetrate or contact mucous membranes) exposed to treatment contamination

        a. Use disposable covers whenever possible (e.g., light handles)

        b. Use sterile forceps, overgloves, or paper towels as bridge between contaminated area and noncontaminated area

    2. Effectiveness of surface disinfectant influenced by

        a. Number and type of microorganisms present

        b. "Bioburden"—Amount of organic matter (blood, saliva, or debris) on item being disinfected

        c. Disinfectant used: intermediate-level, Environmental Protection Agency (EPA) registered, tuberculocidal

        d. Appropriate viricidal and fungicidal activity

        e. Concentration and length of exposure—Follow manufacturer's direction

        f. Proper surface disinfection technique

            (1) Use heavy-duty gloves

            (2) Use approved agents such as iodophors, sodium hypochlorite, or complex phenols soaked in large gauze sponges

            (3) Effectiveness of disinfection includes the physical rubbing and removal of contaminated material and chemical inactivation of microorganisms

            (4) Leave the surface wet to disinfect

3. Use prearranged tray setups/cassettes, unit dose materials

4. Use disposables wherever appropriate

5. Surface barriers (single-use covers) when appropriate

F. Infection control during client care

    1. Reduce splatter, aerosol, and droplets

        a. Preprocedural rinse with antimicrobial mouthrinse

        b. Reduce aerosols during procedures

            (1) Use ventilation system with HEPA filtration

            (2) Use high-volume evacuation

            (3) Position client correctly

    2. Minimize cross-contamination

        a. Designate noncontaminated and contaminated zone

            (1) Use overgloves to go into noncontaminated zones

            (2) Avoid touching unprotected surfaces once gloves have become contaminated

            (3) Protect charts, radiographs from contamination

            (4) Use barriers such as paper towels

            (5) Only equipment and supplies necessary for treatment should be in the noncontaminated area

        b. Waste disposal

            (1) Immediately dispose of contaminated waste on tray in small biohazard bag

            (2) Wipe instruments to minimize bioburden

    3. Major source of healthcare worker (HCW) infection—Needlesticks

        a. Use special precautions when handling syringes and sharps

            (1) Angle sharp end away from HCW

            (2) Do not leave uncapped needles on tray

            (3) Never recap with a two-handed technique

                (a) Use "scoop" one-handed technique

                (b) Use commercially available needle capper

                (c) Hold cap with cotton pliers while recapping

                (d) Use the newer automatic recapping needles

        b. Never bend, break, or manipulate needles by hand

        c. Dispose in approved "sharps" container

        d. Exposure incident protocol

            (1) Treat any percutaneous incident as potentially infectious

(2) Immediately cleanse wound

  (a) Squeeze wound to promote bleeding

  (b) Cleanse under running water using antibacterial soap

  (c) Disinfect with bleach or iodophor

(3) Donor should be tested (same day) for anti-HIV and surface antigens to hepatitis B, hepatitis C—Confidentially should be maintained (only employee informed of results)

(4) Inform employer immediately: responsible for providing follow-up

(5) Exposed HCW tested for HIV, HBV, HCV on day of exposure and counseled regarding postexposure evaluation, vaccinations

(6) Although employer receives written report that employee was counseled, tested, informed of results, and needs further evaluation, findings are confidential

G. Post-treatment procedures

1. Treatment area decontamination

  a. All personal protective equipment (PPE) worn, including puncture-resistant nitrile gloves

  b. Removal of sharps and glass cartridges to approved container

  c. Flush water lines for 20–30 seconds

  d. Seal small biohazard bag, transport immediately to workplace-biohazard waste container

  e. Remove all disposable barriers; avoid contaminating clean surfaces

  f. Close instrument cassette; cover tray to avoid transporting airborne microorganisms

  g. If sterilization is delayed, place in holding solution to prevent bioburden from drying on instruments, sterilize ASAP

  h. Dispose of single-use items

  i. Clean suction tubing by flushing with commercial disinfecting solution

2. Infectious waste

  a. EPA regulates disposal and management of waste sharps, extracted teeth and tissue, blood and blood-soaked or blood-caked items; note: liquid or dried blood, saliva, and other body fluids are classified as other potentially infectious material (OPIM)

  b. State and local regulations may vary from EPA

  c. ADA Council on Government Affairs and Federal Dental Services categorize waste as

  (1) Regulated waste (biohazardous)

    (a) Sharps: needles, disposable syringes, broken instruments, suture needles, scalpel blades, burs, local anesthetic cartridges, soft tissues, teeth, and other body tissues

(b) Blood and blood-soaked items, liquid or semiliquid (OPIM)

(c) Articles caked with dried blood or OPIM

(2) Biomedical waste—Solid medical waste, disposable items other than items listed above

(a) Masks, gloves

(b) Saliva ejectors, surface barriers

(c) Disinfection wipes, paper towels

(d) Rubber cups, rubber dams

(e) Client cups, bibs

(f) May be disposed of with trash unless there are local or state restrictions to the contrary

d. Waste management

(1) Biohazardous waste must be labeled and separated from other waste

(2) Disposal dependent on regulatory agencies: incineration, burial, sterilization

3. Instrument care

a. Recirculation area should be centrally located for efficiency

b. Handle contaminated instruments with heavy-duty gloves only

c. Processing should flow from contaminated area to noncontaminated area

(1) Receiving area contaminated, presoaking, waste disposal

(a) Precleaning removes organic debris (bioburden) that interferes with sterilization

(2) Decontamination—Rinsing, ultrasonic cleaning, rinsing, drying

(a) Wet instruments interfere with sterilization from ethylene oxide and dry heat

(3) Packaging for sterilization

(4) Sterilization (may have more than one method)

(5) Storage

(6) Dispensing: trays prepared

d. Use separate area from treatment to avoid contamination from splatter

e. Ultrasonic cleaning safest, most efficient

(1) Follow manufacturer's directions

(2) Do not overload

(3) Cover unit to avoid aerosolization

(4) Manual scrub only when ultrasonic would damage equipment

VI. Protecting the Dental Healthcare Worker (DHCW)

A. Immunizations

    1. HBV—OSHA-required by employer to all workers with occupational exposure

        a. Recombinant DNA HB vaccine given in deltoid muscle at 0, 1, 6 months

        b. Postvaccination testing after last injection for presence of anti-HBV is recommended by CDC, but not required by OSHA

    2. Measles, mumps, rubella, tetanus, polio, chicken pox

    3. Optional: influenza, pneumococcal vaccine

    4. Boosters and reimmunization schedules should be maintained

B. Handwashing

    1. Reduces transient and resident microorganisms on skin

    2. Prevents person-to-person transmission

    3. Prevents autogenous infection if skin becomes broken

    4. Resident microorganisms: *Staphylococcus epidermis*, diphtheroids, micrococci

    5. Gloves are NOT a substitute for routine handwashing

    6. Wash before gloving, after carefully removing gloves, and after any break in glove

    7. Use effective liquid antiseptic soap (should be gentle and nonirritating)

        a. Remove any jewelry

        b. Short handwash

            (1) Begin day with two consecutive 15-second handwashes with soap and water

            (2) Wash hands for 15 seconds between clients, before and after eating, using lavatory, or any contamination

        c. Surgical hand scrub—Before surgical procedures with protocol posted

            (1) Five-minute scrub of hands, arms to elbow, with repeated scrub and rinse using antimicrobial soap and soft sterile brush

            (2) Dry with sterile towel

    8. Intact skin is a natural defense; use brush prudently

    9. Use foot control for sink, or use paper towels to turn on and off

    10. Keep nails short and cuticles groomed to avoid breaks in skin

    11. Personnel with weeping dermatitis or lesions with exudate should avoid contact with saliva and blood

    12. Recommended antimicrobial soaps

        a. Chlorhexidene gluconate 2% or 4%, with isopropyl (Bactoshield, Hibiclens)—Has substantivity

      b. Parachlorometaxylenol 3% (Banique 3, Derm-septic)

      c. Povidone iodine 7.5–10.00% (Betadine)

      d. Triclosan

C. Gloves

    1. Provide protection for client and oral health care worker

    2. Prevent direct contact with potentially infectious materials

    3. Cover abrasions and cuts that could be portals of entry for pathogenic microorganisms

    4. Documented cases of transmission of HIV, HBV, herpes viruses transmitted from DHCW who did not wear gloves

    5. Protocol for glove use

      a. Wear whenever anticipated contact with potentially infectious materials

      b. Wash hands before and after glove use

      c. Do NOT wash gloves with antiseptics; causes "wicking"

      d. Double gloving is NOT recommended

    6. Types of gloves

      a. Single-use nonsterile gloves (examination gloves) adequate for most procedures, fits both hands, sized extra-small to extra-large

        (1) Latex: powdered or unpowdered

        (2) Vinyl

        (3) Nonvinyl (hypoallergenic)

      b. Single-use plastic overgloves ("food-handler gloves")

        (1) Nontreatment

        (2) Worn over treatment gloves to prevent contamination

        (3) Plastic

      c. Heat-resistant gloves for handling hot items

    7. Latex hypersensitivity

      a. Providers should be aware of symptoms, associated risks

        (1) *Immediate hypersensitivity*—Eye itching, watering, coughing, wheezing, drop in blood pressure, anaphylaxis may occur within minutes of exposure (use epinephrine 1:1000 to treat anaphylaxis)

        (2) *Delayed hypersensitivity* (Type IV)—Most common; occurs 48 hours later; dry, cracked, irritated, or "weeping" skin (use diphenhydramine 50 mg to treat hypersensitivity)

      b. Document in medical/dental records

      c. Provide latex-free gloves and armamentarium

D. Protective barriers for mucous membranes

   1. Prevent exposure to droplets, aerosols, and splatter of potentially infectious particles (PIP)

   2. Masks—Prevents inhalation and direct contact with PIP and aerosols

      a. Effective masks filter 95% of particles 3.0–3.2 mcm with minimal leakage

      b. Types

         (1) Glass fiber

         (2) Synthetic fiber

         (3) Dome

         (4) Tie-on

         (5) Ear loop

      c. Disposable particulate respirator (PRM) for use in treating infectious tuberculosis

         (1) Tight face seal to protect against inhalation of droplet nuclei

         (2) Greater filtration—99% for particles larger than 1 micron

      d. Minimizing contamination

         (1) Use new mask for each client or if mask becomes wet (wicking)

         (2) Put mask on before handwash

         (3) Adjust mask to fit tightly against face

         (4) Avoid touching mask, protect from exposure to chemicals

         (5) Keep mask on after procedure to avoid inhaling aerosols

         (6) Remove mask overhead, touching only elastic or ties

   3. Protective eyewear is worn during treatment, disinfection, sterilization, and laboratory procedures

      a. Risk of exposure of eyes to harmful chemicals, debris, potentially infectious materials

      b. Eyewear must cover entire orbit (top and side shields)

      c. Face shields provide most protection, used as an adjunct to glasses and masks for aerosol-producing procedures

      d. Protective eyewear should be routinely provided to clients during treatment; be able to withstand immersion disinfection

      e. During treatment using ultraviolet radiation, special eyewear is needed

E. Protective clothing

   1. Provides coverage to skin and street clothes from potentially infectious materials such as blood and saliva

2. May be disposable or reusable

3. Isolation gown is prototype

    a. Covers street clothing completely

    b. Long-sleeved, high collar, fits closely at neck, wrists

    c. Should be fluid resistant

4. Do not wear outside practice setting

5. Work shoes should be kept in practice area

6. Additional coverage such as plastic aprons, head covers, and shoe covers may be utilized during invasive procedures generating splash and splatter

7. Laundry

    a. Handle sparingly, outside client treatment area

    b. Transport for laundry or disposal in sealed, leakproof bag

    c. Launder separately at temperatures of 60–70°C or more, normal bleach

    d. Dry at high temperature (100°C)

➤ DISEASE TRANSMISSION

I. The Infectious Disease Process

  A. Reservoir of infection

    1. Potential sources of disease agents

    2. Active disease cases, animals (zoonosis), water, food, soil

  B. Portal of exit—Mechanism for infectious agent to escape host (e.g., feces)

  C. Routes of transmission

    1. Direct contact

    2. Indirect contact (fomites, contamination)

    3. Accidental innoculation with instrument or needle

    4. Arthropods—Vectors such as ticks, fleas, spiders

II. The Immune System

  A. Nonspecific resistance

    1. Normal and indigenous flora (e.g., *S. epidermis*)

    2. Natural barriers: intact skin, mucous membranes, nasal hairs, stomach acid, cough reflex, secretions such as tears, mucus, vaginal fluids

    3. Blood components such as leukocytes

    4. Lymphatic system—Transports WBCs and removes foreign cells and debris via lymphatic vessels, lymph fluid, lymphocytes, and reticuloendothelial system

Review of Blood Components

Formed Elements (Cellular Components)

1. Erthryocytes (RBCs)—Function in oxygen transport through hemoglobin; disposal of CO_2, mature RBC has no nucleus
2. Leukocytes (WBCs)—Function in immune and inflammatory response; antigen–antibody response; phagocytosis—ingestion and disposal of invader by certain leukocytes
   a. Granular leukocytes
      - Polymorphonuclear neutrophils (PMNs)*
        No color when stained
        Most numerous inflammatory cell in any stage of infection
        55–65% of WBCs in blood, few in tissue
        First line of defense, first to respond, phagocytic
        Short-lived scavenger cell with powerful bacteriocidal enzymes: collagenase, lysozyme
      - Basophils (1% of WBCs in circulation)
        Stain blue
        Rich in granules of histamine, heparin, serotonin-released in allergic reaction
        React with IgE on sensitized surface of mast cells (in connective tissue of respiratory and GI tract)
      - Eosinophils*
        Stain red
        Mediate allergic response
        Reject parasitic worms
   b. Nongranular leukocytes
      - Monocytes
        3–8% of WBCs in normal circulating blood
        Lifespan of a few hours
        Migrate into tissue and become macrophages
        Take on characteristics of specific tissues, may live for months or years
        Macrophages attack pathogens, participate in immune response
      - Lymphocytes—Small cells, slightly larger than RBC, large nucleus with small amounts of cytoplasm
        Originate from blood-forming stem cells in bone marrow
        Each type of lymphocyte has cluster designation marker (epitopes) or CD markers expressed on their cell membrane (e.g., CD4+ helper cell)
        B lymphocytes or B cells—Bursa-derived cell, precursors of plasma cells that produce antibodies, concentrated in lymphoid tissue, participates in humoral immunity
        T lymphocytes or T cells—Thymus-derived cell that participates in cellular immunity
        Helper T cells—Help other immune cells to increase efficiency; presents macrophage with antigen to B cell, release lymphokines (chemicals that signal immune system)

(continued)

Cytotoxic T cells—Kills cells infected with viruses, intracellular bacterial pathogens, some tumors

Suppressor T Cells—Regulates immune response

Natural killer cells—Lymphocytes without membrane surface markings on B or T cells

Kill certain types of tumor and virus-infected cells

3. Thrombocytes (platelets)—Involved in blood coagulation

Fluid Portion of Blood

Plasma—90% water, 10% proteins (albumin, globulins, fibrinogen, nonprotein nitrogenous material, carbohydrates and fats, inorganic salts, and bicarbonate buffers)

*Indicates cell with phagocytic abilities

5. Inflammation

    a. The sum of the body's reaction to injury or invasion of pathogenic organisms

    b. The process by which repair and regeneration of damaged tissue takes place

    c. Some damage to host cell is directly related to inflammatory by-products

        (1) For example, collagenase released by PMNs to destroy invading bacteria also destroys collagen of principal gingival fibers as secondary result.

    d. Cardinal signs of inflammation—Usually related to effects of vasodilation

        (1) Heat

        (2) Redness or erythema

        (3) Edema

        (4) Pain

        (5) Loss of function

    e. Sequence of events during inflammatory process

        (1) Injury or introduction of invader

        (2) Immediate constriction of microcirculation

        (3) Dilatation of small blood vessels

        (4) Increased permeability of small blood vessels

        (5) Exudate leaves small blood vessels

        (6) Blood viscosity increases, causing microcirculation to decrease

        (7) Margination and pavementing of WBCs on edge of blood vessels

(8) WBCs go into tissue and phagocytose foreign material

(9) Cellular and tissue debris is removed

6. Antimicrobial substances produced by the body

    a. Lysozyme—Nonspecific enzyme found in tears, saliva that digests peptidoglycan of gram-positive bacteria

    b. Interferon—Antiviral protein produced on exposure to viruses, inhibits viral replication

    c. Complement—Group of proteins that function in a cascading series of immunological reactions, stimulated by antigen–antibody activity

    d. Interleukins—Lymphokyine produced by white blood cells that act on other white blood cells; important in cellular immunity

B. Specific resistance: immunity—A condition under which an individual is protected from disease, specific to individual disease-causing organism

    1. Active immunity—Developed after antigens enter the body and the antibody is produced in response

        a. *Naturally acquired*—Result of exposure to disease or developing illness (e.g., "catching chickenpox")

        b. *Artificially acquired*—Development of antibodies after intentional exposure to antigens (e.g., HBV immunization)

    2. Passive immunity—Antibodies enter body from an outside source

        a. *Naturally acquired* (congenital immunity)—Antibodies pass into fetal circulation from mother's bloodstream via the placenta; lasts 3–6 months

        b. *Artificially acquired*—Intentional injection of antibody-rich serum into circulation (e.g., gamma globulin)

    3. Cell-mediated immunity (CMI): protects against viral infections, fungi, some tumor cells, causes transplant rejection

        a. T lymphocytes produce cytokines (such as macrophage-activating factor) in response to altered cell surface

        b. T lymphocyte works with macrophages, B lymphocytes

        c. Responsible for delayed hypersensitivity response (Type IV)

    4. Humoral—Antibody-mediated immunity (AMI)

        a. Good against bacterial infections

        b. Upon stimulation, activated B lymphocytes transform into plasma cells

        c. Plasma cells produce antibodies

        d. Antibodies react with specific antigen

        e. Antigen–antibody complex activates complement, which destroys in the following ways

        (1) Bacteria are lysed

(2) Bacteria are more susceptible to phagocytosis

(3) Chemotaxis attracts PMNs and macrophages

(4) Histamine is released, amplifying inflammatory response

f. Five classes of immunoglobins (Ig) used interchangeably with "antibody"

(1) IgM—Largest, first to appear in circulation; starts agglutination and bacteriolysis

(2) IgA—Primary defense on exposed mucosal surfaces, secretory IgA in saliva, body cavities

(3) IgE—Major role in allergic reactions; sensitizes mast cells and basophils to release histamine, heparin starting Type I reactions

(4) IgG—Classic gamma globulin; 75% of circulating antibodies, "maternal antibody"; crosses placenta

(5) IgD—Trace antibody, probably regulator

C. Errors in the immune response

1. Hypersensitivity reactions—Exaggerated or inappropriate response that causes tissue damage, initiating antigen termed *allergen*

a. Type I—Classic, immediate, anaphylactic, IgE antibody mediated

(1) Mast cells, basophils, release of histamines, prostaglandins, heparin

(2) Genetic, affects 10% of population

(3) Asthma, urticaria, angioedema, "hay fever," anaphylaxis

(4) Allergens—Pollen, dust, pets, foods, medications

b. Type II—Cytotoxic, antibody reacts with cell surface antigen, causing cell death

(1) Complement activates

(2) Rh incompatibility: hemolytic disease of the newborn

(3) Blood transfusion reactions

c. Type III—Immune complex reactions, antibody reacts with soluble antigen, fixes complement, activating an "immune complex"

(1) Usually complexes adhere to macrophages and are destroyed

(2) If remain in circulation, cause blood vessel permeability, damage to blood vessels, tissue destruction results (Arthus reaction)

(3) May be cause of autoimmune diseases such as systemic lupus erythematosus

(4) Examples: serum sickness, farmer's lung, bacterial endocarditis

d. Type IV—Cell-mediated, delayed hypersensitivity

(1) Sensitized T lymphocyte interacts with antigen

(2) Lymphokines released, adversely affecting body cells

(3) Usually 48 hours after exposure to antigen

(4) Examples: contact dermatitis, TB skin test, poison ivy

(5) NO antibody involved

2. Autoimmune diseases (autoallergic)—Body usually recognizes itself and does not attack its own tissues

    a. Autoimmune disorders—Body attacks tissue as "nonself"

    b. Examples: rheumatoid arthritis, lupus erythematosus, Graves' disease

3. Immunosuppression—Increased susceptibility to infection due to defective functioning of immune system

    a. Examples

        (1) Drug induced: corticosteroids, cyclosporine; infections common

        (2) Acquired immunodeficiency syndrome (AIDS)—Irreversible disease caused by a defect in cell-mediated immunity that allows development of opportunistic infections and cancers, with a high mortality rate

           (a) Etiology—Lentivirus of human retrovirus family

           (b) Infects lymphocytes (especially CD4+ helper T cells), macrophages, and other immune defense cells

           (c) CDC definition—T-lymphocyte count < 200 cells or CD4+ < 14%, and any of the following conditions: candidiasis of bronchi, trachea, lungs, and esophagus; invasive cervical cancer, coccidiomycosis, cryptococcosis, cytomegalovirus, HIV-related encephalopathy, chronic herpes simplex, disseminated or extrapulmonary histoplasmosis, isoporiasis, Kaposi's sarcoma, Burkitt's or immunoblastic lymphoma, lymphoma of the brain, *Mycobacterium tuberculosis, M. avium, Pneumocystis carinii* pneumonia, recurrent pneumonia, progressive multifocal leukoencephalopathy, recurrent *Salmonella* septicemia, toxoplasmosis of the brain, and HIV wasting syndrome

           (d) Transmission: exposure to infected blood, sexual contact, perinatal, with cofactors such as genital herpes increasing transmission rate

           (e) Oral manifestations

                i) Kaposi sarcoma: neoplastic vascular, pigmented lesion of mucous membrane or skin (blue, purple, brown)

                ii) Oral and esophageal candidiasis

                iii) Herpetic lesions

                iv) Hairy leukoplakia

v) Linear gingival erythema, necrotizing ulcerative periodontitis

vi) Human papillomavirus

vii) Lymphoma

viii) Recurrent aphthous ulcers

(f) No known cure, treated with antiviral agents (synthetic nucleotide analogs such as azidothymidine (AZT), dedeoxyinosine (ddI), dedeoxycytidine (ddC), and protease inhibitors

D. Factors that affect immune response (host state)

1. Abnormal physical conditions

a. Congenital defects of heart, kidney

b. Trauma, burns, surgery, infection, or inflammatory condition

(1) Entrance for pathogenic microorganism

(2) Altered physiological defense

2. Systemic diseases

a. Alcoholism

b. Diabetes mellitus

c. Neoplasms such as leukemia

d. Immunosuppressive disorders such as HIV

e. Malnutrition

f. Genetic disorders such as chemotactic leukocyte defect

3. Prostheses and transplants

a. Nidus for infection

b. Therapy may include suppression of normal immune response to avoid transplant rejection

4. Drug therapy

a. Steroids suppress immune response

b. Chemotherapeutic agents suppress immune response

5. Extreme youth or age

a. Infant dependent on maternal antibodies for first 3–6 months

b. Decreased immune response in elderly

➤ INFECTIOUS DISEASES SPECIFIC TO THE DENTAL HEALTH PROVIDER

Infections of Epithelial Tissues

I. Viral Infections

A. Herpes simplex

   1. Etiological agent—Herpes simplex viruses HSV 1 (oral) and HSV 2 (genital), even in health it is present in saliva

   2. Transmitted through oral or ocular secretions and also through fomites

   3. Retrovirus establishes latent infection in nerve ganglion; reactivates on stress, sunlight, illness

   4. Acute herpetic gingivostomatitis in children

      a. Fever, malaise, localized lymphadenopathy, anorexia, numerous yellow vesicles that rupture and ulcerate, leaving erythemic margins

      b. Painful, duration 7 days, palliative treatment, usually self-limiting

   5. Herpetic whitlow—Infection of fingers

   6. Herpes labialis—"Cold sores, fever blisters," erythematous base with vesicles; prodromal burning and tingling

   7. Ocular herpes—May cause blindness; attacks conjunctiva and cornea

   8. Treatment—Antiviral agents such as acyclovir

B. Varicella zoster virus—Etiological agent for chickenpox, herpes zoster (shingles)

   1. Chickenpox—Mode of transmission: mucosa of upper respiratory tract via droplets

      a. Highly infectious childhood disease

      b. Clinical symptoms—Fever, malaise, rash with vesicle formation

      c. Oral lesions may occur

      d. Vaccine available

   2. Shingles—Reactivation of latent virus in dorsal root ganglion of sensory nerves

      a. Follows nerve pathway—Thoracic area most commonly affected, ophthalmic division of trigeminal nerve second most common

      b. Same etiology as chickenpox, different manifestation of infection

      c. Primarily affects adults: malaise, fever, severe pain with rash and vesicles

      d. Occurs along nerve trunk

C. Measles

   1. Etiology—Rubeola virus

   2. Mode of transmission—Respiratory droplets spreading to lymphoid tissue

    3. Virus is spread throughout epithelial body surfaces

        a. Koplik's spots—First clinical sign; small spots on buccal mucosa

        b. Skin rash follows, fever, may have secondary bacterial infections

    4. Vaccine available

  D. Rubella virus (German measles)

    1. Mode of transmission—Respiratory droplets

    2. Clinical findings—Malaise, low-grade fever, rash, lymphadenopathy

    3. Vaccine available

  E. Mumps (infective parotiditis)

    1. Etiology—Paramyxovirus

    2. Mode of transmission—Respiratory droplets

    3. Inflammation of parotid gland, meninges, testicles

    4. Vaccine available

  F. Infectious mononucleosis

    1. Etiology—Epstein-Barr virus; also causes hairy leukoplakia (HIV+), chronic fatigue syndrome, Burkitt's lymphoma (HIV+), and some nasopharyngeal tumors

    2. Mode of transmission—Direct contact with saliva

II. Bacterial Infections

  A. Lyme disease

    1. Etiological agent—Spirochete *Borrelia burgdorferi*

    2. Mode of transmission—Deer tick bites

    3. Neurological and arthritic problems caused by antigen–antibody complex (type III hypersensitivity reaction)

    4. Clinical findings—Bulls-eye lesion, headaches, fever, myalgia, lymphadenopathy, cardiac disease, neurological problems, arthritis

    5. Vaccine available

  B. Tetnus

    1. Etiology—*Clostridium tetani*

    2. Mode of transmission—Spores enter anaerobic wound site, produce tetanus toxin (usually "puncture wound")

    3. Clinical findings: Trismus or "lock-jaw," facial muscle spasms, dysphagia, breathing difficulty

    4. Vaccine available

C. Streptococcal infections

  1. Etiology—*Streptococcus pyogenes* (group A beta-hemolytic)

  2. Mode of transmission—Rapidly spreads from portal of entry

  3. Clinical findings

    a. Scarlet fever—Acute upper respiratory tract inflammation; bright red oral mucosa; sequelae include rheumatic fever and hemorrhagic glomerulonephritis

    b. Erysipelas—"Invasive strep," angry skin eruptions

D. Staphylococcal infections

  1. Etiology—*Staphylococcus aureus*

  2. Mode of transmission—Entry into wound

  3. Clinical findings—Furuncles (boils), carbuncles, impetigo, "scalded baby syndrome"

  4. Carried in anterior nares, fomites such as stethoscopes

  5. Most strains resistant to penicillin—Methicillin-resistant *Staphlylococcus aureus* (MRSA); serious problem in hospitals

  6. Common nosocomial infection

E. *Pseudomonas aeruginosa* infections

  1. Common in water supplies and dental unit water lines

  2. Pathogenic in immunocompromised client, burn victims, common nosocomial infection

  3. Clinical findings—External ear infections, rash associated with hot tubs, swimming pools

III. Fungal Infections

A. Candidiasis

  1. Etiology—*Candida albicans,* normal part of flora of skin, mucosa

  2. Opportunistic infection manifested in immunocompromised patients

  3. Predisposing factors—Use of broad-spectrum antibiotics, immunological defects (HIV), diabetes mellitus, pregnancy, and malnutrition

  4. Clinical findings

    a. Intraoral lesions

    b. Angular chelitis (perleche)—Infection at corner of mouth; may be secondarily infected with *S. aureus*

➤ RESPIRATORY TRACT INFECTIONS

I. Upper Respiratory Tract Infections

A. "Common cold"

  1. Etiology—Rhinovirus, adenovirus, coronavirus, respiratory syncyntial virus

  2. Clinical findings—Nasal obstruction, "runny nose," sore throat, cough, dyspnea

  3. Self-limiting, palliative treatment only

B. Diphtheria

  1. Etiology—*Corynebacterium diphtheriae*

  2. Pathogenesis—Droplets carry bacteria into mucous membrane; damage caused by systemic toxin

   a. Edema, lymphadenopathy of neck

   b. Pseudomembrane on tonsils; blocks airway

  3. Vaccine available

  4. Detected with Schick test

C. Streptococcal pharyngitis ("strep throat")

  1. Etiology—*Streptococcus pyogenes*

  2. Mode of transmission—Respiratory droplets, ingestion of contaminated substance

  3. Clinical findings—Severe inflammation of throat and tonsils, pain, fever

II. Lower Respiratory Tract Infections

A. Tuberculosis (TB)

  1. Etiology—*Mycobacterium tuberculosis*

  2. Mode of transmission—Inhalation of droplet nuclei, direct inoculation, ingestion of contaminated food or water. Long incubation period: 28–47 days

  3. Risk factors—Immunocompromised patient, chronic alcoholism, diabetes mellitus, HIV, poor nutrition, prolonged contact with those with disease

  4. Clinical symptoms—Early: low-grade fever, weight loss, fatigue, slight cough; later: elevated temperature in afternoon, night sweats, weakness, persistent cough (may be bloody)

  5. Diagnosis—Positive purified derivative (PPD) of TB injected subcutaneously as Mantoux skin test; reaction to test indicates need for chest x-ray

   a. Positive skin test indicates antibodies exist, not necessarily active TB

   b. HIV patients with TB may test negatively due to anergy

  6. Multidrug resistant TB occurs when medication is not taken properly

7. T-cell-mediated, HIV patients at high risk due to lack of T-cell response

8. Granulomas called tubercles; tissue destruction: caseous necrosis

B. Pertussis or "whooping cough"

    1. Etiology—*Bordetella pertussis*

    2. Clinical findings—Paroxysmal cough

    3. Vaccine available

C. Pneumonia—Inflammation of lungs, caused by many species of microorganisms

    1. Bacterial

        a. Pneumococcal pneumonia

           (1) Etiology—*Streptococcus pneumoniae*

           (2) Spread by droplets, carrier state exists

           (3) Risk factors—Extremes of age, lowered resistance, bacteremia

           (4) Clinical findings—Sudden onset of high fever, chills, chest pain, dry cough

           (5) Vaccine available

        b. *Klebsiella pneumoniae*—More serious; common in alcoholics; immunocompromised

    2. Mycoplasmal pneumonia, or "walking pneumonia"; mild presentation

    3. Fungal—*Pneumocystis pneumonia*

        a. Spores inhaled

        b. Disease occurs in immunocompromised (e.g., HIV)

    4. *Chlamydia pneumoniae*—Intracellular organisms

    5. Viral pneumonia—Many viruses implicated

D. Legionnaire's disease

    1. Etiology—*Legionella pneumonphilia*

    2. Mode of transmission—Inhalation of contaminated aerosols

    3. Clinical findings—Influenza-like disease with pneumonia, GI hemorrhage, respiratory failure

    4. Multiplies in municipal water supplies; cultured from dental unit water lines

E. Influenza

    1. Etiology—Rapidly mutating virus

    2. Mode of transmission—Airborne droplets, contact with contaminated object

    3. Clinical findings—Body aches, fever, headaches, dry cough, malaise

    4. Secondary bacterial infections may lead to more serious illness

    5. Vaccine available, recommended for DHCW

F. Histoplasmosis

    1. Etiology—Fungus: *Histoplasma capsulatum*

    2. Mode of transmission—Inhalation of spores carried in feces of birds and bats

    3. Clinical findings—Skin lesions, meningitis

    4. Indigenous to Mississippi River valley; common infection among farmers

G. *Hantavirus* pulmonary virus

    1. Etiology—*Hantavirus*

    2. Mode of transmission—Inhalation of deer mice excretions

    3. Clinical findings—Severe respiratory distress, rapid onset, hemorrhage of lungs

H. Cytomegalovirus (CMV)

    1. Etiology—Cytomegalovirus (herpes virus)

    2. Mode of transmission—Congenital, contact with body fluids, inhalation of respiratory droplets, especially in children in day-care settings

    3. Clinical findings—Infectious mononucleosis, pneumonitis, severe disease manifestations in the fetus; including fetal death, prematurity, retardation, blindness, chronic liver disease

    4. Serious complications in the immunodeficient patient

➤ INFECTIONS OF THE GASTROINTESTINAL TRACT

I. Viral Infections (Table 4-3■)

A. Hepatitis A (HAV)

    1. Mode of transmission—Oral-fecal route due to contaminated food or water, personal contact in unsanitary conditions, blood transfusions in early stage of active disease (rare)

    2. Clinical findings—Disease occurs much more frequently in children, who present with few if any signs and symptoms

        a. Preicteric phase—Abrupt onset of influenza-like illness, fever, headaches, vomiting, nausea, abdominal pain, tender, palpable liver

        b. Icteric phase—Rare in children, continuation of symptoms for days to a month; anicteric form (without jaundice) two to three times more prevalent; 90% of patients recover completely

        c. Immunity—Anti-HAV detectable in blood within 2 weeks of onset

            (1) Immunity follows infection

            (2) No carrier state

            (3) Vaccine (Havrix) available; early immunization recommended

                (a) Food handlers, travelers to foreign countries, children

                (b) Administered 2 weeks before expected exposure; booster for adults

TABLE 4-3   COMPARISON OF HEPATITIS VIRUSES

Etiological Agent	Incubation (I) and Communicable Period (C)	Vaccine

Hepatitis A (HAV)	I—15–50 days
	C—2–3 weeks before jaundice
		Havrix
		    Given to children
		    Foreign travelers
		    Military
		    Food handlers
		    Day care workers

Hepatitis B (HBV)	I—45–160 days
	C—presence of HbsAg
	Carrier state: 5–10%
		Genetically engineered vaccine
		Recombivax
		    Children
		    Healthcare workers
		    Military

Hepatitis C (HCV)	I—2–26 weeks C—chronic in 50–85%/carrier	None exists
Hepatitis D (HDV)	I—uncertain C—uncertain	Vaccine for HBV confers immunity
Hepatitis E (HEV)	I—15–60 days C—duration of illness	None
Hepatitis G	Unknown	None

B. Hepatitis B

  1. Mode of transmission—Blood-borne pathogen, percutaneous and permucosal exposure, infected blood transfusions (screened since 1985), exposure to infected body fluids or contaminated needles, and perinatal transmission

  2. Terms to know

   a. Hepatitis B surface antigen (HBsAg) (Australian antigen)—Surface marker in acute, chronic, and carrier states of HBV

   b. Antibody to hepatitis B surface antigen (anti-HBsAg)—Represents immunity

   c. Hepatitis B e antigen (HBeAg)—High titer indicates high infectivity or development of chronic liver disease and carrier state

   d. Antibody to hepatitis B e antigen (anti-HBeAg)—Indicates low infectivity

   e. Hepatitis B core antigen (HBcAg)—Indicates acute, chronic, or resolved state

f. Antibody to HBcAg (anti-HBcAg)—Indicates prior HBV infection

g. IgM class antibody to hepatitis B core antigen (IgM anti-HBc)—Indicates recent HBc infection

3. Clinical findings

   a. HBV infection (does not occur in response to vaccine)

   b. Similar to HAV, although slower onset and longer duration

   c. Most patients asymptomatic, but jaundice and acute disease do occur

   (1) Symptoms described above with some skin rashes, itching, joint pain

   (2) End of icteric phase corresponds with recovery

   (3) 5–10% will develop carrier state

   (a) HbsAg detectable after 6 months

   (b) Carriers usually asymptomatic and undetected

   (c) High incidence of cirrhosis or hepatocellular carcinoma (cancer of liver)

4. Immunity

   a. Serologic presence of anti-HBsAg indicates immunity

   b. Vaccines available

   (1) Early vaccine derived using inactivated HBsAg from plasma of chronic HBV carriers (Heptavax)

   (2) Recombinant DNA HB vaccine: uses recombinant DNA technology to synthesize HBsAg in yeast culture (Recombivax HB)

   (a) 99% immunity in children, drops to 95% in adults

   (b) Three doses: 0, 1, 6 months; postvaccination testing within 1 month for high-risk groups, including DHCW

   (c) Better response when injection is given in deltoid muscle rather than buttock

   (3) Passive immunization for postexposure prophylaxis—Hepatitis B immune globulin given within 24–48 hours of exposure

C. Hepatitis C (formerly known as transfusion-associated non-A, non-B hepatitis)

   1. Mode of transmission—Percutaneous exposure to contaminated blood and plasma products (blood now tested in the United States), IV drug use, sexual transmission, perinatal exposure

   2. Clinical findings—Insidious onset, few or no clinical symptoms, some patients develop abdominal discomfort, nausea and vomiting, few develop icteric phase; chronic liver disease develops in 50–85%, progresses to liver cancer or cirrhosis

   3. Prevention—Universal precautions, testing of donated blood

D. Hepatitis D (formerly delta hepatitis)

    1. Mode of transmission—HDV cannot cause infection without presence of HBV

        a. Occurs after multiple exposures to HBV such as IV drug users or patients with hemophilia

        b. Similar transmission to HBV: contaminated blood, body fluids, contaminated needles, sexual contact, perinatal transfer

    2. Clinical findings—Severe infection (coinfection or superinfection of HBV), abrupt onset, may cause fulminant hepatitis

E. Hepatitis E (formerly known as enterically transmitted non-A, non-B hepatitis)

    1. Mode of transmission—Oral-fecal, enteric, outbreaks associated with contaminated water sources, inadequate sewage disposal

    2. Clinical findings—Nausea, vomiting, high mortality in pregnant women

    3. Prevention—Proper sanitation, handwashing before food handling

F. Hepatitis G

    1. Mode of transmission—Bloodborne, coinfection with HCV

    2. Disease modality still unknown

II. Bacterial Infections

A. Food poisoning agents (often toxin producing)

    1. Botulism

        a. Etiology—*Clostridium botulinum*

        b. Mode of transmission—Contaminant of food products (improperly cooked or preserved)

        c. Clinical findings—Toxin produced; nerve damage causes speaking difficulties, inability to swallow, heart failure, respiratory paralysis

        d. Sudden infant death syndrome may be linked to infant botulism

    2. Staphylococcal food poisoning

        a. Etiology—Staphylococci (usually *S. aureus*) produced toxin from unrefrigerated foods

        b. Clinical findings—Violent vomiting, diarrhea 1–8 hours after ingestion of enterotoxin

➤ OTHER IMPORTANT DISEASES

I. Sexually Transmitted Diseases

A. Syphilis

    1. Etiology—*Treponema pallidum* (anaerobic spirochete)

2. Mode of transmission—Primarily by sexual contact with skin or mucous membranes

3. Spirochete crosses the placenta—Congenital syphilis occurs

4. Spirochete can pass through break in skin, intact mucous membranes

5. Organisms spread rapidly through lymphatic system and bloodstream, affecting all organs

6. Clinical findings

    a. Primary stage: single granulomatous lesion at point of contact ("chancre")

        (1) Asymptomatic

        (2) Highly contagious

        (3) Lasts 3–5 weeks, heals spontaneously with no scar

    b. Secondary stage—Patient may be asymptomatic for 2–6 months before symptoms occur

        (1) Flulike symptoms

        (2) Shallow, painless ulcers—"Mucous patches" on lips, soft palate, and tongue that are highly contagious

        (3) Swollen lymph nodes

        (4) Maculopapular rashes on face, hands, feet

    c. Tertiary stage—May take years to develop

        (1) "Gumma"—Inflammatory granulomatous lesions on tongue, perforating palate, facial bones

        (2) Gumma is not contagious, usually asymptomatic

        (3) Central nervous system (CNS) involvement leads to loss of fine motor coordination, personality changes

        (4) Major cause of death—Cardiovascular system involvement

    d. Congenital syphilis: Hutchinson's triad

        (1) Tooth development affected

            (a) Hutchinson's incisors—Notched, "screwdriver" appearance

            (b) "Mulberry molars"—Irregular first molars

        (2) Cranial nerve damage

            (a) Deafness

            (b) Impaired vision

            (c) Meningitis

        (3) Poor formation of long bones

        (4) High infant mortality rate

B. Gonorrhea

    1. Etiology: *Neisseria gonorrhoeae,* a gram-negative, aerobic diplococcus

    2. Mode of transmission—Sexual contact spreads microorganism throughout genitourinary tract into reproductive system, causing pelvic inflammatory disease (PID)

    3. Clinical findings

        a. Women at higher risk than are men

            (1) Usually asymptomatic

            (2) May have vaginal discharge, backache, abdominal pain

        b. Men may experience frequent, painful urination

        c. Gonoccoccal glossitis, pharyngitis

            (1) Oral infection including pharyngitis, glossitis, stomatitis

            (2) May include areas of ulceration, tissue sloughing

        d. Gonococcal ophthalmia—newborn's eyes may become infected during birth, treating eyes with 1% silver nitrate prevents blindness

        e. Complications include sterility, meningitis, disseminated infections

C. Chlamydia (chlamydial urethritis or nongonococcal urethritis (NGU)

    1. Etiology—*Chlamydia trachomatis*

    2. Mode of transmission—Sexual contact (grows only in living tissue)

    3. Clinical findings—Gonorrhea-like symptoms, although milder

        a. Leading cause of PID, sterility in women

        b. Called "silent epidemic," affecting 3–5 million women annually in United States

    4. Chlamydial ophthalmia—Disease affecting eyes of infant born to an infected mother; requires erythromycin therapy to prevent blindness

    5. Chlamydial pneumonia—Develops in exposed infants, implicated in myocardial infarctions in adults

D. Human papillomavirus (HPV)

    1. Etiology—HPV are a diverse group of DNA-based viruses that infect the skin and mucous membranes of humans

    2. Mode of transmission—Typically transmitted through sexual contact and infect the anogenital region

    3. Clinical findings

        a. HPV infection is a necessary factor in the development of nearly all cases of cervical cancer

        b. Genital warts—The most easily recognized sign of genital HPV infection

        c. HPV-1 and HPV-2 cause *common* skin warts

4. Human papillomavirus (HPV) vaccine targets certain sexually transmitted strains of human papillomavirus that are associated with the development of cervical cancer and genital warts; the only HPV vaccine currently on the market is Gardasil; a second vaccine, Cervarix, is currently in clinical trials

II. Diseases of the Circulatory System

A. Rheumatic fever

1. Etiology: beta-hemolytic group A streptococcus

2. Mode of transmission—Hypersensitivity reaction developing after streptococcal infection; inflammation of heart valves, abnormal growth of connective tissue, valve scarring occurs

3. Clinical findings—Fever, polyarthritis, malaise, inflammation of heart (carditis)

4. Sequelae of carditis

   a. Defective heart valves

      (1) Narrowing of valve opening—Stenosis

      (2) Failure of valve to close completely—Valvular insufficiency

B. Infective endocarditis (bacterial endocarditis, subacute bacterial endocarditis)

1. Etiology—Microbial invasion of heart valves or endocardium, usually associated with normal flora of respiratory or intestinal tract

   a. Usually streptococci (α-hemolytic) and staphylococci

   b. Yeasts, fungi, and viruses have also been implicated

2. Mode of transmission—Dental procedures may introduce microorganisms into bloodstream (bacteremia), and they lodge on defective heart valves

3. Risk factors

   a. Cardiac abnormalities such as heart valves damaged by rheumatic fever, congenital heart defects, prosthetic heart valves, and arteriosclerosis

   b. Intravenous drug users

   c. Infections at portals of entry; poor oral hygiene, trauma to oral tissues (dental procedures)

   d. Individuals with compromised immune response

4. Clinical findings

   a. Symptoms appear within 2 weeks

   b. Fever, malaise, anemia, weakness, arthralgia, muscle weakness, and heart murmur

   c. Vegetative clusters of microorganisms lead to emboli, diminished heart function

   d. High mortality rate, susceptibility to reinfection

5. Consult with physician, prophylactic antibiotic premedication required

6. Stress importance of oral health to prevent nidus of infection

III. Infections of the Nervous System and Sensory Organs

A. Meningitis—Inflammation of the covering of the brain

    1. Etiology—Variety of causes, high mortality rate

        a. Aseptic meningitis—Caused by viruses, bacteria, chemicals, mycoplasms, and chlamydias

           (1) Acute onset, stiff neck, severe headache, fever

        b. Meningococcal meningitis—*Neisseria meningitidis*

           (1) Mode of transmission—Inhalation of respiratory droplets

           (2) Headache, stiff neck, vomiting, coma within hours

        c. Haemophilus meningitis—*Haemophilus influenzae b*

           (1) Mode of transmission—Inhalation of respiratory droplets

           (2) Respiratory disease, stiff, arched neck, headache

           (3) Primarily affects children, HIB vaccine available

B. Rabies

    1. Etiology—Rabies virus

    2. Mode of transmission—Bite of rabid animal

    3. Incubation period of 4–6 weeks

    4. Clinical findings—Painful throat spasms, inability to swallow, convulsions, respiratory paralysis, and death

C. Poliomyelitis

    1. Etiology—Poliomyelitis virus

    2. Mode of transmission—Oral route into intestines

    3. Clinical findings—Destruction of motor neurons in spinal cord, leading to flaccid paralysis (may be mild to severe)

    4. Vaccine available

D. Toxoplasmosis

    1. Etiology—*Toxoplasma gondii*

    2. Mode of transmission—Contact or inhalation of contaminated cat feces, raw meat, soil, rodents, or through placenta to fetus

    3. Clinical findings—Age dependent

        a. Adults—Resembles infectious mononucleosis

        b. Congenital infection—Stillbirth, severe psychomotor defects, blindness, deafness

    E. Cryptococcoses

        1. Etiology—*Cryptococcus neoformans*

        2. Mode of transmission—Inhalation of dehydrated fungus from bird droppings (especially pigeons)

        3. Clinical findings—Meningitis common in immunocompromised patients; disseminated disease affects skin, lungs, and other organs

    F. Conjunctivitis—Inflammation of eye, various causes

        1. Etiology

            a. Bacterial: *Haemophilus aegyptius*—Common in warm climates, purulent discharge from eyes

            b. Viral

                (1) Chlamydia *trachomatis* (trachoma)

                    (a) Associated with poor sanitation and personal hygiene

                    (b) Inflammation of conjunctiva: scarring, secondary infection, partial or complete blindness

                (2) Coxsackievirus A 24—Hemorrhagic conjunctivitis

                (3) Ocular herpes

                    (a) Herpetic keratoconjunctivitis; corneal ulcers

                    (b) May recur

                    (c) May cause blindness

                    (d) Use of safety glasses has greatly reduced incidence in health care workers

➤ MICROORGANISMS OF THE ORAL CAVITY

I. Normal Oral Environment

    A. Composition of oral flora influenced by many factors

        1. Nutrients available

            a. Nutrients—Fermentable carbohydrates and amino acids required

                (1) Exogenous sources—Dietary sugars from host's diet provide acid and extracellular, insoluble carbohydrates (dextrans, glucans) that provides adhesion mechanism to tooth surface

                (2) Endogenous sources such as gingival exudate, saliva, epithelial cells and leukocytes, and metabolic by-products from other bacteria

        2. pH requirements—Dietary sugars provide an acidic medium

            a. Bacteria that are *aciduric* (tolerant of low pH values) and *acidogenic* (acid producing) become predominant

                (1) *Mutans Streptococcus* and related strains of streptococci

                (2) Lactobacilli

b. Lactic acid produced by breakdown of fermentable carbohydrates (primarily sucrose); starches implicated to a lesser extent

c. If acidogenic plaque is exposed to sugar, immediate acid production may cause pH to drop low enough to decalcify tooth surface in minutes

(1) Below 4.5 for enamel, 6.0–6.7 for root surfaces

(2) Depending on salivary flow and amount of plaque, pH remains low for 20–120 minutes after each sugar exposure

3. Concentration of oxygen—Plaque is predominantly a Gram-positive, facultative mass, even on exposed surfaces

4. Saliva flow

a. Adequate flow rate is necessary to decrease susceptibility to caries

(1) Needed to buffer salivary acids

(2) Flow helps remove bacteria from oral structures

b. Provides components for bacterial attachment to teeth; components may also inhibit bacterial growth or attachment to teeth

(1) Glycoprotein's high molecular weight inhibits adherence

(2) Secretory IgA inhibits microbial attachment

(3) Antibacterial components (lysosyme, lactoperoxidase)

B. Composition of oral microbiota

1. Mucous membranes—Type of surface affects type and number of microorganisms present

a. Cheek—Predominantly *S. sanguis, S. salivarius*

b. Gingival crevice—Predominantly *B. melaninogenicus*

c. Tongue—*S. salivarius*

d. Streptococci most common species in healthy mouth, make up over 50% of mass

2. Saliva—Organisms derived from plaque and tongue (e.g., *S. salivarius*)

3. Tongue, large surface area provided by papilla

4. Gingival sulcus—As cleaning ability decreases, bacteria proliferate, gingival crevicular fluid increases, pathogenicity increases

a. As the periodontal pocket deepens, flora changes from gram-positive, motile aerobes to predominately gram-negative, nonmotile anaerobes

b. Periodontal pocket primary source of periodontal pathogens

5. Tooth surface plaque (* indicates ability to cause caries)

a. Smooth surfaces—*S. sanguis* first colonizer, will be replaced by *Mutans Streptococcus*

b. Most strongly cariogenic bacteria in animals, *S. milleri**, *S. mitior*, and *S. sobrinus** as plaque remains undisturbed on tooth surface

  (1) *Mutans Streptococcus* requires hard surface, will disappear with extractions, reappears with denture placement

   (a) Homofermentive lactic acid former

   (b) Produces insoluble glucans as attachment mechanism to tooth

   (c) High-sucrose diet associated with increase in *Mutans Streptococcus*

  (2) *Mutans Streptococcus* most closely associated with caries in epidemiological studies

c. Occlusal pits and fissures—Morphology allows plaque to remain undisturbed; common caries site; causative organisms include

  (1) *Mutans Streptococcus**

  (2) Acidogenic lactobacilli* (increase as sugar intake increases)

   (a) Causative role in caries not as strong as other species

   (b) Carious lesions act as retention sites

   (c) Found mainly in fissures

d. Interproximal surfaces—Difficulty in access in cleansing allows plaque to proliferate; *Mutans Streptococcus** most common species

e. Root surfaces—Apical migration of the gingival margin exposes cementum

  (1) Extremely susceptible to caries

  (2) *Mutans Streptococcus* (also causative organism in root surface caries)

  (3) *Actinomyces viscosus, A. naeslundii* ferment glucose to lactic acid; primary species implicated in root caries

f. Prerequisites for caries formation

  (1) Cariogenic bacteria

  (2) Nutrient source (fermentable carbohydrates) of substrate for acid production; increase in dietary sucrose will increase cariogenic bacteria

  (3) Ability to produce extracellular, insoluble glucans for adhesion to tooth structure

  (4) Susceptible host

C. Supragingival plaque

  1. Thin layer of 1–20 cells

  2. Mostly gram-positive facultative anaerobic organisms

   a. *S. sanguis, A. viscosus, A. naeslundii* predominate

   b. Other species include *A. israelii, Mutans Streptococcus, Veillonella, Fusobacterium,* and *Treponema capnocytophaga*

D. Subgingival plaque results from apical migration of supragingival plaque

    1. Early in the disease, supragingival plaque influences the subgingival population

    2. As periodontal disease progresses, the flora changes to more anaerobic, gram-negative, nonmotile forms

II. Microbiology of Periodontal, Periapical, and Oral-Facial Diseases

A. *Gingivitis*—Gingival inflammation in response to bacterial plaque and its metabolic by-products; reversible as compared with:

    1. Early stages

        a. Plaque up to 100 times thicker than in health, and is more complex

        b. Predominated by *Actinomyces* species and Gram-positive organisms

    2. Chronic—Increase in Gram-negative, anerobic organisms

        a. Rods predominate

        b. *Actinomyces, Fusobacterium, Bacteroides,* and spirochetes present

B. *Chronic periodontitis*—Inflammatory changes extend into deeper periodontal structures, resulting in loss of alveolar bone

    1. Deepening periodontal pocket provides favorable environment for bacteria

    2. May be multiple diseases with similar characteristics, having different bacterial populations

    3. Progression is usually episodic, dependent on effectiveness of host response

    4. Microorganisms include

        a. *Prevotella intermedia*

        b. *Porphyromonas gingivalis*

        c. *Fusobacterium* species

        d. Spirochetes

        e. *Eubacterium* species

        f. *Bacteroides forsythus*

        g. *Campylobacter rectus*

C. Aggressive periodontitis (formerly "Early-Onset Periodontitis," prepubertal and juvenile periodontitis)—Associated with immune defects; neutrophils or monocytes have defective chemotaxis or impaired function

    1. Genetic or familial tendency

    2. Prepubertal disease may affect primary teeth

    3. Disease may be localized or generalized

        a. Localized lesions affecting permanent first molars and/or incisors

        b. Generalized disease results in rapid overall pattern of bone loss

    4. Atypical—Sparse amounts of thin plaque

     5. Microbiota present

        a. *Capnocytophaga* species (invades tissue, rare in children)

        b. *Actinobacillus actinomycetemcomitans*

        c. *Prevotella intermedius, Eikenella corrodens*

        d. *Porphyromonas gingivalis*

     6. Gram-negative, anaerobic bacteria predominate

     7. Host defense defective, usually impaired neutrophil function

     8. Associated with rapid loss of alveolar bone

  D. Necrotizing periodontal diseases—Acute anaerobic infection causing ulceration of gingival margins; may progress to destruction of gingiva and underlying bone

     1. Interproximal areas affected first; may result in loss of cratering of interdental papilla

     2. Predisposing factors include smoking, stress, poor nutrition, and poor oral hygiene

     3. Symptoms include foul odor, extreme pain, sloughing of gingiva

     4. Predominant microorganisms

        a. *P. intermedia*

        b. Intermediate-sized spirochetes (*Treponema* species)

        c. *Fusobacterium* species

     5. Such rapid destruction of periodontal attachment and bone occurs that pocketing is not present, alveolar bone may be exposed with sequestration

     6. Localized or generalized

     7. Occurs in HIV-infected person—Does not respond well to therapy

  E. Pregnancy and hormonally related gingivitis

     1. *P. intermedia*

     2. Bacteria are black pigmented

  F. Linear gingival erythema (formerly HIV gingivitis)

     1. May have similar presentation to ANUG, but does not respond well to local therapy

     2. Fiery, discontinuous, red outline of free gingival margin; extensive, spontaneous bleeding

     3. Painful, with progression to periodontitis without treatment

     4. Occurs in patients infected with HIV

  G. Factors influencing progression of disease

     1. Invasion of tissue by bacteria (e.g., spirochetes, *Capnocytophaga* species)

2. Bacterial products may cause destruction of tissue

    a. Endotoxins (lipopolysaccharides) activate complement, produce fever and shock, and interfere with normal function of blood homeostasis; associated with Gram-negative bacterial cell walls

    b. Exotoxins are soluble substances secreted by Gram-positive cells that are very toxic to other organisms (e.g., botulism)

    c. Enzymes (lysozyme, collagenase, hyaluraonidase) cause destruction of oral tissue and interfere with normal immune function

3. Plaque bacteria present an antigenic challenge; some local destruction results from inflammatory process (e.g., immune complex, cell-mediated)

4. Humoral immunity

    a. Lymphocytes, plasma cells present in area of plaque

    b. Plasma cells produce antibodies

    c. Complement is activated by bacterial endotoxin, or bacterial antigen–antibody complexes

5. Cellular immunity

    a. Cell-mediated immunity causes release of lymphokines or osteoclast-activating factor

    b. The progression of periodontal disease may be due to these components of cellular immunity

H. Infections of the periapical and oral-facial tissues

    1. Infections may include

        a. Periodontal and periapical abscesses

        b. Endodontically involved infections

        c. Postsurgical and extraction wound infections, including alveolar osteitis (dry socket)

        d. Sinus tract (draining fistulas) infections

        e. Cellulitis (Ludwig's angina)

        f. Injuries as a result of trauma

        g. Osteomyelitis

        h. Pericoronitis

        i. Infections of periodontal origin

    2. Bacteria cultured from these infections are predominantly Gram-negative bacilli such as *Prevotella* and *Porphyromonas*

    3. Acute endodontic infections harbor obligate anaerobic bacteria (e.g., *P. intermedia*)

4. Ludwig's angina
  a. May be caused by normal oral flora gaining access through abscessed tooth
  b. Aerobic or facultative organisms along with anaerobic microorganisms
  c. Rapidly spreading, diffuse swelling of the floor of the mouth and neck
  d. Blockage of airway becomes life-threatening
  e. Infected mandibular molars, thin lingual cortical plate of mandible are predisposing factors

5. Actinomycosis—Opportunistic infection after injury that introduces contaminated debris into tissue
  a. Etiology—*A. israellii, A. naeslundii* (Gram-positive member of normal oral microbiota)
  b. Facial swelling below angle of jaw, chronic superficial mass, abscess with sinus, and chronic discharge

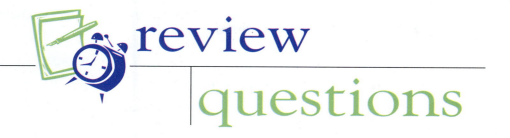
review questions

DIRECTIONS Each of the questions or incomplete statements below is followed by suggested answers or completions. Select the **one** answer that is best in each case.

1. All of the following are nonspecific host defenses against disease EXCEPT one. Which one is the EXCEPTION?
   A. Intact skin or mucous membranes
   B. Saliva, tears, and vaginal fluids
   C. Antibody–antigen complex
   D. Antagonism by resident microbiota
   E. pH of the stomach

2. Immunoglobins are classified as:
   A. Carbohydrates
   B. Complex proteins
   C. Lipids
   D. Simple amino acid chains

3. The immunoglobin found in saliva and in other body secretions is:
   A. IgE
   B. IgD
   C. IgA
   D. IgM
   E. IgG

4. The predominate cell found in acute inflammatory reactions is:
   A. Macrophage
   B. Neutrophil
   C. Lymphocytes
   D. Basophils

5. Chemotaxis is a function of which of the following cell types?
   A. Lymphocytes
   B. Erythrocytes
   ✓C. Neutrophils
   D. Plasma cells

6. Passive immunity is BEST defined as:
   A. Species immunity
   B. A state of temporary insusceptibility to an infectious agent
   C. Individual immunity
   D. An immunity mediated by hormones

7. Which of the following markers indicates immunity to HBV?
   A. Hepatitis B surface antigen
   B. Antibody to Hepatitis B surface antigen
   C. Presence of Delta agent
   D. Hepatitis B "e" antigen

8. The presence of antibodies to HBeAg represents:
   A. Infectivity
   B. Acute infection
   D. A carrier state
   E. Low infectivity

293

9. Contact dermatitis exemplifies which of the following types of hypersensitivity?
   A. Type I
   B. Type II
   C. Type III
   D. Type IV

10. Which of the following parts of an antibody combine with the antigen?
    A. Fc
    B. Fab
    C. Hinge region
    D. Polypeptide

11. Which of the following cells synthesize antibodies?
    A. Mast
    B. Stem
    C. Plasma
    D. Fibroblast

12. Which of the following genera are Gram-negative, comma-shaped rods?
    A. *Treponema*
    B. *Actinomyces*
    C. *Vibrio*
    D. *Staphylococcus*

13. Which of the following bacteria are carried on the skin, in the anterior nares, and are responsible for the transmission of many nosocomial infections?
    A. *Mutans streptococcus*
    B. *Staphylococcus aureus*
    C. *Treponema pallidum*
    D. *Actinomyces naeslundii*

14. Hepatitis B represents which type of immunity?
    A. Active naturally acquired
    B. Artificially acquired passive
    C. Naturally acquired passive
    D. Artificially acquired active

15. What is the immunoglobin that predominates in a Type I hypersensitivity reaction?
    A. IgA
    B. IgE
    C. IgG
    D. IgD
    E. IgM

16. Which of the following indicates the effectiveness of sterilization?
    A. Change of color on autoclave tape or bag
    B. Live spore test
    C. Following time and temperature requirements exactly
    D. Monitoring patients for disease

17. Introduction of a pathogen from a species other than human is termed:
    A. Heterozygous
    B. Homozygous
    C. Zoonosis
    D. Autogenous

18. RNA and DNA are found in which cell organelle?
    A. Mitochondria
    B. Endoplasmic reticulum
    C. Nucleus
    D. Ribosomes

19. In which type of plaque is *Actinobacillus actinomycetemcomitans* found?
    A. Thin Gram-negative
    B. Thin Gram-positive
    C. Thick Gram-negative
    D. Thick Gram-positive

20. The varicella zoster virus is responsible for which ONE of the following diseases?
    A. Herpes simplex I
    B. Shingles
    C. Measles
    D. Infectious mononucleosis

21. All of the following increase the virulence of a pathogen EXCEPT one. Which one is the EXCEPTION?
    A. Endotoxins
    B. Pili
    C. Capsules
    D. Microtubules
    E. Enzyme production

22. Tissue grafted from one species to another is termed:
    A. Autocraft
    B. Homograft
    C. Heterograft
    D. Homoplastic

23. The microorganisms MOST likely to be found in a microscopic plaque sample of a patient with ANUG would be:
    A. Spirochetes and *Prevotella intermedia*
    B. *Fusobacterium*
    C. *Actinobacillus actinomycetemomitans*
    D. *Porphyromonas gingivalis* and *Prevotella intermedia*

24. The FIRST cells that travel to the site of injury are:
    A. B lymphocytes
    B. T lymphocytes
    C. Polymorphonuclear neutrophils
    D. Thrombocytes

25. The bacteria type MOST likely to be seen in mature plaque is:
    A. Gram-positive cocci and a few rods
    B. Gram-negative cocci and rods
    C. Vibrios and spirochetes
    D. Filamentous forms and fusobacterium

26. Which of the following bacteria are predominate in pregnancy gingivitis?
    A. *S. salivarius*
    B. *Prevotella intermedia*
    C. *Porphymonas gingivalis*
    D. *Mutans streptococcus*

27. Affinity for the hard tooth surface is characteristic of:
    A. *S. mitior* and *S. pyogenes*
    B. *Mutans streptococcus* and *S. salivarius*
    C. *Mutans streptococcus* and *S. sanguis*
    D. *Lactobacillus* and *Mutans streptococcus*

28. Bacteria that have the ability to initiate caries on smooth surface enamel must be able to:
    A. Produce mucin
    B. Produce proteolytic enzymes
    C. Produce extracellular insoluble glucans
    D. Survive in a high pH environment

29. Which of the following acids is formed in large quantities after degradation of sucrose by *Mutans streptococcus?*
    A. Lactic
    B. Acetic
    C. Linoleic
    D. Lipoteichoic

30. The principal site for the growth of spirochetes, fusobacteria, and other anaerobes is:
    A. Supragingival dental plaque
    B. The gingival margin
    C. The gingival sulcus
    D. Saliva

31. The most likely species of microorganism to predominate in a necrotic root canal is:
    A. *S. salivarius*
    B. *Mutans streptococcus*
    C. *P. intermedia*
    D. *S. sanguis*

32. Cells that phagocytize microorganisms are which of the following types?
    A. Neutrophils
    B. Macrophages
    C. Lymphocytes
    D. B and C only
    E. A and B only

33. The cell wall of gram-positive microorganisms may include all of the following EXCEPT:
    A. Lipopolysaccharides
    B. Lipoteichoic acids
    C. Petidoglycans
    D. Penicillin binding proteins
    E. Teichoic acids

34. Microbiological safety equipment for protection of healthcare workers recommended in OSHA standards includes:
    A. Gloves
    B. Face mask or shield
    C. Eye goggles
    D. Gowns and aprons
    E. All of the above

35. The only "cold sterilizer" solution capable of destroying bacterial spores, viruses, and vegetative bacteria is:
    A. 90% isopropyl alcohol
    B. 2% glutaraldehyde
    C. Chlorhexidine
    D. Iodophors
    E. Quaternary ammonium

36. Autoclave efficiency should be checked regularly by using:
    A. Heat-activated autoclave tapes that change colors
    B. Plastic strips designed to melt at 121°C
    C. Culture plates of viable bacteria
    D. Vials of culture media containing a pH indicator and a thermophilic spore-forming bacteria
    E. Vials with different acid and base chemical indicators

37. The best method for sterilizing cutting instruments is:
    A. Autoclave for 15 minutes at 15 pounds of pressure at 121°C
    B. Benzalkonium chloride
    C. Boiling water
    D. 10% hypochlorite
    E. 70% ethyl alcohol

38. Which of the following is a Gram-negative anaerobic rod?
    A. *Fusobacterium nucleatum*
    B. *Clostridium prefringens*
    C. *Peptostreptococcus*
    D. *Candida albicans*
    E. *Neisseria meningitides*

39. Herpes zoster is thought to be the adult counterpart of which of the following diseases?
    A. Chickenpox
    B. Measles
    C. Mumps
    D. Smallpox
    E. Rubeola

40. An anaerobic *Streptococcus* is classified as a member of genus:
    A. *Neisseria*
    B. *Peptostreptococcus*
    C. *Hemophilus*
    D. *Lactobacillus*
    E. *Enterococcus*

41. *Lactobacillus acidophilus* is a:
    A. Gram-positive coccus
    B. Gram-positive rod
    C. Gram-negative coccus
    D. Gram-negative rod
    E. Gram-variable spiral bacteria

42. Viruses that infect bacteria are known as:
    A. Saprophytes
    B. Commensals
    C. Protoplasts
    D. Bacteriophages
    E. Spheroplasts

43. A substance that helps prepare bacteria for phagocytosis is a(n):
    A. Bacteriolysin
    B. Interferon
    C. Antitoxin
    D. Opsonin
    E. Hemolysin

44. Chemotaxis is a function of which of the following cells?
    A. Erythrocytes
    B. Leukocytes
    C. Epithelial
    D. Endothelial
    E. All of the above

45. Ethylene oxide has which of the following action on bacteria?
    A. Bacteriostatic
    B. Antiseptic
    C. Disinfects
    √D. Sterilizes
    E. Sanitizes

46. Immuniglobulins are produced by which of the following cell types?
    A. Neutrophils
    B. Macrophages
    C. T lymphocytes
    D. B lymphocytes
    E. Basophils

47. Active immunity may BEST be described as:
    A. The inability of a host to react to a battery of common skin test antigens
    B. An immunity passed from one animal species to another species
    C. An altered state of immune reactivity or hypersensitivity
    D. Acquired by deliberate introduction of an antigen into a responsive host
    E. Normal species immunity acquired genetically

48. The most infectious stage(s) of syphilis is (are) the:
    A. Primary stage
    B. Secondary stage
    C. Latent phase
    D. Tertiary stage
    E. Both A and B

49. Acquired immunodeficiency syndrome (AIDS) is caused by a single-stranded RNA virus known as a(n):
    A. Retrovirus
    B. Tumor virus
    C. Adenovirus
    D. Arbovirus
    E. Parvovirus

50. Treponema pallidum is responsible for which of the following diseases?
    A. Gonorrhea
    B. Pneumonia
    C. Measles
    D. Chicken pox
    E. Syphilis

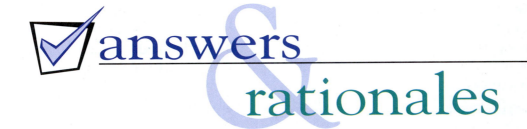

answers & rationales

1.

C. Antibodies are a host defense made in response to specific antigens. Each antibody is specifically designed to fit the surface markers on a specific antigen. Intact skin and mucous membranes are nonspecific host defenses that act as a barrier to harmful substances or organisms. Saliva, tears, and vaginal fluids are nonspecific host defenses that contain IgA to inactivate pathogens. They also serve as a mechanism to flush the invaders away. Resident microflora are nonspecific host defenses that compete for nutrients and surface area. *S. epidermis* is a harmless microorganism that may inhibit the growth of pathogenic *S. aureus* on the skin's surface. The pH of the stomach is extremely low, due to the presence of hydrochloric acid. This nonspecific host defense kills most microorganisms on contact.

2.

B. Immunoglobins are a class of structurally related proteins, with an important role in specific host defense. Immunoglobins are not carbohydrates, lipids, or simple amino acid chains.

3.

C. Saliva and other body secretions contain the immunoglobin IgA. It is considered the secretory antibody. IgE is the immunoglobulin that is responsible for Type I hypersensitivity reactions. IgE combines with the surface of the antigen, activating basophils, and mast cells to release histamine and other inflammatory products. IgD is a trace antibody responsible for regulating the antibody–antigen process. IgM appears only in the bloodstream. It is the first antibody to appear and starts agglutination and bacteriolysis. IgG is the main immunoglobin in the blood, composing up to 75% of the total defense. It is able to cross the placental barrier to protect the fetus.

4.

B. Neutrophils or polymorphonuclear neutrophils (PMNs) are the first line of defense in the inflammatory response and are the most numerous inflammatory cell in any stage of infection. Macrophages are larger phagocytic cells than neutrophils and are present in chronic and acute infections, but not in the same numbers. Lymphocytes may be either T or B lymphocytes and are activated by the presence of PMNs, monocytes, and macrophages. Basophils are a granulocytic WBC that increase in number in myeloproliferative diseases.

5.

B. Neutrophils are attracted to the site of invasion by chemotaxis (chemical attraction). Failure of the chemotactic factor plays a role in diseases of host response such as juvenile periodontitis. Lymphocytes are presented to the antigen by macrophages. Erythrocytes are red blood cells, and are not involved in chemotaxis. Plasma cells are produced by B lymphocytes and are the precursors to antibodies. They are not involved in chemotaxis.

6.

B. Passive immunity is a state of temporary insusceptibility to an infectious agent, due to the introduction of antibodies from another source. These antibodies may be passed from mother to fetus, or may be given in the form of immunoglobin injection of preformed antibodies. Species immunity is that immunity a whole species has toward a certain pathogen and is not considered passive. Individual immunity is protection from a specific pathogen, due to the formation of antibodies. Hormones have no specific relation to immunity.

7.

B. Formation of antibodies to the hepatitis B surface antigen indicates immunity. The presence of both hepatitis B surface and "e" antigens indicate infectivity. The presence of the delta agent indicates coinfection with hepatitis D.

8.

E. The presence of antibodies to HBeAg indicates low infectivity, but not necessarily complete elimination of the disease. The presence of HBeAg indicates infectivity. The presence of HBsAg indicates acute infection, whereas the presence of antibodies to HBsAg indicates immunity. The presence of HBsAg may indicate a carrier state, if it persists longer than 6 months.

9.

D. Contact dermatitis is a type of delayed hypersensitivity or Type IV reaction. This type of reaction usually occurs 2–3 days after exposure to the allergen and is mediated by the T lymphocyte. Type I indicates immediate hypersensitivity, mediated by the antibodies

produced by IgE. Examples are anaphylactic reactions, asthma, and hay fever. Type II hypersensitivity reactions are cytotoxic reactions such as blood transfusion reactions and hemolytic disease of the newborn. Type III hypersensitivity reactions are immune complex reactions that may be responsible for autoimmune diseases such as systemic lupus erythematosus. Both Type II and III are antibody mediated.

10.

B. The Fab or fragment antigen-binding portion of the antibody combines with the antigen. These consist of variable regions with two chains that are responsible for the specificity of the antibody. The Fc (fragment crystallizable) fragment of the antibody contains sites where immune cells of the host will bind. The hinge region is the area where the Fab and the Fc fragments combine. The antibody is a "y"-shaped molecule with a light polypeptide chain and a heavy polypeptide chain; however, these chains are not the antigen attachment site.

11.

C. Plasma cells found in the bone marrow and connective tissue, synthesize antibodies. Mast cells release histamine, serotonin, and heparin when activated by IgE. Stem cells manufacture T or B lymphocytes, and fibroblasts manufacture collagen.

12.

C. *Vibrio* is a genus of gram-negative, comma-shaped bacterial rods. *Treponema* are spiral-shaped bacteria or spirochetes. *Actinomyces* are rod-shaped bacteria, whereas Staphylococci are grape-shaped clusters of round bacteria.

13.

B. *Staphylococcus aureus* is a common microscopic resident of skin, and resides in the anterior nares. It is easily spread from hospital workers to patients through careless infection control practices. In addition, once established, it is resistant to many common antibiotics. It is one of the most common causes of nosocomial or hospital-transmitted infections. *Mutans Streptococcus* is the primary bacterium implicated in the transmission of human caries. *Treponema pallidum* is the causative organism of syphilis in humans. *Actinomyces naeslundii* is the primary bacterium implicated in human root caries.

14.

A. Vaccination represents active-acquired immunity since it is artificial stimulation of the body's production of antibodies to the hepatitis B virus. Acquired passive immunity is the artificial introduction of antibodies in response to a disease threat. Natural active immunity is achieved when the body is exposed to a disease and produces antibodies in response to the immunological challenge. Natural passive immunity is a short-lived immunity that is transferred from one organism to another, such as fetal antibodies crossing the placenta.

15.

B. IgE is the antibody that predominates in a Type I hypersensitivity (classic allergic) reaction. IgA is the antibody that is present in body secretions and on mucous membranes. IgG is the primary antibody in the blood. IgD is a trace antibody, responsible for regulating antibody-producing cells. IgM is the first antibody to appear in the bloodstream and starts the process of agglutination and bacteriolysis.

16.

B. The live spore test is the only definitive test to measure effective sterilization. The change in color of tape or markings on the bag indicates only that the proper temperature was reached, not that all microor-ganisms were killed. Even when time and temperature requirements are followed, there still can be ineffective pressure or temperature achieved to kill all microorganisms. Monitoring patients would be extremely difficult and therefore not conclusive proof that sterilization had been achieved, especially when patients do not report illnesses.

17.

C. A zoonosis is the introduction of a pathogen from another species, especially the animal family. Heterozygous is defined as having different allelic genes at one locus, which may result in the manifestation of a recessive genetic condition. Homozygous is defined as having the same allelic genes at one locus, resulting in dominance of a manifestation of a gene's expression. An autogenous infection is the introduction of the patient's own microflora into injured tissue, causing a local or systemic post-treatment infection.

18.

C. The nucleus is the site of genetic determination and metabolic functioning for the cell and contains chromosomes, DNA, and the nucleolus, which holds RNA. The mitochondria are responsible for the production of the cell's energy, via adenosine triphosphate (ATP). The endoplasmic reticulum is responsible for protein and lipid synthesis and packaging. Rough endoplasmic reticulum contains the tiny granules of RNA in the form of ribosomes, which manufacture proteins. Smooth endoplasmic reticulum contain enzymes that synthesize lipids, especially those used to make membranes. Ribosomes are a granule of ribonucleoprotein, which is the site of protein synthesis as directed by mRNA.

19.

A. *Actinobacillus actinomycetemcomitans* is a small Gram-negative coccoid facultative organism. It is uncommon in that it thrives in thin plaque layers, and may cause diseases such as juvenile periodontitis in relatively clean mouths.

20.

A. Herpes simplex I is a virus that presents as vesicles typically found above the waist and around and in the mouth. It is caused by a different virus in the *Herpesviridae* family. The varicella zoster virus, a member of the herpes virus family, is responsible for two different manifestations of the same etiological agent. In children, the virus presents itself as a common childhood illness called chickenpox, usually a mild vesicular disease. In adults, the latent virus in dorsal root ganglions is reactivated, closely following areas of innervation, and producing an extremely painful rash and vesicles along the nerve trunk. Measles is caused by the rubeola virus. Infectious mononucleosis is caused by the Epstein-Barr virus.

21.

D. Microtubules are protein structures within flagella and are responsible for movement, as well as functioning in the spindle apparatus of the cellular division process of mitosis. They do not increase the virulence of pathogens. Endotoxins, or lipopolysaccharides, are part of the Gram-negative cell wall and increase the virulence of those microorganisms. They have the ability to activate, complement, or disrupt cellular homeostasis, and lead to the destruction of the periodontal attachment apparatus. Pili and fimbrae are attachment mechanisms for microorganisms that allow them to adhere to body structures, usually mucous membranes. Pili also function as a means of exchange of genetic material (important in the transference of drug resistance between species) and as a receptor site for viruses. Bacteria with pili are more pathogenic than those of the same genera without pili. Capsules, or slime layers, are protective mechanisms for bacteria and aid in their virulence. Bacteria that are able to synthesize polymers with a well-defined outer limit that attaches to the cell wall are said to have capsules. If the outer limit is not as well defined, it is called a slime layer or glycocalyx. Bacteria able to synthesize these structures are more virulent and more pathogenic. *Mutans Streptococcus* are able to produce a capsule that allows for adherence to tooth structure. Enzyme production by bacteria allows for greater virulence and tissue destruction.

22.

C. Heterograft (xenograft) is the correct term for tissue grafted from another species. Autograft is the term to define tissue grafted from one's own body. Homograft (allograft) refers to tissue grafted from the same species. Hemoplastic is another term for homograft and allograft.

23.

A. Spirochetes and *P. intermedia* are the predominant bacteria found in ANUG. Fusobacterium are also found in ANUG, but not as commonly as spirochetes and *P. intermedia*. *A. actinomycetemomitans* is not usually found in ANUG. *Porphyromonas gingivalis* and *Prevotella intermedia* are commonly found in adult periodontitis.

24.

C. Polymorphonuclear neutrophils (PMNs) are the first cells to respond to immunological challenge or injury. B lymphocytes must be activated by complement and macrophages. T lymphocytes must be activated by complement and macrophages. Thromocytes or platelets are involved in blood clotting.

25.

C. Vibrios and spirochetes are the bacterial markers for the maturation of plaque, appearing as early as 4–7 days in the rapid plaque formers. Gram-positive cocci and a few rods occur in early plaque. Few gram-negative cocci exist in plaque. Filamentous forms and *Fusobacterium* occur in the early to middle stages of plaque development.

26.

B. *Prevotella intermedia* predominates in all types of hormonal gingivitis. *S. salivarius* are not linked to the development of gingivitis. It is a common inhabitant of saliva. *Porphymonas gingivalis* are common in all types of periodontal disease, but are not considered the primary etiological agent in pregnancy gingivitis. *Mutans Streptococcus* are implicated as the primary etiological agent in human caries.

27.

C. *Mutans Streptococcus* and *S. sanguis* are considered colonizers of tooth structure. Both of these bacteria need to adhere to a hard surface. *S. mitior* and *S. pyogenes* are found on both soft and hard tissues of the oral cavity. *Mutans Streptococcus* do require hard tooth surfaces, but *S. salivarius* are commonly found in saliva and soft oral tissues. *Lactobacillus* causes caries but has no ability to adhere to hard tooth surfaces. It must inhabit a pit, fissure, or existing lesion.

28.

C. "Colonizers" such as *Mutans Streptococcus* and *S. sanguis* are able to adhere to tooth structure due to their ability to produce extracellular insoluble glucans. This allows them to remain in contact with the surface long enough to initiate caries. Mucin is produced by salivary glands and used for lubrication. Proteolytic enzymes may break down the fibrous structure of the periodontal attachment, but do not initiate caries. Bacteria capable of initiating caries do so by producing acid and thereby lowering the pH of the oral environment.

29.

A. Lactic acid is produced by the degradation of sucrose by *Mutans Streptococcus* and the *Lactobacillus* sp. Acetic acid, or vinegar, is not produced by *Mutans Streptococcus*. Linoleic acid is an essential fatty acid, and not produced by *Mutans Streptococcus*. Lipoteichoic acid is a component of Gram-positive cell walls and is not produced by *Mutans Streptococcus*.

30.

C. Spirochetes, *Fusobacterium*, and other anaerobes thrive in the low oxygen environment of the gingival sulcus. Supragingival plaque is heavily populated with Gram-positive facultative anaerobes. The gingival margin is heavily populated with Gram-positive facultative anaerobes. Saliva is primarily populated with Gram-positive facultative anaerobes.

31.

C. *P. intermedia* is consistently found in necrotic root canals. *S. salivarius* is found primarily in saliva and in those soft tissue surfaces coated with saliva. *Mutans Streptococcus* are facultative anaerobes that usually do not dominate the microbiota in a necrotic root canal. *S. sanguis* is an early colonizer of hard tooth structure and is not found in necrotic root canals.

32.

E. Two cell types are involved in phagocytosis; the polymorphonuclear neutrophil and macrophage. Neutrophils are present in the bloodstream and are short-lived cells. Macrophages, on the other hand, are long-lived cells present throughout the connective tissue and around the basement membrane of small blood vessels. Both cell types migrate to sites of inflammation to engulf bacteria and discharge granules consisting of microbicidal substances.

33.

A. Lipopolysaccharide (or endotoxin) is the most significant structure in the cell wall of Gram-negative bacteria. It accounts for a variety of immunological reactions.

34.

E. All body fluids from patients should be considered potentially infectious. The healthcare worker should exercise precautions as mandated by OSHA by using personal protective equipment, which includes gloves, goggles, face shields, gowns or lab coats, and aprons.

35.

B. A solution of 2% glutaraldehyde is an alkalying agent highly lethal to essentially all microorganisms if sufficient contact time is provided and there is absence of extraneous organic material. It is effective for sterilizing apparatuses that cannot be heated. Other products such as alcohols, iodophors, chlorhexidine, and quaternary ammonium compounds are disinfectants.

36.

D. Autoclaves should be quality controlled to ensure that the appropriate temperature, pressure, packing, and timing are correct. A thermophilic microorganism, usually *Bacillus stearothermophilus*, is used as a biological indicator. These organisms are supplied with vials of culture medium containing a pH indicator. The vial is placed in the autoclave with the load and the autoclave is run under normal conditions. The vial is removed and the culture medium is released to mix with the thermophilic microorganisms. The vial is placed in an incubator for a specified period of time and then checked for growth of the organism. If no organisms grow, the autoclave was effective. If the organisms grow in the culture media, the autoclave did not render the contents of that load sterile.

37.

A. Autoclaves are usually operated at 121°C, which is achieved at a pressure of 15 psi for 15 minutes. Under these conditions, spores are killed. The velocity of the killing increases logarithmically with a steam temperature of 121°C and is more effective than 100°C or boiling.

38.

A. *Fusobacterium nucleatum* is a Gram-negative non-spore-forming anaerobic rod. *Clostridium prefingens* is a Gram-positive spore-forming rod. *Candida albicans* is a yeast. *Neisseria meningitides* is a member of the aerobic Gram-negative cocci. *Peptostreptococcus* is a Gram-positive cocci.

39.

A. Reactivation of the varicella-zoster virus, the agent of chickenpox seen most commonly in children, is associated with herpes zoster. It increases in frequency with age and is seen most commonly in adults.

40.

B. An anaerobic *Streptococcus* is classified as a member of genus *Peptostreptococcus*.

41.

B. *Lactobacillus acidophilus* is a Gram-positive rod commonly found in the oropharyngeal flora. It is believed to play some role in the pathogenesis of dental caries.

42.

D. Viruses are capable of reproduction only inside living cells. Those that grow inside bacteria are known as bacteriophages.

43.

D. Substances that prepare bacteria for phagocytosis are known as opsonins. They attach to the surface of the microbe and activate the complement pathway. The complement fragment C3b and a calcium-dependent mannose-binding protein are examples of opsonins.

44.

B. Some bacteria produce chemical substances known as chemotaxins, which directionally attract leukocytes. The adherence of bacteria to the leukocyte activates the membrane and initiates engulfment.

45.

D. Ethylene oxide is an alkylating agent that is an effective sterilizing agent for heat-liable devices that cannot be treated at the temperatures achieved in the autoclave.

46.

D. The role of lymphocytes in the production of antibodies was established many years ago. It is now known that lymphocytes of a subset known as B lymphocytes are programmed to make a single, specific antibody that can be found on the outer surface of the cell to act as a receptor.

47.

D. Primary active immunity is induced prior to exposure to the biological agent. Active immunity or immunization may be acquired with living or dead microorganisms or recombinant proteins.

48.

E. The most infectious stages of syphilis are the primary stage, when a syphilitic chancre has numerous spirochetes present, and the secondary stage, when mucocutaneous lesions with spirochetes are distributed over various areas of the body.

49.

A. The most important human retrovirus infection is acquired immunodeficiency syndrome (AIDS), caused by one of two groups of retroviruses termed human immunodeficiency virus (HIV-1 and HIV-2). Retroviruses are enveloped, single-stranded RNA viruses. They encode reverse transferage (an RNA-dependent DNA polymerase) that copies their genome into proviral double-stranded DNA.

50.

E. The organism *Treponema pallidum* is responsible for syphilis. Syphilis causes disability and death mainly when the heart, blood vessels, and nervous system become affected. Any organ, however, can become affected.

5 Oral Pathology

T he study of oral pathology focuses not only on diseases that affect the oral cavity, but also on systemic diseases that may exhibit oral manifestations.

chapter objectives

After completion of this chapter, the learner should be able to:

- ➤ Describe the terminology related to general and oral pathology
- ➤ Describe the inflammatory process
- ➤ Discuss regeneration and repair
- ➤ List and describe the anomalies of the oral cavity
- ➤ List and describe cysts of the oral cavity
- ➤ List and describe benign neoplasma
- ➤ Describe bacterial infectious diseases
- ➤ Describe viral infectious diseases
- ➤ Describe fungal diseases
- ➤ Describe vesiculoerosive diseases
- ➤ Discuss blood dyscrasias
- ➤ Describe endocrine disorders
- ➤ Discuss oral cancer

I. Terminology and Definitions

A. Terminology based on appearance and consistency

1. Color

a. Pink or coral pink—Color of normal mucosa

b. Erythematous—Implies red or inflamed

c. Leukoplakia—Implies white lesion; does not rub off

d. Blue-black or reddish-purple—Implies amalgam, melanin, or a vascular lesion

2. Nodule—Small, firm, palpable lesion above or below surrounding surface level

a. Pedunculated—Narrow base that grows on a stalk

b. Sessile—Wide base without stalk

c. Hypertrophy—Increase of tissue size due to an increase in cell size

d. Hyperplasia—Increase of tissue size due to an increase in cell numbers

3. Papule—Small, elevated growth usually < 5 mm in diameter

4. Macule—Small, nonelevated lesion usually of a different color

5. Vesicle—Fluid-filled blister < 5 mm in diameter

6. Bulla (plural = bullae)—Fluid-filled blister > 5 mm in diameter

7. Pustule—Vesicle or bulla filled with pus

8. Corrugated—Wavy elevations and depressions, also wrinkled

9. Fissured—Deep grooves with no cracks or ulcerations

10. Papillary—Rough surface with small projections (cauliflower-like)

B. Radiographic terminology

1. Unilocular—Only one radiolucent compartment

2. Multilocular—Several radiolucent compartments with the same or varied sizes

3. Honeycombed—Several radiolucent compartments of the same size

4. Well-circumscribed—Well-defined border with clearly defined margins

5. Diffuse—Poorly identifiable margins that blend into normal tissue

6. Sclerotic—Appears more radiopaque than normal

II. General Pathology

A. Inflammation—Vascular response to injury (Figure 5-1■)

1. Steps in acute inflammatory response

a. Vasoconstriction—First brief inflammatory response

b. Vasodilation—Relaxation of the smooth muscles caused by chemical mediators at time of injury; process known as active hyperemia and is responsible for erythema and heat

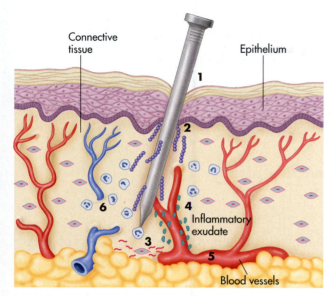

1. Dirty nail punctures skin.
2. Bacteria enter and multiply.
3. Injured cells release histamine.
4. Blood vessels dilate and become permeable, releasing inflammatory exudate.
5. Blood flow to the damaged site increases.
6. Neutrophils (polymorph) move toward bacteria (chemotaxis) and destroy them (phagocytosis).

FIGURE 5-1 ■ Vascular Changes That Occur with Inflammation

c. Exudate—Increased vascular permeability allows fluid and plasma proteins to leave the blood vessels into injured tissues to help dilute the injurious agents

d. Serous exudate—Associated with mild inflammation and composed of plasma fluids, proteins, and a few white blood cells; example: fluid in a blister

e. Fibrous exudate—Rich in protein (fibrinogen); causes the exudates to close due to the formation of fibrin; example: pleurisy—exudates on the surface of lung caused by pneumonia

f. Purulent exudate (suppuration)—Contains many white blood cells— neutrophils (polymorphonuclear leukocytes, or PMNs); example: pus

g. Edema—Exudate escapes from the blood vessels into the tissues

h. Fistula—Exudate drains, forming a passage through the tissue

i. Margination—Movement of white blood cells to the periphery of blood vessels

j. Adhesion (pavementing)—White blood cells become sticky and adhere to walls of blood vessels

k. Emigration—Following adhesion, the white blood cells emigrate from the blood vessels with plasma fluids and enter the injured tissue due to chemotactic factors

l. Chemotaxis—Moving of white blood cells toward the target area for the body's defense against the injury

m. Opsonization—Serum factors called opsonins help neutrophils recognize and attach to the pathogens; enhance phagocytosis

n. Phagocytosis—Ingesting of the foreign substance

2. White blood cells involved in acute inflammatory response (leukocytes)

a. Neutrophil (polymorphonuclear leukocyte, or PMN)

(1) First cell to emigrate to site of injury

(2) Primary cell

(3) Main goal is to kill infectious agent

b. Monocyte (macrophage)

(1) Second cell involved in inflammation

(2) Removes dead and dying cells to help pave the way for fibroblasts to heal wounds

c. Eosinophil and mast cell—Involved in inflammation and immunity

3. Chronic inflammation

a. Results from injury that persists for weeks or months

b. Cells involved are lymphocytes, plasma cells, and macrophages

c. Repair is simultaneous as chronic inflammation proceeds, but cannot be complete until source of injury is removed

d. Granulomatous inflammation—Microscopic grouping of macrophages form granulomas

4. Chemical mediators of inflammation—Chemical agents called chemical mediators that start or amplify the inflammatory response control inflammation; they can be exogenous or endogenous

a. Histamine

(1) Vasoactive amine

(2) Initiate the early phases of acute inflammation, and mediates increased vascular permeability

b. Kinin system

(1) Mediate inflammation by causing increased permeability of the venules

(2) Limited to early phases of inflammation

(3) Bradykinin produces pain

c. Clotting mechanism

(1) Functions to clot blood

(2) Mediates inflammation

(3) Important in repair process

d. Complement system—Mediates vascular response (releases histamine)

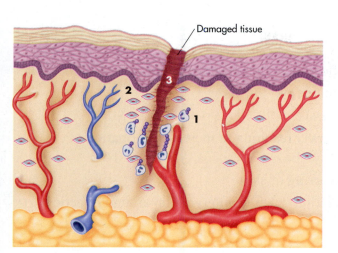

Damaged tissue

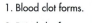

1. Blood clot forms.

2. Dried clot forms scab.

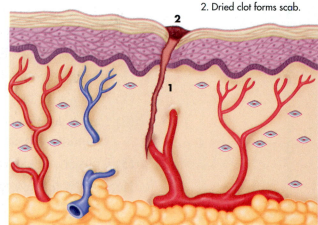

1. Neutrophils phagocytize bacteria.

2. Fibroblasts produce connective tissue fibers.

3. Fibers contract, drawing cut surfaces together.

FIGURE 5-2 ■ Fibroblasts Healing a Wound

B. Regeneration and repair (Figure 5-2■)

    1. Repair—Body's attempt to restore injured tissues by replacing damaged cells with new cells; usually completed within 2 weeks

        a. Day of injury—Clot forms (locally produced fibrin) as blood flows to site of injury

        b. One day following injury

            (1) Neutrophils emigrate to injured tissues

            (2) Phagocytosis of foreign substances

        c. Two days following injury

            (1) Monocytes emigrate to injured tissues

            (2) Macrophages continue phagocytosis

            (3) Neutrophils reduce in number as chronic inflammation proceeds

            (4) Fibroblasts increase in connective tissue and granulation tissue forms in connective tissue

        d. Seven days following injury—Fibrin is digested by tissue enzymes and initial repair is completed

        e. Two weeks following injury

            (1) Granulation tissue forms scar tissue

            (2) Increased number of collagen fibers and decreased vascularity

2. Types of repair

  a. Healing by primary intention

   (1) Healing of tissue with little loss of tissue

   (2) Small clot with little granulation tissue; example: surgical incision

  b. Healing by secondary intention

   (1) Injury with loss of tissue

   (2) Large clot forms, slowly resulting in increased formation of granulation tissue

   (3) Causes extensive scarring of skin

  c. Healing by tertiary intention—Active intervention around infection

III. Anomalies of the Oral Cavity

A. Mucosal anomalies

  1. Abnormalities of the tongue (Table 5-1■)

    a. Ankyloglossia—Tongue-tie; lingual frenum is too short or attached too anteriorly (Figure 5-3■)

    b. Lingual varices—Enlarged tortuous veins on ventral surface of tongue

    c. Fissured (Figure 5-4■)—Deep dorsal surface grooves; usually developmental on adults

    d. Hairy—Proliferation of filiform papillae; *clinical manifestations:* white, black, yellow, or brown filiform papillae due to chromogenic bacteria, smoking, food, and some drugs; most notably caused by antacids, oxygenating rinses, corticosteroids, and systemic antibiotics (Figure 5-5■)

    e. Central papillary atrophy (median rhomboid glossitis)—Raised erythematous rhomboid-shaped area located in midline of tongue, anterior to circumvallate papillae and devoid of filiform papillae; possibly caused by fungal infection from *Candida albicans* (Figure 5-6■)

    f. Geographic (migratory glossitis) (Figure 5-7■)—Erythematous areas devoid of filiform papillae, usually with a yellowish-white border; areas appear to migrate, but in reality one area heals and another appears; most likely an autoimmune response related to stress

    g. Lingual thyroid nodule—Thyroid tissue remnant during developmental stages; may be the only functioning thyroid tissue; *location:* on tongue posterior to circumvallate papillae; *clinical manifestations:* nodular mass; *treatment:* must do thyroid testing before removal

TABLE 5-1 MUCOSAL ANOMALES – ABNORMALITIES OF THE TONGUE				
Lesion	**Description**	**Location**	**Clinical Manifestation**	**Treatment**
Ankyloglossia	Extensive adhesion of the tongue to the floor of the mouth	Floor of the mouth/tongue	Short lingual frenum	Frenctomy
Lingual thyroid	Small mass of thyroid tissue located on the tongue, resulting from failure of thyroid tissue to migrate from its developmental location	Tongue	Smooth nodular mass at the base of the tongue posterior to the circumvallate papillae near the midline	Usually none, surgical removal if large
Lingual varicosities	Prominent lingual veins commonly seen in individuals over 60 years	On ventral and lateral surfaces of the tongue	Multiple, superficial, red-purple nodules	No treatment needed; a varicosity that contains a thrombus may require surgical excision
Fissured tongue	Cause is unknown; may be the result of a genetic defect (polygenic or autosomal dominant); may be due to vitamin deficiency, or chronic dry mouth	Dorsal of tongue	Deep fissures or grooves, blunted filiform papillae, erythematous mucosa	Instruct patient to keep clean to prevent irritation
Median rhomboid glossitis	Possibly caused by fungal infection from *Candida albicans*	In midline of dorsal tongue	Raised erythematous rhomboid-shaped area of papillary atrophy	No treatment needed unless fungal colonization is confirmed; in that case, treat like erythematous candidiasis

(continued)

TABLE 5-1 MUCOSAL ANOMALES – ABNORMALITIES OF THE TONGUE

Lesion	Description	Location	Clinical Manifestation	Treatment
Geographic tongue	Most likely stress related	Dorsal and lateral borders of tongue	Depapillated erythematous patches (map-like appearance) with white borders	No treatment needed
Hairy tongue	Elongation of filiform papillae	Dorsal of tongue	White, black, yellow, or brown filiform papillae due to chromogenic bacteria, smoking, food, and some drugs; most notably caused by antacids, oxygenating rinses, corticosteroids, and systemic antibiotics	Elimination of predisposing factors; cleaning the dorsal tongue with a soft toothbrush

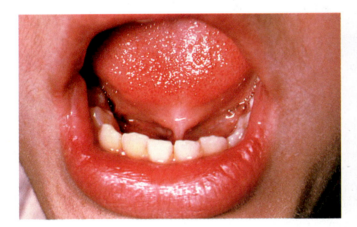

FIGURE 5-3 ■ Ankyloglossia

Source: SPL/Custom Medical Stock Photo, Inc.

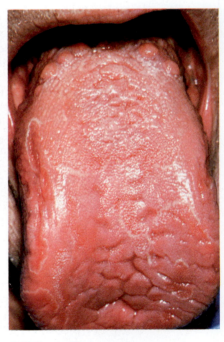

FIGURE 5-4 ■ Fissured Tongue

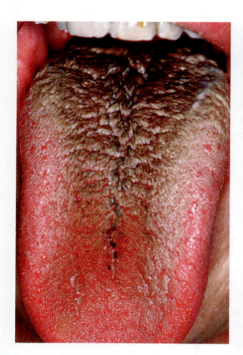

FIGURE 5-5 ■ Hairy Tongue

Source: ISM/Phototake NYC

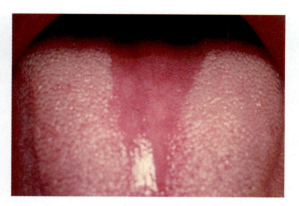

FIGURE 5-6 ■ Median Rhomboid Glossitis

Source: O.J. Staats, MD/Custom Medical Stock Photo, Inc.

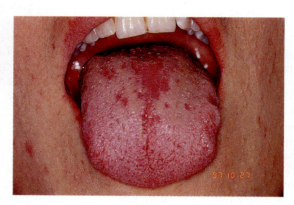

FIGURE 5-7 ■ Geographic Tongue

2. Mucosal tissue variation from normal (Table 5-2■)

    a. Fordyce granules (Figure 5-8■)—Yellowish clusters of ectopic sebaceous glands; *location:* usually on buccal mucosal or vermilion border of the lips, commonly bilateral

    b. Leukoedema—Opalescent (milky) hue of the buccal mucosa resulting from increased intracellular edema

    c. Lip pits—Blind sacs found in the vermillion zone or commissures; cause is usually congenital

    d. Melanin pigmentations—Focal brownish areas that may be racial in origin or indicative of a systemic disease (e.g., Addison's disease or Peutz-Jeghers syndrome)

    e. Retrocuspid papilla—Fibrous elevation lingual to mandibular canines

TABLE 5-2 MUCOSAL ANOMALES – ABNORMALITIES OF OTHER MUCOSAL TISSUE

Lesion	Description	Location	Clinical Manifestation	Treatment
Fordyce's granules	Clusters of ectopic salivary glands	Usually on buccal mucosal or vermilion border of the lips, commonly bilateral	Yellow lobules	No treatment needed
Linea alba	Predominant in patients with clenching or bruxing habit	Buccal mucosa at occlusal plane, usually bilateral	White line that extends from anterior buccal mucosal to posterior buccal mucosa	No treatment needed
Leuko-edema	Benign anomaly common in African Americans caused by thickening of epithelium and the accumulation of edema fluid within epithelial cells	Buccal mucosal, occurs bilaterally	Gray/white film that causes the buccal mucosa to look opaque	No treatment needed
Melanin pigmentation	Prominent in dark-skinned individuals	On gingiva and oral mucosal	Melanin pigment on gingiva and oral mucosa	No treatment needed
Leukoplakia	Specific cause of lesion is unknown	Anywhere in oral cavity	White plaque-like lesion that cannot be rubbed off	Dependent upon histologic diagnosis
Lichen planus	White striae	Skin and oral mucosal lesions; oral mucosa—buccal mucosa, tongue, labial mucosa, floor of mouth gingiva	Oral lesions Wickham's striae Erosive and plaque-like lesions may occur Gingival lesions—desquamative gingivitis	None if asymptomatic Topical corticosteroids such as Kenalog in Orabase or Lidex ointment

f. Leukoplakia—Not a diagnosis; a clinical description of a white lesion that does not rub off (Figure 5-9■)

(1) Etiology—Usually resulting from chronic irritation with hyperkeratosis

(2) Clinical manifestations—May be premalignant with use of high-risk factors (e.g., tobacco or alcohol)

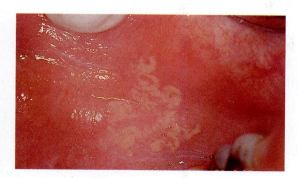

FIGURE 5-8 ■ Fordyce's Granules

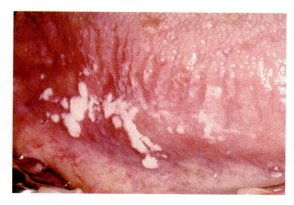

FIGURE 5-9 ■ Leukoplakia

Source: Edward H. Gill/Custom Medical Stock Photo, Inc.

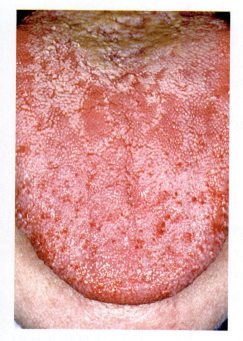

FIGURE 5-10 ■ Oral Lichen Planus

Source: Edward H. Gill/Custom Medical Stock Photo, Inc.

g. Lichen planus—Skin disease (Figure 5-10■)

   (1) Etiology—Unknown

   (2) Oral manifestations

      (a) White or gray thread-like papules in a linear or reticular arrangement (Wickham's striae)

      (b) Plaque-like form (more common on the dorsum of the tongue)

      (c) Bulbous and/or erosive form (see Vesiculoerosive diseases)

(3) Clinical manifestations—More commonly seen in nervous, high-strung individuals

(4) Treatment—None unless symptomatic (e.g., erosive), then corticosteroids are prescribed

h. Linea alba

(1) Predominant in patients with clenching or bruxing habit

(2) Oral manifestations—White line that extends from anterior buccal mucosal to posterior buccal mucosa

(3) No treatment needed

B. Dental anomalies (Table 5-3■)

1. Abnormalities in size and shape of teeth

a. Concresence—Joining of adjacent teeth by cementum only

b. Dens in dente (Dens invaginatus)—Tooth within a tooth; enamel is deposited within the pulp chamber due to the invagination of enamel organ (Figure 5-11■)

c. Dilaceration—Abnormal root curvature caused by trauma during tooth formation (Figure 5-12■)

d. Enamel pearl—Development of excess enamel on root due to misplaced ameloblasts (Figure 5-13■)

e. Macrodont—Denotes large tooth

(1) Relative—Large tooth compared with the rest of dentition

(2) Absolute—Truly enlarged tooth

f. Microdont—Denotes a small tooth (Figure 5-14■)

(1) Relative—Small tooth compared with the rest of dentition

(2) Absolute—Truly small tooth; peg lateral is most common

g. Regional odontodysplasia (ghost teeth on x-ray)—Evidence of thin enamel and dentin with large pulp chambers

h. Talon cusp—Accessory cusp found on the maxillary and mandibular anteriors

i. Taurodontism—Elongated pulp chamber with short roots

TABLE 5-3   ABNORMALITIES IN THE SIZE AND SHAPE OF TEETH

Lesion	Description	Location	Clinical Manifestation	Treatment
Micro-dontia	Developmental; one or more teeth are smaller than normal	Maxillary lateral incisors (peg lateral) is most common, maxillary third molars	*Location: Clinical manifestations:* Tooth is smaller than normal *Radiographic manifestations:* Tooth is smaller than normal	Can restore tooth to resemble normal tooth
Macro-dontia	Uncommon developmental anomaly; teeth are larger than normal	Any tooth	*Clinical manifestations:* Tooth is larger than normal *Radiographic manifestations:* Tooth is larger than normal	No treatment indicated
Talon cusp	Accessory cusp	Cingulum of maxillary or mandibular permanent incisor	*Clinical manifestations:* Cusp that resembles an eagle's talon *Radiographic manifestations:* Increased radiopacity	Removal of talon cusp if it interferes with occlusion
Tauro-dontism	Elongated, large pulp chambers and short roots; "bull-like" teeth	Molars of deciduous and permanent dentitions	*Clinical manifestations:* Normal crown *Radiographic manifestations:* Abnormally short roots, pulp chamber is large and elongated	No treatment indicated
Dens in dente	Tooth within a tooth	Coronal third of the tooth, single tooth, anterior incisors most common (maxillary lateral most frequent and often peg-shaped)	*Clinical manifestations:* Normal shape or malformed crown with deep pit or crevice in area of cingulum, peg-shaped *Radiographic manifestations:* Tooth-like structure appears within tooth	Vital tooth—prophylactic restoration; nonvital tooth—endodontic treatment
Concre-scence	Two adjacent teeth are united by cementum only; may be caused by crowding	Maxillary molars most common; adjacent supernumerary teeth; erupted, unerupted, or impacted teeth	*Clinical manifestations:* Cannot see clinically *Radiographic manifestations:* Roots of adjacent teeth appear connected	No treatment indicated; extraction of involved teeth is difficult

(continued)

TABLE 5-3 ABNORMALITIES IN THE SIZE AND SHAPE OF TEETH				
Lesion	Description	Location	Clinical Manifestation	Treatment
Dilaceration	Abnormal curve or angle in the crown or root of a tooth	Any tooth	*Clinical manifestations:* Cannot see clinically *Radiographic manifestations:* Sharp bend in root of tooth	No treatment required; extraction or endodontic therapy is difficult
Enamel pearl	Small spherical enamel projection located on a root surface	Commonly found on maxillary molars, attached to cementum near the root bifurcation or trifurcation	*Clinical manifestations:* Cannot see clinically *Radiographic manifestations:* Small sphere of enamel	No treatment indicated
Enamel hypocalcification Regional odonto-dysplasia (ghost teeth)	Teeth exhibit reduction of radiodensity, ghost-like appearance, very thin enamel and dentin, teeth are nonfunctional	Several teeth in a quadrant, especially maxillary primary or permanent	*Clinical manifestations:* No eruption or incomplete eruption *Radiographic manifestations:* Thin enamel or no enamel, large pulp chambers, reduced radiodensity	Extraction

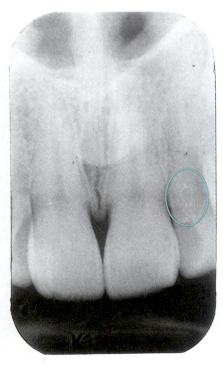

FIGURE 5-11 ■ Dens in Dente

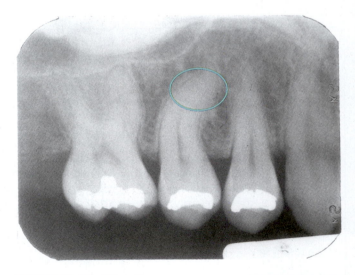

FIGURE 5-12 ■ Dilaceration

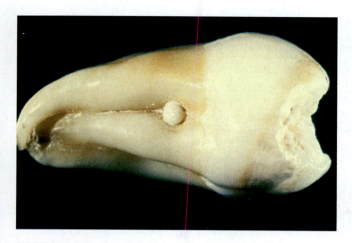

FIGURE 5-13 ■ Enamel Pearl
Source: Edward H. Gill/Custom Medical Stock Photo, Inc.

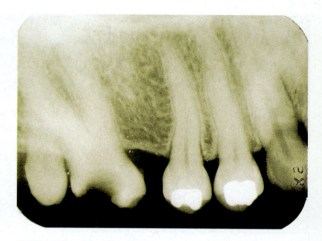

FIGURE 5-14 ■ Microdont
Source: Edward H. Gill/Custom Medical Stock Photo, Inc.

2. Abnormalities in number of teeth (Table 5-4■)

    a. Anodontia (or hypodontia)—Missing teeth; examples include

        (1) Total

        (2) Partial

        (3) Congenital—Failure to develop and may be due to a syndrome (e.g., ectodermal dysplasia)

        (4) Acquired—Through extraction(s)

    b. Fusion—Two teeth are fused into one, resulting in a macrodont; therefore, fewer than normal complement of teeth are present (Figure 5-15■)

    c. Supernumerary (Figure 5-16■)—Extra teeth; mesiodens is most common; usually microdont in size, and may be a result of a syndrome (e.g., cleidocranial dysplasia or dysostosis)

    d. Gemination (twinning) (Figure 5-17■)—Two clinical crowns are evident with usually one root; results in greater than normal number of teeth; usually macrodont in size; result of tooth bud attempting to split

    e. Hypodontia—Lack of one or more teeth, can be any tooth in the dention

TABLE 5-4 ABNORMALITIES IN THE NUMBER OF TEETH

Lesion	Description	Location	Clinical Manifestation	Treatment
Gemination	Incomplete formation of two teeth, paired Gemination = neighboring tooth is present	Primary teeth more common, anterior teeth are more commonly affected	*Clinical manifestations:* Large crown, appears bifid *Radiographic manifestations:* Appears as single root with two crowns joined together	Aesthetic problem, prosthetic treatment
Fusion	Union of two normally separated tooth germs; can be complete or incomplete	Primary teeth more common, anterior region, incisors most common	*Clinical manifestations:* Adjacent teeth appear fused, large crown *Radiographic manifestations:* Large crown with separate fused roots	Aesthetic and occlusal problems; prosthetic treatment
Super-numerary	Extra teeth Mesodens—Most common supernumerary tooth located between maxillary central incisors Distomolar—Second most common supernumerary tooth distal to third molar	Maxillary and mandibular arches, maxillary most common	*Clinical manifestations:* One or more extra teeth, usually smaller than normal *Radiographic manifestations:* One or more extra teeth	Extraction
Anodontia	Congenital lack of teeth	Mandibular and maxillary arches	*Clinical manifestations:* Absence of all primary and permanent dentition *Radiographic manifestations:* All teeth absent	Prosthetic replacement
Hypodontia	Lack of one or more teeth	Any tooth in the dentition, maxillary and mandibular third molars, maxillary lateral incisors, and mandibular second premolars are most common	*Clinical manifestations:* Absence of one or more teeth *Radiographic manifestations:* Absence of one or more teeth	Prosthetic replacement, orthodontic evaluation

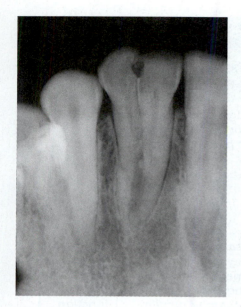

FIGURE 5-15 ■ Fusion

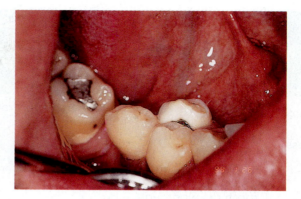

FIGURE 5-16 ■ Supranumerary Teeth

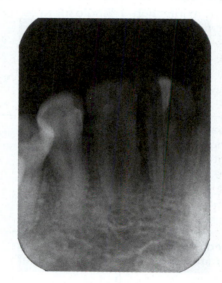

FIGURE 5-17 ■ Gemination

3. Abnormalities in tooth structure (Table 5-5■)

    a. Enamel hypoplasia—Defect in enamel organic matrix formation

        (1) Etiology—Possible factors include

            (a) Genetic (e.g., Amelogenesis imperfecta)

            (b) Environmental (e.g., drug ingestion (fluoride ingestion), fever)

            (c) Metabolic (e.g., vitamin deficiency)

            (d) Febrile illness (e.g., congenital syphilis)

            (e) Trauma or local infection (e.g., infection of decidious teeth)

    b. Enamel hypocalcification—Defect in enamel mineralization

        (1) Etiology—Genetic, environmental, metabolic, or disease

        (2) Oral manifestations—Results in defects in tooth color

        (3) Treatment—None if mild; cosmetic if moderate to severe

TABLE 5-5 ABNORMALITIES OF TOOTH STRUCTURE

Lesion	Description	Location	Clinical Manifestation	Treatment
Enamel hypoplasia Febrile illness or vitamin deficiency	Serious disease such as measles, chicken pox, scarlet fever, or vitamin deficiency (vitamins A, C, and D) that occur during tooth development cause hypoplasia	Permanent central incisors, laterals, cuspids, first molars	Pitting of the enamel, one or more rows of deep pits and stains	
Enamel hypoplasia Local infection or trauma	Occurs from infection of a deciduous tooth	Single tooth re-ferred to as "Turner's tooth"; permanent maxillary incisor and mandibular premolars	*Clinical manifestations:* Yellow to brown enamel, or severe pitting and deformity *Radiographic manifes-tations:* Can be identi-fied before eruption	Restorations for appear-ance or improved function
Enamel hypoplasia Fluoride ingestion	Occurs as a result of large ingestion of concentrated fluoride	All permanent teeth	Mottled (irregular dis-coloration of enamel) discoloration of enamel	Aesthetic— bleaching, bonding, composites, porcelain veneers, crowns
Amelogenesis imperfecta	Inherited conditions affecting the enamel of teeth	All primary and permanent teeth	Random pits on labial and lingual	Asthetic dentistry
Dentino-genesis imperfecta	Hereditary opalescent dentin	All primary and permanent teeth	Bulbous crowns, opalescent brown-bluish color	Asthetic dentistry
Dentinal dysplasia	Abnormal dentin, usually genetic	All primary and permanent teeth	Periapical pathology usually seen on x-ray	Extraction

c. Amelogenesis imperfecta—Abnormal enamel

    (1) Etiology—Genetic or environmental

    (2) Oral manifestations

        (a) Enamel frequently fractures, leaving restorations elevated above the surrounding dentin

        (b) May be an isolated defect or affect several or all teeth

    (3) Clinical manifestations

        (a) Classified according to mode of transmission, appearance, or etiology

(b) Radiographically, teeth exhibit thin, absent, or defective enamel

(4) Treatment—Full coverage restorations

d. Dentinogenesis imperfecta—Abnormal dentin

(1) Etiology—Usually genetic

(2) Oral manifestations—Enamel may fracture due to defective dentinoenamel junction (DEJ)

(3) Clinical manifestations—No pulp chamber or canals are visible on radiographs

(4) Treatment—Full coverage restorations

e. Dentinal dysplasia—Abnormal dentin

(1) Etiology—Usually genetic

(2) Oral manifestations—Roots are short and conical

(3) Clinical manifestations—Periapical pathology is frequently seen on x-ray

(4) Treatment—Usually extraction because of periapical pathology

IV. Cysts

A. Odontogenic cysts (Table 5-6■)

1. Radicular cyst (periapical cyst) (Figures 5-18■ and 5-19■)—Most common intraoral cyst

a. Etiology—Pulpal pathology, which usually results in a nonvital tooth; epithelial lining probably results from rests of Malassez

b. Clinical manifestations—Radiographically, cyst may resemble a periapical abscess or dental granuloma (inflamed granulation tissue with no epithelium)

c. Treatment—Endodontics, apicoectomy, or extraction with bony curettage

2. Residual cyst—Radicular cyst that remains after tooth extraction (Figure 5-20■)

3. Dentigerous cyst (follicular cyst) (Figure 5-21■)—Surrounds crown of unerupted tooth

a. Etiology—Epithelial lining develops from reduced enamel epithelium

b. Clinical manifestations

(1) Cyst attaches at cementoenamel junction (CEJ)

(2) Unilocular radiolucency is evident with well-defined margins

(3) Increased risk of neoplasm forming if left untreated

c. Treatment—Enucleation of cyst, assisted eruption of tooth, or extraction

4. Primordial cyst (Figure 5-22■)—Develops in place of missing tooth

a. Etiology—Epithelial lining develops from remnants of enamel organ

TABLE 5-6 ODONTOGENIC CYSTS RELATED TO TOOTH DEVELOPMENT

Lesion	Description	Location	Clinical Manifestation	Treatment
Dentigerous cyst (also called follicular cyst)	Forms around the crown of an unerupted or developing tooth; epithelial lining originates from the reduced enamel epithelium after the crown has completely formed and calcified	Crown of unerupted or impacted third molar (most common)	*Clinical manifestations:* Can displace teeth if very large *Radiographic manifestations:* Well defined, unilocular radiolucency around crown of unerupted or impacted teeth	Complete removal of cyst and involved tooth
Eruption cyst	Similar to dentigerous cyst	Soft tissue around the crown of an erupting tooth	Soft tissue around crown of an erupting tooth	No treatment needed—tooth erupts through cyst
Primordial cyst	Develops in place of a tooth; originates from remnants of enamel organ; patient history that indicates that a tooth was never present is an important diagnostic tool	Mandibular third molar area; most commonly develops in place of a tooth	Asymptomatic, commonly found in place of third molar or posterior to erupted third molar *Radiographic manifestations:* Well-defined, radiolucent lesion, unilocular or multilocular	Surgical removal of entire lesion
Odontogenic keratocyst	Unique histologic appearance, recurring frequently; lumen is lined with epithelium 8–10 cell layers thick Typically originates from embryologic remnants of the dental lamina	Mandibular third molar region	*Clinical manifestations:* Expansive lesion that can move teeth and resorb tooth *Radiographic manifestations:* Well-defined, multilocular, radiolucent unilocular lesions may also occur	Surgical excision and osseous curettage, high recurrance
Lateral periodontal cyst	Developmental that arises from remnants of the dental lamina	Lateral aspect of tooth usually on mandibular cuspid and premolar area	*Clinical manifestations:* Asymptomatic *Radiographic manifestations:* Unilocular or multilocular radiolucent lesion located on lateral aspect of a tooth root; may cause divergence of adjacent tooth roots	Surgical removal

TABLE 5-6 ODONTOGENIC CYSTS RELATED TO TOOTH DEVELOPMENT (cont.)

Lesion	Description	Location	Clinical Manifestation	Treatment
Gingival cyst	Developmental—develops from epithelial rests of the dental lamina	Soft tissue in mandibular cuspid and premolar area	Swelling of gingival papilla or alveolar mucosa	Local surgical excision
Radicular cyst (periapical cyst)	True cyst—pathologic cavity lined by epithelium; most common cyst in oral cavity Residual cyst—radicular cyst that remains after tooth extraction	Root of nonvital tooth	Most are asymptomatic *Radiographic manifestations:* Well-circumscribed radiolucency attached to the root of the tooth	Root canal, extraction, apicoectomy

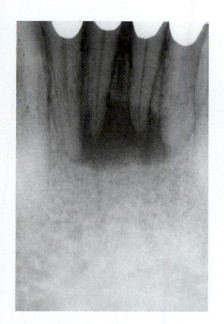

FIGURE 5-18 ■ Radicular Cyst

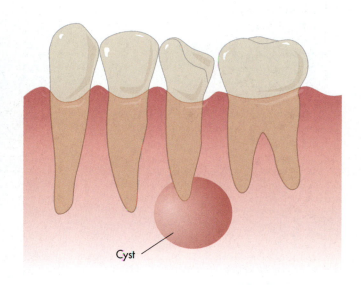

Cyst

FIGURE 5-19 ■ Radicular Cyst

    b. Clinical manifestation—Usually a unilocular radiolucency is evident

    c. Treatment—Surgical removal; enucleation

  5. Eruption cyst—Soft tissue cyst

    a. Etiology—Hematoma in the path of eruption

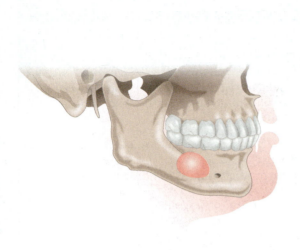

FIGURE 5-20 ■ Residual Cyst

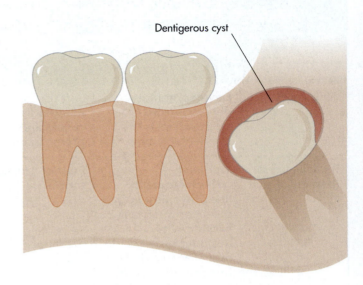

FIGURE 5-21 ■ Dentigerous Cyst

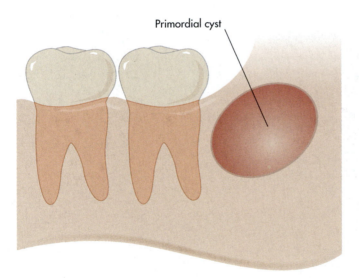

FIGURE 5-22 ■ Primordial Cyst

     b. Clinical manifestations—Usually little or no epithelial lining is evident; fluid buildup is found in path of eruption between crown and soft tissue

     c. Treatment—None or lance overlying gingiva to assist in eruption of tooth

  6. Lateral periodontal cyst—Unilocular or multilocular lucency usually located in mandibular premolar area on lateral aspect of root

     a. Etiology—Epithelial rests in periodontal ligament

     b. Treatment—Surgical removal

7. Gingival cyst—Soft tissue cyst
    a. Etiology—Result of epithelium from rests of Serres (remnants of dental lamina)
    b. Oral manifestations—Swelling usually located on attached gingiva
    c. Treatment—Enucleation, if any
8. Odontogenic keratocyst—Multilocular, rarely unilocular, radiolucency with poorly defined margins
    a. Etiology—Epithelial remnants of odontogenic apparatus
    b. Clinical manifestations—Produces keratin; locally aggressive with a high recurrence rate; and may be indicative of basal cell nevus syndrome
    c. Treatment—Aggressive; complete surgical removal
B. Nonodontogenic cysts (Table 5-7■)
    1. Median palatal cyst (Figure 5-23■)—Unilocular radiolucency in midline of palate
        a. Etiology—Epithelium from rests; remnants are from fusion of palatal shelves
        b. Clinical manifestations—Radiolucency in midline of palate with or without soft tissue swelling
        c. Treatment—Surgical removal
    2. Nasopalatine duct cyst (cyst of the incisive canal)—Located more anteriorly than median palatal cyst
        a. Etiology—Epithelium from rests of nasopalatine duct
        b. Clinical manifestations—Unilocular radiolucency in midline of palate, apical to maxillary centrals (frequently heart-shaped due to superimposed anterior nasal spine)
        c. Treatment—Surgical removal
    3. Median mandibular cyst—Unilocular radiolucency in mandibular midline
        a. Etiology—Epithelium from fusion of rest of mandibular process
        b. Clinical manifestations—Radiolucency in midline of mandible
        c. Treatment—Surgical removal
    4. Globulomaxillary cyst (Figure 5-24■)—Inverted pear-shaped unilocular radiolucency between maxillary canine and lateral incisor
        a. Etiology—Epithelium from fusion rests or odontogenic rests
        b. Oral manifestations—Divergence of roots and convergence of crowns; may exhibit fluctuant soft tissue swelling of gingiva
        c. Treatment—Surgical removal
    5. Simple bone cyst—Pseudocyst of bone with no epithelial lining
        a. Etiology—Considered to be from trauma
        b. Oral manifestations—Unilocular or multilocular lucency that scallops between and around the roots

TABLE 5-7 NONODONTOGENIC CYSTS

Lesion	Description	Location	Clinical Manifestation	Treatment
Nasopalatine duct (incisive canal cyst)	Developmental, arises from epithelial remnants of the nasopalatine duct; commonly seen in adults; when in the papilla, called cyst of the palatine papilla	Nasopalatine canal or the incisive papilla	Asymptomatic, may have pink bulge near apices and between roots of maxillary central incisors on the lingual surface *Radiographic manifestations:* Well-circumscribed radiolucency between maxillary central incisors May cause erosion of the adjacent tooth roots	Surgical removal
Median palatal cyst	Epithelium from remnants from fusion of palatal shelves	Midline of palate	Radiolucency in midline of palate with or without soft tissue swelling	Surgical removal
Median mandibular cyst	Unilocular radiolucency in mandibular midline	Mandibular midline	*Radiographic manifestations:* Radiolucency in midline of mandible	Surgical removal
Globulo-maxillary cyst	Etiology unknown	Between the roots of the maxillary lateral incisor and cuspid	*Clinical manifestations:* Asymptomatic—if a large enough divergence of the roots can result *Radiographic manifestations:* Well-defined pear-shaped radiolucency	Surgical removal
Nasolabial cyst	Soft tissue cyst with no alveolar bone involvement; etiology unknown	Soft tissue of face at nasolabial fold	Swelling in nasolabial fold	Surgical removal
Epidermal cyst	Raised nodule; resembles the epithelium of skin	Skin of the face or neck	Firm, moveable swelling	Surgical removal

			TABLE 5-7 NONODONTOGENIC CYSTS (*continued*)		

Lesion	Description	Location	Clinical Manifestation	Treatment
Dermoid cyst	Soft tissue cyst due to pleuripotential cells derived from ectoderm, mesoderm, and/or endoderm	Floor of the mouth	Fluctuant swelling in floor of mount	Surgical removal
Simple bone cyst	Pseudocyst of bone with no epithelial lining, possibly due to trauma	Mandible	Usually asymptomatic, radiographic scalloping around the roots of teeth	Surgical removal
Aneurysmal bone cyst	Pseudocyst of bone with no epithelial lining considered to be caused from trauma	Posterior maxilla or mandible	Expansion of involved bone, radiographically; honeycomb/soap bubble appearance	Surgical removal, curettage, cryotherapy
Stafne cyst	Pseudocyst (not a true cyst)	Mandible	No bony cavity evident; thinning of mandible; radiographically, well-defined radiolucency inferior to mandibular canal	No treatment needed, variant of normal
Branchial cleft cyst	Soft tissue cyst from trapped rests of branchial clefts	Lateral neck area anterior to sternocleidomastoid muscle, frequently found on ventral side of tongue and floor of mouth	Yellowish nodule	Surgical removal
Thyroglossal duct cyst	Soft tissue cyst; epithelium from remnants of thyroglossal duct (tract)	Midline of neck or posterior portion of tongue	Nodule	Surgical removal

  c. Treatment—Surgery; reveals an empty bony cavity

6. Aneurysmal bone cyst—Pseudocyst of bone with no epithelial lining

  a. Etiology—Considered to be from trauma; histology of blood-filled cavities with peripheral multinucleated giant cells

  b. Clinical manifestations—Multilocular/honeycombed lucency

  c. Treatment—Curettage of bony defect

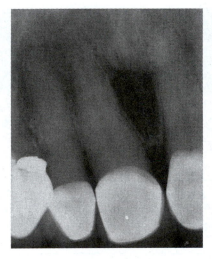

FIGURE 5-23 ■ Median Palatine Cyst

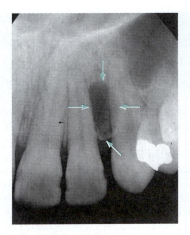

FIGURE 5-24 ■ Globulomaxillary Cyst

7. Stafne cyst (defect)—Pseudocyst

    a. Clinical manifestations

        (1) No bony cavity evident, only thinning of mandible

        (2) Unilocular, well-defined lucency inferior to mandibular canal

    b. Treatment—None; only an anatomical variation

8. Branchial cleft cyst (lymphoepithelial cyst)—Soft tissue cyst in lateral neck area, anterior to sternocleidomastoid muscle

    a. Etiology—Epithelium is from trapped rests of branchial clefts

    b. Oral manifestations—Yellowish nodule frequently found on ventral side of tongue and floor of mouth

    c. Treatment—Surgical removal

9. Thyroglossal duct cyst—Soft tissue cyst in midline of neck or posterior portion of tongue

    a. Etiology—Epithelium is from remnants of thyroglossal duct (tract)

    b. Treatment—Surgical removal

10. Nasolabial cyst—Soft tissue cyst in nasolabial fold or maxillary canine area

    a. Etiology—Epithelium trapped in fusion line of maxillary labial processes

    b. Clinical manifestations—Fluctuant soft tissue swelling inferior and lateral to alae

    c. Treatment—Surgical removal

11. Epidermoid cyst—Soft tissue cyst; contains only tissue derived from ectoderm

    a. Etiology—Trapped epithelium or pleuripotential cells

    b. Clinical manifestation—Skin of the face or neck

    c. Treatment—Surgical removal

12. Dermoid cyst—Soft tissue cyst

    a. Etiology—Pleuripotential cells; contains tissue derived from ectoderm, mesoderm, and/or endoderm

    b. Clinical manifestation—Fluctuant swelling usually found in floor of mouth

    c. Treatment—Surgical removal

V. Benign Neoplasias

A. Nomenclature

1. *Neoplasia* ("new growth")—Implies an uncontrolled growth

2. *Tumor*—Implies swelling; frequently used interchangeably with neoplasm

3. *Benign*—Implies a growth; cannot metastasize (spread to other locations from point of origin); hence, it is not cancer

4. *Malignant*—Has ability to metastasize; therefore, it is cancer

5. *Hyperplasia*—Increase in size resulting from an increase in cell numbers; similar to neoplasia, but is usually a response to stimuli or an irritant

6. *Hypertrophy*—Increase in size resulting from an increase in size of individual cells; mimics neoplasia clinically and is usually a response to stimuli

7. -oma—Suffix added to end of tissue type to imply a benign neoplasm of that tissue (e.g., fibroma, neoplasm of fibrous connective tissue; adenoma, neoplasm of glandular tissue); not all tumors with "oma" suffix are benign (e.g., melanoma is skin cancer)

B. Odontogenic tumors (neoplasms) (Table 5-8■)

1. Ameloblastoma (Figure 5-25■)—Slow-growing, benign, but locally invasive tumor of ameloblasts

    a. Etiology—Ectodermal origin; histologically several types are classified

    b. Oral manifestations—Usually swelling or bony expansion; may be evident only on radiograph

    c. Clinical manifestations

      (1) Multilocular (small unilocular lesions) radiolucency with poorly defined margins

      (2) Peak incidence is in adults, rarely in children

    d. Treatment—Wide surgical excision; recurrence is common

TABLE 5-8 ODONTOGENIC TUMORS

Lesion	Description	Location	Clinical manifestation	Treatment
Amelo-blastoma	Slow-growing aggressive benign tumor, encapsulated and infiltrates into surrounding tissue; can develop from remnants of the dental lamina (rests of Serres), Hertwig's rooth sheath (rests of Malassez), or reduced enamel epithelium lining the dental follicle	Mandible more common; also maxilla	*Clinical manifestations:* Slow-growing expansion of bone, asymptomatic *Radiographic manifestations:* Multilocular honeycombed radio-lucency; may be associated with erosion or divergence of the roots of adjacent teeth	Complete surgical excision
Odontogenic myxoma	Benign non-encapsulated infiltrating tumor; often occurs in young people 10–29 years of age	Mandible more common than maxilla	*Clinical manifestations:* Asymptomatic, expansion of bone *Radiographic manifestations:* Multilocular, honeycombed radio-lucency	Surgical excision
Ameloblastic fibroma	Benign, non-encapsulated tumor of tooth-forming epithelium; more than 90% develop around the crown of an unerupted tooth	Mandibular bicuspid-molar region most common	*Clinical manifestations:* Asymptomatic swelling *Radiographic manifestations:* Well-defined or poorly defined unilocular or multi-locular radiolucency	Surgical removal with extraction of the unerupted tooth
Ontogenic aenomatoid tumor	Encapsulated be-nign tumor sur-rounded by dense fibrous connective tissue; duct-like structures are a distinctive feature, calcifications form in this tumor	70% involve anterior maxilla and mandible	*Clinical manifestations:* Asymptomatic swelling *Radiographic manifestations:* Well-defined radiolucency associ-ated with an impacted tooth; radiopacities within the radiolucency	Enucleation

	TABLE 5-8 ODONTOGENIC TUMORS (*continued*)			
Lesion	**Description**	**Location**	**Clinical manifestation**	**Treatment**
Odontoma	Benign neoplasm composed of mature enamel, dentin, cementum, and dental pulp; two types: compound and complex; most common of odontogenic tumors	Impacted or unerupted teeth, anterior maxilla, posterior mandible most common	*Clinical manifestations:* Failure of permanent tooth to erupt, swelling *Radiographic manifestations:* Compound—cluster of numerous miniature teeth surrounded by radiolucent halo; complex—radiopaque mass surrounded by a thin radiolucent halo	Surgical excision
Cementoma	Hyperplasia of cementum	Anterior portion of mandible at apices	*Radiographic manifestations:* Well-defined and varies from radiolucent to radiopaque, depending on amount of calcified tissue	Surgical excision
Cemento-blastoma	Benign cementum-producing lesion fused to the root of the tooth	Mandibular molars and premolars most common	*Clinical manifestations:* Pain and localized expansion *Radiographic manifestations:* Well-defined radiopaque mass in continuity with the root; mass is surrounded by radiolucent halo	Enucleation of the tumor, removal of involved tooth
Calcifying epithelial odontogenic tumor (Pindborg tumor)	Slow-growing benign tumor of ectodermal origin	Common on mandible but can occur anywhere on maxilla or mandible	Multilocular radioluncency; may be locally invasive; may cause scalloped tooth resorption	Wide surgical excision
Odontogenic myxoma	Slow-growing benign tumor of mesodermal orgin	Anywhere on maxilla or mandible	May cause scalloped tooth resorption Radiographically: Multilocular, honeycombed appearance with poorly defined margins; can cause tooth displacement	Wide surgical excision

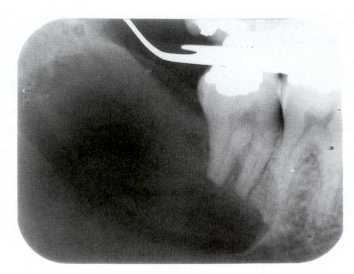

FIGURE 5-25 ■ Ameloblastoma

2. Ameloblastic fibroma—Slow-growing benign tumor made up of ameloblasts and fibroblasts
  a. Etiology—Odontogenic origin (ectodermal and mesodermal components)
  b. Clinical manifestations
    (1) More frequently seen in children and adolescents
    (2) Usually unilocular in form (occasionally multilocular)
    (3) Most have well-defined margins
  c. Treatment—Surgical enucleation; recurrence is unusual
3. Odontogenic adenomatoid tumor (OAT)—Slow-growing benign tumor
  a. Etiology—Ectodermal origin
  b. Oral manifestations—Most frequently found in anterior part of maxilla and may or may not involve impacted teeth
  c. Clinical manifestations
    (1) Early lesions are present as unilocular radiolucencies; older lesions show multiple radiopaque foci
    (2) If an impacted tooth is involved, it is frequently mistaken for a dentigerous cyst (except radiolucency encompasses more than just crown of tooth)
    (3) Usually found in young patients
  d. Treatment—Conservative surgical enucleation; recurrence is rare

4. Calcifying epithelial odontogenic tumor (CEOT)—Also known as Pindborg tumor (slow-growing benign tumor)

    a. Etiology—Ectodermal origin

    b. Clinical manifestations

        (1) May or may not involve unerupted teeth

        (2) Slight tendency for tumor to invade locally

        (3) Radiographs show unilocular or multilocular radiolucency with poorly defined margins and scattered radiopaque foci

        (4) Tumor may produce amyloid

        (5) Usually seen in adults

    c. Treatment—Wide surgical excision; recurrence is common

5. Odontogenic myxoma—Slow-growing benign tumor

    a. Etiology—Mesodermal origin; cell of origin thought to be stellate reticulum

    b. Oral manifestations—May cause scalloped tooth resorption

    c. Clinical manifestations

        (1) Presents itself as a multilocular (small lesion may be unilocular) radiolucency with poorly defined margins

        (2) May be locally invasive

        (3) Usually seen in young adults

    d. Treatment—Wide surgical excision; recurrence is common

6. Odontoma (Figure 5-26■)—Benign tumor that forms enamel, dentin, and cementum

    a. Types

        (1) Compound odontoma—Formation of well-organized microdonts

           (a) Oral manifestations—Most commonly found in anterior teeth

           (b) Treatment—Surgical removal with no recurrence

        (2) Complex odontoma—Disorganized haphazard formation of enamel, dentin, and cementum

           (a) Oral manifestations—Involve no developed teeth; most commonly found in posterior portion of mandible

           (b) Treatment—Surgical removal with no recurrence

7. Cementoma (periapical cemental dysplasia)—Hyperplasia of the cementum

    a. Etiology—Cells probably arise from pluripotential cells in periodontal ligament (PDL)

    b. Oral manifestations—Most commonly found in anterior portion of mandible at apices in females

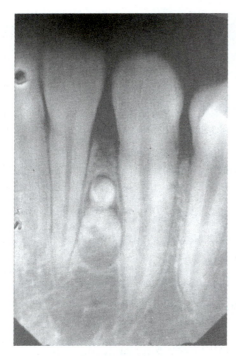

FIGURE 5-26 ■ Odontoma

    c. Clinical manifestations

        (1) Early stages are entirely radiolucent and resemble periapical pathology, but teeth remain vital

        (2) Older lesions become progressively more radiopaque

    d. Treatment—Surgical excision

  8. Cementoblastoma—True neoplasm of cementum

    a. Etiology—Derived from PDL cells

    b. Clinical manifestations

        (1) Usually tumor is all radiopaque with apex of root obliterated on x-ray film

        (2) Usually located in mandibular premolar and molar areas

        (3) Pain may be patient's chief complaint

    c. Treatment—Root amputation (or extraction) and enucleation of tumor

 C. Benign mucosal neoplasms (Table 5-9■)

  1. Fibroma—Most common intraoral soft tissue neoplasm (Figure 5-27■)

    a. Clinical manifestations

        (1) Forms may be sessile, pedunculated, or only hyperplasia in response to stimuli (e.g., irritation = irritation fibroma)

        (2) Color is of normal mucosa unless neoplasm is secondarily ulcerated

TABLE 5-9 BENIGN MUCOSAL NEOPLASMS				
Lesion	**Description**	**Location**	**Clinical Manifestation**	**Treatment**
Fibroma	Most common intraoral soft tissue neoplasm	Anywhere intraorally	Forms may be sellile, pedunoculated, or hyperplasia in response to stimuli Color is of normal mucosa unless neoplasms then secondarily ulcerated	Surgical excision
Pyogenic granuloma	A reactive hyperplasia of vascularized granulation tissue; develops in response to local irritating factors; hormonal changes associated with pregnancy are contributing factor; proliferation of connective tissue; not pus producing; called pregnancy tumor	Gingiva most common area	Ulcerated deep red-purple lesion that bleeds easily	Surgical removal if not resolved
Peripheral giant cell granuloma	A reactive hyperplasia containing osteoclast-like multinucleated giant cells that develops in response to local irritating factors	Occurs exclusively on gingiva or alveolar process anterior to molars	Resembles pyogenic granuloma	Surgical excision; treat local factors (remove bacterial plaque and calculus)
Central giant cell granuloma	A reactive granulomatous proliferation containing multinucleated giant cells; may represent a reparative response to inflammation within the bone; primarily in children and young adults	Occurs within the bone of the maxilla or mandible and primarily in anterior sextants	Asymptomatic; divergence of the roots or teeth adjacent to lesion is common; firm to palpation *Radiographic manifestations:* Most are discovered on routine radiographs, produces radiolucency in the bone	Curettage for smaller lesions Surgical removal for larger lesions

(continued)

TABLE 5-9 BENIGN MUCOSAL NEOPLASMS (continued)

Lesion	Description	Location	Clinical Manifestation	Treatment
Granular cell tumor	Neoplasm of cells exhibiting granular cytoplasm of primitive neural cell origin	Almost exclusively found in adults; most commonly on dorsal portion of tongue but ocassionally occurs elsewhere in oral cavity	Sessile elevation frequently exhibiting a central depression	Surgical excision
Congential epulis	Tumor of gingiva present at birth	Infants; usually occurs on maxillary anterior gingiva but may arise in mandible	Histologically resembles granular cell tumor in adults; soft tissue mass	Surgical excision
Epulis fissuratum	Denture-induced hyperplasia caused from ill-fitting dentures	Elongated folds of tissue along denture flange	Along denture border	Surgical removal of excess tissue, new denture
Papillary hyperplasia	Caused by removable full or partial dentures or orthodontic appliances	On palate	Erythematous papillary projections (cobblestone appearance)	Surgical removal of tissue, new appliance; remove dentures at night
Papilloma	Benign tumor	Soft palate, tongue	Small exophytic pedunculated growth composed of numerous projections that may be white or normal mucosal color "cauliflower-like" appearance	Surgical excision
Lipoma	Benign tumor of mature fat cells	Buccal mucosa, vestibule most common	Yellowish mass	Surgical excision

| | | | Clinical | |
Lesion	Description	Location	Manifestation	Treatment
Chronic hyperplastic pulpitis (pulp polyp)	Excessive proliferation of chronically nflamed pulp tissue in children and young adults	Occurs in teeth with large, open carious lesions; occurs in primary or permanent molars	Red granulation tissue protruding from the pulp chamber fills the cavity of the tooth	Extraction of tooth or endodontic treatment
Cementifying fibroma and ossifying fibroma	Fibroosseous lesion containing cementum and bone	Mandible	Asymptomatic expansion, facial asymmetry Radiographic: Well-defined unilocular lesion, varying degrees of opacities	Surgical excision

Table heading: **TABLE 5-9 BENIGN MUCOSAL NEOPLASMS (*continued*)**

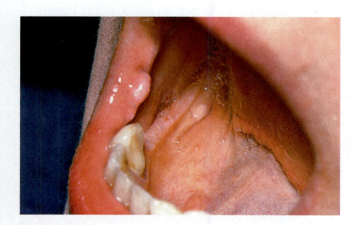

FIGURE 5-27   ■   Fibroma

   (3) Can occur anywhere intraorally

   b. Treatment—Surgical excision with no recurrence

2. Ossifying fibroma—Fibro-osseous lesion that may occur in soft tissue (peripheral ossifying fibroma) or in bone (central ossifying fibroma) (see Neoplasms of the bone)

   a. Etiology

   (1) Odontogenic origin

   (2) Cells of origin are probably from pluripotential cells in PDL

   (3) Histology consists of essentially dense fibrous connective tissue with spicules of vital bone forming with neoplasm

b. Oral manifestations—Development usually occurs on gingiva

c. Clinical manifestations

(1) Peripheral ossifying fibroma mimics fibroma, but texture may be more firm

(2) Form may be sessile or pedunculated

d. Treatment—Surgical excision with no recurrence

3. Cementifying fibroma—Same as ossifying fibroma except it forms cementum within neoplasm instead of bone

a. Etiology—Cells are probably from pluripotential cells in PDL

b. Clinical manifestations—Include a peripheral and central variety (see Neoplasms of the bone)

c. Treatment—None or surgical removal

4. Ossifying-cementifying fibroma (Figure 5-28■)—Same as above except it forms bone and cementum within neoplasm

a. Etiology—Cells are probably from pluripotential cells in PDL

b. Clinical manifestations—Also include a peripheral and central variety (see Neoplasms of the bone)

c. Treatment—None or surgical removal

5. Lipoma (Figure 5-29■)—Neoplasm of adipose (fat) tissue

a. Clinical manifestations—May occur anywhere in oral cavity; form is sessile or pedunculated and of soft texture

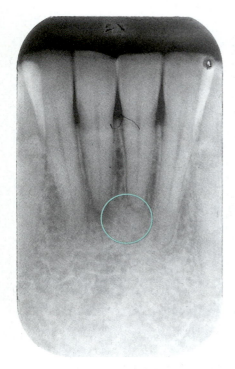

FIGURE 5-28 ■ Ossifying-Cementifying Fibroma

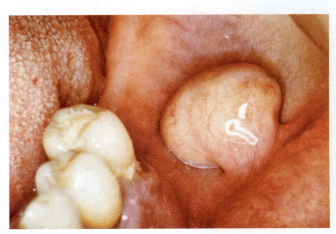

FIGURE 5-29 ■ Lipoma

Source: Edward H. Gill/Custom Medical Stock Photo, Inc.

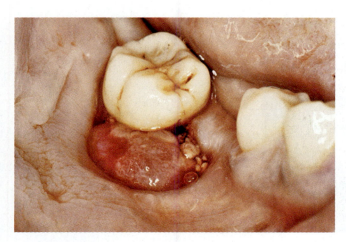

FIGURE 5-30 ■ Pyogenic Granuloma
Source: Edward H. Gill/Custom Medical Stock Photo, Inc.

    b. Treatment—Surgical excision with no recurrence

6. Pyogenic granuloma (Figure 5-30■)—Reactive hyperplasia resulting from a local irritant (usually calculus)

    a. Etiology—Histology consists of inflamed granulation-type tissue with numerous capillaries

    b. Clinical manifestations

        (1) Called granuloma gravidarum (pregnancy tumor) if it occurs in pregnant patient; result of an exaggerated response to hormonal stimuli

        (2) Usually a pedunculated hemorrhagic-colored mass arising from crevicular sulcus

        (3) Bleeds readily on manipulation

        (4) May become quite large or may undergo spontaneous remission

        (5) Older lesions may become sclerotic (fibrous tissue replacement) and eventually resemble a fibroma

    c. Treatment—Surgical excision with removal of irritant; lesion may recur

7. Giant cell tumor (giant cell granuloma) (Figure 5-31■)—Neoplasm of multinucleated giant cells

    a. Etiology—Unknown

        (1) Histology consists of granulation-type tissue with numerous multinucleated giant cells

        (2) Multiple giant cell tumors of bone may be seen in patients with hyperparathyroidism

    b. Clinical manifestations

        (1) Varieties—Peripheral (soft tissue) and central (intraosseous) (see Neoplasms of the bone)

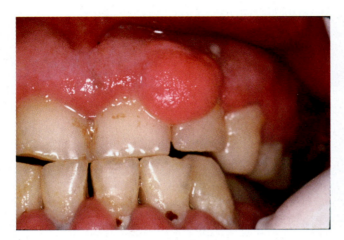

FIGURE 5-31 ■ Peripheral Giant Cell Granuloma

   (2) Similar presentation as a pyogenic granuloma

   (3) Soft tissue lesions tend to be "liver" colored

   (4) Form is pedunculated and tends to grow from crevicular sulcus

  c. Treatment—Surgical excision with recurrence rare

8. Granular cell tumor (granular cell myoblastoma)—Neoplasm of cells exhibiting a granular cytoplasm (myoblastoma—previous terminology used when cell of origin was thought to be a myoblast)

  a. Etiology—Considered to be of primitive neural cell origin

   (1) Histologically, epithelium may proliferate (pseudoepitheliomatous hyperplasia) into underlying lamina propria in 50% of cases, mimicking squamous cell carcinoma, except lesion is benign

  b. Oral manifestations—Most commonly occurs on dorsal portion of tongue, but occasionally occurs elsewhere in oral cavity

  c. Clinical manifestations

   (1) Sessile elevation (nodule), frequently exhibiting a central depression

   (2) Almost exclusively found in adults

  d. Treatment—Surgical excision with no recurrence

9. Congenital epulis (of the newborn)—Tumor of gingiva that is present at birth

  a. Etiology—Unknown

   (1) Histologically resembles granular cell tumor in adults, but cells are thought to be of a different origin

  b. Clinical manifestations—Soft tissue mass; usually occurs on maxillary anterior gingiva, but may arise in mandible

  c. Treatment—Surgical excision with no recurrence

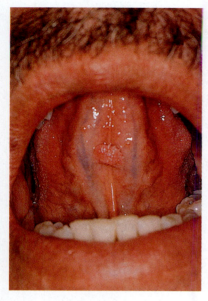

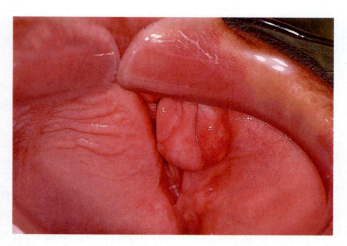

FIGURE 5-33 ■ Epulis Fissuratum

FIGURE 5-32 ■ Papiloma

10. Papilloma (Figure 5-32■)—Epithelial neoplasm induced by papillomavirus

    a. Oral manifestations—Occurs anywhere intraorally as a pedunculated (occasionally sessile) mass with small papillary projections or cauliflower-like surface

    b. Treatment—Surgical excision with recurrence unusual

11. Epulis fissuratum (denture hyperplasia) (Figure 5-33■)—Not a true neoplasm

    a. Clinical manifestations—Reactive hyperplasia caused by an overextended, poor-fitting denture; denture flange sits in groove or crevice created by lesion

    b. Treatment—Surgical excision and remake denture

D. Benign nerve tumors

    1. Neuroma—Neoplasm of neural tissue

        a. Clinical manifestations

            (1) True neoplasm of nerve tissue referred to as plexiform neuroma

            (2) Form may be sessile or pedunculated

            (3) Intraosseous or soft tissue; soft tissue neoplasm exhibits color of normal mucosa; intraosseous form is usually a unilocular radiolucency

            (4) Hyperplasia of neural processes due to trauma is referred to as traumatic neuroma

                (a) Occurs when nerve process is amputated and degenerates while myelin tube (conduit) remains

(b) If scar tissue obstructs myelin conduit as nerve process regenerates, it continues to proliferate, creating a neoplasm of nerve tissue

b. Treatment—Surgical excision with no recurrence

2. Neurofibroma—Neoplasm of neural elements and fibrous connective tissue

   a. Clinical manifestations

   (1) May occur anywhere intraorally

   (2) Multiple neurofibromas may be indicative of von Recklinghausen's syndrome (potential of neurofibromas to undergo malignant transformation)

   b. Treatment—Surgical excision with no recurrence (except von Recklinghausen's syndrome)

3. Neurilemoma (Schwannoma)—Neoplasm of Schwann cells (produce myelin sheath); most often involves the mandible

   a. Forms

   (1) Intraosseous or soft tissue—Usually a unilocular lucency; color is of normal mucosa

   (2) Sessile or pedunculated

   b. Treatment—Surgical excision with no recurrence

E. Vascular neoplasms (Table 5-10■)

1. Hemangioma (Figure 5-34■)—Neoplasm of blood vessels

   a. Etiology—Usually congenital; three types based on histology

   (1) Cellular hemangioma—Composed only of endothelial cells; no vascular channels formed

   (2) Capillary hemangioma—Composed of small vascular channels

   (3) Cavernous hemangioma—Composed of large dilated channels

TABLE 5-10 VASCULAR TUMORS				
Lesion	Description	Location	Clinical manifestation	Treatment
Hemangioma	Benign proliferation of capillaries	Intraoral—tongue most common	Deep red or blue lesions, blanch when pressure is applied	Spontaneous remission
Lymphangioma	Benign tumors composed of lymphatic vessels, present at birth	Intraoral—tongue	Ill-defined mass with pebbly surface	Local surgical excision

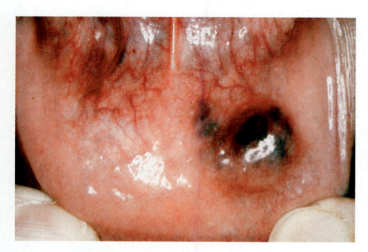

FIGURE 5-34 ■ Hemangioma

    b. Oral manifestation—Most commonly found on tongue

    c. Clinical manifestations

        (1) Enlarges slowly

        (2) Superficial lesions are sessile-red or bluish-red; deeper lesions are of normal color and only palpable or slightly elevated on surface; vascular color not readily detectable in deeper lesions

        (3) May develop in bone as poorly defined multilocular/honeycombed lucencies

    d. Treatment—Use sclerosing agents or surgical excision for small lesions; no recurrence

  2. Lymphangioma (Figure 5-35■)—Neoplasm of lymphatic vessels

    a. Etiology—Usually congenital

    b. Oral manifestations—Most commonly found on tongue

    c. Clinical manifestations

        (1) Cystic hygroma—Congenital lymphangioma in neck

        (2) Sessile in form and color is of normal mucosa

        (3) May only be palpable or cause slight elevation of surface mucosa

    d. Treatment—Use of sclerosing agents or surgical excision with no recurrence

F. Neoplasms of muscle

  1. Rhabdomyoma—Neoplasm of striated (voluntary) muscle

    a. Oral manifestation—Sometimes found on tongue

    b. Clinical manifestations—Lesions are usually sessile in form, deep, and only palpable or cause slight elevation of surface mucosa

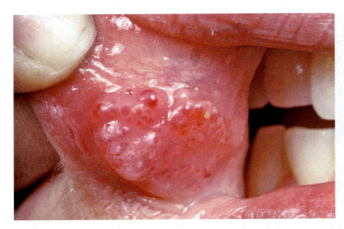

FIGURE 5-35 ■ Lymphangioma

Source: Mediscan

    c. Treatment—Surgical excision with no recurrence

  2. Leiomyoma—Neoplasm of smooth (involuntary) muscle

    a. Etiology—Origin is in smooth muscle wall of blood vessels

    b. Oral manifestations—Rarely found intraorally, usually a uterine fibrous tumor

    c. Clinical manifestations

      (1) Occurs in association with blood vessels

      (2) Sessile in form, palpable, or may cause slight elevation of surface mucosa

    d. Treatment—Surgical excision with no recurrence

G. Salivary gland neoplasms (Table 5-11■)

  1. Pleomorphic adenoma (mixed tumor)—Slow-growing, encapsulated, sessile neoplasm of glandular tissue

    a. Etiology—Consists of ectodermal and mesodermal derivatives (mixed)

    b. Clinical manifestations—Most commonly found in parotid gland extraorally and in minor salivary glands of palate intraorally

    c. Treatment—Surgical excision with chance of recurrence owing to incomplete removal

  2. Monomorphic adenoma—Glandular neoplasm

    a. Oral manifestations—Most commonly found in upper lip

    b. Clinical manifestations

      (1) Consists of one cellular element (monomorphic)

      (2) Sessile form may only be palpable or cause elevation of surface mucosa

    c. Treatment—Surgical excision with no recurrence

TABLE 5-11 SALIVARY GLAND TUMORS

Lesion	Description	Location	Clinical manifestation	Treatment
Pleomorphic adenoma (benign mixed tumor)	Benign tumor that is encapsulated with a mixture of both epithelium and connective tissue	Extraoral—parotid gland; intraoral—palate; can occur wherever salivary gland tissue is present	Slowly enlarging, nonulcerated, painless, dome-shaped mass	Surgical removal; most common salivary gland neoplasm
Monomorphic adenoma	Benign encapsulated salivary gland tumor composed of a uniform pattern or epithelial cells; do not have connective tissue	Most common in the upper lip; can occur anywhere salivary gland tissue is present	Smooth-surfaced mass	Surgical excision
Warthin's tumor	Monomorphic adenoma with two types of tissue: epithelial and lymphoid	Parotid gland often bilaterally and predominantly in adult men	painless, soft, compressible mass	Surgical excision

3. Warthin's tumor (papillary cystadenoma lymphomatosum)—Glandular neoplasm

    a. Etiology—Ductal epithelial proliferation within lymphoid aggregates

    b. Clinical manifestations—Seen predominantly in parotid gland of males, rarely intraorally and occasionally bilaterally; palpable or elevation of the surface

    c. Treatment—Surgical excision with no recurrence

H. Neoplasms of the bone (Table 5-12■)

    1. Exostosis—Hyperplasia of the bone

        a. Oral manifestations

            (1) Frequently seen on alveolar process

            (2) Specific areas, such as palate (midline) and lingual of mandible (premolar areas), are referred to as palatal torus or mandibular tori, respectfully

        b. Clinical manifestations

            (1) Not a true neoplasm of bone (osteoma)

TABLE 5-12 NEOPLASMS OF THE BONE

Lesion	Description	Location	Clinical manifestation	Treatment
Exostosis	Hyperplasia of the bone; not a true neoplasm of the bone	Alveolar process	Consists of a hard texture with color of normal mucosa unless secondarily ulcerated Radiographically, bone is more radioopaque with poorly defined margins	No treatment necessary unless there is interference with speech and mastication
Osteoma	Benign tumor of mature bone that appears normal	Intraosseous	*Clinical manifestations:* Asymptomatic *Radiographic manifestations:* Sharply defined radiopaque mass; may displace adjacent tooth roots	Surgical excision
Chondroma	Neoplasm of cartilage	Rarely found intraorally but may be seen in maxillary anterior or mandibular premolar area		Surgical excision
Osteosarcoma	Malignant tumor of bone-forming tissue (osteoblasts)	Mandible twice as frequent as maxilla	*Clinical manifestations:* Painful swelling, expansion of bone *Radiographic manifestations:* Destructive radiolucent to radiopaque poorly defined lesion; asymmetric widening of periodontal ligament space; "sunburst" pattern	Surgical excision; chemotherapy most common tumor in patients under 40 years of age

      (2) Consists of a hard texture with color of normal mucosa unless secondarily ulcerated

      (3) Large lesions frequently exhibit a lobular shape

      (4) On radiographs, there is evidence of more radiopaque bone with poorly defined margins

      (5) No malignant potential

  c. Treatment—None, unless there is interference with speech and mastication, then surgical excision; occasional slow recurrence

2. Osteoma—Slow-growing neoplasm of bone

  a. Etiology—Arises from periosteum or endosteum

  b. Clinical manifestations

      (1) Almost exclusively found in membranous bones of skull and face in older adults; most commonly found in sinus and on medial surface of ascending ramus or inferior border of mandible

      (2) Detected by palpation or visual asymmetry of area

      (3) Usually sessile in form and occasionally pedunculated

      (4) Radiographically, appears as a solitary mass of dense bone with well-defined margins

      (5) Multiple osteomas may be indicative of Gardner's syndrome (osteomas and intestinal polyps; polyps may undergo malignant transformation)

  c. Treatment—Surgical excision with no recurrence

3. Chondroma—Neoplasm of cartilage

  a. Oral manifestation—Rarely found intraorally, but may be seen in maxillary anterior or mandibular premolar area and at symphysis; locally invasive

  b. Treatment—Surgical excision with rare recurrence

4. Central ossifying fibroma (fibro-osseous lesion of bone)—Same as soft tissue neoplasm, but located within bone

  a. Clinical manifestation—Seen on radiographs as an unilocular radiolucency with varying degrees of radiopacities; usually asymptomatic

  b. Treatment—Surgical removal if symptomatic

5. Central cementifying fibroma—Same as soft tissue neoplasm and central ossifying fibroma stated above, but with spicules of cementum

  a. Treatment—Surgical removal if symptomatic

6. Central cementifying-ossifying fibroma—Same as above, but produces cementum and bone

7. Fibrous dysplasia (monostotic fibro-osseous lesion of the jaws)—Unilateral asymptomatic enlargement of maxilla or mandible

    a. Etiology—Unknown, but trauma and infection are suspected

    b. Oral manifestations—May cause malalignment of teeth

    c. Clinical manifestations

        (1) Considered a neoplasm because of the enlargement

        (2) Radiographs vary from unilocular to multilocular, well-defined radiolucencies to fine trabeculations

        (3) Described as a "ground glass" appearance that blends into surrounding normal bone

    d. Treatment—Removal of lesion and/or recontouring of bone

8. Central giant cell tumor of bone—Similar to soft tissue neoplasm

    a. Clinical manifestations

        (1) Consists of neoplastic, large, multinucleated cells

        (2) Radiographically, a unilocular or multilocular radiolucency is seen with poorly defined margins

        (3) Multiple neoplasms are seen in patients with hyperparathyroidism

    b. Treatment—Surgical removal; treat endocrine disorder if hyperparathyroidism exists

VI. Salivary Gland Pathology

  A. Inflammation and stone formation

    1. *Sialadenitis*—Inflammation of salivary gland tissue

      a. Etiology—May be trauma, mucus retention, or inspissation

      b. Clinical manifestations—May result in enlargement of gland and be acute or chronic

      c. Treatment—Removal or correction of etiology

    2. *Sialodochitis*—Inflammation of salivary gland duct

      a. Etiology—Possible mucus retention or stone formation, but usually trauma

      b. Clinical manifestation—Erythematous oriface of duct; may result in mucus retention if inflammation occludes duct

      c. Treatment—Removal of etiology

    3. *Sialolithiasis*—Stone formation

      a. Etiology—Unknown; may be due to mineralization of mucus plug within the duct

      b. Clinical manifestation—Calcified obstruction may cause mucus retention with swelling; may be palpable and/or visible on radiographs

      c. Treatment—Removal

4. Xerostomia—Dryness of mouth owing to reduced salivary flow

    a. Etiology—Result of inflammation, atrophy, autoimmune disease, or drugs/medications

    b. Clinical manifestation—Oral dryness; may cause mucosal changes

    c. Treatment—Salivary stimulants or saliva substitutes

5. Sjögren's syndrome—Lymphocytic infiltration of salivary glands, resulting in loss of function

    a. Etiology—Autoimmune

    b. Oral manifestations

        (1) Dry mouth (xerostomia)—May lead to erythema of mucosal surfaces

        (2) Tongue may exhibit atrophy of papillae

    c. Clinical manifestations

        (1) Dry eyes (xerophthalmia)—Resulting from destruction of lacrimal glands; results in damage referred to as keratoconjunctivitis sicca

        (2) Frequently other autoimmune processes are characteristic of syndrome

    d. Treatment—Steroids, pilocarpine (stimulates salivary flow), and saliva and tear substitutes

6. Necrotizing sialometaplasia—Necrosis of salivary gland tissue with metaplasia of ducts

    a. Etiology—Caused by infarction of blood supply to the area; amount of destruction is dependent on degree of infarction

    b. Oral manifestation—Necrosis of tissue in palate

    c. Treatment—Palliative, self-limiting

B. Mucous extravasation and retention

    1. Mucocele (Figure 5-36■)

        a. Etiology—Result of trauma to salivary gland duct and extravasation of mucin into surrounding connective tissue; granulation tissue with inflammation surrounds inspissated mucin histologically

        b. Oral manifestations

            (1) Most commonly found in lower lip

            (2) Superficial lesions may present as sessile in form with bluish or translucent swelling; deep lesions may only be palpable or cause elevation of normal-appearing vermillion zone or mucosa

            (3) Swellings may fluctuate in size depending on salivary flow

        c. Treatment—Surgical excision of involved gland and duct

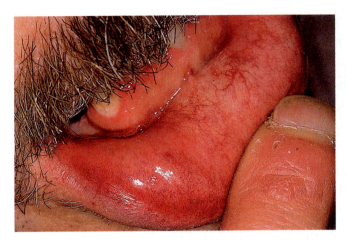

FIGURE 5-36 ■ Mucocele

    2. Mucus retention phenomenon—Same as above without rupture of salivary gland duct

        a. Etiology—Resulting from obstruction of duct by mucus plug or sialolith, resulting in mucin retention without extravasation into surrounding connective tissue

        b. Clinical manifestations

           (1) Extravasation or retention result in similar clinical presentation as stated with mucocele

           (2) Distinction may be evident only histologically

           (3) May occur anywhere minor salivary glands are located

        c. Treatment—Surgical excision

    3. Ranula (Figure 5-37■)—Not a diagnosis, but a clinical description of swelling in floor of mouth

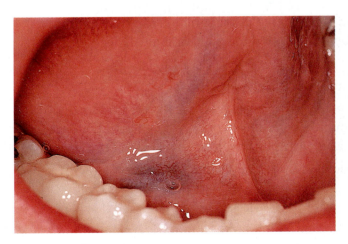

FIGURE 5-37 ■ Ranula

a. Etiology—Frequently resulting from mucus retention as a result of obstruction of submandibular (Wharton's) duct

b. Treatment—Removal of etiology

VII.   Infectious Diseases

A. Bacterial diseases (Table 5-13■)

1. Tuberculosis (TB)—Contagious lung disease

    a. Etiology

        (1) Caused by *Mycobacterium tuberculosis,* a Gram-negative, acid-fast bacillus

        (2) Histologically, classified as granulomatous inflammation with caseous (cheeselike) necrosis and Langerhans giant cells (multinucleated giant cell with nuclei arranged in horseshoe-shaped pattern around periphery of cytoplasm)

    b. Oral manifestations

        (1) Lesions present as progressively enlarging painful ulcerations probably caused by infected sputum

        (2) Oral ulcerations heal as respiratory disease becomes quiescent

    c. Clinical manifestations

        (1) Portal of entry is through respiratory tract

        (2) Lung lesions heal with calcification of necrotic areas visible on chest radiographs

        (3) Chronic cough significant in medical history

        (4) Involvement of nodes in head and neck area are referred to as scrofula

        (5) Involvement of internal viscera referred to as miliary TB

        (6) May involve bone as tuberculous osteomyelitis

        (7) Purified protein derivative (PPD)—Positive test exhibited by erythematous inflammation and induration at injection site within 48 hours

    d. Treatment—Long-term isoniazid, rifampin, or other antituberculous drugs

2. Syphilis—Bacterial disease

    a. Etiology—Caused by *Treponema pallidum*, a spirochete contracted by intimate contact or transplacentally

TABLE 5-13 INFECTIOUS DISEASES: BACTERIAL INFECTIONS

Lesion	Description	Location	Clinical Manifestation	Treatment
Tuberculosis	Infectious chronic granutomatous disease caused by the organism *Mycobacterium tuberculosis*	Lungs—bacteria may spread to other parts of the body; oral lesions are rare and occur on tongue and palate	Oral lesions—painful, nonhealing ulcers	Antituberculosis agents
Actino-mycosis	Infection caused by filamentous bacterium called *Actinomyces israelii*	Skin and oral mucosa	Abscesses that drain bright yellow grains called "sulfur granules"	Antibiotics
Syphilis	Disease caused by spirochete *Treponema pallidum* transmitted from one person to another by direct contact, usually by sexual contact	Primary—oral lesions, mucous membranes Secondary—oral lesions, mucous membranes Tertiary—years after initial infection, involve cardiovascular system and nervous system	Primary—chancre, highly infectious, exhibits piled-up periphery Secondary—mucous patches, grayish-white plaques, most infectious Tertiary—lesion called "gumma", noninfectious	Primary—antibiotics Secondary—antibiotics Tertiary—antibiotics
Acute necrotizing ulcerative gingivitis (ANUG)	Painful erythematous gingivitis, necrosis of the interdental papillae caused by fusiform bacillus and spirochete (*Borrelia cincentii*)	Gingiva	Gingiva is painful and erythematous with foul odor and metallic taste; cratering of interdental papilla *Systemic:* fever, cervical lymphadenopathy	Antibiotics, debridement of necrotic tissues, good oral hygiene

TABLE 5-13 INFECTIOUS DISEASES: BACTERIAL INFECTIONS (cont.)				
Lesion	**Description**	**Location**	**Clinical Manifestation**	**Treatment**
Pericoronitis	Inflammation due to infection by bacteria of mucosal around crown of a partially erupted, impacted tooth; trauma to soft tissue flap (operculum) may also be a cause	Tissue around partially erupted tooth, third molar most common	Swollen, erythematous tissue around partially erupted tooth	Debridement, irrigation, antibiotics
Acute osteomyelitis	Acute inflammation of bone and bone marrow	Bone	Jaw—result from periapical abscess	Drainage, antibiotics
Chronic osteomyelitis	Chronic inflammation of bone, perhaps from inadequate treated acute osteomyelitis	Bone	Painful swollen bone *Radiographic manifestations:* Diffuse and irregular radiolucency that can eventually become radiopaque (chronic sclerosing osteomyelitis)	Debridement/ systemic antibiotics

b. Three stages with characteristic lesions

  (1) Primary stage—Chancre lesion; usually occurs at site of inoculation as a deeply cratered ulceration frequently exhibiting a "piled-up" periphery

   (a) Oral manifestations—Chancres exhibit whitish membrane that may not be diagnostic of syphilis

   (b) Treatment—Antibiotic therapy

  (2) Secondary stage—Evidence of pruritic rash on skin and/or mucous patches on the mucosal surfaces

   (a) Oral manifestations

    i) Lesions are widespread and not associated with site of inoculation

    ii) Skin lesions exude clear fluid when scratched and contains the spirochete

    iii) Mucous patches may also exhibit a whitish membrane teeming with spirochete

(b) Treatment—Secondary stage may recur frequently and requires antibiotic therapy

(3) Tertiary stage—Gumma (gummatous necrosis)

(a) Oral manifestations

i) Occurs years after primary stage

ii) Lesions fatal if they occur in vital structures

(b) Treatment—None

(4) Clinical manifestations of congenital syphilis: Hutchinson's incisors—screwdriver-shaped incisors; mulberry molors—berry-like cusp appearance (Figure 5-38■)

3. Gonorrhea—Sexually transmitted disease

a. Etiology—Caused by *Neisseria gonorrhoeae*, a diplococcus

b. Oral manifestations—Oral lesions are rare, but, if present, resemble nonspecific ulcerations containing microorganisms

c. Treatment—Antibiotics

4. Actinomycosis—Bacterial infection

a. Etiology

(1) Resulting from *Actinomyces israelii*, a normal inhabitant of the oral cavity

(2) Organism causes disease when implanted in the deep wounds or extraction sites protected from free oxygen (anaerobe)

b. Clinical manifestations—Forms fistulae that tend to drain through the skin, exuding colonies of the microorganism as yellowish grit referred to as sulfur granules

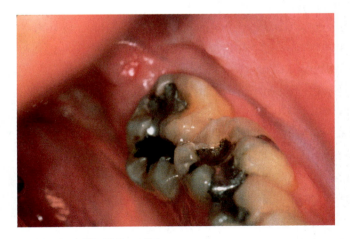

FIGURE 5-38 ■ Mulberry Molar

c. Treatment—Long-term antibiotics

5. Acute necrotizing ulcerative gingivitis (ANUG)—painful erythematous gingivitis, necrosis of the interdental papillae caused by fusiform bacillus and spirochete (*Borrelia cincentii*)

   a. Clinical manifestations—Gingiva is painful and erythematous with foul odor and metallic taste; cratering of interdental papilla; systemic: fever, cervical lymphadenopathy

   b. Antibiotics, debridement of necrotic tissues, good oral hygiene

6. Pericoronitis—Inflammation due to infection by bacteria of mucosa around crown of a partially erupted impacted tooth

   a. Clinical manifestations—Swollen erythematous tissue around partially erupted tooth

   b. Treatment—Debridement, irrigation, antibiotics

7. Acute osteomyelitis—Acute inflammation of the bone and bone marrow

   a. Clinical manifestations—Frequently in jaw resulting from periapical abcess

   b. Treatment—Drainage, antibiotics

8. Chronic osteomyelitis—Chronic inflammation of bone, due to inadequately treated acute oseomyelitis

   a. Painful, swollen bone with radiographically diffuse and irregular radiolucency that eventually becomes radiopaque (chronic sclerosing osteomyelitis)

   b. Treatment—Debridement/systemic antibiotics

B. Viral diseases (Table 5-14■)

1. Herpes simplex (Figure 5-39■)—Two forms: primary and secondary

   a. Primary herpes simplex—First exposure to virus

   (1) Oral manifestations

      (a) Begins as pinpoint vesicles anywhere intraorally and periorally

      (b) Vesicles quickly rupture, leaving small ulcerations

   (2) Clinical manifestations

      (a) Most common in young children; may become endemic in child-care facilities from one infected individual

      (b) Patient may exhibit fever, malaise, or lymphadenopathy; or symptoms may be mild to subclinical

   (3) Treatment—Bed rest, fluids, and no aspirin

   (4) Remission in 10–14 days

TABLE 5-14 INFECTIOUS DISEASES: VIRAL INFECTIONS

Lesion	Description	Location	Clinical Manifestation	Treatment
Verruca vulgaris	Common wart; caused by papillomavirus; skin lesions are more common than oral lesions; may be transmitted from skin to oral mucosa	Intraoral—lips are most common	White, papillary, exophytic lesion	Surgical excision, lesions may recur
Primary herpetic gingivo-stomatitis	Caused by herpes simplex virus type 1, generally seen in children	Lips, gingiva, oral mucosa	Multiple small vesicles that form painful ulcers, swollen painful gingiva, fever, cervical lymphadenopathy	Lesions heal spontaneously in 1–2 weeks
Recurrent herpes simplex infection	Commonly seen on mucosa and in adults; persists in latent state; often occurs following stress, fever, fatigue, menstruation, sunlight Herpetic Whitlow—herpes infection can cause painful infection of the fingers in dentists and dental hygienists	Common on vermilion border of the lips (herpes labialis), hard palate, and gingiva	Tiny vesicles or ulcers that coalesce and form a single lesion	Lesions heal spontaneously in 1–2 weeks
Chicken pox	Highly contagious disease mainly seen in children	Skin and mucous membranes	Vesicular and pustular eruptions	Self-limited disease
Herpes zoster (shingles)	Occurs in adults; transmitted by contaminated droplets	Skin and mucous membranes	Unilateral painful vesicles along a sensory nerve	Antiviral agents, corticosteroids
Herpangina	Generally seen in young children and young adults	Soft palate	Vesicles, fever, malaise	Self-limited
Hand, foot, and mouth disease	Commonly affects children under 5 years of age	Oral mucosa, skin—feet, hands, fingers	Vesicles in mouth	Self-limited
Measles	Highly contagious disease, causes systemic symptoms	Skin primarily, oral mucosa	Oral mucosa—Koplik's spots—erythematous macules with white, necrotic centers	Self-limited

			Clinical	
Lesion	**Description**	**Location**	**Manifestation**	**Treatment**
Mumps	Most common in children	Salivary glands	Painful swelling of salivary glands	Self-limited
Infectious mononucleosis	Epstein-Barr virus, commonly occurs in adolescents and young adults	Systemic disease	Sore throat, fever, lymphadenopathy, malaise, fatigue, enlarged spleen	Self-limited

TABLE 5-14 INFECTIOUS DISEASES: VIRAL INFECTIONS (*continued*)

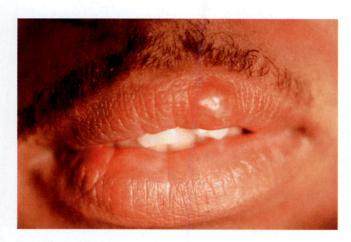

FIGURE 5-39 ■ Herpes Labialis

b. Secondary herpes simplex (recurrent herpes)
(1) Oral manifestations
(a) Most intraoral lesions occur on attached mucosa as small pinpoint vesicles that quickly rupture, leaving small pinpoint ulcerations; several ulcerations may coalesce to form larger ulcerations
(b) Most common site is on hard palate lingual to first molars
(c) Lip lesions (herpes labialis) occur frequently
(2) Clinical manifestations
(a) Transmission is by direct contact
(b) Virus resides in trigeminal ganglia, then migrates down nerve process when immunity is compromised or stressed (usually occurs in same location with each outbreak)
(c) Prodromal tingling may precede eruption of vesicles

(d) Herpetic eczema (skin) is uncommon

(e) Herpetic whitlow (finger) was common in dentistry before wearing gloves

(3) Treatment—Palliative only; antiviral drugs demonstrate efficacy and heal without scarring in 10–14 days

2. Herpes zoster (shingles)

a. Etiology—Caused by varicella-zoster virus, the same virus that causes chickenpox

b. Oral manifestations—Lesions present as small vesicles that quickly rupture intraorally and on skin

c. Clinical manifestations

(1) Usually occurs in adults (regardless of prior history of chickenpox)

(2) Lesions are usually unilateral (follow dermatomes) and rarely cross midline

(3) May persist for weeks, while neuralgia may persist for months

(4) Prodromal burning sensation is common

d. Treatment—Antiviral drugs; only viral disease treatable with steroids

3. Hand, foot, and mouth disease—Coxsackievirus disease

a. Oral manifestation—Causes vesicles with ulcerations intraorally

b. Clinical manifestations

(1) Vesicular papules are found on palms of hands and soles of feet

(2) Usually found in young children

(3) Lesions are distributed, which aids in distinguishing hand, foot, and mouth disease from other viral diseases

c. Treatment—Palliative

d. Remission—Spontaneous in 10–14 days

4. Herpangina—Coxsackievirus disease

a. Oral manifestation—Vesicular-ulcerative lesions occur in soft palate and pharyngitis

b. Treatment—Palliative

c. Remission—5–10 days

5. Mononucleosis—Infectious disease

a. Etiology—Caused by Epstein-Barr virus

b. Oral manifestations—Palatal petechiae common in prodromal stages

c. Clinical manifestations—Fever, malaise, pharyngitis, lymphadenopathy, and splenomegaly

d. Treatment—Palliative

6. Mumps—Viral parotitis, but may affect any major salivary gland

   a. Clinical manifestations—Parotids are most commonly affected; frequently causes bilateral, tender enlargement

   b. Treatment—Palliative

7. Measles (rubeola)—Paramyxovirus skin eruption

   a. Oral manifestations—Evidence of occasional oral ulcerations; Koplik's spots (erythematous macules) with necrotic centers are common on buccal mucosa opposite molars; typically precedes skin lesions

   b. Treatment—Palliative

8. German measles (rubella)

   a. Etiology—Viral-induced disease

   b. Oral manifestations—Enamel hypoplasia has been associated with rubella; similar in appearance to rubeola, but without Koplick's spots

   c. Clinical manifestations—Birth defects occur if contracted during first trimester (include blindness, deafness, and cardiovascular abnormalities)

9. AIDS (acquired immunodeficiency syndrome)—HIV (RNA virus with reverse transcriptase) disease causes depletion of CD4 lymphocytes (T-cell) and compromises immune system; results in death as a result of opportunistic infections or malignancies

   a. Routes of transmission

      (1) Intimate contact with fluid exchange

      (2) Contact with contaminated blood or blood products

      (3) Transplacental

   b. Oral manifestations

      (1) Includes unexplained candidiasis (see Fungal diseases)

      (2) Hairy leukoplakia (Epstein-Barr virus induced)—Hyperkeratotic proliferation of papillae on lateral borders of tongue that are usually found bilaterally

      (3) Opportunistic malignancies

         (a) Kaposi's sarcoma (purplish-red macules or papules most commonly found on palate)

         (b) Linear gingival erythema (LGE)—Distinct erythematous line involving marginal gingiva

      (4) Necrotizing ulcerative periodontitis (NUP)—Rapidly progressive periodontal disease without concomitant local factors

    c. Clinical manifestations

        (1) Symptoms—Flu-like within weeks of infection, but may be subclinical

        (2) Incubation period—Highly variable

        (3) Opportunistic infections are evident

    d. Treatment—Multiple drug regimens without cure at this time

10. Verruca vulgaris—Common wart caused by papillomavirus

    a. Clinical manifestations—White, papillary, exophytic lesion most commonly on lips

    b. Treatment—Surgical excision

C. Fungal diseases (Table 5-15■)

    1. Candidiasis (thrush, moniliasis)

        a. Etiology—Caused by *Candida albicans*, which is frequently part of the normal oral flora

        b. Forms

            (1) White curds—Rub off (pseudomembranous)

            (2) Localized erythematous (Figure 5-40■)—Found especially under removable prostheses (denture sore mouth)

            (3) Leukoplakic areas—Do not rub off (hypertrophic candidiasis), but heal with antifungal medications

        c. Oral manifestation—Angular cheilitis frequently occurs due to *Candida*

        d. Clinical manifestations

            (1) Opportunistic organism evident especially with antibiotic, steroid, chemotherapy use and diabetes mellitus

            (2) Any unexplained candidiasis causes suspicion for compromised immunity (e.g., HIV)

        e. Treatment—Antifungal medications with possible recurrence

    2. Histoplasmosis—Infectious disease

        a. Etiology—Caused by *Histoplasma capsulatum*; histology shows histiocytes and macrophages with organisms in cytoplasm exhibiting a clear halo (mucopolysaccharide capsule)

        b. Oral manifestations

            (1) May cause ulcerations and/or granulomatous inflammation

            (2) Lesions occur as a result of infected sputum

        c. Clinical manifestation

            (1) Portal of entry is through respiratory tract and inhalation of dust (especially bird droppings) containing spores

            (2) Endemic in Ohio and Mississippi River valleys

TABLE 5-15 INFECTIOUS DISEASES: FUNGAL INFECTIONS				
Lesion	**Description**	**Location**	**Clinical Manifestation**	**Treatment**
Candidiasis	Result of an overgrowth of yeast-like fungus *Candida albicans*; most common oral fungal infection	Oral mucosa	Depends on type (see below)	Antifungal medication
Histoplasmosis	Caused by *Histoplasm capsulatum*	Oral mucosa	Ulcerations and granulomatous inflammation	Long-term therapy with amphotericin B and other antifungals
Coccidioido-mycosis	Caused by *Coccidioides immitis*	Oral mucosa	Lesions are not common but when present consist of ulceration and granulomatous	Amphotericin B or Ketocona-zole
Pseudo-membranous candidiasis	Overgrowth of *candida albicans*	Oral mucosa	White curd-like material on mucosal surface, underlying mucosa is erythematous	Antifungal treatment
Erythematous candidiasis	Overgrowth of *candida albicans*	Oral mucosa	Erythematous painful mucosa, may be localized or generalized	Antifungal treatment
Chronic atrophic candidiasis	Overgrowth of *candida albicans*	Palate and maxillary alveolar ridge	Erythematous mucosa limited to mucosa covered by a full or partial denture	Antifungal agents; most common type affecting the mucosa, also known as den-ture stomatitis
Chronic hyper-plastic candidiasis, candidal leukoplakia, hypertrophic candidiasis	Overgrowth of *candida albicans*	Oral mucosa	White lesions that do not wipe off	Antifungal agents
Angular chelitis	Candida organ-isms often cause angular cheilitis	Labial commissures	Erythema or fissures at labial commissures; frequently occurs with intraoral candidiasis	Antifungal agents

(continued)

	TABLE 5-15 INFECTIOUS DISEASES: FUNGAL INFECTIONS (*continued*)			
Lesion	**Description**	**Location**	**Clinical Manifestation**	**Treatment**
Median rhomboid glossitis	Has been associated with candidiasis, and many lesions disappear with antifugal treatment; however, the response to antifungal agents is inconsistent and cause is unknown	Midline of the posterior dorsal tongue	Erythematous, rhombus-shaped flat to raised area	Antifungal agents

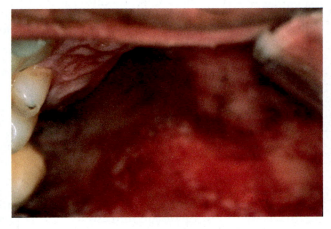

FIGURE 5-40 ■ Erythematous Candidiasis

    d. Treatment—Long-term therapy with amphotericin B and other antifungals with possible recurrence

3. Coccidioidomycosis

    a. Etiology—Caused by *Coccidioides immitis*

    b. Oral manifestations

        (1) Lesions are not common, but when present consist of ulcerations and granulomatous

        (2) Inflammation is present resulting from infected sputum

    c. Clinical manifestation

      (1) Portal of entry is through respiratory tract by inhalation of spores

      (2) Endemic in southwestern United States

    d. Treatment—Use of amphotericin B or ketoconazole with possible recurrence

VIII. Vesiculoerosive Diseases

A. Viral-induced (see Infectious diseases, viral)

    1. Herpes simplex—Also classified as a vesiculoerosive disease because of clinical presentations of small vesicles

      a. Clinical manifestations—Vesicles rupture to leave small areas of ulceration

      b. Treatment—Bed rest, fluids, and no aspirin

    2. Herpes zoster—Classified also as a vesiculoerosive disease

      a. Clinical manifestation—Vesicles rupture, leaving small areas of ulceration

      b. Treatment—Antiviral drugs, the only viral disease treatable with steroids

    3. Hand, foot, and mouth disease—Coxsackievirus

      a. Clinical manifestations

        (1) Predilection to cause vesicles in soft palate, pharynx, and cutaneous areas of hands and feet in young children

        (2) Short duration

      b. Treatment—Palliative

    4. Herpangina—Coxsackievirus

      a. Clinical manifestations

        (1) Predilection for vesicular eruptions of soft palate and pharynx

        (2) May be confused with primary herpetic stomatitis

        (3) Short duration

      b. Treatment—Palliative

    5. Measles

      a. Clinical manifestations

        (1) Intraoral vesicles possible

        (2) Koplik's spots may occur on buccal mucosa

      b. Treatment—Palliative

B. Autoimmune (Table 5-16■)

    1. Recurrent aphthous ulcers (RAU)—Minor aphthae

      a. Etiology—Unknown, but immune dysfunction is suspected; often triggered by some manner of irritation

TABLE 5-16 AUTOIMMUNE DISEASES

Lesion	Description	Location	Clinical Manifestation	Treatment
Recurrent aphthous ulcers	Immune dysfunction suspected, causing painful ulcerations	Most frequently found on freely movable portion of mucosa	Painful lesions with shallow yellow fibrinous center with an erthematous non-elevated margin; single or in crops	Steroid therapy; topical tetra-cycline
Behçet's syndrome	Multisystem disease usually presenting with ocular, oral, and genital herpes	Ocular, oral, genital	Oral: resemble recurrent apthous ulcer tend to occur in crops Ocular–uveitis and/or conjunctivitis Genital: painful ulcerations	Steroid therapy
Major aphthae	Sutton's disease, considered to be an immune dysfunction	Oral mucosa	Large, cratered ulcerations of mucosal surfaces with "piled-up" erthematous margins of long duration	Steroid therapy
Erythema multiforme	Disease affecting skin and mucous mem-branes; etiology un-known; suspected immune dysfunction; infections or drugs	Oral mucosa Skin	Multiple RAU type or larger ulceration; classic skin lesion presents as multiple concentric circles of erythema and normal color skin "Bull's eye lesion"	Steroid therapy
Stevens-Johnson syndrome	Multisystem disease of erythema multiforme	Ocular, oral, and genital regions	Oral and gential: lesions exhibit erythema multi-forme Ocular: conjunc-tivitis or uveitis	Steroid therapy
Sjögren's syndrome (refer to salivary gland pathology)	Autoimmune disease that affects the sali-vary and lacrimal glands, resulting in a decrease in the amount of saliva and tears	Oral cavity and eyes, major and minor salivary glands	Xerostomia → erythe-matous mucosa, oral discomfort, cracked and dry lips, atrophy of fili-form and fungiform papillae, bilateral parotid gland enlarge-ment, decreased lacrimal flow	Nonsteroidal anti-inflammatory agents, corti-costeroids, saliva and tear substitutes; good oral hygiene

Lesion	**Description**	**Location**	**Clinical Manifestation**	**Treatment**
Systemic lupus erythematosus	Acute and chronic inflammatory auto-immune disease—predominantly in women	Multiple involvement	Skin lesions—erythematous rash is most common; classic "butterfly" rash over bridge of nose; erythematous lesions on fingertips	Anti-inflammatory and immuno-suppressive agents; anti-biotic premed-ication prior to dental treat-ment may be necessary
Pemphigus vulgaris	Severe progressive autoimmune disease that affects the skin and mucous membranes	Skin and mucous membranes	Oral lesions—painful ulcers, vesicles, bullae Bullae rupture → epi-thelium remains as gray membrane Positive Nikolsky's sign Skin lesions—erythema, vesicles, bullae, erosions, ulcers	Corticosteroids, immuno-suppressive drugs

TABLE 5-16 AUTOIMMUNE DISEASES   (*continued*)

b. Oral manifestations

   (1) Painful lesions are evident that are usually < 5 mm in dimension

   (2) Have a shallow yellow fibrinous center with an erythematous nonelevated margin

   (3) Lesions are usually single, but may occur in crops

   (4) Adjacent lesions may coalesce to form larger areas of ulceration

   (5) Usually heal in 7–10 days without scarring

   (6) Multiple and multisystem lesions may be suggestive of Behçet's syndrome or some manner of intestinal disorder (i.e., Crohn's)

   (7) Most frequently found on freely moveable portion of mucosa

c. Treatment—Palliative

   (1) Multiple and frequent recurrence may respond to supervised steroid therapy

   (2) Topical tetracycline reduces likelihood of secondary bacterial infection

   (3) Recurrence is likely

2. Behçet's syndrome—Multisystem disease usually presenting with ocular, oral, and genital lesions

   a. Etiology—Suspected to be autoimmune

b. Clinical manifestations

(1) Oral lesions—Resemble RAU and tend to occur in multiple crops

(2) Ocular lesions—Include uveitis and/or conjunctivitis

(3) Genital lesions—Also exhibit painful ulcerations

c. Treatment—Supervised steroid therapy, but may undergo spontaneous remission

3. Reiter's syndrome—Multisystem disease

a. Etiology—Unknown, but autoimmune dysfunction is suspected

b. Clinical manifestations—Frequently manifesting ocular, oral, and genital lesions

(1) Oral lesions—Resemble multiple RAU

(2) Ocular lesions—Include uveitis or conjunctivitis

(3) Genital lesions—Include balanitis, nongonococcal urethritis

(4) Patients frequently exhibit arthritis

c. Treatment—Anti-inflammatory drugs

4. Major aphthae—Periadenitis mucosa necrotica recurrens (PMNR); Sutton's disease

a. Etiology—Considered to be an immune dysfunction

b. Oral manifestations

(1) Large, cratered ulcerations of mucosal surfaces with "piled-up" erythematous margins of long duration

(2) Ulcers heal in weeks to months, usually with scarring

c. Treatment—Supervised steroid therapy

5. Erythema multiforme—Disease affecting skin and mucous membranes (Figure 5-41■)

a. Etiology—Unknown, although an immune dysfunction is suspected and infections or drugs may precipitate onset

b. Oral manifestations

(1) Lesions may exhibit multiple RAU-type or larger ulcerations

(2) Vesicles may occur early or exist at margins of ulcers

c. Clinical manifestations—Classic skin lesion presents as multiple concentric circles of erythema and normal color skin; "Bull's eye lesion"

d. Treatment—Supervised steroid therapy with possible recurrence

6. Stevens-Johnson syndrome—Multisystem disease of erythema multiforme; usually involves ocular, oral, and genital regions; most severe form of erythema multiforme

a. Clinical manifestations

(1) Oral and genital lesions exhibit erythema multiforme

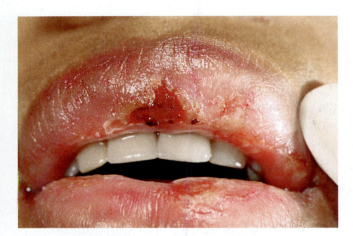

FIGURE 5-41 ■ Erythema Multiforme
Source: Mediscan

       (2) Ocular lesions consist of conjunctivitis or uveitis

    b. Treatment—Supervised steroid therapy with possible recurrence

7. Systemic lupus erythematosus—Chronic skin or systemic disease

    a. Etiology—Considered to be autoimmune

    b. Types

       (1) Chronic discoid—Affects the skin and mucous membranes

       (2) Systemic—Multisystem disease that is occasionally fatal

    c. Oral manifestations

       (1) Lesions present as erythematous plaques or erosions affecting buccal mucosa, gingiva, palate, and vermillion zone

       (2) Ulcerations are seen frequently

    d. Clinical manifestations

       (1) Antibodies are formed against cell nucleus or other cytoplasmic antigens

       (2) "Butterfly" rash is frequently seen, affecting the malar processes; bilaterally connects across bridge of nose

       (3) Females are affected more frequently than males

       (4) Patients complain of malaise, weakness, and an occasional low-grade fever

       (5) Increased sensitivity to ultraviolet radiation is not uncommon

    e. Treatment—Long-term steroids and antimalarial drugs

8. Erosive (bullous) lichen planus (see Anomalies of the oral cavity, Anomalies of other mucosal tissue)—Skin disease affecting basal layer of epithelium

    a. Etiology—Suspected to be autoimmune

   b. Forms

   (1) Erosive and bullous—Least common; exhibits erythematous erosions and ulcerations most common on posterior buccal mucosa and attached gingiva

   (2) Bullous lichen planus—Variant of erosive in which vesicles or bullae precede ulcerations

   (3) Wickham's striae—May be visible at periphery of lesion; may or may not accompany skin lesions

   c. Treatment—Steroid therapy; may undergo spontaneous remission with possible recurrence

9. Pemphigus (*Pemphigus vulgaris, Pemphigus vegetans*) —Skin disease (Figure 5-42■)

   a. Etiology—Autoimmune; histologically an intraepithelial separation (above the basal cell layer) with Tzanck cells (free-floating epithelial cells)

   b. Oral manifestations

   (1) Lesions present as aphthae-like ulcerations or large irregular ulcerations with erythematous margins

   (2) Vesicles or bullae may precede ulcerations

   c. Clinical manifestations

   (1) Antibodies are directed against desmosomes, resulting in acantholysis (loss of cell-to-cell adhesion)

   (2) Individuals may exhibit a positive Nikolsky's sign (sloughing of epithelium after minor trauma)

   (3) May have ethnic or genetic predisposition

   d. Treatment—Steroids

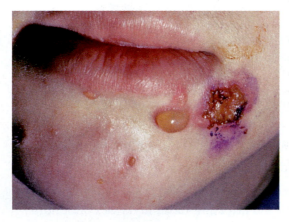

FIGURE 5-42 ■ Pemphigus
Source: Phototake NYC

10. Pemphigoid (benign mucous membrane pemphigoid, cicatricial [scar-forming] pemphigoid)—Autoimmune disease that affects basal layer membrane area; antibodies are directed against hemidesmosomes, resulting in subepithelial separation

   a. Oral manifestations

   (1) Lesions exhibit painful ulcerations with erythematous margins on any mucosal surface

   (2) Desquamative gingivitis—Clinical description of possible pemphigoid; positive Nikolsky's sign is frequently noted

   b. Clinical manifestations—Bullous pemphigoid is considered a variant of cicatricial pemphigoid, but autoimmune findings are not consistent

   c. Treatment—Steroids; may undergo periods of remission and exacerbation

IX. Blood Dyscrasias

A. Vocabulary

   1. *Purpura*—General term for submucosal, subcutaneous bleeding

   2. *Petechiae*—Small, pinpoint, nonelevated red spot of submucosal bleeding

   3. *Ecchymosis*—Purple or purplish-red, nonelevated area of submucosal bleeding, larger than a petechia

   4. *Hematoma*—Purple or purplish-red, elevated area of submucosal bleeding

   5. *Epistaxis*—Spontaneous nose bleed

   6. *Hematuria*—Blood in urine

   7. *Hemoptysis*—Coughing up blood

   8. *Hemolysis*—Rupture of erythrocytes with loss of hemoglobin

   9. *Erythropenia*—Decrease in circulating red blood cells (RBCs)

   10. *Leukopenia*—Decrease in circulating white blood cells (WBCs)

   11. *Thrombocytopenia*—Decrease in circulating platelets

B. Clotting disorders

   1. Thrombocytopenia (idiopathic thrombocytopenic purpura)—Disease of platelets resulting in a decrease in numbers

   a. Etiology

   (1) Idiopathic—Unknown

   (2) Secondary thrombocytopenic purpura—Drugs, chemicals, or radiation

   (3) Immune thrombocytopenic purpura—Autoimmune

   b. Oral manifestations

   (1) Include spontaneous gingival bleeding, ecchymoses, petechiae, or purpura

(2) Invasive procedures, including a prophylaxis, are contraindicated while platelet count is depressed

c. Clinical manifestations—Correlate with decreased platelets (e.g., bruise easily, hematuria, and epistaxis)

d. Treatment

(1) Primary—May undergo spontaneous remission or transfusion, steroids, and splenectomy

(2) Secondary—Elimination of etiology, if possible, and again patient may undergo spontaneous remission, transfusion, steroids, or splenectomy

2. Nonthrombocytopenic purpura—Spontaneous bleeding

a. Etiology

(1) Capillary fragility or defect in platelet function (e.g., aspirin ingestion, nonsteroid anti-inflammatory drugs, and autoimmune disease)

(2) Von Willebrand's disease—Genetic form of nonthrombocytopenic purpura

b. Treatment—Same as for thrombocytopenia

3. Hemophilia—Genetic disease resulting in a deficiency of a clotting factor

a. Types

(1) Hemophilia A—Factor VIII deficiency (X-linked transmission)

(2) Hemophilia B—Factor IX deficiency (X-linked transmission)

(3) Hemophilia C—Factor XI deficiency (questionable transmission)

b. Oral manifestations

(1) Include spontaneous gingival bleeding, purpura, petechiae, ecchymoses, and epistaxis

(2) Invasive procedures including prophylaxis is contraindicated until missing factor is replaced

c. Treatment—Replace missing factor

C. Disorders of red blood cells

1. Anemia—Disorder of oxygen-carrying capability either in RBCs or defect in hemoglobin molecule

a. Etiology—May be a result of dietary deficiencies, genetic or autoimmune

b. Oral manifestations—Angular cheilitis, atrophy of oral mucosa, erythema of tongue (with or without burning), and loss of filiform and fungiform papillae in severe or chronic cases

c. Clinical manifestations—Pallor and fatigue

d. Treatment—Replace deficiency; with pernicious anemia, B_{12} injections are given to bypass gastrointestinal tract where intrinsic factor is missing

e. Types

  (1) Dietary

    (a) Iron-deficiency anemia

    (b) Pernicious anemia—Deficiency in vitamin B_{12} (cobalamin) caused by a loss of intrinsic factor; may have an autoimmune component

    (c) Folate deficiency—Also referred to as megaloblastic anemia

  (2) Genetic

    (a) Thalassemia autosomal dominant—Results in an amino acid change in hemoglobin molecule

      i) Thalassemia major—Severe form that results from homozygous inheritance

      ii) Thalassemia minor—Milder form that results from heterozygous inheritance

    (b) Sickle cell anemia

      i) Autosomal dominant disease that affects predominantly blacks and individuals of Mediterranean descent

      ii) Defect is also an amino acid substitution in hemoglobin molecule, causing RBCs to assume a sickle shape and leading to congestion within capillaries and ischemia of the tissue

      iii) Sickle cell disease is most severe form, resulting from homozygous inheritance

      iv) Sickle cell trait is a milder form, resulting from heterozygous inheritance

2. Aplastic anemia—Results in a severe decrease of all circulating blood cells including RBCs, WBCs (leukopenia), and platelets (thrombocytopenia)

  a. Etiology

    (1) Primary aplastic anemia—Unknown

    (2) Secondary aplastic anemia—Chemical or radiation

  b. Clinical manifestations—Primarily suggestive of leukopenia and thrombocytopenia, which include infections and spontaneous hemorrhage

  c. Treatment

    (1) Primary aplastic anemia—Supportive, but usually fatal

    (2) Secondary aplastic anemia—Remove etiology

3. Polycythemia—Abnormal increase in RBC count; either absolute or relative

  a. Etiology

    (1) Neoplastic (primary polycythemia)

    (2) Decrease in oxygen (secondary polycythemia)

(3) Decreased plasma volume (relative polycythemia)

b. Oral manifestations—Evidence of red to purple mucosa, submucosal ecchymoses, petechiae or hematoma, and spontaneous bleeding

c. Treatment—Chemotherapy and/or removal of etiology

D. Disorders of white blood cells

1. Agranulocytosis—Severe reduction in circulating granulocytes, especially neutrophils, resulting from either a defect in production or accelerated destruction

a. Etiology

(1) Primary form—Unknown

(2) Secondary form—Drugs, chemicals, or radiation

b. Clinical manifestations—Severe infections with fever, malaise, and necrotizing ulcerations

c. Treatment—Antibiotics and transfusions

2. Cyclic neutropenia—Periodic cycles of neutrophils decrease with cycles of normal count, usually over 3–4 weeks

a. Etiology—Genetic and autosomal dominant

b. Oral manifestations—Severe infections, ulcerations, gingival, and periodontal infections

c. Treatment—Antibiotics and transfusions

X. Endocrine Disorders

A. Diabetes mellitus—Disease involving utilization of glucose primarily because of insulin deficiency or resistance

1. Etiology—Genetic, autoimmune, viral, and environmental factors

2. Types

a. Type 1 (IDDM)—Insulin-dependent, caused by insulin insufficiency; juvenile onset

(1) Characteristics—Islets of Langerhans cells are destroyed (possibly autoimmune) or cease to produce adequate insulin

(2) Oral manifestations—Increased susceptibility to infection, xerostomia, gingival and periodontal complications, with severe bone loss in uncontrolled cases

(3) Clinical manifestations—Polydipsea (increased thirst), polyuria (increased urination), and polyphagia (increased appetite), but with loss of weight

(4) Treatment—Insulin replacement

b. Type 2 (NDDM)—Non-insulin-dependent; most common form of diabetes; adult-onset; insulin secreted, but ineffective in controlling glucose metabolism

   (1) Characteristics—Healing time prolonged

   (2) Oral manifestations—Can be same as with Type 1

   (3) Clinical manifestations—Can be same as with Type 1

   (4) Treatment—Diet modifications, exercise, and oral hypoglycemics

B. Hyperthyroidism—Excessive thyroid hormone secretion (Graves' disease)

   1. Etiology—Hyperplasia or tumor of the pituitary gland

   2. Oral manifestations—Bone loss, premature eruption of teeth, and early development of periodontal disease

   3. Clinical manifestations—Exophthalmus (protruding eyes), weakness, and unusual reddish hue to skin

   4. Treatment—Surgery, medication, radiation of thyroid, or radioactive iodine

C. Hypothyroidism—Decreased thyroid hormone secretion

   1. Etiology—Autoimmune, lack of dietary iodine, drugs, and pituitary dysfunction

   2. Types

      a. In children—Referred to as cretinism

      b. In adults—Referred to as myxedema

   3. Oral manifestations—Thickened lips, delayed tooth eruption; in children, macroglossia; in adults, primarily macroglossia

   4. Treatment—Supplemental thyroid hormone

D. Hyperparathyroidism—Multisystem disease; increased secretion of parathyroid hormone

   1. Etiology—Usually owing to parathyroid adenoma

   2. Oral manifestations

      a. Increased radiolucency of bone

      b. Cystic-like spaces in maxilla and mandible

      c. Tendency to develop multiple central giant cell tumors

   3. Clinical manifestations—Weakness, anorexia, polyuria, polydipsea, fatigue, constipation, hypercalcemia, calcifications in internal organs (especially kidneys and pancreas), gastric ulcers, and bone demineralization

   4. Treatment—Removal of adenoma and possible removal of one or more parathyroids

E. Addison's disease—Inadequate production of adrenal steroids

1. Etiology—Autoimmune, malignancy, or necrosis of adrenal tissue

2. Oral manifestations—Paraoral and intraoral pigmentation

3. Clinical manifestation—Bronzing of skin; facial pigmentation

4. Treatment—Steroid replacement therapy

XI. Oral Cancer

A. Soft tissue

1. Squamous cell carcinoma (Figure 5-43■)—Most common primary intraoral malignancy

a. Etiology (risk factors)—Sun exposure (lips, paraoral), tobacco and alcohol use

b. Oral manifestations

(1) Especially with high-risk factors, leukoplakic plaques (those with premalignant potential), and erythroplakia (red lesions)

(2) Speckled leukoplakia (red and white combination)

(3) *Exophytic* ulcerative mass

(4) Most commonly found in floor of mouth, ventral and lateral borders of tongue, soft palate, paraphyrangeal area, and retromolar pad

c. Clinical manifestations—Locally invasive with metastasis to regional nodes, liver, and lungs

d. Treatment—Surgery, radiation, and chemotherapy

2. Verrucous carcinoma—Variant of squamous cell carcinoma

a. Etiology (risk factors)—Primarily tobacco use

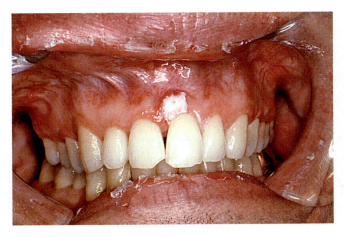

FIGURE 5-43 ■ Squamous Cell Carcinoma

Source: Centers for Disease Control & Prevention

b. Oral manifestations—Slow-growing exophytic red and white mass exhibiting a pebbly surface; locally invasive, but low potential for metastasis

c. Treatment—Surgical excision

3. Basal cell carcinoma (Figure 5-44■)—Epithelial malignancy rarely seen intraorally

a. Etiology (risk factors)—Considered to be sun exposure; cells of origin are basal layer of epithelium

b. Clinical manifestations

(1) Slightly elevated nodule, frequently evidenced with a central depressed area or ulceration that refuses to heal

(2) Low metastatic potential

(3) Basal cell nevus syndrome—Autosomal dominant syndrome manifested by multiple odontogenic keratocysts, multiple basal cell carcinomas, and other skeletal anomalies

(4) Most commonly found on face

c. Treatment—Surgical removal

4. Fibrosarcoma—Malignancy of fibroblasts

a. Oral manifestations—Rapidly growing soft tissue mass with induration; rarely seen intraorally

b. Treatment—Surgery and radiation therapy

5. Rhabdomyosarcoma—Malignancy of skeletal muscle; rapidly growing submucosal mass with induration

a. Oral manifestations—Rarely occurs intraorally, but may occur on tongue and floor of mouth

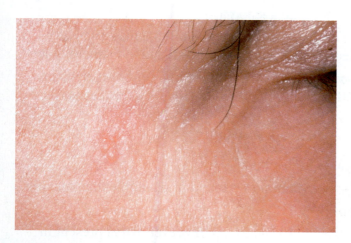

FIGURE 5-44 ■ Basal Cell Carcinoma

b. Treatment—Primarily surgical removal

B. Salivary gland

  1. Mucoepidermoid carcinoma—Malignancy composed of epidermoid cells and mucin-secreting cells

    a. Oral manifestations—Slow-growing, enlarged submucosal or intraglandular mass with indistinct margins

    b. Clinical manifestations

      (1) Most commonly found in parotid gland

      (2) Also seen, but less frequently, in submandibular, sublingual, and minor salivary glands

      (3) Low metastatic potential

    c. Treatment—Surgical excision

  2. Adenoid cystic carcinoma—Slow-growing malignancy most commonly found in minor salivary glands

    a. Oral manifestations

      (1) Firm, unilobular mass within a major salivary gland with some tenderness on palpation

      (2) Slow-growing mass intraorally with indistinct borders, induration, and a propensity for mucosal ulceration

    b. Clinical manifestations

      (1) May be locally invasive with predilection for neural and bony invasion and metastasis to lungs

      (2) Usually found to be well advanced at time of diagnosis

    c. Treatment—Surgical excision

  3. Malignant pleomorphic adenoma—Malignancy arising from a preexisting, long-standing, benign pleomorphic adenoma

    a. Oral manifestations—Firm, unilobular mass within a major salivary gland, with accelerated growth, tenderness, pain, and indistinct borders

    b. Clinical manifestations—Epithelial, mesenchymal (or both) elements may undergo malignant transformation with tendency for metastasis

    c. Treatment—Surgical removal

C. Bone

  1. Osteosarcoma—Malignant tumor of bone

    a. Oral manifestations—More commonly found in mandible than maxilla

    b. Clinical manifestations

      (1) Most common in the 25–40 age group; however, when present in younger age group, it is most commonly found in long bones

        (2) Poorly defined radiolucent and/or radiopaque lesions are evident

        (3) May present as a "starburst" appearance on occlusal films

        (4) Pain may be present if peripheral nerves are involved

    c. Treatment—Chemotherapy and/or surgery

  2. Ewing's sarcoma—Bone malignancy

    a. Etiology—Disputed origin

    b. Clinical manifestations

        (1) Most commonly found in younger age group

        (2) Irregular diffuse radiolucency of the jaws is evident

        (3) May show "onion-skin" appearance (multiple layers) on occlusal films

    c. Treatment—Radiation and/or surgery; prognosis is poor

  3. Multiple myeloma—Malignancy of plasma cells affecting bone

    a. Clinical manifestations

        (1) Radiographs exhibit several sharply punched-out radiolucent areas

        (2) Lateral skull films are frequently involved

    b. Treatment—Chemotherapy

  4. Chondrosarcoma—Malignancy of cartilage resulting in bone lesions

    a. Oral manifestations—Mandible and maxilla are affected with poorly defined radiolucencies

    b. Clinical manifestations

        (1) Occasional scattered calcifications may be seen

        (2) Occurs in any age group

    c. Treatment—Wide surgical excision; prognosis is poor

D. Blood (Table 5-17■)

  1. Leukemias—Group of disorders characterized by proliferation of atypical white blood cells; classified according to the type of cell (e.g., monocytes, lymphocytes, granulocytes) or onset of disease (e.g., acute or chronic)

    a. Types

        (1) Acute—More common in young age group

        (2) Chronic—More common in young adults and older

    b. Oral manifestations—Range from gingival engorgement, spontaneous hemorrhage, ulcerations, to opportunistic infections

    c. Treatment—Radiation and chemotherapy

			TABLE 5-17 TUMORS OF BLOOD	
Lesion	**Description**	**Location**	**Clinical Manifestation**	**Treatment**
Leukemia	Overproduction of atypical white blood cells where normal bone marrow is replaced by immature white blood cells	Gingiva	Gingival enlargement and persistent bleeding	Chemotherapy, radiation, corticosteroids
Non-Hodgkin's lymphoma	Malignant tumor of lymphoid tissue	Intraoral—tonsillar area most common	Gradual enlargement of lymph nodes	Radiotherapy, surgery, chemotherapy

    2. Lymphomas (non-Hodgkin's lymphoma)—Malignancy of lymphocytes more common in lymphatic system, but may spill over into general circulation; classified according to microscopic appearance

        a. Clinical manifestations—Usually presents as a lymphadenopathy; occasionally involves soft tissues and bone

        b. Treatment—Radiation, surgery, chemotherapy

  E. Metastic disease

    1. Metastic tumors

        a. Etiology—Histologically, metastasis resembles primary tumor

        b. Clinical manifestations

            (1) Lesions exhibit poorly defined radiolucencies and ragged resorption of roots

            (2) Most common lesions are found in lungs, prostate, breast, thyroid, and kidneys (prostate, breast, and lung lesions may exhibit foci of calcifications within radiolucency)

            (3) Occasionally metastatic site may be first manifestation (occult metastasis)

            (4) Tumors may metastasize to jaw

        c. Treatment—Dependent on primary tumor and extent of spread

XII. Syndromes

A. Basal cell nevus syndrome—Autosomal transmission

1. Clinical manifestations

a. Include multiple odontogenic keratocysts (OKC), multifocal basal cell carcinoma, hypertelorism, palmar pitting, palmar and plantar keratosis, and bifid ribs

b. Not all manifestations are seen in all patients

c. Multiple OKC and basal cell carcinomas are most consistent

B. Behçet's syndrome (see Vesiculoerosive diseases)—Chronic, autoimmune disease producing ocular, oral, and genital lesions

C. Cleidocranial dysplasis (dysostosis)—Autoimmune dominant transmission

1. Oral manifestations—Underdeveloped premaxilla and multiple supernumerary teeth, frequently impacted owing to crowding

2. Clinical manifestations—Results in enlarged skull, long neck, sloping shoulders, and ability to approximate shoulders because of nondevelopment or partial absence of one or both clavicles

D. Cyclic neutropenia—Autosomal dominant condition exhibiting recurring cycle of neutrophil depletion and regeneration

1. Oral manifestations

a. Severe gingivitis that may progress to periodontitis with recurring attacks

b. Bone loss does not repair between episodes

2. Clinical manifestations—Symptoms are related to neutropenia and include fever, malaise, and pharyngitis

3. Treatment—Management of neutropenia and antibiotic coverage

E. Down syndrome—Chromosomal abnormality (extra or partial excess of chromosome 21)

1. Oral manifestations

a. Macroglossia with protrusion of tongue

b. Fissured tongue

c. High-arched palate

d. Enamel hypoplasia

e. Microdontia

f. Early periodontal disease

2. Clinical manifestations

a. Broad, flat face

b. Open cranial sutures

c. Epicanthal folds

      d. Open mouth

      e. Prognathism

      f. Cardiac abnormalities

      g. Mental retardation

F. Ectodermal dysplasia—X-linked recessive transmission

    1. Etiology—Abnormalities of tissues derived from ectoderm, especially the hair, skin, nails, teeth, and adnexal glandular structures

    2. Oral manifestations—Partial or complete congenital anodontia with teeth conical in shape when present

G. Fibromatosis gingivae (idiopathic gingival fibromatosis)—Suspected autosomal dominant trait

    1. Oral manifestations—Dense, diffuse, smooth, or nodular fibrous enlargement of gingiva with or without inflammation

    2. Treatment—Gingival resection; recurrence is common

H. Gardner's syndrome—Autosomal dominant transmission

    1. Oral manifestations—Multiple impacted and/or supernumerary teeth

    2. Clinical manifestations

      a. Polyps of the colon, osteomas of the bones, and sebaceous cysts of the scalp and back

      b. Polyps may undergo malignant transformation

I. Papillon-Lefèvre syndrome—Autosomal recessive transmission

    1. Oral manifestations—Premature destruction of periodontium

    2. Clinical manifestations—Exhibits reddish-white scaly hyperkeratosis of palmar and plantar surfaces

    3. Treatment—Aggressive periodontal therapy; prognosis is poor

J. Peutz-Jeghers syndrome—Autosomal dominant transmission

    1. Oral manifestations—Oral pigmentations; pigmented macules involve buccal mucosa, gingiva, and hard palate

    2. Clinical manifestations—Intestinal polyposis; polyps have a moderate risk of malignant transformation

K. Reiter's syndrome (see Vesiculoerosive diseases)

    1. Etiology—Unknown

    2. Oral manifestations—Ulcerations resembling recurrent apthous ulcers

    3. Clinical manifestations—Arthritis, urethritis, balanitis, and conjunctivitis

L. Stevens-Johnson syndrome (see Vesiculoerosive diseases)—Chronic disease exhibiting ocular, oral, and genital lesions of erythema multiforme

M. Von Recklinghausen's disease—Autosomal dominant transmission

    1. Oral manifestations—Tumors are most common on lateral borders of tongue, but can occur anywhere

    2. Clinical manifestations

        a. Multiple nerve tissue tumors on skin, brain, and internal viscera

        b. Café au lait ("coffee with cream") pigmentation is common on skin

N. White sponge nevus (Canon's disease)—Autosomal dominant transmission

    1. Oral manifestations—Thick, corrugated, white appearance on buccal mucosa bilaterally

    2. Clinical manifestations—May be present at birth or develop around puberty

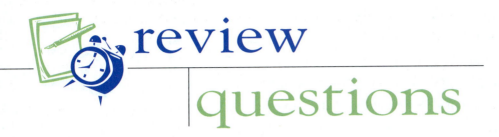
review questions

review questions

DIRECTIONS Each of the questions or incomplete statements below is followed by suggested answers or completions. Select the **one** answer that is best in each case.

1. Which of the following terms defines a fluid-filled lesion usually less than 5 mm in its greatest dimensions?
   A. Bulla
   B. Pustule
   C. Vesicle
   D. Papule
   E. Macule

2. All the following are mucosal anomalies of the oral cavity EXCEPT one. Which one is the EXCEPTION?
   A. Fissured tongue
   B. Concresence
   C. Ankyloglossia
   D. Hairy tongue
   E. Central papillary atrophy

3. White threadlike papules in a linear or reticular pattern—frequently found on the buccal mucosa—are MOST likely:
   A. Leukoedema
   B. Lichen planus
   C. Fordyce granules
   D. Pemphigus
   E. Hyperkeratosis

4. A tooth root exhibiting an unusual curvature is referred to as a(n):
   A. Concresence
   B. Dilaceration
   C. Taurodontism
   D. Anodontia
   E. Macrodont

5. A tooth exhibiting two clinical crowns with usually one root is probably the result of:
   A. Fusion
   B. Concresence
   C. Dens in dente
   D. Gemination
   E. Amelogenesis imperfecta

6. Dentinogenesis imperfecta is a condition with abnormal dentin. On radiographs, it frequently appears with the absence of pulp chambers and canals.
   A. The first statement is TRUE, the second statement is FALSE.
   B. The first statement is FALSE, the second statement is TRUE.
   C. Both statements are TRUE.
   D. Both statements are FALSE.

7. All of the following are odontogenic cysts EXCEPT one. Which one is the EXCEPTION?
   A. Primordial
   B. Residual
   C. Dentigerous
   D. Nasopalatine duct
   E. Radicular

8. Which of the following cysts is frequently the oral manifestation of basal cell nevus syndrome?
   A. Globulomaxillary
   B. Primordial
   C. Odontogenic keratocyst
   D. Periapical
   E. Incisive canal

9. Which of the following terms implies an increase in cell size, but not cell numbers?
   A. Hyperplasia *increase of # cells*
   B. Neoplasia
   C. Hamartoma
   D. Hypertrophy *cell increase*
   E. Choristoma

10. An odontogenic tumor, in which cells arise from the inner enamel epithelium and demonstrate locally invasive potential, is a(n):
    A. Odontogenic adenomatoid tumor
    B. Compound odontoma
    C. Odontogenic myxoma
    D. Ameloblastoma

11. All of the following odontogenic neoplasms are derivatives of ectoderm EXCEPT one. Which one is the EXCEPTION?
    A. Ameloblastoma
    B. Odontogenic myxoma *mesoderm*
    C. Odontogenic adenomatoid tumor
    D. Calcifying epithelial odontogenic tumor

12. Which of the following odontogenic tumors, MOST commonly present at the apices of mandibular anteriors, consists of varying radiolucencies and radiopacities?
    A. Ameloblastoma
    B. Odontogenic myxoma
    C. Cementoma
    D. Odontogenic keratocyst
    E. Calcifying epithelial odontogenic tumor

13. The MOST common intraoral soft tissue neoplasm is a(n):
    A. Cementoma
    B. Lipoma
    C. Papilloma
    D. Epulis fissuratum
    E. Fibroma

14. Which of the following neoplasms manifests as a hemorrhagic, pedunculated mass and is usually an exaggerated response to a local irritant?
    A. Pyogenic granuloma
    B. Fibroma
    C. Lipoma
    D. Epulis fissuratum
    E. Peripheral giant cell tumor

15. Which of the following neoplasms is viral induced?
    A. Pyogenic granuloma
    B. Lipoma
    C. Papilloma
    D. Epulis fissuratum
    E. Peripheral giant cell granuloma

16. A neoplasm of cells that produces myelin is defined as:
    A. Neuroma
    B. Neurilemoma *Schwann cells*
    C. Neurofibroma
    D. Hemangioma

review questions

17. A purplish-red neoplasm, found on the dorsum of the tongue, MOST likely is a:
    A. Lymphangioma
    B. Fibroma
    C. Rhabdomyoma
    D. Pyogenic granuloma
    E. Hemangioma

18. The MOST likely origin of a leiomyoma neoplasm is in the:
    A. Intrinsic muscles of the tongue
    B. Extrinsic muscles of the tongue
    C. Mylohyoid muscle
    D. Striated muscles of the pharynx
    E. Smooth muscles surrounding blood vessels

19. All of the following are common salivary gland tumors found in the parotid EXCEPT one. Which one is the EXCEPTION?
    A. Warthin's
    B. Pleomorphic adenoma
    C. Mixed
    D. Monomorphic adenoma

20. Which bone lesion is occasionally seen in patients with hyperparathyroidism?
    A. Chondroma
    B. Osteoma
    C. Exostosis
    D. Fibrous dysplasia
    E. Central giant cell tumor

21. Inflammation of a salivary gland duct is known as:
    A. Sialadenitis
    B. Sialodochitis
    C. Sialolithiasis
    D. Sialometaplasia

22. The etiology of necrotizing sialometaplasia is due to a(n):
    A. Infarction of blood supply to that portion of the gland
    B. Stone formation in the duct of the involved gland
    C. Inflammation in the gland proper
    D. Obstruction in the glandular duct

23. Which of the following is a clinical description, not a diagnosis, of swelling in the floor of the mouth?
    A. Mucocele
    B. Mucus duct cyst
    C. Ranula
    D. Mucus retention phenomenon
    E. Mucus extravasation phenomenon

24. Tuberculosis may manifest oral ulcerations. These ulcerations heal as the disease becomes quiescent.
    A. The first statement is TRUE, the second statement is FALSE.
    B. The first statement is FALSE, the second statement is TRUE.
    C. Both statements are TRUE.
    D. Both statements are FALSE.

25. The cutaneous manifestation of secondary syphilis is a:
    A. Mucus patch
    B. Mucosal ulceration
    C. Gummatous necrosis
    D. Pruritic rash

26. "Sulfur granules" may be a manifestation of:
    A. Tuberculosis
    B. Gonorrhea
    C. Syphilis
    D. Shingles
    E. Actinomycosis

27. The MOST frequent intraoral site of recurrent herpes is the:
    A. Floor of the mouth
    B. Dorsum of the tongue
    C. Buccal mucosa
    D. Labial mucosa
    E. Gingival and hard palate

28. Shingles is also known as:
    A. Herpes simplex
    B. Herpes zoster
    C. Herpangina
    D. Rubeola
    E. Hand, foot, and mouth disease

29. Which of the following diseases may exhibit prodromal Koplik's spots?
    A. Shingles
    B. Rubeola
    C. Herpangina
    D. Herpes simplex
    E. Rubella

30. Epstein-Barr virus is implicated as the etiology in which of the following conditions?
    A. Thrombocytopenia
    B. Mononucleosis
    C. Herpangina
    D. Pernicious anemia

31. Periadenitis mucosa necrotica recurrens is known as:
    A. Major aphthae
    B. Minor aphthae
    C. Behçet's syndrome
    D. Reiter's syndrome
    E. Stevens-Johnson syndrome

32. Which of the following diseases demonstrates antibodies against desmosomes?
    A. Pemphigoid
    B. Erythema multiforme
    C. Lupus erythematosus
    D. Pemphigus
    E. Erosive lichen planus

33. All of the following are multisystem diseases EXCEPT one. Which one is the EXCEPTION?
    A. Dentinogenesis imperfecta
    B. Enamel hypoplasia
    C. Dentinal displasia
    D. Amelogensis imperfecta

34. Which of the following bleeding disorders is a result of a deficiency of factor IX?
    A. Hemophilia A
    B. Hemophilia B
    C. Hemophilia C
    D. Thrombocytopenia
    E. Erythroblastosis fetalis

35. A term that specifically implies a spontaneous nose bleed is:
    A. Hematoma
    B. Hemoptysis
    C. Purpura
    D. Petechiae
    E. Epistaxis

36. Aplastic anemia is a disease exhibiting deficiencies in which of the following circulating blood counts?
    A. Red blood cells
    B. Granulocytes
    C. Agranulocytes
    D. Hemoglobulin
    E. All blood cells

37. Which of the following diseases manifests episodes of infections and normality?
    A. Cyclic neutropenia
    B. Agranulocytosis
    C. Aplastic anemia
    D. Polycythemia
    E. Thrombocytopenia

38. Which of the following diseases may manifest bronzing of the skin?
    A. Basal cell nevus syndrome
    B. Peutz-Jeghers syndrome
    C. Addison's disease
    D. Hyperparathyroidism
    E. Diabetes mellitus

39. Cancer of the glandular tissue is appropriately defined as:
    A. Liposarcoma
    B. Lymphangiosarcoma
    C. Glandular sarcoma
    D. Adenocarcinoma

40. A cyst located in the midline apical to the maxillary central incisors would MOST likely be a:
    A. Nasopalatine duct
    B. Thyroglossal duct
    C. Globulomaxillary
    D. Branchial cleft
    E. Median mandibular

41. Radiographically, a periapical cyst and a periapical granuloma:
    A. Show different peripheral remodeling characteristics
    B. Are distinguished by the presence of lamina dura
    C. Are indistinguishable
    D. Contain foci of calcification

42. A specific presentation of oral candidiasis, sometimes seen in otherwise healthy patients, is:
    A. Fissured tongue
    B. Geographic tongue
    C. Benign migratory glossitis
    D. Hairy tongue
    E. Median rhomboid glossitis

43. Antibiotics prescribed for a dental infection may cause:
    A. Oral candidiasis
    B. Oral hairy leukoplakia
    C. Median rhomboid glossitis
    D. Geographic tongue
    E. Desquamative gingivitis

44. Xerostomia is related to which of the following?
    A. Peutz-Jeghers syndrome
    B. Antibiotic therapy
    C. Sjögren's syndrome
    D. Benign tumors of the parotid gland
    E. Multiple mucoceles

45. The state of teeth joined together only by cementum is diagnosed as:
    A. Fusion
    B. Concrescence
    C. Budding
    D. Germination

46. Two tooth buds are joined together during development and may appear clinically as a macrodont. The probable diagnosis is:
    A. Budding
    B. Fusion
    C. Germination
    D. Concrescence
    E. Dilacerations

47. A radiograph shows that the roots of a lower molar are severely curved to almost 90 degrees. This is diagnosed as:
    A. Turner's tooth
    B. Hypoplasia
    C. Teratology
    D. Hutchinson's tooth
    E. Dilacerations

48. Which of the following is the MOST common site for a supernumerary tooth?
    A. Between the mandibular incisors
    B. Distal to the maxillary third molar
    C. Between the mandibular premolars
    D. Between the maxillary central incisors
    E. Between the maxillary premolars

49. A patient has lost enamel on the anterior teeth because of a lemon-sucking habit. The diagnosis is:
    A. Chemico-attrition
    B. Attrition
    C. Erosion
    D. Abrasion

50. A common benign neoplasm originating from surface epithelium is:
    A. Verruca vulgaris
    B. The fibroma
    C. The teratoma
    D. The papilloma
    E. Neurofibromatosis

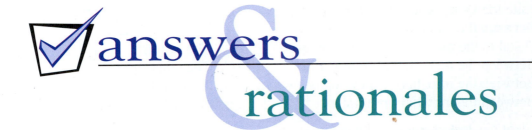
answers & rationales

1.

C. A vesicle is a small fluid-filled lesion usually less than 5 mm in diameter. A bulla, by definition, is a large fluid-filled lesion usually greater than 5 mm in diameter. A pustule is a lesion filled with pus—a more specific fluid content. Papules and macules are lesions that are not filled with fluid.

2.

B. Concresence is a dental anomaly characterized by the joining of adjacent teeth by cementum only. Fissured and hairy tongue, ankyloglossia, and central papillary atrophy are mucosal anomalies of the oral cavity.

3.

B. Lichen planus is an autoimmune disease that frequently exhibits white threadlike papules in a linear pattern (Wickham's striae). Leukoedema is a term that refers to a milky opalescent hue to the buccal mucosa due to increased intracellular edema. Fordyce granules are a yellow submucosal aggregate of sebaceous glands. Pemphigus is an autoimmune skin disease exhibiting oral ulcerations. Hyperkeratosis is a general term implying increased keratin production with no linear pattern.

4.

B. Dilaceration refers to a root that exhibits unusual curvature. Concresence implies adjacent teeth joined together only by the cementum. Taurodontism describes abnormally elongated pulp chambers. Anodontia refers to the absence of one or more teeth—congenital or acquired. A macrodont is a large tooth.

5.

D. Gemination implies twinning of a tooth. Fusion is the joining of two teeth to form one tooth—usually one less than the normal number. Concresence does not affect the crowns since joining is accomplished by cementum only. Dens in dente implies a tooth within a tooth—enamel is within a pulp chamber. Amelogenesis imperfecta is abnormal enamel formation and does not affect tooth numbers.

6.

C. The etiology of dentinogenesis imperfecta is usually genetic, clinically manifesting no pulp chambers or canals.

7.

D. A nasopalatine duct cyst is nonodontogenic. It is a unilocular radiolucency found in the midline of the palate, apical to the maxillary central incisors. Primordial, residual, dentigerous, and radicular cysts are all odontogenic.

8.

C. Multiple odontogenic keratocysts are frequently seen in basal cell nevus syndrome. These multilocular cysts are radiolucent with poorly defined margins. A globulomaxillary cyst is found between the maxillary lateral incisor and canine. The primordial cyst is intraosseous and found in place of a missing tooth. Periapical cyst is another term for radicular cyst involving a nonvital tooth. An incisive canal cyst is developmental and located in the incisive canal.

9.

D. Hypertrophy implies a cellular enlargement only. Hyperplasia implies an increase in cell numbers. Neoplasia implies a tumorous growth owing to an increase in cell numbers. Hamartoma is a neoplasia of cells native to a given area and choristoma is a neoplasia of cells foreign to a given area.

10.

D. Ameloblastoma is a slow-growing benign neoplasm of ameloblasts that arises from the inner enamel epithelium. Odontogenic adenomatoid tumor is noninvasive of odontogenic origin. Compound odontoma is a noninvasive tumor-forming tooth structure. Odontogenic myxoma is a tumor arising from cells of the stellate reticulum.

11.

B. Odontogenic myoxoma is a slow-growing benign tumor of mesodermal origin. Ameloblastoma, odontogenic adenomatoid, and calcifying epithelial odontogenic tumors are entirely from ectodermal derivation.

12.

C. Cementomas are commonly found at the apices of mandibular incisors. The lesion can be entirely radiolucent, then mixed radiolucent/radiopaque to entirely radiopaque in older lesions. Ameloblastoma is not commonly found at the apices of the mandibular incisors and shows no variation in radiolucencies or radiopacities. Odontogenic myxoma is not commonly found at the apices of mandibular incisors and is entirely radiolucent. An odontogenic keratocyst is not an odontogenic tumor, but a cyst. A calcifying epithelial odontogenic tumor is not dependent on existing teeth and not commonly found at the apices of mandibular incisors.

13.

E. Fibroma is the most common intraoral soft tissue neoplasm. A cementoma is not a soft tissue neoplasm, but composed of intraosseous cementum. A lipoma is a neoplasm of adipose tissue not commonly found intraorally. A papilloma is an epithelial neoplasm, but not as common as the fibroma. Epulis fissuratum is a fibrous hyperplasia due to a poor-fitting denture and is not as common as the fibroma.

14.

A. Pyogenic granuloma is a reactive hyperplasia of granulation-type tissue. It is usually pedunculated in response to a local irritant. Fibroma is usually not hemorrhagic in appearance. Lipoma is a neoplasm of adipose tissue and not hemorrhagic in appearance. Epulis fissuratum is a reactive neoplasm that develops in response to a poor-fitting denture and is not hemorrhagic in appearance. Peripheral giant cell tumor is usually liver color in appearance when it is present in the soft tissue.

15.

C. The etiology of papilloma is the human papillomavirus. Pyogenic granuloma is a reactive neoplasm in response to a local irritant. Lipoma is a neoplasm of adipose tissue and not viral-induced. Epulis fissuratum is a reactive neoplasm in response to a poor-fitting denture. Peripheral giant cell granuloma has an unknown etiology; however, it is not suspected as being viral-induced.

and exostosis (bony neoplasm) are not associated with hyperparathyroidism. Fibrous dysplasia is a fibrous and bony proliferation and not associated with hyperparathyroidism.

16.
B. Neurilemoma is a neoplasm of Schwann cells, which produces myelin sheath. Neuroma is a neoplasm of neural tissue. Neurofibroma is a neoplasm of neural elements and fibrous connective tissue. Hemangioma is a neoplasm of blood cells.

17.
E. A hemangioma is most commonly found on the tongue, frequently hemorrhagic in nature. Lymphangioma is a common neoplasm found on the tongue, but not discolored. Fibroma is usually the color of normal mucosa, unless secondarily inflamed. Rhabdomyoma is a neoplasm of striated muscle usually the color of normal mucosa as well. Pyogenic granuloma is not normally found on the tongue and usually arises from the crevicular gingiva.

18.
E. Leiomyoma is sessile in form, palpable, and may cause slight elevation of the surface mucosa. Its origin intraorally is in the smooth muscle walls of blood vessels. The remaining striated muscles may involve rhabdomyoma, a neoplasm of voluntary muscles.

19.
D. Monomorphic adenoma is a glandular neoplasm most commonly found in the upper lip. Warthin's tumor is almost exclusively found in the parotid gland. Pleomorphic adenoma (another name for mixed tumor) is most commonly found in the parotid gland.

20.
E. It is not unusual to find a central giant cell tumor in patients with hyperparathyroidism. Chondroma (cartilaginous neoplasm), osteoma (bony neoplasm),

21.
B. Sialodochitis implies inflammation of a gland duct. Sialadenitis implies inflammation of a gland proper. Sialolithiasis implies salivary gland stone formation. Sialometaplasia implies histological glandular epithelium changes.

22.
A. The etiology of necrotizing sialometaplasia is from interruption of the blood supply. Stone formation, inflammation in the glandular proper, and obstruction and inflammation of the glandular duct do not cause necrosis in the salivary gland.

23.
C. Ranula is only a clinical description and does not imply etiology. Mucocele is a generic diagnosis of either mucous extravasation or retention. Mucous duct cyst implies an obstruction with the duct epithelium, forming a cyst-like lesion. Mucous retention phenomenon implies obstruction of a duct with mucus retention. Mucous extravasation phenomenon implies rupture of a duct with mucus spillage into surrounding connective tissue.

24.
C. Tuberculosis is a disease involving the respiratory system. Symptoms include chronic coughs and occasionally oral ulcerations resulting from coughing up infected sputum.

25.
D. Cutaneous implies skin and pruritic implies itching. Mucous patch and mucosal ulceration are mucous manifestations, not cutaneous manifestations. Gummatous necrosis is a manifestation of tertiary syphilis.

26.

E. Actinomycosis is a bacterial disease that produces pus with granules. The granules appear yellow, similar to a grain of sulfur, but actually are colonies of the microorganism. Tuberculosis, gonorrhea, syphilis, and shingles do not produce pus-containing "sulfur granules."

27.

E. It is common on vermilion border of the lips (herpes labialis), hard palate, and gingiva.

28.

B. Herpes zoster is frequently referred to as shingles. Herpes simplex is also referred to as "fever blisters." Herpangina is seasonal pharyngitis. Rubeola is measles, and hand, foot, and mouth disease are seasonal vesicles in the appropriate sites, respectively.

29.

B. With rubeola, there's evidence of erythematous macules located near the parotid papillae before the measles rash. Shingles, herpangina, herpes simplex, and rubella show no evidence of Koplik's spots.

30.

B. Epstein-Barr is implicated in mononucleosis as well as hairy leukoplakia of AIDS. Thrombocytopenia is a bleeding disorder caused by inadequate or missing platelets. Herpangina is a coxsackievirus disease. Pernicious anemia results from a lack of intrinsic or extrinsic factors associated with vitamin B_{12} deficiency.

31.

A. Periadenitis mucosa necrotica recurrens are large ulcers also known as major aphthae. Minor aphthae are small ulcers. Behçet's syndrome involves ocular, oral, and genital minor aphthae. Reiter's syndrome also involve the ocular, oral, and genital with lesions,

but not aphthae. Stevens-Johnson syndrome involves ocular, oral, and genital erythema multiforme.

32.

D. Pemphigus is an autoimmune disease that destroys desmosomes. Pemphigoid is an autoimmune disease that destroys hemidesmosomes. Erythema multiforme is an autoimmune disease causing "target lesions" on the skin. Lupus erythematosus is an autoimmune disease with antinuclear antibodies. Erosive lichen planus is a disease affecting the basement membrane.

33.

D. Amelogenesis imperfecta is a dental defect resulting in severe hypoplasia or hypocalcification of the enamel. Behçet's, Reiter's, and Stevens-Johnson syndromes are multisystem diseases.

34.

B. Hemophilia B is a bleeding disorder as a result of a deficiency of factor IX. Hemophilia A is a deficiency of factor VIII. Hemophilia C is a deficiency of factor XI. Thrombocytopenia is a deficiency in platelets and erythroblastosis fetalis notes Rh incompatibility.

35.

E. Epistaxis is a spontaneous nose bleed. Hematoma is an elevated area of submucosal bleeding. Hemoptysis refers to coughing up blood. Purpura is a general term for submucosal bleeding. Petechiae is a small, pinpoint, nonelevated area of submucosal bleeding.

36.

E. Aplastic anemia results in a severe decrease in red blood cells, white blood cells, and platelets—not just circulating red blood cells, granulocytes, agranulocytes, and hemoglobin.

37.

A. Cyclic neutropenia is a disorder of the white blood cells that exhibits cycles between normal blood counts and deficiencies of neutrophils. Agranulocytosis has a severe reduction in circulating granulocytes, especially neutrophils. Aplastic anemia results in a severe decrease of all circulating blood cells. With polycythemia, there is an abnormal increase in red blood cells. With thrombocytopenia, there is an abnormal decrease in circulating platelets.

38.

C. With Addison's disease, there is frequently evidence of a bronze discoloration of the skin. Basal cell nevus syndrome manifests skin cancers, skeletal abnormalities, and multiple OKCs. Peutz-Jeghers syndrome manifests oral and perioral pigmentations with intestinal polyps. Hyperparathyroidism is a multisystem disease that manifests bone demineralization. With diabetes mellitus, skin discoloration is not commonly encountered.

39.

D. "Adeno" implies glandular. Carcinoma implies a malignancy of ectodermal origin from which glandular tissue originates. Liposarcoma is a malignancy of adipose tissue, a mesodermal derivative. Lymphangiosarcoma is a malignancy of lymphatic tissue, also a mesodermal derivative. Glandular sarcoma is a malignancy of ectodermal origin, therefore designated as a carcinoma.

40.

A. A nasopalatine duct cyst is unilocular and develops in the incisive canal. A thyroglossal duct cyst develops in the neck and a branchial cleft cyst develops in the lateral part of the neck. A globulomaxillary cyst develops between the maxillary lateral incisor and canine. A median mandibular cyst develops in the midline of the mandible.

41.

C. A periapical cyst and a periapical granuloma are indistinguishable radiographically.

42.

E. Median rhomboid glossitis is a presentation of candidiasis in which a central area on the mid-dorsal surface is devoid of papillae.

43.

A. Use of antibiotics is one of the many predisposing factors that may lead to the development of oral candidiasis

44.

C. Xerostomia (dry mouth) is related to Sjögren's syndrome, an autoimmune process that often includes rheumatoid arthritis and result in the destruction of the salivary glands.

45.

B. The condition of teeth joined together only by cementum is termed concrescence. It is thought to arise as a result of traumatic injury. Concrescence may occur before or after the teeth have erupted.

46.

B. Fusion of teeth is a condition produced when two tooth buds are joined together during development and appear as a macrodont. This is not to be confused with true macrodontia in which all teeth are larger than normal.

47.

E. The condition in which the roots of mandibular molars are severely curved to almost 90 degrees is termed dilacerations. This is thought to be caused by trauma during tooth development. Dilacerated teeth can present problems at the time of extraction.

48.

D. The most common site for supernumerary teeth is between maxillary central incisors. Supernumerary teeth have a 2:1 predilection for males. Supernumerary teeth may closely resemble the teeth of the group to which they belong.

49.

C. Erosion is the wearing away of the teeth due to a chemical process. Lemon-sucking is a frequent cause of erosion. Additionally, erosion is a common clinical finding in patients with bulimia. Eroded areas of the teeth occur most frequently on the facial and lingual surfaces.

50.

D. A very common benign neoplasm originating from oral epithelium is the papilloma. It is often confused with the fibroma, yet each has definite characteristics. The papilloma is an exophytic growth made up of numerous, small, fingerlike projections that result in a roughened verrucous or "cauliflower-like" surface.

6 Pharmacology

Pharmacology is the study of drugs and their effects on living organisms. A *drug* is a chemical substance used for the diagnosis, prevention, or treatment of a disease or condition.

chapter objectives

After completion of this chapter, the learner should be able to:

➤ Discuss drug action and termination

➤ Discuss adverse reactions of drugs

➤ Discuss drug interactions

➤ Describe mechanisms of drug interactions

➤ Describe drugs used in dentistry and their clinical uses, pharmacological effects, toxic reactions, drug interactions, and contraindications

I. Drug Action and Termination

A. Receptors—Macromolecules located on or within cell membranes that the drug must bind with to be effective; lock-and-key fit (specific drug binding with specific receptor) (Figure 6-1■)

   1. Agonist—Drug has affinity for receptor, which produces an effect

   2. Antagonist—Drug has affinity for the receptor; produces no effect

   a. Competitive antagonist—Interacts with same receptor site as agonist and competes with the agonist for the receptor site (reversible binding)

   b. Noncompetitive antagonist—Binds to a receptor site different from the binding site for the agonist but reduces the maximal response of the agonist (irreversible binding)

B. Drug-binding forces—The chemical binding of a drug to a receptor site

   1. Covalent bonds—Sharing of an electron by a pair of atoms; strong bond, often irreversible (tetracycline to dentin)

   2. Ionic bonds—An electrostatic attraction between ions of opposite charge (most common mechanism for drug binding); reversible, easily made, and easily broken

   3. Hydrogen bonds—A special type of attractive interaction that exists between an electronegative atom and a hydrogen atom bonded to another electronegative atom

   4. Van der Waals forces—Weak interactions that develop when two atoms are placed in close proximity

C. Log-dose effect curve—Log of the dose (*x*-axis) versus the intensity of response (*y*-axis) (Figure 6-2■)

   1. Potency—Amount of a drug needed to produce desired therapeutic effect

   2. Affinity—Tendency for a drug to bind to a receptor site

   3. Efficacy—The desired therapeutic response obtained from a drug when a sufficient amount of drug is administered; not related to potency

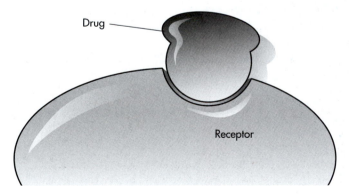

Drug

Receptor

FIGURE 6-1 ■ Drug-Receptor Interaction

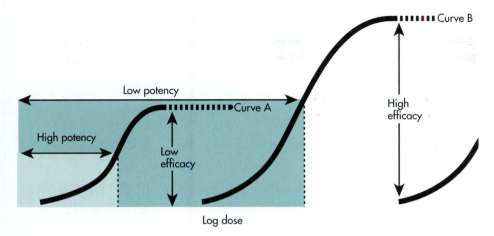

FIGURE 6-2 ■ Log-Dose Effect Curve

4. Ceiling effect (plateau)—Therapeutic effect cannot be increased with a higher dose of the drug

5. Effect dose (ED50)—Dose that produces a therapeutic response in 50% of the subjects given the drug

6. Lethal dose (LD50)—Dose of the drug that produces death in 50% of the subjects given the drug

7. Therapeutic index (TI)—Ratio of the median lethal dose (LD50) to the median effective dose (ED50); expresses the safety of the drug; the greater the TI, the safer the drug

D. Factors altering drug's effect

1. Placebo effect—A perceived effect that occurs after taking an inactive substance; can also have a placebo effect with an active substance given at a dose that is lower than what is needed to produce a therapeutic effect

2. Patient noncompliance—Incorrect or improper use of a medication

3. Drug interaction—Drug action of one or more drugs with concurrent use

E. Routes of administration—Affects drug onset and duration of response

1. Enteral—Placed directly into the gastrointestinal (GI) tract by oral or rectal administration

   a. Oral (PO)—By mouth, slower onset of action, may be affected by presence of food in the GI tract

   b. Rectal—Given as suppositories, creams, enemas for local (hemorrhoids) or systemic (antiemetic) effects; slower onset of action

2. Parenteral—Bypasses the GI tract and includes various injection routes

   a. Intravenous (IV)—Placed directly into the blood; rapid, predictable response; route of choice for emergencies

   b. Intramuscular (IM)—Placed directly into the muscle

     c. Subcutaneous (SC, SQ)—Under the skin (e.g., insulin, local anesthetic)

     d. Intradermal—Into the dermis; small amounts of drugs (e.g., tuberculin skin test)

     e. Intrathecal—Injected into the spinal subarachnoid space; used for treatment of certain forms of meningitis

     f. Intraperitoneal—Into the peritoneal cavity (e.g., dialysis)

     g. Inhalation (INH)—Inhaled into the lungs (gaseous, microcrystalline, volatile drugs, nitrous oxide, and bronchodilators)

     h. Topical—Includes local application to oral mucous membranes, skin, and other epithelial surfaces for local or systemic effects (e.g., anesthetic)

     i. Transdermal—Provides continuous controlled release of medication through semipermeable membrane after application to intact skin (e.g., estrogen/nicotine patches)

     j. Sublingual route (e.g., nitroglycerine)—under the tongue

F. Pharmacodynamics—Study of the biochemical and physiological effects of drugs and the mechanisms of drug action and the relationship between drug concentration and effect; pharmacodynamics is the study of what a drug does to the body, whereas pharmacokinetics is the study of what the body does to a drug

G. Pharmacokinetics—Study of what happens to a drug once it enters, circulates, and leaves the body; what factors influence absorption, distribution, metabolism, and excretion (ADME) (Figure 6-3■)

  1. Absorption—process by which drug molecules are transferred from the site of administration to circulating fluids

     a. Transport mechanism

       (1) Simple diffusion—Substance moves from high concentration to low concentration

       (2) Active transport—Substance is transported against gradient across a biological membrane by "carriers" that furnish energy for transportation of drug

       (3) Facilitated diffusion—Drug is transported down the concentration gradient at a greater rate than passive diffusion; bound to specific carrier proteins

     b. Effects of ionization

       (1) More ionized (water-soluble); increases and facilitates absorption over the surface area

       (2) pH of the tissues at site of administration and dissociation characteristics of the drug determine ease with which the drug will travel through the tissues

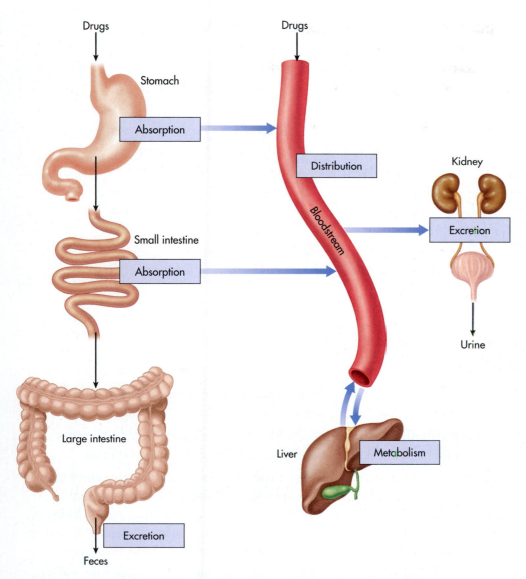

FIGURE 6-3 ■ Four Processes of Pharmacokinetics: Absorption, Distribution, Metabolism, and Excretion

    c. Lipid solubility—The more lipid-soluble (nonionized), the more readily the drug crosses biological membranes

2. Distribution—Drug is distributed throughout the body by plasma proteins in blood

    a. Protein binding—Drug is bound reversibly to plasma proteins, a storage site; a bound drug is not free to exert its action (bound = active) (Figure 6-4■)

    b. Unbound drug—Can cross membranes to site of action, bind to cell receptor; causes an action (free form of drug = active)

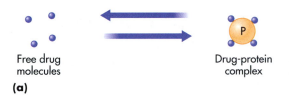

Free drug
molecules

Drug-protein
complex

(a)

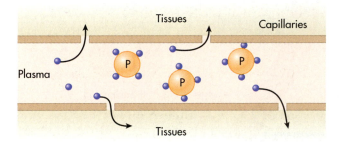

Tissues

Capillaries

Plasma

Tissues

(b)

FIGURE 6-4 ■ Plasma Protein Binding and Drug Availability: (a) Drug exists in a free state or bound to plasma protein. (b) Drug-protein complexes are too large to cross membranes.

    c. Constant equilibrium—Drugs remain in constant equilibrium between the unbound and bound form

    d. Redistribution—Drugs move from the target site of action to other chambers of the body, where they may be able to exert effects

  3. Metabolism (biotransformation)—Process of chemically converting a drug to a form that is usually more easily removed from the body—most common site is liver; body changes the drug to be excreted by the kidneys; microsomal enzyme-dependent (most common: converts lipid-soluble drug to water-soluble metabolite to allow for excretion by kidneys)

  4. Excretion—Drugs and their metabolites eliminated via urine, bile, sweat, saliva, lungs, tears, and milk; kidney is the major organ of drug excretion

II. Adverse Reactions—Undesirable Reactions of Drug Effects

  A. Toxic effect—Exceeds the amount of desired effect; dose-related, predictable (dose causes permanent damage at microscopic level)

  B. Side effect—A dose-related reaction not part of the desired therapeutic outcome; occurs when the drug acts on a target or nontarget organ (undesired effect)

  C. Idiosyncratic reaction—Unexpected reaction to drug, not predictable

  D. Drug allergy—Varies from a mild rash to anaphylaxis; antigen–antibody reaction; not dose-related and not predictable; can be divided into four types of reactions depending on the type of antibody or cell-mediated reaction

E. Interference with natural defense mechanism—Certain drugs may reduce the body's ability to fight infection

F. Teratogenic—Adverse effect of a drug on the fetus, producing deformities

III. Drug Interactions—A drug interaction is a situation in which a substance affects the activity of a drug (i.e., the effects are increased or decreased, or they produce a new effect that neither produces on its own)

A. Definitions

  1. Potentiation—Interaction of two or more drugs resulting in a greater-than-expected effect

  2. Antagonism—Clinical response is reduced by administration of second agent

  3. Summation—Combined activities of two or more drugs that elicit identical or related pharmacological effects; effect is not greater

  4. Synergism—Combination of two or more agonists producing an effect greater than can be achieved by the maximum dose of one of those drugs

B. Mechanisms of interaction

  1. Pharmacokinetic

   a. Absorption alterations

    (1) Absorbed on large surface area—Altered pH may affect disintegration or dissolution (Figure 6-5■)

    (2) Bound or chelated drugs may decrease effect

    (3) Altered GI tract motility may increase or decrease absorption

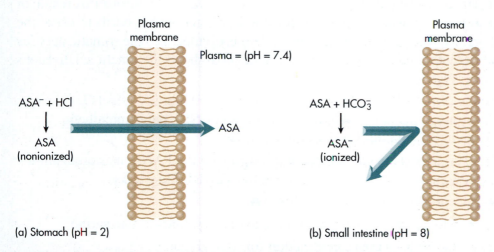

(a) Stomach (pH = 2)   (b) Small intestine (pH = 8)

FIGURE 6-5 ■ Effect of pH on Drug Absorption: (a) In an acidic environment, a weak acid such as aspirin (ASA) is in a nonionized form and absorption occurs. (b) In a basic environment, aspirin is mostly in an ionized form and absorption is prevented.

b. Distribution alterations

(1) Plasma–protein binding—Affected by other drugs with greater affinity, causing second drug to have greater unbound (free) form in the circulation

(2) Blood–brain barrier (BBB)—Some drugs cannot cross the central nervous system (CNS) tissue membranes (protective); drug molecule size is an important variable; if it crosses the BBB it produces CNS effects

c. Metabolism alterations

(1) A drug may induce hepatic microsomal enzyme production and result in a lessened effect of another drug

(2) A drug may decrease microsomal enzymes, resulting in accumulation of another drug, increasing pharmacological effect

d. Excretion alterations

(1) Bound drugs and lipid-soluble drugs cannot be filtered in glomerulus, remain in circulation

(2) Tubular reabsorption may be affected by altered pH

2. Pharmacodynamic—Study of the biochemical and physiological effects of drugs and the mechanisms of drug action and the relationship between drug concentration and effect; sympathetic and parasympathetic nervous system possess sites for drug interactions to occur; have opposite effects

IV. Drugs Used in Dentistry

The nervous system has two major divisions: the central nervous system (CNS) represents the largest part of the nervous system, including the brain and the spinal cord; the peripheral nervous system consists of the nerves and neurons that reside or extend outside the central nervous system (the brain and spinal cord) to serve the limbs and organs. The peripheral nervous system is divided into the somatic nervous system and the autonomic nervous system. Figure 6-6■ shows the functional divisions of the nervous system.

A. Autonomic drugs—Drugs that exert stimulating or inhibiting effects on one or both divisions of the autonomic nervous system (ANS): parasympathetic (PANS) and sympathetic (SANS) (Figure 6-7■)

1. Cholinergic or parasympathetic drugs stimulate the PANS; neurotransmitter is acetylcholine and the termination is by acetylcholinesterase

a. Receptors (Figure 6-8■, Table 6-1■)

(1) Muscarinic—Postsynaptic tissue that responds to muscarine

(a) Eye—Miosis, contraction for near vision

(b) Heart—Bradycardia, decreased blood pressure

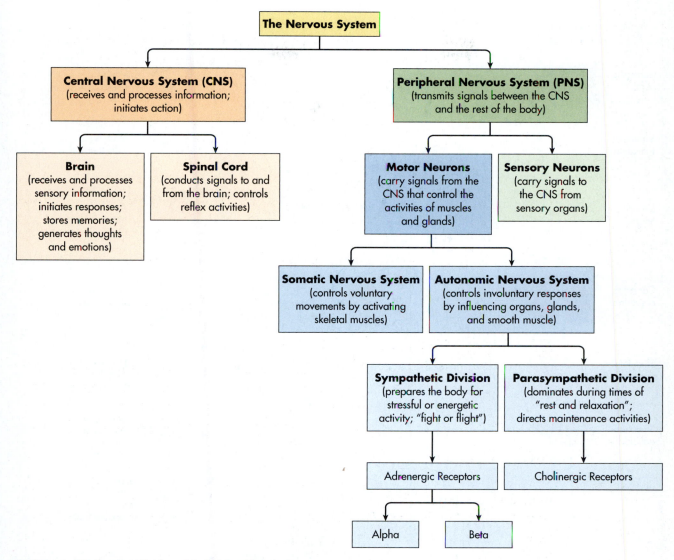

FIGURE 6-6 ■ Functional Divisions of the Peripheral Nervous System

    (c) Lungs—Bronchoconstriction, increase respiratory secretions

    (d) Uterus—Contraction

    (e) Urinary bladder—Contraction (allows for urination)

    (f) Nasopharyngeal—Increased secretions

    (g) GI tract—Increased motility (digestion)

  (2) Nicotinic—Ganglia stimulated by nicotine

    (a) All autonomic ganglia—Stimulation of post-ganglionian neuron

    (b) Skeletal muscle—Contraction

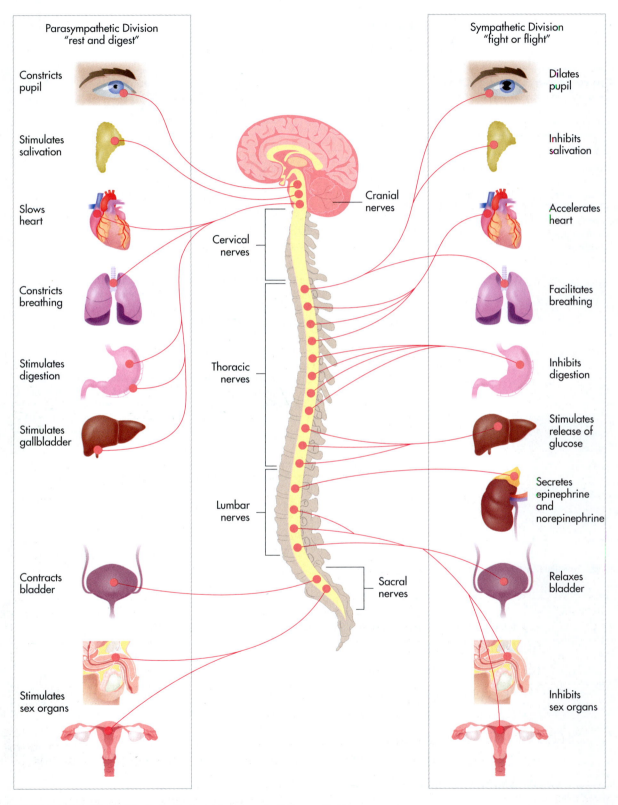

FIGURE 6-7 ■ Effects of the Sympathetic and Parasympathetic Nervous System

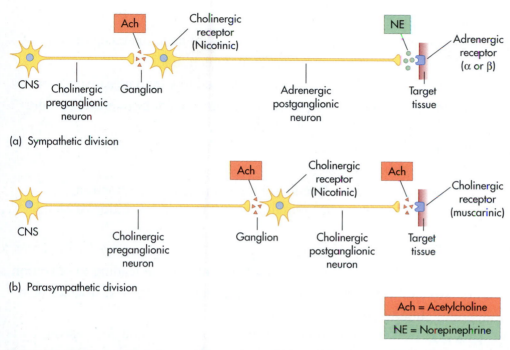

FIGURE 6-8 ■ Receptors in the Autonomic Nervous System: (a) Sympathetic Division; (b) Parasympathetic Division

TABLE 6-1 TYPES OF AUTONOMIC RECEPTORS

Neurotransmitter	Receptor	Primary Locations	Responses
Acetylcholine (cholinergic)	Muscarinic	Parasympathetic target organs other than the heart	Stimulation of smooth muscle and gland secretions
		Heart	Decreased heart rate and force of contraction
	Nicotinic	Postganglionic neurons and neuromuscular junctions of skeletal muscle	Stimulation of smooth muscle and gland secretions
Norepinephrine (adrenergic)	Alpha$_1$	All sympathetic target organs except the heart	Constrict blood vessels, dilate pupils
	Alpha$_2$	Presynaptic adrenergic nerve terminals	Inhibit release of norepinephrine
	Beta$_1$	Heart and kidneys	Increased heart rate and force of contraction; release of renin
	Beta$_2$	All sympathetic target organs except the heart	Inhibition of smooth muscle

Source: Adams, M.P., Josephson, D.L., & Holland, L.N. (2005). *Pharmacology in Nursing: A Pathophysiologic Approach.* Used by permission of Pearson Education, Inc., Upper Saddle River, New Jersey.

b. Mechanism
   (1) Direct action—Drug acts like acetylcholine at the receptor site
      (a) Choline esters—Bethanechol (Urecholine)
      (b) Other—Pilocarpine (Salagen), used to stimulate salivary flow
   (2) Indirect action—Drug inhibits the enzyme cholinesterase, causing acetylcholine buildup at receptor site
c. Pharmacological effects
   (1) Cardiovascular system
      (a) Direct effect—Decreased force and rate of contraction; decreased cardiac output; smooth muscle relaxation of blood vessels
   (2) GI system
      (a) Direct effect—Excitation of smooth muscle leading to salivation
      (b) Indirect effect—Lacrimation, urination, increased stomach acid production, and diarrhea
   (3) Eye—Accommodation for near vision, miosis, and decrease in intraocular pressure
d. Adverse reactions—Extensions of pharmacological effects
e. Treatment of overdose
   (1) Pralidoxime (2-PAM, Protopam) regenerates acetylcholinesterase
   (2) Atropine—Antimuscarinic, does not block nicotinic effects
f. Dental use of pilocarpine—Treatment of xerostomia when functional salivary gland tissue is present

2. Anticholinergic (parasympatholytic)—Inhibits the effects of the PANS; blocks muscarinic receptors throughout the body and nicotinic receptors at high doses
a. Pharmacological effects
   (1) CNS—Low doses, sedation; high doses, stimulation
   (2) Cardiovascular system—Low doses, bradycardia; high doses, tachycardia
   (3) Eye—Increases in intraocular pressure, cycloplegia, mydriasis, glaucoma
   (4) Smooth muscle—Relaxation of the respiratory and GI smooth muscle
   (5) Exocrine glands—Reduction of secretions in the respiratory, GI, and genitourinary tracts
b. Adverse reaction—Extension of the drug's pharmacological effects
c. Contraindications—Patients with glaucoma, prostatic hypertrophy, constipation, urinary retention, and cardiovascular disease

d. Clinical uses

    (1) Preoperative medication

        (a) Dries up secretions

        (b) Blocks the vagal slowing of the heart resulting from general anesthesia

    (2) GI disorders—Reduces increased motility and acid secretions

    (3) Ophthalmologic examination—Full visualization of the retina and relaxation of the lens

    (4) CNS—Treatment of motion sickness, sleep aid, treatment of Parkinson-like symptoms for antipsychotic drugs

e. Examples of drugs

    (1) Atropine (Sal-Tropine)—Prototype agent to decrease salivary flow and respiratory secretions, increase heart rate, and dilate pupils

    (2) Scopolamine (Transderm Scōp)—Antimotion sickness

3. Adrenergic (sympathomimetic)—Stimulates the effects of the SANS (fight or flight)

a. Neurotransmitter—Norepinephrine (NOR)

    (1) Synthesis and inactivation—NOR released from nerve endings, inactivation occurs through dissipation, reuptake by presynaptic nerve terminals or enzymatic breakdown (MAO and COMT)

b. Receptors—Effects on organs and tissues

    (1) alpha (α)

        (a) Eye (iris)—Mydriasis

        (b) Arteries—Vasoconstriction

    (2) beta (β)

        (a) β_1 (heart)—Increased force and rate of contraction

        (b) β_2 (eye)—Relaxation of distant vision

        (c) β_2 (lungs)—Bronchodilation

        (d) β_2 (skeletal smooth muscle)—Contraction

        (e) β_2 (uterus)—Relaxation

        (f) β_2 (bladder)—Contraction of sphincter, urinary retention

c. Mechanism

    (1) Direct action—NOR, epinephrine, and isoproterenol (not used anymore) produce effects directly on a receptor site by stimulating the receptor

    (2) Indirect action—Agents (amphetamine) release endogenous NOR, which then produces a response

(3) Mixed action—Agents (ephedrine) can stimulate the receptor directly or release endogenous NOR to cause a response

d. Pharmacological effects

(1) CNS—Stimulate excitation, alertness, anxiety, apprehension, restlessness, and tremors (at higher doses)

(2) Cardiovascular system

(a) Heart—Increases the force (inotropic) and rate of contraction (chronotropic); increases blood pressure

(b) Vessels

i) Vasoconstriction of smooth muscle (α), which increases total peripheral resistance

ii) Vasodilation of skeletal muscle arteries (β_2), which decreases total peripheral resistance

(c) Blood pressure—Increases

(d) Eye—Decreases in intraocular pressure

(e) Respiratory system—Bronchial relaxation

(f) Metabolic effects—Hyperglycemia (glycogenolysis), decreased insulin release

(g) Salivary glands—Decreases salivary flow

e. Toxic reactions—Extensions of pharmacological effects of anxiety, tremors, palpitations, and arrhythmias

f. Uses

(1) Vasoconstriction

(a) Prolonged action—Added to local anesthetic solutions

(b) Homeostasis—Topically or infiltrated locally to stop bleeding

(c) Decongestion—Incorporated into nose drops or sprays

(2) Cardiac effects—Treatment of shock is controversial; treatment of cardiac arrest

(3) Bronchodilation—Treatment of asthma or anaphylaxis

(4) CNS stimulation—Treatment of attention-deficit hyperactivity disorder (ADHD) and narcolepsy

g. Examples of adrenergic agents

(1) Epinephrine (adrenaline)

(a) Receptor stimulated: α, β

(b) Use: acute asthma attack, anaphylaxis, vasoconstrictor in local anesthesia

(2) Levonordefrin

(a) Receptor stimulated: α

(b) Use: vasoconstrictor added to local anesthesia

(3) Phenylephrine (NeoSynephrine)

(a) Receptor stimulated: α

(b) Use: OTC nose drops or sprays

(4) Isoproterenol (Isuprel)

(a) Receptor stimulated: β

(b) Use: treatment of asthma

(5) Pseudoephedrine (Sudafed)

(a) Receptor stimulated: β

(b) Use: OTC products for common cold

(6) Dopamine (Inotropin)

(a) Receptor stimulated: α, β

(b) Use: treatment of shock

(7) Amphetamine

(a) Receptor stimulated: α, β

(b) Use: treatment of attention-deficit hyperactivity disorder (ADHD) (Ritalin)

h. Dental concerns—Patients who use OTC medications may not inform health care provider; drugs interact with vasoconstrictor added to local anesthetic and increase risk of hypertensive crisis; these drugs interact with many other drugs. Always take blood pressure on patients prior to injecting local anesthetics with epinephrine. Pseudoephedrine increases pulse rate and blood pressure. Decongestants are added to many allergy medications.

4. Adrenergic blocking agents (sympatholytic)—Inhibits the effects of the SANS; blocks all adrenergic receptors (a combination of receptors, or may block only α, β_1, or β_2 receptors)

a. Clinical uses—Hypertension, angina, cardiac arrhythmias, myocardial infarction, glaucoma, prophylactic treatment of migraine headaches, Raynaud's disease

b. Examples

(1) α blocking agents—Tolazoline (Priscoline), prazosin (Minipress), phentolamine (Regitine)

(2) β blocking agents (note -*olol* in generic names)

(a) Nonselective—Affects the heart and lungs; propranolol (Inderal) and nadolol (Corgard); dental concern: use caution when injecting patients with local anesthetics containing epinephrine, nonselective beta blockers increase the pressor response

      (b) Selective—Affects the heart; metoprolol (Lopressor) and atenolol (Tenormin)

   (3) α and β blocking agents end in *-alol*

      (a) Labetalol—Used for hypertension

B. Nonopioid analgesics—General considerations of pain; perception, the physical component, involves a message carried through nerves to the cerebral cortex; and reaction, the psychological component, involves the patient's emotional response.

  1. Salicylates (aspirin)

    a. Site of action—Primarily at peripheral nerve endings

    b. Mechanism—Ability to inhibit the enzyme cyclooxygenase and thereby inhibits prostaglandin synthesis

    c. Pharmacological effects

      (1) Analgesia—Mild to moderate pain

      (2) Antipyretic—Reduces elevated body temperature owing to ability to block prostaglandin synthesis in hypothalamus

      (3) Anti-inflammatory—Reduces inflammation levels to treat mild to moderate pain

      (4) Uricosuric—Decreases excretion of uric acid

      (5) Antiplatelet—Prevents platelets from sticking to each other

    d. Adverse reactions

      (1) GI—Simple dyspepsia, vomiting, or gastric ulceration

      (2) Bleeding altered

         (a) Platelet adhesion—Irreversibly interferes with clotting mechanism; effect lasts for the life of the platelet (7–10 days)

         (b) Hypoprothrombinemia—Inhibits prothrombin synthesis

      (3) Reye's syndrome—May cause hepatoxicity and encephalopathy when used in children with viral infections (e.g., chickenpox or influenza)

      (4) Hypersensitivity—Cross-hypersensitivity exists between aspirin and nonsteroidal anti-inflammatory agents (aspirin triad in asthmatics)

      (5) Aspirin overdose (salicylism)—Tinnitus, headache, nausea, vomiting, dizziness, dimness of vision

    e. Drug interactions—Many interactions caused by aspirin binding to plasma proteins

      (1) Warfarin—An increased risk for bleeding and hemorrhaging

      (2) Probenecid—Interferes with uricosuric effect (only with high dosages of aspirin)

(3) Methotrexate—Can cause increased serum concentration, resulting in toxicity

(4) Sulfonylureas—Can cause a hypoglycemic effect

(5) Antihypertensives—Reduces the effect of angiotensin-converting enzyme (ACE) inhibitors, beta blockers, and loop diuretics (requires several doses over a few days)

2. Nonsteroidal anti-inflammatory agents/drugs (NSAIAs/NSAIDs)

  a. Site of action—Same as aspirin

  b. Mechanism—Same as aspirin

  c. Pharmacological effects: analgesia, antipyretic, anti-inflammatory

  d. Adverse reactions

   (1) Gastrointestinal—GI irritation, pain, ulceration problems

   (2) CNS—Sedation, dizziness, confusion, mental depression, headache

   (3) Blood clotting—Reversibly inhibits platelet aggregation

   (4) Oral—Ulcerative stomatitis, gingival ulcerations, xerostomia, lichenoid drug reaction

   (5) Nephrotoxicity—A poisonous effect of some substances, both toxic chemicals and medications, on the kidney

  e. Therapeutic uses

   (1) Pain control—Greater than aspirin, equal to or greater than some opioids (propoxyphene); useful for dental pain

   (2) Anti-inflammatory—Rheumatoid arthritis and osteoarthritis; useful in dental pain

   (3) Dysmenorrhea—Reduces excess of prostaglandin in uterine wall that produces painful contractions

  f. Examples

   (1) OTC NSAIDs

    (a) Ibuprofen (Motrin, Advil)—Most common, oldest OTC and can be prescription

    (b) Naproxen sodium (Aleve)—Longer in duration of action

    (c) Ketoprofen (Orudis KT)—Similar to ibuprofen

   (2) Prescription NSAIDs

    (a) Ketorolac (Toradol)—Oral and injectable dose form; useful for short-term management of moderate to severe pain

    (b) Naproxen (Naprosyn)

3. Acetaminophen (N-acetyl para-aminophenol [NAPAP])—Tylenol

  a. Pharmacological effects—Analgesic (mild, integumental pain), antipyretic

b. Adverse reactions

(1) Hepatic necrosis—Massive doses or usual doses over a long period have been reported to cause liver damage (do not exceed 4,000 mg per day)

(2) Nephrotoxicity—Associated with long-term consumption; risk is further increased if also taking aspirin or NSAID

c. Drug interactions—Major drug interaction is with alcohol

C. Opioid analgesics and antagonists

1. Classification—Narcotic from poppy plant

a. Mechanism of action at receptor site—Agonist, mixed agonist/antagonist

b. Chemical structure—Useful when allergies are present

c. Potency—Based on amount of pain relief needed, type of pain, and degree of severity of pain (visceral, moderate-severe)

2. Mechanism—Bind to receptors located in CNS, producing altered perception of and response to pain (Figure 6-9■)

a. Mu (μ)—respiratory depression, euphoria, analgesia

b. Kappa (κ)—miosis, sedation, analgesia

c. Sigma (σ)—dysphoria, hallucinations, anxiety, respiratory and vasomotor situation

3. Pharmacological effects

a. Analgesia—Depends on strength of agent; morphine, strongest; codeine, weakest

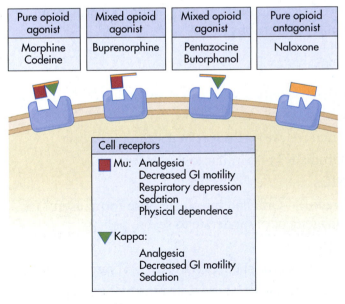

FIGURE 6-9 ■ Opioid Receptors

    b. Sedation and euphoria—Not main effect; produce sedation by κ-receptor stimulation; potentiates analgesia and relieves anxiety

    c. Cough suppression—Depresses cough center in medulla, producing antitussive effect (codeine, found in prescription antitussives)

    d. GI effects—Constipation, nausea and vomiting; used to treat diarrhea symptomatically (paregoric)

4. Adverse reactions

    a. Respiratory depression (outcome of narcotic overdose)—Reduces rate and depth of respiration; produces vasodilation, increasing intracranial pressure; should not be used in patients with head injuries

    b. Nausea and emesis—Stimulates chemoreceptor trigger zone (CTZ) in brain

    c. Constipation—Tonic contraction of the GI tract; slows GI motility; tolerance to this effect does not develop

    d. Miosis—Pinpoint pupils; tolerance to this effect does not develop

    e. Urinary retention—Increase smooth muscle tone

    f. CNS effects—Anxiety, restlessness, nervousness

    g. Abuse—Can occur with all opioids (risk for dependency)

5. Examples (Table 6-2■)

    a. Agonists

        (1) Morphine—Prototype

        (2) Meperidine (Demerol)

        (3) Hydromorphone (Dilaudid)—Orally effective for severe pain

        (4) Methadone—Treatment of opioid addicts and for analgesia

        (5) Oxycodone (Percodan)—Combined with aspirin or acetaminophen (Percocet) for synergistic effect on moderate to severe pain

        (6) Codeine (Empirin #3, Tylenol #3—most commonly prescribed narcotic by dentists)—Weak compared with morphine, combined with nonopioid agent for synergistic effect

    b. Agonist/antagonist

        (1) Pentazocine (Talwin)—Produces analgesic sedation and respiratory sedation

    c. Antagonists

        (1) Naloxone (Narcan)—Pure narcotic antagonist; drug of choice for treating agonist or mixed opioid overdose; reverses opioid-induced respiratory depression

        (2) Naltrexone (ReVia)—Maintenance of opioid-free state; dental pain must be treated with nonopioid analgesics in patients taking this drug

TABLE 6-2 OPIOIDS FOR PAIN MANAGEMENT	
Drug	**Route and Adult Dose (max dose where indicated)**
Opioid Agonists with Moderate Efficacy	
codeine	PO; 15–60 mg qid
hydrocodone bitartrate (Hycodan)	PO; 5–10 mg q4–6h prn (max 15 mg/dose)
oxycodone hydrochloride (OxyContin); oxycodone terephthalate (Percocet-5, Roxicet, others)	PO; 5–10 mg qid prn
propoxyphene hydrochloride (Darvon)	PO; 65 mg (HCl form) or 100 mg (napsylate form) q4h
propoxyphene napsylate (Darvon-N)	prn (max 390 HCl/day; max 600 mg napsylate/day)
Opioid Agonists with High Efficacy	
hydromorphone hydrochloride (Dilaudid)	PO; 1–4 mg q4–6h prn
levorphanol tartrate (Levo-Dromoran)	PO; 2–3 mg tid to qid prn
meperidine hydrochloride (Demerol)	PO; 50–150 mg q3–4h prn
methadone hydrochloride (Dolophine)	PO; 2.5–10 mg q3–4h prn
morphine sulfate (Astramorph PF, Duramorph, others)	PO; 10–30 mg q4h prn
oxymorphone hydrochloride (Numorphan)	SC/IM; 1–1.5 mg q4–6h prn PR; 5 mg q4–6h prn
Opioids with Mixed Agonist-Antagonist Effects	
buprenorphine hydrochloride (Buprenex)	IM/IV; 0.3 mg q6h (max 0.6 mg q4h)
butorphanol tartrate (Stadol)	IM; 1–4 mg q3–4h prn (max 4 mg/dose)
dezocine (Dalgan)	IV; 2.5–10 mg (usually 5 mg) q2–4h IM; 5–10 mg (usually 10 mg) q3–4h
nalbuphine hydrochloride (Nubain)	SC/IM/IV; 10–20 mg q3–6h prn (max 160 mg/day)
pentazocine hydrochloride (Talwin)	PO; 50–100 mg q3–4h (max 600 mg/day) SC/IM/IV; 30 mg q3–4h (max 360 mg/day)

TABLE 6-2 OPIOIDS FOR PAIN MANAGEMENT (continued)	
Drug	**Route and Adult Dose (max dose where indicated)**
Opioid Antagonists	
nalmefene hydrochloride (Revex)	SC/IM/IV; Use 1 mg/ml concentration; nonopioid dependent; 0.5 mg/70 kg; opioid dependent; 0.1 mg/70 kg
naloxone hydrochloride (Narcan)	IV; 0.4–2 mg; may be repeated every 2–3 min up to 10 mg if necessary
naltrexone hydrochloride (Trexan, ReVia)	PO; 25 mg followed by another 25 mg in 1 hour if no withdrawal response (max 800 mg/day)

Source: Adams, M.P., Josephson, D.L., & Holland, L.N. (2005). *Pharmacology in Nursing: A Pathophysiologic Approach.* Used by permission of Pearson Education, Inc., Upper Saddle River, New Jersey.

D. Anti-infective agents

    1. General principles

        a. Therapeutic indications—Acute dental pain with fever; treatment of abscesses and certain periodontal diseases; prophylaxis

        b. Patient—Best defense against a pathogen is host response

        c. Infection—Virulence, number of organisms present, and invasiveness of the microorganism are important in deciding acuteness, severity, and spreading tendency of infection

        d. Anti-infective administration carries risks; benefits versus risks must be weighed

        e. Definitions

            (1) Anti-infective—Acts against or destroys infections

            (2) Antibacterial—Acts against bacteria

                (a) Bactericidal—Kills bacteria

                (b) Bacteriostatic—Inhibits or retards growth of bacteria

            (3) Antibiotic agents—Produced by another microorganism to kill or inhibit the growth or multiplication of bacteria

            (4) Antimicrobial—Acts against microorganisms

            (5) Antiviral—Acts against viruses

            (6) Antifungal—Acts against fungi

            (7) Blood level—Concentration of anti-infective agent present in blood serum

            (8) Minimum inhibitory concentrations (MIC)—Lowest concentration needed to inhibit visible growth of an organism on media after incubation for 18 to 24 hours

(9) Resistance—Occurs when microorganisms are unaffected by an antimicrobial agent; may be natural (always has been resistant) or acquired (develops resistance)

(10) Spectrum—Range of action of a drug

(11) Superinfection, suprainfection—Infection caused by the overgrowth of microbes different from the causative microorganism (e.g., *Candida* infection after antibiotic therapy)

(12) Culture and sensitivity—All infections not responding to antimicrobial therapy should be cultured and sensitivity tests performed (application of antimicrobial agent to culture to determine effective antibiotic); also cases of serious infections and infection in compromised patients

(13) General adverse reactions

    (a) Superinfection

    (b) Allergic reactions—ranges from mild to fatal anaphylaxis

    (c) Drug interactions

        i) Oral antibiotics—Reduced effectiveness of oral contraceptives

        ii) Oral anticoagulants—Increase the effect of the anticoagulant

        iii) Other anti-infective agents—Antibodies may compete for same receptor and should not be given together (erythromycin and clindamycin); a bacteriostatic agent may stop the organism from growing so that the bactericidal does not work effectively (erythromycin and penicillin)

    (d) GI—Nausea, vomiting

    (e) Pregnancy—Risk to the fetus must be considered

    (f) Rule—Use agent with a narrow spectrum that is susceptible to microorganism causing infection or for prophylaxis

2. Antibiotics (Figure 6-10■)

  a. Penicillins (Table 6-3■)

    (1) Mechanism—Inhibits cell wall synthesis; bactericidal

    (2) Groups

      (a) Penicillin G/penicillin V—Narrow spectrum

      (b) Penicillinase—**Beta-lactamase** is a type of enzyme produced by some bacteria that is responsible for their resistance to beta-lactam antibiotics such as penicillins, cephalosporins, cephamycins, and carbapenems. These antibiotics have a common element in their molecular structure: a four-atom ring known as a beta-lactam. The lactamase enzyme breaks that ring

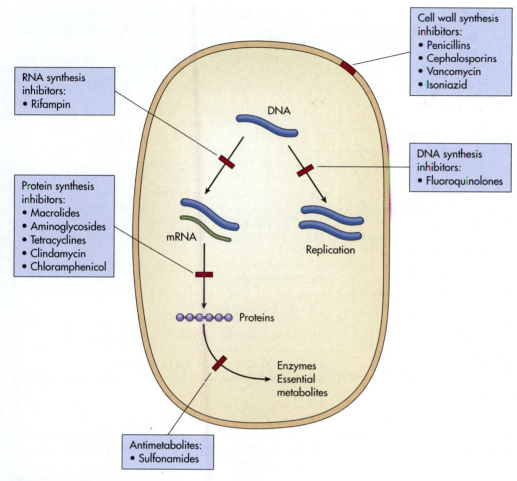

RNA synthesis
inhibitors:
• Rifampin

Cell wall synthesis
inhibitors:
• Penicillins
• Cephalosporins
• Vancomycin
• Isoniazid

DNA

Protein synthesis
inhibitors:
• Macrolides
• Aminoglycosides
• Tetracyclines
• Clindamycin
• Chloramphenicol

DNA synthesis
inhibitors:
• Fluoroquinolones

mRNA

Replication

Proteins

Enzymes
Essential
metabolites

Antimetabolites:
• Sulfonamides

FIGURE 6-10 ■ Mechanisms of Action of Antimicrobial Drugs

open, deactivating the molecule's antibacterial properties. Penicillinase is a particular type of β lactamase, showing specificity for penicillins, again by hydrolysing the beta-lactam ring

  (c) Ampicillin/amoxicillin

  (d) Extended-spectrum penicillin

(3) Pharmocokinetics

  (a) Administered orally or parenterally but not topically due to allergy sensitization potential

  (b) Peak blood levels—Immediately when used intravenously, 30 minutes to 1 hour if given orally or intramuscularly (amoxicillin peaks 2 hours after oral administration, which is the justification for the premedication regimen)

  (c) Half-life—30 minutes to 1 hour

TABLE 6-3 PENICILLINS

Drug	Route and Adult Dose (max dose where indicated)
Narrow Spectrum/Pencillinase Sensitive	
penicillin G benzathine (Bicillin)	IM; 1.2 million units as a single dose
penicillin G procaine (Crysticillin, Wycillin)	IM; 600,000–1.2 million units qd
penicillin G sodium/potassium (Pentids)	PO; 400,000–800,000 units qd
penicillin V (Pen-Vee K, Veetids, Betapen)	PO; 125–250 mg qid
Narrow Spectrum/Penicillinase Resistant	
cloxacillin (Tegopen)	PO; 250–500 mg bid
dicloxacillin (Dynapen)	PO; 125–500 mg qid
nafcillin (Nafcil, Unipen)	PO; 250 mg–1 g qid (max 12 g/day)
oxacillin (Prostaphlin, Bactocill)	PO; 250 mg–1 g qid (max 12 g/day)
Broad Spectrum (Aminopenicillins)	
amoxicillin (Amoxil, Trimox, Wymox)	PO; 250–500 mg tid
amoxicillin-clavulanate (Augmentin)	PO; 250 or 500 mg tablet (each with 125 mg clavulanic acid) q8–12h
ampicillin (Polycillin, Omnipen)	PO; 250–500 mg bid
bacampicillin (Spectrobid)	PO; 400–800 mg bid
Extended Spectrum	
carbenicillin (Geocillin, Geopen)	PO; 382–764 mg qid
mezlocillin (Mezlin)	IM; 1.5–2.0 g qid (max 24 g/day)
piperacillin sodium (Pipracil)	IM; 2–4 g tid-qid (max 24 g/day)
piperacillin tazobactam (Zosyn)	IV; 3.375 g qid over 30 min
ticarcillin (Ticar)	IM; 1–2 g qid (max 40 g/day)

Source: Adams, M.P., Josephson, D.L., & Holland, L.N. (2005). *Pharmacology in Nursing: A Pathophysiologic Approach.* Used by permission of Pearson Education, Inc., Upper Saddle River, New Jersey.

(d) Metabolized—Kidney, excreted in urine virtually unchanged

(e) Acid stability—Penicillin G is unstable in acid environment of the stomach and is administered parenterally; penicillin V is acid-stable and given orally

(4) Adverse reactions

(a) Gastrointestinal upset

(b) Allergic reactions—Mild to anaphylactic

(5) Penicillin G/penicillin V

(a) Spectrum—Includes Gram-positive cocci and certain Gram-negative cocci; not resistant to penicillinase; 90% of oral infections are Gram-positive

(b) Penicillin G—Prototype, parenteral; potassium salt given IV produces most rapid and highest blood level; given IM, produces intermediate blood levels (used to treat STDs)

(c) Penicillin V—Well absorbed with oral administration; used in the treatment of dental infections because it kills resident microorganisms in 90% of dental infections

(d) Examples

  i) Penicillin G

  ii) Penicillin G procaine (Crysticillin)

  iii) Penicillin G benzathine (Bicillin L-A)

  iv) Penicillin V (Pen-Vee K, V-Cillin K)

(6) Penicillinase—Resistant penicillins

(a) Reserved for use only against penicillinase-producing staphylococci

(b) Prototype—Dicloxacillin (Dynapen, Dycill)

(7) Ampicillin/amoxicillin

(a) Spectrum—Gram-positive cocci, some enterococci; not penicillinase resistant

(b) Amoxicillin—A relative of ampicillin, preferred for higher blood levels (better absorbed); less frequent dosage; absorption not impaired by food

  i) Drug of choice in American Heart Association (AHA) antibiotic prophylaxis regimen, to prevent infective endocarditis and in antibiotic prophylaxis for selected total joint replacement (2 grams 1 hour before procedure)

(c) Augmentin—Amoxicillin plus clavulanic acid (inhibits B-lactamases produced by bacteria); has been used in treatment of mixed periodontal infection

(d) Examples

  i) Ampicillin (Polycillin, Omnipen)

  ii) Amoxicillin (Amoxil, Trimox)

(8) Extended spectrum penicillin

  (a) Spectrum—Broader than penicillin G; both Gram-positive and Gram-negative; special activity against *Pseudomonas aeruginosa;* not penicillinase-resistant

  (b) Used parenterally to treat systemic infections

  (c) Examples

   i) Carbenicillin

   ii) Piperacillin

   iii) Ticarcillin

b. Macrolides (Table 6-4■)

  (1) Mechanism—Inhibits bacterial protein synthesis at the 50 S subunit, bacteriostatic

  (2) Adverse reactions

   (a) GI—Abdominal cramps, nausea, vomiting, and diarrhea

   (b) *Cholestatic jaundice*—Primarily seen with estolate but also with ethyl succinate

  (3) Therapeutic uses—Drug of choice in penicillin-allergic patient in medicine, other specific infections, not effective against the anaerobic species in dental infections (in dentistry only use alternative macrolides; erythromycin is not used in dentistry given resistance with most oral organisms; dangerous drug interations, and poor compliance)

  (4) Spectrum

   (a) Erythromycin—Works primarily against Gram-positive organisms; similar to penicillin V

TABLE 6-4 MACROLIDES	
Drug	**Route and Adult Dose (max dose where indicated)**
azithromycin (Zithromax)	PO; 500 mg for one dose, then 250 mg qd for 4 days
clarithromycin (Biaxin)	PO; 250–500 mg bid
dirithromycin (Dynabac)	PO; 500 mg qd
erythromycin (E-Mycin, Erythrocin)	PO; 250–500 mg bid or 333 mg tid

Source: Adams, M.P., Josephson, D.L., & Holland, L.N. (2005). *Pharmacology in Nursing: A Pathophysiologic Approach.* Used by permission of Pearson Education, Inc., Upper Saddle River, New Jersey.

(b) Azithromycin (Zithromax)

    i) Mild to moderate infections of upper/lower respiratory tract

    ii) May have activity against some anaerobes

    iii) Adverse reactions—Stomatitis, candidiasis, dizziness, vertigo, nausea, vomiting, hepatoxicity

    iv) Recommended for use in antibiotic prophylaxis in people who are allergic to penicillin

(c) Clarithromycin (Biaxin)

    i) Similar effects, uses, and adverse reaction as azithromycin

    ii) Used to kill *Helicobacter pylori* in gastric ulcers

    iii) Adverse reactions—linked to pseudomembranous colitis, which is an infection of the colon

(5) Pharmacokinetics

    (a) Broken down in gastric fluid, therefore has enteric coating (erythromycin)

    (b) Administer 2 hours before or 2 hours after meals; blood levels peak 1–4 hours after ingestion

(6) Examples

    (a) Erythromycin base (E-Mycin)

    (b) Erythromycin stearate (Erythrocin)

    (c) Erythromycin ethylsuccinate (E.E.S., Pediamycin)

    (d) Erythromycin estolate (Ilosone)

c. Tetracyclines (Table 6-5■)

(1) Mechanisms of action—Inhibits bacterial protein synthesis at 30 S subunit, bacteriostatic

(2) Pharmacokinetics—Given orally, rapid absorption, kidney excretion mainly; doxycycline excreted in feces

(3) Spectrum—Considered broad-spectrum antibiotics; effective against wide variety of Gram-positive and Gram-negative bacteria, both aerobes and anaerobes; cross-resistance can occur

(4) Adverse reactions

    (a) GI—Anorexia, nausea, vomiting; related to local irritation from altered flora

    (b) Effects on teeth and bones—Should not be used during pregnancy or in children up to 9 years of age; forms covalent bond with enamel, causing intrinsic staining (teratogenic)

    (c) Hepatoxicity—Increases with IV use

    (d) Superinfection—Overgrowth of *C. albicans* (thrush, vaginitis)

    (e) Photosensitivity—Exaggerated sunburn with exposure to sun

TABLE 6-5 TETRACYCLINES

Drug	Route and Adult Dose (max dose where indicated)
demeclocycline (Declomycin)	PO; 150 mg q6h or 300 mg q12h (max 2.4 g/d)
doxycycline (Vibramycin, others)	PO; 100 mg bid on day 1, then 100 mg qd (max 200 mg/day)
methacycline (Rondomycin)	PO; 600 mg/day in 2–4 divided doses
minocycline (Minocin, others)	PO; 200 mg as one dose followed by 100 mg bid
oxytetracycline (Terramycin)	PO; 250–500 mg bid-qid
tetracycline (Achromycin, others)	PO; 250–500 mg bid-qid (max 2 g/day)

Source: Adams, M.P., Josephson, D.L., & Holland, L.N. (2005). *Pharmacology in Nursing: A Pathophysiologic Approach.* Used by permission of Pearson Education, Inc., Upper Saddle River, New Jersey.

      (5) Drug interactions

          (a) Cations—Decreased intestinal absorption, include dairy products, antacids, and mineral supplements

               i) Doxycycline (Vibramycin)—Can take with food

          (b) Enhanced effect of drugs—Oral sulfonylureas

          (c) Reduced tetracycline effect—Barbiturates and phenytoin

          (d) Reduce effectiveness of oral contraceptives, bactericidal antibiotics

      (6) Uses

          (a) Medical—Acne, pulmonary infections in patients with chronic obstructive pulmonary disease (COPD)

          (b) Dental—Periodontal infections

      (7) Examples

          (a) Tetracycline (Achromycin V, Sumycin)

          (b) Doxycycline (Vibramycin)

          (c) Minocycline (Minocin)

    d. Clindamycin (Cleocin)

      (1) Mechanism—A lincosamide antibiotic used in the treatment of infections caused by susceptible microorganisms; it inhibits bacterial protein synthesis at 50 S subunit, bacteriostatic

      (2) Pharmacokinetics—Orally well absorbed; topically, IM or IV more than 90% bound to plasma proteins; drug excreted as inactive metabolite in urine and feces

(3) Spectrum—Effective against Gram-positive organisms and some anaerobe species; cross-resistance between clindamycin and erythromycin

(4) Adverse reactions

    (a) GI effects—Diarrhea, pseudomembranous colitis (PMC), potentially fatal

    (b) Other effects—Superinfections, allergy, neutropenia, thrombocytopenia, agranulocytosis

(5) Uses

    (a) Oral infections caused by bacteroides species, some staphylococcus infections, acne

    (b) An alternative regimen for antibiotic prophylaxis in penicillin-allergic patients

    (c) Good for bone infections

    (d) Drug of choice in penicillin-allergic patient for orofacial infections

e. Metronidazole (Flagyl)

(1) Mechanism—Trichomonacidal, bactericidal

(2) Pharmacokinetics—Well absorbed orally with peak blood levels 1–2 hours after ingestion; 60–80% excreted in urine

(3) Spectrum—Effective against trichomonacidal, ambicidal, and obligate anaerobes such as bacteroides species

(4) Adverse reactions

    (a) GI effects—Disulfiram-like reaction if taken with alcohol; avoid use with alcohol-containing mouthrinses

    (b) Oral effects—Metallic taste

    (c) CNS effects—Headache, dizziness

(5) Uses

    (a) Sexually transmitted diseases and serious anaerobic infections of abdomen, skeleton, and female genital tract

    (b) Dental—anaerobic periodontal infections

f. Cephalosporins

(1) Mechanism—Chemically related to the penicillins; inhibits bacterial cell wall synthesis

(2) Pharmacokinetics—Administered orally, IM, or IV; well absorbed, excreted in urine

(3) Spectrum—effective against most Gram-positive cocci, penicillinase-producing staphylococci, some Gram-negative

bacteria; four generations of agents, extent of antimicrobial action depends on generation; first and second generations primarily used in dentistry (increasing generations increase spectrum of kill)

(4) Adverse reactions

 (a) GI effects—Diarrhea, nausea, vomiting, and abdominal pain; minimized if taken with food or milk

 (b) Other—Nephrotoxicity, superinfection

 (c) Allergy—Cross-sensitivity with penicillin (percentage of patients with cross-sensitivity have IgE-mediated reaction to penicillin)

(5) Uses

 (a) Respiratory infection, sexually transmitted diseases, or various mixed infection used parenterally in hospitals

 (b) Dental use limited to treatment of infection resistance to penicillin

 (c) Alternative antibiotic in antibiotic prophylaxis, often preferred for orthopedic patients requiring premedication

(6) Examples

 (a) First generation

  i) Cephalexin (Keflex)

  ii) Cefadroxil (Duricef)

  iii) Cefazolin (Ancef)

 (b) Second generation—Cefaclor (Ceclor)

 (c) Third generation—Cefixime (Suprax)

 (d) Fourth generation—Cefepime (Maxipime)

g. Aminoglycosides

(1) Mechanism—Inhibits bacterial protein synthesis at 30 S subunit; bactericidal; broad antibacterial spectrum

(2) Pharmacokinetics—Only administered IV or IM; plasma blood levels must be monitored

(3) Spectrum—Effective against most Gram-negative bacilli; resistance to agents can be rapid

(4) Adverse reactions

 (a) Ototoxicity—Toxic to 8th cranial nerve

 (b) Nephrotoxicity—Concentrates in the renal cortex

 (c) Neuromuscular blockade—If given in combination with general anesthetic or skeletal muscle relaxant, it can produce apnea

(5) Uses

 (a) Treatment of aerobic gram-negative infections when other agents are ineffective

 (b) Treatment of hospitalized patients with serious gram-negative infections

 (c) Topically for ear infections

(6) Examples

 (a) Gentamicin

 (b) Neomycin

h. Sulfonamides (Table 6-6■)

(1) Mechanism—Competitive antagonist of para-aminobenzoic acid (PABA); antimetabolite, bacteriostatic

(2) Pharmacokinetics—Given orally with varying absorption depending on agent given; metabolites or free drug excreted in urine

(3) Spectrum—Many gram-positive and some gram-negative bacteria; chlamydia

(4) Adverse reactions—Photosensitivity, allergic reactions, renal crystallization (crystalluria); patient should increase fluid intake

TABLE 6-6 SULFONAMIDES	
Drug	**Route and Adult Dose (max dose where indicated)**
sulfacetamide (Cetamide, others)	Ophthalmic; one to three drops of 10%, 15%, or 30% solution into lower conjunctival sac q2–3h, may increase interval as patient responds or use 1.5–2.5 cm (0.5–1.0 in.) of 10% ointment q6h and at hs
sulfadiazine (Microsulfon)	PO; Loading dose 2–4 g; maintenance dose 2–4 g/d in four to six divided doses
sulfamethizole	PO; 2–4 g initially followed by 1–2 g qid
sulfidoxine-pyrimethamine (Fansidar)	PO; 1 tablet weekly (500 mg sulfidoxine, 25 mg pyrimethamine)
sulfamethoxazole (Gantanol)	PO; 2 g initially followed by 1 g bid-tid
sulfisoxazole (Gantrisin)	PO; 2–4 g initially followed by 1–2 g qid
trimethoprim-sulfamethoxazole (Bactrim, Septa)	PO; 160 mg TMP/800 mg SMZ bid

Source: Adams, M.P., Josephson, D.L., & Holland, L.N. (2005). *Pharmacology in Nursing: A Pathophysiologic Approach.* Used by permission of Pearson Education, Inc., Upper Saddle River, New Jersey.

(5) Uses—Urinary tract infection, otitis media; not used in dentistry

(6) Examples

(a) Sulfamethoxazole

(b) Trimethoprim (Septra, Bactrim)

(c) Sulfamethizole (Thiosulfil)

i. Quinolones (Fluoroquinolone)

(1) Mechanism of action—Inhibits nucleic acid (i.e., DNA) synthesis, bactericidal

(2) Pharmacokinetics—Well absorbed, half-life of 4 hours; antacids interfere with its absorption

(3) Broad spectrum—Wide range of gram-negative and gram-positive organisms

(4) Adverse reactions—GI effects, hypersensitivity

(5) Uses

(a) Indicated for lower respiratory tract, skin, bone and joint, urinary tract infections

(b) Not used in dentistry because the spectrum does not match that of the oral flora

(6) Examples—Generic name "floxacin"

(a) Ciprofloxacin (Cipro), Ofloxacin (Floxin)

(b) Lomefloxacin (Maxaquin)

(c) Norfloxacin (Noroxin)

3. Antifungal agents—Seen more frequently in the immunocompromised patient; fungal infections managed in the dental office are mucocutaneous (affecting skin or mucosa); topical antifungal treatment is preferred to systemic antifungals (ADA recommends to avoid systemics), given serious drug interactions and emergence of resistant fungal organisms (systemics should be "reserved" medications for infections that do not respond to topical drugs)

a. Nystatin (Mycostatin, Nilstat)

(1) Mechanism—Binds to sterols in the fungal cell membrane; changes membrane permeability

(2) Spectrum—Fungicidal and fungistatic against a variety of yeasts and fungi

(3) Dosage forms—Aqueous suspension (contains 50% sucrose), pastille (also contains sugar); dental hygienist should recommend fluoride rinse after therapy

(4) Uses—Treatment and prevention of oral candidiasis

b. Clotrimazole (Mycelex)

  (1) Mechanism—Alteration of cell membrane permeability; cellular constituents lost

  (2) Spectrum—Tinea species and *Candida* species

  (3) Dosage forms—Troches (dissolves in mouth 5x/day for 2 weeks)

  (4) Uses—Local treatment of oropharyngeal candidiasis

c. Ketoconazole (Nizoral)

  (1) Mechanism—Alters cellular membrane and interferes with intracellular enzymes

  (2) Spectrum—Wide variety of fungal infections including many systemic fungal infections

  (3) Pharmacokinetics—Absorbed systemically; requires an acid environment

  (4) Dosage forms—Oral tablets

  (5) Adverse reactions

    (a) GI—Nausea and vomiting

    (b) Hepatoxicity

    (c) Pregnancy and nursing—Teratogenic potential; risk to benefit must be considered

    (d) Drug interactions—H_2 blockers, anticholinergic agents, antacids, warfarin, and cyclosporine

d. Fluconazole (Diflucan)

  (1) Mechanism—Prevents synthesis of ergosterol in the fungal cell by inhibiting fungal cytochrome P450 enzymes

  (2) Dosage forms—Oral tablets or IV

  (3) Uses

    (a) Treatment of cryptococcal meningitis or pharyngeal and esophageal candidiasis

    (b) Serious systemic *Candida* infections

    (c) Prophylactic agent against candidiasis in immunocompromised patients

    (d) Treatment of *Candida* that does not respond to other agents

4. Antiviral agents—Obligate intracellular organisms that use DNA/RNA from host's cells; killing virus often requires harming host cell; the herpes virus of most interest to dentist; immunocompromised patients may have oral symptoms

a. Acyclovir (Zovirax)

  (1) Mechanism—Interferes with DNA polymerase and inhibits DNA replication

(2) Spectrum—Herpes simplex viruses, papilloma viruses

(3) Dosage forms—Oral, topical, IV

(4) Adverse reactions—Burning, nausea, CNS effects

(5) Uses

    (a) Topical—Initial herpes genitalis, limited non-life-threatening initial and recurrent mucocutaneous herpes simplex

    (b) Oral—Initial and management of viral lesions in immunocompromised and nonimmunocompromised patients

    (c) Parenteral—Severe initial herpetic infections in immunocompromised patient

    (d) New agents

        i) Famciclovir (Famvir)

b. Valacyclovir (Valtrex)

(1) Antiviral drug used to treat herpes viruses such as shingles, genital herpes, and oral herpes

(2) Works by inhibiting the replication of viral DNA that is necessary when a virus reproduces itself

(3) Valacyclovir is a so-called pro-drug, which means that it isn't active in itself; valacyclovir converts to acyclovir, which attacks the herpes virus; the duration of valacyclovir is longer than acyclovir, which means that it doesn't need to be taken as often

c. Penciclovir (Denavir)

(1) Available topically for primary and recurrent herpes simplex

(2) Shown to reduce pain and duration of lesions

(3) Advantage—Higher concentration so it stays in the cells longer

5. Antituberculosis agents (Table 6-7■)

a. Patients with tuberculosis are difficult to treat because of their inadequate defense mechanisms

b. Tubercle bacilli develop resistant strains easily, have long periods of inactivity (multiple-drug-resistant strains)

c. Most drugs not bactericidal; high dose cannot be used owing to toxicity

d. Multiple drug combinations frequently required

(1) Isoniazid (INH)

    (a) Mechanism—Bactericidal only against growing tubercle bacilli

    (b) Adverse reactions—CNS effects, hepatoxicity, hepatitis (many drug interactions)

    (c) Uses—Alone as prophylaxis, in combination with rifampin and pyrazinamide (PZA) or other agents

TABLE 6-7 ANTITUBERCULOSIS DRUGS	
Drug	**Route and Adult Dose (max dose where indicated)**
First Line Agents	
ethambutol (Myambutol)	PO; 15–25 mg/kg qd
isoniazid (INH, others)	PO; 15 mg/kg qd
pyrazinamide (PZA)	PO; 5–15 mg/kg tid-qid (max 2 g/day)
rifampin (Rifadin, Rimactane)	PO; 600 mg qd
rifapentine (Priftin)	PO; 600 mg twice a week for 2 mo, then once a week for 4 mo
rifater: combination of pyrazinamide with isoniazid and rifampin	PO; six tablets qd (for patients weighing 121 lb or more)
streptomycin	IM; 15 mg/kg up to 1.0 g/day as a single dose
Second Line Agents	
amikacin (Amikin)	IM; 5–7.5 mg/kg as a loading dose, then 7.5 mg/kg bid
capreomycin (Capastat Sulfate)	IM; 1 g/d (not to exceed 20 mg/kg/d) for 60–120 d, then 1 g two to three times/wk
ciprofloxacin (Cipro)	PO; 250–750 mg bid
cycloserine (Seromycin)	PO; 250 mg q12h for 2 wk, may increase to 500 mg q12h (max 1 g/day)
ethionamide (Trecator-SC)	PO; 0.5–1.0 g/d divided q8–12h
kanamycin (Kantrex)	IM; 5–7.5 mg/kg bid-tid
ofloxacin (Floxin)	PO; 200–400 mg bid

Source: Adams, M.P., Josephson, D.L., & Holland, L.N. (2005). *Pharmacology in Nursing: A Pathophysiologic Approach.* Used by permission of Pearson Education, Inc., Upper Saddle River, New Jersey.

(2) Rifampin (Rifadin)
  (a) Mechanism—Inhibition of DNA-dependent RNA polymerase
  (b) Adverse reactions—GI irritation
  (c) Uses—In combination with other antitubercular agents
(3) Ethambutol (Myambutol)
  (a) Uses—Synthetic tuberculostatic agent effective against *Mycobacterium tuberculosis;* resistance develops very rapidly when used alone; used in combination therapy
  (b) Adverse reactions—Optic neuritis

TABLE 6-8 SELECTED LOCAL ANESTHETICS

Chemical Classification	Drug
Esters	benzocaine (Americaine, Solarcaine, others)
	chloroprocaine (Nesacaine)
	cocaine
	procaine (Novocain)
	tetracaine (Pontocaine)
Amides	articaine (Septodont)
	bupivacaine (Marcaine)
	dibucaine (Nupercaine, Nupercainal)
	etidocaine (Duranest)
	levobupivacaine (Chirocaine)
	lidocaine (Xylocaine)
	mepivacaine (Carbocaine)
	prilocaine (Citanest)
	ropivacaine (Naropin)
Miscellaneous agents	dyclonine (Dyclone)
	pramoxine (Tronothane)

Source: Adams, M.P., Josephson, D.L., & Holland, L.N. (2005). *Pharmacology in Nursing: A Pathophysiologic Approach.* Used by permission of Pearson Education, Inc., Upper Saddle River, New Jersey.

E. Local anesthetics (LA)—drugs that produce a loss of sensation in a localized area of the body (Table 6-8■)

   1. General principles

      a. Two groups—Esters and amides (Figure 6-11■)

      b. Structure

         (1) Aromatic nucleus (lipophilic)

         (2) Linkage (ester or amide followed by an aliphatic chain)

         (3) Amino groups (hydrophilic)

      c. Site of action—Nerve membrane

      d. Mechanism of action (Figure 6-12■)

         (1) Reduces transient increase in sodium flow into nerve membrane

         (2) Binds water-soluble ionized form of LA to calcium ion receptor site

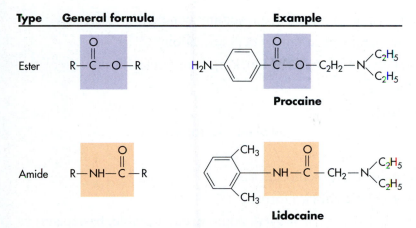

FIGURE 6-11 ■ Chemical Structures of Ester and Amide Local Anesthetics

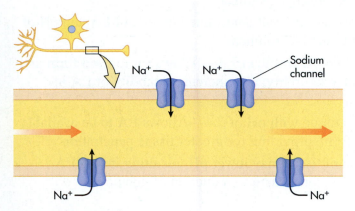

(a) Normal nerve conduction

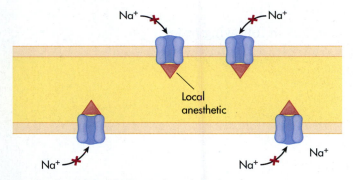

(b) Local anesthetic blocking sodium channels

FIGURE 6-12 ■ Mechanism of Action of Local Anesthetics

        (3) Receptor channel is blocked and sodium conduction decreases

        (4) Results in a decrease in rate of depolarization

        (5) Prevents nerve conduction in blocking pain threshold

    e. Ionization factors

        (1) LAs are weak bases

        (2) LAs occur in equilibrium between two forms

           (a) Lipophilic free base

           (b) Hydrophilic hydrochloride salt

           (c) Characteristics of two forms

               i) Free base—Uncharged, nonionized, unstable, basic, and fat-soluble (lipophilic)

               ii) Hydrochloride salt—Charged, ionized, stable, acidic, and water-soluble (hydrophilic)

           (d) Proportion of base and salt determined by pK_a of LA and pH of surrounding tissue environment

           (e) Dental cartridge pH less than 7.4—Allows for ionized form and increases water solubility; also increases stability of LA in cartridge

           (f) Injection into tissue with pH of 7.4—Allows LA to be available in free base form, providing for greater tissue penetration

           (g) Inflammation of tissue may lower pH, resulting in less LA absorbed; slower onset action, reduction of potency

2. Pharmacology

    a. Reversibly blocks peripheral nerve condition of small unmyelinated fibers

    b. Loss of nerve function occurs in following order

        (1) Autonomic

        (2) Cold

        (3) Warmth

        (4) Pain

        (5) Touch

        (6) Pressure

        (7) Vibration

        (8) Proprioception

        (9) Motor response

    c. Nerve function returns in reverse order

3. Pharmacokinetics

    a. Absorption—Rate dependent on tissue vascularity and route of administration

        (1) Warmth and massage increase vasodilatory activity; cold temperature decreases vasodilatory ability

        (2) Spread over area affected by degree of ionization

    b. Distribution

        (1) Distributed throughout body

        (2) Higher vascular organs, higher concentrations of anesthetics

        (3) Lipid solubility of a particular local anesthetic affects potency of agent

    c. Metabolism

        (1) Esters

            (a) Hydrolyzed by plasma pseudocholinesterase and liver esterases

            (b) Procaine—Hydrolyzed to para-amino benzoic acid (PABA)

        (2) Amides

            (a) Metabolized by liver

            (b) Prilocaine metabolized to orthotolidine, which can produce methemoglobinemia if given in large doses (see Chapter 9)

    d. Excretion—Metabolites and some unchanged drug esters and amides excreted by the kidneys

4. Adverse reactions

    a. Factors influencing toxicity

        (1) Drug

        (2) Concentration

        (3) Route of administration

        (4) Rate of injection

        (5) Vascularity

        (6) Patient's weight

        (7) Rate of metabolism and excretion

    b. CNS effects—Restlessness, tremors, convulsions (initial CNS stimulatory, CNS depressant in overdose)

    c. Cardiovascular effects—Myocardial depression and cardiac arrest

    d. Local effects—Hematoma, tissue soreness, necrosis, trismus, injection technique or excessive volume administered

    e. Malignant hyperthermia (see Chapter 9)

f. Pregnancy and nursing—Use elective dental treatment; usual doses of LA given to nursing mothers will not affect health or normal nursing infant

g. Allergy—Rash to anaphylactic shock

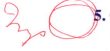

(1) Esters—More allergic potential than amides because metabolized to PABA, only used topically in dentistry because of allergic potential

(2) Alternative drug—Diphenhydramine (Benadryl)

(3) Other ingredients may produce allergic reactions—Sulfite agents, which is the preservative used to prevent oxidation of vasoconstructors added to local anesthetis

5. Composition of LA solutions

a. Vasoconstrictor—Epinephrine, levonordefrin (Neo-Cobefrin); retards absorption, prolongs duration of action of local anesthetic, promotes hemostasis

b. Antioxidant—Sodium metabisulfite, sodium bisulfite, acetone sodium bisulfite; retards oxidation (allergy to these substances is common)

c. Alkalinizing agent—Sodium hydroxide; adjusts pH of solution to between 6 and 7

d. Sodium chloride—Makes solution isotonic

6. Topical anesthetics

a. Lidocaine—Amide

b. Benzocaine—Ester, 20% concentration for professional use and OTC products for oral pain

c. Tetracaine—Ester, longest duration of action (45 minutes)

F. Antianxiety agents—Referred to as either sedative-hypnotic or antianxiety drugs; some patients may require agents before dental appointment

1. Definitions

a. Sedative—A small dose will produce mild CNS depression, causing reduction of activity and anxiety

b. Hypnotic—A large dose will produce greater CNS depression, resulting in sleep

c. Minor tranquilizers—Action similar to sedative hypnotics

d. Major tranquilizers—Antipsychotic activity

2. Benzodiazepines (Table 6-9■)

a. Mechanism—Exerts effects in CNS

b. Pharmacokinetics

(1) Well absorbed orally

(2) Available in many forms

TABLE 6-9 BENZODIAZEPINES FOR ANXIETY AND INSOMNIA	
Drug	**Route and Adult Dose (max dose where indicated)**
Anxiety Therapy	
alprazolam (Xanax)	For anxiety: PO 0.25–0.5 mg tid For panic attacks: PO 1–2 mg tid
chlordiazepoxide (Librium)	Mild anxiety: PO 5–10 mg tid or qid; IM/IV 50–100 mg 1 hr before a medical procedure Severe anxiety: PO 20–25 mg tid or qid; IM/IV 50–100 mg followed by 25–50 mg tid or qid
clonazepam (Klonopin)	PO; 1–2 mg/day in divided doses (max 4 mg/day)
clorazepate (Tranxene)	PO; 15 mg/day at hs (max 60 mg/day in divided doses)
diazepam (Valium)	PO; 2–10 mg bid; IM/IV 2–10 mg, repeat if needed in 3–4 hr
halazepam (Paxipam)	PO; 20–40 mg tid or qid
lorazepam (Ativan)	PO; 2–6 mg/day in divided doses (max 10 mg/day)
oxazepam (Serax)	PO; 10–30 mg tid or qid
Insomnia Therapy	
estazolam (Prosom)	PO; 1 mg at hs, may increase to 2 mg if necessary
flurazepam (Dalmane)	PO; 15–30 mg at hs
quazepam (Doral)	PO; 7.5–15 mg at hs
temazepam (Restoril)	PO; 7.5–30 mg at hs
triazolam (Halcion)	PO; 0.125–0.25 mg at hs (max 0.5 mg/day)

Source: Adams, M.P., Josephson, D.L., & Holland, L.N. (2005). *Pharmacology in Nursing: A Pathophysiologic Approach.* Used by permission of Pearson Education, Inc., Upper Saddle River, New Jersey.

      (3) Highly protein bound, nonionized, lipid soluble, crosses blood–brain barrier easily

      (4) Metabolized by oxidation; duration of action varies with agent

   c. Effects

      (1) Behavioral—Anxiety reduction at low doses; drowsiness and sleep at higher doses

      (2) Anticonvulsant—Prevention of seizures associated with local anesthetic toxicity (drug of choice for treatment of status epilepticus)

    d. Adverse reaction

      (1) CNS effect—Fatigue, drowsiness, muscle weakness, ataxia

      (2) Amnesia—Episodes can last several hours (usually at time of dosing)

      (3) Visual effects—Contraindicated in angle-closure glaucoma

      (4) Dental—Xerostomia

      (5) Phlebitis—When given parenterally

      (6) Pregnancy and lactation—Increased risk of congenital malformation when taking agent in first trimester; Food and Drug Administration (FDA) pregnancy categories D and X (Avoid)

      (7) Abuse—Less than other sedative-hypnotic agents

      (8) Overdose—Flumazenil (Romazicon) benzodiazepine antagonist

    e. Drug interactions—Additive with other CNS depressants, including alcohol

    f. Uses

      (1) Anxiety control

      (2) Insomnia management

      (3) Treatment of epilepsy—Diazepam drug of choice for status epilepticus; convulsions from local anesthetic overdose

      (4) Treatment of alcoholism

      (5) Control of muscle spasms

      (6) Medication before surgery

      (7) Uses in dentistry

        (a) Anxiety reduction

        (b) Preoperative sedation

        (c) Oral sedation

        (d) Seizure management (office emergency kit, valium 10 mg, IM or IV)

    g. Examples—Diazepam (Valium), lorazepam (Ativan), Alprazolam (Xanax)

3. Buspirone (BuSpar)

    a. Mechanism—Binds to serotonin and dopamine receptors

    b. Pharmacological effect—Anxioselective; produces less CNS depression

    c. Two to four weeks to be effective—Not for dental anxiety

4. Barbiturates (Table 6-10■)

    a. Mechanism—Interacts with gamma-aminobutyric acid (GABA) receptor

TABLE 6-10 BARBITURATES FOR SEDATION AND INSOMNIA

Drug	Route and Adult Dose (max dose where indicated)
Short acting	
pentobarbital sodium (Nembutal)	Sedative: PO; 20–30 mg bid or qid Hypnotic: PO; 120–200 mg, 150–200 mg IM
secobarbital (Seconal)	Sedative: PO; 100–300 mg/day in three divided doses Hypnotic: PO/IM; 100–200 mg
Intermediate acting	
amobarbital (Amytal)	Sedative: PO; 30–50 mg bid or tid Hypnotic: PO/IM; 65–200 mg (max 500 mg)
aprobarbital (Alurate)	Sedative: PO; 40 mg tid Hypnotic: PO; 40–160 mg
butabarbital sodium (Butisol)	Sedative: PO; 15–30 mg tid or qid Hypnotic: PO; 50–100 mg at hs
Long acting	
mephobarbital (Mebaral)	Sedative: PO; 32–100 mg tid or qid
phenobarbital (Luminal)	Sedative: PO; 30–120 mg/day IV/IM; 100–200 mg/day

Source: Adams, M.P., Josephson, D.L., & Holland, L.N. (2005). *Pharmacology in Nursing: A Pathophysiologic Approach.* Used by permission of Pearson Education, Inc., Upper Saddle River, New Jersey.

b. Pharmacokinetics—Well absorbed orally and rectally; short and intermediate-acting, metabolized by liver; long-acting, renal excretion as free drug

c. Pharmacological effects

   (1) CNS depression

      (a) Small dose, sedation

      (b) Large dose, disinhibition and euphoria

      (c) At high doses, anesthesia with respiratory and cardiovascular depression, finally cardiac arrest

   (2) Anticonvulsant—Long-acting used in treatment of epilepsy

    d. Adverse reactions

      (1) Sedation or hypnotic doses—Exaggerated CNS effect in elderly and debilitated patients with liver or kidney impairment

      (2) Anesthetic doses—High concentration used for intubation or very short procedure; no significant analgesic effects (does not block reflex response to pain)

    e. Acute poisoning—Cause of death for overdose is respiratory depression

    f. Contraindications—Absolutely contraindicated in patients with intermittent or positive family history of *porphyria*

    g. Drug interactions—Potent stimulators of liver microsomal enzyme production, involved in many drug interactions

    h. Uses—Determined by duration of action

      (1) Ultrashort—IV for induction of general anesthesia; thiopental (Pentothal)

      (2) Short and intermediate—Little use; abused; replaced by benzodiazepines; Secobarbital (Seconal)

      (3) Long-acting—Used for treatment of epilepsy; phenobarbital (Luminal)

5. Nonbarbiturate sedative hypnotic—Offers no advantage over barbiturates

    a. Examples

      (1) Chloral hydrate (Noctec)

        (a) Rapid onset, short duration of action

        (b) Used for preoperative sedation for children in dentistry (easy to overdose)

        (c) Produces gastric irritation

      (2) Meprobamate (Equanil, Miltown)

        (a) Minor tranquilizer for daytime sedation; has anticonvulsant action

        (b) Some muscle relaxant properties

6. Centrally acting muscle relaxants

    a. Action affects the CNS, causing skeletal muscle relaxation

    b. Two common examples, methocarbamol (Robaxin) and cyclobenzaprine (Flexeril), exert effects indirectly on the CNS

    c. Indicated or adjunct to rest and physical therapy for relief of muscle spasm associated with acute painful musculoskeletal conditions

G. General anesthetics

1. General considerations

    a. Anesthesia produced by group of chemical substances that are potent CNS depressants

   b. Produce reversible loss of consciousness and insensitivity to painful
      stimuli

   c. Administered in hospital operating rooms; used also by oral and
      maxillofacial surgeons in hospital or in office; nitrous oxide used in
      dental office to allay patient anxiety (conscious sedation)

2. Stages and planes of anesthesia

   a. Stage I—Analgesia

   b. Stage II—Delirium or excitement; move through smoothly and quickly

   c. Stage III—Surgical anesthesia; four planes, most treatment in this phase

   d. Stage IV—Respiratory or medullary paralysis; reverse stage
      immediately or patient will die; stage not used (overdose = patient too
      deep)

3. Classification of anesthetic agents

   a. Inhalation anesthetics

      (1) Gases—Nitrous oxide; used in Stage I or to produce conscious
          sedation

      (2) Volatile liquids—Halogenated hydrocarbons, ethers

   b. Intravenous agents

      (1) Barbiturates

      (2) Opioids

      (3) Neuroleptics

      (4) Benzodiazepines

4. Examples

   a. Nitrous oxide–oxygen (N_2O–O_2)

      (1) Colorless gas with little or no odor; least soluble in blood of all
          inhalation anesthetics—Used for conscious (*moderate sedation*)
          anesthesia during dental treatment

      (2) Cannot be used alone to give surgical anesthesia because of low
          potency

      (3) Normal concentration of N_2O—10–50% (average 35%)

      (4) Advantages

          (a) Rapid onset

          (b) Easy to administer

          (c) Rapid recovery

          (d) Acceptable for children

      (5) Pharmacological effects

          (a) CNS effects—Analgesia and amnesia

          (b) Circulatory effects—Minimal; peripheral vasodilation

(c) GI—Patient should be warned to avoid a large meal within 3 hours of appointment time to prevent vomiting

(6) Adverse reactions/contraindications

(a) Faulty equipment—Could pose a hazard for dental team members (spontaneous abortion, genetic effect)

(b) Respiratory obstruction—Upper respiratory obstruction (e.g., stuffy nose) or infection

(c) Chronic obstructive pulmonary disease (COPD)—Respiration driven by lack of oxygen, could cease to breathe with high oxygen levels (e.g., emphysema, chronic bronchitis)

(d) Emotional instability—Patients taking psychotherapeutic medication should be evaluated before use

(e) Pregnancy—Use at all is questionable; first trimester critical; incidence of spontaneous abortion increased in female operating personnel

(f) Abuse—Chronic abuse may result in neuropathy

b. Halogenated hydrocarbons—There are many drug interactions with halogenated anesthetics

(1) Halothane (Fluothane) is nonirritating to bronchial mucous membranes

(2) Possible occurrence of postanesthetic hepatitis; popularity diminished

c. Halogenated ether

(1) Enflurane (Ethrane) induction and recovery rapid; depresses respiration; alteration in encephalographic activity; reduced blood pressure, muscle relaxation

(2) Isoflurane (Forane)—Same as other halogenated ethers; useful and popular

d. Ultra short-acting barbiturates

(1) Examples—Methohexital sodium (Brevital), thiopental sodium (Pentothal)

(2) Rapid onset, short duration—Does not provide analgesia

(3) Used for rapid induction to stage III anesthesia

(4) Adverse reaction—Laryngospasm and bronchospasm

(5) Contraindication—Status asthmaticus, porphyria, and known hypersensitivity

e. Ketamine (Ketalar)

(1) Produces dissociative anesthesia—Disrupts association pathways in brain

        (2) Given IV or IM with rapid onset of action

        (3) May produce delirium and hallucinations during recovery

    f. Opiates

        (1) Used as adjunctive drugs to general anesthesia in preanesthetic medication and also to provide analgesia

        (2) Examples

            (a) Morphine

            (b) Fentanyl (Sublimaze)

    g. Benzodiazepine

        (1) Midazolam (Versed)—Useful for induction of anesthesia

H. Emergency drugs—See Chapter 9 for more information

  1. General considerations

    a. Choice of drugs for dental office emergency; kit depends on individual circumstance, experience, and personal preference

    b. Some drugs may only be used by those with advanced cardiac life support (ACLS) training (state practice acts dictate required drugs for emergency kits if dentist administers sedation)

  2. Drugs

    a. Epinephrine

        (1) Actions—Cardiac stimulation, vasoconstriction, bronchial dilation, elevation of blood glucose; indicated for cardiac arrest, severe allergic reaction, circulatory collapse

        (2) Dosage—0.3–0.5 ml of 1:1000 dilution every 5–20 minutes as needed, up to three doses, IM or SQ

    b. Diphenhydramine (Benadryl)

        (1) Actions—Antihistamine used in the treatment of some allergic reactions

        (2) Dosage—50 mg IM, IV of 10 mg/ml

    c. Diazepam (Valium)

        (1) Action—Drug of choice for most convulsions if drug is needed, indicated for toxic reaction to local anesthetic

        (2) Dosage—5–10 mg IV

    d. Naloxone (Narcan)

        (1) Action—Drug of choice for opioid-induced apnea

        (2) Dosage—0.4 mg (1 ml) IV, may be given SQ or IM, onset of action 2 minutes by IV

    e. Oxygen

        (1) Action—Restoration of oxygen saturation of hemoglobin

(2) Dosage—100% via nasal inhalation if spontaneous breathing; must use with positive-pressure ventilation if respiration arrested

f. Aromatic ammonia spirits

(1) Action—Irritation of respiratory mucosa; stimulation of respiratory muscle movement; mobilization of venous return

(2) Dosage—0.3 ml

g. Glucose

(1) Action—Restoration of blood glucose level for maintenance of brain function; indicated for hypoglycemia

(2) Dosage—Operator judgment, quick onset time, use oral form of sucrose (soft drink, juice) in conscious patient; also supplied as viscous solution in tubes (glutose 15)

h. Morphine

(1) Action—Given patient who has suffered an acute infarction to relieve pain and allay apprehension

(2) Dosage—10 mg/ml

i. Methoxamine

(1) Action—Adrenergic agonist with a-adrenergic properties, produces mild increase in blood pressure (not typical drug in dental kits)

(2) Dosage—10 mg/mL

j. Nitroglycerin (Nitrostat)

(1) Action—Relaxation of vascular smooth muscle; reduced cardiac work; indicated for angina pectoris

(2) Dosage—0.3–0.4 mg every 5 minutes, up to 3 doses

(3) Caution—Orthostatic hypotension may occur; onset of dose occurs with 2–4 minutes; if chest pain returns or worsens, assume myocardial infarction

k. Hydrocortisone (Solu-Cortef)

(1) Action—Corticosteroid used for allergic reactions, anaphylaxis, and adrenal crisis

(2) Dosage—50 mg/mL

l. Dextrose

(1) Action—Used IV to manage hypoglycemic episodes when diabetic is unconscious and cannot swallow

m. Albuterol

(1) β_2-adrenergic agonist useful in management of bronchoconstriction

(2) Dosage—Two puffs

V. Drugs That May Affect Patient Treatment

A. Cardiovascular drugs

1. Cardiovascular disease—disease of heart and blood vessels

    a. Hypertension, angina, stroke, atherosclerosis, congestive heart failure

    b. Leading cause of death in the United States

    c. Hypertension most common CV disease, African Americans at high risk

    d. Stress during dental treatment major factor in causing emergency

2. Dental implications

    a. Contraindications to treatment—MI within 6 months; unstable angina, uncontrolled congestive heart failure (CHF), arrhythmia; uncontrolled hypertension

    b. Vasoconstrictor limitation in local anesthesia (1:100,000, aspirating technique); epinephrine dose not to exceed 0.04 mg in patient with cardiovascular disease (2.2 carpules = 1:100,000; 4.4 carpules = 1:200,000)

    c. Risk factors for infective endocarditis (see Chapter 7 for new American Heart Association guidelines); require antibiotic premedication

    d. Precautions with pacemaker patient (vitalometer, electrosurgical unit, electromagnetic ultrasonic scaler)

3. Cardiac glycosides

    a. Causes failing heart muscle to contract more efficiently; increases cardiac output, oxygenation of tissues

    b. Right-sided CHF, edema in extremities; left-sided CHF, edema in lungs

    c. Digoxin—Digitalis-type drug (foxglove plant)

        (1) Increases force and efficiency of cardiac muscle contraction

        (2) Reduces edema by increasing glomerular filtration rate

        (3) Reduces heart rate

        (4) Indicated for treatment of CHF, arrhythmia

        (5) Adverse reactions of digitalis-type drugs

            (a) GI—Nausea, vomiting, salivation, gagging (overdose), anorexia

            (b) CV—Arrhythmia (overdose)

            (c) CNS—Headache, sedation, visual disturbances, weakness, confusion (blue-green vision)

        (6) Drug interactions—Diuretics, sympathomimetic drugs (arrhythmia); tetracycline, erythromycin (digoxin toxicity)

        (7) Dental management

            (a) Observe for signs of toxicity; if present, refer to physician

(b) Use epinephrine with caution, low doses, aspirating syringe

(c) Monitor pulse for bradycardia, arrhythmia

(d) Semisupine or upright chair position—Pulmonary congestion, GI side effects

4. Antiarrhythmic agents

a. Heart rhythm—Sinoatrial (SA) node (right atrium); arteriovenous (AV) node (Purkinje fibers, ventricles)

b. Major drugs used for arrhythmia (abnormal rhythm pattern)

(1) Quinidine—Myocardial depressant, both direct and indirect actions

(2) Lidocaine—Emergency use primarily, ventricular tachycardia

(3) Beta blockers

(4) Calcium channel blockers (verapamil)

(5) Side effects—Nausea, vomiting, hypotension; allergy— thrombocytopenia

(6) Management—Monitor vital signs

5. Antianginal drugs (Table 6-11■)

a. Angina—Pain, heavy feeling, discomfort in chest area; referred pain to jaw or arms due to lack of oxygenation of heart muscle; precipitated by stress

b. Major drugs—Nitrites, nitrates, beta blockers, calcium channel blockers

(1) Nitroglycerin—Acute episodes; sublingual administration; use patient's medications

(2) Amyl nitrite—Emergency use, inhalation (banana oil smell); abused drug

(3) Beta blockers (propranolol, nadolol, metoprolol, atenolol)—Block adrenergic stimulation to heart, slows heart rate, reduces work of the heart; prophylactic use

(4) Calcium channel blockers (verapamil, diltiazem, nifedipine, amlodipine)—Inhibits calcium binding during contraction; reduces workload on heart muscle; increases vasodilation of cornoary arteries; vasodilation in periphery; prophylactic use

c. Action—Reduces oxygen requirement of cardiac muscle, vasodilation

d. Dental implications of treating a patient with angina

(1) Medical history follow-up questions on control, vital signs

(2) Check expiration date on patient nitroglycerin prescription

(3) Manage side effects of agents—Hypotension, xerostomia; gingival hyperplasia (calcium channel blockers, except amlodipine, isradipine)

TABLE 6-11 DRUGS FOR ANGINA, MYOCARDIAL INFARCTION, AND CEREBROVASCULAR ACCIDENTS

Drug	Route and Adult Dose (max dose where indicated)
Organic Nitrates	
amyl nitrite	Inhalation; 1 ampule (0.18–0.3 ml) PRN
isosorbide dinitrate (Iso-Bid, Isordil, Sorbitrate, Dilatrate)	PO; 2.5–30 mg qid
isosorbide mononitrate (Imdur, Ismon, Monoket)	PO; 20 mg qid
nitroglycerin (Nitrostat, Nitro-Dur, Nitro-Bid, others)	SL; 1 tablet (0.3–0.6 mg) or 1 spray (0.4–0.8 mg) q3–5min (max three doses in 15 min)
pentaerythritol tetranitrate (Duotrate, Pentylan, Peritrate, others)	PO; 10–20 mg tid or qid
Beta-adrenergic Blockers	
atenolol (Tenormin)	PO; 25–50 mg qd (max 100 mg/day)
metoprolol (Lopressor, Toprol XL)	PO; 100 mg bid (max 400 mg/day)
propranolol (Inderal, Inderal LA)	PO; 10–20 mg bid-tid (max 320 mg/day)
timolol maleate (Betimol, Blocadren, Timoptic, Timoptic XE)	PO; 15–45 mg tid (max 60 mg/day)
Calcium Channel Blockers	
amlodipine (Norvasc)	PO; 5–10 mg qd (max 10 mg/day)
bepridil (Vascor)	PO; 200 mg qd (max 360 mg/day)
diltiazem (Cardizem, Dilacor XR, Tiamate, Tiazac)	PO; 30 mg qid (max 360 mg/day)
nicardipine (Cardene)	PO; 20–40 mg tid or 30–60 mg SR bid (max 120 mg/day)
nifedipine (Adalat, Procardia)	PO; 10–20 mg tid (max 180 mg/day)
verapamil (Calan, Covera-HS, Isoptin, Verelan)	PO; 80 mg tid-qid (max 480 mg/day)
Glycoprotein IIb/IIIa Inhibitors	
abciximab (ReoPro)	IV; 0.25 mg/kg initial bolus over 5 min then 10 µg/min for 12 hr
eptifibatide (Integrilin)	IV; 18g/kg initial bolus over 1–2 min then 2 µg/kg/min for 24–72 hr
trofiban HCL (Aggrastat)	IV; 0.4 µg/kg/min for 30 min then 0.1 µg/kg/min for 12–24 hr

Source: Adams, M.P., Josephson, D.L., & Holland, L.N. (2005). *Pharmacology in Nursing: A Pathophysiologic Approach.* Used by permission of Pearson Education, Inc., Upper Saddle River, New Jersey.

6. Antihypertensive agents (Figure 6-13■)

a. Types of hypertension—Essential, secondary, malignant; etiology—usually unknown; 140/90 hypertension

b. Stepped-care regimen—Reduced alcohol, reduced salt, no smoking; exercise program, weight reduction, combination drug therapy

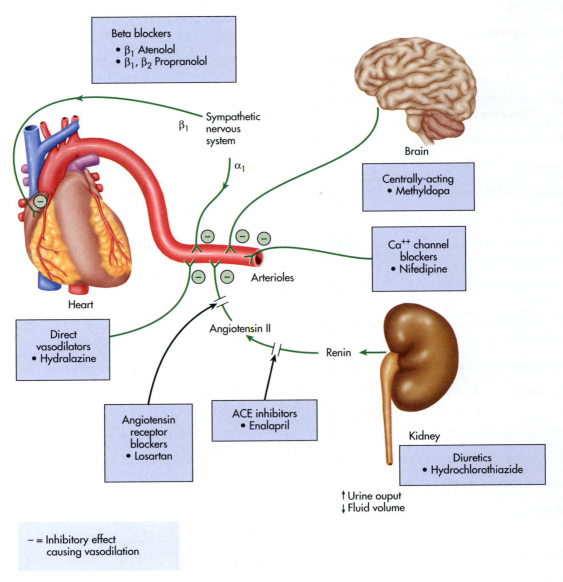

FIGURE 6-13 ■ Mechanism of Action of Antihypertensive Drugs

   c. Major drugs used—Diuretics, beta-blocking agents, ACE inhibitors, calcium channel blockers (Tables 6-12■, 6-13■, 6-14■, 6-15■)

      (1) Action of thiazide, loop and potassium-sparing diuretics—Diuresis

      (2) Action of adrenergic-blocking drugs—Vasodilation, decrease peripheral resistance, decrease heart rate

      (3) Action of calcium channel blockers—Coronary vasodilation

      (4) Action of angiotensin-converting enzyme inhibitors—Prevents formation of angiotensin II that causes vasoconstriction, results in vasodilation, diuresis

      (5) Agents for severe hypertension—Clonidine, guanethidine, reserpine, hydralazine (centrally acting drugs)

   d. Side effects of antihypertensives—Postural hypotension, xerostomia, blood dyscrasia, dizziness; gingival hyperplasia (calcium channel blockers such as nifedipine, verapanil, diltiazen, amlodipine)

   e. Dental implications of treating a hypertensive patient

      (1) Measure vital signs each appointment, stress reduction protocol

      (2) Teach patients to comply with medications

      (3) Manage side effects as needed

      (4) Avoid opioids (caution: increased sedation)

      (5) Limit vasoconstrictor in local anesthetics (healthy person, maximum 0.2 mg; cardiac patient, maximum 0.04 mg with epinephrine)

7. Anticoagulants (Figure 6-14■)

   a. Use of anticoagulants—Prevent blood clots, thin blood consistency

      (1) Indication—Stroke, thromboembolic disease, myocardial infarction

   b. Drugs used by injection—Heparin, enoxaparin

      (1) Action of heparin—Dissolves blood clots, whereas warfarin prevents synthesis of clotting factors in liver

   c. Drug used by oral administration—Warfarin (Coumadin)

      (1) Action of warfarin—Vitamin K antimetabolite, interferes with synthesis of clotting factors

   d. Dental management

      (1) Caution in dental procedures causing bleeding; direct pressure, apply oxidized cellulose; use local, topically applied clotting agents as needed (e.g., Hemodent)

TABLE 6-12 DIURETICS FOR HYPERTENSION

Drug	Route and Adult Dose (max dose where indicated)
Potassium-sparing Type	
amiloride (Midamor)	PO; 5–20 mg in one to two divided doses (max 20 mg/day)
spironolactone (Aldactone)	PO; 25–100 mg qd (max 200 mg/day)
triamterene (Dyrenium)	PO; 100 mg bid (max 300 mg/day)
Thiazide and Thiazide-like Agents	
benzthiazide (Aquatag, others)	PO; 25–200 mg qd
chlorothiazide (Diuril)	PO; 250–500 mg qd (max 2g/day)
chlorthalidone (Hygroton)	PO; 50–100 mg qd (max 100 mg/day)
hydrochlorothiazide (HydroDIURIL, HCTZ)	PO; 12.5–100 mg qd (max 5 mg/day)
indapamide (Lozol)	PO; 2.5–5.0 mg qd
metolazone (Diulo, others)	PO; 5–20 mg qd
polythiazide (Renese)	PO; 1–4 mg qd
trichlormethiazide (Diurese, others)	PO; 1–4 mg qd
Loop/High Ceiling Type	
bumetanide (Bumex)	PO; 0.5–2.0 mg qd (max 10 mg/day)
furosemide (Lasix)	PO; 20–80 mg qd (max 600 mg/day)
torsemide (Demadex)	PO; 4–20 mg qd

Source: Adams, M.P., Josephson, D.L., & Holland, L.N. (2005). *Pharmacology in Nursing: A Pathophysiologic Approach.* Used by permission of Pearson Education, Inc., Upper Saddle River, New Jersey.

TABLE 6-13 ADRENERGIC AGENTS FOR HYPERTENSION

Drug	Route and Adult Dose (max dose where indicated)
Beta-blockers	
atenolol (Tenormin): $beta_1$	PO; 25–50 mg qd (max 100 mg/day)
bisoprolol (Zebeta): $beta_1$	PO; 2.5–5 mg qd (max 20 mg/day)
metoprolol (Toprol, Lopressor): $beta_1$	PO; 50–100 mg qd-bid (max 450 mg/day)
propranolol (Inderal): Prototype: $beta_1$ and $beta_2$	PO; 10–30 mg tid or qd (max 320 mg/day) IV; 0.5–3.0 mg every 4 h prn
timolol (Betimol, others): $beta_1$ and $beta_2$	PO; 15–45 mg tid (max 60 mg/day)
$Alpha_1$-blockers	
doxazosin (Cardura)	PO; 1 mg hs; may increase to 16 mg/day in one to two divided doses (max 16 mg/day)
prazosin (Minipress)	PO; 1 mg hs; may increase to 1 mg bid-tid (max 20 mg/day)
terazosin (Hytrin)	PO; 1 mg hs; may increase 1–5 mg/day (max 20 mg/day)
$Alpha_2$-adrenergic Agonists	
clonidine (Catapres)	PO; 0.1 mg bid-tid (max 0.8 mg/day)
guanabenz (Wytensin)	PO; 4 mg bid; may increase by 4-8 mg/day q1–2 weeks (max 32 mg bid)
methyldopa (Aldomet)	PO; 250 mg bid or tid (max 3 g/day)
$Alpha_1$-and Beta-blockers (Centrally Acting)	
carteolol (Cartrol, Ocupress)	PO; 2.5 mg qd; may increase to 5–10 mg if needed (max 10 mg/day)
labetalol (Trandate, Normodyne)	PO; 100 mg bid; may increase to 200–400 mg bid (max 1200–2400 mg/day)
Adrenergic Neuron Blockers (Peripherally Acting)	
guanadrel (Hylorel)	PO; 5 mg bid; may increase to 20–75 mg/day in two to four divided doses
guanethidine (Ismelin)	PO; 10 mg qd; may increase by 10 mg q5–7d up to 300 mg/day (start with 25–50 mg/day in hospitalized patients, increase by 25–50 mg q1–3d)
reserpine (Serpasil)	PO; 1.5 mg qd initially, may reduce to 0.1–0.25 mg/day

Source: Adams, M.P., Josephson, D.L., & Holland, L.N. (2005). *Pharmacology in Nursing: A Pathophysiologic Approach.* Used by permission of Pearson Education, Inc., Upper Saddle River, New Jersey.

TABLE 6-14 ACE INHIBITORS AND ANGIOTENSIN II RECEPTOR BLOCKERS FOR HYPERTENSION

Drug	Route and Adult Dose (max dose where indicated)
ACE Inhibitors	
benazepril (Lotensin)	PO; 10–40 mg in one to two divided doses (max 40 mg/day)
captopril (Capoten)	PO; 6.25–25 mg tid (max 450 mg/day)
enalapril (Vasotec)	PO; 5–40 mg in one to two divided doses (max 40 mg/day)
fosinopril (Monopril)	PO; 5–40 mg qd (max 80 mg/day)
lisinopril (Prinivil, Zestoretic, Zestril)	PO; 10 mg qd (max 80 mg/day)
moexipril (Univasc)	PO; 7.5–30 mg qd (max 30 mg/day)
quinapril (Accupril)	PO; 10–20 mg qd (max 80 mg/day)
ramipril (Altace)	PO; 2.5–5 mg qd (max 20 mg/day)
trandolapril (Mavik)	PO; 1–4 mg qd (max 8 mg/day)
Angiotensin II Receptor Blockers	
candesartan (Atacand)	PO; Start at 16 mg qd (range 8–32 mg divided once or twice daily)
eprosartan (Teveten)	PO; 600 mg qd or 400 mg PO qid-bid (max 800 mg/day)
irbesartan (Avapro)	PO; 150–300 mg qd (max 300 mg/day)
losartan (Cozaar)	PO; 25–50 mg in one to two divided doses (max 100 mg/day)
olmesartan medoxomil (Benicar)	PO; 20–40 mg qd
telmisartan (Micardis)	PO; 40 mg qd; may increase to 80 mg/day
valsartan (Diovan)	PO; 80 mg qd (max 320 mg/day)

Source: Adams, M.P., Josephson, D.L., & Holland, L.N. (2005). *Pharmacology in Nursing: A Pathophysiologic Approach.* Used by permission of Pearson Education, Inc., Upper Saddle River, New Jersey.

TABLE 6-15 CALCIUM CHANNEL BLOCKERS FOR HYPERTENSION	
Drug	**Route and Adult Dose (max dose where indicated)**
Selective: for Blood Vessels	
amlodipine (Norvasc)	PO; 5–10 mg qd (max 10 mg/day)
felodipine (Plendil)	PO; 5–10 mg qd (max 20 mg/day)
nicardipine (Cardene)	PO; 20–40 mg tid (max 120 mg/day)
nifedipine (Procardia, Adalat)	PO; 10–20 mg tid (max 180 mg/day)
Nonselective: for Both Blood Vessels and Heart	
diltiazem (Cardizem, Dilacor, Tiamate, Triassic)	PO; 60–120 mg sustained release bid
isradipine (DynaCirc)	PO; 1.25–10 mg bid (max 20 mg/day)
nisoldipine (Nisocor)	PO; 10–20 mg bid (max 40 mg/day)
verapamil (Calan, Isoptin, Verelan)	PO; 80–160 mg tid (max 360 mg/day)

Source: Adams, M.P., Josephson, D.L., & Holland, L.N. (2005). *Pharmacology in Nursing: A Pathophysiologic Approach.* Used by permission of Pearson Education, Inc., Upper Saddle River, New Jersey.

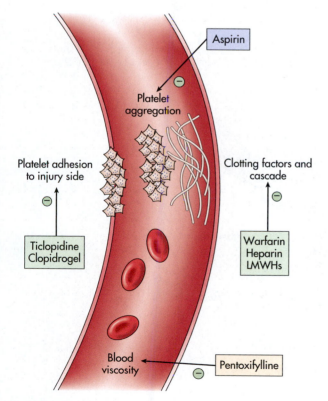

FIGURE 6-14 ■ Mechanisms of Action of Anticoagulants

(2) Use acetaminophen for analgesia, not aspirin or NSAIDs

(3) Physician consult for international normalized ratio (INR) or prothrombin time (INR is the preferred test, okay to treat in dentistry if INR = 2–3, and 3.5 for artificial heart valves)

(4) Antibiotics can potentiate effects of warfarin

    e. Antiplatelet drugs—Ticolpidine, clopidrogel (Plarix), aspirin with dipyridamole (Aggrenox)

    f. Other blood-altering agents—Ticlopidine, dipyridamole, pentoxifyline

8. Antihyperlipidemics (Figure 6-15■)

    a. Drugs indicated to lower cholesterol—Cholestyramine, gemfibrozil, niacin, lovastatin, simvastatin, probucol

    b. Dental implications for patient taking antihyperlipidemics

(1) Monitor vital signs; at risk for cardiovascular disease

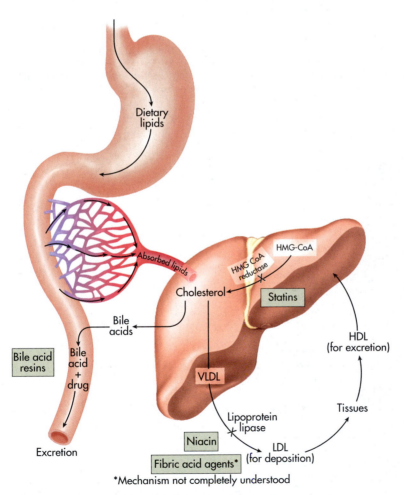

FIGURE 6-15 ■ Mechanisms of Action of Lipid-Lowering Drugs

(2) Monitor liver function if prescribing drugs

(3) Postural hypotension possible with niacin

9. Dental implications of cardiovascular disease

    a. Consider contraindications to dental treatment

    b. Observe situations indicating physician consultation

    c. Stress reduction protocol

    d. Vasoconstrictor limitation, postural hypotension

B. Anticonvulsant agents—Used for prevention or control of two types of seizures

    1. Types of generalized seizures (loss of consciousness in both) (Table 6-16■)

        a. Absence (petit mal)

           (1) Drug therapy—Ethosuximide or valproic acid

           (2) Absence—Does not fall to floor

        b. Tonic–clonic (grand mal)

           (1) Drug therapy—Valproic acid, phenytoin, phenobarbital, carbamazepine

TABLE 6-16 DRUGS USED FOR THE MANAGEMENT OF SPECIFIC TYPES OF SEIZURES

	Partial Seizures	Generalized Seizures		
	Simple or Complex	Absence	Atonic, Myoclonic	Tonic-clonic, Status Epilepticus
Benzodiazepines				
diazepam (Valium)				✓
lorazepam (Ativan)				✓
Phenytoin-like				
phenytoin (Dilantin)	✓			✓
carbamazepine (Tegretol)	✓			✓
valproic acid (Depakene)	✓	✓	✓	✓
Succinimide				
ethosuximide (Zarontin)		✓	✓	

Source: Adams, M.P., Josephson, D.L., & Holland, L.N. (2005). *Pharmacology in Nursing: A Pathophysiologic Approach.* Used by permission of Pearson Education, Inc., Upper Saddle River, New Jersey.

(2) Associated with "aura"

(3) Jerking movements

(4) Status epilepticus—Continuous seizures; emergency treatment is diazepam injection

2. Partial seizures—Simple or complex (psychomotor)

a. Seizures last minutes versus seconds in absence type

b. Aura can occur in complex partial seizures

c. Drug therapy—Carbamazepine, phenytoin, phenobarbital, primidone

3. Drugs used to treat seizures—CNS depressants (Table 6-16)

a. Action—Prevent spread of abnormal electric discharges in brain; drugs used depend on seizure type

b. Adverse reactions relevant to dental treatment

(1) CNS depression results in impaired learning

(2) Opioid drugs—Reduce dose if prescribed by dentist

(3) Nausea, vomiting, anorexia—Consider semisupine chair position

(4) Blood dyscrasis—Reduced healing, low host resistance

c. Numerous drug interactions—Consult with physician before prescribing

d. Types of CNS depressants

(1) Barbiturates—Phenobarbital most common type, used in tonic–clonic and partial seizures

(a) Used alone or in combination with other anticonvulsants

(b) Sedation, excitement, confusion common

(c) Stomatitis—Refer to physician, drug therapy needs changing

(2) Hydantoins—Phenytoin (Dilantin) most common type, used in tonic–clonic and partial seizures

(a) 50% of patients develop gingival hyperplasia

   i) Anterior interproximal, facial—Initial enlargement

   ii) Fibrotic, does not bleed easily, surgical removal

   iii) Strict plaque control necessary to minimize overgrowth

(b) Has narrow therapeutic index—Adverse reactions, drug interactions common

   i) Nausea, vomiting, confusion, dizziness, skin reactions possible

   ii) Vitamin D and folate deficiency—Oral mucosal ulceration, glossitis

(3) Valproic acid (Depakene) and divalproex sodium (Depakote)—All seizure types

(a) Indigestion, nausea, vomiting frequent

    (b) Prolonged bleeding, anticoagulation possible—Blood tests needed before dental procedures causing bleeding; avoid prescribing aspirin, NSAIDs

    (c) Excessive CNS depression with other CNS depressant drugs

   (4) Carbamazepine (Tegretol)—Structurally related to tricyclic antidepressants, anticonvulsant activity

    (a) Used to treat trigeminal neuralgia (tic douloureux)

    (b) Serious blood dyscrasias—Aplastic anemia, agranulocytosis; report petechia, infection, poor healing to physician

    (c) Adverse reactions—Nausea, dizziness, confusion, xerostomia, skin reactions, blood pressure changes; chewable tablet contains sugar, suggest home fluoride for caries control

    (d) Drug interactions frequent—Antibiotics, analgesics

   (5) Ethosuximide (Zarontin)

    (a) Drug of choice for absence seizures

    (b) Side effects include GI upset, drowsiness, blood dyscrasias, gingival enlargement, glossitis

   (6) Benzodiazepines—Oral forms and parenteral forms

    (a) Clonazepam (Klonopin), chlorazepate (Tranzene)—Oral route

    (b) Diazepam (Valium), lorazepam (Ativan)—Parenteral for status epilepticus

    (c) GI, CNS side effects possible—Oral side effects of xerostomia, coated tongue, thirst, painful gingiva

 4. Management of dental patients with seizures

  a. Detailed medical history review—Seizure history; drug effects, interactions

  b. Management of systemic and oral side effects of drugs

  c. Stress management plan, observe for tonic–clonic signs—Move patient to floor if possible, tilt head to side, remove objects from mouth, do not insert gauze-wrapped tongue blade (bright dental light and loud, sudden sounds may trigger seizures)

C. Psychotherapeutic drugs

 1. Types of psychiatric disorders—Organic or functional

  a. Organic—Congenital or caused by injury or disease

  b. Functional—Psychotic disorders, no biochemical abnormality

   (1) Schizophrenia—Loss of perception of reality

   (2) Depression—Loss of self-worth, associated with decreased serotonin

(3) Bipolar disorder—Alternating periods of elation and depression

2. Types of psychotherapeutic drugs

  a. Antipsychotic drugs indicated for schizophrenia

    (1) Phenothiazines are most frequently used

      (a) Chlorpromazine (Thorazine)—Sedation, xerostomia side effects

      (b) Thioridazine (Mellaril), trifluoperazine (Stelazine), prochlorperazine (Compazine), other phenothiazines used

    (2) Action—Calm emotions, antiemetic effect (Figure 6-16■)

    (3) Adverse reactions (Table 6-17■)—Sedation, orthostatic hypotension, extrapyramidal effects (parkinsonism, akathisia, tardive dyskinesia); anticholinergic effects (xerostomia, blurred vision, constipation); blood dyscrasias

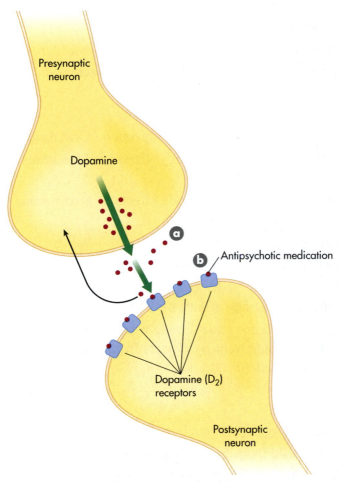

FIGURE 6-16 ■ Mechanism of Action of Antipsychotic Drugs: (a) Overproduction of Dopamine; (b) Antipsychotic medication occupies D2 receptor, preventing dopamine from stimulating the postsynaptic neuron.

TABLE 6-17 ADVERSE EFFECTS OF CONVENTIONAL ANTIPSYCHOTIC AGENTS

Effect	Description
Acute dystonia	Severe spasms, particularly the back muscles, tongue, and facial muscles; twitching movements
Akathisia	Constant pacing with repetitive, compulsive movements
Parkinsonism	Tremor, muscle rigidity, stooped posture, and shuffling gait
Tardive dyskinesia	Bizarre tongue and face movements such as lip smacking and wormlike motions of the tongue; puffing of cheeks, uncontrolled chewing movements
Anticholinergic effects	Dry mouth, tachycardia, blurred vision
Sedation	Usually diminishes with continued therapy
Hypotension	Particularly severe when quickly moving from a recumbent to an upright position
Sexual dysfunction	Impotence and diminished libido
Neuroleptic malignant syndrome	High fever, confusion, muscle rigidity, and high serum creatine kinase; can be fatal

Source: Adams, M.P., Josephson, D.L., & Holland, L.N. (2005). *Pharmacology in Nursing: A Pathophysiologic Approach.* Used by permission of Pearson Education, Inc., Upper Saddle River, New Jersey.

  (4) Drug interactions—Potentiate CNS depressants (decrease dose of opioids); epinephrine safe for dental use; anticholinergic agents (increased effects)

  (5) Temporomandibular joint (TMJ) pain can result from extrapyramidal effects, tardive dyskinesia can make oral procedures difficult

  (6) Dental management relates to drug side effects, medication compliance

  b. Antidepressants—Drugs used may be prescribed for other conditions; question patient about reason for use (Table 6-18■)

  (1) First-generation agents (tricyclic agents, others) (Figure 6-17■)

    (a) Examples—Amitriptyline (Elavil), doxepin (Sinequan), imipramine (Tofranil), amoxapine, desipramine, nortriptyline (Pamelor); monoamine oxidase inhibitors (MAOIs) (tricyclics and MAOIs both raise norepinephrine level)

TABLE 6-18 ANTIDEPRESSANTS	
Drug	**Route and Adult Dose (max dose where indicated)**
MAO Inhibitors (MAOI)	
isocarboxazid (Marplan)	PO; 10–30 mg/day (max 30 mg/day)
phenelzine (Nardil)	PO; 15 mg tid (max 90 mg/day)
tranylcypromine (Parnate)	PO; 30 mg/day (give 20 mg in A.M. and 10 mg in P.M.); may increase by 10 mg/day at 3-week intervals up to 60 mg/day
Tricyclic Antidepressants (TCAs)	
amitriptyline (Elavil)	Adult: PO; 75–100 mg/day (may gradually increase to 150–300 mg/day) Geriatric: PO; 10–25 mg at hs (may gradually increase to 25–150 mg/day)
amoxapine (Asendin)	Adult: PO; begin with 100 mg/day (may increase on day 3 to 300 mg/day) Geriatric: PO; 25 mg at hs; may increase every 3–7 days to 50–150 mg/day (max 300 mg/day)
desipramine (Norpramin)	PO; 75–100 day; may increase to 150–300 mg/day
doxepin (Sinequan)	PO; 30–150 mg/day at hs; may gradually increase to 300 mg/day
imipramine (Tofranil)	PO; 75–100 mg/day (max 300 mg/day)
maprotiline (Ludiomil)	Mild to moderate depression: PO; start at 75 mg/day; gradually increase every 2 weeks to 150 mg/day; Severe depression: PO; start at 100–150 mg/day; gradually increase to 300 mg/day
nortriptyline (Aventyl, Pamelor)	PO; 25 mg tid or qid; may increase 100–150 mg/day
protriptyline (Vivactil)	PO; 15–40 mg/day in three to four divided doses (max 60 mg/day)
trimipramine (Surmontil)	PO; 75–100 mg/day (max 300 mg/day)
Selective Serotonin Reuptake Inhibitors (SSRIs)	
citalopram (Celexa)	PO; Start at 20 mg/day (max 40 mg/day)
escitalopram oxalate (Lexapro)	PO; 10 mg qd; may increase to 20 mg after 1 week
fluoxetine (Prozac)	PO; 20 mg/day in the A.M. (max 80 mg/day)
fluvoxamine (Luvox)	PO; Start with 50 mg/day (max 300 mg/day)

Drug	Route and Adult Dose (max dose where indicated)
paroxetine (Paxil)	Depression: PO; 10–50 mg/day (max 80 mg/day)
	Obsessive-compulsive disorder: PO; 20–60 mg/day
	Panic attacks: PO; 40 mg/day
sertraline (Zoloft)	Adult: PO; start with 50 mg/day; gradually increase every few weeks to a range of 50–200 mg
	Geriatric: start with 25 mg/day
Atypical Antidepressants	
bupropion (Wellbutrin)	PO; 75–100 mg tid (greater than 450 mg/day increases risk for adverse reactions)
mirtazapine (Remeron)	PO; 15 mg/day in a single dose at hs; may increase every 1–2 weeks (max 45 mg/day)
nefazodone (Serzone)	PO; 50–100 mg bid; may increase up to 300–600 mg/day
trazodone (Desyrel)	PO; 150 mg/day; may increase by 50 mg/day every 3–4 days up to 400–600 mg/day
venlafaxine (Effexor)	PO; 25–125 mg tid

TABLE 6-18 ANTIDEPRESSANTS *(continued)*

Source: Adams, M.P., Josephson, D.L., & Holland, L.N. (2005). *Pharmacology in Nursing: A Pathophysiologic Approach.* Used by permission of Pearson Education, Inc., Upper Saddle River, New Jersey.

(b) Adverse effects of tricyclics—CNS (sedation, tremors), xerostomia, orthostatic hypotension, myocardial toxicity (MI, CHF, tachycardia) with overdose

   i) Dental implications—Used in dentistry to treat chronic facial pain, which produces analgesia; use epinephrine with caution (hypertension); xerostomia (home fluoride, saliva substitutes), tremors (electric toothbrushes); increases the effect of vasoconstrictors used in local anesthetics, must decrease dose for patients taking tricyclics

   ii) MAOIs (phenylzine (Nardil), tranylpromine (Parnate) isocarboxazid (Marplan)—Numerous drug interactions, food interactions (aged cheese, wine, fish) precipitating hypertensive crisis; used for depression associated with diseases of aging, Alzhemier's, Parkinson's, as well as posttraumatic stress syndrome and phobias; inhibit the biodegration of vasopressors and are capable of potentiating the actions of vasopressors. Decrease dose of vasoconstrictors used in local anesthetics.

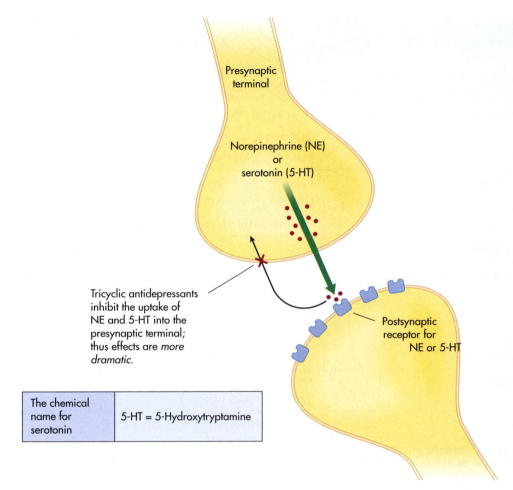

FIGURE 6-17 ■ Tricyclic antidepressants produce their effects by inhibiting the reuptake of neurotransmitters into presynaptic nerve terminals. The neurotransmitters particularly affected are norepinephrine and serotonin.

(2) Second-generation agents (Figure 6-18■)

(a) Examples—Selective serotonin reuptake inhibitors (SSRIs): fluoxetine (Prozac), sertraline (Zoloft), paroxetine (Paxil), fluvoxamine (Luvox)

(b) Other second-generation agents—Trazodone (Desyrel), nefazodone (Serzone), bupropion (Zyban and Wellbutrin used in dentistry for smoking cessation); avoid with alcohol, may produce seizure)

(c) Adverse reactions of SSRIs—Tremors (fluoxetine), nausea, xerostomia, taste changes, orthostatic hypotension, behavioral change, suicidal tendency in adolescents.

(d) Adverse reactions of bupropion—GI distress, constipation, dry mouth, headache, tremors, agitation, dizziness, risk of seizures

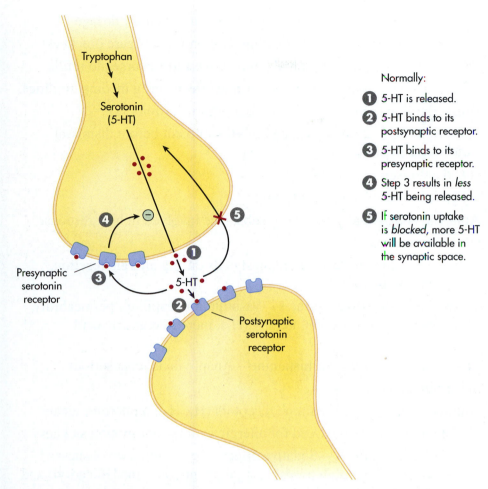

Normally:

❶ 5-HT is released.

❷ 5-HT binds to its postsynaptic receptor.

❸ 5-HT binds to its presynaptic receptor.

❹ Step 3 results in *less* 5-HT being released.

❺ If serotonin uptake is *blocked*, more 5-HT will be available in the synaptic space.

FIGURE 6-18 ■ SSRIs block the reuptake of serotonin into presynaptic nerve terminals. Increased levels of serotonin induce complex changes in pre- and post-synaptic neurons of the brain. Presynaptic receptors become less sensitive, while postsynaptic receptors become more sensitive.

(rare); risk increases with alcohol use or abrupt withdrawal from chronic alcohol use

(3) Lithium (Eskalith, Lithobid)

  (a) Disorders treated

    i) Anxiety

    ii) Phobia

    iii) Bipolar disorder—drug of choice

    iv) Obsessive–compulsive disorder

  (b) Adverse effects—Tremors, thirst, nausea, vomiting; use NSAIDs with caution (decreased clearance of lithium)

  (c) Management consideration during treatment

    i) Communication problems—Patient behavior problems

      ii) Ensure patient has taken medication, check dosage

      iii) Depression can affect motivation for self-care practices

      iv) Narcotics for dental pain—Give short course, no refills

3. Dental management implications for adverse effects, drug incompatibilities

  a. Home fluoride (xerostomia), electric toothbrush (tremors)

  b. Sit upright for 1–2 minutes at end of appointment before dismissal (orthostatic hypotension)

D. Autacoid and antihistamine drugs

  1. Pathophysiology of histamine response

    a. Autacoid is a naturally occurring substance involved in host response

      (1) Host response

        (a) Histamine released from mast cells during allergic reaction, inflammation

        (b) Pharmacological effects—Vasodilation, capillary permeability, bronchoconstriction, itching (H_1), increased gastric acid secretion (H_2)

        (c) Adverse effects of histamine—Anaphylaxis most serious

  2. Antihistamine drugs

    a. Antihistamines block histamine receptors (H_1, H_2), numerous agents

      (1) Older H_1 blockers—Used for allergic rhinitis, antimotion sickness

        (a) Adverse effects—Sedative effects, dry mouth, nervousness, convulsions (high doses) (e.g., diphenhydramine [Benadryl] and Zyrtec)

      (2) Newer nonsedating H_1 blocking agents—Loratadine (Claritin), fexofenadine (Allegra)

      (3) H_2 receptor blockers—Cimetidine (Tagamet); most drug interactions: famotidine (Pepcid), ranitidine (Zantac); fewest drug interactions: nizatidine (Axid) (used to treat GI disorders)

  3. Pharmacological effects of prostaglandin (PG), thromboxanes, leukotrienes, kinins

    a. Produced in response to inflammation, injury

    b. Smooth muscle contraction or relaxation—Depends on type of PG

    c. Platelet adhesiveness affected (increases platelet adhesion [clotting])

    d. Increase body temperature, heart rate, capillary permeability

    e. Liberated as part of the periodontal inflammation process—Role in erythema, edema, alveolar bone resorption

      (1) Leukotrienes are derived from arachidonic acid; play role in asthma and seasonal allergies

(2) Kinins formed by proteolytic enzymes—Role in periodontal inflammation, shock, chronic allergy, anaphylaxis

(3) Substance P—Peptide acts as neurotransmitter in brain, hormone in intestines; causes vasodilation, hypotension, pain transmission, and perception

E. Adrenocorticosteroid drugs—Hormones secreted by adrenal cortex (corticosteroids), which include both glucocorticoids and mineralocorticoids

  1. Major glucocorticoid—Cortisol (hydrocortisone), most frequently used (stress hormone)

    a. Indication—Addison's disease, asthma, systemic inflammatory disease, emergency uses (shock)

    b. Dose forms—Topical, oral, parenteral, inhalational

      (1) Systemic effects—Oral, parenteral mainly

        (a) Prednisone, most common oral form

        (b) Topical forms used in dentistry—Triamcinolone (Kenalog ointment), fluocinonide (Lidex)

      (2) Inhalational forms (used for respiratory distress)—Oral candidiasis may result (rinse mouth and expectorate after use)

  2. Physiology of adrenal cortex function—Fight-or-flight mechanism

    a. Hydrocortisone released by adrenal cortex in response to stress

    b. Steroids (hydrocortisone) inhibit release of adrenocorticotropic hormone (ACTH)

      (1) Therapeutic use—Anti-inflammatory effect, suppression of allergic reactions

      (2) Long-term exogenous steroid therapy—Suppresses adrenal function

        (a) Adrenal crisis triggered by stress—Supplemental steroids; may be indicated prior to stressful and/or invasive dental procedures (consult patient's doctor)

      (3) Adverse reactions proportional to dosage, prolonged therapy

        (a) Abnormal fat distribution—Moon face, buffalo hump, hyperglycemia, weight gain, muscle wasting

        (b) Increased infection, masked infection

        (c) Personality, behavior changes; peptic ulcer

        (d) Impaired wound healing, osteoporosis, glaucoma, cataracts

        (e) Fluid retention, hypertension, adrenal crisis (hypoglycemia, profuse sweating, hypotension, weak pulse, leads to circulatory collapse and shock)

  3. Medical and dental uses of glucocorticoids

    a. Topical—Oral ulcerations, desquamative gingival lesions

  b. Injectable—TMJ arthritis

  c. Chronic systemic diseases—Asthma, COPD, autoimmune diseases

4. Synthetic corticosteroid products

  a. Equivalent doses of products compared with hydrocortisone

  b. Topical products classified by potency—Hydrocortisone weakest, betamethasone most potent (triamcinolone most common steroid used in dentistry—use of topical for more than 2 weeks can cause adrenal suppression)

5. Dental implications and management

  a. Avoid aspirin—GI effects, peptic ulcer possibility

  b. Monitor blood pressure

  c. Examine oral tissues for masked infection, osteoporosis, delayed wound healing

  d. Possibility of adrenal crisis in stressful dental procedures

  e. Stress reduction protocol: reduce fear and anxiety; good pain control is most critical; fear and anticipation of surgery and pain raises cortisol more than actual procedure

F. Hormones

1. Pituitary hormone—Desmopressin—Treats diabetes insipidus, clotting disorders (hemophilia A, von Willebrand's disease)

2. Thyroid hormone—Thyroxine, levothyroxine (Synthroid)—Treats hypothyroidism (myxedema, cretinism)

  a. Effects on physiological function—Needed for growth and development, regulates basal metabolic rate; goal of treatment, bring to euthyroid state

  (1) Oral—Edema in tongue, face, delayed eruption, exfoliation

  (2) Thyroid hormone requires iodine for synthesis

  (3) Goiter is hypertrophy of hypofunctioning thyroid gland—No dental treatment until physician consultation completed

  b. Drug interaction—Use CNS depressants; lower dose of opioids, sedative, and antianxiety drugs

  c. Hyperthyroidism (Graves' disease)—Oversecretion of thyroid hormone

  (1) Epinephrine contraindicated; stress can precipitate thyroid storm

  (2) Excessive sweating, protruding eyes, heart palpitations, hyperventilation; need physician consult before stressful dental procedure

  (3) Treatment: thyroidectomy or antithyroid drugs (radioactive iodine), beta blockers

3. Pancreatic hormones—Glucagon and insulin are produced and secreted by the beta cells in the islets of Langerhans

    a. Diabetes mellitus—Hyperglycemia, glycosuria, severe periodontal disease

        (1) Type 1 (formerly IDDM)—Decrease production/secretion of insulin, insulin injections

            (a) Etiology—Heredity, virus-induced autoimmune response; onset in youth

            (b) Types of insulin—Rapid, intermediate, long (zinc for extended effect), characterized by duration of action

                i) Injected before breakfast—If meal not consumed, risk of insulin shock

                ii) Treatment—Give sugar, juice if conscious

        (2) Type 2 (formerly NIDDM)—defective insulin receptor function

            (a) Etiology—Heredity, obesity; usually adult onset, increased prevalence in children due to obesity

            (b) Drug treatment oral hypoglycemic drugs, if controlled may also require insulin

                i) Sulfonylureas—Tolbutamide, glyburide, glipizide (second-generation agents); increase insulin secretion by beta cells

                ii) Alpha-glucosidase inhibitors (acarbose, miglitol)—Slows breakdown of carbohydrates in intestines; can antagonize treatment for insulin shock

                iii) Biguanide-metformin (Glucophage)—Increases insulin secretion and treats insulin resistance

                iv) Meglitinides (repaglinide, nateglinide)—Stimulates insulin secretion

                v) Thiazolidinediones (pioglitazone, rosiglitazone)—Increases insulin receptor sensitivity

            (c) Drug interactions—Aspirin, sulfonamides, barbiturates

4. Female sex hormones—Estrogens, progesterone, used in hormone replacement therapy, contraceptives

    a. Secreted primarily by ovaries

    b. Indications for treatment: Oral contraception, menstrual disturbances, osteoporosis, hysterectomy, or menopause

    c. Types of estrogen—Conjugated estrogens (Premarin), estradiol, ethinyl estradiol, esterified estrogens

        (1) Side effects—Gingival bleeding, exaggerated inflammation, nausea, hypertension, dry socket

(2) Management—Good plaque control, semisupine position, monitor vital signs

d. Progestins—Progesterone (parenteral), medroxyprogesterone (oral), levonorgestrel (oral)

(1) When uterus is intact, added to estrogen hormone replacement therapy to prevent uterine cancer

e. Oral contraceptives can contain combinations of estrogens and progestins

(1) Drug interactions with oral contraceptives—Antibiotics, high doses of acetaminophen, benzodiazepines

(2) Instruct to use additional form of birth control if antibiotics prescribed until start of next mestrual cycle

f. Estrogen receptor inhibitor—Tamoxifen (treatment of breast cancer)

g. Selective estrogen receptor modulations—raloxifene (Erista)—osteoporosis

5. Male sex hormones—Testosterone, anabolic steroids

a. Medical use—Treatment of breast cancer, hormone replacement therapy

b. Anabolic steroids are Schedule III–controlled drugs—Illicit use to build muscle mass

c. Bisphosphonates—Used clinically for the treatment of osteoporosis, osteitis deformans (Paget's disease of the bone), bone metastasis (with or without hypercalcemia), multiple myeloma, and other conditions that feature bone fragility

G. Respiratory drugs—Used to treat asthma, COPD, bronchoconstriction

1. Pathophysiology of asthma—Allergic response characterized by reduced expiratory airflow, increased mucus secretions, airway restriction (Figure 6-19■)

a. Drugs for asthma—β_2 adrenergic agonists, corticosteroids, theophylline, ipratropium bromide, cromolyn, leukotriene inhibitors (newest)

b. Action—Produce bronchodilation or reduce symptoms

(1) Adrenergic drugs—Epinephrine, albuterol, metaproterenol, pirbuterol, salmeterol

(2) Corticosteroids—Triamcinolone, flunisolide, beclomethasone; dosing: intranasal or inhalation; may require systemic use

(3) Cromolyn (OTC); Intal (prescription)—Used for seasonal allergies, not for acute asthma symptoms

(4) Theophylline—Bronchodilator (asthma, COPD); drug interacts with erythromycin (theophylline toxicity), Ciprofloxacin, Ketoconazole, and other systemic azole antifungals

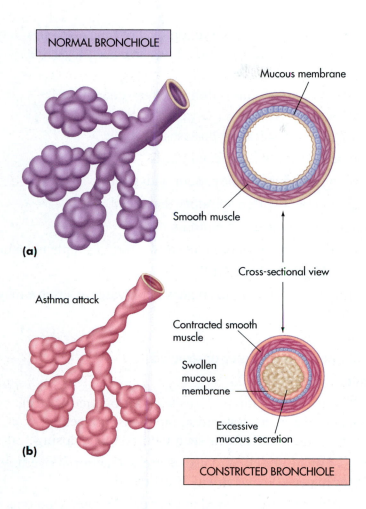

NORMAL BRONCHIOLE

Mucous membrane

Smooth muscle

(a)

Cross-sectional view

Asthma attack

Contracted smooth muscle

Swollen mucous membrane

Excessive mucous secretion

(b)

CONSTRICTED BRONCHIOLE

FIGURE 6-19 ■ Changes in Bronchioles during an Asthma Attack: (a) Normal Bronchiole; (b) Bronchiole during an Asthma Attack

(5) Ipratropium bromide (Atrovent), inhalation route, bronchodilator (asthma, COPD); drug of choice for emphysema

2. COPD—Irreversible airway obstruction from chronic bronchitis or emphysema

3. Other drugs to treat respiratory diseases

a. Nasal decongestants (pseudoephedrine)—Constrict blood vessels of nasal membranes

(1) Chronic use—Rebound swelling and congestion

(2) Side effects—Increased adrenergic effects (tachycardia, hypertension)

b. Expectorants and mucolytics—Promote removal of mucus from respiratory tract; agents—guaifenesin (Robitussin), acetylcysteine (Mucomyst)

c. Antitussives—Cough suppressant action; agents—codeine, dextromethorphan

4. Side effects of drugs to treat respiratory diseases

a. Dry mouth, adrenergic stimulation, candidiasis

b. Nitrous oxide is contraindicated for patient with COPD

5. Management of dental patient with respiratory diseases

a. Stress reduction to prevent acute symptoms

b. Physician consultation for determining need for steroid supplementation

c. Nitrous oxide contraindicated in COPD

d. Aspirin and sulfite preservative in local anesthetic/vasoconstrictor may cause asthma attack

e. Monitor vital signs

f. Semisupine chair position if airway obstructed

6. Metered dose inhalers

a. Advantages—Medications go directly to site of action (act locally), good bronchodilator effect, accurate dose, rapid onset of action, convenient to carry, limits side effects seen with systemic dosing

b. Disadvantages—Difficult for child to use, decreased action if overused, β_2 agonist risk for hyperreflexive airway if overused

H. Gastrointestinal drugs—Actions of drugs used to treat or alleviate symptoms of GI disease

1. Neutralize gastric HCI (antacids)—Acute gastritis, ulcers

a. Sodium bicarbonate, calcium carbonate, aluminum and magnesium salts, magnesium-aluminum hydroxide gel, sucralfate (e.g., Tums)

b. Interactions—Alters absorption of tetracyclines

2. Prevent release of acids (H_2-blockers, proton pump inhibitors, prostaglandin)—Ulcers, GERD (gastroesophageal reflux disease)

a. Cimetidine (Tagamet), ranitidine (Zantac), famotidine (Pepcid)—H_2-receptor antagonists nizatidine (Axid)

(1) Interactions—Antacids, smoking

(2) Side effects affecting dental treatment—Confusion, dry mouth, taste alteration, blood dyscrasias; delayed drug metabolism of drugs metabolized by P450 pathway (cimetidine, ranitidine)

b. Omeprazole (Prilosec)—A proton pump inhibitor

c. Misoprostol (Cytotec)—Prostaglandin

3. Promote intestinal movement (laxatives, GI stimulants)—Constipation, GERD, gastric stasis

    a. Laxatives—Bulk (cellulose), lubricants (mineral oil), stimulants (bisacodyl), stool softeners, saline laxative (magnesium sulfate)

    b. GI stimulants—Metoclopramide, affects upper GI tract

4. Minimize fluid and electrolyte imbalance (antidiarrheals)

    a. Kaolin and pectin (Kaopectate)—Adsorbent action

    b. Opioids—Diphenoxylate (Lomotil) and loperamide (Imodium), decrease GI peristalsis

5. Prevent vomiting (antiemetics)

    a. Anticholinergics/antihistamines—Dimenhydrinate (Dramamine), diphenhydramine (Benadryl), hydroxyzine (Atarax)

    b. Trimethobenzamide (Tigan)—Acts on chemoreceptor trigger zone in brain

    c. Prochlorperazine (Compazine), promethazine (Phenergan)—Phenothiazine antipsychotic drugs

    d. Cannabinoid drugs—Dronabinol (Marinol), marijuana substance

6. Management of dental patient with GI disease

    a. Sodium agents—Contraindicated in patient on sodium-restricted diet

    b. Be aware of potential drug interactions

    c. GI disease symptoms may require semisupine chair position

    d. Manage side effects (dry mouth, sedation, dizziness) as needed

I. Antineoplastic drugs—Cancer chemotherapy agents that interfere with the cell cycle to destroy malignant cells

    1. Agents—A group that depends on mechanism and site of action

        a. Alkylating agents—Nitrogen mustard, nitrosoureas, miscellaneous agents

        b. Antimetabolites—Methotrexate, fluorouracil, mercaptopurine; effective in rapidly growing neoplasms

        c. Others—Plant alkaloids, antibiotics, hormones

            (1) Tamoxifen (Nolvadex)—Blocks estrogen receptors in breast

            (2) Paclitaxel (Taxol)—Used for ovarian cancer, Kaposi's sarcoma

    2. Oral complications of antieoplastic agents—Poor healing, bleeding, blood dyscrasias, xerostomia, mucositis (oral ulceration), taste disturbances

        a. Before initiation of chemotherapy—Eliminate dental disease

        b. Management—prescription-strength fluoride products, palliative rinse for oral pain control (topical anesthetic rinses mixed with coating agents; e.g., liquid Benadryl with Mylanta), ulceration, strict plaque control, warning to prevent injury in self-care methods, chlorhexidine, ice chip (shown to reduce severity of mucositis)

c. Physician consult, WBC, platelet count before dental procedures

d. Dental appointment during week before chemotherapy

3. Adverse drug effects

a. Bone marrow depression—Leukopenia, agranulocytosis, thrombocytopenia, anemia

b. GI sloughing—Bloody diarrhea, stomatitis (mucositis), vomiting

c. Immunosuppression—Poor healing, inability to fight infection

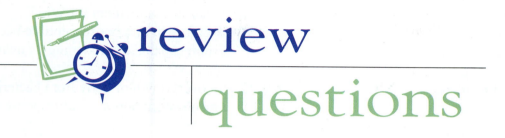

review questions

DIRECTIONS Each of the questions or incomplete statements below is followed by suggested answers or completions. Select the **one** answer that is best in each case.

1. Which of the following describes the degree of attraction between a drug and a receptor site?
   A. Intrinsic activity
   B. Affinity
   C. An antigen/antibody reaction
   D. Acceptor binding

2. Which of the following binds to a receptor and interferes with binding of an agonist?
   A. Placebo
   B. Displacing ion
   C. Antagonist
   D. Full agonist

3. When is oral administration of a drug contraindicated?
   A. Respiratory inflammation is present
   B. Immediate onset of action is necessary
   C. The stomach is full
   D. Sterile technique is required

4. Where does biotransformation of drugs primarily occur?
   A. Bloodstream
   B. Kidney
   C. Liver
   D. Stomach

5. A dental patient becomes sleepy after administration of an antihistamine. This effect would be termed a(n):
   A. Toxic effect
   B. Hyperreaction
   C. Contraindication
   D. Idiosyncracy
   E. Side effect

6. A drug is available to bind to a receptor when it is in a(n):
   A. Plasma protein-bound form
   B. Unbound form
   C. Nonionized form
   D. Ionized form

7. Action of norepinephrine is terminated by being:
   A. Broken down by acetylcholinesterase
   B. Reabsorbed by the adrenergic nerve terminal
   C. Metabolized
   D. None of the above

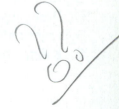

8. Under the effects of the sympathetic nervous system, a person will experience:
    A. Increased energy
    B. Increased respiration
    C. Increased blood pressure
    D. Increased heart rate
    E. All of the above

9. Which route of administration is used MOST often in emergencies?
    A. Oral
    B. Rectal
    C. Sublingual
    D. Intravenous
    E. Intramuscular

10. In dentistry, cholinergic drugs are used to:
    A. Produce a dry field for taking impressions
    B. Calm an anxious patient before a dental procedure
    C. Increase salivary flow to treat xerostomia
    D. Reduce the chance of getting an infection
    E. Potentiate a local anesthetic agent

11. Aspirin is contraindicated in the dental patient with a medical history of:
    A. Heart failure
    B. Ear surgery
    C. Adult-onset diabetes
    D. Mental psychoses

12. Overdose of narcotic analgesics usually produces death from:
    A. Convulsions
    B. Respiratory depression
    C. Brain abscess
    D. Liver failure
    E. Kidney failure

13. A superinfection is defined as:
    A. A massive or virulent infection
    B. Overgrowth of a nonsusceptible bacterium capable of producing its own infection
    C. An overgrowth of body flora bacteria as a result of immunological response to disease
    D. None of the above

14. What is the drug of choice for orofacial infections?
    A. Penicillin
    B. Erythromycin
    C. Tetracycline
    D. Nystatin

15. If the patient is allergic to penicillin G and has an oral infection, the indicated antibiotic is:
    A. Penicillin V
    B. Ampicillin
    C. Tetracycline
    D. Clindamycin

16. Which of the following is the MOST common side effect of erythromycin?
    A. Gastrointestinal
    B. Dermatological
    C. Hematological
    D. Allergenic

17. The patient needs a broad-spectrum antibiotic such as tetracycline. The patient should be cautioned not to use Fem-iron tablets.
    A. The first statement is TRUE. The second statement is FALSE.
    B. The first statement is FALSE. The second statement is TRUE.
    C. Both statements are TRUE.
    D. Both statements are FALSE.

18. Sulfonamides are not considered to be antibiotics because they:
    A. Are semisynthetic chemicals
    B. Only inhibit bacterial growth
    C. Are not produced by microorganisms
    D. Are organic chemicals

19. Which of the following drugs is important in treating candidiasis?
    A. Nystatin
    B. Amphotericin B
    C. Candicidin
    D. Griseofulvin
    E. Flucytosine

20. The major organ for elimination of drugs is the:
    A. Intestines
    B. Bowels
    C. Kidney
    D. Lungs
    E. Skin

21. The mechanism of action of local anesthetics is to:
    A. Block nerve synapses
    B. Coagulate nerve protein reversibly
    C. Depolarize the nerve membrane
    D. Prevent nerve depolarization

22. Drug allergy is an adverse reaction resulting from a:
    A. Previous sensitization to a drug
    B. Failure to apply topical anesthetic before injection
    C. Contact with a nonspecific protein
    D. Drug interaction from a competitive blocking agent
    E. Drug interaction on a plasma ion

23. A local anesthetic with epinephrine is an example of a favorable drug reaction called:
    A. Potentiation
    B. Competitive antagonist
    C. Intrinsic activity
    D. Affinity

24. A patient taking diazepam regularly to treat generalized anxiety disorder is MOST likely to complain of:
    A. Ptyalism
    B. Xerostomia
    C. Palatal petechia
    D. Gingival hyperplasia
    E. Buccal mucosal keratinization

25. All of the following drugs are used for sedation EXCEPT one. Which one is the EXCEPTION?
    A. Equanil
    B. Miltown
    C. Librium
    D. Valium
    E. Coumadin

26. Nitrous oxide is contraindicated for use in which of the following conditions?
    A. Diabetes
    B. Emphysema
    C. Hypertension
    D. Heart disease

27. When considering Guedel's classification of general anesthetics, stage II includes:
    A. Regular respiration
    B. Bradycardia
    C. Loss of vomiting reflex
    D. Hypotension
    E. Unconsciousness

28. The drug of choice for emergency treatment of status epilepticus is:
    A. Phenobarbital
    B. Phenytoin
    C. Trimentadione
    D. Hydantoin
    E. Diazepam

29. The single most useful agent in resuscitative procedures is:
    A. Aromatic ammonia spirits
    B. Antihistamine tablets
    C. Epinephrine by injection
    D. Oxygen

30. Contraindications to dental treatment for the cardiovascular patient include all of the following EXCEPT one. Which one is the EXCEPTION?
    A. Within 6 months after myocardial infarction
    B. Within 6 months after cardiac transplant
    C. Presence of unstable angina pectoris
    D. Presence of uncontrolled arrhythmias
    E. Presence of uncontrolled, severe hypertension

31. Which one of the following statements describes the major effect of digoxin on the failing heart?
    A. Increases the force and efficiency of myocardial contraction
    B. Suppresses parasympathetic effects that slow heart rate
    C. Blocks formation of messenger chemicals that promote vasoconstriction and cardiac edema
    D. Acts synergistically with sympathetic nervous system to reset sympathetic tone of SA node

32. Physician consultation to determine the international normalized ratio (INR) is required before treating the patient taking which of the following drugs?
    A. Nifedipine (Procardia XL)
    B. Ibuprofen (Motrin)
    C. Warfarin (Coumadin)
    D. Menadiol (Synkayvite)

33. Of the following barbiturates, which is indicated for tonic–clonic seizures?
    A. Ethosuximide (Zarontin)
    B. Phenobarbital (Solfoton)
    C. Phenytoin (Dilantin)
    D. Clonazepam (Klonopin)

34. Which of the following drugs might be included in the drug history of a patient being treated for schizophrenia?
    A. Chlorpromazine (Thorazine)
    B. Trifluoperazine (Stelazine)
    C. Thioridazine (Mellaril)
    D. Prochlorperazine (Compazine)
    E. All of the above

35. Which of the following second-generation drugs is most commonly used to treat major depression?
    A. Lithium (Eskalith)
    B. Fluoxetine (Prozac)
    C. Amtriptyline (Elavil)
    D. Bupropion (Wellbutrin)

36. Of the following adverse reactions, which is associated with prolonged hydrocortisone therapy?
    A. Osteoporosis
    B. Desquamative gingival lesions
    C. Abnormal weight loss
    D. Toxic goiter

37. During stressful procedures, adrenal crisis should be anticipated in which of the following situations?
    A. 10 mg hydrocortisone/day within 2 years of appointment
    B. 5 mg prednisone/day for 2 weeks within 2 years of appointment
    C. 5 mg cortisone for 2 days within 2 years of appointment
    D. Twice daily topical application of triamcinolone for 2 years before appointment

38. Which of the following drugs is a proton pump inhibitor used in combination with antibiotics for treating peptic ulcer?
    A. Cimetidine (Tagamet)
    B. Bismuth subsalicylate (Pepto-Bismol)
    C. Kaolin and pectin (kaopectate)
    D. Omeprazole (Prilosec)

39. Drug allergy may manifest itself in many ways; which of the choices below is a severe life-threatening drug allergy?
    A. Anaphylaxis
    B. Localized dermatitis
    C. Photosensitivity
    D. Urticaria

40. If a medication is to be prescribed to be taken at bedtime, the abbreviation used is:
    A. p.o.
    B. a.c.
    C. b.i.d.
    D. h.s.

41. In understanding a prescription, the instructions stating "Take one tablet every 6 hours" may also be written as:
    A. q3h
    B. t.i.d.
    C. q.i.d.
    D. stat

42. A healthcare worker develops a positive reaction to a tuberculin skin test. After proper medical evaluation, the worker may be placed on long-term dosage of:
    A. Insulin
    B. Rifampin
    C. Isoniazid (INH)
    D. Vancomycin

43. In using nitrous oxide–oxygen analgesia, one must keep in mind that:
    A. The patient is put to sleep during the analgesia
    B. Local anesthetic is most often used to supplement the analgesia
    C. At most, a concentration of 10% nitrous oxide and 90% oxygen is sufficient for most analgesia
    D. In no way does nitrous oxide analgesia relax the patient

44. Which of the following is a pharmacologic property of nitrous oxide gas?
    A. An irritant
    B. Lighter than air
    C. Colorless
    D. An organic solvent

45. A drug that is used for the treatment of epilepsy and that may produce excessive gingival enlargement is:
    A. Pheonobarbital
    B. Lincomycin
    C. Dilantin (phenytoin)
    D. Nystatin

46. If a patient complained of chest pain and then placed a white tablet beneath his or her tongue, it might be concluded that it was:
    A. Sugar
    B. Phenoxypenicillin
    C. Nitroglycerin for angina pectoris
    D. Diphenylhydantoin sodium (phenytoin)

review questions

47. Dental patients may be seen who are on long-term cortisone therapy and may develop hyperglycemia and glycosuria. Therefore, caution should be used in cortisone therapy for patients with:
   A. Hypertension
   B. Diabetes
   C. Peptic ulcer
   D. Tuberculosis

48. Another name for mepivicaine hydrochloride is:
   A. Prilocaine
   B. Carbocaine
   C. Xylocaine
   D. Procaine

49. The topical cortisone MOST commonly used in treating oral ulceration is:
   A. Triamcinolone acetonide (Kenalog)
   B. Orabase
   C. Promethazine hydrochloride
   D. Oxycodone hydrochloride

50. If a patient is allergic to salicylates (aspirin), which of the following may be prescribed?
   A. Demerol
   B. Darvon
   C. Tylenol
   D. Codeine

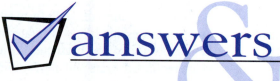

answers & rationales

1.

B. The degree of attraction between a drug and receptor is called affinity. Intrinsic activity refers to the ability of a drug molecule to stimulate the receptor and produce an effect. Receptors that cannot initiate a response are known as acceptors. An antigen/antibody response is a host immune response.

2.

C. The antagonist produces its effect by preventing an agonist from occupying its receptor site. The result is no intrinsic activity. An agonist is a drug capable of binding to a receptor, simulating it, and producing a response. A placebo is an inert substance given in place of a drug.

3.

B. Drugs given orally must be absorbed through the stomach or intestines and also into the hepatic portal circulation, resulting in a much slower onset of action. Food in the stomach is sometimes required for the absorption of the drug. Many drugs that are used to treat respiratory disease are administered by use of a metered-dose inhaler.

4.

C. The liver is the most important organ for drug biotransformation. Other organs play a special role in metabolism, but the liver is the most important organ.

5.

E. A side effect is a dose-related reaction that is not part of the desired therapeutic outcome. A toxic reaction is an extension of the pharmacologic effect on the target organ, resulting in an excessive effect. An idiosyncratic reaction is a genetically related abnormal drug response. A contraindication refers to a reason for not prescribing a drug.

6.

B. A drug that is bound is unavailable to go to the site of action; therefore, a drug must be in its unbound form to get to the site of action and bind to the receptor to produce an effect. Nonionized and ionized forms will affect a drug's absorption.

7.

B. Norepinephrine is terminated principally by its reuptake into the nerve ending, removing it from the site of action. The enzymes monoamine oxidase and catechol-O-methyltransferase play a minor role in the metabolism of norepinephrine and epinephrine. Acetylcholine is metabolized by acetylcholinesterase to yield inactive substances.

8.

E. The SANS effects will increase energy, respiration, blood pressure, and heart rate.

9.

D. IV administration produces the most rapid drug response because the injection is made directly into the blood. Oral administration of drugs must be absorbed through the small intestine, delaying its onset of action. Drugs given rectally are poorly and irregularly absorbed. Sublingual administration of drugs is a topical route and generally used for localized effects. The intramuscular route may be used for drugs that are irritating or for suspensions.

10.

C. Cholinergic drugs stimulate gland cell secretion, resulting in increased salivary flow. Anticholinergic can be used to produce a dry field before some dental procedures. Cholinergic drugs are not used to treat anxiety. Cholinergic drugs are not used to prevent infection or to increase the effect of local anesthetics.

11.

C. A combination of aspirin and sulfonyloreas can cause a hypoglycemic effect. Aspirin may be used to prevent unwanted clotting in heart failure. Aspirin does not affect those patients with a history of ear surgery or mental psychoses.

12.

B. The usual cause of death from an overdose is respiratory depression. This is related to a decrease in the sensitivity of the brainstem to carbon dioxide, which reduces the rate and depth of respiration. A narcotic may adversely affect the kidney and liver, but failure is not usually the cause of death. Convulsions or brain abscesses are not the usual cause of death from an overdose of narcotics.

13.

B. A superinfection is an infection caused by the proliferation of microorganisms different from those causing the original infection. An immunological response of the host does not result in an overgrowth of bacteria. A virulent infection is not the definition of superinfection.

14.

A. Penicillin is often used for the treatment of dental infections because of its bactericidal potency, lack of toxicity, and spectrum action, which includes many oral flora. Erythromycin is active against the same aerobic microorganism as penicillin. It is the drug of first choice against these microorganisms in penicillin-allergic patients, but it is not effective against the anaerobic *Bacteroides* species and would not be effective for infections caused by those microorganisms. In aerobic gram-positive infections, penicillins offer a clear advantage over tetracyclines, but they are rarely the drug of choice for a specific infection. Nystantin is an antifungal agent.

15.

D. The drug of choice against infections in penicillin-allergic patients is clindamycin. Penicillin V and ampicillin are from the same family as penicillin G. Tetracycline is a broad-spectrum antibiotic and is rarely the drug of choice for a specific infection.

16.

A. Side effects most often associated with erythromycin administration are gastrointestinal. Dermatological and hematological effects are not problems. Allergic reactions to erythromycin are uncommon.

17.

A. Fem-iron tablets have cations in them. Divalent and trivalent cations decrease the intestinal absorption of tetracycline by chelating with it. These products should not be taken within 2 hours of ingesting tetracycline.

18.

C. Sulfonamides cannot be classified as antibiotics because they are not produced by living organisms. Penicillin G is the only naturally occurring penicillin. All others are semisynthetic. The sulfonamides are bacteriostatic against many Gram-positive and some Gram-negative bacteria.

19.

A. Nystantin is used for both the treatment and prevention of oral candidiasis in susceptible cases. Amphotericin B, griseofulvin, and flucytosine are used in other types of fungal infections.

20.

C. The most important organ of excretion is the kidney. However, drugs may be removed from the body by any organ that makes contact with the outside environment.

21.

D. After combining with the receptor, local anesthetics block the conduction of nerve impulses by decreasing the permeability of the nerve cell membrane to sodium ions, preventing nerve depolarization.

22.

A. For a drug to produce an allergic reaction, it must act as an antigen and react with an antibody in a previously sensitized patient. The reaction is not dependent on the dose nor is it predictable.

23.

A. Potentiation is the interaction of two or more drugs resulting in an effect that is greater than expected. A competitive antagonist is a drug that has affinity for or combines with the receptor and produces no effect. Intrinsic activity refers to the ability of a drug molecule to stimulate the receptor and produce an effect. Affinity refers to the degree of attraction between a drug and the receptor.

24.

B. Benzodiazepines have been reported to cause xerostomia. Benzodiazepines do not cause excessive salivation, palatal petechia, gingival hyperplasia, or lichen planus.

25.

E. Coumadin is an anticoagulant. Equanil, Miltown, Librium, and Valium may all be used for sedation.

26.

B. Nitrous oxide is contraindicated for patients with respiratory obstruction, COPD, emotional instability, and pregnancy. Diabetes, hypertension and heart disease are not contraindications.

27.

E. Stage II begins with unconsciousness and is associated with involuntary movement and excitement. Sympathetic stimulation produces tachycardia and hypertension. Respiration becomes irregular and emesis and incontinence can occur. Stage II can be uncomfortable for the patient and so should be passed through quickly.

28.

E. Diazepam (Valium) is the drug of choice for the treatment of status epilepticus. Phenobarbital, phenytoin, trimethadione, and hydantoin are used to treat seizures but are not the drug of choice for this situation.

29.

D. Oxygen is the most important drug in the emergency kit. It is indicated in most emergencies, especially if respiratory difficulty is a problem.

30.

B. There is no specific time frame for cardiac transplant recipients to receive dental treatment after transplantation. The time depends on the progress of the individual patient and requires a physician consult.

31.

A. The major effect of digoxin on the failing heart is to increase the force and efficiency of the myocardial contraction. As digoxin increases the cardiac output, the sympathetic tone is decreased, with a decrease in the heart rate as the end result.

32.

C. Warfarin's action is to decrease synthesis of clotting factors and requires the INR to determine the patient's clotting ability; the other agents do not work by the same mechanism.

33.

B. Phenobarbital (Solfoton) is the only barbiturate listed as a choice. Clonazepam (Klonopin) is a benzodiazepine derivative. Phenytoin (Dilatin) is the prototype for the hydantoin group. Ethosuximide (Zarotin) is an anticonvulsant of a miscellaneous group used to treat absence (petit mal) seizures.

34.

E. All of these drugs could be used to treat schizophrenia.

35.

B. Prozac is the only drug listed that is among the top 20 most prescribed drugs.

36.

A. A major risk factor for osteoporosis is long-term prednisone therapy. Hydrocortisone does not cause desquamative gingival lesions but may be used to treat them. It is not used in the treatment of toxic goiters. Long-term use causes weight gain, not weight loss.

37.

B. This distractor follows the "rule of twos" in adrenal drug therapy, the other distractors do not.

38.

D. Omeprazole is the only proton pump inhibitor listed. Cimetidine is an antihistamine. Bismuth subsalicylate is an antidiarrheal. Kaolin is an antidiarrheal combination product.

39.

A. Anaphylaxis is an acute, life-threatening emergency that most frequently occurs after intravenous injection of a drug. Anaphylaxis is characterized by hypotension, bronchospasm, laryngeal edema, and cardiac arrhythmias. Fatal anaphylaxis is rare, but has occurred after a single oral dose of penicillin in highly sensitive individuals.

40.

D. The abbreviation h.s. means at bedtime or hour of sleep. The abbreviation p.o. means by mouth. The abbreviation a.c. means as desired. The abbreviation b.i.d. means twice a day.

41.

C. The abbreviation q.i.d. means 4 times a day. This can also be interpreted as "Take every 6 hours." The abbreviation q3h means once every three hours. The abbreviation t.i.d means three times a day. The abbreviation stat means immediately.

42.

C. Healthcare workers or anyone who develops a positive tuberculin skin test may, after proper chest radiography and medical consultation, be placed on prophylactic long-term (generally 1 year) Isoniazid therapy.

43.

B. Relative analgesia primarily employs the use of nitrous oxide–oxygen, but pain control must be given concomitantly with local anesthetic. Nitrous oxide offers comfort to the dental patient and an increased patient acceptance of dental procedures. Because of increased patient acceptance, the treatment administration is more relaxed.

44.

C. Nitrous oxide is a nonirritating, colorless gas. It has little or no odor. It is stored in a blue cylinder at 750 psi.

45.

C. Phenytoin (Dilantin) produces excessive gingival enlargement in some patients who are treated with this drug. It is a highly effective anticonvulsant drug. The severity of the gingival enlargement differs. It is not seen in every patient taking this drug.

46.

C. When a nitroglycerin tablet is placed beneath the tongue of a patient suffering pain from angina pectoris, it relieves the pain by reducing the workload of the heart and producing a dilation of the blood vessels. Angina pectoris is a syndrome of chest pain or discomfort that results from inadequate blood supply to a segment of the mycocardium.

47.

B. Long-term cortisone therapy produces an enhancement of gluconeogenesis and is contraindicated for patients who have diabetes mellitus. Corticosteroids decrease the resistance to infections because they cause a general depression of the inflammatory response. Most frequently, corticosteroids are used for their anti-inflammatory and anti-allergic actions.

48.

B. The trade names for mepivicaine hydrochloride are Carbocaine and Isocaine. The trade name for procaine is Novacain. The trade names for lidocaine are Xylocaine and Octocaine. The trade names for prilocaine are Citanest and Citanes Forte.

49.

A. Triamcinolone acetonide (Kenalog) has been used to treat some acute and chronic lesions of the oral mucosa, such as recurrent ulcerative stomatitis. As with all corticosteroids, triamcinolone acetonide is entirely suppressive, but not curative. It does not prevent recurrence of any oral lesions.

50.

C. Tylenol (acetaminophen) may be substituted for aspirin when allergy is a problem. Acetaminophen has the same analgesic properties and antipyretic effects as aspirin. It does not, however, have the anti-inflammatory activity of aspirin.

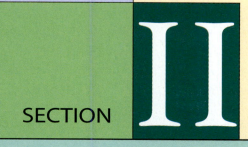

SECTION

II

Provision of Clinical Dental Hygiene Services

7 Assessing Patient Characteristics

Patient assessment is defined as the critical analysis and evaluation or judgment of a particular condition, situation, or other subject of appraisal.

chapter | objectives

After completion of this chapter, the learner should be able to:

➤ Discuss the components of patient assessment

➤ Discuss the procedure and assessment of vital signs

➤ Discuss premedication guidelines

➤ Discuss the gathering of the dental history

➤ Describe the dental examination

➤ Describe the occlusal examination

➤ Describe the periodontal assessment

➤ Discuss nutritional counseling

➤ Describe testing techniques

➤ Discuss preventive dentistry

➤ Describe plaque and calculus development

➤ Describe the removal of bacterial plaque

➤ Describe the types of dentifrices

➤ Discuss stains

➤ Discuss fluoride

➤ Discuss mouth rinses

➤ Describe pit and fissure sealants

➤ PATIENT ASSESSMENT

I. Components

A. Social history—Gathering personal information about the patient such as the essential data for an appointment and legal implications (e.g., care of a minor)

B. Health history—Incorporates subjective and objective information to obtain comprehensive medical data; may include the following information:

1. Status of patient's general health—Indication of how patient will handle dental appointment

   a. Conflicting information from this question compared to information on the history may indicate the patient is overly concerned about health and well-being or unable to understand seriousness of reported conditions

   b. Modifications may be considered of patient who reveals a significant disability, medical, or psychological condition

   c. Estimate medical risk of patient to receive dental care according to the American Society of Anesthesiologists, or ASA (Table 7-1■)

      (1) ASA I: Normal, healthy patient with no apparent systemic disease

      (2) ASA II: Patient with a mild systemic disease

      (3) ASA III: Patient with a severe but no incapacitating systemic disease

      (4) ASA IV: Patient with a life-threatening, incapacitating systemic disease

      (5) ASA V: Patient not expected to survive 24 hours (not applicable in dentistry)

      (6) If an emergency situation exists, add an E before the ASA classification

2. Medical examinations

   a. Is patient currently under the care of a physician?

      (1) Dates and reason for most frequent examinations

      (2) Laboratory tests and results

      (3) New prescriptions and refill prescriptions, reasons for prescriptions

      (4) Anticipated surgeries

      (5) Medical consult may be necessary

      (6) Recommended care modifications considered for a patient with a medically compromising condition

TABLE 7-1 PATIENTS FOR ASA CLASSIFICATION

ASA Classification	Examples of Patients
ASA II	1. Well-controlled NIDDM, epilepsy, asthma, hyper- and hypothyroid disorders (with normal thyroid function) 2. Healthy pregnant women 3. Healthy patients with allergies, especially to drugs 4. Healthy patients with extreme dental fears 5. Healthy patients over 60 years old 6. B.P. between 140 and 160 mmHg systolic and/or 90 and 94 mmHg diastolic
ASA III	1. Stable angina pectoris 2. Well-controlled IDDM 3. Exercise-induced asthma 4. Symptomatic hyper- and hypothyroid disorders 5. Status post-CVA and postmyocardial infarction more than 6 months before treatment with no residual signs and symptoms 6. Emphysema or chronic bronchitis 7. B.P. between 160 and 200 mmHg systolic and/or 94 and 114 mmHg diastolic
ASA IV	1. Unstable angina pectoris 2. CVA within the past 6 months 3. Uncontrolled IDDM and epilepsy 4. Severe CHF or COPD 5. B.P. greater than 220 mmHg systolic or 115 mmHg diastolic
ASA V	End-stage • Cancer • Cardiovascular disease • Hepatic disease • Infectious disease • Renal disease • Respiratory disease

NIDDM = Noninsulin-dependent diabetes mellitus; B.P. = Blood pressure; IDDM = Insulin-dependent diabetes mellitus; CVA = Cardiovascular accident; CHF = Congestive heart failure; COPD = Chronic obstructive pulmonary disease

3. Serious illnesses, hospitalization, surgeries

    a. Seek information regarding any medical conditions that might be of significance to planned dental treatment

    b. Course of healing: normal or abnormal

    c. Stress reduction protocols implemented for patients with medical conditions that could be exacerbated by stress/anxiety from dental hygiene care.

4. Medications prescribed by physician and over-the-counter medications

    a. Relation to dental care

b. Drug interactions

c. Patient's regularity of taking medication

5. History of allergic reactions

a. Penicillin or other antibiotics

b. Local anesthetics

c. Sulfa drugs

d. Barbiturates, sedatives

e. Aspirin, ibuprofen

f. Iodine (Betadine contains iodine)

g. Codeine or other narcotics

h. Latex (*must* use latex-free products when providing treatment)

i. Avoid dispensing medication that may cause an allergic reaction or patient discomfort

6. Current diseases/conditions

a. Bleeding problems

(1) Bleeding associated with previous dental appointments

(2) Anticoagulant medications

(3) Coagulation problems

(4) Aspirin use

(5) Review laboratory test for bleeding time

(6) May need special measures for treatment and medical consultation

b. Blood transfusion

(1) Risk of communicable diseases

c. Damaged heart valve, artificial heart valves, heart murmur, rheumatic fever, or prosthetic devices (joints, valves)

(1) Cardiologist or physician of record should be contacted if the patient is unsure about premedication

(2) Determine type of valve or murmur

(3) Minimize number of appointments for those who take antibiotic premedication to prevent antibiotic resistance

(4) During instructions, link need for good oral hygiene and oral health to minimize bacteremic exposures and risk of further heart disease.

d. Cardiovascular disease (heart trouble, heart attack, angina, high blood pressure, hardening of the arteries, stroke)

(1) Chest pain

(2) Shortness of breath

(3) Ankle swelling

(4) Congenital heart defects

(5) Pacemaker

(6) Stress reduction protocols implemented for patients with cardiac conditions that could be exacerbated by stress/anxiety from dental hygiene care

(7) Review prescribed medications

(8) Has patient been taking prescribed medication?

(9) Monitor vital signs

(10) Assess degree of heart failure and determine ASA classification; follow ASA classification for treatment modifications; may require physician consultation

(11) Supplemental oxygen may be indicated for patients with significant heart damage

(12) Physician consultation necessary for patients who report significant heart damage

(13) Avoid treatment of patients who have had a heart attack within six months of the dental hygiene appointment

(14) Anesthesia—Limit epinephrine to .04 mg maximum

e. Hypertension

(1) Monitor vital signs

(2) Postural hypotension (raise chair slowly)

(3) Review patient medications: diuretics, antiadrenergic agents, vasodilators, calcium channel-blocking agents

(4) Anesthesia—Limit epinephrine to .04 mg maximum

f. Angina pectoris

(1) Prevent stress, morning appointments

(2) Prepare for symptoms: have amyl nitrite, nitroglycerin ready

g. Heart disease

(1) History of disease

(2) Physician consultation

(3) Monitor vital signs

(4) Short, frequent appointments

(5) Pacemakers—Check use of ultrasonics

(6) Review medications: glycosides (digitalis), anticoagulants, antiarrhythmic drugs

h. Fainting spells, seizures, epilepsy or convulsions

(1) Fainting (syncope):

(a) If cause is psychogenic, follow appropriate ASA stress reduction techniques

(b) If fear and/or anxiety has specific cause (e.g., the local anesthetic syringe), avoid exposing client to the cause

(c) Two to three chair adjustments should be performed when returning from supine position to upright position for patient with history or orthostatic hypotension

(d) Other medical conditions or causes should be further explored prior to care planning to determine if physician consultation is indicated or care plan modifications are indicated

(2) Seizures, epilepsy, or convulsions

(a) Epileptic seizures prevented by careful screening at beginning of the appointment; some seizures can be "triggered" by fatigue, recent alcohol consumption, exhaustion, psychological stress, flashing lights, and nitrous oxide–oxygen analgesia; reschedule epileptic patient who reports seizure-triggering factors

(b) Stress reduction protocol recommended for apprehensive epileptic patients

(c) Medications may require alteration in care planning

(d) Valproic acid requires bleeding time test prior to invasive procedures; persons on Dilantin may have drug-influenced gingival enlargement

i. Diabetes

(1) ASA III or IV status may indicate need for antibiotics after extensive surgical procedures to minimize risk of postoperative infection

(2) Avoid scheduling appointments during normal eating times

(3) Periodontal disease accelerated

(4) Use short-acting local anesthetic agents to allow patient to eat, thereby raising blood glucose levels, if necessary

(5) Patient with a blood glucose level exceeding 240 mg/dl should be evaluated carefully before treatment

(6) Patient who reports increased hunger, thirst, and weight loss may have uncontrolled diabetes

(7) Physician consultation indicated prior to dental hygiene care

(8) Patient taking diuretics may be predisposed to postural hypotension; use caution when raising patient from dental chair

(9) Prepare for emergency: insulin; apple juice, frosting

j. Hepatitis, yellow jaundice, cirrhosis, or liver disease

(1) Postpone care for patient with active hepatitis A or E infections until physician clearance is obtained

(2) Patient with liver damage or bleeding problems from a past hepatitis infection may need a physician consultation prior to treatment, especially if medications are to be given

(3) Beware of impaired drug metabolism; reduce the amount of amide local anesthetic if liver disease is present, or choose to administer prilocaine, which is predominantly metabolized in lungs

(4) Jaundice can be an indirect indication of hepatitis infection; physician consultation or immediate referral for diagnosis may be required for patients with no specific etiology

(5) Patient with jaundice due to liver conditions will be medically compromised; physician consultation required prior to care, especially if medications are to be given during treatment

k. AIDS or HIV infection

(1) Recognize opportunistic infections and related problems such as candidiasis, mycobacterium avium complex, Kaposi's sarcoma, *Pneumocystis carinii* pneumonia, cytomegalovirus, and neuropathy

(2) Recognize use of protease inhibitors, antiviral drugs, and antiretroviral drugs

(3) Antibiotic premedication is not usually required unless patient's immune system is severely compromised

l. Thyroid problems (goiter)

(1) Postpone care for clinically hypothyroid or hyperthyroid patients

(2) Immediate physician consultation indicated due to potential for life-threatening emergency

(3) Use minimal amount (0.4 mg max) and small dosages of local anesthetic with vasoconstrictor for controlled hyperthyroid patient; aspirate prior to each injection to avoid injection of anesthetic agent into the bloodstream. The use of local anesthesia with vasoconstrictor is contraindicated with the uncontrolled hyperthyroid patient

m. Emphysema

(1) Continuous oxygen ventilation may be needed by patient; avoid ignition of the oxygen source

(2) Avoid use of nitrous oxide–oxygen analgesia

n. Bronchitis

(1) Avoid aerosol production (e.g., use of mechanized instruments and air-abrasion systems)

o. Lung disease

   (1) Raise back of chair for the patient with difficulty breathing in supine position

   (2) Physician consultation required prior to treatment for patient with chronic signs and symptoms of lung condition

   (3) Keep in mind possible link between oral pathogens and respiratory infection

   (4) Avoid the use of prilocaine since it is primarily metabolized in the lungs

p. Arthritis or painful, swollen joints

   (1) Anticoagulant therapy may cause excessive bleeding during dental surgery; physician consultation indicated prior to surgical procedure

   (2) Physical impairments may limit oral hygiene behaviors and require modified oral hygiene aids

   (3) Patient may be more comfortable at mid-morning or afternoon appointments

   (4) May need shorter appointments if having difficulty opening and closing mouth

q. Stomach ulcer, hyperacidity, or other conditions

   (1) Stress-reduction protocols implemented for patients with stress/anxiety from dental hygiene care

   (2) Sedatives and tranquilizers predispose patient to postural hypotension

   (3) Instruct patient in accordance with dietary requirements

   (4) Medications may cause xerostomia

r. Kidney conditions or dialysis

   (1) Patient who has a kidney condition may need physician consultation prior to treatment for possible prophylactic antibiotic premedication or if medications are to be given during dental hygiene care

s. Tuberculosis or positive TB skin test

   (1) Be alert to medications such as isoniazid, rifampin, and pyrazinamide.

   (2) Do not treat active TB

   (3) A complete medical evaluation for a patient being suspected or being treated for TB must include a medical history, a chest x-ray, and a physical examination prior to any dental treatment

t. Anemia or blood disorders

   (1) Avoid administration of articaine and prilocaine local anesthetic agents or application of topical agents benzocaine to prevent

methemoglobinemia in susceptible individuals; may need oxygen to avoid crisis

u. Herpes

    (1) Reschedule dental hygiene care for patients with active oral lesions

    (2) Counsel patient concerning infectious states of a lesion and potential self-infection to other areas of the body or to other people via contact with the lesion

    (3) Recognize use of acyclovir or Abreva

v. Problems with mental health or nerves

    (1) Person may be drowsy or have xerostomia from medications such as antipsychotic, antianxiety, tranquilizers, antidepressants, antiparkinson

    (2) Compliance may be difficult

    (3) Patient may overreact to stress

w. Cancer

    (1) Render dental and dental hygiene care prior to cancer treatment (surgery, radiation therapy, chemotherapy)

    (2) Recognize signs of oral cancer recurrence during oral assessments (e.g., lymphadenopathy)

    (3) Avoid exposure to excess radiation after cancer radiation therapy

    (4) Antibiotic premedication and blood count may be indicated prior to dental hygiene care

    (5) Avoid tissue trauma following oral cancer treatment

    (6) Head and neck radiation destroys salivary glands; salivary replacement therapy and aggressive dental caries prevention is necessary

    (7) Need for customized fluoride mouth trays for head and neck cancer patient

x. Prosthetic devices (joints, valves, hearing aid, implants) other than dentures

    (1) Antibiotic premedication is vital prior to dental procedures associated with significant bleeding

    (2) Minimize number of appointments for patients who take antibiotic premedication to prevent antibiotic resistance

    (3) During instructions, link need for good oral hygiene and oral health to minimize bacteremic exposures

    (4) Gingival bleeding in the absence of other indicators for periodontal disease may be caused by anticoagulant therapy

y. Use of tobacco or snuff products

    (1) Provide tobacco cessation materials, assist with cessation effort, and arrange follow-up

    (2) Instructions on oral and systemic risks of substance abuse

z. Alcoholism

(1) Avoid alcohol-containing products for patients receiving rehabilitation to stop substance abuse or history of abuse, or taking Antabuse

(2) Alcohol consumption in patients with history of epilepsy predisposes them to seizures

(3) Drug/alcohol rehabilitation programs may prohibit use of vasopressor (vasoconstrictor) with local anesthetic administration

(4) Instructions on oral and systemic risks of substance abuse

(5) High consumption of alcoholic beverages may contribute to alcoholism and xerostomia

(6) Half-life of amide-type local anesthetic agent may be prolonged in a person with liver dysfunction associated with alcoholism, thereby risking local anesthetic overdose; determine if liver dysfunction is present

aa. Pregnant or nursing a baby

(1) Patient may be uncomfortable in supine position, especially in later stages of pregnancy

(2) Patient may be prone to orthostatic hypotension

(3) Avoid exposure to nitrous oxide–oxygen analgesia and medications during pregnancy; avoid tetracycline antibiotic therapy to prevent intrinsic tooth staining in offspring

(4) Radiographs can be taken on pregnant women after first trimester and only in an emergency situation

(5) Consider links between periodontal disease and low birth weight

(6) Category B local anesthetics can be administered after first trimester for immediate care needed

bb. Patient who has taken Redux or Ponimi "fen-phen"

(1) Physician consult indicated prior to care to determine need for antibiotic premedication

C. Vital signs—Monitoring and recording blood pressure, pulse, temperature, and respiration; contributes to a proper systemic evaluation of patient in conjunction with a complete medical history

1. Blood pressure—Force at which blood is pumped against the walls of the arteries

a. Diastole

(1) Minimum amount of pressure exerted against the walls of the vessels

(2) Phase of the cardiac cycle in which the heart relaxes between contractions

b. Systole

    (1) Maximum amount of pressure exerted against the walls of the vessels

    (2) Involves contraction or period of contraction during which left ventricle of heart contracts and blood is forced into aorta and pulmonary artery

c. Armamentarium—Sphygmomanometer, manometer, and stethoscope

    (1) Sphygmomanometer—Consists of an inflatable cuff, pressure bulb for inflating the cuff, and a manometer, a device to read the pressure

        (a) Inflatable cuff—Made of a nonelastic material and fastened with Velcro

        (b) Size of cuff is determined by size of patient's arm

        (c) Proper size width is 20% greater than the diameter of the arm (Figure 7-1■)

    (2) Types of manometers

        (a) Mercury—Contains a column of mercury that rises with an increase in pressure as cuff is inflated; includes tabletop and wall-mounted units or free-standing on wheels; most reliable recorder of blood pressure (Figure 7-2■)

        (b) Aneroid—Contains a circular gauge for registering pressure; needle rotates as pressure rises; accurate and less awkward to

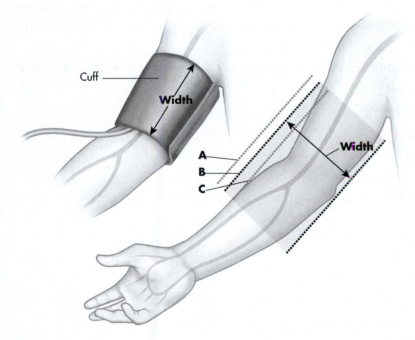

FIGURE 7-1 ■ Selection of Cuff Size: (a) Too Wide; (b) Proper Width—20% Greater than Diameter of Arm; (c) Too Narrow

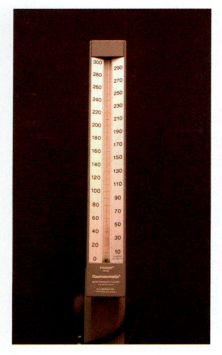

FIGURE 7-2 ■ Mercury Manometer

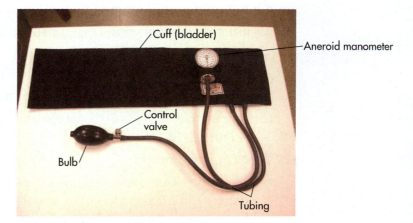

FIGURE 7-3 ■ Parts of the Inflatable Cuff

use than a mercury manometer because gauge is attached to blood pressure cuff (Figure 7-3■)

(c) Electronic—Provides a digital readout on a lit display; does not require a stethoscope like the other two; costly and least likely to give an accurate reading

(3) Stethoscope—Listening aid that amplifies body sounds; components include (Figure 7-4■):

(a) Earpieces

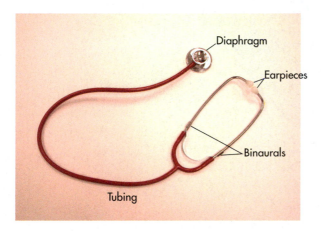

FIGURE 7-4 ■ Parts of the Stethoscope

(b) Binaurals—Connects the earpieces to the tubing

(c) Tubing—Connects the binaurals to the chestpiece

(d) Chestpiece—Amplifies sound; consists of the bell on one side and diaphragm on the other

　　　i) Diaphragm—Flat side covered by a thin plastic disk; best for amplifying high-pitched sounds (i.e., lungs) (Figure 7-5■)

　　　ii) Bell—Cone-shaped side; best for amplifying low-pitched sounds (i.e., heart and vascular)

d. Procedure

(1) Patient preparation

(a) Explain procedure to patient

(b) Seat patient in upright position

(c) Rest patient's arm at level of heart, slightly flexed, and relaxed

(2) Taking blood pressure

(a) Palpate brachial artery in upper arm near inner bend in elbow (Figure 7-6■)

(b) Wrap cuff evenly and snugly around bare upper arm with center of the bladder over brachial artery; lower edge of cuff should be 1 inch above antecubital space where bell of stethoscope will be placed (Figure 7-7■)

(c) Obtain palpatory systolic pressure: Cuff is inflated to point where the circulation has stopped and no pulsations can be felt;

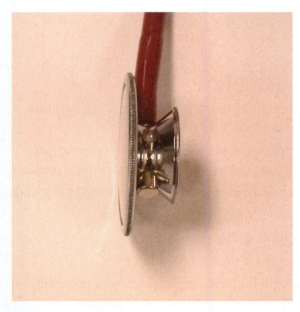

FIGURE 7-5 ■ Stethoscope Diaphragm

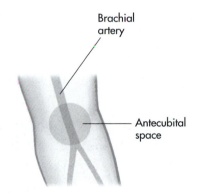

Brachial artery

Antecubital space

FIGURE 7-6 ■ Palpate Brachial Artery

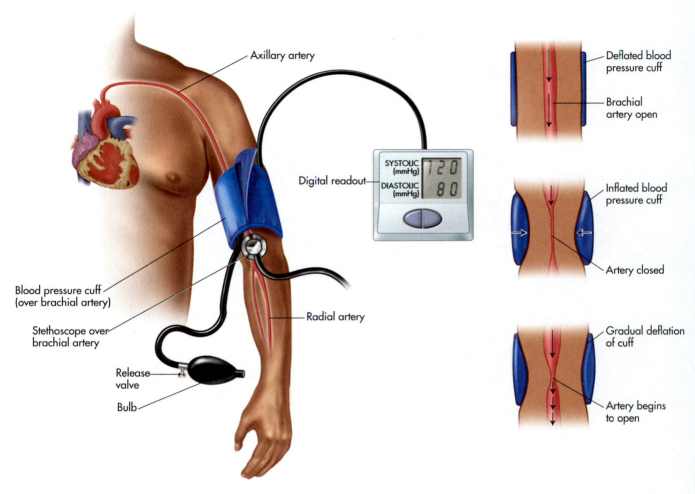

FIGURE 7-7 ■ Application of Blood Pressure Cuff

provides a preliminary estimation of the systolic pressure to ensure an adequate level of inflation

(d) Place the head of the diaphragm over the brachial artery and hold firmly in contact with skin (Figure 7-8■)

(e) Secure the valve and inflate the bladder rapidly to a pressure of 30mm above the previously determined palpatory systolic pressure

(f) Deflate bladder at a rate of 2mm/second, listen for Korotkoff sounds

(g) Record systolic and diastolic readings as a fraction

e. Screening for hypertension (Table 7-2■)

(1) < 140/90—Proceed with routine dental procedures

(2) 140/90–160/95—Recheck blood pressure before dental procedure; if still elevated, refer to physician for evaluation in 3 months

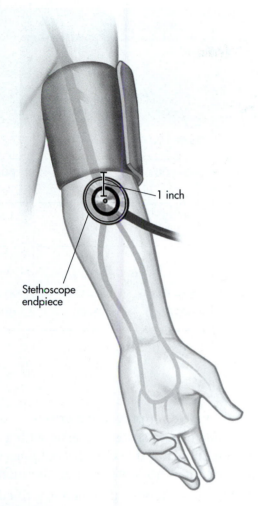

1 inch

Stethoscope
endpiece

FIGURE 7-8 ■ Application of Diaphragm

      (3) 160/95–180/105—Recheck blood pressure before dental procedure; if still elevated, advise patient to see physician in 1 month; call physician before starting treatment

      (4) > 180/105—Recheck blood pressure before dental procedure; if still elevated, refer to physician immediately; DO NOT treat patient

   f. Factors that affect blood pressure

      (1) Increase of blood pressure—Result of exercise, eating, use of stimulants and oral contraceptives

      (2) Decrease of blood pressure—Result of fasting, rest, use of depressants, fainting, loss of blood, or shock

	TABLE 7-2 VITAL STAGES					
	Age					
Vital Signs	**0–1 year**	**1–6 years**	**6–11 years**	**11–16 years**	**Adult**	**Elderly**
Temperature (°F)	96–99.5	98.5–99.5	98.5–99.6	98.6–100.6	98.6–100.6	97.2–99.6
Pulse (beats per minute)	80–160	70–120	70–120	60–100	60–100	60–100
Respirations (per minute)	40–60	25–40	18–25	16–25	16–18	12–25
Blood pressure (mm Hg) Systolic Diastolic	100–150 50–70	74–100 50–80	80–112 54–80	84–120 62–88	94–120 60–90	90–140 60–90

2. Body temperature

    a. Types of thermometers

        (1) Disposable—Single use (effective for preventing cross-contamination); usually made of thin strips of plastic with a specially treated dot or strip indicator that changes color according to temperature; readings are not as accurate as other thermometers

        (2) Mercury—Consists of a thin glass tube with a mercury-filled bulb at the end; mercury is heated by body temperature, causing an expansion in the hollow center of the glass

        (3) Electronic—Provides a digital readout of the temperature; time efficient and decreases cross-contamination

        (4) Tympanic—Placed in ear; measures infrared energy emitted from eardrum (tympanic membrane)

    b. Normal range (Table 7-2)

        (1) Adult—98.6°F–100.6°F

        (2) Child—96°F–100.6°F; higher in infancy and decreases as the child ages

    c. Factors that affect body temperature

        (1) Time of day—Highest in afternoon and early evening; lowest during sleep and early morning

        (2) Increase of temperature—Response to exercise, hot beverages, smoking, infection, dehydration, hyperthyroidism, myocardial infarction, and tissue injury

(3) Decrease of temperature—Response to starvation, hemorrhage, and physiological shock

3. Pulse—Intermittent throbbing sensation felt when fingers are pressed against an artery; indirect measurement of cardiac output

    a. Palpation sites

        (1) Brachial artery—Located in bend of elbow (antecubital space)

        (2) Carotid artery (carotid pulse)—Located at side of neck

        (3) Facial artery—Located at side of face at border of mandible

        (4) Radial artery (radial pulse)—Located at wrist

    b. Normal range (Table 7-2)

        (1) Adult—60–100 beats/minute

        (2) Child—70–105 beats/minute

4. Respirations—Involves inhalation and exhalation; indicates how well the body is providing oxygen to the tissues

    a. Normal range (Table 7-2)

        (1) Adult—12–20 breaths/minute

        (2) Child—16–40 breaths/minute; slows down as the child gets older

D. American Heart Association Guidelines for Premedication—Revised April 2007

    1. Preventive antibiotics prior to a dental procedure are advised for patients with:

        a. Artificial heart valves

        b. A history of infective endocarditis

        c. Certain specific, serious congenital (present from birth) heart conditions, including:

            (1) Unrepaired or incompletely repaired cyanotic congenital heart disease, including those with palliative shunts and conduits

            (2) A completely repaired congenital heart defect with prosthetic material or device, whether placed by surgery or by cathereter intervention, during the first 6 months after the procedure

            (3) Any repaired congenital heart defect with residual defect at the site or adjacent to the site of a prosthetic patch or a prosthetic device

        d. A cardiac transplant that develops a problem in a heart valve; except for the conditions listed above, antibiotic prophylaxis is no longer recommended for any other form of congenital heart defects.

    2. Negligible risk: No antibiotic prophylaxis recommended

        a. Isolated secundum atrial septal defect

        b. Surgical repair of atrial septal defect, ventricular septal defect, or patent ductus arteriosus of more than 6 months' duration

        c. Previous coronary artery bypass graft surgery

     d. Previous Kawasaki disease without valvular dysfunction

     e. Cardiac pacemakers

     f. Implanted defibrillators

     g. Mitral valve prolapse

     h. Rheumatic heart disease

     i. Bicuspid valve disease

     j. Calcified aortic stenosis

     k. Congenital heart conditions such as ventricular septal defect, atrial septal defect, and hypertrophic cardiomyopathy

3. Dental procedures considered for antibiotic prophylaxis in susceptible patients

     a. High-risk category

         (1) Dental extractions

         (2) Periodontal procedures including surgery, scaling, root planing, and probing

         (3) Dental implant placement, reimplantation of teeth

         (4) Endodontic instrumentation or surgery beyond the tooth apex

         (5) Subgingival placement of antibiotic fibers or strips

         (6) Initial placement of orthodontic bands but not brackets

         (7) Intraligamentary local anesthetic injection

         (8) Prophylactic cleaning of teeth or implants with anticipated bleeding

4. Antibiotic prophylactic regimens

     a. Standard prophylaxis

         (1) Amoxicillin—Adults, 2.0 grams; children, 50 mg/kg orally 1 hour before procedure

     b. Patient who cannot use oral medications

         (1) Ampicillin—Adults, 2.0 grams IM or IV; children, 50 mg/kg IM or IV within 30 minutes before procedure

     c. Patients allergic to penicillin

         (1) Clindamycin—Adults, 600 mg; children, 20 mg/kg orally 1 hour before procedure

         (2) Cephalexin or cefadroxil—Adults, 2.0 g; children, 50 mg/kg orally 1 hour before procedure

         (3) Axithromycin or Clarithromycin—Adults, 500 mg; children, 15 mg/kg orally 1 hour before procedure

     d. Allergic to penicillin and unable to take oral medications

         (1) Clindamycin—Adults, 600 mg; children, 15 mg/kg IV 1 hour before procedure

         (2) Cefazolin—Adults, 1.0 g; children, 25 mg/kg IM or IV within 30 minutes before procedure

E. Dental history—Gathering past and present dental information; may include following information

1. Chief complaint, discomfort, and/or pain

2. Previous dental/dental hygiene care, including care from specialists

3. Personal habits, including oral hygiene and grinding

4. Patient's attitude toward dental care and importance of a healthy mouth

5. Sequence of head and neck examination

  a. Overall appraisal—Observe and note abnormalities of posture, gait, general health status; hair and scalp, breathing, state of fatigue, voice, cough, and hoarseness

  b. Face—Observe facial twitching, paralysis; jaw movements during speech, injuries, and signs of abuse

  c. Skin—Observe and note color, texture, blemishes, traumatic lesions, eruptions, swellings, or growths

  d. Eyes—Observe and note size of pupils as well as color of sclera; eyeglasses, protruding eyeballs

  e. Nodes

    (1) Palpate preauricular, occipital, submental/submaxillary, cervical chain, supraclavicular: note indurations, area of tenderness (Figures 7-9■ and 7-10■)

    (2) Interview patient as to history of recent illness or tenderness in the area of concern

  f. TMJ

    (1) Observe and palpate area while patient is opening and closing mouth

    (2) Note limitations or deviations of movement; tenderness, sensitivity, noises (clicking, popping, crepitus)

  g. Lips

    (1) Observe closed, then open

    (2) Look for deviations in color, texture, size, shape; cracks, angular cheilosis; blisters, ulcers; traumatic lesions, irritation from lip biting; limitations of opening, muscle elasticity, muscle tone; evidence of mouth breathing; induration

  h. Breath odor—Note malodors indicating severity, relation to oral hygiene and gingival health

6. Intraoral examination—Observation and palpation of structures within oral cavity

  a. Labial and buccal mucosa

    (1) Systematically examine the vestibule, mucobuccal fold, frena, and opening of Stenson's duct, buccal mucosa

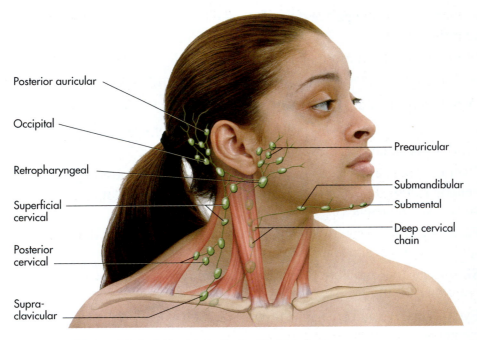

Posterior auricular

Occipital

Retropharyngeal

Superficial
cervical

Posterior
cervical

Supra-
clavicular

Preauricular

Submandibular

Submental

Deep cervical
chain

FIGURE 7-9 ◼ Lymph Nodes Palpated during Head and Neck Examination

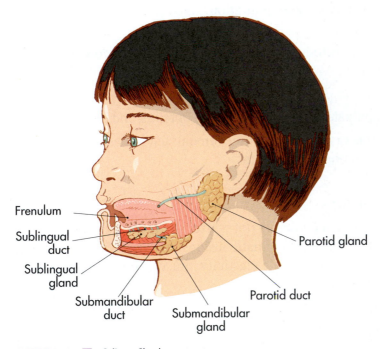

Frenulum

Sublingual
duct

Sublingual
gland

Submandibular
duct

Submandibular
gland

Parotid gland

Parotid duct

FIGURE 7-10 ◼ Salivary Glands

(2) Observe and note deviations from normal in color, size, texture, and contour

(3) Note abrasions, traumatic lesions, cheekbite; effects of tobacco use; ulcers, growths; moistness of surfaces; relation of frena to free gingiva; areas of induration

b. Tongue (Figure 7-11■)

(1) Examine the dorsal ventral surface; lateral borders; base of tongue (retracted)

(2) Observe and note deviations from normal in shape, color, size, texture, consistency; fissures, papilla; coating; lesions—elevated, depressed, flat; indurations

c. Floor of the mouth

(1) Examine ventral surface of tongue, duct openings, mucosa, frena, and tongue action

(2) Observe and note deviations from normal in varicosities; lesions— elevated, depressed, flat, traumatic; indurations; limitation of freedom of movement, frena (ankyloglossia)

d. Saliva—Observe and note deviations from normal in quantity; quality (thick, ropy); evidence of dry mouth; lip wetting; tongue coating

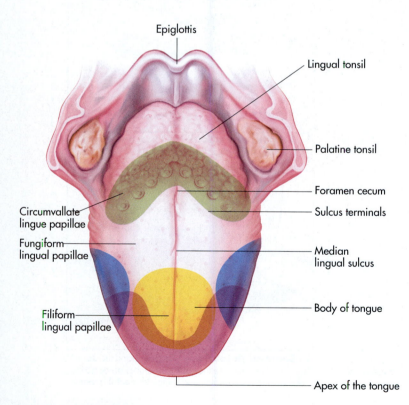

FIGURE 7-11 ■ Parts of the Tongue

  e. Hard palate—Examine and note deviations from normal in height, contour, color; appearance of rugae; tori, growths, ulcers, lesions; surface texture

  f. Soft palate and uvula—Examine and note deviations from normal in color, size, shape; petechiae, lesions, ulcers, growths

  g. Tonsillar region and throat—Examine and note deviations from normal in tonsils (color, size, shape, surface texture); lesions; trauma

7. Extraoral examination—Observation and palpation of structures of the head and neck outside of oral cavity

8. Observation methods of intraoral/extraoral examinations

  a. Palpation (Figure 7-12■)

   (1) Bilateral—Use both hands at same time to examine corresponding structures on opposite sides of body

   (2) Bimanual—Use finger(s) and/or thumb from each hand; apply simultaneously

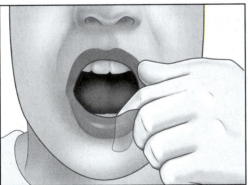

A. Digital palpation—Use index finger. Example—detect the presence of exostosis on the border of the mandible.

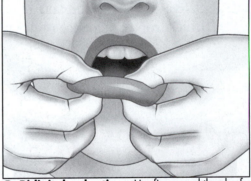

B. Bidigital palpation—Use finger and thumb of same hand. Example—Palpate the lips.

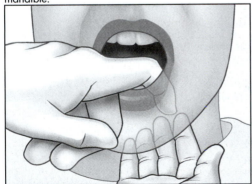

C. Bimanual palpation—Use finger(s) and/or thumb from each hand. Example—palpate floor of mouth.

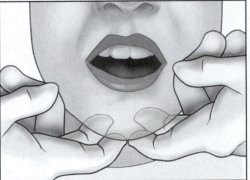

D. Bilateral palpation—Use both hands at same time to examine corresponding structures on opposite sides of body. Example—examine submental nodes.

FIGURE 7-12 ■ Palpation Methods

(3) Digital—Use single finger

(4) Bidigital—Use finger and thumb of same hand

b. Auscultation—Process of listening to body sounds

c. Inspection—Performing a visual examination of body and overall appearance

9. Description of observations (Tables 7-3■ and 7-4■)

a. Size

(1) Record length and width, height of lesion in mm (measure with perio probe)

(2) Elevated lesions may be significant

TABLE 7-3 LESION DESCRIPTORS

Descriptive Colors

pink	red
purple	brown
blue	grey
yellow	black
white	

Descriptive Texture/Consistency Terminology

indurated	soft, spongy
firm	fluctuant
smooth	verrucose
crusted	exophytic
pseudomembranous	fissured
cratered	corrugated

Descriptive Shape Terminology

flat	irregular
elevated (papillary)	depressed (ulcer-like)
pedunculated	sessile
descrete	confluent
lobulated	

TABLE 7-4 LESION CATEGORIES

Lesion Categories

Lesion	Description	Size	Example	
Macule	Circumscribed, change in color without elevation or depression, nonpalpable change in skin color	< 1 cm	Freckle	
Papule	Superficial, solid palpable elevation with circumscribed border	< 1 cm	Mole or elevated freckle	
Nodule	Solid, palpable elevated mass with depth	< 1 cm	Wart, small lipoma, squamous cell carcinoma, fibroma	
Tumor	Solid, palpable elevated mass extending deep into the tissue	> 1 cm	Neurofibroma, large lipoma, carcinoma, and hemangioma	
Wheal	Superficial, elevated area of edema varying in size and shape	varies	Hives, insect bites	

	Description	Size	Example
Plaque	Flat, raised area	> 1 cm	Candidiasis
Vesicle	Circumscribed, fluid-filled elevation	< 1 cm	Herpes labialis
Bulla	Large, fluid-filled elevation containing serum or mucin	> 1 cm	Burn lesion, contact dermatitis
Pustule	Circumscribed, pus-filled lesion	< 1 cm	Acne
Cyst	Encapsulated, fluid-filled mass located in the dermis or subcutaneous tissue	varies	Sebaceous cyst, epidermoid cysts

b. Color—Red, pink, white, and red and white are the most common; also may be blue, purple, gray, yellow, black, or brown

c. Surface texture

　(1) May be smooth or irregular

　(2) Texture may be papillary, verrucous (wart-like), fissured, corrugated, or crusted

d. Consistency—Lesions may be soft, spongy, resilient, hard, or indurated

e. History—Note the length of time the lesion has been present, and whether lesion comes and goes

F. Dental examination

1. Caries—Lesion of hard tissues of teeth that ranges from changes at molecular level to gross tissue destruction and cavity formation

a. Process of caries formation—Pathological process of demineralization and remineralization

　(1) Demineralization—Loss of mineral apatite from tooth structure

　(2) Remineralization—Repair of tooth structure after acidogenic episodes

　(3) Bacterial involvement

　　(a) *Streptococcus mutans*—Associated with coronal caries; appear in large numbers during initial phase of developing carious lesions; have ability to ferment mannitol and sorbitol; mainly produce lactic acid

　　(b) *Lactobacillus* species—Found in greater numbers in more advanced, smooth-surface lesions

　　(c) *L. casei*—Shown to colonize white spot lesions before cavitation

　　(d) *Actinomyces odontolyticus*—Also associated with progression of a lesion

b. Detection of caries

　(1) Direct visual—Includes facial, lingual, and occlusal lesions; may need to utilize mirror for transillumination

　(2) Radiographs—Require proper angulation with no horizontal overlapping; best for viewing interproximal caries

　(3) Explorer—Use for pit and fissure examination; and to follow margin of restorations

　(4) Characteristic changes in the color and translucency of enamel may be seen

　　(a) Chalky white areas of demineralization

　　(b) Grayish-white discoloration of marginal ridges with dental caries of underlying proximal surface

(c) Grayish-white color spreading from margins of restorations caused by recurrent decay

(d) Yellowish-brown to dark brown color of tooth structure with an open carious lesion

c. Classification of caries—G.V. Black's classification (Figure 7-13■)

(1) Class I—Involves pit and fissure surfaces (occlusals of premolars and molars, facials and linguals of molars, and linguals of maxillary incisors)

(2) Class II—Involves proximal surfaces of premolars and molars

(3) Class III—Involves proximal surfaces of incisors and canines, but NOT incisal angle

(4) Class IV—Involves proximal surfaces of incisors and canines, INCLUDING incisal angle

(5) Class V—Involves cervical one-third of facial or lingual surfaces (not pits and fissures)

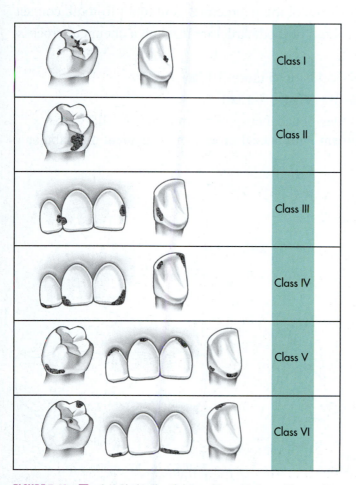

	Class I
	Class II
	Class III
	Class IV
	Class V
	Class VI

FIGURE 7-13 ■ G. V. Black's Classification of Dental Caries and Restorations

(6) Class VI—Involves incisal edges of anterior teeth and cusps of posterior teeth

d. Types of dental caries

(1) Pit and fissure—Involves occlusal surfaces of posterior teeth as well as lingual pits of maxillary incisors

(2) Smooth surface—Involves intact enamel surfaces other than pit and fissure locations

(3) Root surface—Involves any area on the root

(4) Recurrent (secondary)—Involves tooth surface adjacent to an existing restoration

(5) Rampant—Involves rapid and extensive development of cavitation from time of initial incipient lesion

(6) Nursing bottle—Develops from a prolonged exposure to a sugar substance in a bottle; form of rampant decay

2. Abrasion (Figure 7-14■)—Loss of tooth structure from a mechanical cause

3. Attrition (Figure 7-15■)—Loss of tooth structure from tooth-to-tooth contact

4. Erosion (Figure 7-16■)—Loss of tooth structure through a chemical process

G. Occlusal examination

1. Angle's classification of occlusion (Figure 7-17■)

a. Class I—Neutrocclusion (Figure 7-18■)

(1) Molar relation—Mesiobuccal cusp of permanent maxillary first molar is in alignment with buccal groove of permanent mandibular first molar

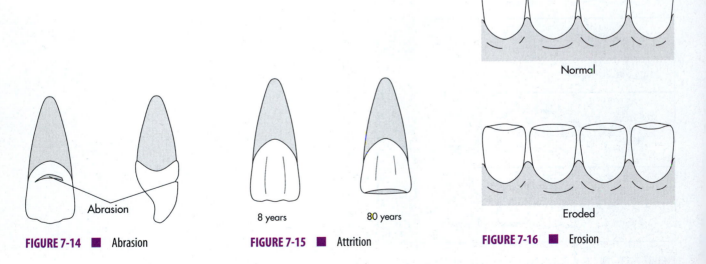

8 years   80 years

Normal

Eroded

FIGURE 7-14 ■ Abrasion   **FIGURE 7-15** ■ Attrition   **FIGURE 7-16** ■ Erosion

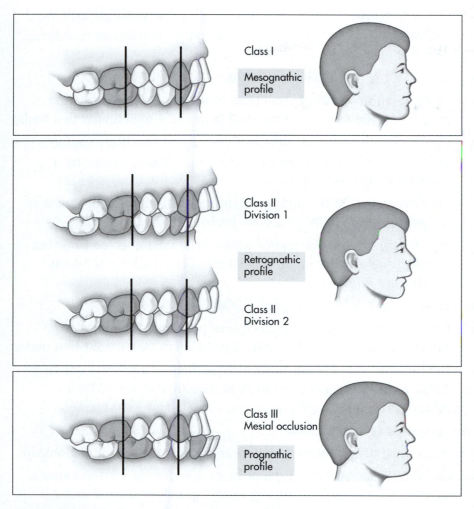

FIGURE 7-17 ■ Occlusal relationships: Class I (*top*): Class II, Division 1 (*middle top*); Class II, Division 2 (*middle bottom*); Class III (*bottom*).

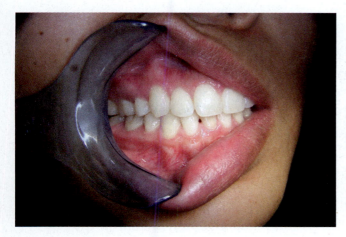

FIGURE 7-18 ■ Class I Occlusion

      (2) Canine relation—Maxillary permanent canine occludes with distal half of mandibular canine and mesial half of permanent mandibular first premolar

   b. Class II—Distocclusion (Figure 7-19■)

      (1) Molar relation—Mesiobuccal cusp of permanent maxillary first molar is mesial to buccal groove of permanent mandibular first molar

      (2) Canine relation—distal surface of permanent maxillary canine is mesial to mesial surface of permanent mandibular canine by a minimum width of half a premolar

         (a) Division I—Molar and/or canine relationship is same, but with permanent maxillary incisors protruded (toward facial)

         (b) Division II—Molar and/or canine relationship is the same but with one or more of permanent maxillary incisors retruded (toward lingual)

   c. Class III—Mesiocclusion (Figure 7-20■)

      (1) Molar relation—Mesiobuccal cusp of permanent maxillary first molar is distal to buccal groove of permanent mandibular first molar

      (2) Canine relation—Mesial surface of permanent maxillary canine is distal to distal surface of permanent mandibular canine by a minimum width of half a premolar

2. Primary dentition (Figure 7-21■)

   a. Flush terminal plane: Primary molars are in an end-to-end relationship

   b. Mesial step: Distal surface of the primary mandibular second molar is mesial to the distal surface of the primary maxillary second molar

   c. Distal step: Distal surface of the primary mandibular second molar is distal to the distal surface of the primary maxillary second molar

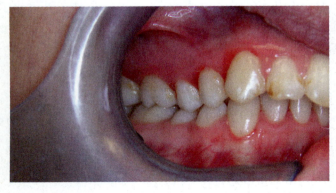

FIGURE 7-19 ■ Class II Occlusion

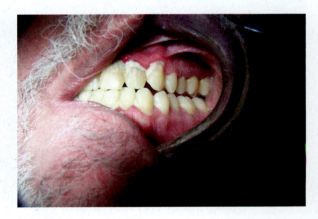

FIGURE 7-20 ■ Class III Occlusion

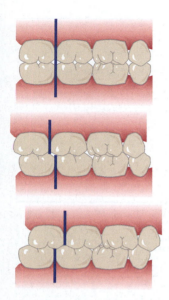

FIGURE 7-21 ■ Occlusal Relationships of the Primary Dentition:
(a) Flush Terminal Plane; (b) Mesial Step; (c) Distal Step

3. Overjet (Figures 7-22■ and 7-23■)—Horizontal distance between labioincisal surface of mandibular incisors and linguoincisal surfaces of maxillary incisors

4. Overbite (Figures 7-22 and 7-24■)—Vertical distance by which maxillary incisors overlap mandibular incisors

   a. Normal overbite—Incisal edges of maxillary incisors are within incisal third of mandibular incisors

   b. Moderate overbite—Incisal edges of maxillary incisors are within middle third of mandibular incisors

   c. Severe (deep) overbite—Incisal edges of maxillary incisors are within cervical third of mandibular incisors

5. Crossbite (Figures 7-22 and 7-25■)—May occur unilaterally or bilaterally

   a. Posterior—Maxillary or mandibular teeth are either facial or lingual to their normal position

   b. Anterior—Maxillary incisors are lingual to mandibular incisors

6. End-to-end (Figures 7-22 and 7-26■)—Cusp-to-cusp occlusion of maxillary and mandibular molars and premolars

7. Edge-to-edge (Figures 7-22 and 7-27■)—Incisal edge-to-incisal edge occlusion of maxillary and mandibular incisors and canines

8. Openbite (Figures 7-22 and 7-28■)—Lack of occlusal or incisal contact between one or more of maxillary and mandibular teeth

Crossbite	A. Unilateral crossbite—right side is normal, left side mandibular teeth facial to normal position; B. Bilateral crossbite 1—mandibular teeth facial to normal position; C. Bilateral crossbite 2— mandibular teeth lingual to normal position; D. Anterior crossbite—maxillary teeth lingual to mandibular teeth.	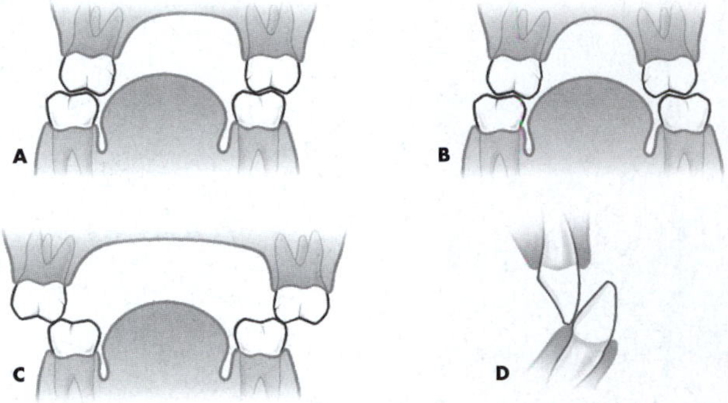
Overbite	Vertical overlap of the maxillary anterior teeth to the mandibular anterior teeth.	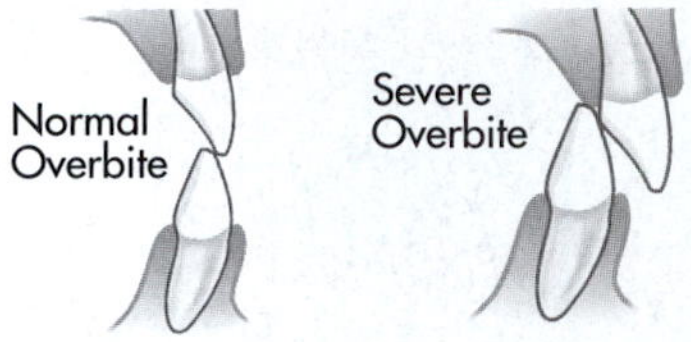
End-to-end	The relationship of the occlusal surface of a maxillary posterior tooth to its corresponding mandibular tooth; occlusal cusp to occlusal cusp.	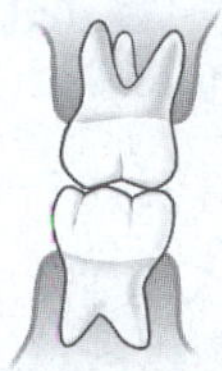
Edge-to-edge	The relationship of the incisal edge of a maxillary anterior tooth to its corresponding mandibular tooth, incisal edge to incisal edge.	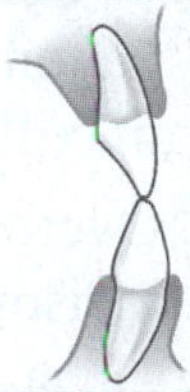
Overjet	The horizontal overlap of the maxillary teeth to the mandibular teeth.	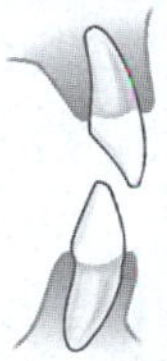
Openbite	Maxillary and mandibular teeth are not in exclusion, may include one or more teeth.	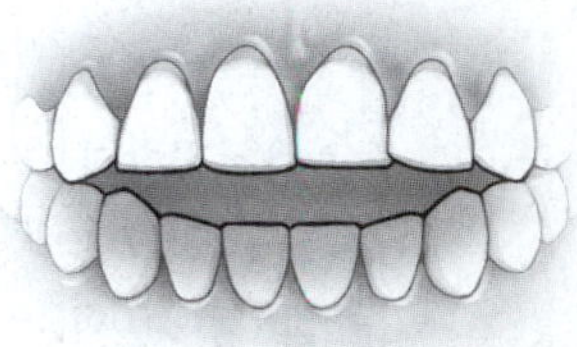

FIGURE 7-22 ■ Malocclusion of Individual or Groups of Teeth

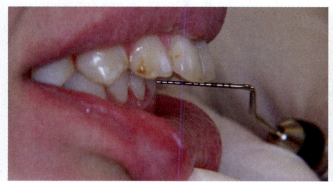

FIGURE 7-23 ■ Overjet of Anterior Teeth

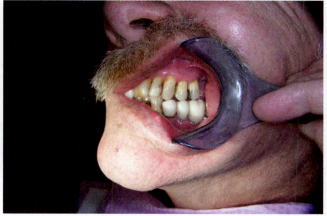

FIGURE 7-26 ■ End to End

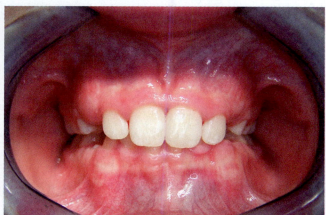

FIGURE 7-24 ■ Overbite

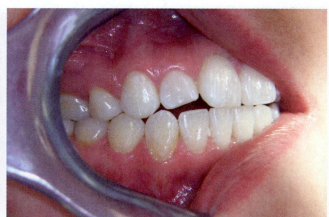

FIGURE 7-27 ■ Edge to Edge

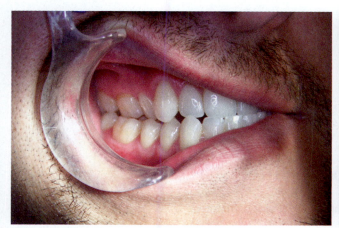

FIGURE 7-25 ■ Anterior and Posterior Crossbite

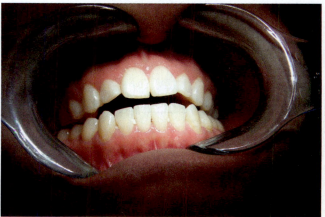

FIGURE 7-28 ■ Openbite

9. Defective restorations—To determine, utilize an explorer to trace around margins of restoration; evidence of a grayish-white color spreading from margins of restorations caused by recurrent decay

10. Demineralized areas—Noted visually as "white spot" lesions

11. Root anatomy—Utilize explorer to detect location of anatomic depressions, root anomalies, calculus, and decay

H. Periodontal assessment—Gathering data involving supporting and surrounding tissues of teeth

1. Sulcus/pocket measurements—Using a periodontal probe, measure from gingival margin to base of sulcus

    a. Definition—Crevice or groove between free gingiva and tooth

    b. Types of pockets (Figure 7-29■)

        (1) Gingival—Gingival margin is coronal to cementoenamel junction (CEJ) because of inflammation of gingival tissues; there is no loss of periodontal attachment

        (2) Suprabony—Base of pocket is coronal to crest of alveolar bone

        (3) Infrabony (intrabony)—Base of pocket is below or apical to crest of alveolar bone

2. Mobility—Movement of tooth

    a. Classification—Includes N, 1, 2, 3 or I, II, III

        (1) N = normal, physiological

        (2) 1 or I = involves slight horizontal mobility, greater than normal

        (3) 2 or II = involves moderate horizontal mobility, greater than a 1 mm displacement

        (4) 3 or III = involves severe mobility and may move in all directions (vertical as well as horizontal)

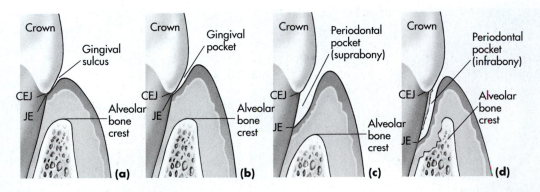

FIGURE 7-29 ■ Types of Pockets: (a) Healthy; (b) Gingivitis; (c) Suprabony; (d) Infrabony

b. Techniques for determining mobility

    (1) Use two single-ended blunt instruments

    (2) Rock the tooth facial-lingually to test for horizontal mobility

    (3) Test vertical mobility by placing blunt end of one instrument on occlusal or incisal surface while depressing tooth

3. Clinical attachment level (Figure 7-30■)

a. Definition—Measure probing depth from CEJ (or other fixed point) to location of probe tip at coronal level of attached periodontal tissues

b. Measurement technique—Select a fixed point on tooth (CEJ is usually used) and measure from that point to base of sulcus/pocket

c. Determine amount of attached gingiva

    (1) On external surface of gingiva, measure from mucogingival junction to gingival margin (determines total gingiva)

    (2) Measure probing depth

    (3) Subtract probing depth from total gingival measurement (amount of attached gingiva)

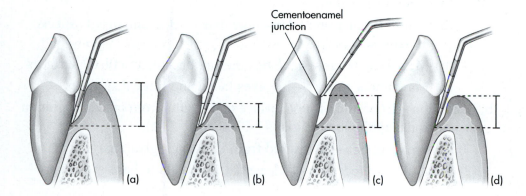

FIGURE 7-30 ■ Loss of Attachment: (a) PPD—Measure from Gingival Sulcus to GM; (b) Recession—Measure from GM to CEJ. (c) GM Covering CEJ—Locate CEJ, Measure Distance to CEJ, then Subtract from Probing Depth; (d) GM at CEJ—Measure from GM to CEJ

4. Loss of attachment—Junctional epithelium migrates toward apex of tooth

  a. Furcation—Involves anatomic area of a multirooted tooth where roots either bifurcate or trifurcate

    (1) Classification (Figure 7-31■)

      (a) Class I—Evidence of early bone loss in furca area; probe can enter furca on either side; can be determined by moving probe from side to side

      (b) Class II—Evidence of moderate bone loss in furcation area; probe can enter furca, but cannot pass between roots

      (c) Class III—Evidence of severe bone loss in furcation area; probe can pass between roots through entire furcation area (not clinically visible)

      (d) Class IV—Same as Class III with exposure resulting from gingival recession (clinically visible)

    (2) Anatomic features

      (a) Bifurcation—Divergence of root trunk into two roots

      (b) Trifurcation—Divergence of root trunk into three roots

    (3) Technique for determining furcation—Furcation probe is instrument of choice used to examine topography of furcation area; accessing furcated areas includes:

      (a) Maxillary first premolars—Involves mesial and distal aspects under contact area

      (b) Maxillary molars—Includes mesial, buccal, and distal surfaces

      (c) Mandibular molars—Involves facial and lingual surfaces

  b. Recession—Exposure of root surface that results from apical migration of junctional epithelium (Figures 7-32■ and 7-33■)

    (1) Visible recession—Measured from CEJ to gingival margin

    (2) Total (actual) recession—Measured from CEJ to base of pocket

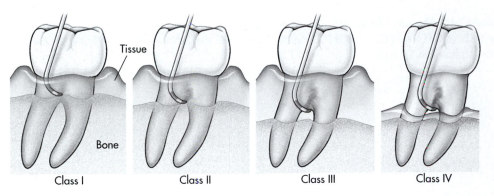

Class I   Class II   Class III   Class IV

FIGURE 7-31 ■ Furcation Classifications

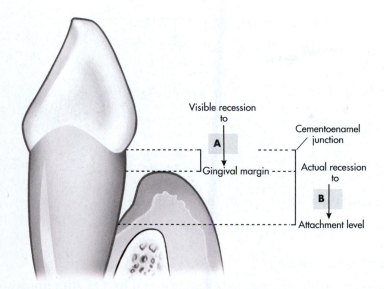

FIGURE 7-32 ■ Gingival Recession: (a) Visible—Measure from CEJ to Gingival Margin; (b) Actual—Measure from CEJ to Base of Pocket

(3) Apparent recession—Exposed root surface that is visible on clinical examination

5. Gingival description—Differentiating among normal, healthy tissues and diseased tissues

   a. Healthy

      (1) Color—Uniformly pink or coral pink

      (2) Contour—Not enlarged, fits tightly around tooth

      (3) Consistency—Firm; attached gingiva firmly bound

      (4) Texture—Free gingiva is smooth; attached gingiva is stippled

   b. Diseased (Figure 7-34■)

      (1) Color—For acute disease, bright red; for chronic disease, a bluish hue (bluish pink or bluish red)

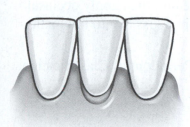

(a) Wide shallow recession

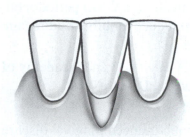

(b) Wide, deep, with narrow attached gingiva

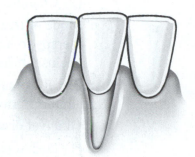

(c) Narrow, deep, with no attached gingiva

FIGURE 7-33 ■ Types of Recession

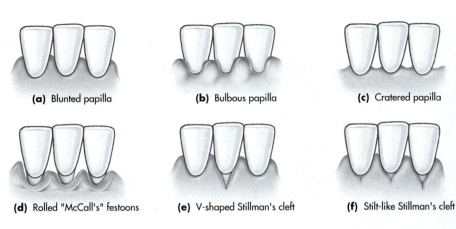

(a) Blunted papilla **(b)** Bulbous papilla **(c)** Cratered papilla

(d) Rolled "McCall's" festoons **(e)** V-shaped Stillman's cleft **(f)** Stilt-like Stillman's cleft

FIGURE 7-34 ■ Diseased Gingiva

    (2) Contour—Enlarged, swollen

    (3) Consistency—For acute disease, soft, spongy, and loss of stippling; for chronic disease, firm, hard, stippled, and fibrotic

    (4) Texture—For acute disease, smooth and shiny; for chronic disease, hard, firm, stippled (sometimes more than normal)

    (5) Bleeding on probing—Indicates diseased gingival tissues; ulcerated pocket wall bleeds on gentle probing

6. Bacterial composition—Made up of pathogenic microorganisms that produce gingivitis and periodontal disease

  a. Healthy—Consists of predominantly gram-positive, aerobic cocci and rods

  b. Diseased—Consists of predominantly gram-negative, anaerobic spirochetes, vibrios, and rods

7. Occlusal trauma—May result from excessive forces and/or lack of bony support

  a. Occlusal forces are transmitted to the periodontal attachment apparatus

    (1) Force can cause changes in bone and connective tissue

    (2) Changes affect tooth mobility and clinical probing depth

  b. Mode of treatment—Establish periodontal health, then apply occlusal therapy to help reduce mobility and regain bone loss due to traumatic occlusal forces

8. American Dental Association and Academy of Periodontics Classification System for Periodontal Disease

  a. Gingival diseases

    (1) Dental plaque-induced gingival diseases

      (a) Gingivitis associated with dental plaque only

        (i) Without other local contributing factors

        (ii) With local contributing factors

(b) Gingival diseases modified by systemic factors

   (i) Associated with the endocrine system:—Puberty-associated gingivitis, menstrual cycle-associated gingivitis, pregnancy-associated gingivitis, pyogenic granuloma, diabetes mellitus-associated gingivitis

   (ii) Associated with blood dyscrasias—Leukemia-associated gingivitis

(c) Gingival diseases modified by medications

   (i) Drug-influenced gingival diseases

   (ii) Drug-influenced gingival enlargements

(d) Gingival diseases modified by malnutrition—Ascorbic acid-deficiency gingivitis

(2) Non-plaque-induced gingival lesions

   (a) Gingival diseases of specific bacterial origin

      (i) *Neisseria gonorrhea*-associated lesions

      (ii) *Treponema pallidum*-associated lesions

      (iiii) Streptococcal species-associated lesions

   (b) Gingival diseases of viral orgin

      (i) Herpesvirus infections—Primary herpetic gingivostomatitis, recurrent oral herpes, varicella-zoster infections

   (c) Gingival diseases of fungal origin

      (i) *Candida*-species infections

      (ii) Linear gingival erythema

      (iii) Histoplasmosis

   (d) Gingival diseases of genetic orgin

      (i) Hereditary gingival fibromatosis

   (e) Gingival manifestations of systemic conditions

      (i) Mucocutaneous disorders—Lichen planus, pemphigoid, pemphigus vulgaris, erythema multiforme, lupus eythematosus, drug-induced

      (ii) Allergic reactions—Dental restorative materials, dental products

   (f) Traumatic lesions—Factitious iatrogenic, accidental

      (i) Chemical injury

      (ii) Physical injury

      (iii) Thermal injury

   (g) Foreign body reactions

b. Chronic periodontitis

(1) Localized

(2) Generalized

c. Aggressive periodontitis—Formerly called early-onset periodontitis

(1) Localized

(2) Generalized

d. Periodontitis as a manifestation of systemic diseases—Several systemic diseases predispose the affected individuals to periodontitis, usually chronic periodontitis

(1) Associated with hematological disorders

(2) Associated with genetic disorders

e. Necrotizing periodontal diseases—Acute inflammation with a distinctive erythema of the supporting structures

(1) Necrotizing ulcerative gingivitis (NUG)

(2) Necrotizing ulcerative periodonitis (NUP)

f. Abscesses of the periodontium—Associated with combinations of pain, swelling, color change, tooth mobility, extrusion of teeth, purulence, sinus tract formation, fever, lymphadenopathy, and radiolucency of the affected bone

(1) Gingival abscess—Localized purulent infection that involves the marginal gingiva or interdental papilla

(2) Periodontal abscess—Localized purulent infection within the tissues adjacent to the periodontal pocket that may lead to the destruction of periodontal ligament and alveolar bone

(3) Pericoronal abscess—Localized purulent infection within the tissue surrounding the crown of a partially erupted tooth

g. Periodonitis associated with endodontic lesions—Infections of periodontal or endodontic orgin may result in periodontitis and may be caused by plaque-associated periodontitis or endodontic infections that enter the periodontal ligament through the apical foramen or accessory canals

(1) Combined periodontic-endodontic lesions

h. Developmental or acquired deformities and conditions

(1) Localized tooth-related factors that modify or predispose to plaque-induced gingival diseases/periodonitis

(2) Mucogingival deformities

(3) Mucogingival deformities and conditions on edentulous ridges

(4) Occlusal trauma

9. Assessment and maintenance of periodontal disease

a. Components of comprehensive periodontal assessment—Examination of the periodontium should occur at each visit and comprehensive exams should be performed on all new patients and at least once a year for established patients; exam includes probing for bleeding, pocket depth, and loss of attachment, mobility, furcation involvement, recession, mucogingival problems, and radiographic bone loss.

b. Phases of patient care

   (1) Care plan—Blueprint or guide that coordinates all treatment procedures and estimates the length of treatment to establish a healthy periodontal environment

   (2) Preliminary phase—Treats emergency needs only; "getting the patient out of pain"

   (3) Phase I—Focuses on controlling the etiological influences responsible for dental disease; includes initial dental hygiene care, self-care education, diet control, removal of plaque-retentive factors, antimicrobial therapy, and dental caries management

   (4) Phase II—Focuses on periodontal surgery, including placement of implants and endodontic therapy

   (5) Phase III—Prosthetic therapy, including the final management of dental caries and exams to evaluate response to restorative procedures

   (6) Phase IV—Maintenance including oral hygiene education, deposit removal, assessment, supportive therapy, and recall interval evaluation

c. Stages of inflammation in the periodontal lesion—Three stages of gingivitis (initial, early, and established) lesion and an advanced lesion of periodontitis

   (1) Stage I (Initial lesion)

      (a) Initial response of tissues to bacterial plaque biofilm; subclinical gingivitis

      (b) Vasodilation, margination, emigration, and migration of PMNs

      (c) Light alteration of the JE

      (d) Increase of gingival crevicular fluid

      (e) 2–4 days, no clinical signs

   (2) Stage II (Early lesion)

      (a) Acute gingivitis

      (b) Continuation of initial lesion

      (c) Chronic inflammatory cells appear

      (d) JE invaginates with rete pegs

      (e) Ulceration in sulcular epithelium

      (f) Destruction of connective tissue fibers

      (g) 4–7 days, clinical signs: redness, swelling, bleeding on probing, loss of tissue tone

   (3) Stage III (Established lesion)

      (a) Chronic gingivitis

          (b) Plasma cells predominate

          (c) Chronic inflammation; blood vessels are congested and blood flow is impaired; increase in enzymes

          (d) Elongated rete pegs in JE extending deep into connective tissue; breakdown of connective fibers

          (e) 14+ days; clinical signs: moderate to severe inflammation, underlying bluish hue, changes in consistency

      (4) Stage IV (Advanced lesion)

          (a) Transition from gingivitis to periodontitis

          (b) Continuation of changes in the established lesion

          (c) Inflammation extends into connective tissue attachment and alveolar bone

          (d) Repair manifests as fibrotic tissue

          (e) Bone resorption by osteoclasts and mononuclear cells

          (f) Time interval: dependent upon host response

          (g) Clinical signs: true periodontal pockets, attachment loss, and bone loss

   d. Goals of periodontal therapy—To eliminate pain, inflammation, and bleeding; to reduce pathologic mobility and tooth loss; to restore function and tissue contour; and to prevent disease recurrence

      (1) Local therapy—Removal of plaque and all plaque retentive factors

      (2) Systemic therapy—Adjunct to control systemic complications that aggravate the disease

   e. Healing processes

      (1) Regeneration—Growth and differentiation of new cells and intercellular substances to form new tissues or parts

      (2) Repair—Healing by scar; restores tissue at the same level on the root as the base of the preexisting pocket by a process of wound healing; may not restore original architecture or function

      (3) Epithelial adaptation—Close apposition of the gingival epithelium to the tooth without complete obliteration of the pocket

      (4) New attachment—Embedding of new periodontal ligament fibers into new cementum and formation of a new gingival attachment

I. Caries/nutritional counseling

   1. Designed to help patient study individual oral problems and understand need for changing habits

   2. Explain specific changes in diet necessary for improved general and oral health

   3. Encourage elimination of sugar-containing foods and substitute low or no-sugar foods

J. Pulp vitality testing—Method used to test a suspected nonvital tooth

    1. Device—Pulp tester (*vitalometer*)

        a. Types

            (1) Battery-operated—Hand-held, battery-operated device

                (a) Advantages—Portable, easy to use

                (b) Disadvantage—Battery can run out

            (2) Plug-in—Requires electrical energy from outlet

                (a) Advantage—More dependable than battery operated

                (b) Disadvantage—Not self-contained

        b. Contraindications—Do not use on patient with a cardiac pacemaker or any electronic life-support device

        c. Technique for use

            (1) Dry teeth to be tested—Isolate teeth with cotton rolls (prevents current from passing to gingiva)

            (2) Moisten tip of tester with a small amount of toothpaste or other electrolyte

            (3) Apply tester tip

                (a) Test at least one tooth other than the one in question (preferably an adjacent tooth) and then same tooth on contralateral side (this determines normal response)

                (b) Place tester (without applying pressure) to middle or gingival third of tooth surface (Figure 7-35■)

            (4) Start with rheostat at zero; advance slowly, but steadily, until patient signals that a sensation is felt

            (5) Test each tooth at least twice and average readings

            (6) Record averaged number of all teeth tested in patient's chart

            (7) Considerations to take when applying tester tip—Avoid contact with gingiva or other soft tissues and metallic restorations

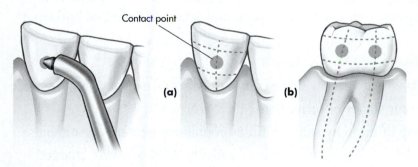

FIGURE 7-35 ■ Position of Pulp Tester: (a) Placement of Pulp Tester in Middle Third of Tooth; (b) Placement of Pulp Tester on Multirooted Tooth

K. Exfoliative cytology

    1. Classification of diagnosis of smears

        a. Class I normal

        b. Class II: minor atypia; no evidence of malignancy

        c. Class III: indeterminate; possible for cancer

        d. Class IV: suggestive of cancer; refer for biopsy

        e. Class V: positive for cancer; refer for biopsy

L. Biopsy

    1. Definition—Removal of tissue from the living organism for the purposes of microscopic examination and diagnosis

    2. Indication for biopsy

        a. Any unusual lesion that cannot be identified

        b. Lesions that do not heal within 2 weeks

        c. Persistent, thick, white, hyperkeratotic lesion that does not break through the surface epithelium

        d. Excisional biopsy—Total excision of small lesion

        e. Incisional biopsy—Small section is removed for examination

M. Toludine blue

    1. Indications for use

        a. Identify lesions that may be malignant

        b. Follow-up for patients treated previously for oral cancer to aid in recognizing early tissue changes

        c. Procedure—Mouth rinse, or applied topically with cotton-tip applicator; post-rinse solution of 1% acetic acid

        d. Results—Lesions that retain the dye are considered suspicious and should be referred for a biopsy

II. Plaque Development (Biofilm)

A. Plaque is a dense, organized bacterial system embedded in an intermicrobial matrix that adheres closely to teeth, calculus, and other structures in oral cavity

B. Life cycle

    1. Acquired pellicle

        a. Organic layer that forms within a couple of hours on a cleaned tooth surface

        b. Includes four stages of formation

            (1) Bathing of tooth by salivary fluids containing protein constituents

            (2) Selective absorption of certain negatively and positively charged glycoproteins

            (3) Loss of solubility of absorbed proteins

      (4) Alteration of glycoproteins by enzymes from bacteria and oral secretions

2. Bacterial colonization—Accumulation of bacterial flora

  a. Types of bacteria

      (1) Supragingival—Consists of a newly formed deposit (contains various gram-positive species) and mature plaque (contains facultative anaerobic microorganisms)

      (2) Subgingival—Contains motile, Gram-negative rods and spirochetes

  b. Timeline of colonization

      (1) Days 1–2—Made up primarily of Gram-positive cocci: *Streptococcus mutans* and *Streptococcus sanguis*

      (2) Days 2–4—Includes predominantly cocci, increasing numbers of gram-positive filamentous forms and slender rods

      (3) Days 4–7—Increase in filaments and more mixed flora with rods, filamentous forms, and fusobacteria; plaque located near gingival margin begins to develop a more mature flora (Gram-negative spirochetes and vibrios)

      (4) Days 7–14—Contains predominantly spirochetes and vibrios, with an increase in white blood cells; more Gram-negative and anaerobic organisms are found

      (5) Days 14–21—Continual increase of spirochetes and vibrios, white blood cells; gram-negative and anaerobic organisms

  c. Supragingival plaque

      (1) Origin—Salivary microorganisms are selectively attracted to glycoproteins from acquired pellicle

      (2) Location—Extends from coronal to margin of free gingiva

      (3) Distribution—Begins on proximal surfaces and other protected areas

      (4) Adhesion

         (a) Attached bacterial plaque—Firmly attach to acquired pellicle, other bacteria, and tooth surfaces

         (b) Unattached (surface) bacterial plaque biofilm—loose; washed away by saliva or during swallowing

      (5) Retention—Found on rough surfaces of teeth or restorations, malpositioned teeth, and carious lesions

      (6) Source—Saliva

  d. Subgingival plaque

      (1) Origin—Downward growth of bacteria from supragingival plaque

      (2) Location—Extends apically to base of sulcus

      (3) Distribution—Shallow pocket; undisturbed area in mouth

        (4) Adhesion

            (a) Attached bacterial plaque biofilm—Includes tooth surface, subgingival pellicle, and calculus

            (b) Unattached (loose) bacterial plaque biofilm—Floats between adherent plaque on tooth and pocket epithelium; unattached plaque is the most toxic

        (5) Retention—Pocket holds plaque against tooth; overhanging margins that extend into sulcus can also hold plaque

        (6) Nutritional sources—Include gingival crevicular fluid, inflammatory exudate, and leukocytes

   3. Bacterial mineralization—Addition of mineral elements, such as calcium and phosphorus, to bacterial plaque biofilm; results in a hardened deposit

      a. Supragingival calculus

        (1) Nutrient source—Saliva

        (2) Color—White, creamy yellow, or gray; may be stained with food and/or beverages, tobacco, and other pigmenting agents

        (3) Distribution—Most commonly found near opening of salivary gland ducts, facial surfaces of maxillary molars, and lingual surfaces of mandibular anterior teeth

      b. Subgingival calculus

        (1) Nutrient source—Gingival crevicular fluid and inflammatory exudate

        (2) Color—Light to dark brown, dark green, or black

        (3) Distributions—Heaviest amount on proximal surfaces, lightest on facial surfaces; occurs with or without associated supragingival calculus deposits

C. Identification methods

   1. Plaque

      a. Disclosing agents—Selective dye in a solution, tablet, or lozenge form used to identify bacterial plaque biofilm on surfaces of teeth

      b. Direct vision—Plaque may be stained with beverages, food, or other pigmented agents, making it easier to view; thick plaque may appear dull, with a furlike appearance

      c. Tactile—Plaque may feel slimy or slippery

   2. Calculus

      a. Visual examination

        (1) If calculus is not stained, it may be necessary to utilize compressed air to "dehydrate" it to view supragingivally; deflect gingival margin for observation subgingivally

(2) Diseased gingival margin does not adapt closely to tooth surface where calculus is present

(3) Transillumination of anterior teeth depicts supragingival calculus as a dark, opaque, shadow-like area on proximal surface

b. Gingival tissue color change—Dark calculus may reflect through gingival tissue

c. Tactile—Utilization of probe or explorer can be used to detect supragingival and/or subgingival calculus deposits

III. Stains

A. Classification of stains

1. Extrinsic stains—External surface of the tooth and can be removed

2. Intrinsic stains—Occur within the tooth and cannot be removed

3. Exogenous stains—Originate from sources outside the tooth; may be extrinsic or intrinsic

4. Endogenous stains—Originate within the tooth and are always intrinsic

B. Extrinsic stains

1. Yellow stain—Dull, yellowish discoloration of teeth associated with dental plaque; usually from food pigments

2. Green stain

a. Light or yellowish green to dark green stain embedded in dental plaque

b. Frequently superimposed by soft yellow or gray debris

c. Composed of chromogenic bacteria and fungi, decomposed hemoglobin, inorganic elements

d. Dark green: may become embedded in surface enamel as exogenous intrinsic stain

e. Demineralization is common under plaque

3. Black line stain

a. Black calculus-like stain that forms near gingival margin

b. Continuous fine line that follows contour of gingival crest

c. Gingiva is firm

d. Teeth are usually clean and shiny

e. Composed of microorganisms, usually Gram-positive rods embedded in intermicrobial substance

f. Mineralization is similar to the formation of calculus

4. Tobacco stain

a. Light brown to dark leathery brown or black

b. Incorporated in calculus deposits

      c. Heavy deposits may become intrinsic

      d. Composed of tar products

5. Other brown stains

      a. Brown pellicle: pellicle stains from various colors

      b. Stannous fluoride: light brown, sometimes yellowish, after repeated use of stannous fluoride

      c. Food sources; tea, coffee, soy sauce

      d. Anti-plaque agents: chlorhexidine, alexidine used in mouthwashes

      e. Betel leaf chewing

6. Orange and red stains

      a. Appear at the cervical third of tooth

      b. Occurrence is rare

      c. Composed of chromogenic bacteria

7. Metallic stains from metal-containing dust of industry

      a. Copper or brass: green or bluish-brown

      b. Iron: brown to greenish-brown

      c. Nickel: green

      d. Cadmium: yellow or golden brown

      e. Industrial workers inhale dust

8. Metallic stains from drugs

      a. Pigment of drug attaches to tooth substance

      b. Black or brown stains

C. Endogenous intrinsic stains

   1. Pulpless teeth

      a. Wide range of colors: light yellow-brown, gray, reddish-brown, bluish-black

      b. Formulated from blood and other pulp tissue elements, root canal treatment, necrosis

   2. Tetracycline

      a. Absorbed by bones and teeth, and can be transferred through the placenta during the third trimester of pregnancy, and to a child in infancy and early childhood

      b. Light green to dark yellow, or a gray-brown

      c. Discoloration depends on dosage, and length of time drug was used

   3. Imperfect tooth development

      a. Amelogenesis imperfecta: yellowish-brown or gray-brown due to incomplete or missing enamel

b. Enamel hypoplasia: teeth erupt with white spots

c. Dental fluorosis: enamel hypomineralization from excessive ingestion of fluoride, teeth erupt with white spots that later become discolored and appear light or dark brown

D. Exogenous intrinsic stains

1. Restorative materials; silver amalgam; gray or black discoloration around restoration

2. Drugs—stannous fluoride topical application: light to dark brown from tin oxide, frequently in occlusal pits and grooves

IV. Fluoride—Salt of hydrofluoric acid; stored primarily in bones and teeth

A. Actions of fluoride

1. Enters dental plaque and affects bacteria by depressing their production of acid, thereby reducing possibility of demineralization of teeth

2. Reacts with mineral elements on surface of tooth to make enamel less soluble to acid end products of bacterial metabolism

3. Facilitates remineralization of teeth that have been demineralized

B. Systemic—Pertaining to or affecting whole body

1. Sources

a. Community water fluoridation

b. Dietary fluoride supplements including fluoride drops, tablets, and lozenges, and vitamins with fluoride

c. Occurs naturally in food

2. Community water fluoridation

a. Fluoride is added to community drinking water supply

b. Most economical method of caries prevention

c. Cost varies depending on size of community and cost of installation and running of a water fluoridation plant; ranges from $0.12 to $5.41/person/year or an average of $0.51/person/year

d. Benefits—Inhibits dental caries in primary and permanent teeth; inhibits coronal and root caries

e. Range—0.7–1.2 ppm; hotter climate = lower end of range, colder climate = higher end of range

3. Dietary supplements—Include liquid drops, tablets, lozenges, and oral rinses; ingested and absorbed into blood system

a. People benefiting from fluoride supplements are those who:

(1) Use a private water supply that does not have natural fluoride and is not practical to fluoridate

        (2) Have access to less than optimum fluoride in the water

        (3) Live in community where water supply has not yet been fluoridated

    b. Method of use

        (1) May be prescribed on an individual basis for use at home or administered to school classroom groups

        (2) If in tablet form, chew first (added topical effect)

        (3) Swish mixture (either liquid or chewed tablet mixed with saliva) for 1 minute

        (4) Do not eat or drink for 30 minutes

C. Topical—Localized; on the surface; pertaining to a particular spot

  1. Professionally applied—Decreases caries by 30–40%

    a. Indications for use

        (1) Primary teeth

        (2) Posteruptive (postmaturation) period—2-year period of maturation after tooth has erupted

        (3) Active caries—New carious lesions at regular maintenance appointment

        (4) Secondary/recurrent caries—Adjacent to previous restorations

        (5) Wearing orthodontic appliances

        (6) Compromised salivary flow

        (7) Teeth supporting an overdenture

        (8) Exposed root surfaces

        (9) Lack of compliance and conscientious efforts for daily bacterial plaque biofilm removal

      (10) Low or no fluoride in drinking water

      (11) Early carious lesions

    b. Types

        (1) Stannous fluoride

           (a) Recommended and approved concentration is 8%

           (b) pH is between 2.4 and 2.8

           (c) Aqueous solutions are not stable due to formation of stannous hydroxide and stannic oxide; solutions must be prepared immediately before use

           (d) Taste is bitter and metallic

           (e) May cause extrinsic brown staining of teeth and gingival irritation

           (f) Consists of 19,360 ppm of fluoride

(2) Sodium fluoride

    (a) Recommended for use in 2% concentration

    (b) Recommended 4 applications be given 1 week apart for children ages 3, 7, 10, and 13

    (c) Has an acceptable taste

    (d) Does not discolor teeth or cause gingival irritation

    (e) pH is 9.2 (basic)

    (f) Consists of 9,040 ppm of fluoride

(3) Acidulated phosphate fluoride

    (a) Recommended for use in 1.23% concentration; generally obtained by use of 2.0% NaF and 0.34% hydrofluoric acid

    (b) Available as an aqueous solution or gel in *thixotropic* base—Gel that is able to liquefy when agitated and revert to a gelatinous state on standing

    (c) pH is between 3.0 and 3.5

    (d) Consists of 12,300 ppm of fluoride

    (e) Causes surface roughening, pitting or etching of porcelain and composite restorations

(4) Varnishes

    (a) Recommended especially for children

    (b) Contains 5% sodium fluoride; treatment usually requires only 0.3–0.5 ml of varnish, which contains 3–6 mg of fluoride

    (c) Retained for 24–48 hours

c. Application methods

  (1) Paint-on technique (solution or gel)

    (a) Isolate teeth utilizing cotton rolls and cotton roll holders—Maxillary and mandibular of one side for adults, maxillary and mandibular separately for children

    (b) Place dry-angle over Stensen's duct opening

    (c) Activate saliva ejector

    (d) Dry teeth

    (e) Moisten all teeth with fluoride, starting with mandibular arch first

    (f) Start timer for appropriate length of time

    (g) Keep surfaces moistened throughout the timing; press solution or gel into interproximal areas

    (h) At end of timing, wipe teeth briefly to remove excess gel or solution

    (i) Instruct patient to expectorate and not swallow

      (j) Proceed to other half of mouth

      (k) Instruct patient not to eat or drink for at least 30 minutes after application

    (2) Tray technique (gel or foam)

      (a) Choose appropriate tray size—Deep enough to cover entire exposed enamel

      (b) Seat patient in upright position

      (c) Load fluoride into tray—2 ml maximum for children and 2.5 ml maximum for adults (avoid overfilling)

      (d) Dry teeth thoroughly with air syringe

      (e) Insert mandibular tray and press against teeth

      (f) Insert maxillary tray and press against teeth

      (g) Insert saliva ejector between trays

      (h) Place cotton roll between trays on opposite side to prevent dislodging of trays

      (i) Leave in place for appropriate amount of time

      (j) Remove trays and request patient to expectorate, making sure patient does not swallow fluoride

      (k) Remove remaining fluoride with suction device

      (l) Instruct patient not to eat or drink for at least 30 minutes

2. Self-applied—Includes prescription and over-the-counter products

  a. Application methods

    (1) Custom tray—Fill tray with appropriate amount and type of fluoride (APF 0.5%, NaF 1.1%, and SnF_2 0.4%) and leave in mouth for designated amount of time

    (2) Rinse—Patient swishes for 1 minute with appropriate amount of fluoride and then expectorates

    (3) Toothbrushing—Fluoride gel or paste is used two or three times daily

  b. Types

    (1) Stannous fluoride—Daily rinse (0.63%) and brush-on gel (0.4%) forms

    (2) Sodium fluoride—Daily (0.05%) and weekly (0.2%) rinses, and 1.19% gel applied in tray

    (3) Acidulated phosphate—0.5% brush-on or gel applied in tray

  c. Indications for use

    (1) Stannous fluoride

      (a) 0.63% daily rinse—Use for high susceptibility to root surface caries and dentinal hypersensitivity

      (b) 0.4% brush-on gel—Use for high caries rate and hypersensitivity

(2) Sodium fluoride

    (a) 0.05% daily rinse—Use on children over 6 years of age and adults with caries susceptibility

    (b) 0.2% weekly rinse—Use for school-based programs

    (c) 1.19% gel in a tray—Use for rampant caries and when patient is undergoing radiation therapy

(3) Acidulated phosphate fluoride—0.5% brush-on gel or applied in tray for rampant caries

3. Toxicity—State or quality of being poisonous

  a. Acute fluoride toxicity—Rapid intake of an excess dose over a short time; average lethal dose is 4–5 grams; *note:* Generally death from acute fluoride toxicity occurs within 4 hours of ingestion

    (1) Signs

      (a) Nausea (caused by formation of hydrofluoric acid in the stomach)

      (b) Vomiting

      (c) Hypersalivation

      (d) Abdominal pain

      (e) Diarrhea

      (f) Cramping of arms and legs due to drop in blood calcium

      (g) Bronchospasm

      (h) Cardiac arrest

      (i) Ventricular fibrillation

      (j) Fixed and dilated pupils

      (k) Hyperkalemia and hypocalcemia

    (2) Treatment—Urgency of treatment is based on number of multiples of 5 mg/kg of fluoride ingested; *note:* The blood reaches its maximum level 1/2 to 1 hour after ingestion of fluoride

      (a) Induce vomiting (e.g., ipecac syrup or digital stimulation)

      (b) Ingest fluoride-binding agents (e.g., milk, lime water, liquid or gel antacids that contain aluminum or magnesium hydroxide)

      (c) Seek medical attention, if needed (maintain blood calcium levels with intravenous calcium, gastric lavage, and/or blood dialysis)

  b. Chronic—Long-term ingestion of fluoride in amounts that exceed approved therapeutic levels

    (1) Factors that increase severity of chronic fluoride toxicity

      (a) Increase in consumption of naturally fluoridated water

      (b) Elevated intake of fluoride in food

      (c) Nutritional diseases

(d) Low-calcium diets

c. Dental fluorosis—Developmental defect of enamel that occurs when an excessive amount of fluoride is ingested during period of enamel formation

(1) Hypomineralized fluorotic region appears as matte white or opaque

(2) Usually symmetrical in mouth

(3) Different clinical degrees of fluorosis include

(a) Normal—No fluorosis

(b) Questionable—Few white flecks or white spots (snow-capping); usually involve incisal edges of anterior teeth or cusps of posterior teeth

(c) Very mild—Small opaque areas involving < 25% of surface

(d) Mild—White opacities are more extensive, but involve < 50% of surface

(e) Moderate—All enamel surfaces are affected with frequent brown staining

(f) Severe—Discrete pitting, brown stains are widespread, with all enamel surface affected; teeth are not discolored at time of eruption—discoloration is due to posteruptive uptake of exogenous stains from diet

V. Mouth Rinses

A. Types

1. Cosmetic—Improve appearance of oral cavity (e.g., reduce oral malodor)

2. Therapeutic—Reduce some disease in mouth (e.g., dental caries, bacterial plaque biofilm, gingivitis); *does not* kill all bacteria in mouth; it reduces the number

B. Ingredients

1. Oxygenating agents

a. Purpose—Cleanse by effervescent action; short-lasting antimicrobial effect; only as long as oxygen is being released

b. Adverse effects—Long-term use results in overgrowth of bacteria, resulting in black, hairy tongue

c. Other information—Common ingredients include hydrogen peroxide, sodium perborate, and urea peroxide

2. Chlorhexidine gluconate—0.12% prescription plaque control rinse

a. Purpose

(1) Absorbed into teeth and pellicle

(2) Time-released over 12–24 hours (substantivity), prolonging bacteriocidal effect

(3) Lysis cell wall consisting of gram-positive and -negative microorganisms and fungi

b. Adverse effects

(1) Brown staining of teeth

(2) Temporary loss of taste

(3) Bitter taste

(4) Dryness, soreness, and burning sensation of mucosa

(5) Epithelial desquamation

(6) Discoloration of teeth, tongue, and restorations

(7) Slight increase in supragingival calculus formation

c. Additional information

(1) Available in other parts of world as 0.2% solution

(2) Used as a preprocedural rinse to lower oral bacterial count

(3) Decreases supragingival bacterial plaque biofilm formation and inhibits development of gingivitis

(4) Used for short-term adjunctive therapy after surgical treatment that limits mechanical plaque control

(5) Used on selective patients to control inflammation in necrotizing ulcerative gingivitis

(6) Used on selective patients to encourage and motivate when oral hygiene has been neglected for a period of time

(7) Suppresses growth of *mutans streptococci*

(8) Should not be used immediately before or after regular toothbrushing as it is inactivated by most dentifrice surfactants

(9) Used as a 30-second rinse, twice daily, with 1 oz of solution

(10) Common names include Peridex and Perioguard

3. Essential oils/phenolic compounds

a. Purpose—Antiplaque and antigingivitis compounds

b. Adverse effects—Has a bitter taste

c. Other information

(1) Active ingredients include thymol, menthol, eucalyptol, and methyl salicylate

(2) Original formula contains 26.9% alcohol; other variety contains 21.6% alcohol

(3) Reduces both plaque accumulation and severity of gingivitis by up to 34%

(4) Common name is Listerine

    d. Quaternary ammonia compounds

      (1) Purpose

        (a) Decreases bacterial cell wall permeability and metabolism

        (b) Possesses no substantivity

        (c) Recommended to control halitosis, not gingivitis

    e. Sanguinarine—Alters bacterial cell wall structure and may inhibit bacterial adhesion

    f. Stannous fluoride

      (1) Purpose

        (a) May possess antiplaque properties

        (b) May alter bacterial cell metabolism or cell adhesion properties

        (c) May reduce plaque for a short time; long-term benefits are unknown

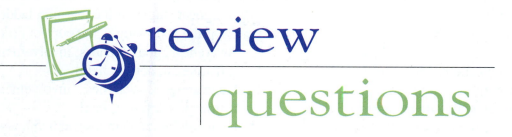
review questions

DIRECTIONS Each of the questions or incomplete statements below is followed by suggested answers or completions. Select the **one** answer that is best in each case.

1. The maximum amount of pressure exerted against the walls of a blood vessel is called
   A. Pulse
   B. Diastolic pressure
   C. Systolic pressure
   D. Cardiac output

2. To determine the proper size of a blood pressure cuff, the width needs to be 20%
   A. Less than the diameter of the upper arm.
   B. Greater than the diameter of the upper arm.
   C. Less than the diameter of the lower arm.
   D. Greater than the diameter of the lower arm.

3. All of the following are types of manometers EXCEPT one. Which one is the EXCEPTION?
   A. Mercury
   B. Aneroid
   C. Titanium
   D. Electronic

4. All of the following factors can INCREASE blood pressure EXCEPT one. Which one is the EXCEPTION?
   A. Fainting
   B. Stimulants
   C. Use of oral contraceptives
   D. Eating

5. All of the following factors can DECREASE body temperature EXCEPT one. Which one is the EXCEPTION?
   A. Starvation
   B. Hyperthyroidism
   C. Hemorrhage
   D. Physiological shock

6. Which of the following arteries is found in the antecubital space?
   A. Radial
   B. Facial
   C. Carotid
   D. Brachial

7. Which of the following palpation methods involves using both hands at the same time to examine corresponding structures on opposite sides of the body?
   A. Bilateral
   B. Bimanual
   C. Digital
   D. Bidigital

8. Using G.V. Black's classification system, which of the following is the correct description of a Class V carious lesion?
   A. Radiographic decay on the mesial of #30
   B. Explorer detectable decay on the occlusal of #30
   C. Explorer detectable decay on the mesial-lingual cusp tip of #30
   D. Explorer detectable decay on the lingual cervical third of #30

9. A patient presents with the following occlusal classification: The mesial surface of the permanent maxillary canine is distal to the distal surface of the permanent mandibular canine by at least the width of a premolar. Which of the following is the patient's occlusal classification?
   A. Class I
   B. Class II, Division I
   C. Class II, Division II
   D. Class III

10. An anterior crossbite involves the maxillary incisors being facial to the mandibular incisors. A posterior crossbite involves the facial cusps of the maxillary posterior teeth being positioned facial to the facial cusps of the mandibular posterior teeth.
   A. The first statement is TRUE, the second statement is FALSE.
   B. Both statements are TRUE.
   C. The first statement is FALSE, the second statement is TRUE.
   D. Both statements are FALSE.

11. A periodontal assessment of #19 reveals 3 mm from the cementoenamel junction (CEJ) to the gingival margin and 4 mm from the gingival margin to the base of the pocket. In millimeters, what is the total (actual) amount of recession?
   A. 1
   B. 3
   C. 4
   D. 7

12. In the principles of learning, from the lowest to highest stages of the learning ladder, which of the following is the correct order?
   A. Awareness, unawareness, involvement, self-interest, action, habit
   B. Unawareness, awareness, involvement, action, self-interest, habit
   C. Unawareness, awareness, self-interest, involvement, habit, action
   D. Unawareness, awareness, self-interest, involvement, action, habit

13. All of the following describe supragingival calculus EXCEPT one. Which one is the EXCEPTION?
   A. Its nutrient sources are gingival crevicular fluid and inflammatory exudate.
   B. Its color can vary depending on agents that pigment it.
   C. It is commonly located on the facial of maxillary molars.
   D. It is commonly located on the lingual of mandibular incisors.

14. All of following are objectives of toothbrushing EXCEPT one. Which one is the EXCEPTION?
   A. Remove calculus and disturb reformation
   B. Remove food debris
   C. Stimulate gingival tissues
   D. Apply therapeutic agents

15. Placing the toothbrush at a 45-degree angle to the apex of the tooth, with part of the brush resting on the gingiva and the other part on the tooth, represents which of the following toothbrushing methods?
   A. Bass
   B. Charters
   C. Fones
   D. Stillman

16. Which of the following factors do NOT need to be considered when recommending a specific toothbrushing technique?
    A. Patient's oral health
    B. Size of toothbrush
    C. Patient's systemic health status
    D. Patient's manual dexterity

17. All of the following patients should be considered when recommending an automatic toothbrush EXCEPT one. Which one is the EXCEPTION?
    A. Elderly
    B. Those who require a large handle
    C. Those with arthritis or poor manual dexterity
    D. Those with orthodontia

18. Which type of dental floss would be MOST appropriate for normal contact areas?
    A. Polytetrafluoroethylene
    B. Tape
    C. Unwaxed
    D. Waxed

19. All of the following indicate use of a single-tufted brush (end-tuft, unituft) EXCEPT one. Which one is the EXCEPTION?
    A. Distal area of the most posterior tooth
    B. Pontics
    C. Irregular gingival margins around migrated or malposed teeth
    D. Interdental cleaning of concave proximal tooth surfaces

20. The action of an oral irrigating device flushes away
    A. Loosely adherent microflora located apical to the gingival margin
    B. Loosely adherent microflora located coronal to the gingival margin
    C. Attached microflora located apical to the gingival margin
    D. Attached microflora located coronal to the gingival margin

21. All of the following are types of therapeutic dentifrices EXCEPT one. Which one is the EXCEPTION?
    A. Fluoride-containing dentifrice
    B. Baking soda–peroxide–fluoride dentifrice
    C. Antimicrobial dentifrice
    D. Antitartar dentifrice

22. Which of the following components of a dentifrice prevents bacterial growth and prolongs shelf life?
    A. Humectant
    B. Preservative
    C. Sweetening agent
    D. Flavoring agent

23. Which of the following active ingredients is found in antitartar dentifrice?
    A. Potassium nitrate
    B. Strontium chloride
    C. Zinc citrate trihydrate
    D. Sodium citrate

24. Where is fluoride primarily stored in the body?
    A. Small intestine *← absorbed*
    B. Kidneys
    C. Bloodstream
    D. Bones and teeth *– stored*

25. Which method of systemic fluoride is MOST economical for caries prevention?
    A. Community water fluoridation
    B. Dietary fluoride supplements
    C. Naturally occurring in food
    D. Professional fluoride treatment

26. What is the appropriate dietary fluoride supplement, in milligrams, for a 3-year-old patient who lives in an area with 0.4 ppm of fluoride in the water?
    A. None
    B. 0.25
    C. 0.5
    D. 1

27. All of the following indicate use of a professional topical fluoride EXCEPT one. Which one is the EXCEPTION?
    A. Wearing orthodontic appliances
    B. Compromised salivary flow
    C. Low community water fluoridation level
    D. Primary teeth

28. For an adult patient, the maximum amount of fluoride recommended for a professionally applied topical treatment (tray technique), in milliliters, is:
    A. 0.2
    B. 0.25
    C. 2
    D. 2.5

29. Which of the following professional topical fluorides has a recommended concentration of 1.23%?
    A. Acidulated phosphate fluoride
    B. Monofluorophosphate
    C. Sodium fluoride
    D. Stannous fluoride

30. What is the first sign of acute fluoride toxicity?
    A. Abdominal pain
    B. Diarrhea
    C. Nausea
    D. Vomiting

31. All of the following factors increase the severity of chronic fluoride toxicity EXCEPT one. Which one is the EXCEPTION?
    A. Increase in consumption of naturally fluoridated water
    B. Swallowing an excess amount of fluoride during a professional fluoride treatment
    C. Elevated intake of fluoride in food
    D. Low-calcium diet

32. In mouth rinses, which of the following ingredients provides cleansing by an effervescent action?
    A. Chlorhexidine gluconate
    B. Essential oils
    C. Oxygenating agents
    D. Stannous fluoride

33. All of the following are adverse effects of chlorhexidine gluconate EXCEPT one. Which one is the EXCEPTION?
    A. Bitter taste
    B. Brown staining of teeth
    C. Epithelial desquamation
    D. White pitting of teeth

34. Which of the following relates to autopolymerization of dental sealants?
    A. Setting time cannot be controlled once catalyst is added
    B. Shorter polymerization time
    C. No mixing of materials
    D. Requires a special curing light

35. While examining the TMJ, the hygienist notes a popping sound. What type of assessment skill is used to hear the sound?
    A. Observation
    B. Palpation
    C. Auscultation
    D. Olfaction

36. While assessing the dentition, the hygienist notices a suspicious area around the margin of an occlusal restoration and radiographically, a radiolucent area is evident. What type of decay is MOST likely?
    A. Incipient
    B. Arrested
    C. Recurrent
    D. Root

37. Upon examining a patient's profile, the hygienist notices that the upper lip is protruded 6 mm to the lower lip. What is the MOST likely occlusal relationship?
    A. Prognathic
    B. Retrognathic
    C. Orthognathic
    D. Normal

38. What is the malrelationship of teeth when vertical space is between the mandibular and maxillary arches?
    A. Openbite
    B. Edge-to-edge
    C. End-to-end
    D. Crossbite

39. A patient demonstrates flossing between teeth #24 and #25. As the floss is moved from #24 to #25, it is kept in a horizontal position, resulting in tissue trauma. Which gingival tissue is involved?
    A. Attached
    B. Gingival margin
    C. Free gingival margin
    D. Interdental papilla

40. When the gingival margin migrates coronally, it is described as:
    A. Recession
    B. A periodontal pocket
    C. Pseudopocket
    D. Bulbous papilla

41. Which of the following permanent teeth are utilized to classify occlusion?
    A. Second molar
    B. Second premolars
    C. First premolars
    D. First molars

42. Which of the following ingredients serves to retain moisture in commercial toothpaste?
    A. Detergent
    B. Humectant
    C. Surfactant
    D. Binder
    E. Surface agent

43. Normal respiration rate for an adult is which of the following?
    A. 14–20 per minute
    B. 25–40 per minute
    C. 30–40 per minute
    D. 60–80 per minute

44. Diastolic pressure represents which of the following?
    A. Aortic pressure
    B. Ventricular relaxation
    C. Heart rate
    D. Ventricular contraction

45. A retrognathic profile is usually associated with which of the following classification of malocclusion?
    A. Class I
    B. Class II
    C. Class III

46. A prognathic profile is usually associated with which of the following classification of malocclusion?
    A. Class I
    B. Class II
    C. Class III

47. A mesial cavity in a mandibular right second premolar is classified as a:
    A. Class I
    B. Class II
    C. Class III
    D. Class IV
    E. Class V

review questions

48. Subgingival calculus differs from supragingival calculus in:
    A. Location
    B. Density
    C. Color
    D. A and C only
    E. A, B, and C

49. Which of the following types of dental stains can become embedded in decalcified surface enamel?
    A. Orange stain
    B. Black line stain
    C. Brown stain
    D. Green stain

50. Oral irrigators (water irrigation devices) are NOT useful for:
    A. Removing bacterial plaque biofilm
    B. Stimulating the gingival
    C. Dislodging debris from orthodontic appliances
    D. All of the above

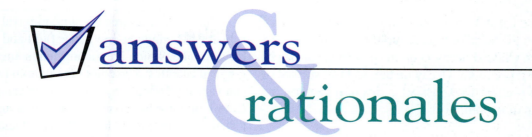

answers & rationales

1.

C. Systolic pressure is the period during which blood is forced into the aorta and pulmonary artery, resulting in the maximum amount of pressure exerted against the walls of the blood vessel. Pulse is the intermittent throbbing sensation felt when the fingers are pressed against an artery. It is an indirect measurement of the patient's cardiac output. The diastolic pressure is the minimum amount of pressure exerted against the walls of the vessels. It is the phase of the cardiac cycle in which the heart relaxes between contractions.

2.

B. The proper size of a blood pressure cuff is 20% greater than the diameter of the arm. If the cuff is too large, the reading will be lower than the actual one. If the cuff is too small, the reading will be higher than the actual one.

3.

C. Titanium is NOT a type of manometer. Mercury, aneroid, and electric are types of manometers.

4.

A. Fainting does NOT cause an increase, but rather a decrease in blood pressure. Use of stimulants and contraceptives and eating cause an increase in blood pressure.

5.

B. Hyperthyroidism is NOT a factor in decreasing temperature. Starvation, hemorrhage, and physiological shock can decrease body temperature.

6.

D. The brachial artery is found in the antecubital space of the elbow. The radial artery is found on the radial portion (thumb-side) of the wrist. The carotid artery is lateral to the larynx. The facial artery is found crossing the border of the mandible.

7.

A. The bilateral palpation technique uses both hands at the same time to examine corresponding structures on opposite sides of the body. The bimanual technique utilizes finger(s) and thumb from each hand simultaneously. Bidigital technique involves the use of a finger and thumb of the same hand. Digital technique involves the use of a single finger.

8.

D. The Class V category involves the cervical third of either the facial or lingual surface—not the pits and fissures. Class II decay is on the proximal surface of any posterior tooth. Decay on the occlusal surface of a tooth is a Class I. Class VI caries is evident on the cusp tip of a tooth.

9.

D. Class III occlusal relationship involves the mesial surface of the permanent maxillary canine located distally to the distal surface of the permanent mandibular canine by at least the width of a premolar. When the maxillary canine occludes with the distal half of the mandibular canine and the mesial half of the mandibular first premolar, it is a Class I occlusion. When the distal surface of the maxillary canine is mesial to the mesial surface of the mandibular canine, by a minimum width of half of a premolar, it is a Class II occlusion.

10.

D. Both statements are false. In an anterior crossbite, the maxillary incisors are located lingually to the mandibular incisors. In a posterior crossbite, the maxillary posterior teeth are located lingual to the respective mandibular posterior teeth.

11.

D. The total amount of recession is 7 mm as a result of the distance measured from the CEJ to the base of the pocket; 3 mm is the amount of recession and 4 mm is the depth of the gingival sulcus.

12.

D. The correct order for the stages of the learning ladder, from lowest to highest, is unawareness, awareness, self-interest, involvement, action, habit (Hint: Unusual Apes Sit In A Hut).

13.

A. The nutrient source for supragingival calculus is saliva, NOT gingival crevicular fluid and inflammatory exudate, which are the nutrient sources for subgingival calculus. The color of supragingival calculus can vary depending on agents, which can pigment it. Common coloring agents include food and bacteria. Calculus is commonly located on the facial of maxillary molars and lingual of the mandibular incisors, adjacent to where salivary glands are located.

14.

A. Calculus cannot be removed with a toothbrush since it is a mineralized deposit. It must be removed with hand or ultrasonic/sonic instrumentation. Objectives of toothbrushing include removing food debris, stimulating gingival tissues, and applying therapeutic agents such as fluoride.

15.

D. The Stillman brushing technique involves placing the brush at a 45-degree angle to the tooth, with part of the bristles on the soft tissue and part on the tooth. The Bass method of toothbrushing involves placing the brush at a 45-degree angle to the apex of the tooth, applying gentle pressure so the bristles enter the sulcus. With the Charters method, the toothbrush is placed at 90 degrees to the long axis of the tooth. The bristles are gently placed between the teeth, but do not rest on the gingiva. The Fones method includes brushing both arches at the same time. The bristles are placed perpendicular to the crown of the tooth and the brush is activated using a large circular motion.

16.

B. The size of the toothbrush does NOT need to be considered when recommending a specific toothbrushing technique, but should be considered when determining which toothbrush to recommend to the patient. The patient's oral health and systemic health status and manual dexterity should be considered when recommending a specific toothbrushing technique.

17.

D. An automatic toothbrush is NOT indicated for orthodontic patients; it is recommended for the elderly, those with arthritis/poor manual dexterity, and those who may require a large handle.

18.

D. Waxed dental floss is most appropriate for normal contact areas. Polytetrafluoroethylene dental floss is made of a synthetic material and is indicated for use in tight contact areas and/or rough tooth surfaces, because it is less likely to shred. Dental tape is broad and flat waxed floss indicated for spaces without tight contact areas. Unwaxed floss is indicated in tight contact areas.

19.

D. A single tufted brush is not used for interdental cleaning of concave proximal tooth surfaces because of its size. The distal of most posterior teeth, pontics, and irregular gingival margins around migrated or malposed teeth are areas indicated for a single-tufted brush.

20.

B. An oral irrigating device flushes away loosely adherent microflora located coronally to the gingival margin. It is efficient in disrupting microflora that is NOT attached to the tooth structure or gingival tissue on the coronal portion of the tooth only.

21.

D. Antitartar dentifrice is NOT a type of therapeutic dentifrice. The ADA considers calculus inhibition a cosmetic benefit. Therapeutic dentifrices containing fluoride, baking soda–peroxide–fluoride, and antimicrobial agents reduce disease in the mouth.

22.

B. The preservative in dentifrice prevents bacterial growth, which prolongs the shelf life of the product.

Humectants retain moisture in a dentifrice and sweetening agents impart a pleasant flavor for patient acceptance. Flavoring agents make the toothpaste desirable and mask other unpleasant flavors.

23.

C. Zinc citrate trihydrate is an active ingredient in antitartar dentifrices. Potassium nitrate, strontium chloride, and sodium citrate are found in antihypersensitivity dentifrices.

24.

D. Fluoride is primarily stored in bones and teeth in the human body. Fluoride is rapidly absorbed by the small intestine, excreted via the kidneys, and can be found in the bloodstream.

25.

A. Community fluoridation is the most economical systemic method for caries prevention. Dietary fluoride supplements and foods that naturally contain fluoride are sources of systemic fluoride, but are not as economical as community fluoridation. Professional fluoride treatment is a topical form of fluoridation.

26.

B. A 3-year-old child would require a supplemental fluoride of 0.25 if the community water supply is < 0.4 ppm of fluoride. However, a 3-year-old may be prescribed 0.5 mg of fluoride if the concentration of community fluoride is less than 0.3 ppm. A supplement of 1 mg would never be prescribed to a 3-year-old.

27.

C. Low community water fluoridation level is NOT an indication for applying professional topical fluoride. However, wearing orthodontic appliances, having a compromised salivary flow, and primary teeth are indications for use of a professional topical fluoride treatment.

28.

D. An adult patient would receive 2.5 ml of fluoride during a professional fluoride treatment. A child fluoride treatment would contain 2.0 ml of fluoride. It is important to administer the correct amount to receive the full benefit of fluoride. Administering too much fluoride could cause acute fluoride toxicity if swallowed.

29.

A. Acidulated phosphate fluoride has a recommended concentration of 1.23%. This is obtained by combining 2.0% sodium fluoride and 0.34% hydrofluoric acid. Monofluorophosphate is found in dentifrices only. Professionally, sodium and stannous fluorides are available at 2.0% and 8.0%, respectively.

30.

C. The first sign of acute fluoride toxicity is nausea. Following nausea, the patient may also experience vomiting, abdominal pain, and diarrhea.

31.

B. Swallowing an excess amount of fluoride during a professional fluoride treatment is an example of acute, not chronic, fluoride toxicity. Factors that increase the severity of chronic fluoride toxicity include an increase in the consumption of fluoridated water, elevated intake of fluoride in food, and a low-calcium diet.

32.

C. Oxygenating agents cleanse the mouth by an effervescent action. Chlorhexidine gluconate is an antimicrobial that has bactericidal effects. Essential oils are the active ingredients in Listerine and have both antigingivitis and antiplaque effects. Stannous fluoride is a therapeutic agent.

33.

D. Chlorhexidine gluconate does NOT produce white pitting of teeth. Bitter taste, brown staining of teeth, and epithelial desquamation are adverse effects of chlorhexidine gluconate.

34.

A. Autopolymerization or self-cured sealants require the mixing of a monomer and a catalyst. Once the catalyst is added, the setting time cannot be controlled. Light cured or photopolymerization involves a shorter polymerization time, no mixing of materials, and a special curing light.

35.

C. The examination skill of auscultation involves listening to the sounds made by various structures and functions. Observation involves the visual deviation of the structures. While palpating the TMJ, the dental hygienist would feel the popping sensation. Olfaction is an examination skill of smell.

36.

C. Recurrent decay is a lesion that occurs at the margin(s) of an existing restoration. An incipient lesion can be arrested before permanent damage to the tooth has occurred. With arrested decay, remineralization has occurred. Root caries are found on the root surfaces, not on the occlusal surfaces.

37.

C. The patient presents with a retrognathic profile, which is associated with a Class II occlusal relationship. Normal occlusion and Class I malocclusion present with an orthognathic profile. Class I malocclusion is differentiated from a normal occlusion because of malposed teeth. Class III malocclusion involves a prognathic facial profile.

38.

A. An openbite is the lack of occlusal or incisal contact between one or more maxillary and mandibular teeth. Edge-to-edge malrelationship involves the anterior teeth only. The teeth meet on the incisal edges. End-to-end malrelationship is similar to edge-to-edge, except it involves the posterior teeth. Crossbite malrelationship is present when the maxillary teeth are positioned lingually to the mandibular teeth.

39.

D. The interdental gingiva is traumatized when the floss is not lifted toward the incisal edge while moving from one tooth to the next. The attached gingiva is not affected by flossing because it is located apical to the interdental gingiva. The gingival and free gingival margins are interchangeable terms describing the tissue closest to the crown of the tooth.

40.

C. Pseudopocket is a term used when the marginal gingiva has moved coronally and produced an artificially deepened sulcus. Recession is the apical migration of the gingival margin. A periodontal pocket results from loss of attachment of gingival tissues. Bulbous papilla is a clinical characteristic of diseased gingiva involving the interdental papilla.

41.

D. The determination of the classification of occlusion is based on the principles of Edward H. Angle. He defined normal occlusion as the normal relation of the occlusal inclined planes of the teeth when the jaws are closed and based his system of classification on the relationship of the permanent first molars.

42.

B. Humectants serve to retain moisture in commercial toothpastes. They comprise 20–40% of the total composition of commercial toothpastes. Commonly used humectants are sorbitol, glycerol, and propylene glycol.

43.

A. Normal respiration rate for adults is 14–20 per minute. For children, rates range from 18–30. Factors that may increase respiration include exercise, excitement, pain, hemorrhage, and shock. Sleep, pulmonary insufficiency, and certain drugs may decrease respiration.

44.

B. Diastolic pressure represents ventricular relaxation. Systolic pressure represents ventricular contraction. Normal adult blood pressure is 120/80.

45.

B. A retrognathic profile is usually associated with Class II occlusion. Class I occlusion is associated with a mesognathic profile. Class III occlusion is associated with prognathic profile.

46.

C. A prognathic profile is usually associated with Class III occlusion. Persons with prognathic profiles have normal maxillas and protruded mandibles. The buccal groove of the mandibular first permanent molar is mesial to the mesiobuccal cusp of the maxillary first permanent molar by at least the width of a premolar.

47.

B. A mesial cavity in a mandibular right second premolar is classified as a Class II. Class II cavities are found in proximal surfaces of premolars and molars.

48.

E. Subgingival calculus differs from supragingival calculus in location, density, and color. Subgingival calculus is harder and more dense than supragingival calculus. Subgingival calculus is usually heaviest on proximal surfaces and lightest on facial surfaces.

49.

D. Dark green stain occasionally becomes embedded in surface enamel. Often the enamel under the stain is decalcified. Green stain results from oral uncleanliness and originates from chromogenic bacteria and fungi.

50.

A. Oral irrigators (water spray devices) are useful for loosening debris from the gingival sulcus and dislodging debris from orthodontic appliances. Oral irrigators will disrupt bacteria plaque, but will not remove it. Use of oral irrigation is sometimes referred to as hydrotherapy.

8 Obtaining and Interpreting Radiographs

The science of oral and maxillofacial radiology is based on principles of physics, chemistry, and biology. Understanding the function and applications of diagnostic imaging modalities used in dentistry and other health care professions is fundamental to the specialty.

chapter objectives

After completion of this chapter, the learner should be able to:

- ➤ Discuss radiation physics
- ➤ Describe the production of radiation
- ➤ Discuss image receptors
- ➤ Describe exposure factors
- ➤ Describe intraoral radiographic techniques
- ➤ Discuss radiation biology and safety
- ➤ Describe radiographic infection control
- ➤ Describe darkroom processing and quality assurance
- ➤ Describe intraoral technical and processing error identification and correction
- ➤ Describe panoramic radiography and error correction
- ➤ Discuss localization techniques
- ➤ Discuss radiographic anatomy
- ➤ Describe film mounting and duplication

➤ INTERPRETATION

I. Radiation Physics

A. Radiation—Transmission of energy through space and matter in the form of waves or particles

B. Types of radiation

    1. Electromagnetic radiation—Transmission of wave energy through space and matter as a combination of electric and magnetic fields

      a. Characteristics

        (1) Have no mass

        (2) No electrical charge

        (3) Travel at the speed of light in a straight but oscillating path

        (4) Exists in a wide range of magnitudes or energy continuum (Figure 8-1■)

        (5) Dualistic nature—Some characteristics best explained by wave theory, some by quantum theory

      b. Wave theory—Radiation propagated in form of waves (Figure 8-2■)

        (1) Wave motion—Wavelength; one wavelength is the distance from crest to crest or valley to valley

        (2) Frequency—Number of crests or valleys per unit of time

        (3) Wavelength and frequency determine energy level; short wavelength and high frequency = high energy level

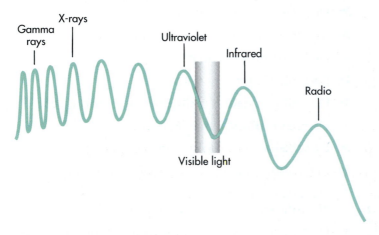

FIGURE 8-1 ■ Electromagnetic Spectrum

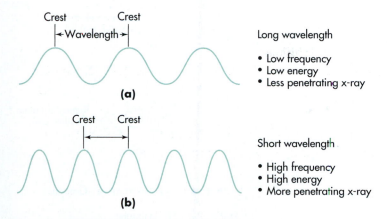

FIGURE 8-2 ■ Differences in Wavelengths and Frequencies

    c. Quantum theory

        (1) Describes electromagnetic radiation as small bundles of energy called quanta or photons

        (2) Transfer of energy occurs as a flux of quanta or photons; each photon travels at the speed of light and contains specific amount of energy

        (3) Quantum theory useful for describing interaction of radiation with atoms and the production of x-rays

    d. Examples

        (1) Long wavelengths—Radar, television, radio

        (2) Short wavelengths—Visible light, ultraviolet light, x-rays

  2. Particulate radiation—Atomic nuclei or subatomic particles that travel at high velocity

    a. Characteristics

        (1) Have mass and energy

        (2) All particles have an electrical charge except neutrons

        (3) Travel in straight lines at high speeds

    b. Examples

        (1) Alpha particles, beta particles, and cathode rays (electrons)

        (2) Nucleons—Protons (+) and neutrons (Figure 8-3■)

C. Properties of x-rays

  1. Are invisible

  2. Travel in straight lines

  3. Travel at speed of light

  4. Have no mass or weight

  5. Have no charge

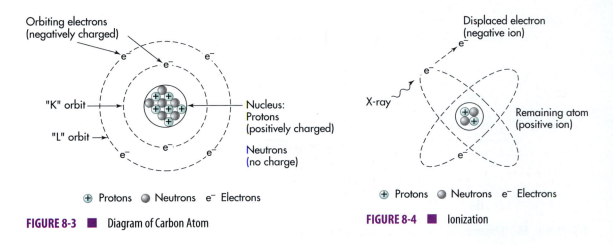

FIGURE 8-3 ■ Diagram of Carbon Atom

FIGURE 8-4 ■ Ionization

6. Interact with matter causing ionization

7. Can penetrate opaque tissues and structures

8. Can affect photographic film emulsion (causing a latent image)

9. Can affect living tissue

D. Ionization—Process by which a neutral atom acquires a positive or negative charge (Figure 8-4■)

1. Electromagnetic radiation and particulate radiation of sufficient energy can interact with atoms and create ion pairs

2. Ion pair: + ion = atom with lost electron, ~ ion = the ejected electron

3. Mechanism by which biological systems are altered or damaged

4. Examples of ionizing radiation

a. Electromagnetic—Ultraviolet light, x-rays, gamma rays

b. Particulate—Alpha particles, beta particles, protons

II. Production of Radiation

A. X-ray generating equipment and components

1. Control panel components (Figure 8-5■)

a. Main on/off switch

b. Milliamperage (mA) selector—Adjusts amount or flow of electrical current

(1) 1 mA = 1/1000 ampere

(2) Typically fixed at a specific mA such as 10 mA

c. Kilovoltage (kVp) selector—Adjusts potential difference or rate of electrical current

(1) 1 kVp = 1,000 volts

(2) Usually fixed at 70 kVp

(3) Variable kVp machines range from 50 to 100 kVp

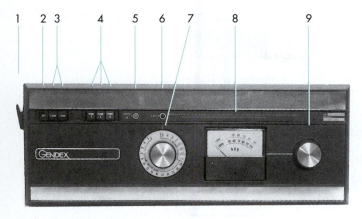

FIGURE 8-5 ■ Control Panel

    d. Timer—Regulates the length of x-ray exposure; calibrated as fraction of a second

      (1) Formats

        (a) Standard fractions of a second (1/2 second)

        (b) Decimal fractions of a second (.50 second)

        (c) Impulses (30 impulses/second)

      (2) Conversion

        (a) To convert exposure time in seconds to impulses, multiply by 60 (1/2 × 60 = 30 impulses)

        (b) To convert impulses to exposure time in seconds, divide by 60 (30 ÷ 60 = 30/60 or 1/2 or .50)

    e. Exposure switch/button—Engages system to produce x-rays

    f. X-ray emission light/audible signal—Indicates when x-rays are being produced

2. X-ray tubehead—Metal encasement housing the x-ray production components (Figure 8-6■)

    a. X-ray tube—Air-evacuated leaded glass tube with unleaded glass window to allow x-rays to leave x-ray tube

    b. Cathode (~) electrode

      (1) Molybdenum metal focusing cup

      (2) Tungsten filament—Thin wire

      (3) Controlled by low-voltage (8–12 volts) electrical circuit

    c. Anode (+) electrode

      (1) Copper metal sheath or rod

      (2) Tungsten metal "target" (focal spot) embedded on the surface of copper rod

      (3) Controlled by high-voltage (50,000–100,000 volts) circuit

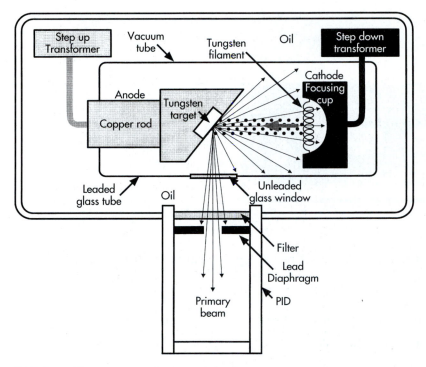

FIGURE 8-6 ■ Components of an X-ray Tubehead

    d. Transformers—Devices used to alter electrical current

        (1) Step-down transformer or low-voltage (mA) circuit; decreases electrical current from 110 or 220 volts to 3–5 volts to heat tungsten filament

        (2) Step-up transformer or high-voltage (kVp) circuit; increases the voltage as required by the technique the radiographer is using from 110 or 220 to 60–90 kVp to produce x-rays

        (3) Autotransformer—Voltage compensator that corrects minor fluctuations in the current flowing through the wires; allows selection of variable kVp settings on x-ray units with a kVp range

    e. Oil—Surrounds x-ray tube and serves to dissipate heat

    f. X-ray filter—Millimeter layers of aluminum metal used to filter x-ray beam

    g. Lead diaphragm or collimator—Device that restricts size of x-ray beam

    h. PID (position indicating device) or x-ray cone—Device that guides the x-ray beam toward patient and receptor

B. Production of x-rays

    1. Turn on the machine and set the exposure factors—mA, kVp, time

    2. Depress the exposure button to activate the system to produce x-rays

    3. Heat the tungsten filament

        a. Controlled by the mA setting via the step-down transformer

    b. Thermionic emission—Occurs whenever a filament is heated to incandescence (glowing red with heat), creating an electron cloud

    c. Provides a source of particles to use for producing x-rays

    d. Once the filament is heated, a time delay switch applies power to the high-voltage circuit

4. Electrons set in motion

    a. + charged anode attracts the electrons from the ~ charged cathode

    b. Speed of the traveling electrons is controlled by the kVp setting via the step-up transformer; the higher the kilovoltage, the greater the speed

5. Anode target bombardment

    a. Cathode electron particles interact with the tungsten target atoms; < 1% (≈ 0.2%) of the interactions produce x-rays

    (1) Bremsstrahlung (general or braking) radiation—Interactions at or near the nucleus that suddenly stop or brake high-speed electrons; major source of x-ray photons

    (2) Characteristic radiation—K, L shell interactions that dislodge an electron, attracting an electron from the next shell to fill the vacancy; minor source of x-ray photons (energy loss is how the x-ray is given off)

    b. Cathode electron particles interact with outer electron shells of tungsten target atoms; > 99% (≈ 99.8%) of the interactions produce heat

6. Heat is conducted via the copper sheath/rod into the oil surrounding the x-ray tube

7. X-rays leave the glass tube via the unleaded glass window

8. Primary x-ray beam

    a. Filtered with aluminum to remove long-wavelength x-rays

    b. Collimated to reduce the size of the x-ray beam

    c. Guided through the PID (x-ray cone) for patient radiography

III. Image Receptors

A. Intraoral radiographic film—Used for direct imaging (x-ray interaction with film emulsion)

    1. Film composition

    a. Film wrappings

    (1) Outer plastic or paper cover—Protects film from light and moisture

    (a) Plain white side directed toward x-ray source

    (b) Colored side indicates film speed and single or double film packet; side placed away from x-ray source

    (2) Inner black paper—Protects film from light and moisture

(3) Lead foil—Located between black paper and outer cover

    (a) Reduces film fog by absorbing secondary radiation scattering back from patient's tissues

    (b) Helps reduce patient exposure by attenuating the primary beam after penetrating the film base

b. Film identification dot—Convex on source side of the film, concave on the other

    (1) Used to determine patient's right and left sides

    (2) Placed coronally on periapicals and toward x-ray source

    (3) Corresponds to white side or exposure side of film

c. Film base and emulsion

    (1) Film base—Polyester plastic material with a blue tint

        (a) Provides stiffness with some flexibility

        (b) Tint reduces eye fatigue

    (2) Film emulsion—Gelatin matrix with a suspension of silver halide crystals

        (a) Silver halide crystals or grains

            i) 95% silver bromide

            ii) Small amount of silver iodide

            iii) Sulfur-containing crystal lattice contaminant (sensitivity speck) increases sensitivity of silver bromide crystals

    (3) Adhesive—Aids in adherence of emulsion to film base

    (4) Supercoating—Gelatin layer over emulsion that helps prevent scratching

2. Film size and purpose (Figure 8-7■)

a. Periapical (sizes 0, 1, 2)—Records entire tooth or group of teeth and surrounding structures

b. Bitewing (sizes 0, 1, 2, 3)—Records interproximals of posterior teeth crowns and supporting alveolar bone

c. Occlusal (size 4)—Records large portion of either maxilla or mandible; used to view broader area or to localize objects (size 2)—Used on pedo patients

d. Surveys—Combination of several periapical and/or bitewing films

3. Film speed—Refers to sensitivity of silver halide emulsion to radiation; the more sensitive the film emulsion, the less x-ray exposure required

a. American National Standards Institute (ANSI) speeds

    (1) A (slowest), F (fastest)

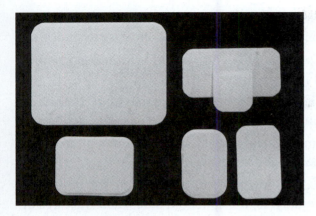

FIGURE 8-7 ■ Intraoral Film: Size 4 Occlusal (*top left*); Size 3 Bitewing (*top right*); Size 0, 1, and 2 Periapicals (*bottom, from L to R*)

(2) Current available speeds—D (Ultraspeed), E (Ektaspeed), and F (Insight); E speed is twice as fast as D and requires half the exposure; F speed requires 20% exposure of E speed film

B. Extraoral radiographic film—Used to examine structures of the skull, the maxilla and mandible, facial bones, and the temporomandibular joint; they can show the extent of a fracture, growth, or malignancy and can be used to study jaw development, tooth eruption, or normal and abnormal conditions (x-ray interaction with intensifying screens)

    1. Sizes and types of extraoral projections

        a. Lateral jaw (5 in. × 7 in.)—Records right or left side of the jaws (Figures 8-8■ and 8-9■)

        b. Panoramic (5 or 6 in. × 12 in.)—Records entire maxilla, mandible, and immediately adjacent structures

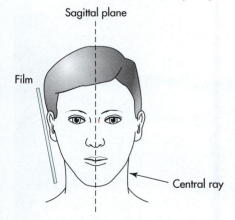

FIGURE 8-8 ■ Lateral Jaw Survey (Lateral Oblique Survey). Note that the central ray is directed at the cassette slightly underneath the opposite side of the mandible.

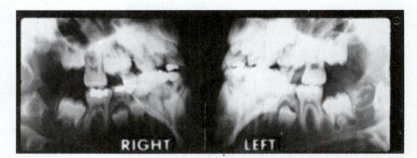

FIGURE 8-9 ■ Typical Lateral Jaw Radiograph of a Child with a Mixed Dentition. This exposure is generally made with 5 × 7 in. (13 × 8 cm) film on adults.

    c. Cephalometric (skull projections) (8 in. × 10 in.)—Record entire skull in various ways to view specific anatomy, symmetry, and disease processes

        (1) Lateral head plate—Common projection used for orthodontics to assess facial growth (Figure 8-10■)

        (2) Waters projection—View useful for examining maxillary sinuses as well as frontal and ethmoid sinuses

        (3) Posteroanterior—Examine facial growth and development, disease, trauma, and developmental abnormalities.

        (4) Submentovertex—Used to show the base of the skull, the position and orientation of the condyles, the sphenoid sinus, and fractures of the zygomatic arch)

2. Cassettes—Film holder for extraoral radiographs that contains two intensifying screens (Figure 8-11■)

3. Intensifying screens (Figure 8-12■)—Screens fluorescence upon exposure to x-rays

    a. Reduces patient radiation dose

    b. Sum of x-rays and fluorescent light emitted by the screen; phosphors exposes the film

    c. Basic components

        (1) Base—Plastic support material

        (2) Reflecting layer—Reflect light emitted from phosphor layer back to the film

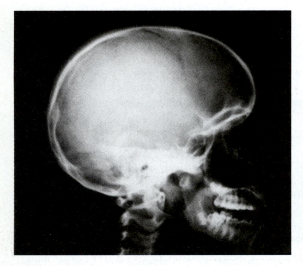

FIGURE 8-10 ■ Lateral Head Plate

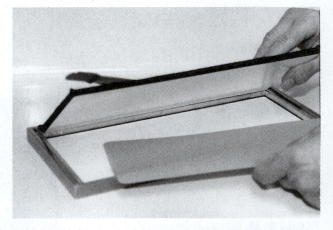

FIGURE 8-11 ■ View of Open Extraoral Cassette. The film is placed between the intensifying screens. The film must be loaded or unloaded in the darkroom with special subdued light.

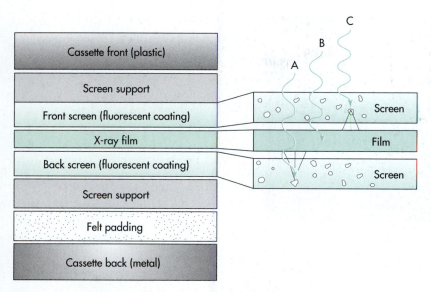

FIGURE 8-12 ■ Cross section of Cassette and Diagram Showing the Effect of X-ray and Fluorescent Light on the Film

        (3) Phosphor layer—Light-sensitive phosphorescent crystals suspended in plastic material

            (a) Calcium tungstate screens—Emit blue and blue-violet light

                i) Must be matched with blue light-sensitive film

                ii) Slower crystals that require more x-ray exposure

            (b) Rare earth screens—Emit green light

                i) Must be matched with green light-sensitive film

                ii) Faster crystals that require at least one-half the x-ray exposure of calcium tungstate screens

IV. Exposure Factors

  A. Visual characteristics (Figure 8-13■)

    1. Density—Overall degree of blackness or darkness on the radiograph

      a. Factors affecting density—Exposure factors (mA, time, kVp), source–film distance, subject (patient) thickness (Figure 8-14■)

    2. Contrast—Difference in densities among various regions on a radiograph (Figure 8-15■)

      a. Factors affecting contrast—kVp, subject contrast (thickness, density, atomic number), film contrast (ability to display differences in subject contrast, film processing)

    3. Sharpness—Ability of a radiograph to define an edge (Table 8-1■)

      a. Factors affecting sharpness—Focal spot size, movement, film emulsion grain size, intensifying screen fluorescence

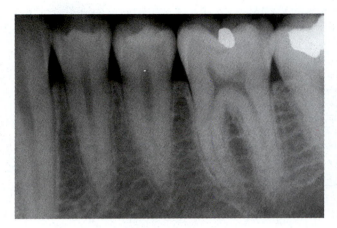

FIGURE 8-13 ■ Acceptable Diagnostic Radiogram

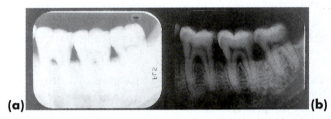

(a) **(b)**

FIGURE 8-14 ■ Radiographic Density. Radiograph (a) is underexposed and appears too light (white). Radiograph (b) is overexposed and appears too dense (dark).

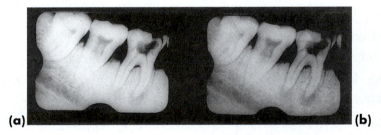

(a) **(b)**

FIGURE 8-15 ■ Radiographic Contrast. Radiograph (a), made using 60 kVp, has high contrast. Radiograph (b), made using 90 kVP, has low contrast.

TABLE 8-1   FACTORS INFLUENCING SHARPNESS

Factors	Modify	Sharpness
Focal spot size	Small focal spot Large focal spot	Increase sharpness Decrease sharpness
Target-fil distance	Long target-film distance Short target-film distance	Increase sharpness Decrease sharpness
Object-film distance	Short object-film distance Long object-film distance	Increase sharpness Decrease sharpness
Movement	No movement Movement	Sharp image Fuzzy image
Screen thickness	Thin screen Thick screen	Increase sharpness Decrease sharpness
Screen-film contact	Close contact Poor contact	Increase sharpness Decrease sharpness
Film crystal size	Small crystals Large crystals	Increase sharpness Decrease sharpness

4. Resolution—Ability of a radiograph to record and demonstrate separate structures that are close together

   a. Factors affecting resolution—Focal spot size, movement, film emulsion grain size, intensifying screen fluorescence

B. Exposure factors

   1. mA—Controls quantity or number of x-rays

      a. Function of tube current, usually fixed at specific mA

      b. Affects film density or degree of film darkening

         (1) Dependent on quantity or number of x-rays reaching the film; more x-rays → dark image, few x-rays → light image

         (2) Low density—Light image from low mA setting; to darken the image, increase the mA setting

         (3) High density—Dark image from high mA setting; to lighten the image, decrease the mA setting

      c. A change in mA changes the quantity or number of x-rays produced; rule of thumb

         (1) An increase of 5 mA will increase the number of x-rays

            (a) To maintain original film density, divide time by 2

            (b) 5 mA @.30 sec. = 10 mA @.15 sec.

(2) A decrease of 5 mA will decrease the number of x-rays

    (a) To maintain original film density, multiply time by 2

    (b) 10 mA @.20 sec. = 5 mA @.40 sec.

2. Exposure time—Controls length of time that x-rays are produced

  a. Most frequently altered exposure factor

  b. A change in time alters quantity or number of x-rays

  c. Affects film density or degree of film darkening

    (1) Dependent on quantity or number of x-rays reaching film; more x-rays → dark image, few x-rays → light image

    (2) Low density—Light image from decreased exposure time setting or premature release of exposure button; to darken image, increase time setting and complete exposure cycle

    (3) High density—Dark image from increased exposure time setting; to lighten image, decrease exposure time setting

3. Milliampere-seconds (mAs)—Combined density factor; product of milliamperage and time

  a. 10 mA × .30 seconds = 3 mA

  b. 15 mA × .20 seconds = 3 mA

  c. Most significant density factor

4. kVp—Controls quality or penetrating power of x-rays; minor factor in controlling quantity of x-rays

  a. Chiefly affects contrast or range of densities on radiograph

  b. Scale of contrast is affected because of altered penetrating power

    (1) Long scale contrast (> 70 kVp)—Many shades of grays, blacks, whites; described as low contrast

    (2) Short scale contrast (≤ 70 kVp)—Few shades, mostly blacks or whites; described as high contrast

  c. A change in kVp will alter the quantity or number of x-rays affecting film density; rule of thumb

    (1) Each 15 kVp increase will increase the number of x-rays

      (a) To maintain original film density, divide time by 2

      (b) 60 kVp @.50 sec. = 75 kVp @.25 sec.

    (2) Each 15 kVp decrease will decrease the number of x-rays

      (a) To maintain original film density, multiply time by 2

      (b) 85 kVp @.15 sec. = 70 kVp @.30 sec.

  d. Altering kVp without adjusting time

    (1) Increasing kVp will increase film density and decrease contrast

    (2) Decreasing kVp will decrease film density and increase contrast

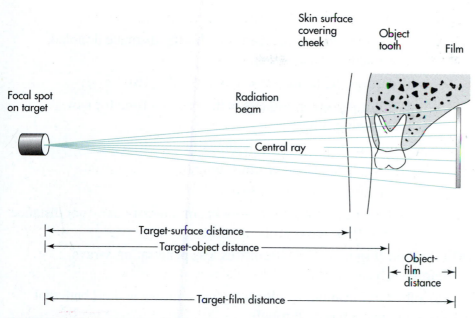

FIGURE 8-16 ■ Distances. Note the relationship among target, skin surface, object (tooth), and x-ray film distance.

5. Source–film distance (Figure 8-16■)—Distance from the source of x-rays to the film affects beam intensity (number and energy of x-rays) and, consequently, film density; a long distance decreases beam intensity and film density, a short distance increases beam intensity and film density

   a. Inverse square law—Intensity of x-ray beam varies inversely with square of the source–film distance

     (1) Formula

$$\frac{I1}{I2} = \frac{D2^2}{D1^2}$$

     (2) Sample problem:

       (a) I1 = .10 sec, D1 = 8″, D2 = 16″

       (b) $\dfrac{I1}{I2} = \dfrac{D2^2}{D1^2}$

     (3) Applications

       (a) PID length changes (Figure 8-16)

       (b) Distance from open end of PID to skin surface

       (c) Radiation safety principle

     (4) Strategies for inverse square law problems

       (a) Determine if problem refers to PID change or operator safety

(b) PID change

    i) Determine distance factor—Has the distance doubled, tripled, or quadrupled?

    ii) Square the factor ($2^2 = 4, 3^2 = 9, 4^2 = 16$)

    iii) Multiply squared factor × the original time for new exposure time

(c) Operator distance and beam intensity

    i) Establish distance from source (6)

    ii) Square the distance (36)

    iii) Invert the distance = x-ray beam intensity at 6-foot distance is 1/36 of the original intensity

(5) Filtration (Figure 8-17■)–Removes less penetrating x-rays, improves beam quality

(a) Inherent filtration—Unleaded glass window and oil bath that x-ray beam passes through

(b) Added filtration—Metal filter, usually aluminum, installed by manufacturer

(c) Total filtration—Sum of inherent and added filtration

    i) 1.5 mm Al @ < 70 kVp

    ii) 2.5 mm Al @ ≥ 70 kVp

(6) Collimation—Restricts size of x-ray beam (Figures 8-17■ and 8-18■)

(a) Collimators

    i) Lead collimator with diaphragm

    ii) Lead-lined PIDs—Preferably long, open-ended, rectangular PIDs; further collimate or restrict the size of x-ray beam (Figure 8-19■)

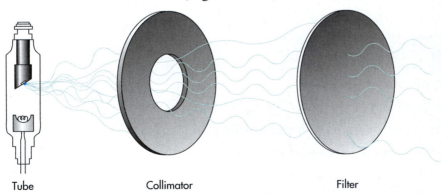

Tube   Collimator   Filter

FIGURE 8-17 ■ Collimator and Filter. The collimator is a lead washer that restricts the size of the x-ray beam. The filter is an aluminum disc that filters (removes) the long wavelength x-rays.

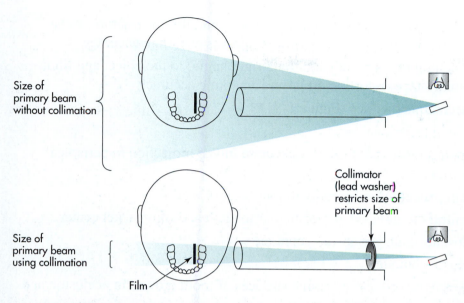

Size of primary beam without collimation

Size of primary beam using collimation

Collimator (lead washer) restricts size of primary beam

Film

FIGURE 8-18 ■ Effects of Collimation on Primary Beam. Lead collimators control the shape and size of the primary beam. The beam is limited to the approximate size of the film.

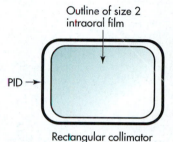

Outline of size 2 intraoral film

PID →

Rectangular collimator

FIGURE 8-19 ■ The rectangular collimator restricts the beam to the approximate size of a #2 film.

iii) Reduces volume of tissue exposed at skin surface

iv) Area of exposure at skin surface should not exceed 2.75 inches or 7 cm in diameter (Figure 8-20■)

V. Intraoral Radiographic Techniques

A. Rules of accurate image formation

1. Use as small focal spot as possible (determined by manufacturer); affects image unsharpness and magnification

2. Place film as close to structure as possible (short object–film distance); minimizes image unsharpness and magnification

3. Use longest source–object distance possible (PID); minimizes image unsharpness and magnification

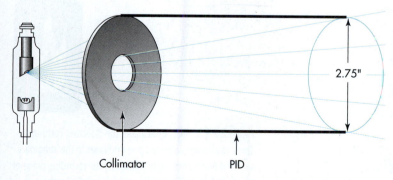

2.75"

Collimator

PID

FIGURE 8-20 ■ The collimator restricts the size of the primary beam to 2.75 in. (7 cm) at the end of the PID.

4. Place film parallel (both vertically and horizontally) to structures to be imaged; minimizes shape distortion, improves anatomic accuracy

5. Direct central ray perpendicular (at a right angle) to the object and film; minimizes shape distortion, improves anatomic accuracy

B. Intraoral technique theories (Figure 8-21■)

1. Paralleling technique

   a. Applies most of the rules of accurate image projection to periapical radiography

   b. Film packet placed parallel to long axes of teeth

   c. Central ray directed perpendicular to teeth and film packet center

   d. Most accurate periapical technique

2. Bitewing technique

   a. Used to record interproximal surfaces of tooth crowns in occlusion and alveolar bone height

   b. Typically used to record posterior tooth crowns; sometimes used to record anterior tooth crowns

   c. Most accurate view of interproximal surfaces and alveolar bone height

3. Bisecting angle technique (Figure 8-22■)

   a. Applies one of the rules of accurate image projection to periapical radiography

   b. Film packet placed against the lingual surfaces of teeth and bone

   c. Based on geometry of equilateral triangles; central ray directed perpendicular to an imaginary line that "bisects" or divides angle formed by long axes of teeth and film packet

   d. Images have shape distortion; not as anatomically accurate in imaging structures as paralleling or bitewing techniques

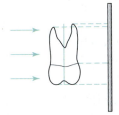
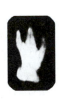

FIGURE 8-21 ■ Principle of Paralleling Technique. The x-ray beam is directed perpendicular to the recording plane of the film, which has been positioned parallel to the long axis of the tooth.
Source: Courtesy of Dentsply/Rinn Corporation

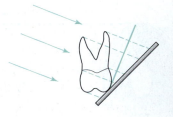
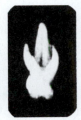

FIGURE 8-22 ■ Principle of the Bisecting Technique. The x-ray beam is directed perpendicular to the imaginary line that bisects the angle formed by the recording plane of the dental x-ray film and the long axis of the tooth.
Source: Courtesy of Dentsply/Rinn Corporation

VI. Radiation Biology and Safety

A. Radiation biology

    1. Definition—Study of effects of ionizing radiation on biological or living systems

    2. Attenuation

        a. Absorption or transfer of x-ray energy to the material or matter through which it passes

        b. X-radiation entering a biological system; begins to lose its energy and can produce various effects

        c. Photon interactions with matter

          (1) Compton scattering

            (a) Occurs when an x-ray photon interacts with outer orbital electron in absorber atom

              i) Photon gives up some of its energy by ejecting an outer electron from shell (recoil ẽ or Compton ẽ;)

              ii) Results in ionization of absorber atom (+ ion), ejected electron (~ ion)

              iii) Colliding photon is scattered in a different direction and continues to give up its energy through further interactions

            (b) 62% of the photons from the dental x-ray beam undergo Compton scattering

              i) 30% of the scatter escapes the patient tissues

              ii) Remainder contributes to film fog

          (2) Photoelectric effect

            (a) Occurs when an x-ray photon of sufficient energy collides with a K shell electron in absorber atom

              i) Photon gives up its energy by ejecting electron from the K shell (recoil ẽ or photoelectron)

              ii) Results in ionization of absorber atom (+ ion), ejected electron (~ ion)

              iii) Vacancy in the K is filled by L shell electron, which releases characteristic radiation; 80% of photoelectron interactions occur at K shell level

            (b) 30% of photons absorbed from the dental x-ray beam are absorbed by the photoelectric effect

              i) Energy is absorbed by patient

              ii) Does not result in film fog

          (3) No interaction—9% of x-rays pass through without any interaction

(4) Coherent scattering (Thompson effect, classical scattering, or unmodified scattering)

   (a) Low-energy photon passes near outer electron in absorber atom
      i) Causes electron to vibrate at same frequency as the photon; excitation
      ii) No x-ray energy is transferred to the atom; no damage done
      iii) Only effect is change in direction of x-ray photon
   (b) Accounts for < 8% of interactions in dental examinations
   (c) Has little effect on film fog

B. Effects of ionizing radiation on living systems

1. Direct effect

   a. Direct alteration of biological molecules such as proteins, carbohydrates, and nucleic acids
      (1) Energy is absorbed by molecule
      (2) Energy transferred between unstable intermediate molecules
      (3) Stable damaged molecules formed
         (a) Rearrangements from dissociation of molecules into free radicals (atoms or molecules with unpaired electrons in valence shell)
         (b) Differ in structure and function from original molecules
   b. Accounts for ≈ 33% of radiation-induced biological damage

2. Indirect effect

   a. Ionization or radiolysis of the H_2O molecule
      (1) Water is predominant molecule in biological system, approximately 80% by weight
      (2) Breakdown of H_2O molecule
         (a) Production of free radicals; hydroxyl free radical believed to be most destructive
         (b) Leads to production of H_2O_2, a major toxin due to its reactivity in achieving ground state
         (c) Reactions result in formation of new molecules with different chemical and biological properties than the original
      (3) Accounts for ≈ 66% of radiation-induced biological damage

3. Linear energy transfer (LET)—Measure of rate at which energy is transferred from incident radiation to tissue along path radiation is traveling

   a. The higher the LET, the greater the tissue damage; protons and alpha particles have high LET and are more damaging than x-rays
   b. X-rays have a relatively low LET and are sparsely ionizing; ionize relatively few atoms and/or biomolecules and less likely to cause a direct biological effect

4. Cell sensitivity

    a. Somatic—All tissues of the body except reproductive

        (1) Somatic effects of radiation are not passed along to future generations

        (2) Include cancer and other disorders that do not involve the reproductive or genetic tissues

        (3) Follow a linear, threshold dose–response; a certain dose is necessary before demonstrable damage occurs

    b. Genetic—Reproductive cells

        (1) Genetic effects of radiation occur only in reproductive cells and can be passed to future generations

        (2) Include alterations of chromosomes that may result in mutations in future generations

        (3) Believed to occur in a linear, nonthreshold, dose–response model; no dose is considered safe

    c. Law of Bergonie-Tribondeau—Describes cells most sensitive to effects of radiation

        (1) Mitotic activity—High mitotic rate and history

        (2) Growth and development—Primitive or immature

        (3) Degree of differentiation—Undifferentiated without specialized function

        (4) Cells with a large nucleus/cytoplasm ratio

    d. Categories of cell/tissue sensitivity—Radiosensitive to radioresistant

        (1) High sensitivity—Small lymphocyte, bone marrow, reproductive cells, intestinal mucosa

        (2) Intermediate sensitivity—Connective tissue, small blood vessels, growing bone and cartilage, salivary glands, lungs, kidneys, liver

        (3) Low sensitivity—Optic lens, mature erythrocytes, muscle, nerve

    e. Target or critical organ concept

        (1) Various somatic tissues are designated as critical organs for radiological health purposes

        (2) Concept based on radiosensitivity and potential effects

        (3) Critical organs include female breast, skin, thyroid, lens of the eye, hematopoietic tissues, genetic tissues

5. Other factors

    a. Area of exposure

        (1) Whole-body—Radiation exposure to entire body

        (2) Localized—Radiation exposure restricted to specific area of the body

       b. Latent period—Time interval between irradiation and development of an observed biological effect

         (1) Short-term, early, or acute effects

           (a) May occur minutes, hours, or weeks after exposure

           (b) Usually result of high dose to whole body

           (c) Ultimate early effect is death

         (2) Long-term, late, or chronic effects

           (a) May occur months, years, or decades after exposure

           (b) Result of low dose received over a long time

           (c) May have no observable effect or result in cancers later in life

       c. Cumulative effect—Residual injury without repair from repeated radiation exposure

C. Units of radiation measurement

    1. Systems

       a. Standard or traditional units (Roentgen, rad, rem)

       b. International units (C/kg, gray sievert)

    2. Exposure dose—Measure of radiation quantity or exposure and refers to the ability of x-rays to ionize air; measure is taken at the skin surface before radiation has penetrated patient's tissues

       a. Roentgen (R)—amount of radiation capable of ionizing 1.6×10^{12} ion pairs per gram of air; $1.0 \text{ R} = 2.58 \times 10^4$ C/kg of air

       b. Coulombs per kilogram (C/kg); $1 \text{ C/kg} = 3.88 \times 10^3$ R (3876 R)

    3. Absorbed dose—Used to measure quantity of any type of ionizing radiation received by a mass of any type of matter including patient's tissues

       a. rad—1.0 rad = .01 gray (divide rad by 100 to equal gray)

       b. gray (Gy)—1 Gy = 100 rads (multiply gray by 100 to equal rad)

       c. Units may be expressed in smaller units such as mR (millirad, .001 R = 1 mR) or cGy (centigray, .01 gray = 1 cGy)

    4. Dose equivalent—Measure used to compare biological effects or damage an exposed individual might expect to occur from (RBE, relative biological effectiveness) different types of radiation

       a. DE = AD (absorbed dose) × QF (quality factor); quality factor for x-rays is 1

       b. rem (Roentgen equivalent man)—1.0 rem = .01 sievert (divide rem by 100 to equal sievert)

       c. sievert (Sv)—1 Sv = 100 rems (multiply sievert by 100 to equal rem)

       d. Units may be expressed in smaller units such as mRem (millirem; .001 Rem = 1 mRem) or cSv (centisievert; .01 sievert = 1 cSv)

D. Radiation safety and protection for dental patients

  1. Guiding principles

   a. ALARA—As Low As Reasonably Achievable

   b. Risk-versus-benefit decision—Determination that the benefit of radiographic examination outweighs risk

   c. Minimize exposure, maximize diagnostic result

  2. Somatic reduction measures

   a. Selection criteria—Guidelines for prescribing dental radiographs; used to determine need, type, and frequency of radiographic examinations

   (1) Based on positive historical findings, positive clinical signs and symptoms, patient risk factors, type of visit (new or recall patient), patient age, and type of dentition

   (2) Produces high-yield, individualized radiographic examinations that influence diagnosis and treatment

   (3) Ensures maximum patient benefit with minimum of patient exposure

   b. Film speed—Using E speed film instead of D speed film produces a 40–50% exposure reduction; F speed film further reduces E speed exposures by 20%

   c. Rare earth intensifying screens for extraoral radiography result in 50% reduction compared with calcium tungstate screens

   d. Correct processing and quality assurance procedures reduce patient exposure by avoiding retakes

   e. Primary beam collimation—Rectangular collimation reduces skin surface dose 60–70%

   f. Aluminum filtration—Estimated 57% reduction in exposure by removing low energy, longer wavelength x-rays

   g. Kilovoltage range

   (1) Lower kilovoltage settings result in higher skin doses than higher kilovoltage settings

   (2) An 80 kVp setting results in a 45% reduction in exposure compared with using 60 kVp

   h. Paralleling technique with film holding devices and beam alignment guides standardize technique and reduce retakes

   i. Lead shields—.25 mm lead minimum

   (1) Thyroid collar—50% exposure reduction to thyroid

   (2) Apron—Aids in shielding bone marrow sites in the chest and abdomen

   (3) Apron—Primary gonadal shield

E. Radiation safety and protection for dental personnel

1. Maximum permissible dose (MPD)

    a. Radiation exposure not expected to cause appreciable bodily injury to a person at any time during life

    b. Whole body dose limit for occupational exposure = 5 rems/year (0.05 Sv or 50 mSv); 1.25 rem/calendar quarter (0.0125 Sv or 12.5 mSv)

    c. Whole body dose limit for pregnant radiation users and nonoccupationally exposed individuals = 0.5 rems (0.005 Sv or 5 mSv); 1/10 occupational MPD

    d. Goal—Achieve an occupational exposure dose as close to 0 as possible by adhering to radiation safety and protection rules

2. Maximum accumulated dose (MAD)—Accumulated lifetime dose limit for occupationally exposed workers

    a. Formula—MAD = N (age) ~ 18 (legal age for radiation worker) × 5 rems/year

    b. Example—MAD for a 35-year-old radiation worker: MAD = (35 ~ 18) × 5 = 85 rems or 850 mSv

3. Radiation sources

    a. Background radiation—Ionizing radiation ubiquitous in the environment and encountered in daily life

        (1) Natural—Radiation exposure from radon (55%), cosmic radiation (8%), terrestrial radiation (8%), and internal source radiation (11%); greatest contributor ≈ 82%

        (2) Artificial or manufactured—Medical x-rays (11%), dental x-rays (.30%), nuclear medicine (4%), consumer products (3%); totals ≈ 18%

        (3) Other sources—Occupational (< .03%), nuclear fuel (< .03%), nuclear fallout (< .03%); totals < .10%

        (4) Average annual effective dose from all sources = 3.60 mSv

    b. Dental sources

        (1) Primary—Radiation generated at target and collimated by PID; used for patient radiography

        (2) Secondary—Scatter radiation produced by interaction of primary radiation with the patient's facial tissues

        (3) Leakage—Radiation emitted from tubehead encasement during exposure

4. Safety rules and protection measures

    a. Avoid primary beam

        (1) Do not stand in or near primary beam or its path

        (2) Do not hold x-ray head, PID, or patient in place

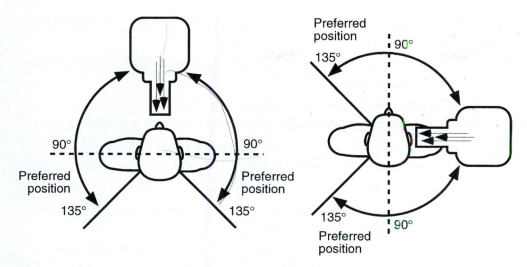

FIGURE 8-23 ■ For optimum operator safety, the clinician should stand 6 feet from the x-ray source, at a 90–135 degree angle to the primary beam.

    (3) Do not hold films in patient's mouth

  b. Distance and position rule (Figure 8-23■)

    (1) Stand 6 feet from source of x-rays

    (2) Preferred operator position—Between 90° and 135° to the primary beam

  c. Barriers

    (1) Primary barrier—Designed to attenuate primary beam; common primary barriers are operatory walls

    (2) Secondary barrier—Intended to absorb secondary and leakage radiation; secondary barriers are ceiling and floor

  d. Radiation monitoring

    (1) Pocket/badge dosimeter worn at chest/waist level

    (2) Monitors MPD for one individual; only for occupational exposure

    (3) Analyzed quarterly—Dentist responsible for evaluation and monitoring of reports

VII.   **Radiographic Infection Control**

  A. Operator protection

    1. Universal precautions recommended—Gloves, masks, eyewear, work attire

  B. Operatory preparation and clean-up

    1. Intraoral x-ray unit

      a. Precleaning and disinfection procedures

        (1) Spray–wipe–spray technique with ADA-accepted water-based surface disinfectant-detergent

(2) Surface disinfectant-detergent must remain in contact with surface for 10 minutes to achieve disinfection

b. Prepare x-ray head, PID, control panel, exposure switch, work surface; cover with plastic barriers

c. Postprocedure clean-up—Use gloves to carefully remove covers, properly dispose of instruments, place clean barriers with fresh gloves

d. If barrier techniques are not used, precleaning and disinfection procedures must be completed between patients

2. Panoramic x-ray machines

a. Preclean, disinfect, and cover control panel, exposure button, chin rest, head, temple support, and handgrips

b. After film exposure, remove gloves and wash hands to handle cassette

c. Postprocedure clean-up—Use gloves to remove covers, properly dispose of bitepiece, place clean barriers with fresh gloves

d. If barrier techniques are not used, precleaning and disinfection procedures must be completed between patients

C. Film handling

1. Organize film and sterile instruments on covered surface away from x-ray source

a. Keep exposed and unexposed film separated

b. Lay out films in survey order; place exposed films in plastic cup

2. Film barriers—Use film barrier bag or commercially covered film packets for daylight loading automatic processors

D. Conventional darkroom processing procedures

1. After completing intraoral procedures, replace soiled gloves with fresh gloves, use paper towel or overgloves to open darkroom door

2. Shell films in safelight conditions—Drop films out on clean paper towel without touching the film

3. Properly dispose of contaminated film wrappings, container, and gloves

4. Wash and dry hands

5. Handle films on edges and insert into processor

E. Daylight loader automatic processors

1. Use film barrier envelopes for film packets

2. With gloves, drop film packets out of barrier into a cup or onto a towel

3. Remove and dispose of contaminated gloves; wash and dry hands

4. Open daylight loader window and cover bottom surface of unit with paper towels or plastic wrap

5. Place film receptacle and powderless gloves into unit, close window

6. Insert hands through sleeves, put on gloves, shell films and insert films into processor

7. Remove gloves, withdraw hands through the sleeves

8. Open window, fold covering materials over waste materials, remove and correctly dispose waste materials

VIII. **Darkroom Processing and Quality Assurance**

  A. Darkroom requirements

    1. Design—Adequate size for processing activities, convenient arrangement of equipment, proper ventilation

    2. White light tight environment

      a. Typical light leaks occur around doorframe, ceiling tiles, vents, wall seams

      b. Seal leaks with black masking tape or weather stripping

    3. Environmental conditions

      a. Temperature—70°F/21°C

      b. Humidity—50–70%

      c. Cleanliness—Essential for quality processing and avoidance of artifacts

    4. Safelight conditions—Adequate darkroom illumination without compromising image quality

      a. Safelight lamps, filters, and bulbs

        (1) Filters white light (green and blue spectrum) to which film is most sensitive

        (2) Filters

          (a) Red filter (GBX-2)—Safe for both intraoral and extraoral film; requires a 15-watt incandescent bulb

          (b) Orange filter (ML-2)—Safe for intraoral film only; requires a 10-watt incandescent bulb

        (3) Working distance and time

          (a) Safelight lamps mounted 4 feet from counter surface

          (b) Five-minute working time under safelight lamps

  B. Processing chemicals

    1. General principles

      a. Wetting—Softens emulsion so developer chemicals can act on emulsion

      b. Development—Transforms latent image into visible image via reduction of exposed silver halide crystals

      c. Rinsing—Stops development and removes excess chemicals from emulsion

    d. Fixation—Removes unexposed silver halide crystals from the emulsion

    e. Washing—Removes all excess chemicals from the emulsion

    f. Drying—Removes the water from the emulsion

2. Developer solution components

    a. Metol (Elon) (reducing agent)—Brings up the gray tones

    b. Hydroquinone (reducing agent)—Brings up the black tones and contrast

    c. Sodium carbonate (activator)—Softens and swells emulsion

    d. Potassium bromide (restrainer)—Prevents reducing agents from developing the unexposed silver halide crystals

    e. Sodium sulfite (preservative)—Prevents rapid oxidation

    f. Water (solvent)—Medium for dissolving chemicals

3. Fixer solution components

    a. Ammonium or sodium thiosulfate (fixing agent)—Clears away the unexposed, undeveloped silver halide crystals

    b. Acetic or sulfuric acid (neutralizer/acidifier)—Stops development by neutralizing developer chemicals

    c. Aluminum chloride (chrome alum) or sulfide (hardener)—Shrinks and hardens the emulsion

    d. Sodium sulfite (preservative)—Prevents chemical deterioration

    e. Water (solvent)—Medium for dissolving chemicals

4. Automatic processing solutions—Formulated for mechanical transport systems and higher temperature processing

    a. Chemical differences

        (1) Phenidone replaces metol for gray tone production

        (2) Hardening agent (gluteraldehyde) and antiswelling agent (sulfide compounds) added to developer to prevent emulsion from sticking to the rollers

        (3) Additional hardening agent added to fixer to prevent emulsion from sticking to the rollers

5. Replenishment—Restores the ability of the processing chemicals to perform their function without changing the entire volume

    a. Ready-to-use developer or fixer solution added daily to solution reservoirs

    b. Replenished solutions should be replaced with fresh chemicals every 2–4 weeks under normal conditions, more frequently when indicated

    c. Solution lifespan is dependent on use factor—Exposure to air, temperature

C. Automatic processing systems

    1. Automatic processing system components

2. Processing solutions—Formulated for mechanical transport systems higher temperature processing

3. Sequence: developer, fixer, rinse, dry

4. Temperature—Ranges from 83°F (28°C) to 105°F (40°C)

   a. Heating element controls the temperature of developer solution

   b. Rollers designed to rotate at a speed compatible with the developer temperature

5. Time—Average processing cycle is 4.5–5.5 minutes

6. Film feed—Insert films slowly, allowing space among films

7. Drying chamber—Blows films dry before exit

8. External film receptacle—Receives finished radiographs

9. Maintenance

   a. Daily

     (1) Replenish each solution with 4–7 ounces of chemicals after the equivalent of 4–6 full mouth or panoramic surveys

     (2) Clean rollers daily by running cleaning sheets through the processor; cleaning sheets should not be reused due to solution contamination potential

   b. Weekly—Rollers should be removed and cleaned

     (1) Rinse under warm water

     (2) Spray with special cleaner and allowed to sit for 10 minutes

     (3) Wipe clean with separate sponges

     (4) Rinse with water and excess water removed before reinstallation

   c. Every 2–4 weeks

     (1) Thorough cleaning of entire machine and roller system

     (2) Replace with fresh chemicals; fill the fixer reservoir first

   d. Monthly

     (1) Inspect moving parts for wear

     (2) Lubricate moving parts as needed

     (3) Check dryer, remove accumulated dust

   e. Use a system cleaner to clean entire processing unit every 3 months

   f. Cleaning procedures should be completed with a protective gown, utility gloves, mask, eyewear, and adequate ventilation

D. Manual processing

1. Equipment

   a. Stainless steel solution tanks, film racks, solution stirrers

   b. Temperature regulator—Mix hot and cold running water

      c. Overflow pipe—Maintains a clean, circulating water bath

      d. Floating thermometer—Determine temperature and development time

      e. Darkroom timer—Used to time the development, fixation, and wash cycles

2. Solution sequence and time (follow manufacturer's directions)

      a. Development—5 minutes @ 68°F (20°C)

      b. Rinse—(30 seconds) stops development

      c. Fixation—10 minutes @ 68°F (20°C)

         (1) Films can be viewed after 3 minutes following a brief 30-second rinse

         (2) Films must be returned to the fixer solution for 7 more minutes to equal a total of 10 minutes

      d. Wash—Running water for 20 minutes @ 68°F (20°C)

      e. Drying cycle—Films can be air dried or placed in a commercial film dryer

3. Temperature and time

      a. Time of development is inversely proportional to temperature of water bath

      b. As temperature increases, time of development decreases

4. Solution maintenance and change

      a. Replenishment

         (1) Replenish each solution with 8 ounces of chemicals (depending on size of tanks); may require some solution to be removed to replenish

         (2) Level of solution should be adequate to cover all films

      b. Change solutions every 3–4 weeks

         (1) Solution reservoirs and master tank should be cleaned with commercial cleaner

         (2) Thoroughly rinse before reassembly

         (3) Fill fixer tank first, then developer

         (4) Fill water bath, stir solutions

      c. Cleaning procedures should be completed with a protective gown, utility gloves, mask, eyewear, and adequate ventilation

E. Quality assurance

1. Action plan used to ensure production of high-quality, diagnostic images while minimizing costs and exposure to personnel and patients

2. X-ray machine

      a. Periodically tested by qualified service representative or radiation physicist per state law requirements

         (1) X-ray output

         (2) Kilovoltage calibration

         (3) Half value layer—Aluminum filtration

      (4) Timer accuracy

      (5) Milliamperage reproducibility

      (6) Collimation

   b. Office maintenance

      (1) Check arm for drifting—Tighten as needed

      (2) Check x-ray head and PID for drifting—Tighten as needed

3. Safelight and darkroom conditions

   a. Check for proper safelight filter and distance

   b. Inspect for light leaks in total darkness

      (1) Mark leaks with chalk

      (2) Eliminate with black masking tape or weather stripping

   c. Coin test

      (1) Place coin on unwrapped film in total darkness; let it remain 5 minutes; process film

      (2) If coin image is present, light leak exists and needs to be eliminated

      (3) After white leaks eliminated, repeat coin test to evaluate safelight conditions

4. Film processing quality control

   a. Stepwedge—Test device with graduated layers of metal, configured similar to a staircase

      (1) Used to produce test images such as reference and/or check films for solution monitoring

      (2) Commercial—Graduated layers of aluminum or copper

      (3) Homemade—Graduated layers of lead foil taped together

   b. With a fresh film, produce a control film or reference radiograph at bitewing exposure time and process in fresh solutions

   c. Expose a check film each day and process as usual

   d. Compare check film to control or reference film—If visible difference between two films, there is a processing problem

   e. Resolve processing problem such as temperature adjustment, replenishment, or solution change before patient films are processed

5. Image receptor quality assurance

   a. Film storage—Cool, dry place away from x-ray source, chemical fumes @ 50°–70°F and 30–50% relative humidity

   b. Cassettes examined monthly for damage and function; replace as needed

      (1) Rigid—Defective hinges, latches

      (2) Flexible—Open seams, defective latch mechanisms

(3) Screens inspected for cracks or defects; clean periodically

    (a) Clean with cotton ball or gauze and special screen cleaner

    (b) Wipe dry with fresh cotton ball or gauze

    (c) Air dry before closing cassette; wet screens will stick together and tear the screens upon opening

6. Viewbox care

  a. Inspect monthly, replace light bulbs when needed

  b. Operatory viewbox—Preclean, disinfect, and cover; place mounted radiographs under clear plastic cover

  c. Change cover between patients

IX. Intraoral Technical and Processing Error Identification and Correction

  A. Technical errors and artifacts

    1. Vertical angulation errors—Deviation from true long axis dimension

      a. Foreshortening—Too much vertical angulation used (Figure 8-24■)

        (1) Shape distortion, resulting in an image shorter than actual structure

        (2) Correction—Decrease the vertical angulation; place film parallel to the teeth long axes

      b. Elongation—Not enough vertical angulation used (Figure 8-25■)

        (1) Shape distortion, resulting in an image longer than actual structure

        (2) Correction—Increase vertical angulation; make sure film is not distorted

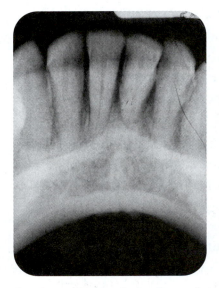

FIGURE 8-24 ■ Foreshortened Image of the Lower Anterior Teeth

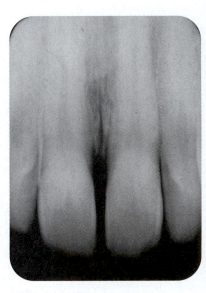

FIGURE 8-25 ■ Elongated Image of the Maxillary Incisor Teeth

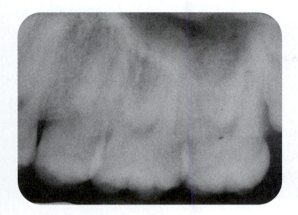

FIGURE 8-26 ■ Horizontal Angulation Error

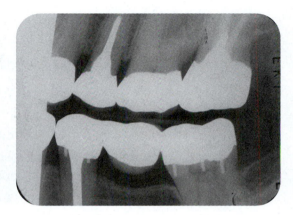

FIGURE 8-27 ■ Cone Cut Error

2. Horizontal angulation errors—Diagonal entry to proximal contacts (Figure 8-26■)

   a. Results in overlapping of interproximal contacts and widening of the image horizontally

   b. Correction—Direct central ray perpendicular to the labial/buccal surfaces of the teeth crowns

3. Cone cut errors—Lack of centering x-ray beam over the film (Figure 8-27■)

   a. Results in partial exposure of film; clear zone with no image

   b. Correction—Direct central ray to film center and central ray entry point

4. Film placement errors—Improper film location or orientation relative to anatomic area

   a. Inadequate coverage of area (periapicals/bitewings)

   b. Inadequate apical coverage (periapicals)

   c. Backward placement of the film packet—Lead foil pattern and opposite orientation of the mounted film

   d. Correction—Follow film descriptions for correct film location; position dot or white side of film toward the x-ray source

5. Film bending errors—Improper film folding, creasing, or crimping, which interferes with image quality

   a. Creasing film before exposure results in white artifacts; creasing or crimping film before and after exposure results in black artifacts

   b. Correction—Limit film bending

     (1) Use appropriate film size

     (2) Use film packet edge cushions to minimize patient discomfort

     (3) Handle films carefully during film holder insertion or removal

B. Exposure errors

    1. Overexposure

        a. Results in high-density or dark film

        b. Correction—Reduce exposure time; check for small patient size

    2. Underexposure

        a. Results in low-density or light film

        b. Correction—Increase exposure time; check for large patient size; make sure exposure button was not released too soon

    3. Double exposure (Figure 8-28■)

        a. Bizarre pattern of superimposed images

        b. High-density appearance

        c. Accompanied by blank, transparent unexposed film

        d. Correction—Separate unexposed film from exposed film

    4. Unexposed film

        a. Results in blank, transparent appearance of film base

        b. Correction—Separate unexposed film from exposed film

C. Patient management and patient preparation errors

    1. Movement—Motion unsharpness

        a. Results in blurred image of recorded structures

        b. Correction—Stabilize film placement and instruct patient to remain still during entire exposure

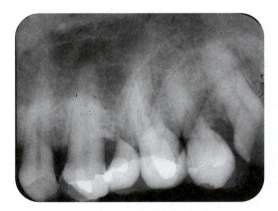

FIGURE 8-28 ■ Double-exposed Film

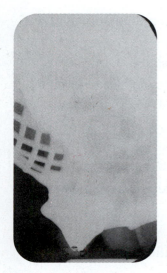

FIGURE 8-29 ■ Radio-opaque
Image of Removable Prosthesis Superimposed over Dental Structures

2. Eyewear and removable prostheses errors (Figure 8-29■)

a. Results in radiopaque images of these items superimposed over dental structures

b. Correction—Instruct patient to remove glasses and removable prostheses before radiographic procedures

3. Thyroid collar and lead apron placement errors

a. Results in lead shield image superimposed over dental structures

b. Correction—Place shields so that they do not interfere with the path of the x-ray beam and film

D. Processing errors and artifacts

1. Film handling errors

a. Emulsion scratches—White areas where emulsion has been removed from film base

b. Black static electricity artifacts—Tree or branchlike in shape, owing to friction or rough film handling

c. Partial or complete white light exposure of film—Black zone or completely black image

d. Correction—Handle the films carefully, separate films gently, and handle on edges in safelight conditions

2. Solution contamination errors

a. Black or gray droplet artifacts or fingerprints from precontamination with developer or fluoride solution

       b. White droplet artifacts or fingerprints from precontamination with fixer solution

       c. Brown-yellow artifacts from inadequate film washing

       d. Corrections—Use clean, dry hands to handle films on clean, covered darkroom working surfaces; allow proper film washing with clean, circulating water

   3. Automatic processing errors

       a. Dark image (also applies to manual processing)

          (1) Overdevelopment owing to high processing temperature without time adjustment

          (2) Overreplenishment

          (3) White light leaks or improper safelight conditions

       b. Light image (also applies to manual processing)

          (1) Underdevelopment owing to low processing temperature without time adjustment

          (2) Underreplenishment

       c. Brown image from exhausted developer solution

       d. Green image from inadequate fixation or exhausted fixer

       e. Streaked image owing to dirty rollers; dirty image from dirty water bath

       f. Film feed artifacts—Film overlapping and gear marks

       g. Corrections—Use time–temperature processing methods with fresh or properly replenished solutions and clean wash water; insert films slowly to allow space between films

   4. Solution sequence errors

       a. Fixer placed in developer reservoir results in a blank, transparent image; fixer removes entire film emulsion, leaving the plastic base

       b. Drain and thoroughly clean and rinse solution reservoirs; replace with fresh chemicals

X. Panoramic Radiography and Error Correction

  A. Criteria for a diagnostic panoramic radiograph

    1. Entire maxilla and mandible recorded including the temporomandibular joints

    2. As anatomy allows, symmetrical display of structures right to left

    3. Slight smile or slight downward curve of the occlusal plane

    4. Good representations of the teeth with minimal over- or undermagnification

    5. Overlapping of posterior interproximal surfaces is expected

    6. Tongue positioned against palate to eliminate palatoglossal air space

    7. Minimal or no cervical spine shadow

8. Acceptable film density and contrast

9. Free of technical, film handling, and processing errors

B. Panoramic imaging concepts

    1. Tomography—Body sectioning method of revealing a depth of tissue or image layer called the focal trough

    2. Focal trough is a predetermined layer or thickness of structures that will be imaged in focus on the film; correct patient positioning is essential for optimal results

    3. X-ray source has a vertical slit aperture and directs the x-ray beam in a lingual to labial direction through structures

    4. Accomplished by simultaneous movement of the x-ray head and film cassette in opposite directions during exposure

    5. Side of the patient's dental arches closest to the film is recorded in focus while the side closest to the x-ray source is blurred out of focus

    6. Resulting image is uniformly magnified owing to the long object–film distance with some posterior contact overlapping

    7. Ghost images or remnant images from the opposite side may superimpose over the desired structures

        a. Structures that ghost tend to be thicker and will not be completely blurred out of focus

        b. Ghost images appear on the opposite side, higher on the film than the original structure, and are magnified and blurred more in the vertical than the horizontal plane

        c. Examples of structures that ghost include the rami, lower border of the mandible, chin rest, some right/left side markers and earrings

    8. Panoramic machines vary in style but operate based on the preceding principles and allow operator to select appropriate mA and kVp; time is fixed

    9. Cassettes—5 or 6 × 12-inch rigid or flexible cassette (type compatible with machine) with intensifying screens

C. Panoramic radiographic technique

    1. Preexposure preparation

        a. Use proper infection control procedures to preclean and disinfect unit and place sterile bitepiece

        b. Load cassette in safelight conditions

        c. Place into cassette holder on machine

        d. Instruct patient to remove all metallic objects from the head and neck region, including earrings, necklaces, barrettes, hairpins, intraoral prostheses, hearing aids, eyeglasses

e. Place panoramic lead apron (long front and back panel), fully clearing the back of the neck region; do not use a thyroid collar

f. Explain procedure to the patient and instruct the patient to remain still during entire exposure

g. Exposure factor considerations—Obesity, large bone structure, racial differences, frail or small bone structure, edentulous; adjust mA and kVp as needed

2. Patient positioning requirements

a. Stands or sits with straight spine

b. Anterior teeth bite end-to-end in bitepiece groove

c. Head planes

(1) Midsagittal (horizontal) plane is positioned perpendicular to the floor

(2) Occlusal (vertical) plane is positioned parallel to the floor; Frankfort and ala-tragus plane also used

(3) Anteroposterior (forward–backward) plane is aligned with a specific landmark per manufacturer

d. Tongue pressed against palate

e. Lips and eyes closed

D. Identification and correction of common errors

1. Patient positioning errors

a. Cervical spine error

(1) Spinal column is slumped

(2) Creates a pyramid to column-shaped radiopacity superimposed over the anterior teeth

(3) Correction—Instruct patient to sit or stand tall with spine erect; make sure chin rest is high enough to maintain straight spine position

b. Midsagittal plane errors

(1) Patient's head tilted to one side

(a) Side tilted toward film is imaged smaller in width, and side toward x-ray source is imaged larger in width; one side is higher than the other

(b) Correction—Center midsagittal plane and align it perpendicular to floor

(2) Patient's head rotated to one side (Figure 8-30■)

(a) Side rotated toward film is imaged smaller in width and side toward x-ray source is imaged larger in width

(b) Correction—Center the midsagittal plane and align it perpendicular to floor

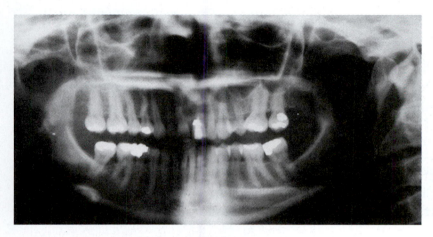

FIGURE 8-30 ■ Panoramic Midsagittal Image Error

c. Vertical head plane errors

    (1) Patient's head is tilted upward

        (a) Upper teeth are blurred and larger in width; hard palate is superimposed over maxillary teeth apices; condyles may be cut off; occlusal plane flat or frowned

        (b) Correction—Move head down and align occlusal plane parallel to floor

    (2) Patient's head is tilted downward (Figure 8-31■)

        (a) Lower teeth are blurred and larger in width with foreshortened apices; condyles may be cut off; severe grin to the occlusal plane

        (b) Correction—Move head up and align occlusal plane parallel to floor

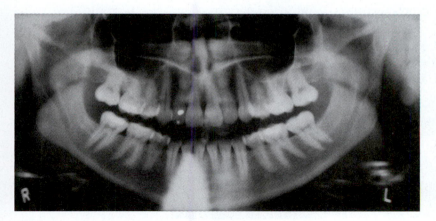

FIGURE 8-31 ■ Panoramic Vertical Head Plane Error

d. Anteroposterior plane errors

(1) Patient is positioned too far forward (Figure 8-32■)

(a) Teeth are blurred and smaller in width; severe overlapping of teeth (especially premolars); spine may be superimposed over the ramus areas

(b) Correction—Move the head back toward x-ray source and align with landmark; make sure teeth are end-to-end in bitepiece groove

(2) Patient is positioned too far backward

(a) Teeth are blurred and larger in width; excessive ghosting of each ramus and spine; image too large for film

(b) Correction—Move head forward toward the film and align with landmark; make sure teeth are end-to-end in bitepiece groove

e. Patient preparation errors—Metallic objects left in place, producing radiopaque artifacts

(1) Objects include earrings, necklaces, napkin chain, eyeglasses, intraoral prostheses, barrettes

(2) Correction—Instruct patient to remove metallic objects from head and neck

f. Patient moves during exposure, causing motion unsharpness

(1) Make sure patient is capable of cooperating with procedure

(2) Correction—Instruct patient to close eyes and remain still during entire exposure cycle

g. Patient does not press tongue against palate

(1) Radiolucent air space artifact is created in maxillary apical region

(2) Correction—Instruct patient to swallow and press tongue against roof of mouth; close lips around bitepiece

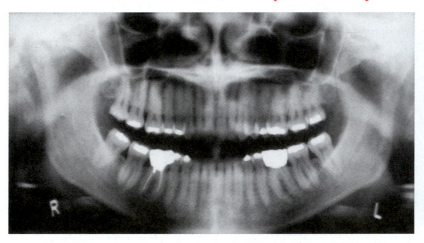

FIGURE 8-32 ■ Panoramic Anteroposterior Plane Error

h. Exposure errors

    (1) Double exposure

        (a) Bizarre pattern of superimposed images with high-density appearance

        (b) Correction—Process film immediately after exposure; be sure to keep unexposed and exposed cassettes separated from each other

    (2) Overexposure

        (a) Results in high-density or dark film

        (b) Correction—Reduce kVp/mA; check for small patient size

    (3) Underexposure

        (a) Results in low-density or light film

        (b) Correction—Increase kVp/mA; check for large patient size

i. Operational errors

    (1) Cassette resistance

        (a) Produces alternating white and black vertical bands or lines from cassette contact with patient's shoulder

        (b) Correction—Make sure patient's spine is straight, head is erect, and shoulders down; avoid placing inferior aspect of cassette against patient's shoulder

    (2) Incomplete exposure

        (a) Results in partially exposed image

        (b) Correction—Maintain constant pressure on exposure button until cycle of machine rotation is complete

XI. Localization Techniques

A. Tube shift technique—Compares change in position of object between two images taken at different horizontal or vertical angulations (Figure 8-33■)

  1. Two-film comparison is required such as two periapicals, a periapical and bitewing, periapical and topographical occlusal

  2. Object movement is compared with movement of x-ray head, not PID or x-ray cone

  3. Alternate terms for this technique—Buccal object rule, Clark's rule, and the SLOB rule

  4. SLOB acronym

    a. S = same; L = lingual; O = opposite; B = buccal

    b. If object moves in same direction as x-ray head, object is lingual in location

    c. If object moves in opposite direction to x-ray head, object is buccal in location

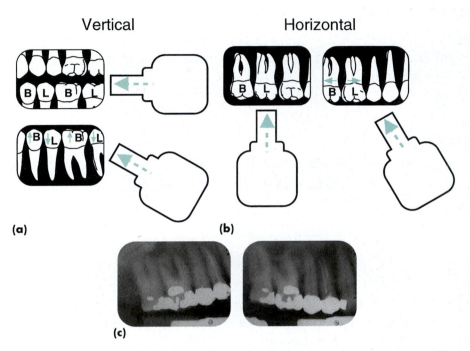

FIGURE 8-33 ■ In the SLOB rule, objects move in a particular direction relative to the movement of the x-ray head. (a) This image illustrates how lingual objects move the same direction as the x-ray head and how buccal objects move opposite the direction of the x-ray head in the vertical plane. (b) This image demonstrates the same pattern of object movement in the horizontal plane. (c) Application of the SLOB rule requires a two-film comparison. Compare the molar and premolar periapical radiographs and observe that the CV amalgam restorations move the same direction as the horizontal movement of the x-ray head. In addition, notice that the filled pulp canals on tooth #5 have become separated. The lingual canal moves forward, the same as the movement of the x-ray head, while the buccal canal moves opposite the x-ray head.

    B. Right-angle technique—Compares position of objects between two images taken at right angles to one another (Figure 8-34■)

        1. Two-film comparison—Central ray (CR) directed perpendicular to film

            a. Paralleling technique periapical—CR perpendicular to long axes of teeth

            b. Cross-sectional occlusal—CR perpendicular to occlusal plane of teeth

        2. Comparison of two films determines location of object(s) in question

XII. Radiographic Anatomy

    A. Radiopaque versus radiolucent

        1. Radiopacities

            a. Structures that are dense structurally and absorb x-rays either fully or partially

            b. Results in little or no change in emulsion

            c. Appear white or shades of white/gray after film processing

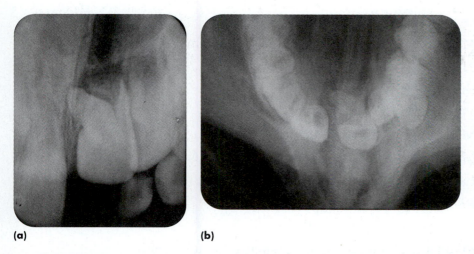

(a)　　　　　　　**(b)**

FIGURE 8-34 ■ The right angle technique of localization compares the position of an object on two films taken at right angles to one another. (a) This anterior periapical was taken with the central ray at a right angle to the teeth long axes. (b) This cross-sectional maxillary occlusal was taken with the central ray directed at a right angle to the incisal/occlusal plane. The comparison of these two films confirms that the mesiodens is impacted lingual to #9.

   2. Radiolucencies

   　　a. Structures that are not dense structurally and allow x-rays to pass through

   　　b. X-rays interact with film emulsion

   　　c. Appear black or shades of black after film processing

B. Maxillary anatomic landmarks (Figure 8-35 a–g■)

   1. Maxillary tuberosity (a)

   　　a. Molar region—Distal to third molar

   　　b. Heel or rounded end of alveolar ridge

   　　c. Radiopaque

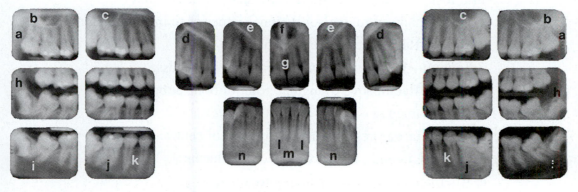

FIGURE 8-35 ■ Anatomic landmarks shown on this full mouth survey include (a) maxillary tuberosity; (b) zygomatic process; (c) maxillary sinus; (d) inverted Y; (e) nasal fossa; (g) incisive foramen; (h) external oblique ridge; (i) mandibular canal; (j) internal oblique ridge; (k) mental foramen; (l) mental ridge; (m) genial tubercles surrounding the lingual foramen; and (n) inferior border of the mandible.

2. Coronoid process of mandible

    a. Molar region—Inferoposterior corner of film

    b. Triangular or thumb-shaped bone

    c. Radiopaque

3. Pterygoid plates

    a. Molar region—Distal to tuberosity

    b. Medial pterygoid plate or pterygoid hamulus—Small, finger-like bone

    c. Lateral pterygoid plate—Thin wing of bone

    d. Both radiopaque

4. Zygomatic process and bone (b)

    a. Molar and premolar region—Superior to molar teeth

    b. Zygomatic process—U-shaped radiopacity above first molar

    c. Zygomatic bone—Broad radiopacity extending away from zygomatic process in posterior direction

    d. Alternate name—Malar process/malar bone

5. Maxillary sinus (c)

    a. Molar, premolar, and canine region—Oblong cavity superior to posterior teeth

    b. Alternate name—Maxillary antrum

    c. Radiolucent body with fine radiopaque borders

6. Inverted Y (d)

    a. Canine and lateral incisor region—Superior to teeth roots

    b. Bony septum between maxillary sinus and nasal fossa

    c. Radiopacity dividing two radiolucent cavities

7. Nasal fossa (e), nasal septum (f), and anterior nasal spine

    a. Lateral and central incisor region—Superior to incisor teeth roots

    b. Fossa—Radiolucent oblong cavities

    c. Septum—Radiopaque vertical band dividing fossa

    d. Spine—Radiopaque triangular point of bone at base of nasal septum

8. Incisive foramen (g)

    a. Central incisor region—Between roots of central incisors

    b. Oval-, diamond-, or heart-shaped radiolucency

    c. Alternate name—Nasopalatine foramen

9. Midpalatine suture

    a. Central incisor region—Midline, between central incisor teeth

b. Thin, vertical linear radiolucency

c. Alternate names—Median palatal, maxillary suture, or intermaxillary suture

C. Mandibular anatomic landmarks (Figure 8-35 h–n■)

  1. External oblique ridge or line (h)

    a. Molar region—Crosses third molar crown

    b. Diagonal outer ridge of anterior ramus

    c. Radiopaque diagonal stripe

  2. Mandibular canal space (i)

    a. Molar and premolar region—Inferior to molar roots

    b. Diagonal radiolucent tube or ribbon with fine radiopaque borders

    c. Alternate name—Inferior alveolar canal space

  3. Internal oblique ridge or line (j)

    a. Molar and premolar region—Crosses molar roots

    b. Diagonal inner ridge of anterior ramus

    c. Radiopaque diagonal stripe

    d. Alternate name—Mylohyoid ridge or line

  4. Mental foramen (k)

    a. Premolar and canine region—Adjacent to premolar roots

    b. Circular radiolucency

    c. Sometimes misinterpreted as periapical pathology

  5. Submandibular fossae

    a. Molar and premolar region—Between internal oblique ridge and lower border of the mandible

    b. Cavity on lingual surface of the mandible for submandibular gland

    c. Poorly defined radiolucency with sparse trabecular pattern

  6. Mental ridge (l)

    a. Canine and incisor region—Inferior to teeth roots

    b. Radiopaque inverted V-shaped or triangular ridge

  7. Genial tubercles (m)

    a. Incisor region—Inferior third of anterior mandible

    b. Radiopaque ring of bone

    c. Alternate name—Mental spines

  8. Lingual foramen

    a. Incisor region—Inferior third of anterior mandible

    b. Pinpoint radiolucency often surrounded by genial tubercles

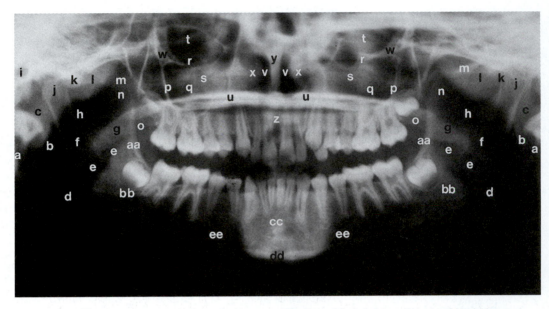

FIGURE 8-36 ■ Anatomic landmarks shown on this panoramic radiograph include (a) cervical spine; (b) styloid process; (c) ear soft tissue; (d) angle of the mandible; (e) oropharyngeal air space; (f) mandibular foramen; (g) soft palate; (h) nasopharyngeal air space; (i) external auditory meatus; (j) mandibular condyle; (k) articular eminence; (l) zygomatic arch; (m) zygomaticotemporal suture; (n) coronoid process; (o) maxillary tuberosity; (p) zygomatic process; (q) maxillary sinus; (r) infraorbital canal; (s) infraorbial foramen; (t) orbit; (u) hard palate; (v) nasal fossa; (w) rim of the orbit; (x) nasal conchae; (y) nasal septum; (z) incisive foramen; (aa) external oblique ridge; (bb) ghost of the opposite ramus and inferior border of the mandible; (cc) genial tubercles and lingual foramen; (dd) inferior border of the mandible; and (ee) mental foramen.

9. Inferior or lower border of mandible (n)
 a. Possible to be seen on any mandibular periapical
 b. Radiopaque horizontal band

D. Anatomic landmarks on panoramic radiographs (in addition to previously described anatomic landmarks) (Figure 8-36■)

 1. Maxillary

  a. Nasal conchae (x)—Radiopaque ovoid bones located on lateral aspects of nasal cavity (turbinates)

  b. Hard palate (u)—Radiopaque, horizontal band superior to maxillary teeth that forms roof of oral cavity

 2. Mandible

  a. Mandibular condyle (j)—Radiopaque, rounded articular process of the mandible

  b. Angle of mandible (d)—Radiopaque intersection of ramus and body of mandible

  c. Mandibular foramen (f)—Radiolucent opening into mandibular canal on medial surface of ramus

3. Adjacent structures
   a. Rim of orbit (w)—Radiopaque bone cavity surrounding orbit (eye socket); orbit (t) is radiolucent
   b. Infraorbital canal (r)—Radiolucent tubular structure with parallel radiopaque borders extending from floor of orbit to infraorbital foramen
   c. Infraorbital foramen (s)—Radiolucent circular external opening of infraorbital canal located on anterior surface of maxilla
   d. Pterygomaxillary fissure (loop between m and w)—Radiolucent inverted teardrop-shaped space between posterior maxilla and pterygoid plates
   e. External auditory meatus (i)—Radiolucent ovoid opening of ear canal
   f. Zygomaticotemporal suture (m)—Radiolucent diagonal junction between zygomatic process (p) of temporal bone and temporal process of zygomatic bone; processes form zygoma
   g. Zygomatic arch (l)—Radiopaque horizontal bony process that attaches to temporal bone
   h. Glenoid fossae (above j)—Radiolucent cavity in temporal bone where mandibular condyle rests
   i. Articular eminence (k)—Radiopaque bony prominence on inferior surface of zygomatic arch anterior to glenoid fossae
   j. Cervical spine (a)—Radiopaque vertebrae in neck region
   k. Styloid process (b)—Radiopaque slender, pointed projection extending downward from temporal bone
   l. Hyoid bone—Radiopaque, U-shaped bone in neck

4. Soft tissues
   a. Nasal soft tissue—Faint radiopacity of tip and ala of nose
   b. Soft palate (g)—Faint radiopacity extending downward from posterior aspect of hard palate
   c. Ear lobes (c)—Faint radiopacity of fleshy part of ear inferior to external auditory meatus
   d. Tongue—Faint radiopacity representing lateral and dorsal surfaces of tongue
   e. Lips—Faint radiopacity of upper and lower lip

5. Air–space images
   a. Nasopharyngeal (h)—Radiolucent airway of pharynx and nasal cavity located above soft and hard palate
   b. Oropharyngeal (e)—Radiolucent airway of pharynx and oral cavity located below soft palate
   c. Palatoglossal (below u)—Radiolucent space between dorsum of tongue and hard palate

XIII.   Film Mounting and Duplication

A. Film mounting procedures

1. Labial mounting—Film dot convexities toward operator, patient's right and left; ADA-accepted standard for film mounting

2. Lingual mounting—Film dot concavities toward operator, operator's right and left

3. Film mount selection

   a. Plastic or cardboard frame material opaque to light

   b. Number of film windows matches orientation and number of radiographs

   c. Organizes film survey to reflect patient's oral cavity

   d. Proper labeling and identification—Include patient's full name, date of survey, dentist's office, and operator

4. Mounting procedure

   a. Orient film dot convexity uniformly

   b. Identify film types

      (1) Bitewings—Crowns in occlusion, horizontal placements (usually), smile appearance of occlusal plane

      (2) Anterior periapicals—Vertical placements of the crowns and apices of canine and incisor teeth

      (3) Posterior periapicals—Horizontal placements of crowns and apices of premolar and molar teeth

      (4) Arrange films in order, then mount with respect to

         (a) Tooth morphology

         (b) Anatomic landmarks

         (c) Natural order and progression of dentition

         (d) Match restorations and missing teeth from film to film

         (e) Check for smile appearance or curve of occlusal plane

B. Film duplication procedures

1. Film duplication—Process of copying radiographs by passing ultraviolet light through an original survey and exposing film designed for duplication

2. Duplication film has a single emulsion

   a. Emulsion side has a light, dull appearance

   b. Nonemulsion side has a dark, shiny appearance

   c. Sheet duplication film does not have a film identification dot

   d. Direct reversal film; whiteness is deposited rather than blackness

3. Light exposure of duplication film is opposite to principles of x-ray film exposure

   a. Low-density or light original radiographs require less light exposure on duplication

   b. High-density or dark original radiographs require more light exposure on duplication

4. Good contact between duplication film and mounted radiographs necessary to prevent blurring and fuzziness of duplicated image

5. Duplication procedure

   a. Place correctly organized radiographs into flat pocket mount

   b. Take survey into darkroom and continue procedures under safelight conditions

   c. Place mounted film survey with front of mount placed toward the duplicator light box surface for labially mounted radiographs

   d. Place emulsion side of duplication film on lingual side of mounted radiographs

   e. Close lid of duplicator, pressing duplication film firmly against the survey, and latch it

   f. Set timer on light box for appropriate amount of light exposure; press timer button and observe exposure

   g. Process exposed duplication film and evaluate results; repeat if necessary

   h. Trim, label, identify right and left sides of finished film using original survey as reference

XIV. Interpretation

A. Viewing conditions

   1. Subdued background lighting

   2. Viewbox used for even light distribution and transillumination

   3. Eliminate excess light around films/mount

   4. Use systematic approach when making observations

   5. Magnification is useful for examining small details

B. Caries (Figure 8-37■)

   1. Cavity preparation and restoration classification

   a. Class I—All pit and fissure cavities

   (1) Occlusals of molars and premolars

   (2) Occlusal two-thirds of facial and lingual surfaces of molars

   (3) Lingual pits of maxillary incisors

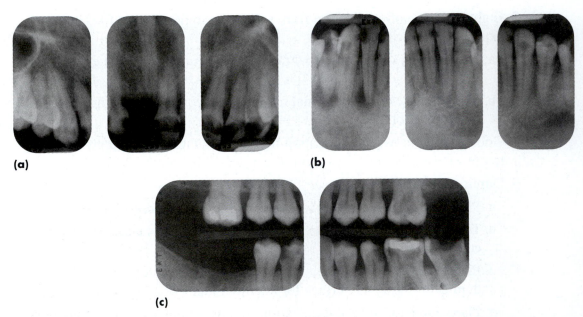

(a)

(b)

(c)

FIGURE 8-37 ■ (a) The maxillary anterior periapicals display the following carious lesions: CIII lesions—#6 mesial, #7 mesial and distal, #9 distal, #10 distal; CIV lesions—#9 mesial, #10, mesial and #11 mesial; CV lesion—#9 facial. (b) The mandibular anterior periapicals display the following carious lesions: CII lesions—#20 distal and occlusal, #21 distal, #28 mesial, occlusal, and distal, #29 mesial and distal; CIII—#22 mesial and distal, #23 mesial and distal, #24 mesial and distal, #25 mesial, #26 mesial and distal, #27 mesial; CIV lesions—#25 distal; CV lesions—#22 facial, #27 facial. (c) The premolar bitewing views display the following carious lesions: CII lesions—#3 mesial and distal, #4 mesial and distal, #5 mesial and distal, #12 mesial and distal, #13 mesial and distal, #14 mesial, occlusal, and distal, #18 mesial, occlusal, distal, buccal, and lingual, #19 mesial and distal, #20 mesial, occlusal, and distal, #21 mesial and distal, #28 mesial, occlusal, and distal, #29 mesial and distal; CIII lesions—distal, #11 distal, #27 distal; CV lesions—#19 buccal, #21 buccal.

    b. Class II—Cavities on proximal surfaces of molars and premolars

    c. Class III—Cavities on proximal surfaces of incisors and canines not involving incisal angle

    d. Class IV—Cavities on proximal surfaces of incisors and canines involving incisal angle

    e. Class V—Cavities on gingival one-third of facial or lingual surfaces of all teeth

    f. Class VI—Cavities on the incisal edge of anterior teeth or the cusp tips on posterior teeth

2. Interproximal caries

    a. Carious lesions that occur just below the contacts of the teeth

    b. Best found radiographically on bitewings

    c. Typical shape—Horizontal V-shaped or triangular radiolucency

    d. Degree classification

        (1) Incipient (Class/Type I)—Lesion has penetrated less than halfway through the enamel layer

      (2) Moderate (Class/Type II)—Lesion has penetrated more than halfway through the enamel layer but does not involve the dentinoenamel junction (DEJ)

      (3) Advanced (Class/Type III)—Lesion has penetrated through the DEJ and spread less than halfway to the pulp

      (4) Severe (Class/Type IV)—Lesion has penetrated through the DEJ and spread more than halfway to the pulp or involves the pulp

3. Occlusal caries

    a. Caries involving the pits and fissures of posterior teeth

    b. Radiographically apparent once through the occlusal enamel layer

    c. Typical shape—Triangular radiolucency with the base broadening as the dentin is invaded

4. Buccal and lingual caries

    a. Caries of the cervical third of the facial or lingual surfaces of the crown

    b. Typical shape—Crescent or dot radiolucency in the cervical third of the crown

    c. May be confused with Class V radiolucent tooth-colored restorations

5. Root caries

    a. Carious involvement of cementum and dentin of exposed root surfaces

    b. Typical shape—Diffuse rounded inner border without lateral tooth edge

    c. May be confused with cervical burnout

      (1) Phenomenon of x-ray penetration of cementoenamel junction (CEJ) anatomy

      (2) Wedge-shaped radiolucency adjacent to CEJ

      (3) Lateral root edge is seen

6. Recurrent caries

    a. Caries that occur around margins of existing restorations

    b. Typical shape—Radiolucent halo below interproximal or occlusal margin

C. Periodontal disease

1. Benefits and limitations of radiographs

    a. Benefits

      (1) Depiction of bone height and density

      (2) Permits evaluation of root length and shape

      (3) View periodontal ligament (PDL) widening

      (4) View normal anatomy relative to bony defects

      (5) Periapical coverage of teeth

      (6) Observe moderate to advanced furcation involvement and local irritants

b. Limitations

(1) Inability to evaluate incipient bone loss

(2) Unable to determine presence or absence of periodontal pockets or level of epithelial attachment

(3) Unable to determine morphology of bone defects, buccal/lingual bone status, mobility, or early furcation involvement

2. Classification of periodontal disease progression

a. Case Type I

(1) Gingivitis

(2) No radiographic changes

(3) Alveolar bone 1.5–2.0 mm from CEJ

b. Case Type II

(1) Early or mild periodontitis

(2) Radiographs may show crestal lamina dura changes, triangulation, 20–30% bone loss

(3) Alveolar bone 3–4 mm from CEJ

c. Case Type III

(1) Moderate periodontitics

(2) Radiographs show mild to moderate bone loss, 30–50%

(3) Alveolar bone 5–7 mm from CEJ

(4) Furcation involvement, bony defects

d. Case Type IV

(1) Advanced periodontitis

(2) Radiographs show severe bone loss, > 50% bone loss

(3) Alveolar bone ≥ 8 mm from CEJ

(4) Severe destruction of periodontal structures, advanced furcation involvement and bony defects

3. Early disease observations

a. Crestal bony changes—Loss of sharp angle between crestal lamina dura and alveolar crest, decreased bone density (radiolucent)

b. PDL widening near bony crests (triangulation)

c. Widened vascular channels

4. Evaluation of bone loss—Determined by comparing bony margins to plane of adjacent CEJs

a. Normal appearance

(1) Bone crests—Anterior crests are pointed, posterior crests are flat and angular

      (2) Normal height—1.5–2.0 mm from CEJ

      (3) Bone crests are radiopaque, with lamina dura extending from lateral root surfaces across crestal bone with trabeculated underlying bone

      (4) Periodontal ligament space—Linear radiolucency (0.25–0.40 mm wide) located between tooth root and lamina dura

  b. Types of bone loss

      (1) Horizontal bone loss—Bony margin is parallel to plane of adjacent CEJs (Figure 8-38■)

      (2) Vertical bone loss—Bony margin is diagonal to plane of adjacent CEJs (Figure 8-39■)

      (3) Localized or generalized condition

      (4) Degree classification—Mild (slight), moderate, advanced (severe)

  c. Evaluation of bony defects—Areas of decreased bone density that vary in size, shape, and location

  d. Local factors and irritants

      (1) Calculus deposits—Radiopaque spurs, rings, ledges

      (2) Faulty restorations—Overhanging margins, poor proximal contours

      (3) Occlusal trauma—May widen PDL or thicken lamina dura or both

      (4) Areas of food impaction

      (5) Root morphology and crown–root ratio

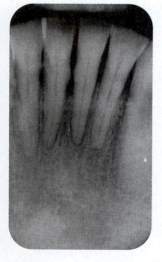

FIGURE 8-38 ■ Horizontal Bone Loss

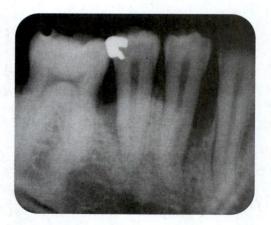

FIGURE 8-39 ■ Vertical Bone Loss

      e. Furcation involvement (Figure 8-40■)

         (1) Advanced bone loss that exposes furcation areas of multirooted teeth

         (2) Radiographic appearance—Area of decreased bone density (radiolucency) within furcation

         (3) Class II and Class III furcation involvement visible radiographically

D. Periapical disease—Most common types

  1. Periapical granuloma

    a. Most common aftermath of pulpitis

    b. Round radiolucency with well-defined radiopaque border

    c. Vary in size; may show some trabeculations within lesion

    d. Nonvital tooth, usually asymptomatic

  2. Periapical cyst

    a. Often sequela of periapical granuloma

    b. Nonvital tooth, usually asymptomatic

    c. Radiographic presentation similar to periapical granuloma

    d. Often larger, more radiolucent with fewer central trabeculations than periapical granuloma

    e. May involve more than one tooth

  3. Chronic periapical abscess

    a. May develop after an acute periapical abscess or in existing periapical granuloma

    b. Radiolucent lesion with diffuse, irregular borders that blend into the bony pattern

    c. Often extends beyond tooth apex and involves lateral aspects of root

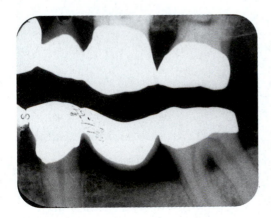

FIGURE 8-40 ■ Class II and Class III Furcation Involvement

     d. Involved tooth usually asymptomatic

     e. Fistulous tract may be found clinically

4. Condensing osteitis or chronic focal sclerosing osteomyelitis

     a. Reaction of bone to infection

     b. Typically involves first molars in young people

     c. Well-circumscribed radiopaque mass surrounding apex or apices of carious or heavily restored tooth

     d. Root outline visible

     e. Sclerotic bone may have distinct or diffuse border

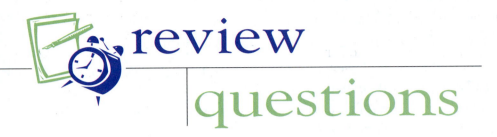

review questions

DIRECTIONS Each of the questions or incomplete statements below is followed by suggested answers or completions. Select the **one** answer that is best in each case.

1. All of the following descriptions are characteristic of electromagnetic radiation EXCEPT one. Which one is the EXCEPTION?
   A. Some types can ionize human tissue
   B. Include visible and ultraviolet light
   C. Travel in an oscillating motion
   D. Include alpha and beta particles *Particulate Rx*
   E. Energies vary in wavelength

2. All of the following descriptions are characteristic of x-ray energy EXCEPT one. Which one is the EXCEPTION?
   A. Form of particulate radiation *Electromagnetic*
   B. Cause certain substances to fluoresce
   C. Produce a latent image on a receptor
   D. Capable of penetrating matter
   E. Differentially absorbed

3. Which of the following accurately describes the anode electrode?
   A. Aluminum focal spot
   B. Source of x-rays
   C. Controlled by low-voltage circuit
   D. Surrounded by molybdenum focusing cup

4. The step-down transformer is responsible for all of the following activities EXCEPT one. Which one is the EXCEPTION?
   A. Supplies current to the cathode electrode
   B. Is operated by the mA switch
   C. Decreases electrical current
   D. Creates a potential difference

5. What is Bremsstrahlung radiation?
   A. Radiation produced by particle interaction at the P or Q shell level of target atoms
   B. X-ray photons generated as a result of particle interaction at or near the nucleus of target atoms
   C. Thermal energy produced by particle interaction at the outer shell levels of target atoms
   D. A minor source of particle energy generated

6. All of the following statements are correct regarding intraoral film EXCEPT one. Which one is the EXCEPTION?
   A. Intraoral film consists of a plastic film base coated with silver halide crystals.
   B. The purpose of the lead foil is to reduce film fog by absorbing scatter radiation.
   C. The color-coded side of the film packet is directed toward the x-ray source.
   D. The outer covering of the film packet is either plastic or paper.

7. Fluorescent light and x-rays produce the latent image on intraoral radiographs. The visible image on an extraoral film is the result of chemical processing of the exposed film.
   A. The first statement is TRUE. The second statement is FALSE.
   B. The first statement is FALSE. The second statement is TRUE.
   C. Both statements are TRUE.
   D. Both statements are FALSE.

8. Which of the following is the most common method of altering film density?
   A. Changing the milliamperage setting
   B. Adjusting the kilovoltage peak
   C. Changing the length of the PID
   D. Altering the exposure time

9. The x-ray machine is set at 10mA, 60 kVp, and .80 second. It is necessary to change the kilovoltage setting to 90 kVp. To maintain the same film density, what would be the new exposure time at 90 kVp?
   A. 1.60 seconds
   B. 1.20 seconds
   C. .40 second
   D. .20 second
   E. .10 second

10. Collimation of the x-ray beam produces all of the following outcomes EXCEPT one. Which one is the EXCEPTION?
    A. Increases intensity of x-ray beam
    B. Restricts size of x-ray beam
    C. Reduces exposure to patient
    D. Minimizes image magnification
    E. Improves image sharpness

11. The x-ray machine is equipped with a short 4-inch PID and the exposure factors are set at 15 mA, 80 kVp, and .10 second. If the PID is changed to a 12-inch length, what should the exposure time be at the new distance?
    A. .20 second
    B. .40 second
    C. .90 second
    D. 1.00 second
    E. 1.60 seconds

12. Which of the following phrases is MOST representative of long-scale contrast?
    A. Produced by reduced x-ray penetration of the involved structures
    B. Described as high contrast with a black or white appearance
    C. Type of contrast preferred for carious lesion diagnosis
    D. Described as low contrast with few shades between black and white
    E. Demonstrates a broad range of densities on the processed radiograph

13. Which of the following phrases does NOT accurately describe x-ray beam filtration?
    A. Amount of required filtration depends on the kilovoltage setting
    B. Includes inherent filtration such as the window and oil
    C. Platinum is the most common filter material
    D. Total filtration includes inherent and added
    E. Improves quality of x-ray beam

14. All of the following phrases are consistent with the paralleling technique EXCEPT one. Which one is the EXCEPTION?
    A. A short position indicating device is used
    B. It is the preferred method for taking radiographs
    C. The film is placed parallel to the long axes of the teeth
    D. The central ray is directed at a right angle to the teeth and film
    E. It produces images with the least unsharpness, magnification, and shape distortion

15. From the list below, select the factor that would BEST achieve the anatomic accuracy of an image.
    A. Focal spot size
    B. Object–film distance
    C. Source–object distance
    D. Object–film parallelism

16. All of the following phrases are descriptive of Compton scattering EXCEPT one. Which one is the EXCEPTION?
    A. Photon interaction occurs with electron in the K shell of absorber atom.
    B. It produces a scattered photon of lower energy called a recoil electron.
    C. 62% of x-ray beam photons undergo Compton scattering.
    D. It results in ionization of the involved absorber atom.
    E. It contributes to film fog.

17. All of the following accurately describe the indirect effects of x-radiation EXCEPT one. Which one is the EXCEPTION?
    A. Ionization event
    B. Production of free radicals
    C. Direct alteration of biomolecules
    D. Radiolysis of water
    E. 66% of induced biological damage

18. Which of the following cells or tissues are NOT highly sensitive to the effects of radiation?
    A. Bone marrow
    B. Small blood vessels
    C. Small lymphocyte
    D. Sperm and ova

19. Which of the following is consistent with the dose equivalent?
    A. Compares biological effects of different types of radiation
    B. Quantifies the radioactivity of x-rays
    C. Measure of ability of x-rays to ionize air
    D. Measure of radiation exposure

20. Using the following would result in patient exposure reduction EXCEPT one. Which one is the EXCEPTION?
    A. Lead-lined thyroid collar
    B. 16-inch PID rather than an 8-inch PID
    C. Rectangular collimation
    D. Rare earth-intensifying screens
    E. A low kilovoltage

21. In the developer, what is the function of the reducing agent hydroquinone?
    A. Removes the unexposed, undeveloped silver bromide crystals *fixing*
    B. Stops development by neutralizing chemical carryover
    C. Reaction provides the black tones and contrast of the image
    D. Softens the film emulsion to speed development

22. Which one of the following quality assurance procedures is NOT accurately described?
    A. The coin test is used to evaluate x-ray machine function such as output, kilovoltage calibration, and milliamperage reproducibility.
    B. Solution monitoring involves the comparison of a control film taken at the time of solution change and a daily check film.
    C. On a monthly basis, inspect cassettes for damage and function and clean the intensifying screens.
    D. Preclean, disinfect, and cover operatory viewboxes in preparation for patient care and replace light bulbs as needed.

23. To correct the technical error of overlapping, it is necessary to
    A. Increase the vertical angulation to reduce the overlapping of the structures
    B. Place the film so that it is parallel to the long axes of the teeth to be recorded
    C. Direct the horizontal angle through the interproximal surfaces of the teeth of interest
    D. Decrease the positive vertical angle and move the x-ray beam in a more posterior direction

24. All of the following descriptions indicate backward placement of an intraoral film packet EXCEPT one. Which one is the EXCEPTION?
    A. The colored side of the film packet was placed toward the x-ray source.
    B. The film identification dot convexity was directed toward x-ray source.
    C. The pattern of the lead foil appears on the processed radiograph.
    D. The processed film has a low-density appearance.

25. Which of the following does NOT cause a high-density radiograph?
    A. White light leaks or improper safelight conditions in the darkroom
    B. Overdevelopment owing to a high processing temperature
    C. Underreplenishment of the processing solutions
    D. Double exposure of a film

26. Panoramic ghost images display certain radiographic features. Which of the following features is NOT characteristic of ghost images?
    A. Typical structures that produce ghosts include the ramus areas and metal earrings.
    B. Ghost images are reversed and appear on the same side as the original structure.
    C. Ghost images appear magnified and blurred in the horizontal plane.
    D. Ghost images appear higher on the film than the original structure.

27. Which guideline does NOT aid in the production of a diagnostic panoramic radiograph?
    A. Place occlusal plane parallel to the floor
    B. Lead apron clears back of the neck
    C. Patient stands or sits with erect spine
    D. Have patient place tongue in floor of mouth

28. Which of the following selections is NOT descriptive of the tube shift method of object localization?
    A. Also referred to as Clark's rule or the buccal object rule, object movement is compared to movement of the PID
    B. Buccal objects move in the opposite direction
    C. Lingual objects move in the same direction
    D. Requires at least a two-film comparison

29. Select the landmark that is radiopaque and recorded on posterior periapicals.
    A. Genial tubercles
    B. Mandibular foreman
    C. Zygomatic bone
    D. Maxillary sinus

30. Compared with intraoral radiographs, all of the following landmarks are found ONLY on panoramic radiographs EXCEPT one. Which one is the EXCEPTION?
    A. External auditory meatus
    B. Cervical spine
    C. Hyoid bone
    D. Coronoid process

31. Which one of the following selections is NOT an accurate description of carious lesions?
    A. Carious lesions that occur on the proximal surfaces of incisors and canines are classified as Class III lesions.
    B. The typical radiographic presentation of a Class V lesion is a crescent or dot radiolucency.
    C. Frequently, a recurrent carious lesion occurs under the proximal margin of a restoration.
    D. Class II lesions are best found radiographically and located just below the contacts of posterior teeth.
    E. An incipient carious lesion is one that is proximal and has penetrated to the DEJ.

32. All of the following selections describe the benefits of radiographs in periodontal disease assessment EXCEPT one. Which one is the EXCEPTION?
    A. Can determine the level of epithelial attachment
    B. Observe periodontal ligament widening
    C. Observe the apical regions of the teeth
    D. Evaluate root length and shape
    E. View bone height and density

33. Which of the following descriptions is NOT consistent with the normal radiographic presentation of periodontal structures?
    A. Anterior bone crests are narrow and pointed
    B. Posterior bone crests are flat and angular in shape
    C. Normal bone height is 1.0–3.0 mm from the CEJ
    D. Bone crests are radiopaque with the lamina dura outlining the bony septa
    E. The periodontal ligament space is a linear radiolucency surrounding the tooth root

34. All of the following radiographic observations are consistent with early periodontal disease EXCEPT one. Which one is the EXCEPTION?
    A. Triangulation
    B. Decreased bone density
    C. Widened vascular channels
    D. Thickening of the lamina dura
    E. Loss of a sharp angle between the crestal lamina dura and bone crest

35. How does the periapical cyst differ from the periapical granuloma?
    A. Usually larger and may involve more than one tooth
    B. Demonstrates central trabeculations within lesion
    C. Round radiolucency with a well-defined border
    D. Tooth usually asymptomatic
    E. Involves a nonvital tooth

36. A radiograph that is too light in density may be caused by
    A. Overdeveloping the film
    B. Using an exhausted developer
    C. Using high kilovoltage
    D. Too much radiation exposure time

37. Yellow-brown stains on radiographs can result from all of the following EXCEPT
    A. Unclean processing tanks
    B. Insufficient fixing
    C. Insufficient washing
    D. Overfixing

38. Image magnification may be minimized by
    A. Using a long cone
    B. Using a short cone
    C. Placing the film as far from the tooth as possible
    D. Shortening the exposure time

39. Radiographic examinations should be made on patients
    A. At least every 2 years
    B. At various intervals depending on their dental history
    C. At least every 3 years
    D. Whenever professional judgment dictates

40. On intraoral radiographs, dark areas around the necks of teeth are sometimes misinterpreted as carious lesions. These areas result from
    A. Attrition
    B. Abrasion
    C. The mach band effect
    D. Cervical burnout

41. Which of the following cells are LEAST sensitive to radiation (radioresistant)?
    A. Epithelial cells of the gastrointestinal tract
    B. Lymphocytes
    C. Nerve cells
    D. Fibroblasts

42. Black lines on a film may be produced by
    A. Fixer spills onto the film prior to processing
    B. High temperature
    C. Static electricity
    D. Air bubbles

43. Panoramic radiographs are very useful for many reasons, but they may NOT accurately depict with of the following?
    A. Interproximal caries
    B. Presence of foreign bodies
    C. The relationship of one intraoral structure to another
    D. Fractures of the mandible

44. Intensifying screens used when extraoral radiographs are made
    A. Aid in decreasing radiation exposure to the patient
    B. Contain silver bromide crystals
    C. Increase radiographic sharpness
    D. Reduce film fog

45. Cone cutting (partial image) on a radiograph is caused by
    A. Pointed plastic cone of radiation
    B. Underexposure
    C. Improper coverage of the film with the primary beam of radiation
    D. Placing the film in reverse to the beam of radiation
    E. All of the above

46. Which of the following is radiolucent restorative material?
    A. Amalgam
    B. Acrylic
    C. Silver points
    D. Gold

47. Processing solutions should be monitored and changed every
    A. Day
    B. Week
    C. 2 weeks
    D. 4 weeks

48. Which form of radiation is known to cause ionization of body tissue cells?
    A. Microwaves
    B. Radar
    C. X-ray
    D. Radio

49. Radiation injury during tooth development *before mineralization* can lead to
    A. Hypocalcification
    B. Tooth bud destruction
    C. Complete anodontia
    D. Radiation caries
    E. hyperplastic enamel

50. A herringbone pattern on the dental radiograph is indicative of
    A. Poor washing technique
    B. Overdevelopment
    C. Inadequate fixation
    D. Film placed backward *(waffle)*
    E. Inadequate development

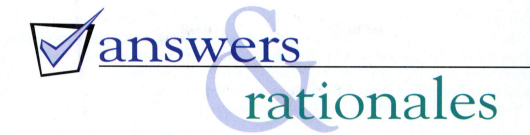
answers & rationales

1.

D. Alpha and beta particles are not electromagnetic radiations. They are considered particulate radiation. Electromagnetic radiation has the following characteristics. It travels in a wave motion and has energies with varied wavelengths. Some types of electromagnetic radiation can ionize human tissue. Visible and ultraviolet light are some familiar examples of this type of energy.

2.

A. X-ray energy is not a form of particulate radiation. X-rays are a form of electromagnetic radiation and are not particles. X-ray energy is classified as causing certain substances to fluoresce, produce a latent image, differentially absorb, and capable of penetrating matter.

3.

B. X-rays are generated by electron bombardment of the anode target. The anode is housed inside the x-ray tube and is composed of a copper rod with a tungsten metal target, controlled by the high-voltage circuit. X-rays are generated by electron bombardment of the anode target. The molybdenum focusing cup is located in the cathode, not the anode.

4.

D. The step-up transformer, rather than the step-down transformer, creates a potential difference between the anode and cathode in the x-ray production system. The step-down transformer is operated by the mA switch, supplies a low-voltage current to the cathode to heat the tungsten filament, and produces free electrons (electron cloud) at the cathode.

5.

B. Bremsstrahlung radiation is produced when high-speed electrons are stopped or slowed down by the tungsten atoms as they collide with the nuclei of the target atoms.

6.

C. This would produce an image error owing to improper placement of the film in relation to the x-ray source. In all instances, the white side of the film packet is directed toward the x-ray source. The intraoral film packet consists of the base, which is coated with halide crystals; the lead foil, which reduces film fog; and the plastic or paper outer covering.

7.

D. In extraoral radiography, it is the sum of the fluorescent light and x-rays that expose the film, rather than x-rays alone as with intraoral radiography. The detail and visibility of a radiograph depends on two independent factors: the radiographic contrast and sharpness.

8.

D. The most common method of altering film density is by changing the exposure time. Some intraoral x-ray machines have fixed milliamperage and kilovoltage settings, only allowing variations in exposure time. Changing the length of the PID isn't a common method of altering film density.

9.

D. The rule of thumb for altering kilovoltage is for every 15 kVp increase, divide the time by 2. In this problem, the kVp was increased from 60 to 90, requiring two reductions in the exposure time.

10.

A. Collimation restricts the primary beam of radiation, reducing the area of exposure at the skin surface. In addition, it keeps the x-rays more parallel to one another and improves image geometry. Intensity is altered when the source–object distance is changed. Optimum collimation infers a 16-inch PID, which would decrease beam intensity and require an increase in exposure time if changed from a shorter PID.

11.

C. In this inverse square law problem, the PID was changed from 4-inch to 12-inch. The law states that intensity varies as the square of the source–film distance. Since the distance tripled, square 3 and multiply the original time by 9 to calculate the new exposure time to equalize the x-ray beam intensity at 12 inches.

12.

E. Long-scale contrast is produced at higher kilovoltage settings by greater beam penetration of structures. This produces many shades of gray on the processed film, lowers contrast, and is preferred for periodontal diagnosis—not carious lesions—because more subtle changes can be observed.

13.

C. The most common filter material used in dental x-ray machines is aluminum. The amount of added aluminum filtration is determined by the kilovoltage setting.

14.

A. The paralleling technique utilizes a long PID rather than a short PID. The longer cone is used to counteract the magnification that occurs from a slightly increased object–film distance as well as to minimize image unsharpness.

15.

D. Anatomic accuracy is best achieved when the film is placed parallel to the teeth of interest, and the central ray is directed perpendicular to the teeth and film. Focal spot size, object–film distance, and source–object distance affect geometric rather than anatomic accuracy of an image.

16.

A. Photon interaction occurs with electron in the K shell of absorber atom. Compton scattering is the result of photon interaction with outer electron shells of the absorber atom.

17.

C. The indirect effects of x-radiation occur through ionization or radiolysis of water molecules and produce free radicals that cause various reactions in the formation of new molecules. It is estimated that 66% of induced biological damage occurs via this process. The direct alteration of biomolecules results when radiation interacts with the DNA of the cells. This does not occur in dental radiation.

18.

B. Small blood vessels are categorized as having intermediate sensitivity rather than high sensitivity to the effects of radiation. Bone marrow, small lymphocytes, and sperm and ova are highly sensitive to the effects of radiation.

19.

A. The dose equivalent is used to compare the biological effects (relative biological effectiveness) of different types of radiation. It does not measure the radiation exposure or ability to ionize air, or quantify the radioactivity of x-rays.

20.

E. Lower kilovoltage produces a higher skin dose than higher kilovoltage. Use of a lead-lined thyroid collar, rectangular 16-inch PID, and rare earth-intensifying screens reduce radiation exposure to the patient.

21.

C. Hydroquinone is the developer reducing agent that generates the black tones and contrast of the radiographic image. In the fixing solution, the sodium thiosulfate removes the unexposed, undeveloped silver bromide crystals. Water stops the developing process. Sodium carbonate softens the film emulsion to speed development.

22.

A. The coin test is a quality assurance procedure for evaluating white light leaks and safelight conditions in the darkroom. Solution monitoring, inspection of cassettes, and infection control for the viewboxes are quality assurance procedures.

23.

C. To correct overlapping, direct the horizontal angle through the interproximal surfaces of the teeth.

24.

B. If the film was placed backward, the film dot concavity was placed toward the x-ray source.

25.

C. Underreplenishment of the processing solutions would produce a low-density image. Overreplenishment of the processing solutions would produce a high-density image. Double exposure, white light, and overdevelopment would produce high-density images.

26.

B. Ghost images are reversed, but they appear on the opposite side of the original structure rather than the same side. Typical structures that ghost are the ramus areas and metal earrings. Ghost images also appear magnified and blurred in the horizontal plane and higher on the film than the original structure.

27.

D. In panoramic radiography, the tongue should be placed on the palate rather than the floor of the mouth and the lead apron should be placed so that it clears the back of the neck. The patient should sit or stand with an erect spine and be positioned with the occlusal plane parallel to the floor.

28.

A. In the tube shift method of object localization, the object movement is compared with the movement of the x-ray head rather than the PID. The tube-shift method of localization is also referred to as Clark's rule or buccal object rule. This means that buccal objects move in the opposite direction, and lingual objects move in the same direction, and at least two films are required for comparison.

29.

C. The radiopaque posterior landmark includes the zygomatic bone. The genial tubercles are radiopaque but appear on a mandibular anterior periapical. The mandibular foramen and maxillary sinus are radiolucent.

30.

D. The coronoid process appears in both intraoral and panoramic films. Of the landmarks listed, the external auditory meatus, cervical spine, and hyoid bone appear only on panoramic films.

31.

E. An incipient lesion is defined as one that has penetrated less than halfway through the enamel and does not involve the DEJ.

32.

A. The epithelial attachment is soft tissue in origin and, therefore, the level of attachment cannot be determined on dental radiographs; however, the remaining selections benefit periodontal disease assessment.

33.

C. The normal alveolar bone height, as measured on dental radiographs, is 1.5–2.0 mm from the CEJ and should not be confused with probing depths. The remaining descriptions are consistent with normal radiographic appearances of periodontal structures.

34.

D. Thickening of the lamina dura is more of a response to occlusal trauma than periodontal disease. Triangulation, decreased bone density, widened vascular channels, and loss of a sharp angle between the crestal lamina dura and bone crest are early radiographic signs of periodontal disease.

35.

A. The periapical cyst is the sequela of the periapical granuloma and is often larger and involves more than one tooth. Both the periapical cyst and periapical granuloma are round radiolucencies with well-defined borders and central trabeculations within the lesion that involve nonvital, asymptomatic teeth.

36.

B. A weakened developer will not fully develop the latent image in the usual time, and the density of the radiograph will be too light. A rough indication of an exhausted developer solution can be obtained by matching a good density radiograph with one taken at a later time. Less density in the more recent radiograph indicates an exhausted developer. A film positioned backward in the patient's mouth will also result in a lack of density due to the attenuation of the primary beam by the lead backing of the film. Additionally, a kVp, mA, exposure time that is too low, or a target film distance (TFD) that is too great results in a film that is too light.

37.

D. Film must be fixed in a fresh solution for an adequate length of time (i.e., 10 minutes), then washed in running water for 20 minutes. Failure to do either of these procedures will result in a lack of removal of processing chemicals. Remaining chemicals on the film will result in discoloration of the image. Additionally, if all the exposed crystals are not removed during processing, they will oxidize over a period of time and stains will result.

38.

A. In panoramic radiography, the tongue should be placed on the palate rather than the floor of the mouth and the lead apron should be placed so that it clears the back of the neck. The patient should sit or stand with an erect spine and be positioned with the occlusal plane parallel to the floor. The paralleling technique requires a target-to-object distance that is as long as possible to remain practical. The technique also requires that the x-rays strike the object and recording surface at right angles, with the x-ray film placed parallel to the long axis of the tooth. The paralleling technique requires wide separation of tooth and film. This lack of contact between tooth and film would produce distortion if a short target-to-film distance cone were used; magnification of the image on the film would occur. There is a reduction in magnification when the extended distance cone is used.

39.

D. Currently there are no specified lengths of time between which radiographs should be made on various types of patients in various age groups. The old description of "routine radiographs" has no place in today's practice of radiation reduction. The decision for radiographic examinations is therefore based on professional judgment as far as dental radiography is concerned.

40.

D. The area of the tooth between the enamel-covered crown and the portion of the root superimposed upon by alveolar bone attenuates fewer photons than the areas superior and inferior to it. As a result, a dark area referred to as cervical burnout is seen on the radiograph.

41.

D. The cells that are the most sensitive to the biological effects of radiation have been found to be those that are least differentiated, immature, and are experiencing or will experience mitotic activity. Con-

versely, cells of nervous tissue and mature bone, which are well differentiated, are the least sensitive.

42.

C. A film packet should never be opened forcefully, especially when the darkroom air is dry. This could produce static electricity, which appears characteristically as dark streaks on the processed radiographs. The film should be held by the edges to prevent crimping or fingernail pressure, which appears as a crescent-shaped dark area. Bending a film can also produce a black line because the emulsion is sensitized to energy.

43.

A. Despite their many advantages (broad coverage, anatomical relationships, the speed and ease with which they are made, and the exposure reduction when compared to a complete mouth survey), panoramic radiographs, as a result of magnification, distation, and interproximal overlap, frequently are not usable for determining the existence and/or extent of interproximal caries.

44.

A. Intensifying screens consist of tiny calcium tungstate crystals bonded in a uniform layer on a firm x-ray–penetrable base material. These screens are generally used in pairs with a double-emulsion base. This method of recording the image of an object requires much less radiation to the patient compared with when the x-ray film alone is used.

45.

C. If the central ray is not directed at the center of the film, cone cutting will result. The unexposed or white part of the film will not be in the path of radiation. Cone cut is the term commonly used to describe a radiograph made when the primary beam of an x-ray does not completely cover the film.

46.

B. The radiopacity of dental materials is contingent on atomic weight. Materials with low anatomic weight, such as acrylic, are radiolucent. Materials with high atomic weight, indicating a greater density, are radiopaque.

47.

D. Processing solutions should be changed every 4 weeks or as recommended by the manufacturer.

48.

C. Any radiation that produces ions is called ionizing radiation. The concern in dental radiography is that possible changes can occur in the cellular structures of the tissues as the ions are produced by the passage of x-rays through the cells.

49.

B. Radiation in children can affect the odontogenic cells. A tooth bud may be completely destroyed if irradiated before mineralization has started. The damage may not appear for several years after radiation exposure. Head and neck irradiation therapy can also cause osteoradionecrosis.

50.

D. A herringbone pattern indicates placement of the packet in the mouth backward with foil next to the teeth. Film exposed prior to processing can produce radiation fog.

9 Planning and Managing Dental Hygiene Care

Medical conditions occur suddenly with little or no warning. Most of these emergency medical conditions are precipitated by physiological or psychological stress like that experienced in a dental office. The dental hygienist will encounter at least one medical crisis during his or her practice lifetime. Actions taken during that time can have a direct impact on the outcome of the crisis.

chapter objectives

After completion of this chapter, the learner should be able to:

➤ Discuss the prevention of a medical emergency

➤ Discuss recognition and provision of emergency situations

➤ Discuss emergency management techniques

➤ Describe unconsciousness, emergency treatment, and management

➤ Describe altered consciousness, emergency treatment, and management

➤ Discuss chest pain and its implications, emergency treatment, and management

➤ Discuss respiratory distress, emergency treatment, and management

➤ Discuss cardiac arrest, emergency treatment, and management

➤ Discuss drug-related emergencies, emergency treatment, and management

➤ Discuss seizures or convulsions, emergency treatment, and management

➤ Discuss planning individualized patient education programs

➤ Describe dental caries

➤ Discuss dietary recommendations to reduce the potential for caries formation

➤ Discuss principles of dietary counseling

➤ Describe primary, secondary, tertiary prevention

➤ Describe principles of planning, teaching, and learning for disease prevention

➤ Discuss methods of removing bacterial plaque (biofilm)

➤ Discuss dentrifrices

➤ Discuss oral cancer

➤ Discuss tobacco cessation

➤ Describe oral habits

➤ Discuss the neurophysiology of local anesthetics

➤ Discuss the pharmacological aspects of local anesthetics and vasoconstrictors

➤ Discuss the indications and contraindications to the use of local anesthetics and vasoconstrictors

➤ Describe the armamentarium used in administering local anesthetics

➤ Discuss the techniques for maxillary and mandibular anesthesia

➤ Discuss the local complications to administering local anesthetics

➤ Discuss local anesthetic emergencies

➤ Discuss nitrous oxide sedation

➤ Discuss indications and contraindications to nitrous oxide sedation

➤ Discuss pharmacology and physiology of nitrous oxide

➤ Describe armamentarium for use of nitrous oxide

➤ Discuss safety features for use of nitrous oxide

➤ Discuss recognition and management of compromised patients

Note: For information on infectious diseases and infection control, see Chapter 4, "Microbiology, Infectious Diseases, and Infection Control."

➤ RECOGNITION OF AND PROVISION FOR EMERGENCY SITUATIONS

I. Prevention

A. Medical Crisis

    1. Awareness of risk factors

    2. Take and carefully evaluate thorough patient history

        a. Identify medical conditions indicative of potential emergency medical risk

        b. Identify drugs taken that are indicative of conditions that may cause potential emergency medical risk

    3. Seek medical consultation if history indicates potential problems or if more information is needed

    4. Take precautions to prevent life-threatening emergencies from occurring, based on the medical history

    5. Avoid complacency about patient's medical risk status

        a. Patient's longevity in the practice or absence of a previous problem, resulting in a lack of a history update or precautions addressed

        b. Must be a first time for the emergency

            (1) Know potential risk of the patient

            (2) Take necessary precautions to avoid medical emergency

            (3) Know what to do to manage the emergency

    6. Recognize physical signs and symptoms of anxiety

        a. Cold, sweaty palms or forehead

        b. Unnaturally stiff posture

        c. "White knuckle syndrome" (tightly gripping the arm of the chair or other objects)

        d. Wringing hands, playing with items in the hands

        e. Increased blood pressure and heart rate

        f. Trembling

        g. Excessive sweating

        h. Dilated pupils

    7. Take precautions or actions appropriate to particular medical status

    8. Reduce anxiety and stress

B. Preparation for potential emergency situations

    1. Staff training—Provides knowledge and skills to respond immediately and appropriately to potentially life-threatening incident

    2. Victim survival is possibly dependent on first few minutes or hours

    3. Know when emergency has occurred and what to do until medical assistance arrives

4. Ideally, all team members should be trained and certified in cardiopulmonary resuscitation; must know and post emergency medical assistance phone number(s)

5. Know contents of emergency kit or crash cart

6. Know roles for a given emergency scenario

7. Emergency practice drills

    a. Necessary to keep staff ready for potential emergencies

    b. Practice to keep skills updated

    c. Become comfortable with individual roles to prevent chaos in crisis situation

8. Need for emergency kit or crash cart

    a. Essential items that are readily and easily accessible

    b. Contents must be regularly checked; nothing should be out-of-date or contents are not useful

    c. Awareness of what team members can or should legally administer

    d. With most emergencies, no drugs are necessary—Mainly first-aid items

    e. Some emergencies require immediate use of drugs—Can make the difference between life and death

    f. Commercially available

9. Considerations for a custom-designed kit

    a. Type of practice

    b. Knowledge and skill of dentist(s) in emergency medicine

    c. Type of emergencies most commonly encountered

    d. Choose only equipment and drugs for which personnel are trained

    e. Select only equipment and drugs legally allowed to be utilized

10. Primary role of auxiliary

    a. Provision of basic life support

    b. Support of dentist in administration of additional supportive therapies until medical emergency personnel arrive

11. Emergency first-aid kit or crash cart basic contents

    a. Resuscitation mask or face shield with one-way valve

    b. Oxygen with positive pressure ventilation capability (e.g., demand/positive pressure valves, or a self-inflating device such as an Ambu bag)

    c. Nitroglycerin tabs 0.3 mg (fresh and unopened) or oral nitroglycerin spray—Coronary vessel dilator used for angina pectoris

    d. Epinephrine (Adrenalin)—At least two preloaded 1:1,000 epinephrine syringes—Antiallergic drugs: to combat undue reactions to drugs such as penicillin or to combat severe asthmatic attack

e. Injectable antihistamine, such as diphenhydramine HCl 10 mg/ml or chlorpheniramine 10 mg/ml—Antiallergic drugs: to combat undue reactions to drugs such as penicillin or to combat severe asthmatic attack

12. Common optional additional drugs and equipment

a. 21-gauge needle

b. Amyl nitrate vaporole—An alkyl nitrite, which acts as a vasodilator, expanding blood vessels and thus lowering blood pressure; it is used medically to treat heart diseases such as angina, and to treat cyanide poisoning

c. Medihaler Ventolin (albuterol)—Antiasthmatic bronchodilator

d. Aromatic ammonia vaporoles—One inhalant, break under nose; irritant: increases respiratory rate

e. Gauze, bandages, and adhesive tape

f. Glucola—Oral sucrose—Used for insulin shock

g. Syringes

h. Tourniquets (3)

13. Additional optional drugs and equipment—Requires additional knowledge and advanced training for safe use; to be added according to ability and desire of the dentist

a. Airways, adult and child; oropharyngeal or nasopharyngeal

b. Analgesic (morphine)—Morphine is a highly potent opiate analgesic drug used for severe pain

c. Anticholinergic (atropine)—Atropine lowers the "rest and digest" activity of all muscles and glands regulated by the parasympathetic nervous system; occurs because atropine is a competitive antagonist of the muscarinic acetylcholine receptors; injections of atropine are used in the treatment of bradycardia (an extremely low heart rate), asystole, and pulseless electrical activity (PEA) in cardiac arrest.

d. Anticonvulsant (midazolam)—A drug that is a benzodiazepine derivative; it has powerful anxiolytic, amnestic, hypnotic, anticonvulsant, skeletal muscle relaxant, and sedative properties.

e. Antihypertensive (nifedipine)—A dihydropyridine calcium channel blocker; its main uses are in angina pectoris and hypertension

f. Corticosteroid (injectable)—Hydrocortisone sodium succinate; used as an immunosuppressive drug, given by injection in the treatment of severe allergic reactions such as anaphylaxis and angioedema, in place of prednisolone in patients who need steroid treatment but cannot take oral medication, and perioperatively in patients on long-term steroid treatment to prevent an Addisonian crisis

g. Cricothyrotomy needle or scalpel—An emergency incision through the skin and cricothyroid membrane to secure a patient's airway during certain emergency situations, such as an airway obstructed by a foreign object or swelling, a patient who is not able to breathe adequately on their own, or in cases of major facial trauma that prevent an airway through the mouth

h. Endotracheal intubation equipment—Endotracheal intubation is the placement of a flexible plastic tube into the trachea to protect the patient's airway and provide a means of mechanical ventilation

i. Narcotic antagonist (naloxone)—Naloxone is a drug used to counter the effects of opioid overdose, for example heroin or morphine overdose; naloxone is specifically used to counteract life-threatening depression of the central nervous system and respiratory system

j. Vasopressor (injectable)—Methoxamine; a vasopressor medicine that produces an immediate and prolonged rise in blood pressure

14. *Good Samaritan statutes*

a. Laws for legal protection of people who willingly give emergency care without accepting anything in return

b. Vary from state to state

c. All require individuals to act as reasonable and as prudent as another person would act under the same conditions

d. Provides for protection of person providing emergency care from being successfully sued and found financially responsible

e. Common sense and reasonable level of skill is expected, but not what is beyond training and legal limitations

f. Standard of care expected is not as strict in an emergency situation as it is in a nonemergency situation

C. Emergency management

1. Need for immediate recognition and action for acutely life-threatening conditions

a. Purpose is to sustain life until medical attention can provide definitive treatment

b. Recognize potential to become threat to life

c. Take action to prevent exacerbation of condition to one of grave potential

2. Basic life support (*BLS*)—Necessary management for most acute medical emergency conditions

a. Terminate any dental care in progress and immediately notify dentist of emergency

b. Place patient in supine position

    (1) UNLESS there is respiratory discomfort and/or chest pain in that position

    (2) As an alternative, patient should be placed in semisupine or upright position

c. Check for consciousness

d. Check for adequate breathing

    (1) If there is an airway obstruction and signs of respiratory difficulty, establish and maintain open airway

    (2) Oxygen may be administered (DO NOT administer oxygen to a person who is hyperventilating)

e. Check pulse

f. In absence of respiration or respiration and pulse, administer basic life support

g. Establish baseline vital signs—Respiration, pulse, blood pressure

h. Call emergency medical service (EMS) and provide information about the emergency

i. Continue to monitor vital signs

j. Do no harm

k. Provide or assist in specific supportive treatment as indicated by the condition

l. Stay calm throughout

D. Terminology

    1. *Allergen*—Antigen that can exhibit allergic symptoms

    2. *Allergy*—Hypersensitive response to allergen

    3. *Anaphylactic*—Life-threatening systemic allergic reaction; also called anaphylactic shock

    4. *Idiosyncrasy*—Peculiar or individual reaction to drugs and/or food substance

    5. *Infarct*—Death of tissue from lack of oxygen

    6. *Pruritus*—Severe itching

    7. *Tachypnea*—Rapid respiration

    8. *Urticaria* (also called hives)—Vascular reaction of skin, characterized by wheals or papules

    9. *Bradycardia*—Slow heart rate

II. Unconsciousness

A. Vasodepressor syncope—Sudden transient loss of consciousness that usually occurs secondary to a period of cerebral ischemia; most common emergency in dentistry

1. Medical history findings

    a. Caused by decreased oxygen flow to brain, most frequently occurring in young adult male patients (16–35 years old) with unexpressed stress or fear

    b. Psychogenic factors—"fight-or-flight response"

    (1) Fright

    (2) Anxiety

    (3) Emotional stress

    (4) Pain

    c. Nonpsychogenic factors

    (1) Hunger

    (2) Exhaustion

    (3) Poor physical condition

    (4) Sitting/standing in upright position

    (5) Hot, humid, and/or crowded environment

2. Common symptoms

    a. Presyncope—Patient reports feeling of warmth with heavy perspiration, faint or dizzy, seeing spots before the eyes, and nausea

    (1) Vital signs—Increase in respiration and heart rate

    b. Syncope—Irregular breathing, jerky, pupils dilate

    (1) Vital signs

        (a) Bradycardia

        (b) Decreased blood pressure

    c. Postsyncope—Patient feels disoriented and confused

3. Dental considerations

    a. Presyncope

    (1) Discontinue procedure as soon as symptoms are noted

    (2) Place patient in supine position—Feet elevated

    (3) Pass ammonia vaporale under patient's nose

    b. Syncope—Assess consciousness

    c. Postsyncope—Do not continue dental treatment

4. Emergency treatment

    a. Terminate dental procedure

    b. Presyncope—Patient in supine position with legs elevated; move legs vigorously

    c. Syncope—Loss of consciousness

        (1) Place patient in supine position

        (2) Assess ABCs (airway, breathing, circulation), may administer oxygen, and monitor vital signs

        (3) If recovery is not within 3–5 minutes, call EMS and perform BMEP

    d. Postsyncope—Do not continue dental treatment; have a friend take the patient home

B. Postural hypotension (orthostatic hypotension)—A sudden fall in blood pressure, typically greater than 20/10 mm Hg, that occurs when a person assumes a standing position, usually after a prolonged period of rest; second leading cause of loss of consciousness

    1. Fall in blood pressure in which patient faints when rapidly brought to an upright position with legs elevated

        a. May be caused by drugs, varicose veins, later stages of pregnancy, prolonged periods of recumbency

        b. Results when there is a pooling of blood in lower extremities that diverts from brain and other vital organs

    2. Medical history findings

        a. Medications—Check for antihypertensives, antidepressants, and narcotics

    3. Common symptoms upon standing or sitting

        a. Light-headedness, pallor, dizziness, sweat, blurred vision

        b. May lose consciousness

        c. Vital signs—Blood pressure is low; heart rate at baseline or above

    4. Dental consideration—To avoid occurrence, return chair slowly to upright position

    5. Emergency treatment

        a. Terminate dental procedure and assess consciousness

        b. Place patient in supine position with feet elevated above the level of heart

        c. Patient may flex thigh muscles to encourage blood flow to return to the brain before raising the chair slowly

        d. Assess ABCs

        e. Administer oxygen, if necessary

        f. Monitor vital signs

        g. Elevate patient slowly and reevaluate vital signs

C. Acute adrenal insufficiency (adrenal crisis)

    1. Sudden lack of sufficient circulating adrenal hormones

        a. Before glucocorticosteroid therapy, was the terminal stage of Addison's disease

        b. Hypersecretion of cortisol is referred to as Cushing's syndrome

        c. Secondary adrenal insufficiency—Produced with the administration of exogenous glucocorticosteroids to a patient with functional adrenal cortices; can produce an adrenocortical hypofunction by producing a disuse atrophy of the adrenal cortex and thereby decreasing the ability of the adrenal cortex to increase corticosteroid levels in response to stressful situations. This leads to the development of signs and symptoms associated with acute adrenal insufficiency.

    2. Medical history findings

        a. History of Addison's disease

        b. Acute withdrawal of steroids after long-term use

        c. Acute adrenal insufficiency is seen in only 0.01–0.7% of normal population

    3. Common symptoms

        a. Mental confusion

        b. Muscle weakness

        c. Intense abdominal pain

        d. Lower back and/or leg pain

        e. Signs of hypoglycemia

        f. Extreme fatigue and weakness

        g. Episodic syncope

        h. Anorexia, weight loss

        i. Hypotension

    4. Dental considerations

        a. Establish treatment plan

        b. Consult physician before beginning dental treatment

        c. Use stress-reduction protocol

        d. Within 2–3 months after discontinuing adrenocortical hormone therapy, patient is susceptible when undergoing trauma to subacute form of adrenal crisis

    5. Emergency treatment

        a. Terminate dental procedure

        b. Position the patient in supine position if patient appears mentally confused and wet and clammy; otherwise, position patient depending on comfort

        c. ABCs (airway, breathing, circulation)

    d. Monitor vital signs

    e. Call EMS immediately

    f. Dentist should administer glucocorticosteroid from patient's kit or office emergency kit if available, or EMT will administer

    g. Transport patient to hospital

III. Altered Consciousness

  A. Cerebrovascular accident (CVA, stroke)—Most common form of brain disease

    1. Types

      a. Hemorrhagic—A form of stroke that occurs when a blood vessel in the brain ruptures or bleeds.

      b. Occlusive—Also known as ischemic stroke; the cause of approximately 80% of strokes, a *blood vessel* becomes *occluded* and the blood supply to part of the brain is totally or partially blocked.

    2. Medical history finding

      a. May have previously experienced transient ischemic attacks (TIA or ministroke)

      b. High blood pressure

      c. Diabetes

      d. Use of oral contraceptives

      e. Cigarette smoking

      f. Age

    3. Common symptoms

      a. Sudden unilateral weakness and numbness or paralysis

      b. Difficulty speaking (aphasia)

      c. Pupils of unequal size

      d. Hemorrhagic CVA may also include

        (1) Sudden severe headache

        (2) Nausea

        (3) Vomiting

        (4) Chills

        (5) Sweating

        (6) Vertigo

        (7) Unconsciousness (indicates grim prognosis)

    4. Dental considerations

      a. Do not schedule for elective treatment within 6 months of episode— Recurrence is greater

  b. Use stress-reduction protocol

  c. Record vitals—Monitor blood pressure and heart rate

  d. Assess bleeding—Patients are often on aspirin or anticoagulant therapy

5. Emergency treatment

  a. Treatments to prevent or limit brain damage are time-sensitive—Call EMS immediately

  b. Monitor vital signs—If blood pressure is markedly elevated, raise head and chest slightly

  c. Administer oxygen

  d. If office is equipped, an IV line should be established using 5% dextrose

B. Hypoglycemic episode in a diabetic patient (insulin shock); normal glucose levels are generally maintained within a range of 70–140 mg/dl for healthy individuals

1. Lack of adequate circulating blood sugar with acute onset of severe symptoms

  a. Can result in death

  b. May be triggered by normal insulin intake and lack of adequate food, overdose of insulin, overexercise, or other physical or emotional stress

2. Medical history findings

  a. Insulin-dependent diabetes mellitus (IDDM)—Type 1

  b. Normal insulin intake with failure to eat normally

3. Common symptoms

  a. Changes in level of consciousness, including

   (1) Less spontaneity of conversation

   (2) Lethargy

   (3) Incoherence

   (4) Dizziness

   (5) Drowsiness

   (6) Confusion

   (7) Diaphoresis

  b. Personality change (sometimes these symptoms are mistakenly assumed to be result of inebriation)

  c. Central nervous system (CNS) involvement includes

   (1) Hunger

   (2) Weakness

   (3) Nervousness

   (4) Trembling

   (5) Cold sweat (symptom that helps distinguish hypoglycemia from hyperglycemia)

    d. Following CNS symptoms are clinical signs of

       (1) Tachycardia

       (2) Pallor

       (3) Sometimes paresthesia (numbness and tingling sensation)

    e. Later stage—Unconsciousness, tonic–clonic movements, hypotension, rapid thready pulse, hypothermia

4. Dental considerations

    a. Be sure patient has tested blood sugar level

    b. Patient has eaten adequate meal before dental visit

    c. Schedule appointments early in day

    d. Avoid use of epinephrine in local anesthesia

    e. Provide stress-reduction protocol

5. Emergency treatment

    a. Terminate dental procedure and if conscious, give patient something with sugar (like orange juice) in it and place patient in upright position

    b. If no response in approximately 5 minutes, call EMS and monitor vital signs

    c. If unconscious

       (1) Call EMS

       (2) Monitor vital signs

       (3) Give basic life support as necessary

    d. If response is immediate, further action may not be necessary

IV. Chest Pain

  A. Myocardial infarction (MI, heart attack)

    1. Result of deficient blood supply to heart muscle, resulting in cellular death

    2. Characterized by sudden severe and prolonged substernal pain

    3. Medical history findings

      a. Coronary heart disease

      b. Hypertension

      c. Obesity

      d. Males (50–70 years)

      e. Survivors are usually receiving medications, such as diuretics, digitalis, aspirin, nitrates

    4. Common symptoms

      a. Severe persistent crushing pain or pressure in sternum that is not relieved by change in position, rest, or nitroglycerin (if it has been previously prescribed)

   b. Patient may clutch at chest with fist (Levine sign)

   c. Pain or pressure may radiate to neck, jaw, and/or arms

   d. Breathing difficulty

   e. Pale, ashen, or cyanotic appearance

   f. Profuse sweating (cold perspiration)

   g. Nausea and vomiting possible when pain is severe

   h. Vital signs appear as blood pressure may be low, respiration rapid and shallow, and heart rate weak, thready, and shallow

5. Dental considerations

   a. DO NOT treat patient within 6 months after MI without cardiology consult

   b. Use stress reduction protocol

   c. Nitrous oxide is highly recommended for sedation

6. Emergency treatment

   a. Terminate dental procedure and call EMS—Survival chances may depend on time it takes to receive definitive care (cardiac arrest may occur at any time)

   b. Help victim to rest comfortably, usually in upright or semiupright position

   c. Monitor vital signs, BLS

   d. Oxygen may be administered; administer nitroglycerin (do not administer in presence of hypotension [i.e., systolic pressure below 100 mm Hg])

   e. Be prepared to provide CPR

B. Angina pectoris

1. Inability of the coronary arteries to supply the myocardium with adequate oxygenated blood

2. Extreme difficulty in breathing caused by weakening or failure of left side of heart

3. Medical history finding—History of angina pectoris

4. Common symptoms

   a. Squeezing, heavy, dull chest pain lasting from 1 to 10 minutes

   b. Vital signs are normal

5. Dental considerations

   a. Use stress reduction protocol

   b. Place patient in comfortable position

6. Emergency treatment

   a. Terminate dental procedure—BLS

   b. Administer vasodilator, nitroglycerin tablet(s)/spray

   c. May administer oxygen (nasal cannula or hood preferred)

d. When episode is over, a decision whether or not to continue dental work is made

e. If the episode does not abate, administer oxygen and a second dose of nitroglycerin (no more than three doses); if pain is not relieved within 15 minutes, treat as MI and call EMS

V. Respiratory Distress

A. Hyperventilation

1. Second most common emergency situation in dental office

2. Prevalent in especially tense and nervous patients 15–40 years of age

3. Common findings

a. Overbreathing (rapid, shallow breathing), confusion

b. Feeling of a lump in the throat (globus hystericus)

c. Lightheaded, giddy (vertigo, dizziness)

d. Increased apprehension

e. Later—Paresthesia of hands, feet, and perioral area, muscular twitching, carpo-pedal spasm (cramping of hands or feet), and unconsciousness

4. Emergency treatment

a. Discontinue dental treatment and position upright, remove materials from mouth, and loosen clothing

b. DO NOT administer oxygen

c. If attempt is unsuccessful, have patient breathe into cupped hands or small paper bag

d. Monitor pulse and assist patient in reducing anxiety by allowing patient to express fears

B. Acute pulmonary edema

1. Rapid accumulation of fluid in alveoli and interstitial tissue of lungs

2. Results in extreme difficulty in breathing caused by weakening or failure of left side of heart

3. Medical history findings

a. Congestive heart failure

b. Possible history of heart disease, hypertension, and/or chronic lung disease

4. Common symptoms

a. Extreme dyspnea (difficulty breathing)

b. Tachypnea (rapid respiration)

c. Cyanosis

d. Frothy pink sputum

   e. Cold extremities

   f. Cough

5. Emergency treatment

   a. Terminate dental procedure, activate EMS, place patient upright to assist breathing

   b. Check ABCs; administer oxygen

   c. Alleviate symptoms of respiratory distress by bloodless phlebotomy (phlebostasia)

   (1) Tourniquets or blood pressure cuffs applied to extremities using just enough pressure to keep blood from entering extremity

   (2) One tourniquet is released for 5 minutes, then reapplied, followed by release of another extremity, continuing this rotation until the patient has been transported by EMS to medical care facility

6. Definitive treatment

   a. Dentist or emergency personnel may administer vasodilator

   b. Patient transported to acute care facility for additional procedures

   c. If office is equipped and dentist is comfortable, administration of either morphine sulfate or meperidine (Demerol) to relieve apprehension and to improve circulatory dynamics is indicated

C. Acute asthmatic episode—Asthma is a chronic disease of the respiratory system in which the airway occasionally constricts, becomes inflamed, and is lined with excessive amounts of mucus, often in response to one or more triggers

   1. Medical history finding

   a. Asthma—Usually with acute asthmatic episodes requiring emergency care or hospitalization

   2. Common symptoms

   a. Dyspnea (difficulty breathing)

   b. Normal inspiration with wheezing exhalation because diameter of bronchial tube has decreased

   c. Tachypnea (increased rate of breathing)

   d. Cyanosis

   e. Chest distension

   f. Nasal flaring

   3. Status asthmaticus—An acute exacerbation of asthma that does not respond to standard treatments of bronchodilators and corticosteroids

   a. Symptoms continue unabated even with treatment

   b. Patient experiences

   (1) Extreme fatigue

   (2) Dehydration

(3) Cyanosis

(4) Peripheral vascular shock

(5) Drug intoxication

(6) Rapid heart rate

4. Emergency treatment

a. Terminate procedure and BLS

b. Position comfortable, usually upright with arms forward

c. Assist patient in administering bronchodilator, if available (his or her own, or from emergency kit)

d. Avoid using barbiturates and narcotics because they may increase risk of bronchospasms

e. If episode continues, administer oxygen and call EMS immediately

D. Emphysema

1. Condition of lungs in which there is decrease in the ability to draw extra oxygen caused by loss of elasticity (increased compliance) of the lung tissue, destruction of structures supporting the *alveoli*, and destruction of capillaries feeding the alveoli.

2. Form of chronic obstructive pulmonary disease (COPD)

3. Decrease in tissue and lung elasticity, (decrease O_2) reserve

4. Common symptoms

a. Undue breathlessness on exertion

b. Can coexist with chronic bronchitis

c. Bronchioles become plugged with mucus

5. Emergency treatment

a. BLS

b. Sit patient in upright position

c. Follow stress-reduction protocol

d. Be cautious about administering oxygen—Could cause patient to go into respiratory arrest (administer 3L or O_2 per minute)

VI. Cardiac Arrest

A. Clinical death

1. Heart stops beating or beats ineffectively in generating a pulse

2. Causes inadequate circulation to brain and other vital organs

3. Common causes

a. Anaphylaxis

b. Drowning

c. Drug overdose

    d. Electrocution

    e. Massive trauma

    f. Suffocation or hypoxia

4. Medical history finding—Cardiovascular disease

5. Common symptoms

    a. No breathing

    b. No pulse

    c. No respiration

6. Emergency treatment

    a. Follow BLS (as a refresher, the steps in cardiopulmonary resuscitation follow; be sure to keep CPR certification current)

        (1) Assess consciousness, shake, and shout

        (2) Call for help

        (3) Position in supine position

        (4) Head tilt–chin lift

        (5) Look, listen, and feel for respiration for 5 seconds

        (6) If no breathing, pinch nose shut and give two rescue breaths (use one-way valve face mask if available) or use Ambu bag or positive pressure oxygen ventilation (watch chest rise)

        (7) Check carotid pulse (5–10 seconds)

        (8) Call for EMS

        (9) If no pulse, find the hand position by

            (a) Locating notch at lower end of sternum with two fingers

            (b) Place heel of other hand on sternum next to fingers

            (c) Remove first hand and place it on hand that is on sternum, keeping fingers off chest

      (10) Position rescuer's shoulders over hands

            (a) Compress victim's chest 1 1/2–2 inches

            (b) Move up and down smoothly

            (c) Always keep hand in contact with chest

      (11) Give 30 compressions

      (12) Give two full breaths and repeat cycle of 30 compressions and two breaths for 1 full minute

      (13) Reassess pulse—If no pulse continue CPR, rechecking pulse every 2 minutes; defibrilation if AED is available

      (14) Do not stop

            (a) Until another trained person takes over

(b) Until EMS personnel arrive and take over

(c) Until person's heart restarts

(d) Unless you are too exhausted to continue

(15) If pulse returns, but breathing does not—Continue rescue breathing

(16) If patient is breathing and has a pulse, maintain airway and monitor vitals until EMS personnel arrive

B. Respiratory arrest

   1. Cessation of breathing due to illness, injury, electrical shock, obstructed airway, or drowning

   2. May possibly follow respiratory distress

      a. Air passages becoming narrow due to swelling

      b. As a result of swelling, adequate air exchange is blocked and respiratory arrest results

   3. Common symptom—Breathing ceases

   4. Emergency treatment

      a. Follow BLS (as a refresher, the steps in rescue breathing follow)

      b. Assess consciousness, shake, and shout

      c. Call for help

      d. Position in supine position (on left side in third trimester of pregnancy)

      e. Head tilt–chin lift

      f. Look, listen, and feel for respiration for 5 seconds

      g. If not breathing, pinch nose shut and give two rescue breaths (use one-way oxygen ventilation)

      h. Check carotid pulse (5–10 seconds)

      i. If pulse, continue rescue breathing once every 5 seconds for adults (every 3 seconds for child)

VII. **Drug-Related Emergencies**

 A. Anaphylactic shock

   1. Severe allergic reaction causing systemic release of histamines and other chemical mediators

   2. Produces acute life-threatening changes involving circulation and bronchioles consistent with shock

   3. Medical history findings—Previous allergic reactions, particularly to drugs and/or materials used in or during dental procedures

   4. Common symptoms—Onset rapidly after contact with allergen and typically, but not always, evolve through four phases

      a. Skin reactions (such as generalized rash, intense pruritus, urticaria, flushing, edema)

    b. Smooth muscle spasm (gastrointestinal reactions such as cramping, abdominal pain, nausea, vomiting, diarrhea)

    c. Acute respiratory distress due to laryngeal edema—Wheezing

    d. Cardiovascular distress and collapse (hypotension, cardiac arrhythmias, tachycardia, cyanosis, circulatory collapse, and cardiac arrest)

5. Emergency treatment—Fatalities may occur in minutes; quick action is necessary

    a. Follow BLS

    b. Definitive treatment—Dentist or emergency personnel should determine dosage, route of administration, and administer epinephrine

        (1) Dose is generally 0.3 to 0.5 ml of 1:1,000 epinephrine intramuscular (IM), intravenous (IV), subcutaneously (SC), sublingual, or directly into tongue

        (2) Have epinephrine ready to administer in preloaded syringe

        (3) If there is no significant improvement within 5 minutes, a second dose of epinephrine is usually administered

    c. Continue to monitor vital signs

    d. Additional drugs that may be administered after clinical improvement are noted (e.g., antihistamine and corticosteroid)

VIII.   Seizures or Convulsions

A. Epilepsy

    1. Grand mal (generalized tonic–clonic)—Most common form

    a. Prodromal phase

        (1) Patient experiences increase in anxiety or depression

        (2) Aura (sensory phenomena) may follow

    b. Preictal phase

        (1) Patient loses consciousness

        (2) Experiences myoclonic jerks

        (3) Epileptic cry occurs

    c. Ictal phase

        (1) Tonic

            (a) Generalized muscle contractions

            (b) Evidence of dyspnea and cyanosis

            (c) Lasts 10–20 seconds

        (2) Clonic

            (a) Generalized relaxation of muscles

            (b) Heavy breathing

(c) Patient may froth at the mouth

(d) Lasts 2–5 minutes

d. Postictal phase

(1) Tonic–clonic movements stop

(2) Breathing returns to normal

(3) Consciousness returns, patient is initially disoriented, confused; patient may fall asleep

(4) Full recovery within 2 hours

2. Petit mal (absence of seizures)

a. Occurs shortly after awakening or during periods of inactivity

b. Brief loss of awareness

c. Patient may stare blankly or experience rapid blinking of eyes

d. History of seizures

3. Common symptoms

a. Momentary altered consciousness

b. Loss of consciousness and bilateral jerking of extremities

c. Sustained muscular contraction

d. Alternating contraction (tonic contractions) and relaxation of muscles (clonic convulsions)

e. Possible aura (sensory phenomena) experienced before seizure

4. Emergency treatment

a. Protect victim from harm by removing objects nearby that could cause injury (do not attempt to restrain or wedge mouth open)

b. Maintain airway if needed

c. Summon EMS only if the following occurs

(1) Seizure lasts longer than 5 minutes

(2) Injury is present

(3) Victim has no previous history of seizure

(4) Victim is pregnant, diabetic, or does not immediately regain consciousness

➤ INDIVIDUALIZED PATIENT EDUCATION

I. Planning Individualized Program

A. Personal background

1. Collect and apply information about the patient

a. Education

b. Attitude regarding oral health care

c. Personal homecare and frequency

d. Dexterity

e. Age and physical, mental abilities

f. Patient motivation

B. First lesson

1. Increase patient awareness to bacterial plaque biofilm

a. Discuss the formation and relationship to periodontal disease and caries formation

b. Develop plaque control program

c. Use illustrations and demonstrations in patient's own mouth to identify inflamed areas; have patient return the demonstration to ensure that they understand the procedure

d. Use disclosing solution to identify masses of plaque; record a plaque score

e. Keep instructions simple: first flossing, then brushing techniques

C. Second lesson

1. Evaluate patient's homecare

a. Evaluate gingiva with patient

b. Apply disclosing solution; compare present with past plaque scores

c. Review and extend knowledge

➤ INSTRUCTION FOR PREVENTION AND MANAGEMENT OF ORAL DISEASE

I. Caries

A. Host factors

1. Food

2. Bacterial plaque biofilm

3. Saliva

4. Tooth factors

5. Caries micoorganisms—*Mutans Streptococcus, Streptococcus sobinus, Lactobacilli*

B. Bacteria

1. *Streptococcus Mutans*—Gram-positive nonmotile bacteria with a spherical or coccoid morphology

2. *Streptococcus sobrinus*

3. *Lactobacilli*—Gram-positive nonmotile rods that do not form spores; grows optimally under anaerobic conditions; metabolically both oxidative and fermentive

C. Critical pH

1. A pH of less than 5.5

2. The pH of dental plaque that results in demineralization of tooth structure and caries formation

D. Time

1. The length of time the pH of bacterial plaque biofilm is less than 5.5

2. After sugar and/or starch is eaten, plaque is below the critical pH for approximately 20–30 minutes

E. Cariogenic foods

1. Have the potential to cause caries

2. Foods that can be fermented by oral bacteria to produce acids, which lower the pH of dental plaque (also called fermentable carbohydrates)

3. Sugars—Sugars (mono- and disaccharides), which include glucose, fructose, maltose, sucrose, and lactose

4. Examples of foods that contain some form of sugar: table sugar, brown sugar, fruit, juices and fruit cocktails, dried fruits such as raisins and apples, white or chocolate milk, ice cream, frozen and fruit-flavored yogurt, honey, baked beans, molasses, syrup, cookies, granola and granola bars, plain and sweetened cereals, potato and corn chips, jams and jellies, pancakes, muffins, cake, icing, biscuits, candies, gum, sodas, ketchup, and many brands of peanut butter

5. Cooked starches—Complex carbohydrates such as flour, pasta, potatoes, cereals, and rice that have been cooked by baking, boiling, or frying

6. Example of foods that contain cooked starch—White and whole wheat bread, pastries, doughnuts, whole-grain cereals, rice, pasta, potato dishes, crackers, pretzels, popcorn, corn and flour tortillas, pizza dough, and rolls

7. Combined foods

   a. Foods that contain cooked starch and one or more types of sugars have a potential to cause dental caries equal to or greater than sucrose

   b. Many of the foods listed under simple sugars fall into this category, such as sweetened cereals, pastries, granola, pancakes, muffins

F. Other factors related to food and caries

1. Quantity

   a. Amount of sugar and/or starch eaten

   b. The greater the amount eaten at each meal or snack, the greater the potential for caries formation

2. Frequency

   a. Number of times sugar and/or starch are eaten during the day

b. The greater the frequency of eating meals and snacks that contain sugar and/or starch, the greater the potential for caries formation

c. The number of times when the pH of plaque is below 5.5

G. Physical form

1. The form in which sugar and starch are eaten

2. Sugars and starches eaten in the form of a solid, along with the stickiness of the food, increases the potential for caries formation

3. Sugar consumed in a liquid form has a lower caries potential

4. The stickiness of a food is related to its ability to be retained on tooth structure

5. Starchy foods such as chips, crackers, and bread are retentive as much or more than foods with just sugar

H. Time of Day

1. What times sugar and/or starch are eaten during the day

2. Where more potential for caries formation exists if sugars and starch are eaten as a snack without fat or protein

3. When sugar and/or starch are eaten during meals containing fat and protein, caries potential is decreased

II. Dietary Recommendations to Reduce the Potential for Caries Formation

A. Limit snacking on foods with sugar and/or starch

B. Eat foods with low amounts of sugars and/or cooked starches

C. Eat sugar with meal

D. Limit the number of meals and snacks

E. Use moderate amounts of sugar substitutes

F. Refer to food labels for the total amount of carbohydrate and sugars in foods

G. Use spices such as allspice, cinnamon, ginger, and nutmeg to enhance the flavor of foods that contain low amounts of sugar

H. Clear mouth with water or unsweetened beverages after eating foods containing sugar and/or starch

I. Brush teeth or chew gum with xylitol if unable to brush

III. Principles of Dietary Counseling

A. Form a treatment plan for dietary assessment and counseling—Assess patient willingness and motivation

B. Obtain a record of food intake

1. Ask patient to keep a record of all food and beverage intake for a specified length of time, usually 3–5 days

2. Have client include the use of cough drops, cough syrup, gum, candy, etc.

C. Review the diet record with the patient

   1. Ask if anything else was consumed at each meal or snack time

   2. Ask about beverage intake and condiment use (ketchup, mustard, mayonnaise, soy sauce, honey, etc.)

D. Code food items

   1. Code each food item according to the food groups of the food guide pyramid

   2. Estimate the number of servings of each food according to food group

   3. Code foods that contain sugar and/or cooked starches

   4. Code foods according to physical form

E. Assess food intake

   1. Tally the number of servings from each food group

   2. Note food groups and/or number of servings that were deficient or excessive

   3. Tally the number and physical form of sugars/starches eaten

F. Counsel patient

   1. Discuss with patient the findings of the dietary assessment

   2. Have patient suggest foods they like that could be added or substituted to make their diet more healthful and to reduce caries potential

   3. Help patient set realistic and measurable dietary goals

   4. Stress making small changes that can be maintained

   5. Reassess diet

      a. Determine time interval for reassessment

      b. Evaluate behavior and dietary changes

      c. Help patient set new goals if needed

➤ PREVENTIVE DENTISTRY

Preventive dentistry includes the management of behaviors to prevent oral disease, the coordination and delivery of primary preventive oral hygiene services, the provision of secondary preventive intervention to prevent further disease, and the facilitation of the patient's access to care and implementation of oral care goals.

I. Prevention

A. Primary prevention—Involves techniques and agents to forestall onset and reverse progress of disease, or arrest disease process before treatment becomes necessary

   1. Examples

      a. Mechanical and chemical plaque (dental biofilm) removal

      b. Use of fluorides

      c. Sugar discipline

      d. Use of pit and fissure sealants

      e. Patient education and health promotion

B. Secondary prevention—Involves routine treatment methods to terminate a disease and restore tissues to as normal as possible

    1. Examples

      a. Deep scaling

      b. Restorations

      c. Periodontal debridement

      d. Endodontics

C. Tertiary prevention—Involves using measures necessary to replace lost tissues and rehabilitate patients so physical capabilities and/or mental attitudes are as near to normal as possible after secondary prevention has failed

    1. Examples

      a. Prosthodontics

      b. Implants

II. Planning

A. Patient needs—Involves inner forces that drive a person to action

    1. Maslow's hierarchy of needs—Developed by Abraham Maslow, humanistic psychologist; includes five levels of basic human needs: physiological (physical), safety (security), love (social), self-esteem/status (ego), and self-actualization (self-fulfillment) (Figure 9-1■)

      a. Physiological needs—Includes those needs necessary to maintain body homeostasis (food, water, oxygen, sleep)

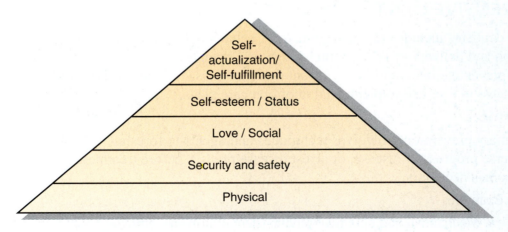

FIGURE 9-1 ■ Maslow's Hierarchy of Needs

    b. Safety (security)—Controls number of hazards that can cause physical and mental damage as well as guaranteeing a stable and predictable environment

    c. Love (social)—Focuses on group acceptance, opportunity to give and receive friendship

    d. Self-esteem (ego)—involves feelings of self-worth including achievement, confidence, competence, and status

    e. Self-actualization (self-fulfillment)—Focuses on a positive tendency for development, growth, and self-enhancement

  2. Health belief model—Based on views that an individual's decision to engage in healthy behavior depends on three components

    a. Patient's chance of susceptibility to disease

    b. If occurrence of disease will have some impact on patient's life

    c. If the benefits of taking action outweigh barriers to that action

B. Priorities—Involves judgments made concerning relative importance of one diagnosis/decision over another

C. Goals of the appointment(s)—Include broad-based statements that identify specific indicators to measure patient performance

  1. Related specifically to dental hygiene diagnosis

  2. Reflects patient's expected outcomes

  3. Guides the dental hygiene and patient interventions required to achieve desired outcome

III. Principles of Learning

A. Concepts

  1. Learning is more effective when an individual is physiologically and psychologically ready to learn

  2. Motivation is essential for learning

  3. Learner has to recognize and understand what is being taught and will learn only what is useful

  4. Learning takes place more rapidly when what is being taught has meaning

B. Learning ladder—Designed to demonstrate how individuals learn in a sequential series of steps (Figure 9-2■)

  1. Unawareness—Possessing limited or inaccurate information

  2. Awareness—Obtaining correct information, but does not possess any personal meaning

  3. Self-interest—Recognizing prospective objective with slight inclination to act

  4. Involvement—Attitude is influenced and action is forthcoming

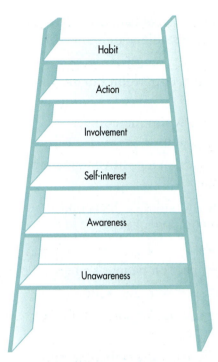

FIGURE 9-2 ■ Learning Ladder

5. Action—New concepts and practices are tested

6. Habit—Commitment is reached in performing behavior

IV. Principles of Teaching

   A. Show, tell, do—Effective in helping children overcome a fearful situation

      1. Show and tell patient what service will be provided

      2. Provide service

V. Removal of Bacterial Plaque (Biofilm)—An essential component of the therapeutic approach in preventing and controlling many dental diseases

   A. Manual toothbrushes

      1. Components

         a. Head—Working end; consists of tufts of bristles that are made of nylon filaments or natural bristles from boar's hair (have open tube and are not recommended due to biofilm development in tubes); all filaments should be soft and end-rounded

         b. Handle—Portion of toothbrush that is grasped

         c. Shank—Section that connects head to handle

2. Characteristics of an effective toothbrush—Includes size, shape, and texture to conform to patient comfort

    a. Size—Should be selected based on size of patient's mouth; large enough to remove plaque effectively, yet small enough to access all areas of the mouth

    b. Shape

        (1) Handle—Modification may include angled, offset, angled and offset, small and narrow, large and wide, rounded, and squared; handle should allow patient to comfortably grasp toothbrush

        (2) Head—May be designed in a diamond style or square; brushing plane may be flat, rippled, dome-shaped, or bilevel

    c. Texture/firmness—Involves bristle resistance to pressure; composition involves tufted or multitufted and diameter of bristle

        (1) Tufted—Five or six tufts long and three tufts across

        (2) Multitufted—10 or 12 tufts in three or four rows; positioned in close proximity allowing for greater force during use

        (3) Diameter—Usual range for adult toothbrush bristles is between 0.007 and 0.015 inches (filament size)

3. Types of toothbrushes

    a. Adult toothbrushes—A soft bristle brush is recommended for most patients; extra-soft are recommended to patients with dentinal hypersensitivity or postperiodontal surgery.

        (1) Soft toothbrush—Bristles 0.007–0.009 inches in diameter

        (2) Medium toothbrush—Bristles 0.010–0.012 inches in diameter

        (3) Hard toothbrush—Bristles 0.013–0.014 inches in diameter

        (4) Extra-hard toothbrush—Bristles 0.015 inches in diameter

    b. Child toothbrush—Bristles are shorter and diameter is reduced to 0.005 inches

4. Toothbrushing

    a. General objectives

        (1) Remove plaque (dental biofilm), disrupt colonization to help prevent reformation

        (2) Clean teeth of food, debris, and stain contained in plaque (dental biofilm)

        (3) Stimulate gingival tissues

        (4) Used to apply dentifrice or therapeutic agents

b. Methods

    (1) Horizontal—Position bristles perpendicular to crown of tooth; brush in a back-and-forth horizontal pattern

    (2) Fones—Position bristles perpendicular to crown of tooth; brush in a circular (rotary) motion (Figure 9-3■)

    (3) Leonard—Up-and-down brushing motion over facial surfaces of closed posterior teeth

    (4) Stillman—Position bristles at a 45-degree angle to apex of tooth, with part of brush resting on gingiva and other part on teeth; move brush using a vibratory motion while applying slight pressure; lift brush and repeat in next area

    (5) Charter—Place brush at a 90-degree angle to long axis of tooth so bristles are gently forced between teeth, but do not rest on gingiva; move brush in several small rotary motions, keeping bristles in contact with gingival margin

    (6) Bass—Place brush at a 45-degree angle to tooth apex; apply gentle pressure so bristles enter sulcus; use a vibratory motion (horizontal jiggle) to activate bristles

    (7) Roll—Position bristles parallel to and against attached gingiva; turn wrist to flex bristles first against gingiva and then facial surface; roll bristles coronally

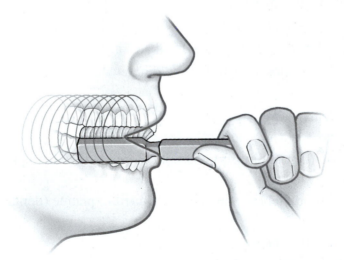

FIGURE 9-3 ■ Fones Method: Circular Motion Extending from Maxillary to Mandibular Gingiva

c. Modified techniques

   (1) Modified Stillman and Charters—Position bristles in same position as original method, then gently begin a vibratory motion; slowly press-roll bristles coronally, continuing vibratory motion during roll (Figure 9-4■)

   (2) Modified Bass—Sulcular brushing is done either before or after use of rolling method (wiggle and roll)

d. General considerations when recommending a specific technique

   (1) Consider patient's oral health status: number of teeth, alignment, mouth size, removable prostheses, orthodontic appliances, periodontal status, and gingival condition

   (2) Review patient's systemic health status, muscular and joint diseases, and mental capabilities

   (3) Patient's age

   (4) Patient's interest and motivation

   (5) Patient's manual dexterity

   (6) Ease and effectiveness in explaining and demonstrating toothbrushing technique

B. Automatic (powered) toothbrushes—Battery or electrical

   1. Components

   a. Head—Usually smaller than manual toothbrushes; removable to allow for replacement; three basic patterns

      (1) Reciprocating—Back-and-forth motion

      (2) Arcuate—Up-and-down motion

      (3) Elliptical—Combination of reciprocating and arcuate motions

   b. Shank—Connects into handle

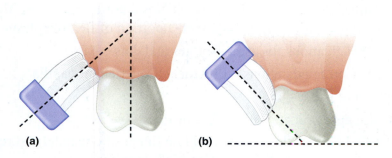

FIGURE 9-4 ■ (a) Stillman Method; (b) Charter's Method

      c. Handle—Contains power device (battery or electric current); portion of toothbrush that is held

   2. Indications for use

      a. Parental brushing of children

      b. Physically and mentally compromised

      c. Elderly

      d. Arthritic and/or poor dexterity

      e. Poorly motivated

      f. Patients who require a large handle

   3. Methods of use—Follow manufacturer's directions

C. Dental floss

   1. Types

      a. Waxed—Contains wax coating

         (1) Indications for use—Normal contact areas, irregular tooth surfaces, defective or overhanging restorations

         (2) Contraindications—Tight contact areas

      b. Unwaxed

         (1) Indications for use—Tight contact areas

         (2) Contraindications—Crowded teeth, heavy calculus deposits, defective or overhanging restorations

      c. Tape—Broad and flat waxed floss

         (1) Indications for use—Interdental space without tight contact areas

         (2) Contraindications—None

      d. Polytetrafluoroethylene—Made of synthetic material

         (1) Indications for use—Tight contact areas and rough proximal tooth surfaces

         (2) Contraindications—None

      e. Tufted floss (Super Floss)—Contains a portion of waxed floss, followed by thicker tufted floss, and then a portion of flexible plastic at the end

         (1) Indications for use—Bridges and diastemas

         (2) Contraindications—Presence of interdental papilla

   2. Method of use

      a. Use approximately 18 inches of floss

      b. Wind bulk of floss around middle finger of one hand and remaining floss lightly around same finger of other hand

      c. Secure floss with thumb and index finger of each hand, leaving 3/4 to 1 inch of floss between hands

       d. Use thumb and index finger to guide floss between teeth using a seesaw motion

       e. Once past contact point, adapt floss to each interproximal surface by creating a C-shape

       f. Move floss in an apical–coronal motion several times

       g. Repeat procedure on adjacent interproximal tooth with care to prevent damage to interproximal papilla

       h. Gently guide floss out of contact area using seesaw motion

       i. Obtain clean area of floss for next tooth

    3. Accomplishments achieved by using floss

       a. Removes plaque and debris that adhere to teeth, restorations, orthodontic appliances, fixed prostheses, interproximal gingiva, and implants

       b. Aids in identifying presence of subgingival calculus, overhanging restorations, and interproximal carious lesions

       c. Reduces gingival bleeding

       d. May be used as a vehicle for applying polishing or chemotherapeutic agents to proximal or subgingival areas

D. Interdental brush—Small, spiral bristle brush; core of brush that holds bristles may be made of plastic, wire, or a nylon-coated wire

    1. Indications for use

       a. Provides plaque removal at interproximal areas, in and around furcations, orthodontic bands, and fixed prostheses with large spaces present

       b. Provides gingival stimulation

       c. Applies chemotherapeutic agents

    2. Contraindications—Avoid using when healthy interproximal papilla is present

    3. Method of use

       a. Moisten brush

       b. Insert at an angle approximating normal gingival contour

       c. Activate by using an in-and-out motion

E. Single-tufted brush—Single-tufted or group of small tufts (e.g., end-tuft and unituft)

    1. Indications for use—Use on regions not easily reached with other devices

       a. Irregular gingival margins around migrated or malposed teeth

       b. Lingual and palatal tissues that elicit a gag reflex with a full-size toothbrush

       c. Distal areas of most posterior teeth

       d. Orthodontic appliances

       e. Pontics

f. Precision attachments associated with crown and bridge or implant abutments

g. Application of chemotherapeutics

2. Contraindications—Avoid using when a normal contact area presents itself with interproximal papilla

3. Method of use

a. Direct end of tuft into proximal area and along gingival margin

b. Combine rotating motion with intermittent pressure

c. Use sulcular brushing stroke

F. Toothpicks—Utilized with a holder, the toothpick can be more effectively applied at proper angle and access hard-to-reach areas (Figure 9-5■)

1. Indications for use

a. Plaque removal at and just beneath gingival margin

b. Interdental cleaning of concave proximal tooth surfaces

c. Exposed furcation areas

d. Orthodontic appliances

e. Application of chemotherapeutics

f. Fixed prostheses

2. Contraindications—Avoid subgingival insertion or vigorous proximal use to prevent gingival damage

3. Method of use

a. Moisten toothpick

b. Apply toothpick perpendicular to gingival margin

c. Using moderate pressure, trace around gingival margin of each tooth

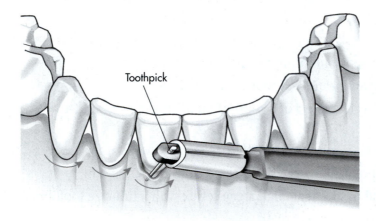

Toothpick

FIGURE 9-5 ■ Use of Toothpick in Holder. Apply toothpick perpendicular to gingival margin and trace gently around the margin.

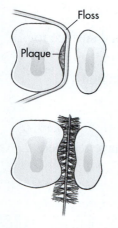
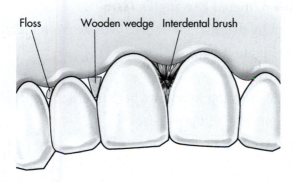

FIGURE 9-6 ■ Use of Wooden Wedge, Interdental Brush, and Floss

G. Wedge stimulators—Plastic or wooden triangular aids used for removing plaque (Figure 9-6■)

    1. Indications for use—Interdental areas with tooth surfaces and no interdental gingiva

    2. Contraindications—Avoid using in presence of interdental gingiva

    3. Method of use

        a. Soften wood

        b. Insert wedge from facial aspect with flat surface of triangular base resting on gingiva and tip of wedge angled coronally

        c. Move wedge in and out while applying moderate pressure and using a burnishing stroke

H. Gauze strips—6-inch piece of gauze bandage (Figure 9-7■)

    1. Indications for use—Proximal surfaces of teeth adjacent to edentulous areas, teeth that are widely spaced, or implant abutments

    2. Contraindications—Interproximal spaces with presence of interdental gingiva

    3. Method of use

        a. Fold in half a 1-inch wide, 6-inch long gauze bandage

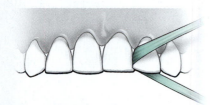

FIGURE 9-7 ■ Gauze strip: Used Adjacent to Endentulous Area, in Interproximal Spaces, or Distal to Posterior Teeth

      b. Place fold toward gingiva

      c. Adapt gauze by wrapping it around the exposed proximal surface to facial and lingual line angles

      d. Activate by using a "shoeshine" stroke from facial to lingual

I. Knitting yarn (Figure 9-8■)

    1. Indications for use

      a. Proximal cleaning in areas where interdental papillae have receded

      b. Abutments of fixed prostheses

      c. Isolated teeth

      d. Teeth separated by diastemas

      e. Distal surface of most posterior teeth

      f. Apply chemotherapeutic agent

    2. Contraindications—Avoid using cotton yarn where interdental gingiva is present

    3. Method of use

      a. Fold yarn in half using approximately 8 inches

      b. Thread and tie approximately 8 inches of dental floss

      c. Insert floss through contact area and draw yarn into embrasure

      d. Clean tooth surface with a facial–lingual stroke

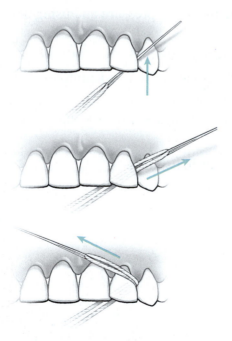

FIGURE 9-8 ■ Knitting Yarn

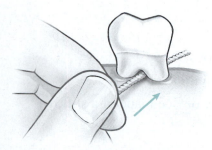

FIGURE 9-9 ■ Pipe Cleaner: Used to Clean Exposed Furcation

J. Pipe cleaner (Figure 9-9■)

    1. Indications for use

        a. Proximal surfaces where interdental gingiva is missing

        b. Open furcation areas

    2. Contraindications—Avoid using on implants and where interdental gingiva is present and furcation areas are not exposed

    3. Method of use

        a. Use one-third of a regular pipe cleaner

        b. Work end of cleaner through space

        c. Activate using an in-and-out motion

K. Rubber tip stimulator—Conical or pyramidal flexible rubber or plastic tip attached to a handle or to end of toothbrush

    1. Indications for use

        a. Cleans debris from interdental area

        b. Stimulate tissue

    2. Contraindications—None

    3. Method of use

        a. Place tip at 90-degree angle to long axis of tooth

        b. Utilize moderate pressure while tracing along gingival margin or use an in-and-out motion in open embrasure area

L. Floss holder—Y-shaped or C-shaped yokes with handle allowing patient to manipulate floss by holding handle

    1. Indications for use for patients who

        a. Have large hands

        b. Are physically challenged

        c. Lack normal dexterity

        d. Have caregivers providing oral care

        e. Prefer not to put hands in mouth

    2. Contraindications—None

    3. Method of use

      a. Tightly secure floss between two prongs of yoke

      b. Use same technique as described for flossing

M. Bridge (floss) threader—Blunt-ended, needle-like device made of a stiff, yet flexible, plastic or a plastic loop where floss is inserted

    1. Indications for use; carries floss

      a. Through embrasure areas under contact points too tight for floss insertion

      b. Between proximal surface and gingiva of abutment teeth of fixed prostheses

      c. Under pontics

      d. Around orthodontic appliances

      e. Under splinting

    2. Contraindications—Avoid using in areas where regular flossing can be utilized

    3. Method of use

      a. Insert floss into threader

      b. Direct end of threader into target area

      c. Disengage floss from threader to adapt to tooth surface

      d. Utilize flossing technique previously described

N. Oral irrigator—Targeted application of a pulsated or steady stream of water or other irrigant used for cleansing and/or therapeutic purposes

    1. Indications for use—Flush away loosely adherent microflora located coronal to gingival margin

    2. Contraindications—Avoid using on patients with a possible risk to subacute bacterial endocarditis

    3. Method of use

      a. Direct jet tip toward interdental area, holding tip at right angle to long axis of tooth

      b. Start on lowest pressure setting, increase slightly over time depending on condition of gingiva and tissue comfort

      c. Lean over sink

      d. Trace around each tooth, spending extra time at interproximal areas

      e. Hold in area for 5–7 seconds for whirlpool effect

VI. Dentrifrices—Substance used with a toothbrush or other applicator to remove bacterial plaque biofilm, materia alba, and debris from gingiva and teeth for cosmetic purposes, and for applying specific agents to tooth surfaces for therapeutic purposes

A. Types

    1. Cosmetic—Improves appearance of teeth (i.e., to remove stain)

    2. Therapeutic—Reduces some disease in mouth

        a. Fluoride-containing dentifrice—Contains up to 260 mg of fluoride; safe and effective fluoride content for over-the-counter dentifrice is 0.22% for NaF, 0.76% for MFP, and 0.4% for SnF_2

        b. Baking soda–peroxide–fluoride dentifrice (e.g., Mentadent)—Combination of 0.75% stable peroxide gel, baking soda, and 1,100 ppm sodium fluoride

        c. Antimicrobial dentifrices

            (1) Chemical compounds used to supplement usual brushing and flossing in mechanical plaque control

            (2) Stannous salts have reported activity against caries, plaque, and gingivitis

                (a) Marketed in United States as Crest Pro Care

                (b) Has shown superior efficacy in antimicrobial, plaque acidogenicity, gingivitis or gingival bleeding, and tartar control

            (3) Triclosan—Broad-spectrum antibacterial agent effective against wide variety of bacteria

                (a) Marketed in United States as Colgate Total

                (b) Approved by FDA in July 1997 as the first dentifrice to help prevent gingivitis, plaque, and caries

                (c) Received ADA's Seal of Acceptance for its benefit in reducing gingivitis, plaque, caries, and tartar

B. Components

    1. Humectants—Retain moisture and prevent drying once exposed to air; help stabilize preparation

    2. Preservatives—Prevent bacterial growth; help prolong shelf life

    3. Sweetening agents—Impart pleasant flavor for patient acceptance

    4. Flavoring agents—Make dentifrice desirable; mask other ingredients that may have a less pleasant flavor

    5. Coloring agents—Enhance attractiveness

   C. Other dentifrices

      1. Antitartar

         a. Tetrasodium phosphate and disodium dihydrogen pyrophosphate (e.g., Crest Tartar Control)

         b. Zinc citrate trihydrate—Tartar control versions for Aim and Close-Up

         c. ADA seal has not been awarded to anticalculus products because ADA considers calculus inhibition a cosmetic effect; seal is awarded due to anticaries effect of these products

      2. Antihypersensitivity—Active agents include potassium nitrate, strontium chloride, and sodium citrate

➤ ORAL CONDITIONS

I. Oral Cancer

   A. Common sites

      1. Lateral border of the tongue

      2. Lower lip

      3. Floor of the mouth

      4. Oropharynx

   B. Common signs of oral cancer

      1. Ulceration—Loss of skin surface

      2. Erythema—Red lesion

      3. Induration—Hard

      4. Fixation—Nonmobile lesion

      5. Chronicity—Failure to heal

      6. Lymphadenopathy—Hardening and enlarged lymph nodes

      7. Adenopathy—Disease of glands

      8. Leukoplakia—White patch

   C. Self-examination—Instruct patient to

      1. Identify sores, swellings, lumps on face, neck, mouth that do not heal within 2 weeks

      2. Report persistent hoarseness

      3. Check facial symmetry

      4. Check for changes in skin color, size of moles

      5. Check cheeks, lips by retracting with fingers, and view for color variations, ulcerations, swellings, lumps

     6. Check under tongue by lifting to roof of mouth; use gauze to grasp tongue and evaluate the sides of tongue

D. Risk factors for oral cancer

    1. Tobacco abuse—Smoking and smokeless tobacco

    2. Alcohol use

II. Tobacco Cessation

A. Four steps of intervention

    1. Ask patient about tobacco use in nonjudgmental manner

    2. Advise patient to stop using tobacco products by clearly stating the consequences

    3. Assist patient in taking the necessary steps to stop by setting a quit date; remove all tobacco products; avoid people who use tobacco

    4. Arrange patient follow-up services

    5. 4 As—Ask, advise, assist, arrange

III. Oral Habits

A. Bruxism

    1. Oral manifestations—Decrease in canine height and flattening of incisal and occlusal surfaces

    2. Suggested patient interventions—Night guard, stress management protocols

B. Thumbsucking

    1. Oral manifestations—Open-bite, tongue thrusting, protruding teeth, anterior overjet, deep narrow palate

    2. Suggested patient interventions—Make child aware of habit, restrict movement of hand to mouth, incentive program, orthodontic evaluation

➤ ANXIETY AND PAIN CONTROL

I. Reduction of Stress

A. Appointment scheduling

    1. New patient—First appointment should be consultation and assessment to build rapport and evaluate level of anxiety

    2. Time of appointment—Plan according to patient health requirements, usually morning appointment when patient is well rested

    3. Waiting time—Minimize waiting time; morning appointments will reduce chance of long waits

4. Eating requirements—Help prevent hypoglycemia and hunger

5. Length of appointment—Limit to patient's durability

B. Medication

1. Premedication—When indicated by physician and dentist

2. Pain control—Topical anesthetics or local anesthetics to reduce pain during treatment

3. Patient's personal medications—Instruct patient to bring medications needed in case of an emergencies

II. Pain Control

A. Definitions

1. Local anesthesia—The loss of sensation in a circumscribed area of the body as a result of the depression of excitation in nerve endings or the inhibition of the conduction process in peripheral nerves; local anesthetic agents used in practice prevent both the generation and conduction of a nerve impulse; provides a chemical roadblock between the source of the impulse (e.g., periodontal abscess) and the brain; the impulse is unable to reach the brain.

2. Pain—A protective mechanism manifested by an environmental change in an excitable tissue.

3. Pain perception threshold—The physioanatomical process by which an impulse is generated following application of an adequate stimulus and transferred to the CNS; differ little between healthy individuals

4. Pain reaction threshold—The physioanatomical process by which an impulse is generated following application of an adequate stimulus and transferred to the CNS; differ little between healthy individuals

5. Stimulus—An environmental change in an excitable tissue

    a. Chemical—Citric acid

    b. Thermal—Hot/cold sensation

    c. Mechanical—Toothbrush/instrument

    d. Electrical—Electrical toothbrushes

6. Impulse—A wave of excitation initiated by a stimulus; electrical message from one part of body to another (it has to be a minimal threshold stimulus)

7. Minimal threshold level (MTL)—Stimulus of sufficient magnitude to stimulate nerve impulse; different nerve fibers (depending on size of fiber) have different MTL

8. All-or-none principle

    a. Once nerve is excited, impulse will travel full length of fiber without additional stimulus

      b. Impulse travels same speed from any stimulus, which exceeds minimum threshold level

B. Physiology of the peripheral nerves

  1. Ions in nerve transmission

      a. Na+ (Sodium)—Predominantly in extracellular fluid

      b. K+ (Potassium)—Predominantly in intracellular fluid

      c. Cl− (Chloride)—Predominantly in extracellular fluid; does not diffuse through the nerve sheath, regardless of the stage of nerve transmission

  2. Nerve conduction (Figure 9-10■)

      a. Resting potential—Balance exists between positive sodium ions on the outside of the nerve membrane and negative potassium ions on the inside of the membrane

      b. Depolarization

         (1) A stimulus, which may be chemical, thermal, mechanical, or electrical in nature (such as pain), that produces excitation of the nerve fiber, which leads to increase in permeability of the cell membrane to sodium ions

         (2) The rapid influx of sodium ions to the interior of the nerve cell causes a depolarization of the nerve membrane from the resting level to its firing threshold

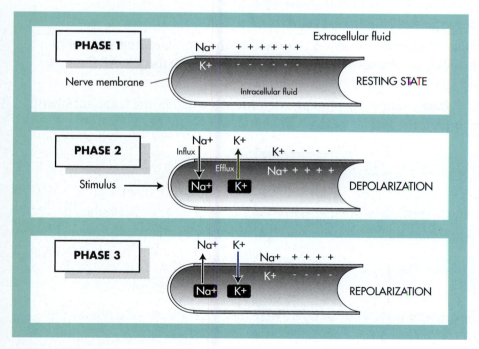

FIGURE 9-10 ■ Nerve Conduction

    c. Repolarization

      (1) The sodium pump actively transports the sodium ions out of the nerve cell while potassium ions diffuse to the inside of the nerve cell

      (2) The nerve's resting potential is reestablished

      (3) Absolute refractory period—Period where nerve will not fire no matter what intensity of stimulus applied

      (4) Relative refractory period—Nerve will fire only if greater than usual stimulus is applied

C. Pharmacology of local anesthetics

  1. Ideal local anesthetics

    a. Potent local anesthesia

    b. Reversible local anesthesia

    c. Absence of local reactions

    d. Absence of systemic reactions

    e. Rapid onset

    f. Satisfactory duration

    g. Adequate tissue penetration

    h. Low cost

    i. Stability in solution (long shelf-life)

    j. Ease of metabolism and excretion

D. Chemical properties (Figure 9-11■)

  1. Aromatic lipophilic group—Composed of the aromatic ring structure; ensures that the anesthetic agent is able to penetrate the lipid-rich nerve membrane where impulse conduction is blocked

  2. Intermediate chain—This linkage determines whether the local anesthetic agent is classified as an ester or an amide

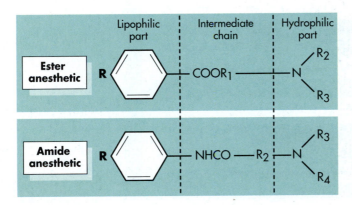

FIGURE 9-11 ■ Chemical Structure of Ester Anesthetic and Amide Anesthetic

3. Hydrophilic amino group—When combined with hydrochloric acid, allows the anesthetic to diffuse through the interstitial fluid in the tissues to reach the nerve

E. Actions of local anesthetics

    1. Interrupt nerve conduction—Block ability of membrane to undergo changes, which occur when nerves fire

    2. Vasodilation

        a. Increase in rate of absorption of the local anesthetic

        b. Increase in blood levels and therefore increase risk of anesthetic toxicity

        c. Decrease duration of action

        d. Increased bleeding at the site of injection

F. Properties and ionization factors

    1. Base form—Lipophilic (fat soluble) and un-ionized (not charged); penetrates the nerve

    2. Hydrophilic (water soluble) and ionized (charged)—Form in cartridge

    3. The salts of local anesthetics exist as both uncharged molecules called the free base (RN) and positively charged molecules called the cation (RNH); Ionization equilibrium depends on pH and pKa

    4. pKa—The proportion of drug in each form is determined by the pKa of the local anesthetic and the pH of the environment

    5. Infection—Acidic environment and lower pH and the amount of free base are reduced; therefore, dental anesthesia is more difficult to attain

G. Pharmacokenetics—The body's handling of local anesthetics

    1. Absorption—First to the site of administration, then to the circulation, which carries it to the body; it is determined by the degree of ionization, and dependant on the vascularity of the tissue.

    2. Distribution—Once absorbed, the drug is distributed throughout the body into the systemic circulation

    3. Metabolism (biotransformation of esters)—Hydrolyzed in the blood by plasma pseudocholinesterase (an enzyme).

    4. Metabolism of amides—Metabolized by the liver; Prilocaine is metabolized predominantly by the lungs and small amounts in liver

    5. Excretion—Kidney is the primary excretory organ for both esters and amides

    6. Influences of adverse reactions and toxicities dependant upon

        a. Nature of the drug

        b. Concentration of the drug and dose

        c. Route of administration

        d. Rate of administration

e. Vascularity

f. Age

g. Weight of patient

h. Health of patient

i. Route and rate of metabolism and excretion

7. Composition

a. Vasoconstrictor—Added to local anesthetic solution to delay absorption, reduce toxicity, and prolong duration

b. Antioxican—Included to retard oxidation of epinephrine (sodium bisulfite or metabisulfite)

c. Sodium hydroxide—Alkalinizes the pH of the solution to between 6 and 7

d. Sodium chloride—Makes solution isotonic

H. Short-acting amide local anesthetics—Pulpal anesthesia for about 30 minutes

1. Lidocaine 2% (Xylocaine)

a. 36 mg/carpule

b. 4.4 mg/kg

c. 300 mg maximum recommended dose (MRD)

2. Mepivacaine 3% (Carbocaine)

a. 54 mg/carpule

b. 4.4 mg/kg

c. 300 mg MRD

3. Prilocaine 4%

a. 72 mg/carpule

b. 6 mg/kg

c. 400 mg MRD

I. Intermediate-acting local amide anesthetics—Pulpal anesthesia about 60 minutes

1. Lidocaine 2% 1:100,000 and 1:50,000 epinephrine

a. 36 mg/carpule

b. 4.4 mg/kg

c. 300 mg MRD

2. Mepivacaine 2% 1:200,000 and 1:20,000 levonordefrin

a. 54 mg/carpule

b. 4.4 mg/kg

c. 300 mg MRD

3. Prilocaine 4% 1:200,000 epinephrine

a. 72 mg/carpule

b. 6 mg/kg

      c. 400 mg MRD

  4. Articaine 4% 1:100,000 and 1:200,000 epinephrine

      a. 72 mg/carpule

      b. 7 mg/kg

      c. 500 mg MRD

J. Long-acting amide local anesthetics—Pulpal anesthesia 90+ minutes

  1. Bupivacaine 0.5% 1:200,000 epinephrine

      a. 9 mg/kg

      b. **1.**3 mg/kg

      c. 90 mg MRD

K. Dosages (MRD)

  1. Determine mg per carpule calculated by concentration of solution

      a. Example: 2% solution

$$2\% = \frac{2\text{ g}}{100\text{ mL}} \implies \frac{2000\text{ mg}}{100\text{ mL}}$$

$$= \frac{20\text{ mg}}{1\text{ mL}} = 20\text{ mg/mL}$$

$$\text{amount in 1 carpule} = \frac{20\text{ mg}}{1\text{ mL}} \times \frac{1.8\text{ mL}}{\text{carpule}} = 36\text{ mg/carpule}$$

Carpule of anesthetic contains 1.8 mL of solution
1 g = 1,000 mg

  2. Determine MRD based on patient's weight in kg

      a. Example: Using Lidocaine 2%, on 125-pound patient

        125 ÷ 2.2 = 57 kg

        57 kg × 4.4 mg/kg = 251 mg MRD

        lbs ÷ 2.2 = kg

        Each local anesthetic has set mg/kg determined by manufacturer

3. Determine maximum number of carpules that can be administered

      a. Example: Using Lidocaine 2%, on 125-pound patient

      Determine MRD, which is 251 mg

      251 mg ÷ 36 mg (mg in one carpule of Lidocaine) = 6.9 carpules

      Divide mg per carpule by MRD

L. Topical local anesthetics

  1. Indications

      a. To provide regional (topical) analgesia at the site of application for patient comfort

    b. Avoid using ester topical anesthetics on patient with a history of allergic reactions to many sources

    c. Patients allergic to ester anesthetics should be given an amide topical anesthetic

2. Agents

    a. Benzocaine—Ester of PABA; Hurricaine gel used in dentistry (20%)

    b. Lidocaine 2–5%—Amide

    c. Tetracaine 2%—Ester of PABA

    d. Oraquix

        (1) Needleless application of local anesthetic in periodontal pockets

        (2) Lidocaine and prilocaine periodontal gel; 25/25 mg per g

        (3) Effective in 30 sec

        (4) Lasts 14–31 minutes; sufficient for scaling and root planning

M. Pharmacology of Vasoconstrictors

1. Role of vasoconstrictors

    a. Increased safely by decreasing reuptake of local anesthetic by blood vessels

    b. Increased duration

    c. Decreased dose required

    d. Increased hemostasis—Less blood because of shutdown of vessels

    e. Counteracts vasodilatation action of local anesthetic

2. Mechanism of action of vasoconstrictor

    a. Exert their action directly on the adrenergic receptors

    b. Counteracts vasodilatation action of local anesthetic—Alpha (α) effects of vasoconstrictors cause constriction of blood vessels, decreasing the amount of blood flow to the site of injection, thereby decreasing systemic absorption of the local anesthetic

3. Systemic effects of vasoconstrictors

    a. Cardiac excitability

    b. Increased heart rate

    c. Increased force of contraction

    d. Increased stroke volume and cardiac output

    e. Increase in diastolic and systolic pressures

    f. Increase in myocardial oxygen consumption

4. Adverse reaction of vasoconstrictors

    a. Anxiety

b. Apprehension

c. Nervousness

d. Increased blood pressure

e. Increased heart rate

5. Inactivation of vasoconstrictors—Major—Termination of drug action takes place primarily due to reuptake of the drug by adrenergic nerves; monoamine oxidase (MAO) and catechol-o-methyltranserage (COMT)

6. Agents

    a. Epinephrine (Adrenalin) Concentrations

        (1) 1:50,000

        (2) 1:100,000

        (3) 1:200,000

    b. Levonordefrine (Neo-cobefrin)—Concentration 1:20,000

N. Dosages of vasoconstrictors

    1. Determine mg per carpule calculated by concentration of solution

    Example: Using 1:100,000 concentration

$$1:100,000 = \frac{1000 \text{ mg}}{100,000 \text{ mL}} = \frac{1 \text{ mg}}{100 \text{ mL}}$$

$$= \frac{0.1 \text{ mg}}{1 \text{ mL}}$$

$$0.1 \times 1.8 \text{ mL/carpule}$$
$$= .018 \text{ mg/carpule}$$ *Dentistry*

Carpule contains 1.8 mL of solution

    2. MRD of vasoconstrictors

    a. Healthy patient, .2 mg

    b. Compromised patient, .04 mg for epinephrine and .2 mg for Levonordephrin

    3. Determine maximum number of carpules

    Example: Epinephrine 1:100,000

    Determine mg per carpule = .018 (as determined above)

    Healthy patient

    .2 ÷ .018 mg = 11.1 carpules

    Compromised patient

    .04 ÷ .018 = 2.2 carpules

    Local anesthetic and vasoconstrictor must be calculated separately and lower of the two maximum doses is MRD, called the limiting factor

O. Medical history review for local anesthetics

    1. Absolute contraindication

        a. Requires that the offending drug not be administered to the individual under any circumstances

        b. The administration of such a drug is contraindicated in all situations because it substantially increases the possibility of a life-threatening risk for the patient

    2. Relative contraindication

        a. Signifies that it is preferable to avoid administration of the suspected drug because there is the increased possibility that an adverse reaction may occur; however, if an acceptable substitute is not available, the drug may be used judiciously; administer the minimal dose that still produces sufficient pain control

P. Vasoconstrictor/drug interations—Epinephrine and other vasoconstrictors should be used with great caution or eliminated entirely when patients are taking the following drugs

    1. Monoamine oxidase inhibitors (MAOIs)

        a. Monoamine oxidase is one of the two enzymes responsible for the inactivation of epinephrine and norepinephrine

        b. If the activity of MAOIs is inhibited by the action of certain drugs, then the systemic effects of epinephrine result

        c. MAOIs are occasionally prescribed for patients with hypertension or psychological depression

        d. Phenylzine (Nardil), tranylpromine (Parnate), isocarboxazid (Marplan)

    2. Tricyclic antidepressants

        a. Prescribed for the treatment of neurotic or psychotic depression; when epinephrine is given to patients taking these drugs, the pressor (blood pressure raising) activity of the epinephrine is potentiated two to four times

        b. If the patient also has arrhythmias, the situation is of even greater concern

        c. Amitriptyline (Elavil), doxepin (Sinequan, Adapin), nortriptyline (Pamelor), imipramine (Tofranil), desipramine (Norpramin, Pertofrane), protriptyline (Vivactil), trimipramine (Surmontil), amoxapine (Asendin)

    3. Antihypertensives (beta blockers)

        a. Like the tricyclic antidepressants, the antihypertensives potentiate the action of epinephrine and other adrenergic amines by increasing the pressor potency two to six times

4. Propranolol (Inderal), metoprolol (Lopressor), atenolol (Tenormin), timolol (Blocadren), nadolol (Corgard), pindolol (Visken)

    a. Cardiac drugs—Digitalis glycosides are used for the treatment of congestive heart failure; the combination of digitalis glycosides and epinephrine increases the potential for cardiac arrythmias

    b. Antidiabetic agents

        (1) Oral hypoglycemic agents—Epinephrine and other sympathomemic amines inhibit the peripheral glucose uptake by the tissues and increase glucose released by the liver

        (2) Hyperglycemia can result; epinephrine is, therefore, an antagonist to antidiabetic agents

        (3) Insulin, chlorpropamide (Diabinese), glyburide (Diabeta), glypizide (Glucotrol)

5. Cocaine—Insulin, chlorpropamide (Diabinese), glyburide (Diabeta), glypizide (Glucotrol)

Q. Ester-derivative local anesthetic drug/drug interactions

  1. Cholinesterase inhibitors

    a. Frequently prescribed for the treatment of myasthenia gravis and glaucoma

    b. Patients taking cholinesterase inhibitors should not be given ester-derivative local anesthetics

    c. Ester derivatives are metabolized primarily in the bloodstream by plasma cholinesterase

        (1) If cholinesterase is inhibited, then the ester derivatives are more slowly broken down and systemic toxicity may result

  2. Sulfonamides

    a. Procaine and other ester-type local anesthetics undergo hydrolysis to para-aminobenzoic acid (PABA), a major metabolic by-product; sulfonamides competitively inhibit PABA in microorganisms

    b. PABA derivatives, therefore, may antagonize the antibacterial activity of sulfonamides, rendering them ineffective

  3. Atypical plasma-cholinesterase

    a. Relative to esters

    b. Slow to metabolize esters

    c. Use amide local anesthetics

R. Amide-derivative local anesthetic drug/drug interactions

  1. Cimetidine (tagamet)—Inhibits hepatic metabolism of amides by decreasing hepatic blood flow, therefore increasing risk of toxic overdose

2. Beta blockers

    a. One type of antihypertensive—Inhibits metabolism of amides by decreasing hepatic blood flow, therefore increasing risk of toxic overdose

    b. Not all antihypertensives behave in this manner; see PDR for specific interactions

S. Other interactions

  1. Cardiovascular disease

    a. No vasoconstrictors—Absolute contraindication if:

      (1) Blood pressure greater than 200/115

      (2) Not after a heart attack or stroke

      (3) Unstable angina (uncontrolled)

      (4) Cardiac arrhythmia—Refractory arrhythmia

      (5) Heart failure (relative)—may not tolerate lying down for treatment; increase risk for toxicity

  2. Liver disease

    a. Relative contraindication to amides

    b. Possible risk of toxicity

    c. Prilocaine can be used because is metabolized primarily in the lungs

  3. Kidney disease—No contraindications; use judiciously

  4. Uncontrolled hyperthyroidism—Absolute contraindication; could cause thyroid crisis, thyroid storm (loss of speech, bulging eyes)

  5. Pregnancy/placental barrier/fetal implications

    a. Relative contraindication

    b. Use as little as possible, try not to use in first trimester

    c. FDA categories

      (1) Category B—Lidocaine, prilocaine; safest choice

      (2) Category C—Mepivacaine, bupivacaine, procaine

  6. Methemoglobinemia—Prilocaine and articaine when administered in large doses, and topical anesthetic benzocaine can cause the inability to carry oxygen and clinical cyanosis occurs, relative contraindication

  7. Malignant hyperthermia

    a. Relative contraindication to amides

      (1) Complications associated with the administration of general anesthesia

      (2) Unusual hereditary condition

      (3) Will cause patient to have high fever during surgery (Dantrolene treats symptom)

8. Age—More susceptible to maximum permissible dose, therefore reduce dose in children and elderly patients

9. Bleeding disorders

a. Hemophiliac patients: need to use caution not to puncture artery; infiltrate instead of block injection

b. Hematoma could be a life-threatening situation

c. Should bleeding occur, use pressure and ice

10. Uncontrolled diabetes—Absolute contraindication to vasoconstrictors; risk of hyperglycemia

11. Pheochromocytoma

a. Absolute contraindication

(1) Tumor in adrenal gland

(2) Produces adrenal insufficiency

(3) Rule of twos: 20 mg cortisone for 2 weeks or longer within past 2 years

III. Local Anesthesia Armamentarium

A. Syringes

1. Breech-loading, metallic, aspirating, cartridge type—Most commonly used syringe for the administration of an intraoral local anesthetic (Figure 9-12■)

2. Pressure-type syringe—Used when administering a periodontal ligament (PDL) injection, which provides pulpal anesthesia to one tooth (Figure 9-13■)

3. Jet injector—Delivers .05–.2 mL of anesthetic agent to the mucous membranes at a high pressure via small openings called jets (Figure 9-14■)

B. Needles (Figure 9-15■)

1. Bevel—The angled surface of the needlepoint that is directed into the tissues

2. Shank—Length of the needle from the point to the hub

3. Hub—Plastic or metal piece that attaches the needle onto the syringe

4. Syringe penetrating end—Punctures the rubber diaphragm of cartridge and tip rests within the cartridge

5. Colored shield—Protects the part of the needle that is inserted into the tissues

6. Gauge

a. Diameter of the lumen of the needle

b. Higher the gauge number, the smaller the diameter of the lumen

c. Most commonly used needles are 25, 27 gauge

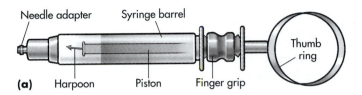

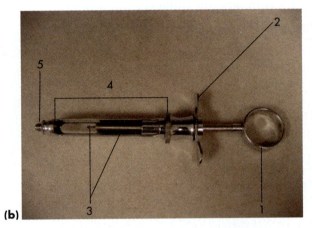

FIGURE 9-12 ■ (a) Breech-loading Aspirating Syringe; (b) Parts of Syringe: 1. Thumb Ring, 2. Finger Grip, 3. Piston with Harpoon, 4. Syringe Barrel, 5. Needle Adapter

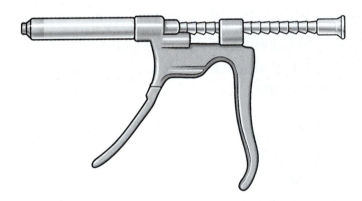

FIGURE 9-13 ■ Pressure-type Syringe

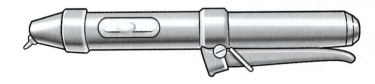

FIGURE 9-14 ■ Jet Injector

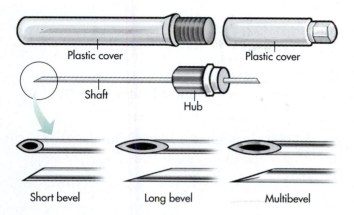

FIGURE 9-15 ■ Parts of Needle and Types of Bevels

    d. Recommended to use 25-gauge needle for those injections that pose a high risk of aspiration or when a significant depth of soft tissue must be penetrated

    e. 27-gauge may be used for all other injections

    f. Advantages of larger-gauge needles

       (1) Less deflection

       (2) Greater accuracy

       (3) Needle breakage less likely to occur

       (4) Aspiration of blood is more reliable through larger lumen

    g. Length (Figure 9-16■)

       (1) Long: 1 5/8 in. or 40 mm measured from hub to the needle tip; preferred for those injections that require penetration of significant soft tissue (inferior alveolar and infraorbital nerve blocks)

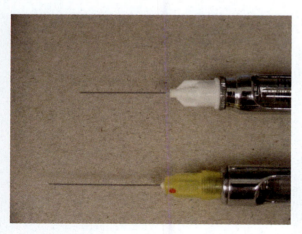

FIGURE 9-16 ■ Needle Lengths. The top needle is short, approximately 20 millimeters from bevel tip to hub. The bottom needle is long, approximately 32 millimeters from bevel tip to hub.

(2) Short: 1 in. or 25 mm; recommended when not penetrating significant tissue

h. Insertions

(1) Needles should not be inserted to the hub

(2) Retrieval is very hard if the needle is embedded in the tissue

(3) The face of the bevel is directed parallel to bone

i. Disposal—Comply with OSHA guidelines, which is to recap the needle utilizing "scoop" method and place in a "sharps" disposal container

j. Pain on insertion

(1) Due to dull needle

(2) Prevention: change needle after 3–4 injections

k. Pain on withdrawal—Due to barbs on needle tip

C. Cartridge—Hold 1.8 mL of local anesthetic solutions (Figure 9-17■)

1. Ingredients

a. Local anesthetic drug

b. Vasoconstrictor drug

c. Preservative for vasoconstrictor (usually sodium bisulfite)

d. Sodium chloride

e. Distilled water

2. Bubbles

a. Small bubbles (1–2 mm in diameter) may at times be seen in a cartridge; this is nitrogen gas that was bubbled into the anesthetic solution during the manufacturing process to preclude oxygen, which destroys the vasoconstrictor; these bubbles are harmless and can be ignored (Figure 9-18■)

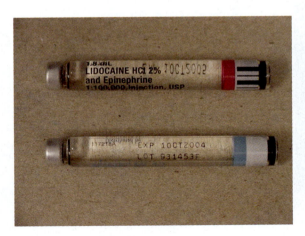

FIGURE 9-17 ■ Anesthetic Carpule

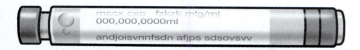

FIGURE 9-18 ■ Small Bubbles in Cartridge

    b. Large bubbles (larger than 2mm) are an indication that the solution has been frozen; because sterility of the solution is no longer guaranteed, the cartridge should not be used (Figure 9-19■)

3. Extruded stopper

    a. Accompanied by a large bubble in the cartridge; is an indication the solution has been frozen and should be discarded

    b. No bubble indicates that the cartridge has probably been stored too long in chemical disinfecting solution; will produce burning sensation upon injection (Figure 9-20■)

4. Sticky stopper—Does not advance smoothly through the glass cylinder when pressure is applied to the thumb ring

5. Corroded cap—May be observed if it has been immersed in quaternary compounds

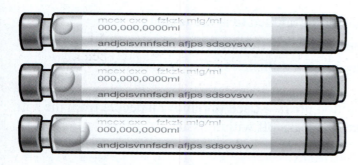

FIGURE 9-19 ■ Large Bubbles in Cartridge

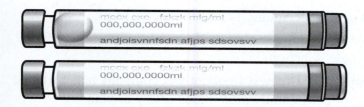

FIGURE 9-20 ■ Frozen Carpule: Large Bubble and Extruded Stopper (top);
(b) Stored in Disinfecting Solution: Extruded Stopper and No Bubble (bottom)

6. Rust on aluminum cap—Signifies that a cartridge has broken or leaked in the metal container

7. Leakage during injection—Off-center perforation of the needle into the diaphragm of the cartridge

8. Burning on injection

    a. Normal response to pH of drug

    b. Cartridge containing sterilizing solution

    c. Overheated cartridge

    d. Vasoconstrictor pH outdated solutions

D. Supplementary armamentarium

    1. Topical antiseptics

       a. Reduce the risk of introducing surface microorganisms into the tissue, which could result in infection

       b. Contain iodine; caution against patients allergic to iodine

    2. Topical anesthetic

       a. Applied to the mucous membrane prior to the initial needle penetration to anesthetize the terminal nerve endings

       b. Concentration is high to facilitate diffusion of the drug through the mucous membranes

       c. Small amounts should be applied to avoid toxicity

       d. Apply to injection site for 1–2 minutes

       e. Most contain ester local anesthetics such as benzocaine; possible allergic reaction to these agents is greater than amide topical anesthetics

    3. Hemostat, forceps, cotton pliers—Used to remove a needle from the soft tissues in case the needle breaks off within tissue

IV. Administering Local Anesthesia

A. Classification of injections (Figure 9-21■)

    1. Nerve block anesthesia

       a. Injection of local anesthetic solution close to a nerve trunk

       b. Has the advantage of blocking sensations from a large portion of the anatomy with a single injection

       c. Disadvantage: major blood vessels frequently accompany nerve trunks, and the possibility of accidentally piercing an artery or vein is significantly enhanced

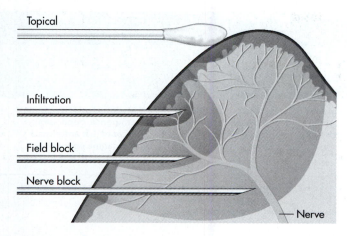

Topical

Infiltration

Field block

Nerve block

Nerve

FIGURE 9-21 ■ Administration Techniques

2. Field block anesthesia—A form of regional anesthesia commonly employed in the maxillary arch; injection of local anesthetic solution close to large terminal nerve branches

3. Infiltration anesthesia

    a. Provides pain relief solely in the area bathed by the drug solution

    b. Only terminal nerve endings are affected by infiltration

    c. Usually employed for soft tissue anesthesia

4. Topical anesthesia—Surface application of a local anesthetic to block free nerve endings supplying the mucosal surfaces

B. Maxillary injections (Table 9-1■); Mandibular injections (Table 9-2■)

TABLE 9-1 MAXILLARY INJECTIONS

Injection	Nerve Anatomy	Spreading of Anesthesia	Penetration Site	Landmarks	
Anterior Superior Alveolar (ASA)	Branch of the infraorbital nerve (Figures 9-22■, 9-23■)	Pulpal anesthesia of maxillary central, lateral, and cuspid; facial periodontium, and bone overlying these teeth (Figure 9-24■)	Height of mucobuccal fold slightly mesial to the canine eminence	Mucobuccal fold, canine eminence, depression located just anterior to the canine eminence	
Middle Superior Alveolar (MSA)	Branch of the infraorbital nerve (Figures 9-22, 9-23)	Pulpal anesthesia of 1st and 2nd maxillary premolars and MB root of maxillary 1st molar in 60% of population; buccal periodontal tissue and bone over same teeth (Figure 9-25■)	Height of mucobuccal fold above apex of maxillary second premolar	Mucobuccal fold, second premolar	
Infraorbital	Forward continuation of maxillary nerve, enters orbit via inferior orbital fissure, passing through infraorbital canal, and exits through infraorbital canal and foramen; carries sensory fibers from lower eyelid and adjacent tissue (Figures 9-22, 9-23)	Pulpal anesthesia of the maxillary central incisor, lateral incisor, and canine, 60% max premolars, MB root of the first molar in 60% of population; lower eyelid, lateral aspect of the nose, upper lip, buccal and labial periodontal tissues, and bone overlying these same teeth (Figure 9-26■)	Height of mucobuccal fold above the first premolar	Mucobuccal fold, infraorbital notch, infraorbital ridge, infraorbital depression, infraorbital foramen	
Posterior Superior Alveolar (PSA)	Given off immediately prior to the nerve entering the infraorbital groove; penetrates posterior of maxillary tuberosity via posterior superior alveolar foramen, travels forward under the mucosa of the maxillary sinus (Figure 9-22)	Pulpal anesthesia of the 3rd, 2nd, and 1st maxillary molars entirely in 60%, MB root anesthetized in 40%; buccal periodontium and bone overlying these teeth (Figure 9-27■)	Height of mucobuccal fold opposite the distal portion of the second molar	Mucobuccal fold, second molar, maxillary tuberosity, maxillary occlusal plane, midsaggital plane	
Nasopalatine	Sensory nerve, leaves the spenopalatine ganglion through the spenopalatine foramen, passing forward and downward on the nasal septum through the incisive canal to the incisive foramen; runs in a posterior direction (Figure 9-28■)	Nasal septum; hard palate and overlying soft tissue of the maxillary anterior teeth bilaterally (Figure 9-29■)	Lateral to the incisive papilla	Maxillary central incisors; incisive papilla	
Greater Palatine	Sensory nerve, leaves the sphenopalatine ganglion and descends through the greater palatine canal to the greater palatine foramen; continues in an anterior direction (Figure 9-28)	Hard palate and overlying soft tissue maxillary 3rd molar; the first premolar on side injected (Figure 9-30■)	Slightly anterior to the greater palatine foramen	GP foramen located at the junction of the maxillary alveolar process and palatine bone distal to the maxillary second molar	

Deposit Location	Depth of Penetration	Technique	Anesthetic Solution	Adverse Effects
Apical region of canine	Short needle 25- or 27-gauge 1/4 of needle	Angle needle from lateral toward the bone above the apex of the cuspid Aspirate	1/3 to 1/2 of cartridge 20–30 seconds to deposit solution	Scrape periosteum from injecting too close to periosteum or too rapidly
Above (3–5 mm) the apical region of the second premolar	Short 25- or 27-gauge 1/4 of the needle length	Parallel to long axis of the 2nd maxillary premolar above the apex Aspirate	1/2 to 2/3 of cartridge 30–45 seconds	Pain from injecting too close to periosteum or too rapid deposition
Upper rim of the infraorbital foramen, the needle should gently contact bone when reaching the deposition site	Long needle 25-gauge, 1/2 the needle length	Locate infraorbital foramen; maintain pressure with your finger over the foramen during injection, massage; bevel toward bone	1/2 to 2/3 cartridge 30–45 seconds	Scrape periosteum from injecting too close to periosteum
Posterior and superior to the posterior border of the maxilla at the PSA nerve foramina	Short needle 3/4 of needle length 25- or 27-gauge	Upward 45 degrees to occlusal plane; inward and backward 45 degrees to midsagittal plane Aspirate	1/2 to 3/4 carpule 30–60 seconds to deposit solution	Needle inserted too far posterior and superior may tear maxillary artery or pterygoid plexus of veins, resulting in hematoma; mandibular anesthesia
Incisive foramen beneath the incisive papilla	No more than 4–6 mm or until bone is lightly contacted 27-gauge short needle	45–90 degrees to tissue at the edge of incisive papilla; watch for blanching of the tissue; use pressure anesthesia Aspirate	Several drops to 1/4 carpule 20–30 seconds	Because of the density of the tissues, the anesthetic solution may appear around the needle penetration site during administration
Greater palatine nerve located between soft tissue and bone of the hard palate	No more than 5–7 mm or until palate is lightly contacted 25- or 27-gauge short	Advance syringe from opposite side of mouth at right angle to target area; use pressure anesthesia, topical and swab	1/4 cartridge 20–30 seconds	

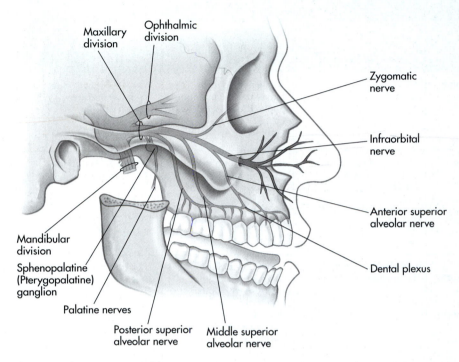

FIGURE 9-22 ■ Divisions of Maxillary Nerve (V$_2$)

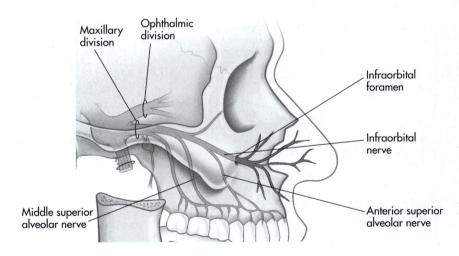

FIGURE 9-23 ■ Branches of Infraorbital Foramen

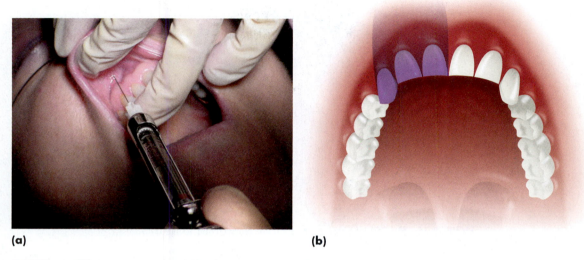

(a)   (b)

FIGURE 9-24 ■ Anterior Superior Alveolar (a) Injection Technique; (b) Spread of Analgesia

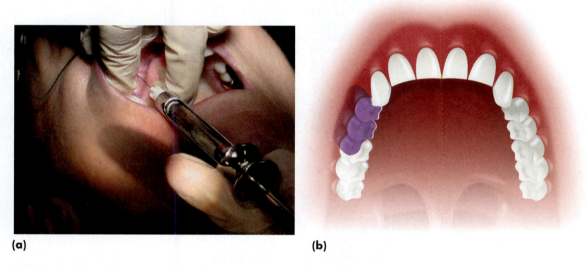

(a)   (b)

FIGURE 9-25 ■ Middle Superior Alveolar (a) Injection Technique; (b) Spread of Analgesia

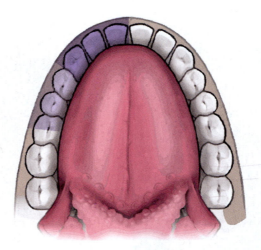

FIGURE 9-26 ■ Darkened area shows anesthesia provided from IO injection.

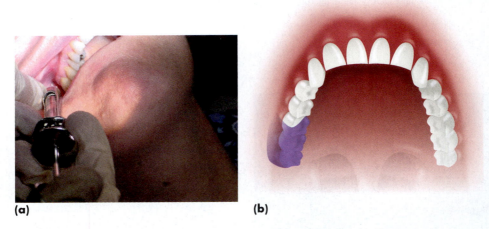

(a)   **(b)**

FIGURE 9-27 ■ Posteror Superior Alveolar (a) Injection Technique; (b) Spread of Analgesia

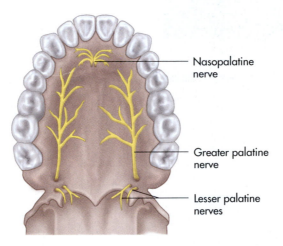

Nasopalatine
nerve

Greater palatine
nerve

Lesser palatine
nerves

FIGURE 9-28 ■ Nasopalatine Nerve and Greater Palatine Nerve

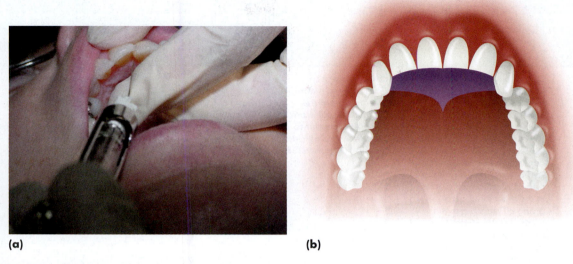

FIGURE 9-29 ■ Nasopalatine (a) Injection Technique; (b) Spread of Analgesia

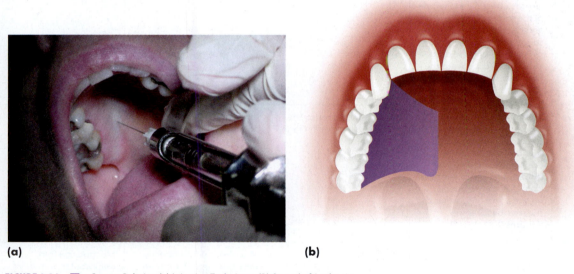

FIGURE 9-30 ■ Greater Palatine (a) Injection Technique; (B) Spread of Analgesia

TABLE 9-2 MANDIBULAR INJECTIONS

Injection	Nerve Anatomy	Spreading of Anesthesia	Penetration Site	Landmarks	
Inferior Alveolar	Largest branch of the mandibular division; sensory nerve; passes downward from the infratemporal fossa below the inferior head of the lateral pterygoid muscle, lateral to the sphenomandibular ligament and medial to the ramus entering the mandibular foramen; travels in the mandibular canal giving off branches to the teeth near the mental foramen it divides into the mental nerve and the incisive nerve (Figures 9-31■, 9-32■).	Mandibular teeth to midline; body of mandible, inferior portion of the ramus, facial tissue from the second premolar to midline, lower lip on side of injection (Figure 9-33■)	Middle of pterygomandibular triangle at the height of the coronoid notch (6–10 mm above the occlusal plane of the mandibular molars)	Anterior border of ramus, external oblique ridge, coronoid notch, internal oblique ridge, pterygomandibular raphe, pterygomandibular triangle, mandibular occlusal plane	
Lingual	Sensory nerve, passes downward with the inferior alveolar nerve, communicating with the chorda tympani of the facial nerve; crosses obliquely to the side of the tongue running in an anterior direction across the submandibular salivary gland and along the tongue to its tip, lying beneath the mucous membrane (Figures 9-31, 9-34■)	Lingual gingival tissue to the midline, anterior 2/3 of the tongue and floor of the oral cavity (Figure 9-31)	Same as IA	Same as IA	
Buccal nerve block	Sensory nerve; travels along the medial side of the ramus of the mandible, crosses the ramus near the anterior border, and sends terminal branches to the buccal mucosa and gingiva up to the mental foramen (Figures 9-31, 9-35■)	Buccal soft tissues to the mandibular molars (Figure 9-36■)	In vestibule, distal and buccal to the most distal molar in the quadrant	Mandibular molars, vestibule, mucobuccal fold	
Incisive	Sensory nerve, continuation of the inferior alveolar nerve within the incisive canal, at the mental foramen, to the midline of the mandible (Figures 9-32, 9-37■)	Teeth anterior to the mental foramen, and the respective periosteum (Figure 9-38■)	Mucobuccal fold directly over the mental foramen	Mucobuccal fold, mandibular premolars, mental foramen	
Mental Nerve	Sensory nerve, branches from the inferior alveolar nerve passing through the mental foramen proceeding toward the midline of the mandible (Figures 9-31, 9-32, 9-37, 9-39■)	Facial soft tissues from the mental foramen anterior to midline, lower lip, skin of chin (Figure 9-38)	Mucobuccal fold directly over the mental foramen	Mucobuccal fold, mandibular premolars, mental foramen	

Depth of Penetration	Deposit Location	Technique	Anesthetic Solution	Adverse Effects
Until bone is lightly contacted 2/3 to 3/4 of the needle length inserted, withdrawal needle 1 mm; long needle 25-gauge	Superior to the mandibular foramen at the inferior alveolar nerve before it enters the foramen	Locate pterygomandibular triangle, place thumb on the greatest depression (coronoid notch), roll your finger medially to locate the internal oblique ridge; the point of penetration is between the internal oblique ridge and the pterygomandibular raphe; syringe barrel rests on premolars of opposite side	.09–1.8 ml approx 60 sec to 2 min to deposit solution	Transient facial paralysis from deposition in parotid gland; hematoma
After depositing solution for IA withdraw needle until 1/2 its length remains in tissues		Same as IA	1/4 cartridge or less	"Shocking" pain if lingual nerve is touched
1–4 mm until bone is lightly contacted	Buccal nerve as it passes over the anterior border of the ramus	Administer after IA; penetrate mucous membrane until bone is contacted	1/8 to 1/4 of cartridge	Trismus of tendonous attachment, of temporalis; ballooning of tissue
1/4 length of short 25-or 27-gauge needle	Directly over mental foramen, usually between the apices of the 1st and 2nd premolars	Locate mental foramen; pull tissue laterally advances needle to level of foramen; massage solution into foramen for 2 min.	1/3 to 1/2 of cartridge	
1/4 length of short 25- or 27-gauge needle	Directly over mental foramen, usually between the apices of the first and second premolars	Locate mental foramen; pull tissue laterally advances needle to level of foramen; do not massage in solution	1/3 to 1/2 of cartridge	

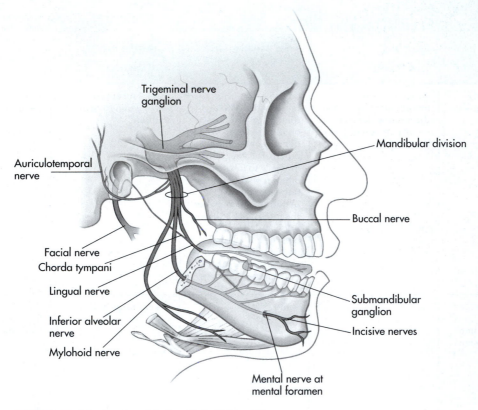

FIGURE 9-31 ■ Branches of the Mandibular Division (V₃)

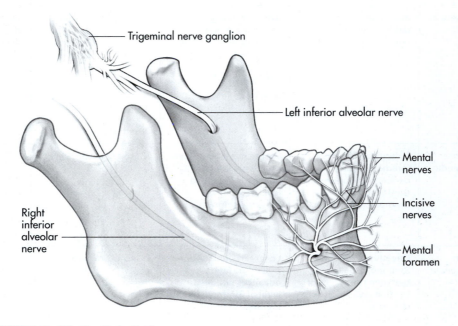

FIGURE 9-32 ■ Mandibular Division

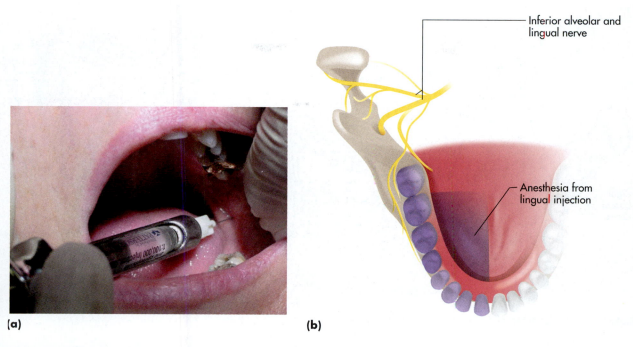

(a)   (b)

FIGURE 9-33 ■ Inferior Alveolar and Lingual (a) Injection Technique; (b) Spread of Analgesia

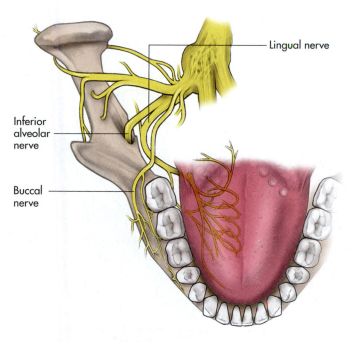

FIGURE 9-34 ■ Mandibular Division

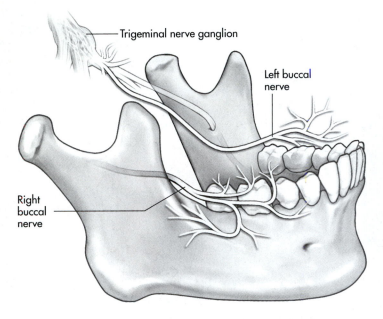

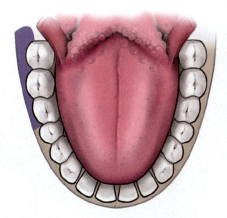

FIGURE 9-36 ■ Darkened area shows anesthesia provided by buccal injection.

FIGURE 9-35 ■ Buccal Nerve (Long Buccal Nerve or Buccinators Nerve)

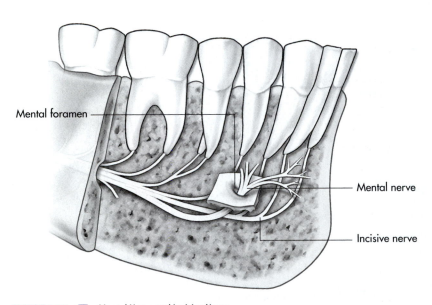

FIGURE 9-37 ■ Mental Nerve and Incisive Nerve

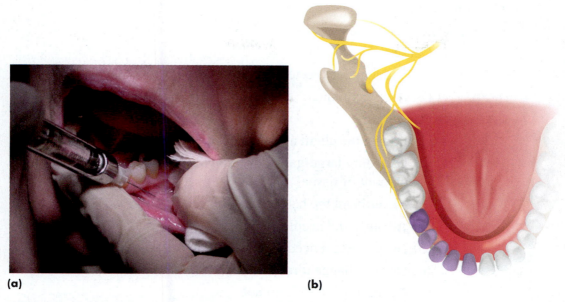

(a)   (b)

FIGURE 9-38 ■ Mental Nerve/Incisive Nerve (a) Injection Technique; (b) Spread of Analgesia

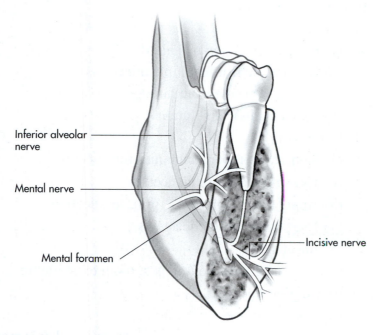

Inferior alveolar nerve

Mental nerve

Mental foramen

Incisive nerve

FIGURE 9-39 ■ Mental Nerve

C. Complications

    1. Needle breakage

        a. Causes

            (1) Sudden, unexpected movement

            (2) Poor technique

        b. Prevention

            (1) Inform the client about the procedure

            (2) Use long, large-gauge needle when penetrating a significant amount of tissue

            (3) Never bend the needle

            (4) Advance the needle slowly

            (5) Never force a needle against firm resistance such as bone

            (6) Do not change direction while needle is embedded in tissue

            (7) Never insert needle to hub

        c. Management

            (1) Remain calm

            (2) Instruct the client not to move; keep your hand in patient's mouth

            (3) Attempt to remove needle fragment if needle is protruding

            (4) If you cannot remove, refer to oral surgeon

            (5) Document incident

    2. Pain during injection

        a. Causes

            (1) Careless injection technique

            (2) Dull needle from multiple injections

            (3) A barbed needle from hitting bone

            (4) Rapid deposit of solution

        b. Prevention

            (1) Adhere to proper techniques for injections

            (2) Use sharp, disposable needles

            (3) Apply topical anesthetic prior to injection

            (4) Use sterile anesthetic agents

            (5) Inject slowly

            (6) Store anesthetic solutions at room temperature

    3. Burning during injection

        a. Causes

            (1) Local anesthetic with a vasoconstrictor that is more acidic than the tissue

        (2) Contamination of anesthetic in disinfecting solution

        (3) Heated cartridge

        (4) Expired solution

        (5) Solution deposited too rapidly

    b. Prevention

        (1) Store cartridge in a dark place at room temperature; do not store in chemical disinfectants

        (2) Check expiration date

        (3) Inject slowly

4. Hematoma—Swelling and discoloration of the tissue resulting from effusion of blood into extravascular spaces

    a. Causes—Inadvertent puncture of blood vessel, particularly an artery, most common after PSA or IA injection

    b. Prevention

        (1) Be attentive to anatomical detail

        (2) Modify injection technique depending on patient's mouth

        (3) Use a short needle for the PSA

        (4) Minimize the number of needle insertions

        (5) Maintain appropriate technique

    c. Management

        (1) If swelling appears, apply direct pressure to the site of bleeding for at least 2 minutes

        (2) Apply ice to the region—Warm the next day

        (3) Inform patient of possibility of soreness and limited movement

        (4) Advise patient that swelling and discoloration will disappear after 7–14 days

        (5) Dismiss patient when bleeding has stopped

5. Facial paralysis—Loss of motor function of the facial expression muscles

    a. Causes

        (1) Parotid gland located on the posterior border of the ramus—Local anesthetic solution deposited into the parotid gland during IA injection where the facial nerves pass

        (2) To avoid—Always contact bone before depositing solution during IA injection

    b. Prevention

        (1) Adhere to techniques recommended for IA

        (2) Needle should always contact bone to avoid depositing solution in parotid gland

    c. Management

        (1) Reassure the patient; paralysis lasts only a few hours

        (2) Instruct patient to remove contact lenses

        (3) Ask the patient to close their eyelid manually to keep cornea lubricated

        (4) Document

6. Paresthesia—Prolonged anesthesia for many hours or days following injection

    a. Causes

        (1) Irritation to nerve following injection of agent contaminated in disinfecting solution

        (2) Edema places pressure on nerve

        (3) Trauma of nerve sheath from needle contacting nerve during injection

        (4) Hemorrhage into or around neural sheath

    b. Prevention

        (1) Store dental cartridges properly

        (2) Avoid placing cartridges in disinfectant

        (3) Follow proper technique

    c. Management

        (1) Reassure patient

        (2) Arrange exam with dentist

        (3) Consultation with oral surgeon

        (4) Record incident

7. Trismus—Spasm of the muscles of mastication that results in soreness and difficulty opening the mouth

    a. Causes

        (1) Trauma to the muscles in the infratemporal space following injection

        (2) Multiple needle insertions

        (3) Contaminated solution with disinfectant

        (4) Depositing large amounts of solution in restricted areas, causing distension of tissues

        (5) Hemorrhage that leads to muscle dysfunction

        (6) Low-grade infection

    b. Prevention

        (1) Store anesthetic properly

        (2) Use sharp, sterile, disposable needles

        (3) Follow appropriate injection control protocol

        (4) Use minimal effective amount of solution and deposit slowly

   c. Management

     (1) Arrange for exam from dentist

     (2) Heat therapy

     (3) Direct patient to open and close mouth and move mandible from side to side for 5 minutes every 3–4 hours

     (4) Infection—Antibiotic treatment

     (5) If severe pain, refer to oral surgeon

     (6) Record incident

8. Infection

   a. Prevention

     (1) Use sterile, disposable needle

     (2) The needle should be sheathed prior to injection and immediately after

     (3) Use appropriate infection control guidelines when handling the anesthetic cartridges

     (4) Store anesthetic in original container, and wipe off diaphragm with disinfectant if necessary

     (5) Use topical antiseptic

9. Edema—Swelling of the tissues

   a. Causes

     (1) Trauma during injection

     (2) Administration of contaminated solution

     (3) Hemorrhage

     (4) Infection

     (5) Allergic response

   b. Prevention

     (1) Follow appropriate infection control protocol when storing and handling components of local anesthetic armamentarium

     (2) Observe guidelines for administering atraumatic injections

     (3) Conduct an adequate preanesthetic patient assessment

10. Tissue sloughing—Surface layers of epithelium may be lost

   a. Causes

     (1) Sterile abscess may develop after prolonged ischemia, usually on palate (vasoconstrictor)

     (2) Tissue irritation caused by topical anesthetic

   b. Prevention

     (1) Use topical anesthetics appropriately—Limit to 1–2 minutes

     (2) Avoid high concentrations of vasoconstrictors

11. Soft tissue trauma

   a. Causes—Lip, tongue, or cheek trauma results when patient inadvertently chews or bites tissues while numb

   b. Prevention

   (1) Select anesthetic agent with duration appropriate for length of appointment

   (2) Warn patient not to eat, drink, or test anesthesia area by biting

   (3) Place cotton roll between teeth and soft tissue

   (4) Use warning stickers on child to remind parent that child is numb

V. Local Anesthetic Emergencies

A. Local anesthetic overdose—Overly high blood levels of a drug in various organs and tissues

   1. Causes of overdose

   a. Biotransformation of the anesthetic is unusually slow

   b. Elimination of the anesthetic from the body through the kidneys is unusually slow

   c. The total dose administered is too large

   d. Absorption of the anesthetic from the site of injection is unusually rapid

   e. The anesthetic is administered intravascularly

   2. Prevention of overdose

   a. Medical history review is very important

   b. Ester LA biotransformed in the blood by enzyme pseudocholinesterase, which causes the drug to undergo hydrolysis to para-aminobenzoic acid

   c. Patients with familial history of atypical pseudocholinesterase may be unable to detoxify the drug

   d. Calculation of maximum permissible dose is very important

   e. Age of patient and physical status (need to adjust dose accordingly)

   f. Addition of a vasoconstricting drug in the local anesthetic solution reduces the systemic toxicity of the anesthetic agent by slowing absorption into cardiovascular system

   g. Limit area of use of topical anesthetics—Topicals are administered in high concentrations

   h. Know your anatomy

   i. Always aspirate

   j. Use 25- or 27-gauge needle

   k. Aspirate in two planes

l. Administer drug slowly

m. Medical history review is very important

3. Clinical manifestations of local anesthetic overdose reactions

  a. Early signs and symptoms

    (1) Talkative, restless, apprehensve, excited

    (2) Tremors or convulsions—If too large a dose or IV injection

    (3) Increased blood pressure and/or pulse rate

  b. Late signs and symptoms

    (1) Convulsions, followed by depression

    (2) Drop in blood pressure

    (3) Weak, rapid pulse or bradycardia

    (4) Apnea

    (5) Unconsciousness

    (6) Death

  c. Treatment of overdose

    (1) Protect patient during the convulsive period (consider 10 mg Valium IV, if convulsive period is prolonged longer than 15 minutes)

    (2) Call paramedics

    (3) Record vitals

    (4) Supportive therapy (oxygen at 6 liter flow, maintain blood pressure)

    (5) Treat bradycardia (0.4 mg Atropine IV)

    (6) Gently restrict limbs; move all instrument trays away and keep hands and materials out of patient's mouth

B. Epinephrine overdose

1. Causes of overdose—More likely to develop if concentrations of epinephrine greater than 1:100,000 are administered, great potential for epinephrine overdose in patients with cardiovascular disease

2. Prevention of overdose

  a. Use the lowest effective concentration of epinephrine needed to produce the desired effect and carefully observe dosage guidelines

  b. Reduce total dose of vasoconstrictor to avoid systemic complications in patients with cardiovascular disease

  c. IV injection may produce an epinephrine overdose

  d. Know drug interactions and decrease dose accordingly

  e. For patients with cardiovascular disease and patients taking drugs that interact with epinephrine, decrease dose to .04 mg

  f. Use the lowest effective concentration of epinephrine needed to produce the desired effect and carefully observe dosage guidelines

C. Clinical manifestations

    1. Fear, anxiety

    2. Tenseness

    3. Restlessness

    4. Throbbing headache

    5. Tremor

    6. Perspiration

    7. Weakness

    8. Dizziness

    9. Pallor

    10. Respiratory difficulty

    11. Palpitations

    12. Sharp elevation in blood pressure

    13. Elevated heart rate

    14. Cardiac dysrhythmias

D. Treatment

    1. Terminate procedure

    2. Position patient upright

    3. Reassure patient

    4. Basic life support, as indicated

    5. Monitor vital signs

    6. Activate EMS, if needed

    7. Administer oxygen, if needed

    8. Allow patient to recover and discharge

E. Allergic reactions

    1. Causes of allergic reaction

        a. Most often in response to ester local anesthetics

        b. Amide allergic reactions are extremely rare

        c. Reports of allergy to sodium bisulfite are numerous

        d. Sodium bisulfite—Preservative in vasoconstrictors

    2. Prevention of allergic reactions

        a. Anesthetic assessment is the primary measure for prevention

        b. Patient with multiple allergies has an increased potential for allergic reactions to medications (avoid ester topical anesthetics)

        c. Medical history is very important to determine true allergic reaction

3. Mild allergic reaction

　　a. Clinical manifestations of mild allergic reaction

　　　　(1) Mild pruritis (itching)

　　　　(2) Mild urticaria (rash)

　　　　(3) Angioedema (localized swelling of extremities, lips, tongue, pharynx, larynx)

　　b. Treatment of mild allergic reaction

　　　　(1) Diphenhydramine (Benedryl) 25–50 mg IV or IM

　　　　(2) Repeat up to 50 mg every 6 hours p.o. for 2 days

4. Severe allergic reactions

　　a. Clinical manifestations

　　　　(1) Severe pruritus

　　　　(2) Severe urticaria

　　　　(3) Mucous membrane rhinitis

　　　　(4) Angioedema—Swelling of lips, eyelids, cheeks, pharynx, larynx; may progress to anaphylactic shock

　　　　(5) Cardiovascular—Fall in blood pressure

　　　　(6) Respiratory—Wheezing, choking, cyanosis, hoarseness

　　　　(7) Dypsnea

　　　　(8) Central nervous system—Loss of consciousness, dilation of pupils

5. Treatment of severe allergic reaction

　　a. Epinephrine 1:1000 0.3–0.5 cc IV, IM or SC (contraindication: severe hypertension)

　　b. Theophylline ethylenediamine (Aminophylline), 250–500 mg IV over 10 minutes (contraindication: hypotension)

　　c. Steroids—Hydrocortisone sodium succinate (Solucortef), 100 mg IV

　　d. Cardiopulmonary resuscitation (if indicated)

　　e. Caution: Since aminophylline may cause hypotension, it should be given with extreme caution to asthmatic patients who are also hypotensive

VI. Nitrous Oxide

A. Inhalation sedation: rationale

　　1. Advantages

　　　　a. Onset of action is more rapid; equal to onset of IV medications

　　　　　　Oral　　30-minute onset

　　　　　　Rectal　30-minute onset

IM	10- to 15-minute onset
IV	20-sec onset (approx. arm-to-brain circulation time); 1–2 min for clinical actions to develop
Inhalation	20-sec pulmonary circulation to brain time; 2- to 3-minute onset for clinical actions to develop

b. Provide peak clinical actions in a time span permitting titration

Oral	60-min peak action
Rectal	60-min peak action
IM	30-min peak action
IV	60-sec to 20-min peak action
Inhalation	3- to 5-min peak action

c. Depth of sedation can be altered from moment to moment

Oral	Cannot easily deepen or lighten sedation
Rectal	Cannot easily deepen or lighten sedation
IM	Cannot easily deepen or lighten sedation
IV	Sedation level may easily be deepened; however, lessening of sedation is difficult to achieve
Inhalation	Sedation levels easily changed either way

d. Duration of action is not fixed

Oral	Fixed duration of action, approx. 2–3 hours
Rectal	Fixed duration of action, approx. 2–3 hours
IM	Fixed duration of action, approx. 2–4 hours
IV	Fixed duration of action, with significant variation by drug, Diazepam, 45 minutes
Inhalation	Duration variable, at discretion of administrator

e. Recovery time is rapid—Because N_2O is not metabolized by the body, the gas is rapidly and virtually completely eliminated from the body within 3–5 minutes

Oral	Recovery not entirely complete even after 2–3 hours
Rectal	Recovery not entirely complete even after 2–3 hours
IM	Recovery not entirely complete even after 2–3 hours
IV	Recovery not entirely complete even after 2–3 hours
Inhalation	Recovery usually complete following 3–5 minutes of inhalation of 100% O_2

f. Titration possible—Ability to administer small, incremental doses of a drug until a desired clinical action is obtained; also with IV

g. Can be discharged with no prohibitions on their activities; others need escort home

h. No injection required

i. Inhalation sedation is safe with few side effects

j. Drugs used in this technique have no adverse effects on the liver, kidneys, brain, or cardiovascular and respiratory systems

k. Can be used instead of local anesthetic in certain procedures

B. Disadvantages

1. Initial cost of equipment

2. Continuing cost of gases (O_2 and N_2O)

3. Nitrous oxide is not a potent agent; when used in combination with at least 20% O_2 there will be a small percentage of patients in whom the technique will fail to produce the desired clinical actions

4. A degree of cooperation is required from the patient

5. All members of the dental staff employing N_2O–O_2 must receive training in its safe and effective use

6. There is a possibility that chronic exposure to trace amounts of N_2O–O_2 is deleterious to the health of dental personnel

C. Contraindications—There are no absolute contraindication to the administration of N_2O–O_2 inhalation sedation as long as the percentage of O_2 administered is greater than 20%; there are several relative contraindications

1. Patients with compulsive personality—Is a "take charge" individual, one who does not like the feeling of losing control; will fight the effects of the drug

2. Claustrophobic patients—Will not be able to tolerate the nasal hood or face mask

3. Children with severe behavior problems—Child must cooperate to breathe gas through nose

4. Patients with severe personality disorders—Should be carefully evaluated prior to administering any sedation

5. Upper respiratory tract infection or other acute respiratory conditions—Must be inhaled through nose

6. Chronic obstructive pulmonary disease (emphysema, chronic bronchitis)

7. Pregnancy

D. Indications—Major indication is the management of fear and anxiety

1. Medically compromised patients

a. Respiratory disease

b. Cerebrovascular disease

c. Hepatic disease

d. Epilepsy and seizure disorders

e. Allergy

f. Diabetes

2. Periodontics and dental hygiene

   a. Initial periodontal examination

   b. Scaling, curettage, and root planing

   c. Management of necrotizing ulcerative gingivitis

   d. Use of ultrasonic instrumentation

   e. Periodontal surgery

E. Pharmacology and physiology

1. Nitrous oxide preparation—Nitrous oxide is prepared commercially through the heating of ammonium nitrate crystals to 240° C, at which point the ammonium nitrate decomposes to N_2O and H_2O

2. Physical properties—N_2O is nonirritating, sweet-smelling, colorless gas; it is the only nonorganic compound other than CO_2 that has any CNS depressant properties and is the only inorganic gas used to produce anesthesia in humans

3. Chemical properties—N_2O is stable under pressure at usual temperatures; marketed in cylinders as a liquid under pressure, N_2O returns to the gaseous state as it is released from the cylinder

4. Solubility

   a. N_2O is relatively insoluble in the blood and is carried in the blood in physical solution only, not combining with any blood elements

   b. The oxygen in the N_2O molecule is not available for use by the tissues because N_2O does not break down in the body

   c. On inhalation these gases rapidly diffuse across the alveolar membrane into the blood; because of their poor blood solubility, only a small quantity is absorbed and the alveolar tension rises rapidly so that the tension of the gas in the blood is also increased quickly

   d. Because of the rich cerebral blood supply, the tension of these gases within the brain also rises rapidly and the onset of clinical actions is quickly apparent

   e. The rate of recovery from sedation or anesthesia produced by these gases is equally rapid once delivery of the anesthetic ceases; N_2O is neither flammable nor explosive

5. Potency—N_2O is the lease potent of the anesthetic gases.

6. Pharmacology

   a. After N_2O is inspired through the mouth and/or nose, the gas is transported through the respiratory tract into alveolar sacs, where it is rapidly absorbed into the pulmonary circulation. N_2O replaces N_2 in the blood, the N_2 being eliminated as the N_2O–O_2 mixture is inhaled.

    b. Primary saturation of the blood and brain with N_2O is accomplished by the displacement of N_2 from the alveoli and the blood, and occurs within 3 to 5 minutes of the onset of N_2O–O_2 administration

    c. N_2O diffuses out of the blood and into the alveoli as rapidly as it diffused into the blood during induction

    d. If the patient is allowed to breathe atmospheric air at this time, a phenomenon known as diffusion hypoxia may develop, which is responsible for most reports of headache, nausea, and lethargy after N_2O administration—a hangover effect; the alveoli of the patient breathing atmospheric air become filled with a mixture of N_2, O_2, CO_2, and N_2O; the adverse effects of diffusion hypoxia may be prevented through the routine administration of 100% O_2 for a minimum of 3–5 minutes at the termination of the procedure

    e. N_2O is nonallergenic

7. Central nervous system—The actual mechanism of action of N_2O is unknown, but almost all forms of sensation are depressed (sight, hearing, touch, and pain); memory is affected to a minimal degree, as is the ability to concentrate or perform acts requiring intelligence; N_2O produces a mild depression of the central nervous system, primarily the cerebral cortex

8. Cardiovascular system—A slight depression of myocardial contraction is produced at a ratio of 80% N_2O:20% O_2 through a direct action of the drug on the heart; the response of vascular smooth muscle to norepinephrine is slightly increased at this level; at levels below this ratio there is no clinically significant effect on the cardiovascular system

9. Respiratory system—N_2O is not irritating to the pulmonary epithelium; it may therefore be administered to patients with asthma with no increased risk or bronchospasm

10. Gastrointestinal tract—N_2O has no clinically significant actions on the gastrointestinal tract or any organs; in the presence of hepatic dysfunction, N_2O may still be used to effect with no increased risk of overdosage or adverse reaction

11. Kidneys—N_2O exerts no significant effects on the kidneys or on the volume and composition of urine

12. Hematopoiesis—N_2O inhibits the action of methionine synthetase, an enzyme involved in vitamin B_{12} metabolism, leading to impaired bone marrow function, producing a picture similar to pernicous anemia in laboratory animals exposed to N_2O for prolonged periods of time; the effects of repeated short-term exposure to N_2O are of greater concern; the vitamin B_{12} deficiency has been reported in dentists using nitrous oxide regularly in their practices and in persons abusing the drug

13. Skeletal muscle—N_2O does not produce relaxation of skeletal muscles

14. Physiological contraindications—There are no contraindications to the use of N_2O in combination with an adequate percentage of O_2; if administered with a minimum of 25% oxygen, it is a safe agent

F. Armamentarium

1. Types of inhalation sedation units

a. Demand-flow units—Do not deliver gas continuously to the patient but instead varies the rate and volume of delivered gas according to the patient's respiratory demands; not commonly used in dentistry

b. Continuous-flow units—Contain flowmeters and are characterized by the continuous flow of gases regardless of the respiratory pattern of the patient; gas continues to be delivered through the machine even as the patient exhales; provides significantly greater accuracy and safety

c. Portable system—Compressed gas cylinders are attached to the inhalation sedation unit at the yoke assembly; this system is used in offices where the frequency of N_2O–O_2 use is low or in situations that the expense of a central storage system is prohibited

d. Central storage system—The supply of N_2O and O_2 is located at a distance from the area in which the gases are delivered to patients; in the treatment area the inhalation sedation unit will be present along with the accessory equipment required for the delivery of the gases; the head is usually mounted on a wall or bracket; gas cylinders are maintained in a storage area and delivered to the treatment area through copper pipes

2. Parts of the units

a. Compressed-gas cylinders—All compressed-gas cylinders are tested by the U.S. Department of Transportation every 5 years to ensure their integrity; the agents used in inhalation sedation, N_2O and O_2, are color-coded light blue and green, respectively; the following are important considerations when handling compressed gas cylinders

(1) Use no grease, oil, or lubricant of any type to lubricate cylinder valves, gauges, regulators, or other fittings that may come into contact with gases; this is extremely dangerous; once the grease or oil ignites, either N_2O or O_2, although nonflammable, will support combustion

(2) Store full cylinders in the vertical position

(3) Store cylinders in an area in which the temperature does not fluctuate; heat in particular should be avoided

(4) Handle cylinders with care; especially avoid dropping them

(5) Open cylinder valves slowly in a counterclockwise direction

(6) Close all cylinder valves tightly when not in use

(7) Cylinders should be "cracked" before attaching them to the sedation machine; the term "cracked" signifies opening the cylinder just

slightly, allowing some gas to escape, thereby blowing out any particles of dust that may have lodged in the orifice of the cylinder

b. Oxygen cylinder—O_2 in a compressed-gas cylinder is present in a gaseous state; because the O_2 cylinder contains only gas, the pressure gauge on the machine yoke reflects the actual contents of the cylinder; as oxygen leaves the cylinder, the pressure within the cylinder will drop accordingly; this is an important factor in the safety of inhalation sedation because if an O_2 cylinder became empty during a procedure while the N_2O cylinder still contained gas, it would be potentially possible to administer 100% N_2O

c. Nitrous oxide cylinder—N_2O cylinders are factory-filled to 90–95% capacity with liquid N_2O; above the liquid in the tank is N_2O vapor; because of the presence of liquid in the N_2O cylinder, the gas pressure gauge on the cylinder will record "full" as long as any liquid remains in the cylinder; once all of the liquid N_2O is gone and only gaseous N_2O remains, the pressure gauge will fall in relation to the pressure of gas now remaining (acting now like the O_2 pressure gauge)

d. Regulators—Also called reducing valves, are located between the compressed-gas cylinder and the flowmeter; the regulator functions to reduce the high-pressure gas coming from the cylinder to a pressure that is safe for the patient; the actual delivery pressure is set by the manufacturer

e. Manifolds (central system only)—Serves to join multiple compressed-gas cylinders together

f. Yokes (portable system only)—Holds the cylinder of compressed gas tightly in contact with the nipples of the portable sedation unit

g. Flowmeters—From the reducing valves the individual gases are carried through low-pressure tubing into the back of the unit; the gases are then directed to the flowmeters, which permit the administrator to deliver a precise volume of either gas to the patient

h. Emergency air intake valve—On the bag tee, above the reservoir bag, an emergency air valve is located; it provides the patient a supply of atmospheric air in the event that the sedation unit ceases to function and gas flow from the machine is terminated; during normal use the emergency air valve remains shut, but it opens automatically once gas flow through the machine is terminated

i. Rubber goods

(1) Reservoir bag—Attaches to the base of the bag tee; a portion of the gas being delivered through the unit to the patient is diverted into the reservoir bag, where it may be used during inhalation sedation to provide a reservoir from which additional gas may be drawn

should the respiratory demands of the patient exceed the gas flow being delivered; it can also be used to monitor respiration; assuming an airtight seal of the nasal hood and no mouth breathing, the reservoir bag will inflate slightly with every exhalation and deflate slightly with each inspiration, allowing the operator to determine respiratory rate

(a) Connecting tubes

(b) Breathing apparatus

    i) Nasal hood—Has one or two tubes entering into it, delivering gases from the inhalation unit; exhaled gases are eliminated into the surrounding environment through an exhaling valve located on top of the nasal hood

    ii) Scavenging nasal hood—Two tubes deliver fresh gases from the sedation unit, the other tubes carrying exhaled gases away from the treatment area to a safe repository; this is preferred to protect dental staff

3. Safety features

  a. Pin index safety system—The pin index safety system makes it physically impossible to attach an N_2O compressed-gas cylinder to the yoke attachment for O_2, which could result in the inadvertent administration of 100% N_2O instead of 100% O_2

  b. Minimum oxygen liter flow—Inhalation sedation units are designed so that once turned on the unit delivers a preset minimum liter flow of O_2 through the flowmeter; the flow of N_2O cannot start until a flow of O_2 has been established

  c. Oxygen fail-safe—In either the portable or central systems the cylinder of O_2 will become depleted before the cylinder of N_2O; the O_2 fail-safe system is designed to prevent this from happening by automatically terminating the flow of N_2O whenever the delivery pressure of O_2 falls below a predetermined level

  d. Emergency air inlet

  e. Oxygen flush button—Permits the rapid delivery of high flows of 100% O_2 to the patient; the button is located on the front of the sedation unit in easy view

G. Inhalation sedation: Techniques of administration

  1. Preparation of the equipment—The cylinders are opened by turning the knob on the top of the cylinder in a counterclockwise direction; start turning the knob only slightly, just barely opening the cylinder, permitting the pressure gauge to rise slowly; once the pressure reaches its maximal level, the knob may be turned freely until fully open

  2. Review medical history, and record preoperative vital signs

3. Patients with contacts should remove them to avoid any irritation that might occur from gas leaks around mask

4. Position patient in a comfortable position

5. Start the flow of O_2 at 6L/min, and place the nasal hood over the patient's nose; remind the patient to breathe through the nose

6. Secure nasal hood

7. Determine proper flow rate for the patient

8. Observe the reservoir bag

9. Begin titration of N_2O

10. Observe the patient

11. Continue titration of N_2O

12. Observe the patient

13. Begin dental treatment

14. Observe the patient and inhalation sedation unit during the procedure

15. Terminate the flow of N_2O and administer O_2 3–4 minutes

16. Discharge the patient

17. Record data concerning the sedation procedure

18. Cleansing of the equipment

H. Signs and symptoms of oversedation

1. Persistent closing of mouth

2. Spontaneous mouth breathing

3. Complaints of nausea and effects of sedation felt as too intense or uncomfortable

4. Failure to respond rationally or sluggish responses

5. Sleepiness

6. Incoherent speech or dreaminess

7. Becomes uncooperative

8. Uncoordinated movements

I. Inhalation sedation complications

1. Excessive perspiration

2. Expectoration

3. Behavioral problems

4. Shivering

5. Nausea and vomiting

J. Current concerns

    1. Chronic exposure to trace anesthetics

        a. Nitrous oxide in dental offices—In the absence of measures for controlling N_2O concentrations, measurable levels of N_2O are found throughout the dental suite in which N_2O–O_2 inhalation sedation is used without scavenging

        b. Methods to minimize

            (1) Testing equipment for leaks

            (2) Venting of waste gases

            (3) Scavenging nasal hoods

            (4) Air-sweep

            (5) Minimizing talking by patient

            (6) Monitoring of air

    2. Recreational abuse of nitrous oxide—The use of N_2O for nonmedical purposes by health professionals

    3. Sexual phenomena and nitrous oxide—In recent years an increasing number of situations have been reported in which a male doctor has been accused of sexual assault by a female patient who received conscious sedation of N_2O during her treatment

➤ RECOGNITION AND MANAGEMENT OF COMPROMISED PATIENTS

I. Patient with diabetes mellitus—Group of metabolic disorders resulting in hyperglycemia (abnormal increase in blood glucose)

  A. Types of diabetes

    1. Type I diabetes

        a. Insulin-dependent diabetes mellitus

        b. Commonly in young children, but may occur at any age

        c. Hereditary, but not as common as Type II

        d. Symptoms—Polyuria, polyphagia, thirst, mimic flu

    2. Type II diabetes

        a. Non insulin-dependent diabetes mellitus

        b. Occurs in adults usually after 40 years of age, but may occur younger

        c. Risk factors—Obesity and poor nutrition

        d. Symptoms—Can have same symptoms as Type I, delayed healing, fatigue

  B. Effects of diabetes related to dental care

    1. Impaired healing

    2. Increases susceptibility to infections

3. Inflammation may increase patient's insulin requirements

4. Insulin reactions

5. Long-term problems—Nephropathy, vascular disease, blindness

C. Dental hygiene treatment considerations

    1. Appointment time should be in morning or alternate, after lunch

    2. Well-controlled patient—No alterations in treatment

    3. Uncontrolled diabetes—Postpone treatment until diabetes is controlled

    4. Be aware of systemic complications related to diabetes and treat appropriately (hypertension, congestive heart failure, angina, renal failure)

D. Oral complications

    1. Accelerated periodontal disease

    2. Xerostomia

    3. Delayed healing

    4. Increased susceptibility to infection

    5. Candidiasis

II. Patients with Cardiovascular Disease

A. Infective endocarditis—Disease caused by microbial infection of the heart valves; infection must be promply controlled or patient may develop heart failure leading to death

    1. Dental management

        a. Complete medical history with specific questions regarding history of congenital heart defects, prosthetic valves, or past occurrences of infective endocarditis

        b. Pretreatment antibiotics

B. Ischemic heart disease—Results from oxygen deprivation to the myocardium as a result of coronary atherosclerosis

    1. Manifestations of ischemic heart disease—Angina pectoris

    2. Dental management

        a. Stress reduction

        b. Myocardial infarction may occur during dental procedure

        c. Premedication with valium 5–10 mg

        d. Terminate procedure if patient becomes fatigued

        e. Nitroglycerin tablet, should angina occur

C. Congestive heart failure—Complex symptoms that can occur from many different specific disease processes; heart failure develops when the heart can no longer function as a pump and causes a collection of fluids in various organs

    1. Dental management

        a. No dental care until patient is under good medical management

b. Upright position during treatment

c. Bleeding and prothrombin times prior to surgery

d. Terminate procedure if patient becomes fatigued

e. If patient is taking digitalis, may be more prone to nausea

f. Anticoagulants should be reduced (takes 3–4 days)

g. Antihypertensive agents—Reduce vasoconstrictor to .04 mg when administering local anesthetics

D. Myocardial infarction—Most serious manifestation of ischemic heart disease; "heart attack"; left coronary artery is most often affected

1. Dental management

a. No routine dental care until at least 6 months following infarction

b. Morning appointments

c. Bleeding tendency if patient is on anticoagulants

d. Terminate procedure if patient becomes fatigued

E. Congenital heart disease—Anomalies of the structure of the heart following irregularities in development during the first 9 weeks in utero

1. Ventricular septal defects

a. Left to right shunt

b. Oxygenated blood from the lung is normally pumped by the left ventricle to the aorta, passes through defect back to right ventricle

c. Small defects—Heart murmur

d. Large defects—Heart enlarges to compensate for overload

e. 80% are located in the membranous septum just below the aortic valve

2. Patent ductus arteriosus

a. Left to right shunt

b. Ductus that connects the pulmonary artery to the aorta usually closes within a few hours of birth; if it does not, there is flow from the aorta into the pulmonary artery, causing blood from the aorta to pass back into the lungs

c. Heart compensates to provide the body with oxygenated blood and becomes overburdened

d. Surgery is recommended before 2 years of age

3. Tetrology of Fallot

a. Right to left shunt

b. Lesion consists of ventricular septal defect, and pulmonary stenosis that causes reduced venous return from the lungs

c. "Blue baby"

4. Pulmonary stenosis—Malformation that obstructs blood flow that leads to right ventricular dilation and hypertrophy

5. Coarctation of the aorta—Localized constriction at or distal to the left subclavian artery from the aorta, resulting in narrowed pulse pressure distal to the obstruction; "absent or weak pulses in lower limbs"

F. Patients with bleeding disorders

   1. Classification of bleeding disorders

   a. Nonthrombocytopenic purpuras

      (1) Infections, chemicals, or certain allergies may alter the structure and function of vascular wall, resulting in bleeding problem

      (2) Platelets may be defective and unable to perform their proper functions, caused by genetic defects, drugs (aspirin, NSAIDs, penicillin, cephalosporins)

      (3) Normal numbers of platelets

   b. Thrombocytopenic purpuras

      (1) Caused by radiation, various systemic diseases (leukemia) and have a direct effect on bone marrow

      (2) Total platelet count is reduced

   c. Disorders of coagulation

      (1) Inherited—Hemophilia

         (a) Acquired—Liver disease (liver produces all the coagulation factors)

         (b) Acquired—Vitamin deficiency; if vitamin K is not produced, will result in decreased plasma level of prothrombin

         (c) Anticoagulation drugs—Heparin, Coumadin

   2. Phases of bleeding control

   a. Vascular phase—Immediately following injury → vasoconstriction

   b. Platelet phase—Platelets become sticky and produce plugs to seal off openings

   c. Coagulation phase—Initiated by two separate mechanisms; extrinsic (outside blood vessel) and intrinsic (within blood vessel)

   3. Dental management

   a. Screen patient for bleeding times

   b. Oral complications—Spontaneous bleeding, prolonged bleeding, petechiae, hematomas

   c. Avoid PSA and IA injections

   4. Laboratory tests

   a. Prothrombin time—Normal = 11–15 seconds

   b. Activated partial thromboplastin time—Normal = 25–35 seconds

      c. Thrombin time—Normal = 9–13 seconds

      d. Bleeding time—Normal = 1–6 minutes

      e. Platelet count—Normal = 140,000–400,000/mm$_3$

G. Patients with liver disease

    1. Stages of alcoholic liver disease

      a. Fatty infiltrate

        (1) Enlargement of the liver

        (2) Completely reversible

      b. Alcoholic hepatitis

        (1) Diffuse inflammatory condition of the liver

        (2) Characterized by destructive cellular changes, some of which may be irreversible, which lead to necrosis

      c. Cirrhosis

        (1) Most serious

        (2) Irreversible condition characterized by abnormal regeneration

        (3) Progressive deterioration of the metabolic and excretory functions of the liver

    2. Dental management of liver disease

      a. Bleeding tendencies

      b. Inability to metabolize and detoxify certain drugs

      c. Limit dose of amide local anesthetic except for Prilocaine

    3. Common dental drugs metabolized by the liver

      a. Local anesthetics

        (1) Amides, except for Prilocaine

      b. Analgesics

        (1) Aspirin

        (2) Tylenol

        (3) Codeine

        (4) Demerol

      c. Sedatives

        (1) Valium

        (2) Barbiturates

      d. Antibiotics

        (1) Ampicillin

        (2) Tetracycline

    4. Hepatitis—See Infection Control section

H. Patients with neurological disorders

    1. Epilepsy

        a. Partial (focal, local)

           (1) Simple partial seizure—Without loss of consciousness

           (2) Complex partial seizure—Simple partial seizure with loss of consciousness

           (3) Partial seizures evolving to general tonic–clonic convulsions

        b. Generalized

           (1) Convulsive seizures—Absence seizures, atypical absence seizures, myclonic seizures, atonic seizures

           (2) Nonconvulsive seizures—Tonic–clonic seizures, tonic seizures, clonic seizures

        c. Signs and symptoms of seizure

           (1) Sudden cry

           (2) Muscle rigidity, uncoordinated beating movements of the limbs

        d. Oral complications

           (1) Phenytoin-induced gingival hyperplasia

           (2) Fractured teeth following grand-mal seizure

           (3) Injury to lips and tongue due to biting during seizure

        e. Dental management

           (1) Prevent occurrence of generalized tonic–clonic seizure by decreasing psychotic stress and apprehension, fatigue, flashing lights, and noises

           (2) Maintain optimal oral hygiene because plaque and gingivitis are complicating factors to phenytoin-induced gingival overgrowth

           (3) Surgical reduction of gingival hyperplasia, if indicated

        f. Anticonvulsant medications

           (1) Phenytoin dilantin

           (2) Carbemazepine (Tegretol)—Drug interaction with propoxphene and erythromycin

           (3) Phenobarbital (Luminal)

           (4) Valproic acid—Drug interaction with aspirin and NSAIDs

    2. Stroke—Result of focal necrosis of brain caused by chronic cerebrovascular disease

        a. Predisposing factors

           (1) Atherosclerosis

           (2) Hypertension

(3) Smoking

(4) Cardiovascular disease

(5) Diabetes mellitus

b. Signs and symptoms

(1) Transient ischemic attack (TIA)—Small strokes that last only a few minutes with no damage as a result of the attack

(2) Sudden and temporary weakness or numbness on one side of the body

(3) Temporary loss of speech

(4) Temporary loss of vision, usually in one eye

(5) Dizziness, unsteadiness, sudden falls

c. Dental management

(1) Short appointment

(2) Bleeding tendencies due to anticoagulant medications

I. Patients with adrenal insufficiency—Hypofunction of the adrenal cortex

1. Adrenal cortex—Produces three adrenal steroids

a. Glucocorticoids

(1) Cortisol—Responsible for regulation of carbohydrates, fat and protein metabolism, vascular reactivity, inhibition of inflammation, maintenance of homeostatis during physical and emotional stress

(2) Responses to stress → hypothalamus releases corticotropin-releasing hormone (CRH) → stimulates pituitary production and secretion of adrenocorticotropic hormone (ACTH) → stimulates adrenal cortex to produce and secrete cortisol

b. Mineralocorticoids

(1) Aldosterone secreted by adrenal cortex to balance extracellular and intercellular sodium and potassium

c. Androgens

(1) Dehydroepiandrosterone secreted by adrenal cortex; effects are the same as testicular androgens but of relatively low importance

2. Primary adrenocortical insufficiency

a. Addison's disease—Progressive destruction of adrenal cortex

3. Secondary adrenocortical insufficiency

a. Most common, resulting from administration of exogenous corticosteroids and inhibits ACTH production, resulting in partial adrenal insufficiency

b. Dependent on dose and duration of administration

4. Dental treatment concerns

a. Inability to tolerate stress

b. Delayed healing

c. Susceptibility to infection

d. Hypertension

5. Dental management

a. Rule of twos

(1) Adrenal suppression should be suspected if a patient has received a glucocorticosteroid therapy:

(a) In a dose of 20 mg or more of cortisone or its equivalent daily

(b) For a continuous period of 2 weeks or longer

(c) Within 2 years of dental therapy

b. Administer exogenous glucocorticosteroids before, during, and possibly after the stressful situation, dependent upon physician evaluation.

J. Patients with thyroid disease

1. Hypothyroidism—Disease caused by insufficient production of thyroid hormone by the thyroid gland; thyroid failure usually caused by disease of the thyroid gland

a. Primary causes of hypothroidism

(1) Autoimmune hypothyroidism

(2) External radiation therapy

(3) Iodine deficiency

(4) Antithyroid drugs

(5) Idiopathic

b. Secondary causes

(1) Pituitary tumor

(2) Infiltrative disease (sarcoid) of pituitary

c. Dental management

(1) Hypothyroid coma may develop if exposed to stressful situations

(2) Untreated patients may be sensitive to narcotics, barbiturates, and tranquilizers

d. Oral complications

(1) Increased tongue size

(2) Delayed eruption of teeth and malocclusion

2. Hyperthyroidism—The result of excess thyroid hormone production, causing an overactive metabolism and increased speed of all the body's processes; also called thyrotoxicosis and may progress into thyroid storm

a. Causes

(1) Graves' disease—Toxic diffuse goiter

(2) Toxic multinodular goiter

(3) Toxic uninodular goiter

b. Dental management

(1) Thyroid storm in untreated patients may be caused by infection, trauma, stress

(2) Untreated patients are sensitive to epinephrine and other pressor amines and are an absolute contraindication

(3) Hypertension risks in untreated patient

(4) Emergency protocol: call EMS; hydrocortisone (100–300 mg), CPR if needed

c. Oral complications

(1) Progressive periodontal disease

(2) Extensive dental caries

(3) Tumors on posterior tongue

K. Patient with cancer

1. Prevention program prior to cancer therapy

a. Plaque control

b. Daily fluoride therapy

c. Dietary instructions

d. Eliminate gross infection

e. Treat carious lesions

2. Effects of radiation on oral cavity

a. Mucositis

b. Candidiasis

c. Xerostomia

d. Loss of taste

e. Trismus

f. Cervical caries

g. Sensitivity to teeth

3. Oral management

a. Brushing with very soft toothbrush

b. Baking soda/saline rinses

c. Chlorhexidine rinses to reduce inflammation

d. Topical anesthetic rinses or ointments prior to eating for pain

e. Xerostomia management

f. Management of radiation caries that are predisposed from xerostomia (intensify prevention procedures with daily fluoride therapy)

g. Management of fungal infections—Candidiasis is most common (treat with antifungal agent that does not contain sugar)

L. Chemotherapy

    1. Oral effects of chemotherapy

        a. Mucositis

        b. Excessive bleeding and spontaneous gingival bleeding

        c. Xerostomia

        d. Infection

        e. Poor healing

    2. Dental management

        a. Determine need for antibiotic coverage if granulocyte count is less than $2,000/mm^3$

        b. Control spontaneous bleeding with gauze, periodontal dressing

        c. Topical fluoride for caries prevention

        d. Xerostomia management

    3. Xerostomia management

        a. Pilocarpine therapy, 5–10 mg

        b. Saliva substitutes

        c. Water and ice chips

        d. Moist food and sugarless gum

        e. Humidifier

M. Patients with HIV/AIDS

    1. HIV—Patient with HIV has a CD4+ cell count of less than $200/mm^3$ or with CD4 percentage less than 14% of total CD4+ cell count regardless of opportunistic diseases

        a. Viral disease

            (1) Virus infects host cell → replicates self → destroys cell functioning → results in cell death

            (2) New viruses released into body → process repeated → CD4+ cells destroyed → immune system malfunctions → death occurs

        b. Blood assays

            (1) Evaluate various cells in the blood

            (2) Lymphocyte subset detects degree to which CD4+ T lymphocytes are destroyed and identifies vulnerability of person developing AIDS; must examine CD4+ cell counts over time to determine immune system dysfunction

    2. CD4+ cell counts and medical concerns

        a. Healthy—CD4+ counts between $500/mm^3$ and $1,500/mm^3$ with average around $1,000/mm^3$

     b. Opportunistic infections like herpes simplex, herpes zoster, and candidiasis—CD4+ cell counts between 500/mm^3 and 800/mm^3

     c. Significant immunodeficiency like toxoplasmosis, PCP, and cryptococcal meningitis—CD4+ cell counts less than 200/mm^3

     d. CD4+ cell counts less than 100/mm^3 at risk of developing lymphoma, cytomegalovirus, and mycobacterium avium complex

     e. Examining CD4+ cell counts only is not an accurate method for determining disease progression; must consider CD4+ cell counts and viral loads over a period of time

  3. Viral loads and medical interventions

     a. Viral loads measure amount of HIV/RNA found in the blood and are good predictors of virus activity/disease progression

     b. Viral load—5,000 copies/mL or less; low level of viral replication; no medical intervention needed unless CD4+ count is less than 350

     c. Viral load—10,000–50,000 copies/mL; significant replication; start medical intervention regardless of CD4+ count

     d. Viral load—Over 100,000 copies/mL; rapid deterioration; therapy needs to be initiated or changed immediately

  4. CD4+ cell counts and viral load

     a. Synergistic relationship between CD4+ cell counts and viral load

     b. High viral load correlates with low CD4+ cell counts and vice versa

N. Common HIV+/AIDS—Related illnesses

  1. Mycobacterium avium complex (MAC)—Bacterial infection caused by organisms found in food, water, or dust; this infection can be life-threatening in persons with AIDS

     a. Symptoms—Fever, night sweats, abdominal pain

     b. Treatment—Clarithromycin or azithromycin and ethambuto

  2. Candidiasis—Fungal infection commonly identified in the oral cavity but can spread to esophagus and sometimes stomach

     a. Symptoms—Scrapable white or red patches on tongue, palate, gingiva; difficulty swallowing and loss of appetite

     b. Treatment—Fluconazole, nystatin, clotrimazole

  3. *Pneumocystis carinii* pneumonia (PCP)—Pneumonia commonly found in persons with AIDS; caused by a protozoal infection

     a. Symptoms—Fever, dry cough, weight loss, difficulty breathing

     b. Treatment—Systemic Bactrim, Septra, Dapsone, or Clindamycin

4. Cytomegalovirus (CMV)—Viral infection that can spread to various parts of the body (i.e., eyes, stomach, lungs) CMV is a member of the herpes viruses and only becomes active once the immune system is weakened

    a. Symptoms—In the eyes—blurry vision; in the esophagus—pain, ulcers, difficulty swallowing; in the lungs—pneumonia

    b. IV or intraocular implants of ganciclovir or foscarnet; some other experimental drugs are also used

5. Kaposi's sarcoma—A fatal, metastasizing, malignant vascular cancer found in 90% of all patients with AIDS (Figure 9-40■)

    a. Symptoms—Purplish lesions found all over the body and often orally

    b. Treatment—Vinblastine, chemotherapy, conventional surgery, laser surgery, or radiation

6. Neuropathy—Pathological changes in the peripheral nervous system; nerve damage that occurs and is possibly a side effect of drugs or HIV infection

    a. Symptoms—Tingling "pins and needles" feeling in the extremities

    b. Treatment—Currently only experimental medications and magnetic treatments are available

7. Oral manifestations associated with HIV+/AIDS

    a. Kaposi's sarcoma—Aggressive vascular, fatal tumor—treatment of chemotherapy, laser surgery, radiation, intralesional injection of vinblastine sulfate

    b. Hairy leudoplakia—Indicates HIV+ and immunosuppression, nonremovable white plaque; location—lateral border of tongue and dorsal surface of tongue; treatment—acyclivor, topical application of Podophyllum 25% (tincture of Benzoin)

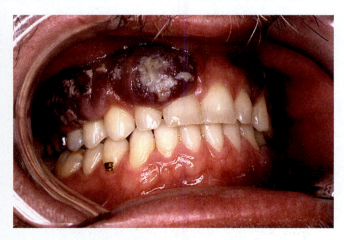

FIGURE 9-40 ■ Kaposi's Sarcoma

Source: Sol Silverman, Jr., DDS/Centers for Disease Control and Prevention

c. Candidiasis—Various types include pseudomembranous (white scrapable plaques), atrophic (fiery red), hyperplastic (nonscrapable white plaques), and angular cheilitis (white plaques on top of fissures and cracks at commisure regions); treatment—fluconazole, nystatin, and clotrimazole (Figure 9-41■)

d. Linear gingival erythema—Confined to soft tissues, generalized, distinctly erythematous; treatment—scale and root plane, oral hygiene instructions, chlorhexidine mouth rinse/irrigation, and 2–3 weeks reevaluation (Figure 9-42■)

e. Necrotizing ulcerative gingivitis—Chronic or acute, punched-out papilla, very painful; treat with debridement, interoffice chlorhexidine irrigation, scale and root plane as able, consider systemic antibiotics and antifungal medication, retreat as needed, and 4–6 week reevaluation

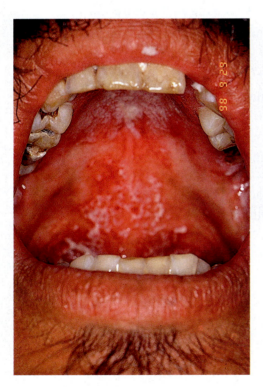

FIGURE 9-41 ■ Candidiasis

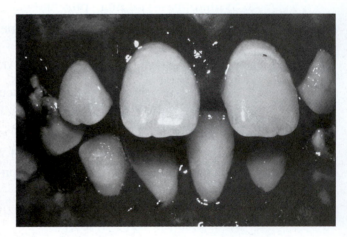

FIGURE 9-42 ■ Linear Gingival Erythema

      f. Necrotizing ulcerative periodontitis—Severe soft tissue destruction, rapid periodontal attachment destruction and bone loss, found in localized areas; treatment—aggressive dental hygiene therapy, chlorhexidine, metronidazole, or amoxicillin to destroy oral bacteria (Figure 9-43■)

O. Side effects of commonly prescribed antiretrovial medications

  1. Nucleoside analogue reverse transcriptase inhibitors

      a. Vides (ddl)—Xerostomia, candidiasis, peripheral neuropathy

      b. Zerit (d4T)—Peripheral neuropathy, neutropenia, and thrombocytopenia

      c. Combivir (AZT and 3TC)—GI upset and peripheral neuropathy

      d. Epivir (3TC)—GI upset and peripheral neuropathy

      e. HIVID (ddC)—Hypertension, renal failure, GI upset, and peripheral neuropathy

      f. Retonivir (AZT, ZDV)—Granulocytopenia, anemia, and GI upset

      g. Ziagen (Abcavir Sulfate)—Renal failure and GI upset

  2. Protease inhibitors

      a. Agenerase (Amprenavir)—Anemia, parasthesia, GI upset, diabetes mellitus, and several drug interactions, specifically with Abacavir

      b. Crixivan (Indinavir sulfate)—Anemia, GI upset, diabetes mellitus, renal insufficiency; patients should avoid nonsteroidal anti-inflammatory drugs

      c. Fortovase (Saquinavir)—Cardiovascular problems, thrombocytopenia, pancytopenia, anemia, GI upset, peripheral neuropathy, diabetes mellitus, and several drug interactions, specifically with clindamycin

      d. Invirase (Saquinavir Mesylate)—Thrombocytopenia, pancytopenia, and GI upset

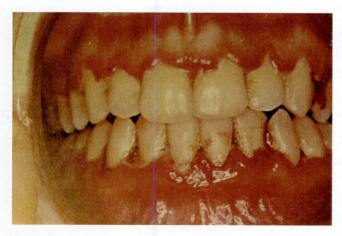

FIGURE 9-43 ■ Necrotizing Ulcerative Periodontitis

e. Norvir (Ritonavir)—Cardiovascular problems, thrombocytopenia, leukopenia, peripheral neuropathy, increased bleeding problems, and parasthesias

f. Viracept (Nelfinavir Mesylate)—Anemia, GI upset, peripheral neuropathy, neutropenia, leukopenia, and increased bleeding

3. Non-nucleoside reverse transcriptase inhibitors

a. Rescriptor (Delvirdine mesylate)—Anemia, GI upset, thrombocytopenia, neutropenia, skin rashes, drug interactions with Amprenavir, Fluconazole, and Indinavir

b. Sustiva (Efavinez)—Cardiovascular problems, GI upset, skin rashes, drug interactions with Amprenavir, Azithromycin, Fluconazole, Indinavir, Nelfinavir, Ritonavir, Saquinavir, and Zidovudine

c. Viramune (Nevirapine)—Decreased hemoglobin, platelets, neutrophils, life-threatening hepatotoxicity, toxic epidermal necrolysis, fever, drug interactions with Amprenavir, Erythromycin, Indinavir, Nelfinavir, Ritonavir, Saquinavir, and Zidovudine

P. Reviewing a patient's CBC results

1. Important blood components

a. Platelets

(1) These cells initiate blood clotting

(2) Low reading indicates increased risk of bleeding

(3) A count of less than 50,000/mcl requires information on partial thromboplastin time (PTT) and prothrombin time (PT)

b. Hemoglobin (Hb or Hgb)

(1) These are red blood cells carrying oxygen

(2) Low reading indicates anemia

c. Hematocrit (HCT)

(1) Another way of measuring hemoglobin in blood

(2) Low reading indicates anemia

d. Red blood cell (RBC) count

(1) Another way of measuring hemoglobin in blood

(2) Low reading indicates anemia

e. White blood cell (WBC) count

(1) These cells fight off infection

(2) High reading indicates infection

f. Absolute neutrophils (AB NTS)

(1) White blood cells

(2) Increased neutrophil reading indicates bacterial infections, hemorrhagia, inflammation, and leukemia

(3) Low neutrophils reading indicate viral infection, TB, and typhoid; medications like Carbimazole and Sulphonamides can cause lower than normal readings in neutrophils

(4) If this reading is below 500, the patient will need to be premedicated with antibiotics

g. Absolute lymphocytes

(1) These cells fight off infection and destroy microorganisms

(2) Increased lymphocyte reading indicates viral infections

(3) Low lymphocyte reading seen in AIDS, steroid therapy, post-chemotherapy, or radiotherapy

h. Absolute eosinophils—Another type of white blood cells; increased reading indicates asthma, parasitic infections, allergic disorders, restrictive cardiomyopathy, and neuropathy

i. Absolute monocytes—Part of white blood cells; increased reading indicates acute and chronic infections like TB and protozoa

j. Absolute basophils—Part of white blood cells; increased reading indicates viral infections

k. CD4+ T lymphocytes and viral load—Should also be examined and included as part of the CBC results; most effective way to determine health of person with HIV/AIDS is to examine a trend in CD4+ cell counts and viral loads over time

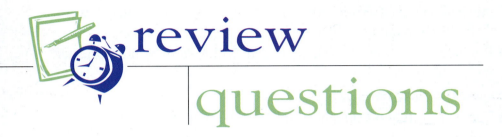

review questions

DIRECTIONS Each of the questions or incomplete statements below is followed by suggested answers or completions. Select the **one** answer that is best in each case.

1. In acute adrenal insufficiency, which of the following hormones is suddenly lacking?
   A. Glucocorticosteroid
   B. Epinephrine
   C. Insulin
   D. Thyroxin

2. Which of the following conditions would contraindicate placing a patient in the supine position during the management of an acute medical emergency?
   A. Unconscious respiratory distress
   B. Second trimester of pregnancy
   C. Syncope
   D. Cerebrovascular accident in a patient with normal blood pressure

3. A 70-year-old man with a history of hypertension and congestive heart failure suddenly experiences tachypnea, extreme dyspnea with cyanosis, and frothy pink sputum. Which of the following conditions is being experienced?
   A. Hyperventilation
   B. Acute asthmatic episode
   C. Cerebrovascular accident
   D. Acute pulmonary edema

4. Which of the following is the MOST acute diabetic problem encountered in the dental office?
   A. Hypoglycemia
   B. Ketoacidosis
   C. Hyperglycemia
   D. Hypoinsulinism
   E. Infection

5. Which of the following would be the MOST appropriate treatment for a hyperventilating patient?
   A. Administer epinephrine
   B. Have patient breathe into a paper bag
   C. Place patient in a supine position
   D. Administer oxygen

6. Bloodless phlebotomy may relieve the symptoms of respiratory distress associated with acute pulmonary edema. Tourniquets are applied to extremities using enough pressure to keep blood from entering the extremity. One tourniquet is released then reapplied and another is released. This rotation is continued. All of the following are true of bloodless phlebotomy EXCEPT one. Which one is the EXCEPTION?
   A. The tourniquet is released on the extremity 10 minutes at a time.
   B. Rotations of release and reapplication of tourniquets are continued until the patient reaches a medical facility for more definitive treatment.
   C. A synonym for bloodless phlebotomy is phlebostasia.

7. The initial treatment for syncope is to
   A. Administer spirits of ammonia
   B. Administer epinephrine
   C. Administer oxygen
   D. Place patient in a supine position with legs elevated

8. A known diabetic patient states she is not feeling well. She is feeling cool, looks pale, and is beginning to slur her speech. Immediate treatment should include administration of
   A. Insulin
   B. Oxygen
   C. Epinephrine
   D. Orange juice or a sugared beverage

9. All of the following patients have an increased chance of orthostatic hypotension EXCEPT one. Which one is the EXCEPTION?
   A. Those with varicose veins
   B. Elderly
   C. Woman in third trimester of pregnancy
   D. Children

10. Angina pectoris is due to
    A. Anxiety
    B. Ischemia
    C. Hyperoxia
    D. Hypercalcemia

11. Emergency treatment of hyperventilation includes all of the following EXCEPT one. Which one is the EXCEPTION?
    A. Have patient breathe into cupped hands
    B. Stop treatment
    C. Position client upright
    D. Administer oxygen

12. In the management of the conscious CVA patient, all of the following procedures apply EXCEPT one. Which one is the EXCEPTION?
    A. Administer oxygen
    B. Call EMS
    C. Place client in supine position
    D. Monitor vital signs

13. Dyspnea refers to
    A. The inability to breathe, except in an upright position
    B. Increased rate of breathing
    C. Difficulty in breathing
    D. No respiratory movement

14. The MOST common breathing change observed in the dental office is
    A. Airway obstruction
    B. Hyperventilation
    C. Hypoventilation
    D. Asthma

15. All of the following are symptoms of asthma EXCEPT one. Which one is the EXCEPTION?
    A. Hyperventilation
    B. Dyspnea
    C. Wheezing
    D. Cyanosis

16. Tachycardia is characterized by an increase in
    A. Pulse rate
    B. Respiration rate
    C. Body temperature
    D. Blood pressure

17. The clinical manifestations of respiratory distress include all of the following EXCEPT one. Which one is the EXCEPTION?
    A. Increased heart rate
    B. Hypoventilation
    C. Abnormal breathing noises
    D. Coughing

18. Which of the following does NOT pertain to managing the patient experiencing a grand mal seizure?
    A. Protect the patient from injury
    B. Call 911
    C. Patient is confused and has a headache during the postictal stage
    D. Move patient to the floor for safety reasons

19. Predisposing factors of hyperventilation occur in all of the following patients EXCEPT one. Which one is the EXCEPTION?
    A. Children
    B. Those with acute anxiety
    C. Those experiencing pain
    D. Those 15–40 years old

20. Which of the following is a predisposing factor of acute myocardial infarction?
    A. Males 70–80 years of age
    B. Females 60–70 years of age
    C. Obesity
    D. Diet high in vitamin C

21. Dental therapy considerations for a patient with a history of angina would include all of the following EXCEPT one. Which one is the EXCEPTION?
    A. Cease treatment if patient is sweating
    B. Give oxygen during treatment
    C. Use nitrous oxide during treatment
    D. Keep patient in supine position if attack is underway

22. Destruction of the alveolar wall and loss of elastic recoil of the lungs are a result of which of the following disease processes?
    A. Emphysema
    B. Asthma
    C. Acute pulmonary edema
    D. Airway obstruction

23. The most common medical emergency in the dental office is
    A. Diabetic coma
    B. Syncope
    C. Myocardial infarction
    D. Drug overdose reaction

24. Exophthalmos, tachycardia, and nervousness are all signs of which of the following conditions?
    A. Hypertension
    B. Hypotension
    C. Hyperthyroidism
    D. Hypothyroidism

25. Which of the following conditions is NOT stress-induced?
    A. Angina pectoris
    B. Epilepsy
    C. Orthostatic hypotension
    D. Syncope

26. The most widely used local anesthetics are
    A. Amides
    B. Esters
    C. Ethyls
    D. Amines

27. Drug toxicity is NOT influenced by:
    A. Nature of drug
    B. Concentration of drug
    C. Rate of injection
    D. Height of patient
    E. Vascularity
    F. All of the above

28. All of the following are reasons for using vasoconstrictors EXCEPT to
    A. Decrease diffusion at the injection site
    B. Slow absorption of the anesthetic into the bloodstream
    C. Increase the vasodilatory affect of the local anesthetic
    D. Decrease bleeding at the site of injection

29. A patient with atypical plasma cholinesterase can be safely administered:
    A. An ester
    B. An amide
    C. Neither an ester or an amide
    D. Procaine

30. A patient with syncope should be treated with
    A. Valium
    B. Talwin
    C. Nitrous oxide
    D. Spirits of ammonia
    E. Benedryl

31. A patient has been given a local anesthetic. He suddenly begins to complain of intense itching. What drug should be administered?
    A. Benedryl
    B. Epinephrine
    C. Hydrocortisone
    D. Aminophyline

32. Which of the following nerves innervates the hard and soft palate?
    A. ASA
    B. PSA
    C. Nasopalatine
    D. Greater palatine
    E. Infraorbital

33. Another name for Mepivacaine is:
    A. Prilocaine
    B. Carbocaine
    C. Xylocaine
    D. Procaine

34. When injecting a complete 1.8 ml carpule of 2% Lidocaine, the patient receives how many milligrams of anesthetic solution?
    A. 15 mg
    B. 36 mg
    C. 1.8 mg
    D. 72 mg

35. Vasoconstrictors used in local anesthetic preparations are sympathomimetic amines.
    A. True
    B. False

36. What is the most common complication associated with dental local anesthetic injections?
    A. Syncope
    B. Drug allergy
    C. Epinephrine overdose
    D. Anaphylaxis

37. Paresthesia:
    A. Cannot be caused by local anesthetic injection
    B. Is usually permanent
    C. Should be followed up every 2 months during the first year
    D. Warrants informing the patient but there is no need to document in chart

38. Which of the following is not caused by epinephrine?
    A. Tremor
    B. Anxiety
    C. Headache
    D. Sleepiness
    E. Palpitations

39. The major cause of a hematoma is:
    A. Poor operator technique
    B. Not aspirating
    C. Tearing the blood vessel

40. The best administration technique to obtain adequate anesthesia in an area of infection is:
    A. Field block
    B. Nerve block
    C. Infiltration
    D. None of the above; you never administer anesthesia if a patient has an infection

41. A healthy 122-pound patient will receive Mepivacaine 3% for a cavity prep. How many carpules of Mepivacaine can she receive?
    A. 3.8
    B. 4.5
    C. 5.6
    D. 2.8

42. Pressure should be applied during the injection with a cotton tip applicator for which of the following injections?
    A. Posterior superior alveolar nerve block
    B. Infraorbital nerve block
    C. Greater palatine nerve block
    D. Anterior superior alveolar nerve block

43. The nasopalatine nerve block anesthetizes:
    A. Soft tissue of the palate of the anterior teeth bilaterally
    B. Soft tissue of the palate from the maxillary third molar through the premolars on side of injection
    C. Soft tissue of the palate of the anterior teeth on side of injection
    D. Soft tissue of the palate from the maxillary third molar through the premolars bilaterally

44. The depth of needle penetration for the posterior superior alveolar injection is:
    A. 3/4 short needle
    B. 3/4 long needle
    C. 1/2 short needle
    D. To the hub of a short needle

45. Which of the following injections should pressure be applied to aid the flow of the anesthetic solution into the foramen?
    A. Greater palatine
    B. Nasopalatine
    C. Posterior superior alveolar
    D. Infraorbital

46. The middle superior alveolar nerve block anesthetizes the pulps of the maxillary third, second, and first molars in 100% of patients.
    A. True
    B. False

47. Following the administration of a right infraorbital injection, a crossover injection can be administered directly at the apex:
    A. Right central incisor
    B. Right lateral incisor
    C. Left lateral incisor
    D. Left central incisor

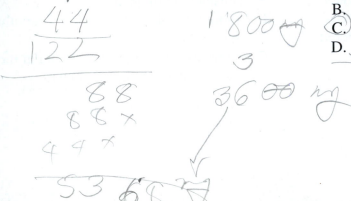

48. Which of the following injections is the needle inserted upward 45 degrees, inward 45 degrees, and backward 45 degrees, until the needle hits bone?
    A. PSA
    B. IA
    C. Mental
    D. Greater palatine

49. The most common adverse reaction for the ASA injection is to scrape the periosteum from injecting too close to the periosteum.
    A. True
    B. False

50. What is the maximum safe dose of epinephrine per appointment for a healthy adult patient of average weight?
    A. 0.02 mg
    B. 0.04 mg
    C. 0.2 mg
    D. 0.4 mg

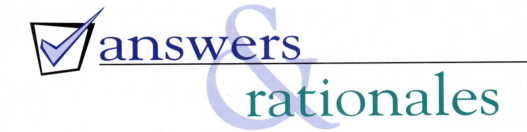

answers & rationales

1.

A. Glucocorticosteroid is the hormone lacking in acute adrenal insufficiency. The adrenal gland is made up of two glands, the cortex and the medulla. Cortisol, a glucocorticosteroid, is the most important product of the adrenal cortex and helps the body adapt to stress. Epinephrine is an adrenal hormone and a synthetic adrenergic vasoconstrictor used to treat asthmatic attacks, bronchospasm, and allergic reactions. Insulin is a hormone released by the pancreas to regulate blood glucose. Thyroxin (T_4) is a hormone of the thyroid gland that influences metabolic rate.

2.

D. A cerebrovascular accident (CVA) patient exhibiting normal blood pressure should be placed in a comfortable sitting position—upright or semiupright. An unconscious respiratory distress patient, a patient pregnant in her second trimester, and a syncope patient can be placed in a supine position.

3.

D. Patients with acute pulmonary edema usually experience symptoms such as tachypnea, extreme dyspnea with cyanosis, and pink frothy sputum. The symptoms of hyperventilation include a feeling of tightness, light-headedness, and palpation of the heart. An acute asthmatic episode is precipitated by non-allergic factors, and the patient usually experiences shortness of breath, wheezing, and coughing. A cerebrovascular accident (CVA) patient may experience the following: headache with blurred vision, aphasia, and altered consciousness.

4.

A. Hypoglycemia is the most common acute problem experienced by a diabetic. Its cause is most commonly due to a patient not eating or not eating enough after injection of insulin. Ketoacidosis, a complication of diabetes, results from an accumulation of ketone bodies as a result of an inadequate carbohydrate metabolism. It is characterized by acetone breath and mental confusion. Diabetics (hyperglycemics) are more prone to infections. Hypoinsulinism is a result of too little insulin.

5.

B. When a patient is hyperventilating, the most appropriate form of treatment is having the patient breathe into a paper bag or cupped hands. Epinephrine is contraindicated; the drug of choice is diazepam. It is also recommended to bring the patient to an upright position. Do not administer oxygen, because the patient needs more carbon dioxide to balance the system.

6.

A. The tourniquets, which are applied to the extremities, should be released 5 minutes at a time—not 10. Rotations of release and reapplication of tourniquets are continued until the patient has reached a medical facility. Phlebostasia is a synonym for bloodless phlebotomy.

7.

D. The initial treatment for syncope is to place the patient in a supine position. The next step is to place ammonia spirits under the patient's nose. Oxygen may be administered, but epinephrine is not recommended. If bradycardia persists, an anticholinergic (atropine) may be administered.

8.

D. The diabetic patient is experiencing signs of hypoglycemia and should be given a substance containing sugar, such as orange juice. A patient should be given insulin when there is evidence of hyperglycemia. Oxygen and epinephrine are not recommended for the treatment of hypoglycemia. The patient will already be experiencing an increase in epinephrine and anxiety activities during the hypoglycemic state.

9.

D. Children usually do not experience orthostatic hypotension. Most generally, causes include prolonged periods of recumbency and convalescence, increased age, varicose veins, and the third trimester of pregnancy.

10.

B. Angina pectoris is due to an insufficient blood supply to the heart muscle. Coronary arteries are not providing the myocardium with an adequate supply of oxygen, causing myocardial ischemia. In treating this patient, the healthcare provider needs to practice stress-reduction protocol to minimize anxiety. Hyperoxia is a condition with abnormally high oxygen tension in the blood. Hypercalcemia refers to a greater amount of calcium in the blood.

11.

D. It is not recommended to administer oxygen to a hyperventilating patient; the patient needs to breathe in a gaseous mixture (7% CO_2 + 93% O_2) instead. As this is not available in most practices, it would be more likely to have the patient breathe into a paper bag or cupped hands. Always stop treatment first and place the patient in an upright position before continuing with the proper management steps.

12.

C. The conscious CVA patient should be placed in a comfortable position—upright or semiupright—instead of in a supine position. Then the vital signs should be taken. It would be appropriate to call the EMS and be ready to administer oxygen.

13.

C. Dyspnea refers to difficulty in breathing. Tachypnea refers to an increased respiratory rate. Orthopnea refers to the inability to breathe, except in an upright position, and apnea refers to no respiratory movement.

14.

B. Hyperventilation is an increase in frequency or depth of respiration. It is a common emergency situation experienced in dentistry because it is triggered as a result of extreme anxiety. With airway obstruction, patients with good airflow may experience a forceful cough, wheezing between coughs, and the inability to breathe. Individuals with poor air exchange may experience a weak cough and absent voice sounds. Hypoventilation does not meet metabolic demands and is common in acute asthmatic attacks.

15.

A. Hyperventilation is not a common symptom for asthmatics. However, they do experience dyspnea, wheezing, coughing, and cyanosis.

16.

A. Tachycardia is an increase in pulse rate. Tachypnea is an increase in respiratory rate. An increase in body temperature and blood pressure result in fever and hypertension, respectively.

17.

B. Hyperventilation, not hypoventilation, is a generalized problem associated with respiratory distress. Wheezing, coughing, and an increased heart rate are also clinical manifestations of respiratory distress.

18.

D. If the seizure occurs while the patient is in the dental chair, do not move the patient—place the chair in a supine position. Moving the patient could be difficult. However, if the patient is not seated and seizure develops, place the patient on the floor in a supine position. If the seizure continues longer than 5 minutes, summon medical assistance. In the meantime, it is important to protect the patient from injury. It is common for the patient to be confused and have a headache in the postictal stage.

19.

A. Hyperventilation rarely occurs in children, because they usually do not hide their fears. However, it can occur from acute anxiety and in individuals experiencing pain, metabolic acidosis, and drug intoxication. It is most generally experienced in adults between the ages of 15 and 40 years.

20.

C. Obesity is a prediposing factor of acute myocardial infarction. Other risk factors include coronary ar-

tery disease, being male (especially those in their 50s–70s), and undue stress. A diet including vitamin C does not cause myocardial infarction.

21.

D. The patient experiencing angina should be placed in an upright position, not supine. If there is evidence of the patient sweating, treatment should cease. It is protocol to use nitrous oxide and oxygen during treatment.

22.

A. With emphysema, there is destruction of the alveolar wall and loss of elastic recoil of the lungs. With asthma, the lungs overdistend. The mucous plugs occlude the smaller bronchi, which results in a decreased size of the airway lumen. In acute pulmonary edema, fluid fills the alveolar spaces of the lungs from the pulmonary capillary bed. With complete airway obstruction, sympathetic outflow increases, causing an increase in blood pressure, heart rate, and respiratory rate.

23.

B. Fainting—a sudden loss of consciousness—is the most common medical emergency that occurs in the dental office. Diabetic coma, myocardial infarction, and drug overdose reaction are not the most frequently occurring medical emergencies in the dental office.

24.

C. Exophthalmos (bug-eyed), tachycardia, and nervousness are common characteristics found in individuals with hyperthyroidism. With hypothyroidism, common characteristics include apathy, fatigue, weak skeletal muscles, and decreased appetite, heart rate, and blood pressure. Hypertension involves an increase and hypotension a decrease in blood pressure.

25.

C. Orthostatic hypotension is a disorder of the autonomic nervous system in which the patient faints when assuming an upright position. It can be caused by prolonged periods of recumbency. Angina pectoris, epilepsy, and syncope are all stress-induced conditions. Therefore, using a stress-reduction protocol when dealing with these patients in the office is mandatory.

26.

A. The amide-type local anesthetics were introduced in the 1940s. Their widespread usage is due to the decrease in the frequency of allergic reactions versus the ester local anesthetic.

27.

D. The height of the patient is not related to drug toxicity. The patient's weight is important to determine maximum permissible dose.

28.

C. Vasoconstrictors counteract the vasodilatory effects of local anesthetics.

29.

B. Atypical plasma cholinesterase is a relative contraindication to the use of esters. Therefore, amides local anesthetics are the choice.

30.

D. The first response to a patient experiencing syncopy is supine positioning. Ammonia spirits can be used if the patient does not respond to the supine positioning.

31.

B. Epinephrine 1:1,000 is the drug of choice for anaphylaxis.

32.

D. The greater palatine nerve innervates the hard and soft palate.

33.

B. Carbocaine is the generic name for Mepivacaine.

34.

B. There are 36 mg of anesthetic in a 2% solution.

35.

A. Vasoconstrictors such as epinephrine are naturally occurring in your body, and are considered sympathomimetic amines.

36.

A. Syncopy is the most common medical emergency following the administration of local anesthetics.

37.

C. Paresthesia should be followed up every 2 months during the first year.

38.

D. Sleepiness is caused by a local anesthetic overdose in the later stages.

39.

C. Hematomas are caused by tearing the blood vessel during the injection. Hematoma can develop even if the clinician uses proper technique.

40.

B. The nerve block is the injection given the furthest away from an infection, so you will have a greater chance of getting anesthesia in that area.

41.

B. A 122-pound patient can receive 4.4 carpules of Mepivacaine.

42.

C. Pressure anesthesia using a cotton-tip applicator is used on palatal injections to increase patient comfort.

43.

C. The nasopalatine injection only anesthetizes the soft tissue and bone underlying the palatal anterior teeth from canine to canine.

44.

A. Three-fourths the depth of a short needle is recommended for the PSA injections; a deeper penetration increases the risk of penetrating the ptergoid plexis of veins.

45.

D. Following the IO injection, the clinician should massage the area to assist the local anesthetic in penetrating the infraorbital foramen.

46.

B. Approximately 65% of the population do not have an MSA nerve.

47.

D. For a crossover injection the clinican gives an infiltration over the central incisor on the opposite side.

48.

A. This is the technique for the PSA injection.

49.

A. A common reaction for the ASA injection is to scrape the periosteum because of the close proximity of the needle to the bone. The bevel of the needle should be toward the bone to assist in patient comfort.

50.

C. A healthy patient can have .2 mg of epinephrine per appointment. A medically compromised patient can only have .04 mg of epinephrine.

10 Performing Periodontal Procedures

Periodontology involves the diagnosis, treatment, and prevention of diseases associated with the periodontium.

chapter objectives

After completion of this chapter, the learner should be able to:

➤ Describe components of gingiva

➤ Discuss periodontal ligament

➤ Describe the types of cementum

➤ Discuss the alveolar process

➤ Understand the risk factors of periodontal disease

➤ Describe the oral factors that affect periodontal health

➤ Understand the systemic factors influencing periodontal disease

➤ Discuss the microbiology of periodontal disease

➤ Describe the clinical assessment of periodontal disease

➤ Understand the American Academy of Periodontology Disease Classification

➤ Describe gingivitis

➤ Describe periodontitis

➤ Discuss the nonsurgical approach to periodontal therapy

➤ Discuss the surgical approach to periodontal therapy

➤ Describe dental implants

➤ Describe the types of periodontal emergencies

➤ Discuss the endpoint objectives of periodontal therapy

➤ Describe the types of dental conditions found in the periodontal patient

➤ Describe the basic instrument design

➤ List and describe the types of assessment instruments

➤ List and describe the types of dental hygiene instruments

➤ Describe the basic principles of instrumentation

➤ Describe the use of the periodontal probe

➤ Describe the use of the explorer

➤ Describe the use of the sickle scaler

➤ Describe the use of the universal curets

➤ Describe the use of the area-specific curets

➤ Discuss the paradigm shift in nonsurgical periodontal therapy

➤ Describe power-driven scalers

➤ Describe ultrasonic procedures

➤ Describe gingival curettage

➤ Describe instrument sharpening

➤ PERIODONTOLOGY

I. Periodontium

  A. Gingiva

    1. Components

      a. Free gingiva—Located at crest of alveolus; not attached, outer boundary of sulcus

      b. Free gingival groove—Located at inferior border of free gingiva, point opposite of alveolar crest, depression

      c. Attached gingiva—Located below free gingival groove; lies over underlying bone

      d. Mucogingival junction—Located where attached gingiva ends

      e. Alveolar mucosa—Located below mucogingival junction

      f. Gingival sulcus—Denotes space between gingiva and tooth

      g. Col—Consists of nonkeratinized tissue located between lingual and facial papilla

    h. Interdental papilla—Denotes tissue that occupies interdental space between two adjacent teeth

    i. Epithelial attachment—Located at base of sulcus, where epithelium attaches to tooth

    j. Epithelium—Contains both keratinized and nonkeratinized tissues

        (1) Keratinized—Consists of oral epithelium

        (2) Nonkeratinized—Consists of sulcular and junctional epithelium

    k. Sulcular (crevicular) fluid—Serum-like fluid that passes from gingival connective tissue through tissues into the sulcus; an inflammatory exudate

        (1) Characteristics

            (a) Less fluid is present in healthy gingiva than in diseased gingiva

            (b) Amount of fluid may be proportionate to severity of inflammation

    l. Connective tissue

        (1) Known as lamina propria

        (2) Vascular and has nerve tissue

        (3) Components

            (a) Fibroblasts—Produce collagen and elastic fibers; collagen gives connective tissue its strength

            (b) Composed of mast cells, macrophages, histiocytes, plasma cells, and lymphocytes

    m. Gingival fiber groups

        (1) Marginal gingiva—Consists of dense fiber bundles made of collagen

        (2) Functions of fibers

            (a) Brace gingiva against tooth

            (b) Assist gingiva to withstand forces of mastication

            (c) Connect free marginal gingiva to cementum and attached gingiva

        (3) Types of fiber groups

            (a) Gingivodental—Located on facial, lingual, and interproximal surfaces

            (b) Circular—Encircles tooth

            (c) Transseptal—Located interproximally and forms horizontal bundles

B. Periodontal ligament (PDL)—Consists of connective tissue fibers (collagen) that surround root and connect tooth to bone

    1. Functions

        a. Transmit occlusal forces to bone

        b. Attach teeth to bone

c. Maintain gingival tissues in their proper relationship to teeth

d. Resist impact of occlusal forces

e. Protect nerves and vessels from injury by surrounding root with soft tissue

f. Supply nutrients to remaining periodontal structures—Bone, cementum, and gingiva

g. Transmit touch, pressure, and pain through sensory nerve fibers

2. Fiber bundles

a. Made of collagen

b. Attach to cementum and bone by Sharpey's fibers

c. Not visible on radiograph, but space where they are located can be seen on radiograph as radiolucent line surrounding root of tooth

d. Principal fibers—Arranged in distinct groups

   (1) Transseptal—Extend interproximally over alveolar crest; embedded in cementum of two adjacent teeth

   (2) Alveolar crest—Located apically to junctional epithelium and extend obliquely from cementum to alveolar crest

   (3) Horizontal—Extend at right angles to long axis of tooth

   (4) Oblique—Extend from cementum in a coronal direction to the bone; largest and most significant fiber group

   (5) Apical—Extend from cementum at root apex to base of tooth socket

   (6) Interradicular—Found only in multirooted teeth; extend from cementum at furcation to bone in furcation area

3. Remodeling

a. Cells found in PDL (e.g., fibroblasts, cementoblasts, osteoblasts) can remodel bone and cementum

b. Fibers adapt to occlusal stimuli and increase in size when occlusal forces increase

C. Cementum—Consists of calcified tissue covering tooth root

1. Types

a. Acellular cementum—Covers cervical one-third to one-half of root

   (1) No cells are present

   (2) Contains calcified Sharpey's fibers

   (3) Plays a significant role in supporting tooth in socket

b. Cellular cementum—Formed after tooth has erupted

   (1) Located more apically than acellular cementum; compensates for lost tooth crown length that occurs with attrition

   (2) Less calcified than acellular

   (3) Fewer Sharpey's fibers present

2. Patterns of formation—Continuous process with periods of greater and lesser activity

a. Arranged in layers or lamellae

b. Form more rapidly at apex

3. Cementoenamel junction (CEJ)—Defines tooth's anatomic crown; useful in assessing attachment loss or bone loss

a. Types

(1) Cementum overlaps enamel—60–65%

(2) Cementum meets enamel, not overlapping—30%

(3) Cementum and enamel do not meet (dentin is exposed)—5–10%

4. Anomalies

a. Hypercementosis—Localized or generalized, prominent thickening of cementum often accompanied with nodular overgrowth at apex; numerous etiologies, including Paget's disease

b. Cementicles—Globular masses of cementum that lie free in PDL or adhere to root surface

D. Alveolar process—Portion of mandible and maxilla that forms and supports tooth sockets; occurs with tooth eruption

1. Disappears after a tooth is lost

2. Bones that make up alveolar process

a. Dense outer plate (cortical bone)—Includes facial and lingual compact bone

b. Socket wall—Made up of compact bone (cortical bone); holds ends of PDL—Sharpey's fibers; lamina dura

c. Cancellous bone—Located between outer cortical plates and socket wall; less dense and spongy; contains trabeculae

3. Parts

a. Alveoli—Tooth sockets

b. Interdental septum—Area of bone between teeth

(1) Composed of facial and lingual cortical plates, socket walls, and underlying cancellous bone

(2) Shape is determined by size and shapes of crowns of approximating teeth

c. Bone coverings—Composed of vascular connective tissue containing osteogenic cells

(1) Periosteum covers outer bone surface

(2) Endosteum covers inner bone surface

4. Bone remodeling

a. Continuous changing of bone

b. Can be removed (resorbed) or added (formed)

c. Function, age, and systemic factors determine changes in bone

II. Risk Factors

A. Definition—Attributes or exposures that increase probability that a disease will occur

B. Causes—Environmental conditions, habits, or other diseases that increase or decrease patient's susceptibility to periodontal infection

C. Identification—Analyze information obtained from oral examination, clinical studies of periodontium, and medical/dental histories

D. Categories

1. Unchanging risk factors

    a. Include gender, genetic factors, congenital immunodeficiencies, past history of periodontal disease, and congenital systemic diseases

    b. Contribute to periodontal problems—Factors include diabetes and conditions or diseases involving reduction of neutrophil numbers or function

    c. Risk factors do not change, even if periodontal health is restored

2. Changing risk factors

    a. Include poor oral hygiene, age, certain medications, tobacco and alcohol use, stress, acquired immune system deficiencies, acquired endocrine diseases, acquired inflammatory diseases, nutritional deficiencies, and tooth restorations, which enhance plaque accumulation or inhibit normal function

    b. Contribute to periodontal problems as well

    c. Risk factors that can be removed or changed

        (1) Poor oral hygiene—Primary factor in gingival and periodontal disease

        (2) Tobacco use

            (a) One of the most significant risk factors in development and progression of periodontal disease

            (b) Users exhibit greater bone loss, increased pocket depths, and calculus formation

            (c) Users exhibit same or less gingival inflammation and same levels of plaque accumulation as nonsmokers

            (d) Nicotine and other toxic substances in tobacco alter host's ability to neutralize infection by reducing neutrophils' effectiveness

            (e) Alters periodontal tissue vasculature; reduces immunoglobulin levels and antibody responses to bacterial plaque biofilm

(3) Nutritional status

  (a) Secondary factor in etiology of periodontal disease

  (b) Deficiencies of nutrient elements associated with wound healing may contribute to gingival and periodontal disease progression

  (c) Nutrients important for wound healing include

    i) Protein—Repairs tissue and increases resistance to infection

    ii) Vitamin C—Promotes collagen formation, tissue synthesis, and wound healing

    iii) Folic acid—Enhances red blood cell maturation, tissue synthesis, and cell proliferation

    iv) Vitamin B_{12}—Enhances red blood cell maturation, tissue synthesis, and cell proliferation

    v) Vitamin A—Increases resistance to infection and promotes tissue synthesis; deficiency affects integrity of epithelium

    vi) Vitamin K—Affects prothrombin formation

    vii) Iron—Promotes red blood cell formation

    viii) Zinc—Enhances connective tissue formation, wound healing, and protein synthesis

(4) Side effects—Certain medications may have impact on gingival/periodontal tissues and their response to periodontal treatment; severity of periodontal reaction to medications varies among patients

  (a) Gingival hyperplasia—Medications associated with gingival hyperplasia include

    i) Phenytoin (Dilantin)

    ii) Calcium channel blockers

      • Diltiazem (Cardizem, Dilacor)

      • Nifedipine (Procardia)

      • Primidone

      • Valproic acid

      • Verapamil (Calan, Isoptin, Verelan)

    iii) Cyclosporine

  (b) Xerostomia—Medication categories associated with xerostomia include:

    i) Anorectics (Dexadrine, amphetamine, dextroamphetamine, Adipex-P, and Pondimin)

    ii) Anticholinergics (Atrovent, Artane, Bentyl)

    iii) Anticonvulsants (Valium)

  iv) Antidepressants (Anafranil, Asendin)

  v) Antihistamines (Seldane, Benadryl)

  vi) Antihypertensives

   • Diuretics (Lasix)

   • Central adrenergic inhibitors (Catapres, Aldomet)

   • Peripheral adrenergic antagonists (Minipres)

   • Calcium-channel blockers (Calan)

   • Angiotensin-converting enzyme (ACE) inhibitors (Capoten, Vasotec, Monopril)

  vii) Antiparkinson (L-dopa, Dopar, Artane)

  viii) Antipsychotics (Clozapine, Clozaril, Haldol)

  ix) Muscle relaxants (Flexeril)

  x) Acne treatment (Accutane)

 (c) Altered host resistance—Medications that may alter host resistance to infection include

  i) Antibiotics

  ii) Insulin

  iii) Oral hypoglycemics

  iv) Systemic corticosteroids

 (d) Abnormal bleeding—Medications that may cause abnormal bleeding include

  i) Aspirin

  ii) Dipyridamole

  iii) Nonsteroidal anti-inflammatory drugs (NSAIDs)

  iv) Phenytoin (Dilantin)

  v) Quinidine

  vi) Methyldopa

(5) Dental restorations, whose design or material contributes to plaque retention, can contribute to development of gingival inflammation and periodontal destruction

(6) Risk factors that demand most attention in management of periodontal disease—Smoking and diabetes

III. Oral Factors Other than Microorganisms that Affect Periodontal Health

 A. Calculus (mineralized plaque)

  1. Sources of minerals are precipitated salts that originate in saliva and sulcular (crevicular) fluid

2. Inorganic content is mainly calcium phosphate, with lesser amounts of calcium carbonate and other organic compounds

3. Deposits are classified by their location (supragingival or subgingival)

a. Supragingival calculus

(1) Attaches coronal to gingival margin

(2) Displays chalky, creamy white appearance

(3) Mineralization results from saliva

(4) Relatively easy to remove

(5) Deposits occur on, but are not limited to, buccal surfaces of maxillary molars, opposite Stensen's duct, and lingual surfaces of mandibular anterior teeth, opposite Wharton's duct

b. Subgingival calculus

(1) Attaches apical to gingival margin

(2) Displays dark brown–black appearance

(3) More difficult to remove than supragingival calculus

(4) Mineralization results from sulcular fluid

(5) Deposits occur on all root surfaces in sulcus or pocket

4. Significant in gingival and periodontal disease because it contributes to bacterial plaque accumulation owing to its porous surface; inhibits plaque removal and is a tissue irritant

B. Plaque control—Primary factor in reduction or elimination of gingival and periodontal disease

1. Conditions that can temporarily or permanently affect plaque control or removal include

a. Faulty restorations

b. Partial dentures

c. Orthodontic appliances

d. Malocclusion

C. Other conditions that can affect periodontal health

1. Unreplaced missing teeth—Increase risk of migration of teeth and loss of bone support

2. Mouth breathing—Dehydrates exposed gingival tissue causing tissue to become enlarged and inflamed; affects maxillary incisal area

3. Excess occlusal forces—Can result in compression and necrosis of periodontal ligament and root, as well as cementum and alveolar process resorption

IV. Systemic Factors Influencing Periodontal Diseases

A. Periodontitis associated with systemic diseases

1. General information

   a. Periodontal disease is directly related to presence of microorganisms in periodontal structures

   b. Involves large quantities of pathogenic bacteria

   c. Host response is modified by systemic disease

   d. Composition of microorganisms or host's ability to respond to microorganisms has impact on health of periodontal tissues

   e. Microorganisms affect periodontal tissues and, in some cases, general systemic health of individual

   f. Destruction of tissues results in ulcerated sulcular epithelium—Portal of entry for microorganisms or their toxins to invade circulatory systems, distributing microorganisms systemically

   g. Studies support significant correlation between periodontal diseases and specific systemic diseases

2. Specific systemic diseases

   a. Diabetes

      (1) Uncontrolled diabetics have increased risk of developing periodontal disease, with severity of periodontal disease being greater

      (2) Patients with poorly controlled blood glucose levels have increased risk for developing acute periodontal abscesses and chronic inflammatory periodontal diseases

         (a) Hyperglycemia, associated with uncontrolled diabetes, exacerbates inflammatory destruction, and impairs wound healing

         (b) Metabolic compounds accumulate in tissue and contribute to vascular inflammatory and neural complications

      (3) Diabetics may have impaired polymorphonuclear (PMN) leukocyte function, which will alter the inflammatory response—Exaggerated inflammatory response

      (4) More difficult to control periodontal disease in presence of diabetes

   b. Cardiovascular disease

      (1) Periodontal disease puts individual at increased risk for heart disease including heart attacks and stroke

      (2) Circulating periodontal pathogens may result in small blood clots that can block arteries

   c. Human immunodeficiency virus (HIV) infection

      (1) Periodontal disease associated with HIV infection is a rapid progression of chronic periodontitis

(2) HIV invades T-4 (T-helper) lymphocytes (with CD4 receptor cells)

(3) Virus binds to CD4 lymphocyte cell surface

(4) Number of CD4 lymphocytes decreases

(5) Ultimately, there is a depressed immune function, which is a significant factor in development of HIV-associated periodontal disease

(6) With HIV infection, there may be inadequate function of PMN leukocytes, which will alter the inflammatory response

d. Neutrophil disorders

(1) Significant in development and progression of periodontal diseases because neutrophil function is critical to well-functioning inflammatory response

(2) Primary neutrophil defects or disorders

(a) Agranulocytosis—Acute disease; white blood cell count drops

(b) Cyclic neutropenia—Involves periodic episodes of abnormally low number of neutrophils

(c) Chediak-Higashi syndrome—Inherited metabolic disorder with neutrophils containing perioxidase-positive inclusion bodies

(d) Lazy leukocyte syndrome

(3) Neutrophil defects or impairment secondary to other systemic conditions

(a) Papillon-LeFèvre syndrome

(b) Down syndrome

(c) Inflammatory bowel disease

(d) Addison's disease—Chronic adrenal insufficiency

e. Pregnancy

(1) Evidence suggests that pregnant women with periodontal disease are at increased risk of delivering low-birth-weight infants; circulating inflammatory products and toxins that occur as a result of the periodontal disease may affect fetal development

V. Microbiology of Periodontal Diseases

A. Microorganisms

1. Accumulation around gingival margins is associated with majority of periodontal diseases

2. Found in bacterial plaque (biofilm) in gingival sulcus or pocket

3. Only a small number (approximately 12) found in oral cavity are associated with gingival or periodontal diseases

4. Bacteria associated with gingival or periodontal diseases have properties that are especially damaging or destructive to structures of periodontium—Maintain similar structural or toxic characteristics (e.g., Gram-negative anaerobic)

5. Bacteria cause tissue damage by substances they release or as a consequence of host's inflammatory and immune response (some have tissue-invasion properties; others have enzymes that break down connective tissue)

B. Bacterial characteristics—Use following characteristics to identify or categorize bacteria

1. Morphotypes (shapes)

a. Cocci—Ball-shaped and spherical

b. Rods—Long and thin

(1) Bacilli—Rectangular in shape

(2) Filaments—Threadlike

(3) Fusiforms—Threadlike, with tapered ends

c. Spirochetes—Spiral, with fibrils (little fibers) in cell wall

2. Cell wall—Identifying characteristic of bacteria

a. Characteristics

(1) Contains receptor proteins that contribute to bacteria's adherence

(2) Lipopolysaccharides are destructive endotoxins that cause inflammatory or immune host response

(3) May have fimbriae or pili (projections of cell wall) contributing to bacterial adhesion to tooth or other bacteria

(4) Contains polysaccharides—Long-chained, sticky carbohydrates

(a) Glucans help bacteria stick together

(b) Salivary enzymes destroy peptidoglycan found in bacterial wall

b. Gram stain properties

(1) Gram-positive bacteria will pick up Gram stain (a violet stain) in cell wall

(2) Gram-negative bacteria will *not* pick up Gram stain in cell wall

3. Oxygen needs influence where bacteria can survive

a. Aerobic—Require oxygen to survive

b. Anaerobic—Do not survive in an oxygen-rich environment

c. Facultative anaerobe—Can use oxygen, but can survive if no oxygen is present

4. Bacterial metabolism

    a. Fermentors—Gram-positive bacteria metabolize carbohydrates, including saccharides, resulting in fermentation

    b. Nonfermentors—Food source includes proteins (amino acids or peptides)

C. Classification of periodontal bacteria—Bacteria associated with periodontal disease are generally Gram-negative, anaerobic

  1. Supragingival plaque

    a. Formation begins shortly after plaque is removed

      (1) Pellicle—Acellular, organic layer is deposited on tooth surface within minutes after tooth surface is cleaned

        (a) Aids in attachment of bacteria

        (b) Provides receptors for bacteria to adhere

        (c) Allows initial layer of bacteria to attach

      (2) Bacterial attachment

        (a) After first layer of bacteria attaches, many other bacterial species will accumulate in colonies

        (b) Composition varies among individuals and as plaque matures

        (c) Mature plaque is allowed to accumulate on tooth surface for extended period

    b. Types of bacteria

      (1) Gram-positive species—Accumulate in new plaque; cocci are predominant

      (2) Facultative anaerobic microorganisms increase in number as plaque matures; these create environment that is suitable for anaerobic bacteria to colonize

  2. Subgingival plaque

    a. Accumulates in layers on tooth surface and also as loosely adhered plaque close to sulcular tissue *after* supragingival plaque is established

    b. In these areas, motile, Gram-negative rods and spirochetes will increase

    c. Tissue-associated plaque (loosely adherent) is free-floating in sulcus or pocket

    d. More toxic than attached plaque—Significant factor in periodontal destruction

    e. Types of bacteria frequently associated with periodontal disease

      (1) Most frequently implicated microorganisms

        (a) *Porphyromonas gingivalis* (*P. gingivalis*)

        (b) *Actinobacillus actinomycetemcomitans* (*Aa*)

        (c) *Prevotella intermedia* (*P. intermedia*)

(2) Other microorganisms, with lesser significance

(a) *Bacteroides forsythus*

(b) *Fusobacterium* sp.

(c) *Peptostreptococcus micros*

(d) *Campylobacter rectus*

(e) *Treponema denticola*

(f) Enteric rods

(g) *Streptococcus* sp.

(h) *Actinomyces* sp.

D. Virulence of periodontal pathogens

1. Tissue destruction

a. Depends on pathogenicity or virulence of microorganisms and host's ability to protect body from destructive nature of microorganisms

b. May occur as a result of direct invasion of bacteria into inflamed sulcus and because of substances that are components of bacteria or bacterial by-products

c. Bacteria may also trigger inflammatory or immune response

d. Methods of destruction may vary because microorganisms have different destructive characteristics

2. Bacterial infection with *Aa*, *P. gingivalis*, and *P. intermedia* have greatest significance

3. Nature of bacterial plaque is significant; sulcular ulceration allows bacteria and/or by-products to invade gingival connective tissue

4. Host response is significant

5. Tobacco, alcohol, stress, or systemic conditions alter immune response

6. Pathogenic bacteria can produce

a. Proteolytic enzymes

(1) Collagenase degrades collagen

(2) Hyaluronidase can increase tissue permeability and contribute to bone resorption

(3) Chondroitinase can increase tissue permeability

(4) Proteases break down noncollagenous proteins and increase capillary permeability

b. Bacterial waste products—Include hydrogen sulfide

c. Toxins

(1) Leukotoxin disturbs PMN leukocytes

(2) Endotoxin is found in cell wall of Gram-negative bacteria

    (a) Include lipopolysaccharides, which can cause tissue necrosis and initiate inflammation and immune response

    (b) Some stimulate bone resorption

E. Microbial plaque

  1. Emphasis is on control of plaque formation and retention

  2. Periodontal microflora

    a. Gingival health—Includes Gram-positive cocci and short rods

    b. Gingivitis—Includes Gram-negative bacteria—*Fusobacterium nucleatum, Veillonella parvula, Actinomyces viscosus, P. intermedia*

    c. Adult periodontitis—Includes *A. actinomycetemcomitans, P. gingivalis, P. intermedia, B. forsythus, Eikenella corrodens, F. nucleatum, C. rectus, Treponema* sp.

    d. Refractory adult periodontitis—Includes variety of microorganisms, but not limited to *B. forsythus, F. nucleatum, C. rectus, P. gingivalis, P. micros*

    e. Generalized and localized juvenile periodontitis—Includes *A. actinomycetemcomitans, Prevotella* sp., *P. gingivalis, Capnocytophaga sputigena, E. corrodens, Eubacterium* sp.

    f. Generalized prepubertal gingivitis—Includes *P. intermedia, A. actinomycetemcomitans, E. corrodens, C. sputigena*

    g. Localized prepubertal periodontitis—Includes *F. nucleatum, Selenomonas* sp., *C. rectus, B. forsythus, Capnocytophaga* sp.

    h. Acute necrotizing ulcerative gingivitis and necrotizing ulcerative periodontitis—Includes *P. intermedia, F. nucleatum, Borrelia vincentii,* and spirochetes

    i. HIV-associated gingivitis and periodontitis—Includes *Candida albicans, P. gingivalis, P. intermedia, A. actinomycetemcomitans, F. nucleatum, C. rectus*

    j. Rapid progressive periodontitis—Includes *A. actinomycetemcomitans, P. gingivalis, P. intermedia, Bacteroides capillus, B. forsythus, E. corrodens, C. rectus*

F. Immune response

  1. Inflammation—Results from tissue response to irritation or injury

    a. Vessels become permeable to certain phagocytic cells (e.g., PMN leukocytes and macrophages)

    b. Phagocytic cells travel to area of injury

      (1) Bacterial invaders are engulfed by the phagocytic cells and destroyed by enzymatic activity

(2) Bacterial breakdown products attract antibodies that facilitate immobilization and destruction of invader cells

c. Mast cells release histamine-producing vasodilatation, which tends to cause swelling and increase bleeding when tissue surface is interrupted

d. Certain lymphocytes produce elements capable of inducing bone resorption

e. Plasma cells travel to area of injury and produce immunoglobulins, which have ability to neutralize enzymes and toxin produced by bacteria

VI. Clinical Assessment

A. Periodontal assessment

1. Appearance of gingival tissues can provide information about past or present gingival disease

2. Clinical attachment loss

　　a. Identifies distance from CEJ to base of sulcus or pocket

　　b. Best indicator of damage to periodontium

　　c. Increase in attachment loss indicates progression of periodontal disease

3. Furcation—Identification and measurement

　　a. Loss of attachment on multirooted teeth results in exposure of root furca to oral environment

　　b. Use furcation probe (Nabers) or explorer to detect furcation involvement

　　c. Access to furcation varies depending on number of tooth roots

　　　　(1) Mandibular molars—two roots; access from buccal and lingual

　　　　(2) Maxillary molars—three roots; access from buccal, mesial, and distal

4. Tooth mobility—Degree a tooth is able to move in horizontal or apical direction; some mobility is physiological and not due to periodontal disease

5. Tooth positioning—Malposed teeth may increase plaque retention, resulting in increase in periodontal destruction

6. Lost tooth—Increases risk of pathological migration of teeth (teeth may drift or tip away from their physiological position, resulting in occlusal trauma and increased bone destruction)

7. Dentition assessment

　　a. Caries—Harbor bacteria

　　b. Restoration status—Restorations should be intact without defective margins; margins that promote plaque retention increase risk of tissue inflammation and recurrent caries

　　c. Proximal contact relationships—Open contacts allow for food impaction and debris accumulation; tight contacts make flossing difficult

d. Unusual wear patterns on teeth may suggest occlusal trauma

e. Tooth anomalies, such as hypoplastic areas or extra cusps, can increase risk of plaque retention

8. Radiographic examination

a. Provides information about calcified structures, such as bone and tooth

b. Full mouth radiographs and periapical and vertical bitewings are valuable for periodontal assessment

c. Assists in recognizing both normal and abnormal structures

d. Used to detect caries, bone and periapical pathology, and calcified deposits

e. Aids in identifying integrity of margins of restorations

f. Used for periodontal assessment

(1) Normal bone patterns

(a) Height or crest of alveolar bone should be 1–2 mm apical to tooth's CEJ

(b) Contour of alveolar bone should follow contour of CEJ

(c) Lamina dura is intact with alveolar ridge—Appears as a white (radiopaque) line that outlines tooth roots and alveolar crest

(d) Periodontal ligament space will be visible as a black (radiolucent) area between tooth root and lamina dura—Width of periodontal ligament space should be uniform from tooth to tooth

(e) Cancellous bone will be radiopaque, but less dense than lamina dura; within cancellous bone are irregular patterns known as trabeculae that surround marrow spaces

(2) Indicators of bone destruction in periodontal disease

(a) Patterns of bone loss can be horizontal or vertical, both of which can be identified on radiographs

(b) Radiographs do not identify initial bone destruction; by the time bone destruction is radiographically identified, disease has progressed

(c) Horizontal bone loss is a reduction of bone height, with distance between bone and CEJ being > 2 mm

(d) Vertical bone loss is an angular loss of bone height that leaves a gap or trough between bone and tooth root surface

(3) Changes in furcation involvement—As a result of bone loss, furcation of multirooted teeth may be exposed and no longer encased in alveolar bone; may not always be visible on radiograph, and if so, it will appear as radiolucent area at furca

(4) Changes in periodontal disease

    (a) Changes in radiodensity of lamina dura—Crest of lamina dura will be less well defined; appearance at crest may have breaks or be fuzzy

    (b) Radiolucent wedges are apparent at alveolar crest adjacent to tooth root surfaces

    (c) Slight radiolucent projections will extend from alveolar crest in apical direction

VII. Guidelines for the Management of Patients with Periodontal Diseases

A. Level 3—Patients who should be treated by a periodontist

  1. Severe chronic periodontitis

  2. Furcation involvement

  3. Vertical/angular bony defect(s)

  4. Aggressive periodontitis

  5. Periodontal abscess and other acute periodontal conditions

  6. Significant root surface exposure and/or progressive gingival recession

  7. Peri-implant disease

B. Level 2—Patients who would likely benefit from co-management by the referring dentist and the periodontist

  1. Early onset of periodontal disease (prior to 35 years of age)

  2. Unresolved inflammation at any site

  3. Pocket depths $\geq$ 5 mm

  4. Vertical bone defects

  5. Radiographic evidence of progressive bone loss

  6. Progressive tooth mobility

  7. Progressive attachment loss

  8. Anatomic gingival deformities

  9. Exposed root surfaces

C. Level 1—Patients who may benefit from co-management by the referring dentist and the periodontist

  1. Any patient with periodontal inflammation/infection and the following systemic conditions—Diabetes, pregnancy, cardiovascular disease, chronic respiratory disease

  2. Any patient who is a candidate for the following therapies who might be exposed to risk from periodontal infection—Cancer therapy, cardiovascular surgery, joint-replacement surgery, organ transplantation

VIII. Gingivitis—Reversible inflammation of the gingiva

A. Accumulation of plaque is directly related to development of gingivitis

B. Chronic plaque-associated gingivitis—An inflammatory response to irritant bacterial plaque; majority of gingivitis falls in this category

C. Other conditions of gingiva may alter its appearance or be caused by microbial infection

    1. Acute necrotizing ulcerative gingivitis (ANUG)—Acute gingival disease that results in destruction and cratering of gingival tissues, especially interdental papilla

        a. Accompanied with severe pain, excess salivation, spontaneous gingival bleeding, and foul breath odor with metallic taste

        b. Associated with *P. intermedia, F. nucleatum, B. vincentii,* and spirochetes

        c. Risk factors include stress, malnutrition, smoking, and immunosuppression

    2. Primary herpetic gingivostomatitis is an acute viral infection that presents with numerous intraoral ulcerations

        a. Etiology—Herpes simplex virus

        b. Patient will be febrile and have oral pain

        c. More common in children than adults

        d. After acute infection subsides, virus remains dormant in a nerve ganglion and may subsequently cause episodes of recurrent or secondary herpes—Most commonly seen as herpes labialis

    3. Hormone-induced gingivitis is exaggerated tissue response to local irritant plaque; may occur when there are fluctuations in hormones, including pregnancy, puberty, oral birth control medication, and steroid therapy

IX. Periodontitis—Inflammation of periodontal tissues and loss of connective tissue

A. Presence or accumulation of plaque may initiate periodontal disease, but it is not the only factor involved in its development and progression

B. Etiology of periodontal diseases is more complex than etiology of gingival disease

C. Nature and severity of the diseases are related to virulence of bacteria and host's ability to resist bacterial invasion

    1. Similar microorganisms do not cause all periodontal diseases, nor does every form of periodontal disease cause same pattern of tissue destruction

    2. Some forms of periodontal disease are easier to treat than others

D. Pathogenesis of periodontitis

    1. Bacterial infection with *Aa, P. gingivalis,* and *P. intermedia* has greatest significance

    2. Nature of bacterial plaque is significant—Sulcular ulceration allows bacteria and/or by-products to invade gingival connective tissue

3. Host response is significant

4. Tobacco, alcohol, stress, or systemic conditions alter immune response

E. Types—Numerous periodontal diseases are identified with unique etiology, characteristics, and age of onset (old nomenclature from the 1989 World Workshop in Clinical Periodontics; for updated nomenclature, see F below).

1. Adult periodontitis

a. Includes gingival inflammation, pocket formation, possible mobility, and bone loss

b. Some contributing factors include ineffective oral hygiene, malposed teeth, and poorly contoured restorations

2. Prepubertal periodontitis

a. Generalized—Affects primary teeth, involves rapid alveolar bone destruction, associated with leukocyte abnormalities, and is accompanied by middle ear, skin, and upper respiratory infections

b. Localized—Affects few teeth, exhibits less gingival inflammation and bone destruction, and is not accompanied by other infections

3. Juvenile periodontitis

a. Localized—Rapid attachment and vertical bone loss at incisors and first molars; minimal plaque is present

b. Generalized—Generalized rapid attachment and bone loss; minimal plaque is present

4. Rapidly progressive periodontitis—Rapid onset, with rapid and severe bone loss; episodic; amount of plaque varies

5. Acute necrotizing ulcerative periodontitis

a. Sudden onset, pain, necrosis, and cratering of interdental papillae and spontaneous bleeding

b. Usually localized in anterior regions

c. Accompanied by foul breath, metallic taste, and excess salivation

6. Refractory periodontitis—Resistant to repeated routine treatment methods

F. Updated nomenclature—November 1999 *Annals of Periodontology* published a new classification system for periodontal diseases and conditions intended to recognize shortcomings in the existing classification system, which came from the 1989 World Workshop in Clinical Periodontics

1. This new system is being incorporated into both clinical practice and education

2. Because literature using the 1989 classification system is still widely used, reference to both 1989 and 1999 classification systems are included

3. In addition to renaming some diseases, and adding others, there is clarification of the designation of periodontitis as a manifestation of systemic diseases; refractory periodontitis has been eliminated

4. Gingival diseases—New category

    a. Dental plaque-induced gingival diseases

        (1) Associated with dental plaque only

        (2) Modified by systemic factors

            (a) Associated with the endocrine system

                i) Puberty-associated gingivitis

                ii) Menstrual cycle-associated gingivitis

                iii) Pregnancy-associated gingivitis, pyogenic granuloma

                iv) Diabetes mellitus-associated gingivitis

            (b) Associated with blood dyscrasias

                i) Leukemia-associated gingivitis

        (3) Gingival diseases modified by medications

        (4) Modified by nutrition

    b. Non-plaque induced gingival lesions

        (1) Gingival diseases of specific bacterial origin

            (a) Neisseria gonorrhea-associated lesions

            (b) Treponema pallidum-associated lesions

            (c) Streptococcal species-associated lesions

        (2) Viral origin

            (a) Herpesvirus infections

        (3) Fungal origin

            (a) Candida-species infections

            (b) Linear gingival erythema

            (c) Histoplasmosis

        (4) Genetic origin

            (a) Hereditary gingival fibromatosis

        (5) Gingival manifestations of systemic conditions

            (a) Mucocutaneous disorders

                i) Lichen planan

                ii) Pemphigoid

                iii) Pemphigus vulgaris

                iv) Erythema multiforme

                v) Lupus erythematosus

                vi) Drug induced

            (b) Allergic reactions

(6) Traumatic lesions (factitious, iatrogenic, accidental)

(7) Foreign body reactions

(8) Not otherwise specified (NOS)

5. Chronic periodontitis—Replaces term adult periodontitis

    a. Localized

    b. Generalized

6. Aggressive periodontitis—Replaces term early-onset periodontitis

    a. Localized

    b. Generalized

7. Periodontitis as a manifestation of systemic diseases

    a. Associated with hematological disorders

        (1) Acquired neutropenia

        (2) Leukemia

    b. Associated with genetic disorders

        (1) Familial and cyclic neutropenia

        (2) Down syndrome

        (3) Leukocyte adhesion deficiency syndromes

        (4) Papillon-LeFèvre syndrome

        (5) Chediak-Higashi syndrome

        (6) Histiocytosis syndromes

        (7) Glycogen storage disease

        (8) Infantile genetic agranulocytosis

        (9) Cohen syndrome

       (10) Ehlers-Danlos syndrome

       (11) Hypophosphatasia

8. Necrotizing periodontal diseases—Replaces term necrotizing ulcerative periodontitis

    a. Necrotizing ulcerative gingivitis (NUG)

    b. Necrotizing ulcerative periodontitis (NUP)

9. Abscesses of the periodontium—New category

    a. Gingival abscess

    b. Periodontal abscess

    c. Pericoronal abscess

10. Periodontitis associated with endodontic lesions—New category

11. Developmental or acquired deformities and conditions—New category

    a. Localized tooth-related factors that modify or predispose to plaque-induced gingival diseases/periodontitis

      b. Mucogingival deformities and conditions around the teeth

         (1) Gingival/soft tissue recession

         (2) Lack of keratinized gingiva

         (3) Decreased vestibular depth

         (4) Aberrant frenum/muscle positions

         (5) Gingival excess

         (6) Abnormal color

      c. Mucogingival deformities and conditions on edentulous ridges

      d. Occlusal trauma (primary and secondary)

X. Nonsurgical Periodontal Therapy (soft tissue management)—Provided by dental professional

A. Objectives

    1. Remove bacterial plaque to restore periodontal health

    2. Slow or stop progression of periodontal disease

    3. Prepare tissues for surgical therapy

B. Definitions of nonsurgical periodontal therapies

    1. Scaling—Removal of calculus and stain from surfaces of teeth with hand-activated instruments and/or sonic and ultrasonic scalers

    2. Root planing—Smoothing of root surfaces, including removal of rough cementum or dentin that is impregnated with calculus and endotoxins

    3. SRP—Combines scaling and root planing

    4. Periodontal debridement—Nonsurgical removal of tooth surface irritants

    5. Prophylaxis—Involves mechanical plaque control procedures that can be performed by dental hygienist or dentist to prevent and control periodontal diseases, such as scaling, polishing, and flossing

    6. Coronal polishing—Removal of stains and bacterial plaque (nonmineralized deposits) from surface of teeth with a hand or rotary instrument; frequently accomplished using a rubber cup with polishing agent on a slow-speed handpiece

    7. Selective polishing—Polishing only surfaces of teeth that have extrinsic stain and visible plaque

    8. Gingival curettage—Removal of epithelial lining of periodontal pocket by scraping surface with an instrument, such as a curet

C. Goals of nonsurgical periodontal therapy—Correct and preserve dentition in state of health, comfort, and function with appropriate esthetics throughout lifetime of individual

    1. Treatment goals

      a. Eliminate and control etiological factors causing disease

    b. Maintain periodontal health

    c. Prevent recurrence of disease

  2. Specific nonsurgical treatment objectives

    a. Establish conditions conducive to reattachment of connective tissue and healing of periodontal tissues

    b. Eliminate microorganisms, calculus, and other irritants on and within tooth surface to reduce inflammation

    c. Promote connective tissue regeneration

    d. Make root surface biologically acceptable to gingival tissues

D. Techniques—Use of hand-activated instrumentation and sonic/ultrasonic scalers

E. Antibiotics in the treatment of periodontal disease—Used because mechanical removal (scaling, debridement) may not always be effective

  1. Certain periodontal situations benefit from use of antibiotics when used in conjunction with mechanical debridement

  2. Treatment is intended to alter subgingival bacterial flora

  3. Antibiotics may be provided systemically or locally

    a. Systemic antibiotics—Selection must be determined based on nature of pathogen

      (1) Tetracycline (minocycline, doxycycline)—Proved successful for treatment of certain periodontal diseases (a low dose of doxycycline hyclate [Periostat] is an effective enzyme suppressor, including collagenase)

        (a) Can accumulate in high concentrations in gingival sulcus

        (b) Blocks production of collagenase

        (c) *Aa* is highly susceptible to tetracycline

      (2) Metronidazole (Flagyl, MetroGel, Protostat)

        (a) Useful for oral soft tissue infections resulting from gram-negative bacilli (*Bacteroides*) and gram-positive spore-forming bacilli (*Clostridium*)

        (b) Targets anaerobes

        (c) Used in combination with other antibiotics (e.g., Helidac [metronidazole and tetracycline])

        (d) Useful for patients with ANUG or HIV

      (3) Penicillin—Not considered effective in treatment of periodontal disease

        (a) Periodontal pathogens are resistant to penicillin

        (b) Enzymes produced by periodontal pathogens tend to break down the penicillin, making it ineffective

        (c) Augmentin (amoxicillin and clavulanic acid) has been found helpful for treating *Bacteroides* infections

b. Local delivery—Places antibiotic or antimicrobial at site of infection; occurs after mechanical care (scaling, root planing, debridement)

   (1) Tetracycline embedded fiber (Actisite)—Placed in periodontal pocket

      (a) Delivers high level of antibiotic directly to diseased site

      (b) Fiber is left in pocket for 10 days, then removed

   (2) Chlorhexidine contained in gelatin strip (PerioChip) (Figure 10-1■)

      (a) Biodegradable in 10 days

      (b) Useful in treating adult periodontitis and maintenance patients

      (c) Used in pockets > 5 mm

      (d) Low risk of antibacterial resistance

   (3) Doxycycline gel (Atridox) (Figure 10-2■)

      (a) Injected into periodontal pocket

      (b) Conforms to periodontal pocket and solidifies

      (c) Biodegrades in 7 days

      (d) Low risk of antibacterial resistance

   (4) Antimicrobial rinse irrigation at periodontal pocket; chlorhexidine may have short-term beneficial effect

   (5) Minocycline powdered microspheres (Arestin)

      (a) Premixed, premeasured powder injected into periodontal pocket

      (b) Effective against periodontal pathogens

      (c) Microspheres are bioresorbed

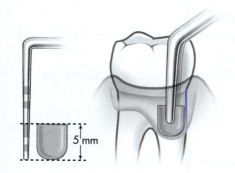

FIGURE 10-1 ■ Application of Chlorhexidine Chip

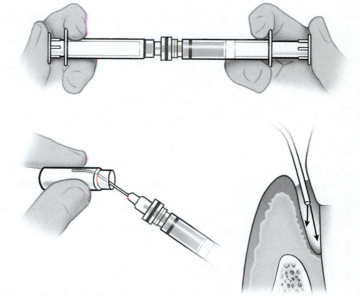

FIGURE 10-2 ■ Application of Doxycycline Polymer

XI. Periodontal Surgery—Treatment alternative if nonsurgical therapy does not produce expected end results

A. Advantages or outcomes

1. Attain shallow probing depths that are easier to maintain and more conducive to microbial flora of periodontal health

2. Reestablish or regenerate form and function of bone

3. Enhance gingival anatomy to facilitate supragingival plaque removal and resist both periodontal breakdown and caries

4. Facilitate restorative procedures where clinical crown length is inadequate for prosthetic care or where restorative margins would invade biological attachment level

B. Procedures

1. Gingivectomy

   a. Excision or removal of diseased gingiva

   b. Establishes healthy gingival contour

   c. Indications—Fibrous gingiva, deep bony pocket, gingival enlargements, and crown lengthening

2. Gingivoplasty

   a. Reshaping gingiva to increase physiological contours

   b. Not intended to eliminate pockets

3. Periodontal flap surgery—Provides visibility and access to root surfaces and bone

4. Mucogingival surgery

   a. Corrects gingival–mucous membrane relationships

   b. Creates or widens zone of attached gingiva

5. Gingival grafts—Borrows gingival tissue from one location to be placed at a gingival defect

6. Frenectomy—Releases or removes labial frenum that is impinging on gingival tissue

7. Bone graft—Fills bony defect

8. Guided tissue regeneration

   a. Creates environment where desirable cells are allowed to grow and undesirable cells are inhibited from growing

   b. Uses a barrier membrane—Polytetrafluoroethylene membrane (ePTFE) and polylactic acid with citric acid membrane

9. Osteoplasty—Reshapes bone without removing tooth supporting bone

10. Osteoectomy

    a. Removes tooth supporting bone

    b. Corrects exostosis, craters, and ledges

C. Healing—Wound heals in series of physiological steps that are part of inflammatory process; restores integrity of injured tissue

    1. Healing sequence

        a. Clot formation—Initial response to tissue wound; contains platelets that initiate and regulate clot formation

        b. Granulation tissue development—Highly vascular connective tissue, containing capillaries, fibroblasts, and inflammatory cells; fibroblasts create extracellular matrix on which wound repairs occur

        c. Epithelialization—Epithelial cells cover wound, allowing underlying granulation tissue to mature to connective tissue

        d. Collagen formation—Strengthens wound

        e. Regeneration—Vascular granulation tissue is replaced by original cell types

        f. Maturation—Wound healing is complete

D. Periodontal dressings—Substance applied to cover gingival wounds during healing, which provides patient comfort by protecting the healing wound

    1. Periodontal dressing placement

        a. Most dressings are activated by mixing two equal amounts of material (zinc oxide and resins with fatty acids) (Figure 10-3■)

        b. Lubricate fingers and roll mixture into the length needed to cover the surgical site, dry the site, and place dressing at the gingival margin over the surgical site; use finger pressure to adapt the material and press it interproximally, trim the dressing around each tooth so it follows the CEJ and does not interfere with occlusion; advise patients to not brush the dressing or eat coarse foods that may dislodge it; they should rinse with salt water to remove debris; patient should not worry if small parts

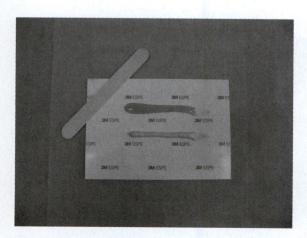

FIGURE 10-3 ■ Dispense equal amounts of tube 1 (paste) and tube 2 (gel) onto a mixing pad.

of the dressing come off but should return if all of the dressing comes off in the first day or two or if they are having discomfort (Figures 10-4■ and 10-5■)

2. Periodontal dressing removal—Gently insert a curet or cotton pliers under the border of dressing and pry it away from the teeth (watch for sutures); use a curet to remove any attached pieces of dressing, debride soft tissue with a cotton swab soaked in hydrogen peroxide, and have patient rinse with warm water

E. Suture removal—Periodontal dressing should be removed and the teeth, tissue, and sutures cleansed before removing the sutures; there are two types: interrupted and continuous

1. Removal of interrupted sutures

a. Placement is from facial to lingual in a single interproximal space

b. Removal is done by locating the knot with cotton pliers and the suture is cut between the knot and the tissue

c. Grasp the knot with cotton pliers and gently pull the suture out of the tissue

2. Removal of continuous sutures

a. Continuous sutures are placed from facial to lingual in an interproximal space and continued around the adjacent tooth to the next interproximal space

b. Removal is accomplished by cutting the suture between the knot and the tissue and the vertical loops of suture material, where it enters the tissue in each interproximal space, facial and lingual

c. Using cotton pliers, withdraw each strand by pulling on the portion that is wrapped around the buccal and lingual surface of each tooth

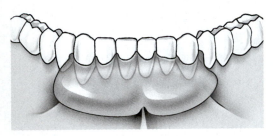

FIGURE 10-4 ■ Placement of Periodontal Dressing

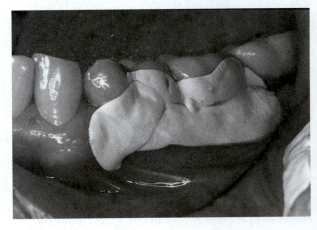

FIGURE 10-5 ■ Periodontal Dressing

XII. Dental Implants

  A. Patient selection—Factors include good oral hygiene, positive dental and medical histories including reasonable ability to heal, adequate bone for implant placement, and motivated patient

  B. Implant surgery—Usually accomplished in several phases with long periods of healing after each surgery before prosthesis is placed

  C. Implant success

  1. Osseointegration—Biological anchorage or contact that is established between implant surface and bone; bone forming in and around implant

  2. Clinical signs of success

  a. No clinical mobility

  b. Ability to bear load (have a functioning prosthesis)

  c. Comfortable

  d. Intact adjacent structures

  e. No evidence of peri-implant radiolucency

  f. Minimal loss of bone height

  D. Implant failure

  1. Recognition of implant failure—Lack of osseointegration

  a. Implant mobility

  b. Feeling of discomfort

  c. Peri-implant radiolucency

  d. Inability to support prosthesis

  2. Treatment—Remove implant

XIII. Periodontal Emergences

  A. Periodontal abscess—Localized, purulent inflammatory process

  1. Associated with periodontal pockets and furcation involvement

  2. Involves a blocked or occluded sulcus, preventing drainage of bacteria

  3. Can result in periodontal destruction

  a. Acute—Sudden onset may resolve quickly

  b. Chronic—Slow to develop, may be present for a long time, sometimes becomes acute

  4. Signs and symptoms

  a. Pain (more common with acute)

  b. Swelling of soft tissues

  c. Tenderness to percussion

  d. Tooth extruded from socket

  e. Mobility of affected tooth

5. Treatment

    a. Establish drainage at gingival margin of pocket or at point of swelling

    b. Use warm salt water rinses and antibiotics

    c. Eliminate pocket surgically

6. Differentiating between endodontic and periodontal abscess

    a. Endodontic abscess is an infection of the tooth pulp; tooth will be nonvital

    b. Periodontal abscess is associated with periodontal structures primarily, not pulp; tooth may be vital

B. Gingival abscess

    1. Acute localized infection at marginal gingiva or interdental papilla

    2. Evidence of purulent area in connective tissue

    3. Etiology—Wedged or embedded debris or food at gingival margin (e.g., popcorn hull)

    4. Not associated with periodontal disease

C. Pericoronitis

    1. Occurs at partially erupting or impacted tooth, often third molars; areas not easily cleaned where food or debris are wedged under gingival tissue

    2. Gingival tissue (operculum) partially covering erupting tooth creates environment for bacterial growth to occur

    3. Signs and symptoms

        a. Red, swollen gingival tissues at site of erupting tooth; swelling may extend to angle of jaw, ear, and cervical lymph nodes

        b. May be painful to touch

    4. Treatment

        a. Establish drainage

        b. Irrigate with saline, antimicrobial rinse, or warm salt water rinses

        c. Follow-up treatment may include tooth extraction or surgical removal of operculum

D. Acute necrotizing ulcerative gingivitis (ANUG)—Acute, destructive condition of gingival tissues

    1. Associated with presence of several microorganisms

    2. Not considered contagious

    3. Bacterial plaque biofilm is primary etiological factor—Host–parasite imbalance

    4. Contributing factors to development of ANUG—Stress, cigarette smoking, alcohol consumption, low socioeconomic status, poor nutrition, age, general debilitated state

    5. Additional factors contributing to ANUG—Calculus, operculum, overhanging margins, improper tooth contacts, malposed teeth, and food impaction

6. Signs and symptoms

    a. Sudden severe pain of teeth or gingiva, gingival bleeding (sometimes spontaneous), and fetid breath odor

    b. Ulcerated marginal gingiva and interdental papilla—Described as punched-out areas or craters

    c. Ulceration may occur on other soft tissues, including tongue and lips

    d. Evidence of fever, headache, loss of appetite, and lymphadenopathy

7. Treatment

    a. Remove debris as soon as possible to reduce risk of permanent loss of papilla

    b. Use ultrasonic instrumentation for both debridement and irrigation

    c. Emphasize plaque control and home care

    d. Use antibiotics, when indicated

    e. Schedule multiple treatment visits

E. Acute herpetic gingivostomatitis—An acute, viral infection of the oral mucosa; 7- to 10-day duration

  1. Etiology—Herpes simplex virus

  2. Signs and symptoms

    a. Clinical appearance of small yellow ulcers with raised, red margins

    b. May be present on tongue, gingiva, lips, buccal mucosa, palate, pharynx, and tonsils

    c. Sore mouth, often too sore to eat or drink

  3. Treatment

    a. Palliative; keep patient comfortable; use warm water rinses and soft diet

    b. Emphasize fluid intake and topical anesthetic rinses

XIV. Endpoint Objectives of Periodontal Therapy

A. Specific objectives

  1. Resolution of inflammation

    a. No bleeding on probing

    b. No suppuration

    c. Gingival contours—Color, texture, and form are within normal limits

    d. Gingival attachment is resistant to recurrent disease

B. Supportive periodontal treatment (SPT)

  1. Following definitive treatment and post-treatment evaluation, schedule patient for SPT at 3-month intervals

  2. SPT visit—Evaluate signs of disease activity (e.g., bleeding and/or suppuration on probing, increase in probing depths, and gingival atypia)

      3. Direct therapeutic application to sites reflecting recurrence of disease or periodontal breakdown

      4. Assess plaque control motivation

  C. Periodontal maintenance

      1. Once periodontal health has been established, goal of further care centers on maintaining periodontal health

      2. Without continued periodontal maintenance, there is little value in therapeutic periodontal care

XV. **Dental Conditions in the Periodontal Patient**

  A. Root caries

      1. Prevalence

         a. Incidence is increasing as population is keeping their teeth longer

         b. Once established, may progress rapidly

      2. Risk factors

         a. Periodontal disease—Because of exposed root surfaces

         b. Lack of fluoridated water

         c. Dry mouth (xerostomia)

         d. Oral hygiene deficits

         e. Cariogenic diet

      3. Etiology—*Actinomyces viscosus*

      4. Clinical detection

         a. Root caries color ranges from light yellow to dark brown/black

         b. Explorer will stick

         c. May be subgingival

      5. Prevention

         a. Fluoride therapy (including home fluoride regimen)

         b. Oral hygiene improvement

         c. Diet modification

  B. Dentin hypersensitivity

      1. Associated with periodontal disease because it frequently is related to exposed root surfaces

      2. Commonly seen in individuals who have periodontal disease or who have had treatment for periodontal disease; result of root surfaces open to the oral environment

      3. Most frequently found on facial surfaces of teeth at cervical margins

      4. Pain transmission

         a. Caused by mechanical, chemical, thermal, or bacterial stimuli to exposed dentinal tubules

b. Sweets, acids, sour substances, acidic plaque, temperature changes (especially cold), and drying or desiccation of exposed dentin can be painful

c. Pain is localized and sharp; usually disappears quickly when stimulus is removed

5. Hydrodynamic theory of hypersensitivity—Current theory

a. Dentinal tubules are open channels extending from pulp chamber

b. Tubules are fluid-filled and may have odontoblasts extending from pulp into tubule

c. Fluid within dentinal tubules flows both outward and inward depending on pressure variations in surrounding tissues

d. Rapid movement of fluid in open dentinal tubules may disrupt odontoblasts, eliciting transmission of pain-causing stimulus

e. Pain is detected by myelinated A-delta fibers in pulp

6. Contributing factors

a. Loss of tooth structure from occlusal wear, toothbrush abrasion, enamel erosion, and parafunctional habits

b. Exposure of root surface to oral environment because of gingival recession, aging, chronic periodontal disease, periodontal surgery, incorrect toothbrushing habits, and root surface preparation for dental restorations

7. Management—Related to covering, sealing, or blocking tubules because pain is related to open dentinal tubules; tubules can also close naturally

8. Numerous products are available with variable results

a. Active ingredients include potassium nitrate, sodium citrate, potassium oxalate, strontium chloride, and fluoride

b. Varnishes, resins, sealants, glass ionomers; composite restorations can be used

➤ PERFORMING PERIODONTAL PROCEDURES

I. Basic Instrument Design

A. Parts (Figure 10-6■)

1. Handle—Designed for holding instrument; identify instrument by design name and number stamped on handle; available in various weights, diameters, and surface textures

a. Weight—Hollow metal handle is lighter in weight than solid metal handle; increases tactile sensitivity, reduces hand fatigue, and helps prevent repetitive strain injury (RSI)

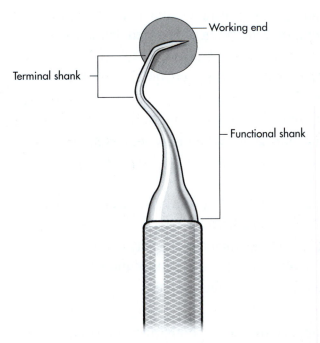

Working end

Terminal shank

Functional shank

FIGURE 10-6 ■ The functional shank is the portion of the instrument between the handle and working end. The terminal shank is adjacent to the blade.

    b. Diameter—Easier to control handle with a larger diameter; reduces muscle cramping and helps prevent RSI

    c. Surface texture—Easier to control in a wet environment if handle is knurled (serrated); helps prevent RSI

2. Working end—Performs function (work) of instrument; consists of face, back, lateral surfaces, and cutting edges; has three sections—Heel, middle, and tip (or toe)

3. Shank—Metal rod between handle and working end that extends instrument length

    a. Types

        (1) Simple—Designed for instrumentation of anterior teeth; shank is bent in one plane only

        (2) Complex—Designed for subgingival instrumentation of posterior teeth; shank is bent in two planes

        (3) Functional—Encompasses entire shank from working end to handle

            (a) Short—Accesses coronal surfaces of teeth

            (b) Long—Accesses coronal and root surfaces of teeth

        (4) Terminal (lower)—Section of shank nearest to working end; begins below working end and extends to first shank bend; it is an

important reference point when determining the correct working end for instrumentation

b. Flexibility—Determined by function of instrument

(1) Flexible—Provides most tactile information; needed for detection of subgingival calculus and removal of light calculus and endotoxins (e.g., explorers and area-specific curets such as "finishing" Graceys)

(2) Moderately flexible—Provides some tactile information; needed for removal of small or medium-sized calculus deposits (e.g., universal curets)

(3) Rigid—Provides little tactile information; needed for removal of large calculus deposits (e.g., sickle scalers and rigid curets)

B. Types

1. Mouth mirror—Assessment instrument

a. Functions

(1) Retracts patient's cheek or tongue for improved visibility and patient protection

(2) Provides indirect vision of surfaces that cannot be viewed directly

(3) Reflects light onto a dark area in mouth, indirect illumination

(4) Provides transillumination to reflect light (e.g., through an anterior tooth)

b. Description

(1) Working end is round

(2) Used in all phases of dental hygiene procedures

(3) Fogging is minimized by gently rubbing mirror against buccal mucosa or dipping in commercial mouth rinse

2. Explorer—Assessment instrument

a. Function—Provides superior tactile information in locating supragingival and subgingival calculus deposits, tooth surface irregularities and defects, overhanging margins and other defects in restorations, and decalcification and caries; available in a variety of designs

b. Description

(1) Fine, wirelike working end that terminates to a sharp point

(2) Types include Shepherd hook, straight, pigtail, cowhorn, Orban-type, and 11/12 (Figures 10-7■, 10-8■)

3. Periodontal probe—assessment instrument

a. Functions

(1) Assesses periodontal health

(2) Measures lesions and overjets

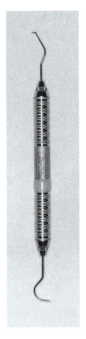

FIGURE 10-7 ■ Straight Explorer or Shepherd's Hook

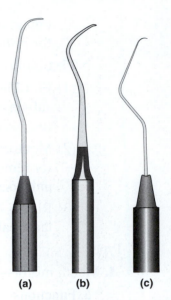

(a) **(b)** **(c)**

FIGURE 10-8 ■ Types of Calculus-Detecting Explorers: (a) 11/12; (b) Pigtailed or Cowhorn; (c) Orban-Type

b. Description—Blunt, rod-shaped working end marked in millimeter units

    (1) Calibrated—Straight probe is available in plastic or metal in several different designs and calibration patterns, color-coded styles, as well as computerized pressure-sensitive

        (a) Used to measure sulcus and pocket depths, recession, clinical attachment levels, and width of attached gingiva

        (b) Assesses consistency of gingival tissue

        (c) Evaluates presence of bleeding and suppuration (purulent exudate)

        (d) Measures other oral structures

    (2) Furcation—Curved probe (Nabers probe) is used to detect extent of attachment loss in furcated areas; extent of furcation is denoted as a classification, not a millimeter measurement

    (3) Examples (Figure 10-9■)—PSR probe (used for periodontal screening and recording), Marquis, UNM, Michigan O, Williams, Novatech series (right-angle tip) and Nordent PCL JB 2–4 (color coded)

4. Periodontal file

  a. Functions

    (1) Crushes large supragingival or subgingival calculus deposits

    (2) Roughens burnished calculus to facilitate deposit removal with another instrument

    (3) Also used to smooth margins of amalgam restorations

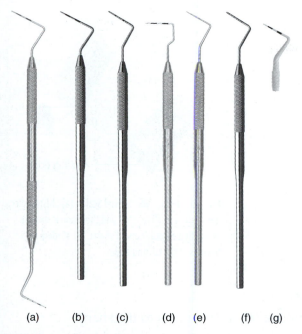

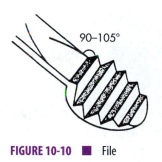

90–105°

FIGURE 10-10 ■ File

(a) (b) (c) (d) (e) (f) (g)

FIGURE 10-9 ■ Types of periodontal probes: (a) PSR (lower end); (b) Marquis; (c) UNC; (d) Novatech; (e) Michigan O; (f) Williams; (g) PCV 12 pt. (colorvue)
Source: Courtesy of Hu-Friedy Manufacturing Company

b. Description (Figure 10-10■)

    (1) Rigid shanked instrument with a working end that is thin in width and either rounded, oblong, or rectangular in shape

    (2) Has multiple straight-cutting edges that are at 90- to 105-degree angles to the shank

    (3) Used with a pull stroke

c. Designs

    (1) Paired working ends—Consists of four working ends that are needed to instrument all surfaces of a tooth—mesial, distal, facial, and lingual

    (2) Double-ended—Designed for use on facial/lingual surfaces or mesial/distal surfaces; each working end offers a single-surface application

d. Examples—Hirschfield 3/7, 5/11, 9/10 and Orban 10/11 and 12/13

5. Hoe

a. Functions

    (1) Used to remove large, heavy supragingival calculus

    (2) Subgingival use is limited by design (in current practice, sonic and ultrasonic scalers are generally used for this purpose)

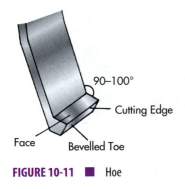

90–100°

Cutting Edge

Face   Bevelled Toe

FIGURE 10-11 ■ Hoe

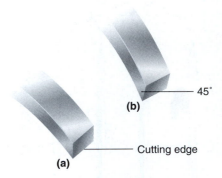

45°

(b)

Cutting edge

(a)

FIGURE 10-12 ■ Chisel Scaler. (a) Chisel scaler has a single cutting edge and the blade is continuous with a slightly curved shank. (b) 45-degree bevel is at the cutting edge.

  b. Description (Figure 10-11■)

   (1) Single cutting edge angled at 90–100 degrees to the shank

   (2) Designed like the periodontal file in that four working ends are needed to instrument each surface of a tooth (see Periodontal file)

   (3) Used with a pull stroke

 6. Chisel

  a. Functions—Used to dislodge heavy calculus, particularly from exposed proximal surfaces on mandibular anteriors; use is limited

  b. Description (Figure 10-12■)

   (1) Double-ended push instrument with either a straight or curved shank

   (2) Blade is continuous with shank

   (3) Cutting edge is formed with tip beveled at a 45-degree angle

   (4) Used only in a horizontal direction with a push stroke

 7. Sickle scaler

  a. Functions

   (1) Used to remove heavy supragingival calculus deposits from all aspects of tooth crown (facial, lingual, mesial, distal)

   (2) Design not recommended for subgingival use because of possible soft tissue trauma and excessive removal of cementum (Figure 10-13■)

  b. Description

   (1) Working end has pointed back and is triangular in cross section

   (2) Two cutting edges on each working end meet at a point called the tip

   (3) Cutting edges are at same level and may be straight or curved

   (4) Face is perpendicular (90-degree angle) to terminal shank

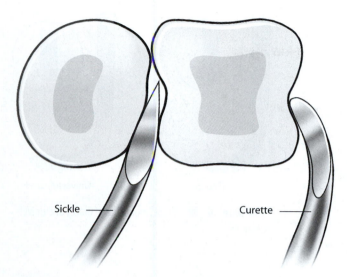

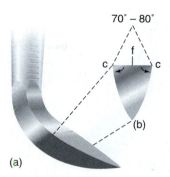

FIGURE 10-14 ■ Straight Sickle Scaler. (a) The straight blade converges to a point where the two cutting edges meet at the tip. (b) A cross section of the scaler shows the face, the two cutting edges, and the 70- to 80-degree internal angles. This type of sickle scaler is also known as the jacquette scaler.

FIGURE 10-13 ■ The triangular-shaped tip of a sickle scaler cannot adapt to subgingival root concavities.

(5) Straight-shank sickle (anterior instrument) is often single-ended because same end may be used on mesials and distals

(6) Bent-shank sickle may be used on anteriors and/or posteriors and is usually double-ended, with one end designed for mesials and other end for distals

c. Examples (Figures 10-14■ and 10-15■)

(1) Anterior sickle scalers—OD1, Jacquette-30, Jacquette-33, Towner-U15, Goldman-H6, Goldman-H7, H 6/7, Whiteside-2

(2) Posterior sickle scalers—Jacquette 14/15, Jacquette 31/32, Jacquette 34/35, Mecca 11/12, Ball 2/3, Catatonia 107/108, 204 SD, IPFW 204

8. Curet

a. Function—Used to remove deposits supragingivally and subgingivally on crown and root surfaces

b. Description

(1) Designed with a long or short, rigid or flexible, simple or complex, functional shank

(2) Designed with paired mirror-image working ends (available as one double-ended curet or a pair of single-ended curets)

(3) Working ends have rounded backs and are semicircular in cross section; curves upward toward a rounded toe

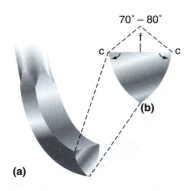

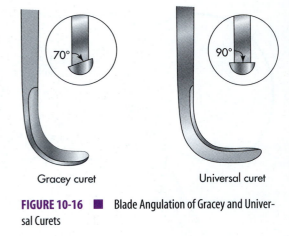

FIGURE 10-15 ■ Curved Sickle Scaler.
(a) The curved blade terminates to a point.
(b) A cross section shows the face and the two cutting edges formed where the lateral surfaces meet the face at 70- to 80-degree angles.

FIGURE 10-16 ■ Blade Angulation of Gracey and Universal Curets

c. Types (universal, area-specific, and finishing curets) (Figure 10-16■)

(1) Universal curet—Implies that one double-ended working end can be used on all anterior and posterior tooth surfaces

(a) Function—Designed to remove light or moderate supragingival and subgingival calculus

(b) Description (Figure 10-17■)—Lateral surfaces form two parallel cutting edges that curve upward toward rounded toe and are at the same level (cutting edge is not self-angulated)

i) Each working end has two cutting edges—Both cutting edges are used

ii) Face is perpendicular to terminal shank

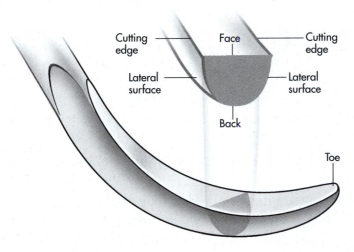

FIGURE 10-17 ■ Characteristics of a Universal Curette

      iii) Terminal shank is not parallel with handle

      iv) Functional shank designs vary in length and rigidity

(c) Examples—Columbia 2R/2L, 4R/4L, 13/14; Barnhart 1/2, 5/6; Younger-Good 7/8; Langer 1/2, 3/4, 5/6; Rule 3/4; Indiana University 13/14; HU 1/2; Bunting 5/6; Mallery 1/2

(d) Suggested applications

      i) Columbia 13/14—Works well in anterior areas or areas with slight to moderate probing depths

      ii) Columbia 4R/4L—Has longer terminal shank than Columbia 13/14; works well in deeper pockets in posterior areas

      iii) Columbia 2R/2L—Has longer terminal shank than Columbia 4R/4L and is ideal for use in deep facial or lingual pockets

(2) Area-specific curet (Table 10-1■)—Implies that a single area-specific curet can be applied only to certain tooth surfaces and areas of mouth

(a) Function

      i) Depending on the rigidity of shank, it is designed to remove light to moderate supragingival and subgingival calculus and endotoxins

      ii) Ideal for adapting to root morphology

TABLE 10-1 OTHER GRACEY CURETS	
Gracey 15/16 Curet	Modification of Gracey 11/12 for superior access to mesial surfaces of posterior teeth
Gracey 17/18 Curet	Modification/Gracey 13/14 with accentuated angles for superior access to distal surfaces of posterior teeth
Gracey Mesial-Distal Curet	Modification/combination of Graceys 11, 12, 13, and 14 on double-ended instruments; G11/14 and G12/13 allow clinician to complete all surfaces on either the facial or lingual aspect of a sextant without changing instruments
Gracey Prophy Series	Shorter and more rigid shank than the Standard series
Rigid Gracey Series	Standard length, but with a more rigid shank and working end
Hu-Friedy After-Five Series	Thinner working end; terminal shank is 3 mm longer than standard Gracey series
Hu-Friedy Mini-Five Series	Thinner working end shortened to half the length of standard Gracey series; terminal shank is also 3 mm longer than standard Gracey series

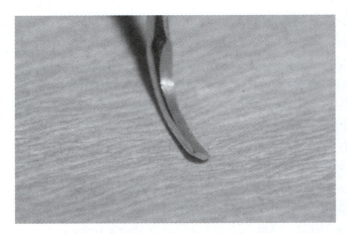

FIGURE 10-18 ■ The curved face tilts toward the tooth surface.

(b) Description (Figure 10-18■)—Lateral surfaces form two cutting edges that curve upward toward rounded toe

  i) Face is offset or tilted at a 60- to 70-degree angle to terminal shank and cutting edges are at different levels (cutting edge is self-angulated)

  ii) Only one cutting edge (lower, longer cutting edge) per working end is used

  iii) Designed with longer terminal shanks for access to middle- and apical-third of root

  iv) Functional shank is more complex and varies in length and rigidity

(c) Examples of area-specific curets—Standard Gracey series, Hu-Friedy After-Five Series, Hu-Friedy Mini-Five series, Hu-Friedy Vision Curvette series, Kramer-Nevins series, Turgeon series, and Nordent SC GR 1-2 MDC

(3) Finishing curet (Gracey)—Has flexible shank and is intended for light scaling

II. Basic Principles of Instrumentation

A. Grasp—Recommend modified pen grasp

B. Fulcrum (finger rest)—Acts as a support beam for hand and wrist to pivot on during instrumentation; common error in instrumentation technique is a weak fulcrum, resulting in poor stroke control and tissue trauma

  1. Intraoral

   a. Hold ring finger straight with tip resting on incisal, occlusal, or occlusolingual/occlusofacial line angles of tooth

   b. Ideal fulcrum is established on a stable tooth in the same arch and as close as possible to tooth being instrumented (1–4 teeth away)

2. Advanced

    a. Use if basic intraoral fulcrum is not effective or possible

    b. Useful in achieving parallelism for deep pocket access or when edentulous areas preclude use of basic fulcrum

    c. Includes extraoral fulcrum on chin or cheek, cross-arch fulcrum, opposite-arch fulcrum, modified intraoral fulcrum, finger-on-finger fulcrum, piggy-back fulcrum, and stabilized fulcrum

C. Adaptation—Place lead third (toe) of cutting edge in contact with tooth surface in preparation for stroke, roll instrument to adapt to curved tooth surfaces

D. Angulation (Figure 10-19■)

  1. Establish correct angle between instrument face and tooth surface (< 90-degree angle and > 45-degree angle)

  2. Ideal angulation for scaling is 60–80 degrees

  3. Incorrect angulation > 90 degrees may result in trauma to epithelial lining of pocket

  4. Incorrect angulation of < 45 degrees may result in burnished calculus deposits

E. Insertion (Figure 10-19)

  1. Insert face at a 0-degree angulation to tooth surface until working end is positioned at base of pocket

  2. Establish a 60- to 80-degree face-to-tooth angulation before initiating a stroke

F. Lateral pressure—Use index finger or thumb to press inward against handle to engage cutting edge and apply pressure to tooth before and during activation of stroke

G. Motion activation

  1. Move instrument to produce an oblique, circumferential (horizontal), or vertical stroke

  2. Hand, wrist, and arm should move as a single unit and rotate to produce each stroke

  3. Avoid fatiguing finger-powered strokes

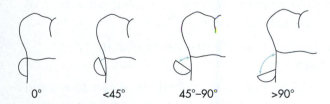

0°   <45°   45°–90°   >90°

FIGURE 10-19 ■ Scaling should be done by adapting the lower 1/3 of the instrument, inserted subgingivally by closing the blade (face toward the tooth at 0 degrees), and the angle between the face of the blade and the tooth surface should be between 45 and 90 degrees.

H. Handle roll

    1. Roll instrument handle between and during strokes, as strokes progress around tooth to reestablish correct adaptation of leading third of cutting edge to tooth

    2. This is particularly important at line angles, depressions, furcations, and root concavities

I. Assessment stroke (exploratory or placement stroke)

    1. Use relaxed grasp and feather-light pressure

    2. Apply many overlapping, long, flowing, sweeping strokes

    3. Apply multidirectional strokes and cover entire root surface to detect calculus, overhanging restorations, and other tooth surface irregularities

    4. Use with explorers, curets, thin sonic, and ultrasonic tips

    5. Perform with curets, sonic, and ultrasonic instruments during periodontal debridement to determine if working strokes have been successful in deposit removal

    6. Use explorer to evaluate for complete removal of deposits

J. Working stroke—Use appropriate pressure and stroke to debride tooth surfaces

    1. Calculus removal work stroke—Use with sickle scalers, curets, sonic and ultrasonic tips to remove calculus deposits

        a. Hand-activated instruments—Use firm pressure and limited short, controlled, scraping, pull strokes beginning beneath deposit and proceeding coronally

        b. Sonic and ultrasonic instruments—Use light pressure and sweeping, brushlike push–pull strokes in an erasing motion

    2. Root surface debridement work stroke (formerly called root planing)—Use with area-specific curets and slim sonic and ultrasonic tips to remove residual calculus granules and endotoxins from root surfaces

        a. Apply long multidirectional, controlled overlapping strokes (by using a vertical stroke series followed by oblique and circumferential series) with very light even pressure

        b. Work in long, narrow sections or tracts beginning each stroke at base of pocket and ending at cementoenamel junction (CEJ)

        c. Avoid firm pressure and too many strokes that may result in unnecessary removal of cementum

        d. Know pocket topography and root anatomy (locations of furcations and root concavities) to help facilitate thorough root surface debridement

        e. Refer to comprehensive periodontal charting and radiographs often during instrumentation

III. Use of Periodontal Probe

A. Sulcus and pocket depth measurement—Measure distance, in millimeters, from base of pocket to gingival margin

    1. Use basic probing technique with a calibrated probe

    2. Position probe parallel to long axis of tooth

    3. Gently insert probe to base of pocket

    4. Work around entire circumference of tooth in strokes 1–2 mm apart

    5. Chart six measurements per tooth (three depths on facial aspect and three on lingual aspect), recording deepest measurement in each area

    6. Slant probe slightly under contact to assess interdental col area

B. Extent of inflammation—Evaluate presence of bleeding and/or purulent exudate (suppuration) on probing

C. Calculus detection—Use probe to detect location of calculus deposits

D. Recession—Use calibrated probe to measure distance from gingival margin to exposed CEJ

E. Clinical attachment level (attachment level; probed level of attachment)

    1. Use calibrated probe to measure distance from CEJ to junctional epithelium

    2. Best clinical indicator of bone support because bone level is approximately 2 mm apical to junctional epithelium

    3. Methods used to determine attachment level

        a. Gingival margin is at CEJ—Measure distance from base of pocket to CEJ

        b. Gingival margin is receded apically to CEJ—Measure distance from base of pocket to CEJ

        c. Gingival margin is 1 mm or greater coronal to CEJ—Measure distance from base of pocket to gingival margin (overall measurement), then measure distance from CEJ to gingival margin and subtract from overall measurement

F. Width of attached gingiva—Determine by measuring with a calibrated probe

    1. On external surface of gingiva, measure distance from gingival margin to mucogingival junction to obtain total width of gingiva

    2. Insert probe into sulcus and measure probing depth

    3. Subtract probing depth from total width of gingiva

G. Gingival consistency—Determine by placing length of calibrated probe against the free gingiva and applying gentle pressure

    1. Slight indentation and blanching of tissue will quickly disappear if it is healthy

    2. Tissue will remain blanched and indented for a few seconds if edematous

    3. Tissue will not exhibit blanching and indentation if fibrotic

H. Size of lesions or deviations—Use calibrated probe to measure and document width, length, height, or depth of lesion, or other deviation from normal

I. Classification of furcation involvement

    1. Use furcation probe (Nabers probe) to detect and classify extent of furcation involvement

    2. Attempt insertion of probe into buccal, lingual, mesial, and distal furcations to determine extent of bone loss and classify

    3. Classifications

        a. Class I: Slight bone loss in furcation area; furcation concavity can be detected but probe cannot be inserted into furcation

        b. Class II: Partial bone loss in furcation area; furcation probe can be inserted into furcation but does not pass through it

        c. Class III: Complete bone loss in furcation area; furcation probe passes between roots completely through furcation

        d. Class IV: Same as Class III but furcation is exposed clinically due to gingival recession

J. Assessing mobility

    1. Horizontal mobility

        a. Place blunt handle ends of two single-ended instruments (e.g., mirror and probe) to opposite sides of each tooth

        b. Apply alternating pressure from the facial and lingual aspects and assess facial–lingual mobility

    2. Vertical mobility—Apply vertical pressure with end of blunt handle to occlusal or incisal

    3. Classifications

        a. N = normal physiological mobility (all teeth exhibit slight normal mobility)

        b. Grade I = slight mobility; up to 1 mm horizontal displacement in facial–lingual direction

        c. Grade II = moderate mobility; > 1 mm horizontal displacement in facial–lingual direction

        d. Grade III = severe mobility; > 1 mm displacement in both vertical and horizontal directions

IV. Use of Explorer

A. Shepherd hook and straight explorers—Each is an unpaired explorer with strong rigid shank ideally suited for caries detection in the following areas:

    1. Pit and fissures—Explore posterior occlusal surfaces and anterior lingual cingulum areas

    2. Smooth surfaces—Explore facial, lingual, and proximal aspects of crowns

    3. Root surfaces caries—Explore exposed roots commonly found in geriatric patients owing to gingival recession

    4. Recurrent decay—Explore along restorative margins

B. Orban-type explorer—Unpaired explorer best suited for use in deep, narrow pockets of anterior teeth or facial and lingual surfaces of posterior teeth

C. 11/12 Explorer—Paired explorer with mirror-image working ends

  1. Description—Universal instrument

    a. Adapts to all anterior and posterior surfaces

    b. Well suited to adapt in deep pockets, especially on proximal surfaces of posterior teeth and in other limited-access areas owing to its long, complex functional shank

  2. Determine correct working end as follows

    a. Use on anterior teeth

      (1) Begin with a stable fulcrum

      (2) Position terminal (lower) shank parallel to long axis of anterior tooth surface and adapt working end to tooth

      (3) Tip of correct working end will curve toward tooth

      (4) Use one working end on all surfaces toward operator from a given aspect (facial or lingual); opposite end is used on all surfaces away from operator from the same aspect (facial or lingual)

    b. Use on posterior teeth

      (1) Correct working end is established when terminal (lower) shank is parallel to proximal surface

      (2) Use one working end on distobuccal, buccal, and mesiobuccal surfaces of each tooth in a sextant; opposite working end is used on distolingual, lingual, and mesiolingual surfaces of teeth in same sextant

D. Pigtail and cowhorn explorers

  1. Each is paired with mirror-image working ends and is a universal instrument, adapting to all anterior and posterior surfaces

  2. Best suited for use in normal sulci or shallow pockets

  3. Operated same as 11/12 explorer

V. Use of Sickle Scaler

A. Use of anterior sickle (single-ended)

  1. Design—Two cutting edges on a single working end; one cutting edge is used on all surfaces toward operator, opposite cutting edge on same working end is used on all surfaces away from operator

  2. Strokes (application)

    a. Begin with stable fulcrum at midline on facial or lingual surface of tooth

    b. Adapt leading third of cutting edge

    c. Establish 60- to 80-degree face-to-tooth surface angulation

   d. Activate pull strokes working toward proximal surface

B. Use of posterior sickle (double-ended)

   1. Design—Two cutting edges per working end

      a. Use one cutting edge from distofacial line angle to just past center of distal surface; use opposite cutting edge of same working end from distofacial line angle to just past center of mesial surface

      b. Use both cutting edges of one working end on entire facial aspect of the posterior sextant; use the two cutting edges of opposite working end on the entire lingual aspect of the same sextant

   2. Strokes (application)

      a. Begin with stable fulcrum and position terminal shank parallel to the long axis of tooth and adapt working end to proximal surface

      b. Adapt correct cutting edge

      c. Begin strokes at distofacial line angle with tip pointed distally

      d. Adapt leading third of cutting edge

      e. Establish 60- to 80-degree face-to-tooth surface angulation

      f. Activate pull strokes to just past center of distal surface

      g. Lift and turn instrument so leading third of opposite cutting edge of same working end is adapted at distofacial line angle with tip pointed mesially

      h. Establish 60- to 80-degree face-to-tooth surface angulation

      i. Activate oblique strokes to just past center of mesial surface

VI. Use of Universal Curets—One double-ended universal curet can be applied to all anterior and posterior tooth surfaces; each working end has two cutting edges

   A. Use of universal curet on anterior surfaces

      1. Strokes (application)

         a. Begin with stable fulcrum and position terminal (lower) shank parallel to long axis of tooth and adapt working end

         b. Establish correct cutting edge, accomplished when instrument face tilts toward tooth

         c. Use one working end on all surfaces toward operator and opposite working end on all surfaces away from operator

         d. Adapt leading third of cutting edge

         e. Insert at midline on facial or lingual surface of tooth

         f. Establish 60- to 80-degree face-to-tooth surface angulation

         g. Activate pull strokes working toward proximal surface

   B. Use of universal curet on posterior surfaces—Technique is same as posterior sickle scaler

VII. Use of Area-Specific Curets—Use only one cutting edge (lower, longer cutting edge) on each working end

    A. Use of an area-specific curet on anterior surfaces

        1. Strokes (application)

          a. Select one double-ended, area-specific curet appropriate for anterior teeth

          b. Begin with stable fulcrum and position terminal shank parallel to anterior tooth and adapt a working end

          c. Establish correct working end (face of blade will tilt toward tooth)

          d. Use one working end on all surfaces toward operator; use opposite working end on all surfaces away from operator

          e. Adapt leading third of lower cutting edge

          f. Insert at midline on facial or lingual surface of tooth

          g. Establish 60- to 80-degree face-to-tooth surface angulation

          h. Activate pull strokes working toward proximal surface

    B. Use of area-specific curet on posterior surfaces

        1. Strokes (application)

          a. Select curet appropriate for surface (e.g., Gracey 13 or 14 for distal surface, Gracey 11 or 12 for mesial surface)

          b. Adapt lower cutting edge to a proximal surface—Correct curet and cutting edge are adapted when terminal shank is parallel to proximal surface

          c. Insert by adapting leading third of lower cutting edge to tooth surface at angles to ensure overlapping strokes

          d. Establish 60- to 80-degree face-to-tooth surface angulation and activate pull strokes across surface—Mesial curets can be used from distofacial or distolingual angle to midline of mesial surface

          e. Use at least four area-specific curets (e.g., Gracey 11, 12, 13, and 14) or two double-ended Gracey curets (e.g., Gracey 11/12 and 13/14) to complete facial and lingual aspects of a posterior sextant

          f. Debride each root as if it were a single-rooted tooth, if furcation involvement is present

VIII. Paradigm Shift in Nonsurgical Periodontal Therapy

    A. Old paradigm includes scaling and root planing

        1. Treatment objectives

          a. Complete mechanical removal of plaque, calculus, and cementum

          b. Achieve hard, glassy, smooth root surfaces

          c. Promote effective daily plaque control by patient

2. Instrumentation

    a. Scaling—Use firm pressure with hand-activated instruments for calculus removal

    b. Root planing—Use moderate to firm pressure with hand-activated instruments to remove residual calculus and necrotic, altered cementum

    c. Ultrasonic and sonic instrumentation—Use of hand-activated instrumentation preferred over ultrasonic and sonic instrumentation; concept that ultrasonic or sonic instrumentation must be followed by root planing with hand instruments for complete removal of deposits and altered cementum

3. Misconceptions

    a. Belief that endotoxins are firmly bound and absorbed into cementum; therefore this "altered" cementum and all residual calculus must be eliminated with extensive root planing before healing can occur

    b. Removal of cementum is an essential component of nonsurgical periodontal therapy

    c. Evaluate success of therapy immediately following instrumentation; based on calculus removal and attainment of smooth root surfaces

B. New paradigm involves periodontal debridement

  1. Treatment objectives

    a. Establish an environment favorable to periodontal health and maintenance

    b. Mechanically remove all detectable plaque and plaque-retentive factors such as calculus deposits

    c. Mechanically remove endotoxins from root surfaces (specifically complex lipopolysaccharides [LPS] found in cell walls of gram-negative bacteria)

    d. Facilitate shift in oral flora from disease-related to health-related organisms

    e. Stimulate patient's immune response

    f. Promote effective daily plaque control

    g. Reevaluate healing response after initial therapy to identify areas of persistent inflammation that may need additional nonsurgical treatment; determine whether surgical treatment is necessary

    h. Stop progress of disease and allow for tissue healing

    i. Institute maintenance program to maintain periodontal health

  2. Instrumentation

    a. Supragingival and subgingival debridement—Use appropriate pressure with hand-activated instruments to remove the type of calculus present

    b. Root surface debridement

       (1) Use light, overlapping strokes with hand-activated or power-driven instruments for removal of all plaque and endotoxins (LPS) from entire root surface

       (2) Root surface debridement does NOT include purposeful and aggressive cementum removal

       (3) Cementum is intentionally conserved

    c. Ultrasonic and sonic instrumentation

       (1) As a result of advances in ultrasonic tip design and a new approach to periodontal therapy, ultrasonic instrumentation is no longer restricted to supplemental role of gross calculus removal

       (2) Primary role in periodontal instrumentation since the late 1980s

       (3) Modern units with modified tips have proven equally effective as hand scaling in periodontal debridement

       (4) Some clinical research suggests ultrasonics may be more effective than hand-activated instruments in deep pockets and furcations (majority of practitioners, however, continue to rely on hand instrumentation)

3. Antimicrobial adjuncts—Use antimicrobial agents and antibiotics as needed to control disease (e.g., use of antimicrobial irrigation devices and/or rinses, antimicrobial solution vs. water in ultrasonic unit, systemic antibiotics, and tetracycline fibers)

4. Assessment of host response—Assess factors influencing immune response (e.g., neutrophil deficiencies, smoking, pregnancy, medications, diabetes and other systemic illnesses)

5. New concepts

    a. Complete calculus removal is extremely challenging, especially in deeper pockets

    b. Healing can occur in spite of residual calculus

    c. Endotoxins are not incorporated into cementum and do not "alter" cementum; they loosely adhere to cementum and are easily removed

    d. Excessive removal of cementum is not necessary and may be detrimental to the periodontium; therefore, debridement techniques should not include intentional removal of cementum

    e. Key to successful treatment involves restoration of delicate balance between oral flora and host immune response

    f. Success of treatment is *not* evaluated by root smoothness, but is determined by absence of inflammation and infection, healing and repair of damaged periodontal tissues, and cessation of progress of periodontal disease

IX. Power-Driven Scalers

A. Involve a rapidly vibrating water-cooled tip that fractures and dislodges calculus deposits and flushes debris from pockets

B. Types—Units are classified as ultrasonic or sonic

    1. Ultrasonic instruments (Figure 10-20■)

        a. Magnetostrictive (Figure 10-21■)

            (1) Description of unit

                (a) Houses electric generator in a portable unit with power and water adjustment controls

                (b) Includes handpiece with a variety of insert (tip) designs (Figure 10-22■)

                (c) Connects to electrical and water outlets

                (d) Activates power by using foot control

            (2) Mechanism of action

                (a) Converts electrical energy into mechanical energy in the form of vibrations

                (b) Electrical current creates a magnetic field and expansion and contraction of metal stacks in handpiece insert; causes vibration of tip

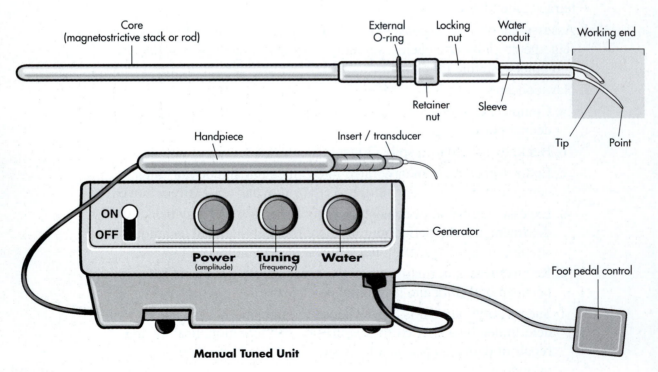

Manual Tuned Unit

FIGURE 10-20 ■ Parts of Ultrasonic Unit

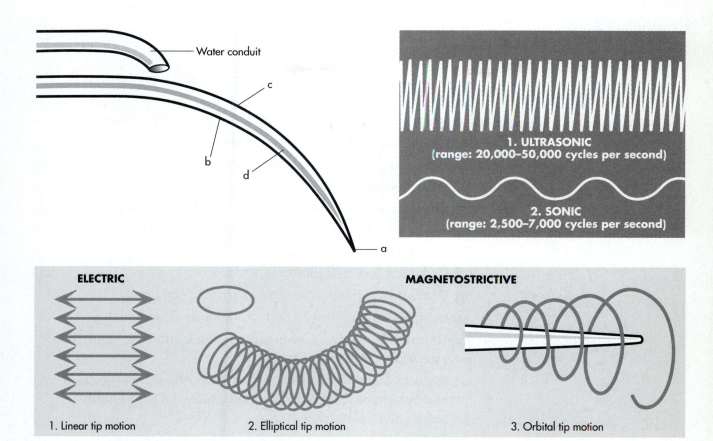

FIGURE 10-21 ■ Magnetostrictive Tips

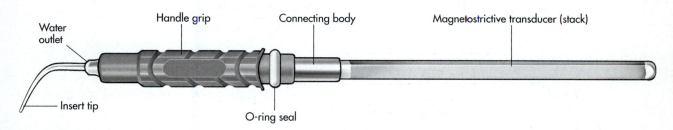

FIGURE 10-22 ■ Components of a Magnetostrictive Unit

(c) Generates heat; therefore water flow through tip serves as coolant and water lavage

(3) Vibrations—Range from 25,000 to 35,000 cycles/second

(4) Tip (insert)—Moves in elliptical pattern; all four surfaces of tip are active, which permits debridement with the most easily adapted tip surface (back, sides, or front)

   b. Piezoelectric (piezoceramic)

   (1) Description of unit

      (a) Houses electric generator in a portable unit with power and water adjustment controls

      (b) Includes handpiece with a variety of insert (tip) designs

      (c) Connects to electrical and water outlets

      (d) Activates power by using foot control

   (2) Mechanism of action

      (a) Converts electrical energy into mechanical energy in the form of vibrations via quartz or metal alloy crystal transducer

      (b) Produces no magnetic field

      (c) Generates less heat than magnetostrictive types

      (d) Water flow through tip serves as coolant and lavage

   (3) Vibrations—Range from 25,000 to 50,000 cycles/second

   (4) Tip (insert)—Moves in a linear pattern (back and forth); only two surfaces of tip (both sides) are active

      (a) Reduces hammering through linear movement, but limits number of active surfaces; thus adaptation of tip-to-tooth morphology is restricted

      (b) Use of tip-tightening and loosening tool is necessary

2. Sonic instruments

   a. Description—Small, air-driven scaler handpiece that attaches directly to dental unit

   (1) Screw working tips onto handpiece

   (2) Turn water switch of dental unit to ON

   (3) Activate power by using dental unit rheostat

   b. Mechanism of action

   (1) Driven by compressed air rather than electrical current

   (2) Produces vibrations by air pressure passing over metal rod contained within handpiece

   (3) Generates no heat

   (4) Reduces frictional heat at tip-to-tooth interface and provides water lavage with water coolant

   c. Vibrations—Ranges from 2,000 to 6,300 cycles/second; slower rate of vibration results in lowered capacity for heavy calculus removal; light to moderate calculus can be effectively removed

   d. Tip

   (1) Movement of tip is elliptical or orbital

(2) All four surfaces of tip are active

(3) Requires use of tip-loosening tool

C. Advantages of ultrasonic and sonic instrumentation

   1. Modified tip designs—As effective as hand-activated instrumentation for periodontal debridement

     a. Resemble periodontal probe, thinner in diameter than standard ultrasonic and sonic tips, and are significantly smaller than hand-activated curets

     b. Provide greater tactile sensitivity and maximum access to deep, narrow pockets and superior adaptation to root anatomy including furcations and root concavities (standard Gracey curets are too large to enter 50% of all molar furcations)

     c. Inserts easily beneath tight gingival margins

     d. Removes less cementum than standard ultrasonic tips or hand-activated instruments and provides more conservative approach to periodontal therapy

   2. Less soft tissue trauma—Tips having no cutting edge; results in faster healing rates

   3. Flushing action (water lavage)

     a. Penetrates to base of pockets and flushes out blood and loosened debris (plaque, calculus, endotoxins)

     b. Improves visibility during instrumentation

     c. Provides antibacterial effect through acoustic streaming and cavitation

       (1) Acoustic streaming—Continuous stream of water creates pressure within confines of pocket and removes bacteria from pockets; gram-negative motile rods are particularly sensitive to acoustic streaming

       (2) Cavitation—Spray of tiny bubbles is released at instrument tip; bubbles collapse and produce shock waves referred to as cavitation, which tears apart bacterial cell walls at treatment site; promotes flushing of pocket debris

   4. Reduces instrumentation time—Removes heavy calculus and stain in less time than with hand-instrumentation

   5. Increases patient comfort—Reduces instrumentation pressure and time, which is less fatiguing for patient

   6. Reduces operator fatigue—Decreases effort in removing heavy calculus and stain; offers a lighter grasp and pressure than with hand instrumentation

   7. May reduce chance of injury to clinician because tips do not have cutting edges

   8. Overhang removal—Special tips are available for safe, effective removal of amalgam overhangs

9. Cement removal—Accomplishes removal of excess crown, bridge, or orthodontic cement

D. Disadvantages of ultrasonic and sonic instrumentation

   1. Aerosol production

     a. Releases oral microorganisms, blood, saliva, and debris into air in form of an aerosol

     b. Can be minimized through

       (1) Using antimicrobial pretreatment mouth rinse

       (2) Positioning patient properly (supine with head turned to side)

       (3) Using high-volume evacuation

       (4) Cupping cheeks or lips for water containment

       (5) Reducing water flow slightly

       (6) Using focused-spray ultrasonic inserts

   2. Impeded visibility from water spray

     a. Problem can be minimized by

       (1) Keeping mirror face thoroughly wet

       (2) Using high-volume evacuation

       (3) Reducing water flow slightly

   3. Contraindications for some patients—Use is not recommended on patients with any of the following conditions

     a. Communicable diseases that can be transmitted via aerosols (e.g., tuberculosis, hepatitis, strep throat, flu, respiratory infections)

     b. Unshielded cardiac pacemaker—Magnetostrictive ultrasonic instruments should not be used on or near these patients

     c. High susceptibility to infection—Includes patients who are debilitated, have organ transplants, uncontrolled diabetes, or immunosuppression from disease or chemotherapy

     d. Respiratory or pulmonary disease or difficulty in breathing (e.g., asthma, emphysema, cystic fibrosis, mouth breathing)—Because of high infection risk and danger of aspiration of bacterial plaque

     e. Difficulty in swallowing or compromised gag reflex (e.g., muscular dystrophy, paralysis, multiple sclerosis)

     f. Young age—Primary and newly erupted teeth have large pulp chambers that are more susceptible to injury from vibrations and heat from ultrasonic instruments

     g. Certain dental conditions

       (1) Avoid use on demineralized tooth surfaces, dentinal hypersensitivity, porcelain crowns, laminate veneers, composite resin restorations, and titanium implant abutments

   (2) Amalgam and gold restorations may also be potentially damaged

   (3) Avoid close and prolonged contact with restorations

E. Treatment modifications for contraindications from dental conditions

 1. Use plastic ultrasonic and sonic tips on titanium implant abutments

 2. Reduce volume of water on magnetostrictive systems on patients sensitive to cold water—Warmer water increases patient comfort

 3. Use dentin desensitizing treatments or local anesthestic for sensitive patients who need ultrasonic instrumentation

F. Armamentarium

 1. Types of tips (inserts)

  a. Sonic tips are available in sickle, universal, and probe-shaped designs

  b. Ultrasonic tips are available in a wide variety of designs resembling periodontal probes, chisel scalers, sickle scalers, and curets, as well as a ball-ended furcation and concavity design

 2. Tip selection

  a. Select larger, stronger standard tips for heavy or tenacious calculus removal

  b. Select modified thin tips for deplaquing and removing light to moderate calculus and endotoxins—Thin tips are available in "straight" or "right and left" curved designs resembling a furcation probe

   (1) Modified (thin) straight tip designs—Used primarily for preventive care and deplaquing; thin straight tips can be used on any surface in any quadrant and are well suited for patients with case type I gingivitis, exhibiting 3–4 mm gingival pockets with bleeding and inflammation, and minimal to no bone loss

   (2) Modified (thin) curved right and left tip designs—Well suited for negotiating periodontal pockets > 4 mm deep; use for instrumenting periodontal case types II, III, and IV

    (a) Right tip is designed for use on all surfaces on mandibular right facial, mandibular left lingual, maxillary right lingual, and maxillary left facial

    (b) Left tip is designed for use on all surfaces on mandibular right lingual, mandibular left facial, maxillary right facial, and maxillary left lingual

    (c) Both right and left tips are needed to completely instrument a quadrant

 3. Work area—Use of barriers, surface disinfection, and laminar airflow systems are particularly important because of aerosol production

 4. Operator protection

  a. Wear gown with high neck and long sleeves

b. Cover hair

c. Wear high bacterial filtration efficiency (HBFE) face mask, protective eyewear, face shield, and gloves; change face mask every 20 minutes in an aerosol-producing environment to prevent moisture penetration

5. Patient protection

a. Drape patient with plastic drape, towel or bib, and tissues

b. Place protective eyewear and cover hair

c. Request patient to turn off hearing aid(s)

G. Ultrasonic procedures

1. Flush water lines—Connect sterilized ultrasonic handpiece to connector tubing; flush over sink for 5 minutes at beginning of day and for 3 minutes between patients

2. Select tip(s)—Base selection of tip shape on patient's health or disease status, root anatomy (including furcations and concavities), and type and location of deposits to be removed

3. Insert tip into ultrasonic handpiece—Hold handpiece upright and fill with water; release foot pedal and insert sterilized tip until it snaps into place (process must be repeated each time tip is changed)

4. Adjust frequency, water, and power settings—Make adjustments while holding tip over sink; correct settings ensure maximum instrument efficiency and comfort for operator and patient

a. Frequency—Involves number of cycles per second (cps)

(1) Controls speed of movement of tip—Higher the frequency, faster the vibration and increased ability to remove tenacious deposits (more heat is also generated at higher frequencies)

(2) Units may have either manual or automatic frequency control (manual tuning or autotuning)

(a) Manual tuning units—Require frequency adjustments for each tip

(b) Tuning frequency also controls pattern of water spray from tip

(c) Unit is correctly tuned when a fine mist with a rapid drip is produced at tip—obtained by adjusting power setting

b. Water setting

(1) Adjust water volume so a maximum mist or "halo" surrounds the tip with no excessive dripping of water; once set, water control needs little adjustment

(2) Deliver water coolant to tip through internal or external water supply

(3) Maintain water stream directly over tip; insufficient water can result in instrument overheating and damage to dental pulp

       (4) Use antimicrobial solution in place of water irrigation, when indicated and if unit permits

   c. Power (length of stroke [amplitude])—Controls distance tip travels in a single vibration; higher the power, longer the stroke, and greater the "chipping" action of tip

       (1) Higher power settings—Increase deposit removal ability and are best suited for initial debridement of moderate to heavy calculus or tenacious deposits using general-purpose rigid tips; greater damage to tooth surfaces is associated with higher power settings

       (2) Low to medium power settings—Appropriate for sulcular and pocket debridement and light instrumentation using modified thin tips; use of low power with smaller, shorter strokes are needed for root surface debridement

       (3) Basic power setting principle—Avoid high settings; with thinner tip, lower the power setting needed; use lowest power setting possible at which a particular tip functions properly

       (4) Power boost feature—Some units have a manual or automatic feature that can override manual power settings to temporarily boost power as needed

5. Position patient in supine position—Turn patient's head to right while instrumenting treatment areas on patient's right side and left while instrumenting treatment areas on left side

6. Position high-speed suction—Place on lowest side where water pools; operator working alone may link saliva ejector to high-speed suction and request patient's assistance with suctioning

7. Establish grasp and fulcrum—Use light, relaxed pen or modified pen grasp with light intraoral or extraoral fulcrum

8. Activate tip—Position tip near tooth surface and activate tip before adaptation and insertion

9. Select active tip surface—Use active tip surface that best conforms to tooth surface being instrumented; back and sides of tip are primarily used

10. Adapt tip to tooth (Figure 10-23■)—Adapt last several millimeters of an active tip surface

   a. Direct tip apically with length parallel to long axis of tooth or at no more than a 15-degree angle with tooth surface (similar to placement of a periodontal probe)

   b. Utilize convex curvature of back of tip in furcation anatomy

   c. Direct point of tip away from tooth and toward tissue (opposite of hand instrumentation principles); *never* use point of tip on tooth surfaces— dull point may still damage tooth structure

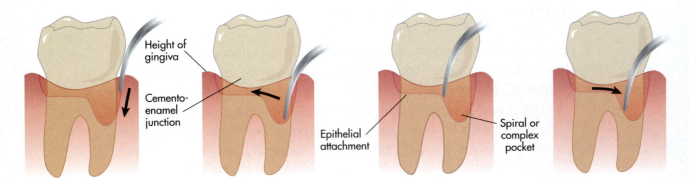

FIGURE 10-23 ■ Using Ultrasonic Tip to Debride in Deep Pocket

    d. Slant tip or assume a perpendicular relationship to long axis of tooth when instrumenting proximal surface to ensure adequate coverage under contact

11. Plan sequence—Review location of calculus with an explorer; plan systematic sequence to minimize number of times tips must be changed

12. Activate strokes—Use light overlapping strokes in sweeping or erasing-type motion

    a. Keep tip in constant motion in continuous looping pattern (avoid using heavy pressure that can damage or remove tooth structure)

    b. Apply multidirectional strokes to cover entire root surface

    c. Release foot pedal to aid in water control or to allow patient a brief rest

13. Evaluate

    a. Periodically explore/evaluate debrided areas with inactive tip

    b. Evaluate a completed quadrant or sextant with explorer

H. Sonic procedures

1. Flush water lines—Switch dental unit water to ON position; hold dental handpiece line over sink and activate a steady stream of water for 5 minutes at beginning of day and for 1 minute between patients to flush system

2. Connect sterilized sonic handpiece to dental unit line and turn dental unit water OFF

3. Insert sterilized sonic tip—Hand-tighten tip (be careful of sharp point)

    a. Do not tighten tip with sonic handpiece wrench

    b. Lock tip onto handpiece by stepping on dental unit rheostat

    c. Turn dental unit water back ON

4. Adjust water

    a. Hold handpiece tip over sink in a vertical position

    b. Activate power with dental unit rheostat

    c. Adjust dental unit water control until fine mist appears at tip

  5. Establish patient position, clinician's grasp and fulcrum, adaptation and instrumentation technique—Similar to those for an ultrasonic instrument (see steps 5–13 on pp. 795–796)

  6. Change tips—Position handpiece horizontally over sink

    a. Remove tip with sonic handpiece wrench while activating rheostat

    b. Select new tip, hand-tighten, and activate rheostat to lock into place

X. Gingival Curettage—Involves debriding soft tissue wall of periodontal pocket

A. Inadvertent (incidental) curettage—Unintentional (accidental) removal of soft tissue lining of periodontal pocket with hand or ultrasonic instruments during normal subgingival instrumentation; different from intentional curettage

B. Intentional curettage

  1. Description

    a. Deliberate removal of diseased soft tissue lining of periodontal pocket

    b. Includes removal of junctional and pocket epithelium and immediate subadjacent connective tissue

    c. Accomplished with sharp hand-activated curet, ultrasonic instrument, or with use of chemicals

  2. Rationale

    a. May be included after periodontal instrumentation in attempt to promote pocket reduction through tissue shrinkage and new connective tissue attachment

    b. Necessity for and additional benefits of curettage are currently highly questioned

  3. Procedure with hand-activated curet

    a. Anesthetize soft tissues

    b. Activate a sharp curet with face of blade at a 70-degree angle to soft tissue pocket wall

    c. Apply digital pressure to outer surface of facial or lingual gingiva to provide support against instrument; move along pocket wall to remove epithelial lining

  4. Post-treatment procedures

    a. Irrigate site with normal saline solution

    b. Apply pressure with sterile gauze moistened in normal saline to facilitate readaptation of tissue, stop bleeding, minimize clot thickness, and promote healing

    c. Apply periodontal dressing as needed

XI. Dental Implants

A. Osseointegrated dental implant—Stable functional replacement for a single tooth, several, or all teeth; consists of an anchor, abutment, and prosthetic crown; bridge, fixed, or removable denture; restores natural tooth function

    1. Parts

        a. Anchor—Metal fixture inserted into bone

        b. Abutment—Metal attachment connected to anchor by center screw; acts as a connection between implant anchor and prosthetic appliance

        c. Implant—Anchor and abutment; titanium is preferred material owing to its biocompatibility with bone; others include vanadium, vitallium, ceramic, cobalt alloys, or aluminum

B. Candidate selection criteria

    1. Need for tooth replacement

    2. Good physical, mental, and oral (periodontal) health

    3. Consistent and effective daily plaque control

    4. Adequate manual dexterity to ensure daily plaque control procedures

    5. Sufficient quantity and quality of alveolar bone to retain dental implant

    6. Cooperation and communication with dental team

    7. Signed informed consent

C. Benefits

    1. Improve function (mastication and speaking), appearance, self-confidence, and self-esteem

    2. Enhance patient comfort

    3. Decrease alveolar bone resorption, tissue ulceration, and pressure

    4. Eliminate direct forces on gingiva and alveolar crest

    5. Preserve remaining alveolar bone

    6. Increase retention of prosthetic appliance

D. Risks

    1. Improper patient selection

    2. Development of dehiscence (a hole in the buccal or labial plate of alveolar process) as a result of placing implant in area of insufficient bone

    3. Improper control of immediate stress or load resulting from pressure placed on implant too soon after initial surgery

    4. Rejection of implant—Inability of body to accept metal implant

    5. Inadequate time allowed for healing and interface development

    6. Failure to osseointegrate—Inadequate fusion of bone to implant anchor

7. Development of periimplantitis—Involves inflammation and infection in periimplant tissues (gingiva around implant abutment) resulting from inadequate personal or professional oral hygiene care

8. Inadequate manufactured quality of dental implant or prosthetic design

E. Types of dental implants

    1. Endosseous implant (Figure 10-24■)

        a. Most widely used

        b. Implant is placed within bone

        c. Abutment posts protrude through oral tissues to support removable prosthetic overdenture (attached to abutment by magnets, O-rings, or clips), dentist-retrievable denture (attached to abutment with tiny screws), or fixed prosthetic crown or bridge

        d. Procedure involves two surgeries

           (1) First surgery

              (a) Implant anchor (blade, screw, or cylinder) is inserted through an intraoral incision into a hole drilled in bone

              (b) Periosteum is sutured closed over anchor

              (c) Tissues are allowed to heal and osseointegrate for 4–6 months in maxilla and 3–6 months in mandible

              (d) In osseointegration, bone cells grow around and directly fuse to metal anchor—success of implant is dependent on osseointegration

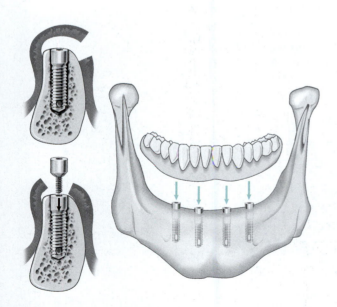

FIGURE 10-24 ■ Endosseous Implant

(2) Second surgery

(a) Top of anchor is surgically reexposed and abutment is attached onto anchor by a center screw

(b) Periosteum is sutured so abutments protrude through periosteum

(c) Healing caps are temporarily placed on abutments

(d) Gingival tissues heal in 3 weeks in maxilla and 1 week in mandible

(e) Biological seal forms and attaches healthy periimplant soft tissues to implant abutment

e. Prosthetic phase—Fixed or removable dental appliance is fabricated and attached to implant abutments

2. Subperiosteal implant (Figure 10-25■)

a. Metal framework is placed over bone and under periosteum

b. Metal posts on framework protrude through oral tissues to support prosthesis

c. System used when width or depth of bone is insufficient for endosseous implants

d. Procedure involves two surgeries

(1) First surgery

(a) Intraoral incision is made to expose alveolar bone

(b) Impression is taken of alveolar bone

(c) Surgical site is closed

(d) Dental laboratory fabricates metal framework from impression and model

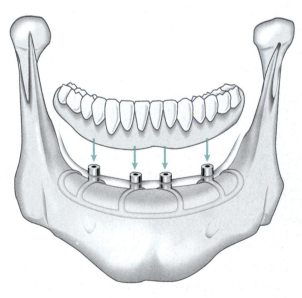

FIGURE 10-25 ■ Subperiosteal Implant

(2) Second surgery

    (a) After surgical reexposure, metal framework is placed over alveolar bone and under periosteum

    (b) Surgical site is closed

    (c) Metal posts on framework protrude through gingiva to attach a fixed or removable prosthetic appliance

    (d) No osseointegration occurs with this type of implant

3. Transosteal implant—Metal framework is placed through mandible

    a. Rarely used and, when so, strictly on mandible (cannot be placed in maxilla)

    b. Used when patient has an atrophic edentulous mandible or a congenital or traumatic deformity of mandible

    c. Procedure involves drilling holes in chin through an extraoral incision and inserting an implant consisting of five to seven parallel pins into mandible—two terminal pins protrude through gingiva and act as abutments to attach dental appliance

F. Professional implant maintenance procedures—Involves working with dentist and patient to maintain gingival health and bone support for implant

  1. Assessment—Collect, analyze, and document following patient data

    a. Changes in medical history

    b. Location of implants—Prudent to ask new patients if they have any dental implants; it may not be evident without radiographs

    c. Conditions of oral mucosa

    d. Discomfort, pain, swelling, inflammation, or infection associated with implants

    e. Color, texture, consistency of periimplant tissues

    f. Periodontal probing depths

      (1) Routine probing of implants is controversial because of possibility of disturbing the biological seal, leading to local infection and implant failure

      (2) Current consensus—Probing should *not* be performed routinely on implants; probe only when problem is suspected, using a plastic probe

    g. Bleeding on probing (if performed)

    h. Presence of exudate in sulci around implant abutments

    i. Amount of plaque and calculus accumulation

    j. Salivary percolation at periimplant sulcus—Breakdown of biological seal is indicated if bubbles form at sulcus on application of vertical pressure to implant

    k. Mobility of implant or implant prosthesis—Check screw retention, horizontal and vertical mobility of implant; loose screw can cause mobility of dental prosthesis and implant

    l. Results of microbiological monitoring tests

    m. Marginal bone height surrounding implant anchor—Determined by radiographs taken at appropriate intervals, and as needed

    n. Oral hygiene knowledge, beliefs, and habits

2. Periodontal debridement of implants

    a. Periimplant irrigation

      (1) Precede and follow scaling with antimicrobial solution such as 0.12% chlorhexidine gluconate, particularly when periimplantitis is present

      (2) Deliver solution to periimplant sulcus with either a plastic disposable syringe or powered oral irrigation unit

    b. Materials contraindicated for use on implant abutments—Avoid the following materials that may scratch or alter abutment surface:

      (1) Metal sonic and ultrasonic tips, scalers, probes, explorers, and other metal instruments—Metal easily scratches abutments

      (2) Prophylaxis cup or brush polishing with abrasive paste or flour of pumice

      (3) Air polishing device—Use is controversial

      (4) Acidulated phosphate fluoride—Corrodes titanium implant abutments

    c. Materials indicated for use on implant abutments

      (1) Plastic probe

      (2) Plastic, plastic-tipped, Teflon-coated, and wood-tipped scalers—Used safely for calculus removal (use of graphite and gold-tipped scalers is controversial)

      (3) Plastic ultrasonic or sonic scaler tips

      (4) Rubber cup, rubber point, or porte polisher with gel dentifrice or tin oxide

      (5) Low concentration of neutral sodium fluoride

    d. Plaque and calculus removal—Supragingival calculus formation is more common than subgingival calculus on implant abutments

      (1) Lateral pressure—Apply little pressure to remove calculus from implants; attachment of calculus to implant is weak; occasional tenacious deposits can be removed with plastic ultrasonic or sonic tips

      (2) Apply basic skills—Use basic operator and patient positioning, grasp, and fulcrum; *avoid* fulcruming on implant

      (3) Activation of strokes—Apply light pressure with hand-activated and ultrasonic scaling strokes

      (4) Direction of scaling strokes—Apply strokes in vertical, oblique, or horizontal direction away from periimplant tissues

      (5) Variety of implant scalers—Includes standard sickle, universal, and Gracey curet designs, as well as the following:

         (a) Universal—Used on apical portion of prosthetic framework; activate strokes in facial-to-lingual direction

         (b) Lingual—Used on lingual aspect of abutment; activate vertical strokes

         (c) Facial—Used on facial aspect of abutment; activate vertical strokes

         (d) Wrench-type—Wraps around mesial and distal aspects of abutment; activate vertical strokes

      (6) Stain removal—Not routinely performed on dental implants; porte polisher is instrument of choice for polishing implants; polish gently with nonabrasive agent when selective stain removal is indicated

      (7) Plaque removal—Remove plaque on implant abutments and underneath prosthetic appliance by buffing with G-Floss, Postcare Implant Flossing Cord, Super Floss, dental floss and/or tape used with a floss threader, moistened ribbon, yarn, or gauze

      (8) *Caution:* Care must be taken not to scratch implant or disrupt biological seal while scaling or polishing

3. Planning patient's disease-control program

    a. Designing a home care plan

      (1) Tailor to patient's preference, motivation, compliance, and dexterity

      (2) Consider implant abutment length and position, and prosthetic design

      (3) Access for plaque removal between appliance and gingival tissue and health of periimplant tissues

    b. Providing home care instructions

      (1) Provide oral/written instructions and educational pamphlets to patient

      (2) Demonstrate self-care procedures and observe patient practice

      (3) Instructions must be reinforced and modified as appropriate at recall visits

4. Continuing care schedule

    a. Oral hygiene instruction—Give immediately after implant abutment insertion and at each recall visit

    b. Recall maintenance visits—Schedule every 3 months for first year, then every 3–4 months thereafter

    c. Radiographic evaluation—X-ray study of implant, bone, and periodontal structures every 3 months for first year, then annually thereafter unless otherwise indicated

d. Removal of fixed prosthetic appliances (e.g., dentist-retrievable denture)—Dentist removes fixed prosthesis to check implant stability, assess gingival health, and clean appliance annually at recall maintenance appointment

e. Visits to dentist or oral surgeon—Schedule annual follow-up visits with practitioner who placed implant

f. Follow-up for signs of infection—Return to general dentist in 10–14 days or refer to specialist

G. Patient oral physiotherapy aids and procedures

1. Patient warnings

a. Caution patient never to use safety pin, paper clip, or other metal objects to self-clean implants or abutments

b. Warn against using hard bristle brushes that can damage implant abutment surface and lead to gingival and periimplant recession

c. Avoid conventional metal-wired interdental brushes

2. Disclosing agent—Use disclosing agent with magnifying intraoral mirror, face mirror, and pen light to evaluate plaque control on implant abutment, dental appliances, restorations, and natural teeth twice weekly

3. Brushes—Use combination of soft-bristle toothbrushes as needed to remove plaque from implant abutment, dental appliances, restorations, and natural teeth

a. Small, compact head toothbrush—For general use and on appliances; direct bristles at a 45-degree angle toward soft tissues; use two to three times daily

b. Uni-tuft interspace brush—Tapered or flat; especially useful for reaching facial and lingual surfaces of implants; use two to three times daily

c. Plastic nylon-coated interdental brush (Figure 10-26■)—Tapered or flat; especially useful for reaching interproximal surfaces of implants; use at least once daily

d. Motor-powered rotary brushes—Recommend to patients with limited manual dexterity; use on LOW power, one to two times daily

4. Implant abutment floss aids

a. Types

(1) G-Floss

(2) Postcare Implant Flossing Cord (red = thick; green = thin)

(3) Super Floss (Figure 10-27■)

(4) Dental floss and/or tape used with a floss threader

(5) Moistened ribbon, yarn, or gauze

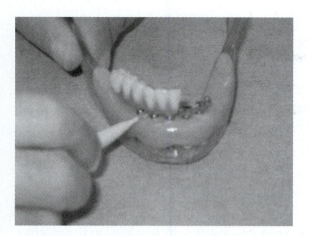

FIGURE 10-26 ■ Using Interdental Brush to Clean Implant

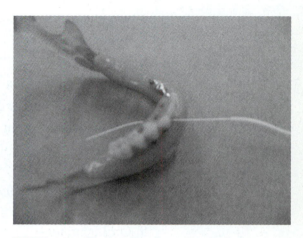

FIGURE 10-27 ■ Using Superfloss to Clean Implant

b. Instruction for use

   (1) Loop aid around implant abutment

   (2) Crisscross and pull back and forth in a shoeshining motion

   (3) Wrap in a C-shape and use in back-and-forth polishing motion to clean around accessible natural teeth and under fixed bridges, connecting bars, or implant overdenture

   (4) Use at least once daily

5. Rubber tip stimulator (Figure 10-28■)

   a. Tapered

   b. Use to remove debris from all tooth surfaces and gingival sulcus

   c. May also use to stimulate and massage periimplant tissue once daily

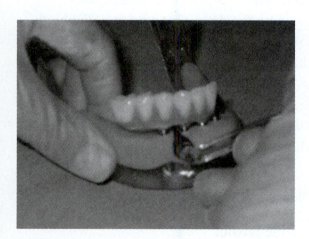

FIGURE 10-28 ■ Using a Rubber Tip Stimulator to Clean Implant

6. Wooden wedge stimulator, wooden pick, or porte polisher—Use for plaque removal as needed

7. Dentifrice

　　a. Recommend use of fine abrasive or gel anticalculus dentifrice twice daily

　　b. Use of abrasive dentifrice can alter implant abutment surface

8. Antimicrobial agent

　　a. Recommend a 30-second rinse with 0.12% chlorhexidine gluconate twice daily for 5–7 days immediately after abutment connection surgery

　　b. Thereafter, apply as needed to specific sites with cotton swabs, brushes, or other oral hygiene aids

9. Oral irrigator—Use as indicated when periimplant inflammation is present

　　a. Use with caution and never at implant junction

　　b. Use only with horizontal tip and flow placed on *low* setting

　　c. Use solutions such as phenolic, plant alkaloid, or 0.12% chlorhexidine gluconate mouth rinse

　　d. Use only as needed

XII.　Polishing

A. Purpose

　　1. Removes extrinsic stains from surfaces of teeth

　　2. Superficial polishing of crowns considered a cosmetic procedure with minimal therapeutic benefits (stains are not etiological factors for any disease or destructive process)

　　3. Selective procedure not needed by every patient, especially on a routine basis

B. Selective polishing

　　1. Perform after scaling and other periodontal treatment is completed

　　2. Assess for presence of unsightly stains and determine need to polish teeth, restorations, and removable prostheses

　　3. Polish only selected surfaces where objectionable stain is noted

C. Effects of polishing

　　1. Beilby (polish) layer—Removes and redeposits surface material; fine scratches and surface irregularities are filled in by fine particulate being removed

　　2. Bacteremia—Antibiotic premedication indicated for risk patients

　　3. Aerosol production

　　　　a. Accompanies polishing with handpiece and prophylaxis angle as well as air polishing

　　　　b. Porte polisher produces very little aerosol

　　　　c. Aerosols contraindicate polishing for patients with, and who are highly susceptible to, infection via contaminated aerosols (e.g., asthma, emphysema, other respiratory diseases, breathing or swallowing difficulties, and immunosuppression)

4. Spatter of polishing agent and contaminants—Patient and operator need protective eyewear

5. Removal of tooth structure—Removes fluoride-rich surface layer of enamel

    a. Loss of enamel from repeated polishing over time can be significant

    b. Rapid removal of cementum and dentin occurs owing to softness and porosity

    c. Avoid polishing newly erupted teeth (they are more porous and less mineralized), areas of thin enamel (e.g., amelogenesis imperfecta, areas of abrasion) demineralization, and exposed cementum and dentin

6. Increased roughness of tooth surfaces—Can create grooves and scratches

7. Heat production

    a. May cause pain or discomfort and damage to dental pulp from frictional heat of rubber cup

    b. Primary teeth, which have large pulp chambers, are particularly susceptible to heat damage

8. Trauma to gingival tissues—Gingival epithelium can be abraded by rubber cup polishing at too high a speed, extended application of rubber cup with abrasive agent, or incorrect air-polishing technique

9. Reaction to abrasive particles—Polishing agent and microorganisms can be forced into tissues by rotation of rubber cup, which can result in inflammation and/or delayed healing; polishing is contraindicated immediately after subgingival instrumentation in patients with deep periodontal pockets and for patients with soft, spongy gingiva

10. Increased tooth sensitivity—Abrasive agent uncovers dentinal tubules ends and thus increases sensitivity; avoid areas of existing dentinal hypersensitivity

11. Surface damage to restorative materials—Application of abrasive polishing agents can roughen surfaces of gold, amalgam, composite, and porcelain restorations, as well as titanium implants, and is therefore contraindicated for restored root surfaces

D. Indications for polishing (by any method)

1. Removal of unsightly stains—Remove stains not otherwise removed during toothbrushing or periodontal instrumentation

2. Prepares teeth for sealants, restorative procedures, or orthodontic bonding

3. Patient motivation—Encourages patient to maintain improved appearance

E. Procedures common to all polishing methods

1. Clinician preparation—Wear gown with high neck and long sleeves, cover hair; wear mask, protective eyewear, faceshield, and gloves

2. Patient preparation

    a. Administer antibiotic premedication for all patients at risk

    b. Use antimicrobial pretreatment mouthrinse

    c. Use plastic drape, towel or bib, protective eyewear, and hair covering

    d. Coat lips with nonpetroleum lip lubricant

    e. Give patient extra tissues

3. Patient position—Place in normal supine with head turned to right or left

4. Moisture containment—Cup patient's cheeks and lips to contain water, saliva, and abrasive agent

5. Modified pen grasp—Rest handpiece in "V" between thumb and index finger

6. Fulcrum—Use extraoral or intraoral fulcrum (same or opposite arch)

7. Initial stain removal

    a. Remove stains incorporated in plaque and calculus along with deposits during scaling

    b. Remove thick, heavy stains with ultrasonic and/or hand-activated instruments to avoid excessive polishing

        (1) Select ultrasonic tip that is more rounded and broad (vs. thin and pointed) for greater coverage and less tooth surface damage

        (2) Use hand-activated hoe, sickle, and curet—Curet adapts well to stained curvatures of teeth

8. Use of coarser polishing agents

    a. When coarser polishing agent is needed for moderate stain removal, follow up with a fine polishing agent

    b. Use fresh rubber cup or wooden point with fine polish

9. Interproximal stains

    a. Use dental tape with abrasive agent to remove interproximal stains remaining after polishing (avoid use of abrasive in contact area)

    b. Use finishing strips for interproximal stain removal only when all other methods fail

10. Floss—Rinse and floss to remove debris and abrasive particles retained between teeth

F. Power-driven polishing with rubber cup and bristle brush

    1. Selection of polishing agent

        a. Use least abrasive agent first, moving to more abrasive agent if first fails to remove stain

        b. Use of over-the-counter toothpaste may be ample for professional use when stain is minimal—May also be used when stain is absent and patient requests polishing in spite of selective polishing education

2. Abrasive agents available for polishing structures

   a. Enamel—Super-fine silex (silicon dioxide), zirconium silicate, calcium carbonate (chalk or whiting), pumice flour or superfine pumice, and tin oxide

   b. Metallic restorations—Pumice flour or superfine pumice, calcium carbonate, tin oxide, and levigated alumina

   c. Composite restorations—Aluminum oxide (alumina)

   d. Porcelain restorations—Diamond polishing paste

   e. Laboratory use only—Use rouge on gold and precious metal alloys; use coarse (lab) pumice on mouthguards

3. Commercial polishing preparations—Contain an abrasive (e.g., pumice), water, humectant (e.g., glycerin), binder (e.g., agar), artificial sweetener, and flavoring agent

4. Application principles for abrasives

   a. Rate of tooth surface abrasion and generation of frictional heat are increased by greater quantities of abrasive in polishing agent, speed of application, and pressure

   b. Therefore, use wet agents, low speeds, and light, intermittent pressure

5. Polishing equipment

   a. Handpiece—Autoclavable, belt-driven, or motor-driven slow (low) speed handpiece; 6,000–10,000 rpm; three basic designs: straight, contra-angle, and right angle

   b. Prophylaxis angle—Disposable or autoclavable, contra- or right-angle attachment

   c. Rubber cup, rubber tip, and bristle brush attachments—Disposable; three basic types: threaded stem for threaded right angle, snap-on for button-end right angle, and mandrel stem for latch-type contra-angle

6. Procedures for using prophylaxis angle

   a. Switch dental unit water to OFF position

   b. Use high-volume suction

   c. Fill cup with abrasive agent and almost bring into contact with tooth surface (but not touching) before activating handpiece; keep abrasive moist to reduce frictional heat

   d. Apply steady pressure with toe to rheostat to produce even, low speed

   e. Apply light pressure with rubber cup so edges flare slightly

   f. Use intermittent, light pressure (1–2 seconds contact) in small dabbing, circular strokes

   g. Turn entire handpiece to adapt cup to distal, facial/lingual, and mesial aspects

    h. Work from gingiva toward incisal or occlusal of each tooth

    i. Adapt cup rim to tooth concavities (e.g., lingual fossa of anterior teeth)

    j. Keep rubber cup filled with polishing agent to prevent frictional heat buildup in the tooth

    k. Keep working end moving at all times

    l. Restrict use of bristle brush to occlusal surfaces—Soften bristles in hot water before use

    m. Use rubber tip on occlusal surfaces or under orthodontic wires

G. Air-powered polishing

    1. Description—Also called airpolishing, air-powder polishing, air-abrasive polishing, and airbrasive polishing

       a. Air-powered device delivers slurry of warm water, sodium bicarbonate powder, and air through a handpiece

       b. System includes air, water, power lines, foot control, autoclavable handpiece sheath, nozzle, and wire nozzle-cleaning tool

       c. Available in combination ultrasonic scale/airbrasive units

    2. Advantages of air polishing

       a. Removes plaque and stain as effectively as rubber cup polishing and requires less time

       b. Effective on chlorhexidine, tobacco, and coffee stains

       c. Effective on stain in difficult access areas (e.g., occlusal pits and fissures)

       d. Less abrasive than rubber cup polishing with traditional prophylaxis pastes

       e. Efficiently removes plaque, stain, and debris from teeth with orthodontic appliances

       f. Effective for root detoxification on periodontally diseased roots

    3. Disadvantages of air polishing

       a. Aerosol production—Once a significant problem; can be nearly eliminated by use of disposable aerosol-reduction device fitted on nozzle of air polisher and connected to suction

       b. Use of mirror for indirect vision—Not usually possible unless aerosol-reduction device is used

       c. Spray may be uncomfortable for patient and inconvenient for clinician unless aerosol-reduction device is used

       d. Contraindications for use includes

          (1) All contraindications for polishing in general as with any method

             (a) High susceptibility to infection transmissable via aerosols

             (b) Difficulty swallowing or breathing

      (c) Communicable diseases transmissable via aerosols

      (d) Patients at risk for bacteremia require premedication

      (e) Exposed cementum or dentin

      (f) Areas of hypersensitivity and demineralization

      (g) Thin enamel

      (h) Soft, spongy gingiva

      (i) Immediately after instrumentation in deep pockets

      (j) Primary or newly erupted teeth

      (k) Restored tooth surfaces

      (l) Titanium implants

   (2) Patients on restricted sodium diet—Including patients with controlled hypertension

   (3) Patients with end-stage renal disease

   (4) Use on acrylic denture materials

   (5) Use on most restorative materials may

      (a) Cause pitting and wear of composite resins, porcelain, and dental cements

      (b) Erode cement and damage margins of dental castings

      (c) Wear dental sealants

      (d) Result in matte finish with prolonged or excessive use on polished metal surfaces

      (e) Remove and alter surface titanium on dental implants (use is controversial on implants)

4. Procedures for air polishing

  a. Connect water and air lines—Use caution not to switch air and water lines; unit will malfunction

  b. Flush water line—Flush line for 2–5 minutes before first use each day

  c. Use three foot control positions

   (1) OFF offers a continuous air spray

   (2) First position releases water spray only for rinsing teeth and tongue

   (3) Second position releases cleaning slurry

  d. Powder and water delivery

   (1) Adjust amount of powder delivered by turning indicator on top of chamber (12:00 maximum; 6:00 minimum)

   (2) Adjust water volume with water control

  e. Direct nozzle tip *slightly* apically at the following angles:

   (1) Anterior facial and lingual surfaces—60 degrees to surface

        (2) Posterior facial and lingual surfaces—80 degrees to surface

        (3) Posterior occlusal—90 degrees to surface

    f. Direct center of spray onto middle third of tooth surfaces; *avoid* directing into sulcus

    g. Use constant circular motion, keeping nozzle 3–4 mm from tooth surface

    h. Limit application time to 1–2 seconds per surface

    i. Clean 4–6 tooth surfaces, then rinse with water-only foot control position

    j. Use both hands to cup and shield spray unless using aerosol-reduction device

    k. Place gauze over lip and cheek to protect from spray unless using aerosol-reduction device

H. Cleaning removable dentures—Basic methods

  1. Ultrasonic cleaning—Procedure of choice

    a. Use solution designated for stain and calculus removal and follow manufacturer's directions

    b. Rinse with warm (never hot) water

    c. Use moderately stiff brush to scrub free solution and loosened debris

  2. Combination manual and power-driven

    a. Remove calculus by scaling, being careful not to scratch denture

    b. Polish only external surfaces (polishing internal surface of denture may alter fit)

    c. Soften bristle brush in hot water and use to polish nonmetal parts with very wet superfine pumice

    d. Polish metal parts with rubber cup and tin oxide

    e. Rinse thoroughly with warm (never hot) water

  3. Dental lathe in laboratory

    a. Polish nonmetal parts with wet rag wheel and fine pumice

    b. Polish metal parts, other than clasps, with separate wet rag wheel and tin oxide

    c. Use porte polisher and tin oxide on clasps

    d. Rinse thoroughly with warm (never hot) water

XIII. Instrument Sharpening

  A. Advantages

    1. Reduces number of strokes required for deposit removal and therefore saves time

    2. Reduces operator fatigue in fingers, hand, and wrist

      3. Provides greater instrument control owing to less pressure required for deposit removal

      4. Reduces possibility of burnishing deposits and scratching or grooving roots

      5. Increases tactile sensitivity

B. Stationary instrument–moving stone technique

      1. Determine design characteristics of the instrument-working end

         a. Face and lateral surface of the sickle scaler, universal curet, and area-specific curet meet in internal angle of 70–80 degrees

         b. Sharp cutting edge is a line—Has length, but no width

         c. Dull cutting edge is rounded—Has length and width

      2. Lubricate stone (optional)

         a. Reduces frictional heat

         b. Use sterile oil for natural and synthetic sharpening stones

      3. Grasp instrument handle in palm of hand, rest hand on countertop, and position working end

         a. Point toe (tip) directly toward operator

         b. Position face parallel to countertop

            (1) Universal curet—Lower shank is perpendicular to countertop

            (2) Area-specific curet—Lower shank is *not* perpendicular to countertop

      4. Grasp lower portion of stone and initially position stone perpendicular to instrument face

      5. Tip lower portion of stone toward instrument's lateral surface and establish 70- to 80-degree angle between stone and instrument face

      6. Move stone in short up-and-down strokes and finish in downward stroke

      7. Sharpen cutting edge in sections (heel, middle, and toe thirds)

      8. Sharpen one cutting edge (lower) per working end on area-specific curet

      9. Sharpen two cutting edges per working stroke end on universal curet and sickle scaler

    10. Continue sharpening strokes to round back of working end of curet

    11. Use semicircular strokes to round back of working end of curet

    12. Hone the face to remove wire edges

    13. Evaluate sharpness of cutting edge(s) with plastic sharpening test stick

➤ PERIODONTOLOGY

Etiology and Pathogenesis of Periodontal Diseases

Definitions

- Scaling—Instrumentation of the crown and root surfaces of the teeth to remove plaque and calculus
- Oral prophylaxis—Supra- and subgingival scaling and selective polishing combined to remove plaque, calculus, and stain from teeth
- Root planing—Definitive procedure designed for the removal of cementum and dentin that is rough and/or permeated by calculus, or contaminated by toxins and microorganisms
- Deplaquing—Removal or disruption of bacterial plaque and its toxins subgingivally after debridement has been completed
- Periodontal debridement—Removal of all subgingival plaque and its by-products, clinically detectable plaque retentive factors (calculus and overhangs), detectable calculus-embedded cementum to finish the root surface during periodontal instrumentation while preserving as much of the tooth surface as possible
- Periodontal maintenance procedures (PMP)—An extension of periodontal therapy that involves continuing periodic assessment and preventive treatment of the periodontal structures to allow for early detection and treatment of new or recurring periodontal disease
- Active therapy—Nonsurgical and/or surgical therapy
- Initial therapy—First phase of treatment performed to eliminate or suppress infectious microorganisms and to establish an environment that promotes health of the periodontal tissues

I. Tissues of the Periodontum

  A. Gingiva

    1. Components

      a. Free gingiva—Located at crest of alveolus; not attached, outer boundary of sulcus

      b. Free gingival groove—Located at inferior border of free gingiva, point opposite of alveolar crest, depression

      c. Attached gingiva—Located below free gingival groove; lies over underlying bone

      d. Mucogingival junction—Located where attached gingiva ends

      e. Alveolar mucosa—Located below mucogingival junction

      f. Gingival sulcus—Denotes space between gingiva and tooth

      g. Col—Consists of nonkeratinized tissue located between lingual and facial papilla

h. Interdental papilla—Denotes tissue that occupies interdental space between two adjacent teeth

i. Epithelial attachment—Located at base of sulcus, where epithelium attaches to tooth

j. Epithelium—Contains both keratinized and nonkeratinized tissues

  (1) Keratinized—Consists of oral epithelium

  (2) Nonkeratinized—Consists of sulcular and junctional epithelium

k. Sulcular (crevicular) fluid—Serum-like fluid that passes from gingival connective tissue through tissues into the sulcus; an inflammatory exudate

  (1) Characteristics

    (a) Less fluid is present in healthy gingiva than in diseased gingiva

    (b) Amount of fluid may be proportionate to severity of inflammation

l. Connective tissue

  (1) Known as lamina propria

  (2) Vascular and has nerve tissue

  (3) Components

    (a) Fibroblasts—produce collagen and elastic fibers; collagen gives connective tissue its strength

    (b) Composed of mast cells, macrophages, histiocytes, plasma cells, and lymphocytes

m. Gingival fiber groups

  (1) Marginal gingiva—Consists of dense fiber bundles made of collagen

  (2) Functions of fibers

    (a) Brace gingiva against tooth

    (b) Assist gingiva to withstand forces of mastication

    (c) Connect free marginal gingiva to cementum and attached gingiva

  (3) Types of fiber groups

    (a) Gingivodental—Located on facial, lingual, and interproximal surfaces

    (b) Circular—Encircles tooth

    (c) Transseptal—Located interproximally and forms horizontal bundles

B. Periodontal ligament (PDL)—Consists of connective tissue fibers (collagen) that surround root and connect tooth to bone

  1. Functions

    a. Transmit occlusal forces to bone

    b. Attach teeth to bone

    c. Maintain gingival tissues in their proper relationship to teeth

    d. Resist impact of occlusal forces

     e. Protect nerves and vessels from injury by surrounding root with soft tissue

     f. Supply nutrients to remaining periodontal structures—bone, cementum, and gingiva

     g. Transmit touch, pressure, and pain through sensory nerve fibers

2. Fiber bundles

     a. Made of collagen

     b. Attach to cementum and bone by Sharpey's fibers

     c. Not visible on radiograph, but space where they are located can be seen on radiograph as radiolucent line surrounding root of tooth

     d. Principal fibers—Arranged in distinct groups

        (1) Transseptal—Extend interproximally over alveolar crest; embedded in cementum of two adjacent teeth

        (2) Alveolar crest—Located apically to junctional epithelium and extend obliquely from cementum to alveolar crest

        (3) Horizontal—Extend at right angles to long axis of tooth

        (4) Oblique—Extend from cementum in a coronal direction to the bone; largest and most significant fiber group

        (5) Apical—Extend from cementum at root apex to base of tooth socket

        (6) Interradicular—Found only in multirooted teeth; extend from cementum at furcation to bone in furcation area

3. Remodeling

     a. Cells found in PDL (e.g., fibroblasts, cementoblasts, osteoblasts) can remodel bone and cementum

     b. Fibers adapt to occlusal stimuli and increase in size when occlusal forces increase

C. Cementum—Consists of calcified tissue covering tooth root

  1. Types

     a. Acellular cementum—covers cervical one-third to one-half of root

        (1) No cells are present

        (2) Contains calcified Sharpey's fibers

        (3) Plays a significant role in supporting tooth in socket

     b. Cellular cementum—Formed after tooth has erupted

        (1) Located more apically than acellular cementum; compensates for lost tooth crown length that occurs with attrition

        (2) Less calcified than acellular

        (3) Fewer Sharpey's fibers present

2. Patterns of formation—Continuous process with periods of greater and lesser activity

   a. Arranged in layers or lamellae

   b. Form more rapidly at apex

3. Cementoenamel junction (CEJ)—Defines tooth's anatomic crown; useful in assessing attachment loss or bone loss

   a. Types

   (1) Cementum overlaps enamel—60–65%

   (2) Cementum meets enamel, not overlapping—30%

   (3) Cementum and enamel do not meet (dentin is exposed)—5–10%

4. Anomalies

   a. Hypercementosis—Localized or generalized, prominent thickening of cementum often accompanied with nodular overgrowth at apex; numerous etiologies, including Paget's disease

   b. Cementicles—Globular masses of cementum that lie free in PDL or adhere to root surface

D. Alveolar process—Portion of mandible and maxilla that forms and supports tooth sockets; occurs with tooth eruption

   1. Disappears after a tooth is lost

   2. Bones that make up alveolar process

   a. Dense outer plate (cortical bone)—Includes facial and lingual compact bone

   b. Socket wall—Made up of compact bone (cortical bone); holds ends of PDL—Sharpey's fibers; lamina dura

   c. Cancellous bone—Located between outer cortical plates and socket wall; less dense and spongy; contains trabeculae

   3. Parts

   a. Alveoli—Tooth sockets

   b. Interdental septum—Area of bone between teeth

   (1) Composed of facial and lingual cortical plates, socket walls, and underlying cancellous bone

   (2) Shape is determined by size and shapes of crowns of approximating teeth

   c. Bone coverings—Composed of vascular connective tissue containing osteogenic cells

   (1) Periosteum covers outer bone surface

   (2) Endosteum covers inner bone surface

4. Bone remodeling

   a. Continuous changing of bone

   b. Can be removed (resorbed) or added (formed)

   c. Function, age, and systemic factors determine changes in bone

II. Risk Factors

A. Definition—Attributes or exposures that increase probability that a disease will occur

B. Causes—Environmental conditions, habits, or other diseases that increase or decrease patient's susceptibility to periodontal infection

C. Identification—Analyze information obtained from oral examination, clinical studies of periodontium, and medical/dental histories

D. Categories

   1. Unchanging risk factors

   a. Include gender, genetic factors, congenital immunodeficiencies, past history of periodontal disease, and congenital systemic diseases

   b. Contribute to periodontal problems—Factors include diabetes and conditions or diseases involving reduction of neutrophil numbers or function

   c. Risk factors do not change, even if periodontal health is restored

   2. Changing risk factors

   a. Include poor oral hygiene, age, certain medications, tobacco and alcohol use, stress, acquired immune system deficiencies, acquired endocrine diseases, acquired inflammatory diseases, nutritional deficiencies, and tooth restorations, which enhance plaque accumulation or inhibit normal function

   b. Contribute to periodontal problems as well

   c. Risk factors that can be removed or changed

      (1) Poor oral hygiene—Primary factor in gingival and periodontal disease

      (2) Tobacco use

         (a) One of the most significant risk factors in development and progression of periodontal disease

         (b) Users exhibit greater bone loss, increased pocket depths, and calculus formation

         (c) Users exhibit same or less gingival inflammation and same levels of plaque accumulation as nonsmokers

         (d) Nicotine and other toxic substances in tobacco alter host's ability to neutralize infection by reducing neutrophils' effectiveness

(e) Alters periodontal tissue vasculature; reduces immunoglobulin levels and antibody responses to bacterial plaque biofilm

(3) Nutritional status

    (a) Secondary factor in etiology of periodontal disease

    (b) Deficiencies of nutrient elements associated with wound healing may contribute to gingival and periodontal disease progression

    (c) Nutrients important for wound healing include

        i) Protein—Repairs tissue and increases resistance to infection

        ii) Vitamin C—Promotes collagen formation, tissue synthesis, and wound healing

        iii) Folic acid—Enhances red blood cell maturation, tissue synthesis, and cell proliferation

        iv) Vitamin B_{12}—Enhances red blood cell maturation, tissue synthesis, and cell proliferation

        v) Vitamin A—Increases resistance to infection and promotes tissue synthesis; deficiency affects integrity of epithelium

        vi) Vitamin K—Affects prothrombin formation

        vii) Iron—Promotes red blood cell formation

        viii) Zinc—Enhances connective tissue formation, wound healing, and protein synthesis

(4) Side effects—Certain medications may have impact on gingival/periodontal tissues and their response to periodontal treatment; severity of periodontal reaction to medications varies among patients

    (a) Gingival hyperplasia—Medications associated with gingival hyperplasia include

        i) Phenytoin (Dilantin)

        ii) Calcium channel blockers

            • Diltiazem (Cardizem, Dilacor)

            • Nifedipine (Procardia)

            • Primidone

            • Valproic acid

            • Verapamil (Calan, Isoptin, Verelan)

        iii) Cyclosporine

    (b) Xerostomia—Medication categories associated with xerostomia include:

        i) Anorectics (Dexadrine, amphetamine, dextroamphetamine, Adipex-P, and Pondimin)

      ii) Anticholinergics (Atrovent, Artane, Bentyl)

     iii) Anticonvulsants (Valium)

     iv) Antidepressants (Anafranil, Asendin)

      v) Antihistamines (Seldane, Benadryl)

     vi) Antihypertensives

- Diuretics (Lasix)
- Central adrenergic inhibitors (Catapres, Aldomet)
- Peripheral adrenergic antagonists (Minipres)
- Calcium-channel blockers (Calan)
- Angiotensin-converting enzyme (ACE) inhibitors (Capoten, Vasotec, Monopril)

    vii) Antiparkinson (L-dopa, Dopar, Artane)

   viii) Antipsychotics (Clozapine, Clozaril, Haldol)

     ix) Muscle relaxants (Flexeril)

      x) Acne treatment (Accutane)

(c) Altered host resistance—Medications that may alter host resistance to infection include

      i) Antibiotics

     ii) Insulin

    iii) Oral hypoglycemics

    iv) Systemic corticosteroids

(d) Abnormal bleeding—Medications that may cause abnormal bleeding include

      i) Aspirin

     ii) Dipyridamole

    iii) Nonsteroidal anti-inflammatory drugs (NSAIDs)

    iv) Phenytoin (Dilantin)

     v) Quinidine

    vi) Methyldopa

(5) Dental restorations, whose design or material contributes to plaque retention, can contribute to development of gingival inflammation and periodontal destruction

(6) Risk factors that demand most attention in management of periodontal disease—Smoking and diabetes

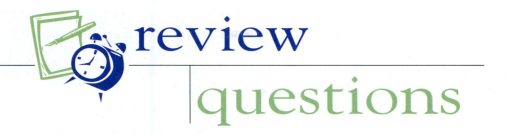

review questions

DIRECTIONS Each of the questions or incomplete statements below is followed by suggested answers or completions. Select the **one** answer that is best in each case.

1. Characteristics of the outer surface of gram-positive bacteria include all of the following EXCEPT one. Which one is the EXCEPTION?
   A. Vesicles or blebs, which contain endo-toxins
   B. Retained crystal violet (purple) stain
   C. A slime layer or glycocalyx
   D. A thick peptidoglycan layer, which is composed of repeating amino sugar units

2. The subgingival bacteria MOST closely associated with periodontal destruction
   A. May be moving freely close to the sulcus wall, but not attached to the plaque matrix
   B. Are incorporated in the plaque's inter-cellular matrix
   C. Will be Gram-positive cocci, such as *Mutans Streptococcus*
   D. Will have high oxygen needs for survival

3. Of the following, which is LEAST likely to be associated with plaque bacteria found on a patient with healthy gingiva?
   A. Most organisms will have fimbriae
   B. Most will be aerobic or facultative anaerobic bacteria
   C. *Actinomyces* sp. is often found
   D. Gram-positive will be more prevalent than Gram-negative bacteria

4. Gram-negative rods, associated with peri-odontitis, include all of the following EXCEPT one. Which one is the EXCEPTION?
   A. *Porphyromonas gingivalis*
   B. *Campylobacter rectus*
   ✓ C. *Treponema denticola*
   D. *Prevotella intermedia*
   E. *Bacteroides forsythus*

5. The "attachment apparatus" includes all of the following periodontal tissues EXCEPT one. Which one is the EXCEPTION?
   A. Gingiva
   B. Periodontal ligament
   C. Cementum
   D. Alveolar bone

6. Of the following risk factors, the MOST significant in the development of periodon-tal disease is
   A. Alcohol consumption
   B. Diet
   C. Cigarette smoking
   D. Low income
   E. Increased age

7. Lipopolysaccharides or endotoxins associated with Gram-negative bacteria are known to
   A. Cause spontaneous bleeding at the marginal gingiva
   B. Stimulate osteoclast-mediated bone resorption
   C. Stimulate corticosteroid formation
   D. Decrease the production of sulcular fluid
   E. Increase the quantity of albumin in the cementum

8. The current regimen for prophylactic antibiotic premedication, before invasive dental procedures in patients at risk of endocarditis, is
   A. 3 grams of penicillin 1 hour before dental procedure, then 1 gram 6 hours later
   B. 3 grams of E.E.S. 2 hours before dental procedure; 1.5 grams of E.E.S. 2 hours after the dental procedure
   C. 5 grams of amoxicillin 6 hours before dental procedure
   D. 2 grams of amoxicillin 1 hour before dental procedure
   E. 2 grams of tetracycline 1 hour before dental procedure and 1 gram 6 hours later

9. The MOST significant periodontal pathogen based on its numeric presence is
   A. *Porphyromonas gingivalis*
   B. *Bacteroides forsythus*
   C. *Prevotella oralis*
   D. *Treponema denticola*
   E. *Actinobacillus actinomycetemcomitans*

10. Rapid and progressive periodontal disease is more likely to occur in all of the following systemic conditions EXCEPT one. Which one is the EXCEPTION?
    A. Agranulocytosis
    B. Down syndrome
    C. HIV infection
    D. Neurological disorders, including epilepsy
    E. Diabetes

11. Factors to be evaluated in determining a tooth's periodontal prognosis include all of the following EXCEPT one. Which one is the EXCEPTION?
    A. Intrinsic stain
    B. Mobility
    C. Furcation involvement
    D. Pocket depths
    E. Root anatomy

12. Mouth rinses containing phenolic compounds are effective in reducing plaque by
    A. Altering the bacterial cell wall
    B. Degrading the bacteria's genetic code
    C. Inactivating the mitochondria
    D. Nourishing the Gram-positive bacteria
    E. Prohibiting pellicle formation

13. In gingival health, which of the following oral structures would NOT be keratinized or parakeratinized?
    A. Attached gingiva
    B. Palatal mucosa
    C. Sulcular epithelium
    D. Interdental or papillary gingiva

14. The fusion of cementum to alveolar bone occurs through
    A. Cementicles
    B. Hemidesmosomes
    C. Hypercementosis
    D. Ankylosis
    E. Cementoids

15. Clinically, the labial attached gingiva is identified coronally by the free gingival groove and apically by the
    A. Lamina dura
    B. Basal lamina
    C. Junctional epithelium
    D. Mucogingival junction
    E. Lamina propria

16. The portion of the periodontal ligament anchored in the cementum includes
    A. Osteocytes
    B. Sharpey's fibers
    C. Cementoid
    D. Cancellous bone
    E. Osteoid

17. In the initial stage of gingivitis, the cell type MOST closely associated with the inflammatory response is
    A. Fibroblast
    B. Neutrophil
    C. Plasma cell
    D. Erythrocyte
    E. Osteoclast

18. Gingival recession is a risk factor for all of the following EXCEPT one. Which one is the EXCEPTION?
    A. Occlusal caries
    B. Loss of cementum
    C. Tooth sensitivity
    D. Increased interproximal plaque accumulation
    E. Loss of tooth structure

19. An essential clinical feature in detecting the presence of periodontitis is
    A. Bone loss
    B. Pocketing
    C. Bad breath
    D. Presence of calculus and plaque
    E. Presence of pain

20. The MOST reliable clinical sign of gingival inflammation is the presence of
    A. Neutrophils in the connective tissue and junctional epithelium
    B. Plasma cells infiltrating the connective tissue of the sulcus
    C. Increased production of fluid in the gingival sulcus
    D. Bleeding on probing at the gingival sulcus
    E. Subgingival plaque accumulation

21. An oral side effect of Dilantin is
    A. Gingival abscesses
    B. Squamous cell carcinoma
    C. Papilloma
    D. Pyogenic granuloma
    E. Gingival hyperplasia

22. Periodontal tissue innervation is by the following nerve(s):
    A. Cranial VII—facial
    B. Cranial V—trigeminal
    C. Cranial III and Cranial V
    D. Cranial XII
    E. Cranial VII and Cranial VI

23. The MOST common position of the cementum in relation to the enamel is
    A. Enamel overlaps cementum
    B. Cementum meets the enamel, with no overlap
    C. Enamel stops 0.5 mm short of the cementum
    D. Cementum slightly overlaps the enamel

24. The diagnostic sign associated with localized juvenile periodontitis is
    A. Bleeding on probing
    B. Pain and abscess formation
    C. Presence of diastema
    D. Vertical bone loss at molars and incisors
    E. Pocket formation and presence of calculus at affected teeth

25. The MOST plentiful inorganic component of calculus is
    A. Brushite
    B. Mucopolysaccharides
    C. Magnesium phosphate
    D. Calcium phosphate

26. The MOST accurate method to detect furcation involvement is through
    A. Interviewing the patient
    B. Radiographic examination
    C. Clinical probing
    D. Testing for fremitus
    E. Presence of suppuration

27. Antibiotic premedication before invasive dental treatment is advised for the patient with a pathological heart murmur to reduce risk of
    A. Myocardial infarction
    B. Cerebrovascular accident
    C. Bacterial endocarditis
    D. Pyogenic granuloma

28. Increased tissue redness associated with gingival inflammation is caused by
    A. Hyperkeratosis
    B. Fluid exudation
    C. Capillary proliferation
    D. Gingival bleeding
    E. Increased sulcular fluid

29. A previous episode of necrotizing ulcerative gingivitis (NUG) may result in which of the following alterations of the interdental papillae?
    A. Edema
    B. Atrophy
    C. Cratering
    D. Recession
    E. Hyperplasia

30. Occlusal forces on the teeth
    A. Should be directed axially
    B. Should not be directed axially because the force will destroy the apical area of the socket
    C. Will result in the narrowing of the PDL if the force is excessive
    D. Will result in osteoblast activity at the area with the most pressure
    E. Causes erosion on the teeth

31. Fetid breath odor, pseudomembranous ulceration at the marginal gingiva and interdental papillae, gingival bleeding, and the presence of spirochetes and fusiform bacteria are associated with
    A. Periapical abscess
    B. Herpes simplex I
    C. Necrotizing ulcerative gingivitis (NUG)
    D. Aphthous ulceration
    E. Pericoronitis

32. The two earliest signs of gingival inflammation preceding established gingivitis are
    A. Increased collagen fibers and vascularity
    B. Increased gingival fluid and bleeding on probing the sulcus
    C. Gingival recession and increased bleeding on probing the sulcus
    D. Presence of calculus and bone loss
    E. Gnawing discomfort and ulceration of the marginal gingiva

33. The valley-like depression of the gingiva, connecting the facial and lingual interdental papillae, is the
    A. Mucogingival junction
    B. Furcation
    C. Col
    D. Gingival sulcus
    E. Free gingival groove

34. Which of the following fibers embeds in the cementum of the tooth to the adjacent tooth over the alveolar crest?
    A. Transseptal
    B. Circular
    C. Alveolar crest
    D. Interradicular
    E. Oblique

35. The removal of a periodontal pocket's gingival wall with a Gracey 11/12 curet or similar instrument with the intent of removing diseased soft tissue is known as
    A. Gingivoplasty
    B. Root planing
    C. Gingival curettage
    D. Gingivectomy

36. Most of the solid material in the composition of plaque consists of
    A. Calcium phosphate
    B. Desquamated epithelial cells
    C. Bacteria
    D. Leukocytes and macrophages
    E. Intercellular matrix

37. Which of the following provides the BEST opportunity for improved reattachment of periodontal ligament fibers to the tooth's root surface?
    A. Disintegration of cementum and dentin
    B. Degeneration of Sharpey's fibers
    C. Presence of infection
    D. Excessive tooth mobility
    E. Removal of the junctional epithelium

38. Which of the following is NOT a cardinal sign of inflammation?
    A. Redness
    B. Heat
    C. Infection
    D. Swelling
    E. Pain

39. A normal distance, in millimeters, between the CEJ and the alveolar crest is
    A. 0.5 to 2.0
    B. 3.0 to 4.5
    C. 4.5 to 6.0
    D. 6.0 to 7.0
    E. 7.0 to 7.5

40. The bluish-red appearance of the gingiva with periodontitis is associated with a(n)
    A. Decrease in plasma cells and an increase in neutrophils
    B. Increase in collagen destruction
    C. Endotoxin and desquamated epithelial cells in the periodontal pocket
    D. Increase in the presence of fibrous connective tissue
    E. Circulatory stagnation and deoxygenated blood

41. Xerostomia can be associated with all of the following EXCEPT one. Which one is the EXCEPTION?
    A. Antihypertensive medications
    B. Antidepressant and antianxiety medication
    C. Consumption of acidic foods
    D. Mouth breathing
    E. Vitamin A and B deficiencies

42. Chlorhexidine gluconate is effective as an antimicrobial agent against all of the following EXCEPT one. Which one is the EXCEPTION?
    A. *Streptococcus* sp.
    B. Gram-positive bacteria
    C. Gram-negative bacteria
    D. Viruses

43. The antibiotic "family" that has shown much promise in the management of periodontal disease is
    A. Tetracycline
    B. Sulfa drugs
    C. Erythromycin
    D. Cephalosporine

44. Which of the following instrument designs is LEAST likely to provide tactile sensitivity?
    A. Flexible shank
    B. Moderately flexible shank
    C. Rigid shank
    D. Hollow metal handle

45. All of the following represent functions of a straight, calibrated probe EXCEPT one. Which one is the EXCEPTION?
    A. Assess attachment loss
    B. Evaluate the presence of bleeding
    C. Measure recession
    D. Detect fractures in teeth
    E. Measure lesions

46. Which one of the following instruments is used with a push stroke?
    A. Periodontal file
    B. Chisel
    C. Hoe
    D. Sickle
    E. Curet

47. Which of the following instruments is recommended to remove light subgingival calculus deposits?
    A. Hoe
    B. Chisel
    C. Sickle scaler
    D. Curet

48. Which of the following instruments has a "self-angulated" cutting edge?
    A. Columbia 13/14
    B. Barnhart 1/2
    C. Jacquette-33
    D. Gracey 11/12
    E. Columbia 4R/4L

49. Tooth #30 has a Class III furcation involvement. Which of the following Gracey curets is BEST suited for scaling the distobuccal aspect of the mesial root?
    A. 1/2
    B. 5/6
    C. 7/8
    D. 11/12
    E. 13/14

50. When scaling with a sickle or curet, the IDEAL angulation, in degrees, between the instrument face and tooth surfaces should be
    A. 15
    B. 45
    C. 70
    D. 90

✓answers & rationales

1.

A. The characteristic of vesicles or blebs is noteworthy in Gram-negative bacteria, not Gram-positive. The endotoxin that is contained within the blebs is associated with tissue damage. The retention of Gram stain, a crystal violet stain, by a bacteria's wall is an identifier for Gram-positive bacteria. Slime layer or glycocalyx and a peptidoglycan layer with repeating amino sugar units are associated with Gram-positive bacteria.

2.

A. The layers closest to the soft tissues contain large numbers of flagellated motile bacteria and spirochetes. Studies suggest that some significant periodontal pathogens are in the loosely adherent or freely movable material in the periodontal pocket, rather than being incorporated into the intercellular matrix of adherent plaque. *Mutans streptococcus* is associated with dental decay, not periodontal destruction. The bacteria associated with periodontal destruction are anaerobic.

3.

A. A significant number of bacteria considered periodontal pathogens have fimbriae or hairlike projections on their surface. "Healthy" plaque is composed of Gram-positive rods and cocci, which are aerobic or facultative anaerobes. *Actinomyces* sp. is also commonly found.

4.

C. *Treponema denticola* is a spirochete, not a rod. *Porphyromonas gingivalis, Campylobacter rectus, Prevotella intermedia,* and *Bacteriodes forsythus* are all Gram-negative rods.

5.

A. Gingiva is not considered part of the "attachment apparatus." The attachment apparatus refers to the periodontal ligament's attachment to the tooth (via the cementum) and the alveolar bone.

6.

C. Cigarette smoking has been identified as a significant risk factor in the development and progression of periodontal disease. While alcohol consumption, diet, low income, and increased age may be identified as possible risk factors, studies do not consistently identify them to be as significant as tobacco use.

7.

B. Endotoxin is known to induce tissue inflammatory response and to stimulate osteoclast-mediated bone resorption. Spontaneous bleeding at the marginal gingiva can be seen when the tissue is fragile. Corticosteroids may inhibit osteoclast activity; however, endotoxin does not stimulate its activity. The presence of plaque and its irritants results in gingival inflammation. There will be an increase, not decrease, in the production of sulcular fluid.

8.

D. The American Heart Association regimen was revised in 1997. This regimen for non-penicillin-allergic individuals calls for 2 grams of amoxicillin 1 hour before dental procedure. This current regimen does not indicate a need for a follow-up dose. The remaining regimens are not current for antibiotic prophylaxis.

9.

A. Although a number of Gram-negative microorganisms are implicated in the various periodontal diseases, *Porphyromonas gingivalis* is found in the greatest quantity. *Bacteroides forsythus, Prevotella oralis, Treponema denticola,* and *Actinobacillus actinomycetemcomitans* are all considered periodontal pathogens, but are not found in as great quantity as *Porphyromonas gingivalis.*

10.

D. Rapid and progressive periodontal disease is not associated with neurological disorders. It is seen in numerous systemic conditions including those where wound healing is limited, when there is a defect in the quantity or quality of the neutrophils, and when the immune system is deficient. A defect in quantity or quality of neutrophils, such as in agranulocytosis, is associated with rapidly progressive periodontal disease. Down syndrome may have neutrophil defects or impairment secondary to the systemic disease. There is depressed immune function as a result of the invasion of the HIV virus into T-helper cells. There may

also be inadequate function of PMN leukocytes, which will alter the inflammatory response. Diabetes is associated with poor wound healing, resulting in a greater risk of RPP.

11.

A. Intrinsic stain, which is incorporated into the tooth structure, does not affect the periodontal prognosis. A tooth's prognosis worsens as the mobility increases. Teeth with furcation involvement are more difficult to keep plaque- and calculus-free, worsening their prognosis. Significant increases in pocket depths worsen a tooth's prognosis, as it is harder to keep these teeth plaque-free. Longer, broad roots have more surface area to assist with securing the tooth in the socket. A short, tapered root has less surface area secured in the socket and therefore has a poorer periodontal prognosis.

12.

A. Altering the bacterial cell wall inhibits the bacteria's ability to survive. An example of a mouth rinse containing a phenol compound is Listerine. Currently, no available mouth rinses degrade the bacteria's genetic code. Cell mitochondria are not inactivated by phenolic mouth rinses. Phenolic compounds are not a source of nutrients for Gram-positive bacteria and do not prohibit pellicle formation.

13.

C. Sulcular epithelium is nonkeratinized tissue. This allows for more movement of fluids and pathogens across the sulcular wall. Attached and interdental gingiva and palatal mucosa are keratinized epithelial tissues.

14.

D. Ankylosis is the fusion of cementum to bone. The cause may be related to tooth trauma or infection. Cementicles are abnormal calcified bodies occasionally found in the periodontal ligament. Hemidesmosomes attach the junctional epithelium to the tooth surface.

Hypercementosis is an excess production of cementum on a root surface. Cementoid is the uncalcified matrix that is the first step in cementum formation.

15.

D. The mucogingival junction is the terminal portion of the attached gingiva and the beginning of the alveolar mucosa. Lamina dura is the compact bone that appears as a radiopaque line surrounding the root of the tooth and the alveolar crest. Basal lamina is the amorphous material adjacent to the basal layer of epithelial cells. Junctional epithelium closely adheres to the tooth at the base of the sulcus. Lamina propria is the highly organized connective tissue component of the oral mucosa.

16.

B. Sharpey's fibers are the terminal portion of the PDL. They are the points of attachment to bone and cementum. Osteocytes are bone-forming cells. Cementoid is uncalcified cementum. Cancellous or spongy bone is located between the cortical plates. Osteoid is the uncalcified layer of intercellular substance, which eventually becomes bone.

17.

B. The PMN leukocyte, known as the neutrophil, is the white blood cell associated with the acute inflammatory response. Stage I gingivitis is the initial inflammatory response of the gingival tissue to plaque. Fibroblasts are cells that form connective tissue. Plasma cells produce immunoglobulin and are more commonly seen in chronic inflammation. The erythrocyte or red blood cell (RBC) is not associated with acute inflammatory response. An osteoclast is a bone-forming cell.

18.

A. There is greater risk of root surface caries, not occlusal, with gingival recession. Loss of cementum exposes dentinal tubules, which may cause dentin hypersensitivity. Intact papillae protect the embrasure spaces from plaque accumulation. When the papillae are lost, the embrasure space is now more plaque retentive. Tooth root structure may be lost through caries, abrasion, and erosion.

19.

B. Pocketing, related to attachment loss, is a distinctive factor in evaluating periodontal disease. Pocketing can be detected clinically using a probe. Although bone loss is a distinctive factor in periodontal disease, it may not be detected clinically. Use of radiographs is a better means to detect bone loss. Not all causes of bad breath are related to periodontal disease. It is not an essential clinical feature of periodontitis. Calculus and plaque may be present when there is gingivitis and periodontitis. However, it is possible to have plaque and calculus present with no evidence of disease. Pain is not usually associated with periodontitis.

20.

D. Bleeding on probing is the most reliable clinical sign of gingival inflammation. Neutrophils and plasma cells must be seen microscopically, as they cannot be seen clinically. Gingival inflammation does not result in an increase of sulcular fluid. However, this is difficult to detect and not a reliable clinical sign of gingival inflammation. Subgingival plaque accumulation is not easily detectable and not a good indicator of gingival inflammation.

21.

E. Gingival hyperplasia can be a side effect of the medication Dilantin. This is not an inflammatory response, but an excess growth of gingival tissue. Gingival abscesses are infections and not oral side effects of Dilantin. Squamous cell carcinoma is a malignancy and not an oral side effect of Dilantin. Pyogenic granuloma is an excessive inflammatory response to an irritant often associated with hormonal imbalances.

22.

B. The trigeminal nerve is a mixed motor and sensory nerve. Its branches innervate the periodontal tissues. The facial nerve is a motor nerve that sends impulses to the muscles of mastication. The oculomotor nerve is a motor nerve that sends impulses to muscles that raise the eyelid and move the eyes. The hypoglossal is a motor nerve that sends impulses to muscles that move the tongue. The abducens is a motor nerve that sends impulses to muscles that move the eyes.

23.

D. Cementum overlaps enamel 60–65% of the time. Enamel does not overlap the cementum. Cementum meets the enamel 30% of the time. Enamel stops 0.5 mm short of the cementum 5–10% of the time.

24.

D. The characteristic diagnostic sign of localized juvenile periodontitis is vertical bone loss at first molars and incisors. Bleeding on probing and diastemas are not unique signs for LJP. LJP is not painful and abscess formation is not a common feature. There is not a significant amount of calculus present in LJP.

25.

D. Calcium phosphate makes up approximately 75% of the inorganic content of calculus. Brushite is present in calculus in small quantities. Mucopolysaccharides are organic, not inorganic compounds. Magnesium phosphate is the second largest inorganic component of calculus.

26.

C. The most accurate way to detect furcation involvement is by clinical probing using a specially designed probe, such as the Nabors. A typical patient would not be aware of a furcation involvement, as furcations are not readily seen. Some furcation involvement can be viewed on radiographs. However, because of variations in film and beam placement, furcations may not routinely be detected this way. Fremitus describes the slight movement of a tooth that can be felt when a tooth experiences excess occlusal forces. Although furcations are risk factors for periodontal abscesses, not all furcations will have evidence of suppuration or purulence.

27.

C. Numerous medical conditions may put a patient at risk of bacterial endocarditis, including disease-produced heart murmur or artificial (prosthetic) heart valves and some congenital heart defects. Myocardial infarction results from an occluded coronary artery. Antibiotic premedication will not prevent a heart attack. Cerebrovascular accident or stroke occurs when there is oxygen deprivation to a portion of the brain resulting from an occluded or damaged vessel in the brain. Antibiotic treatment will not prevent a stroke. Pyogenic granulomas are an exaggerated tissue response to a local irritant. They are associated with patients with hormone imbalances, such as occurs during pregnancy. Reducing the local irritant may manage pyogenic granulomas.

28.

C. The tissue redness seen in gingivitis is characteristic of the inflammatory process. It is related to the increase in capillary formation at the inflammatory site. Hyperkeratosis, an increase in the layer of keratinized epithelial (nonvascular) tissue, would cause tissue to have a pale appearance, not red. Exudation is clear and a sign of inflammation. Bleeding on probing will occur when the gingiva is inflamed; however, bleeding does not cause inflammatory redness. The quantity of sulcular fluid increases with gingival inflammation, but it is not red.

29.

C. Tissue destruction evidenced by blunting or cratering of the interdental papillae is a distinct feature of NUG. After the episode of NUG has resolved, the affected tissue would not be edematous or swollen. The interdental papillae will be destroyed through the disease process. They do not atrophy or shrink. Recession is not a significant factor in identifying past history of NUG. Gingival hyperplasia may be associated with intake of specific medications or heredity; however, it is not associated with NUG.

30.

A. Occlusal forces directed axially result in a uniform distribution along the PDL into the surrounding bone. Forces that are not directed axially contribute to tissue destruction, including vertical bone defects. Evidence of excess occlusal forces may appear on a radiograph as widened PDL space. Osteoblast activity occurs at areas of tension in bone. Osteoclasts—cells that remove bone—are present at areas of pressure on the bone. Erosion is the loss of tooth structure that has had contact with a chemical.

31.

C. Necrotizing ulcerative gingivitis has symptoms such as fetid breath odor, gingival bleeding, presence of spirochetes and fusiform bacteria, and pseudomembranous ulcerations at the marginal gingiva and interdental papillae. This condition may be acute or chronic. A periapical abscess occurs with pulp necrosis. There would be signs of this condition at the marginal gingiva or interdental papillae. Herpes simplex I has generalized ulceration on the mucosa, not limited to the marginal gingiva. Pericoronitis is painful inflammation, with probable infection.

32.

B. Bleeding on probing and an increase in sulcular fluid are the two earliest signs of gingivitis. Collagen fibers are destroyed, not increased, in early gingivitis. Gingival recession and bone loss would be noted with periodontitis, not gingivitis. Calculus alone is not an indicator of either gingivitis or periodontitis. Gingivitis is not painful. However, there will be microulceration of the sulcular epithelium as the gingivitis progresses.

33.

C. The col is located in the proximal space between the facial and lingual papillae. The mucogingival junction is the line of demarcation between the attached gingiva and the oral mucous membrane. A furcation involves the area on a multirooted tooth where the roots separate. The gingival sulcus is the space between the root of the tooth and the sulcular wall of the marginal gingiva. The free gingival groove identifies where the marginal gingiva ends and the attached gingiva begins.

34.

A. Transseptal fibers attach from the cementum of one tooth to the cementum of an adjacent tooth. These fibers are also considered a gingival fiber group. Circular fibers are located in the marginal gingiva. Alveolar crest fibers extend obliquely from the cementum apical to the junctional epithelium to the alveolar crest. Interradicular periodontal ligament fibers are found only in multirooted teeth. They extend from the cementum at the furcation to the bone in the same area. Oblique periodontal ligament fibers extend from the cementum in a coronal direction to the bone. This is the largest and most significant fiber group.

35.

C. The intent of gingival curettage is to create a better environment for healing, by removing the diseased pocket wall. Gingivoplasty reshapes the gingiva to improve its contour. Root planing smooths root surfaces. Gingivectomy surgically removes diseased gingiva.

36.

C. The content of plaque solids is 70–80% bacteria. Plaque has very little inorganic material. There will be small quantities of desquamated epithelial cells present in plaque. Leukocytes and macrophages are not present in plaque in any significant quantity. Intercellular matrix holds the plaque together. Its quantity by volume is considerably less than the bacteria present in plaque.

37.

E. The position of the junctional epithelium determines the maximum height at which the PDL fibers can reattach. During the healing process, both the epithelium and the periodontal ligament fibers may heal more coronally if the junctional epithelium is removed. Periodontal ligament fibers are embedded in cementum by Sharpey's fibers. Without cementum there is no point of attachment. A nondiseased environment is required for good healing or reattachment. Tooth mobility inhibits fibers from reattaching.

38.

C. Infection describes the accumulation and proliferation of a microorganism. An infection is pathological, not physiological, and results in an inflammatory response. Redness, heat, swelling, and pain are all cardinal signs of inflammation. Inflammation is a physiological response to tissue injury.

39.

A. A distance greater than 2.0 mm between the CEJ and the crest of the alveolar bone is suggestive of bone destruction associated with periodontal disease.

40.

E. In chronic periodontitis, there is an increased amount of vasculature, but a slowed rate of circulation. The blood stagnates at the point of inflammation. Because the blood is deoxygenated, it has a dark red/purple or less than bright red appearance. The presence of plasma cells, neutrophils, collagen, products in periodontal pockets, and fibrous connective tissue do not create a bluish-red appearance of the gingiva.

41.

C. Consumption of acidic foods, such as lemons and pickles, induces rather than reduces saliva production. Numerous medications, including antihypertensive, antidepressant, and antianxiety, may cause xerostomia. Mouth breathing results in xerostomia, as do deficiencies of vitamins A and B.

42.

D. Chlorhexidine is not effective against viruses, bacterial spores, or acid-fast bacteria. However, it does possess antimicrobial properties for both gram-positive and gram-negative bacteria, as well as yeast.

43.

A. Tetracycline, minocycline, doxacycline, and natural or synthetic tetracycline have been used successfully in the management of several forms of periodontal disease, including juvenile periodontitis and refractory periodontitis. Sulfa drugs, erythromycin, and cephalosporine are not as effective in managing periodontal disease.

44.

C. Shank flexibility is necessary to detect tooth irregularities and subgingival deposits. Rigid shanks provide little tactile information for the clinician. A flexible shank provides the greatest tactile information, whereas the moderately flexible shank provides some tactile sensitivity.

45.

D. The periodontal probe is not the appropriate instrument to use to detect fractures in teeth. However, it is an excellent instrument to use to assess attachment loss, evaluate the presence of bleeding, and measure recession and lesions.

46.

B. The chisel is used only in a horizontal direction with a push stroke to dislodge heavy calculus from the facial, lingual, and interproximal surfaces. The periodontal file, hoe, sickle, and curet are used with a pull stroke.

47.

D. Curets are designed to remove light to moderate supragingival and subgingival calculus. The hoe offers limited use subgingivally, but can be used to remove heavy supragingival calculus. The sickle scaler removes calculus supragingivally.

48.

D. Area-specific curets, such as the Gracey 11/12, have a longer (self-angulated) cutting edge that is used during instrumentation. The Columbia 13/14, Barnhart 1/2, Jacquette-33, and Columbia 4R/4L have cutting edges on both sides.

49.

E. The Gracey 13/14 is designed to be used on distal surfaces of posterior teeth. When furcation involvement is present, each root is debrided as if it were a single-rooted tooth. The Gracey 1/2 is designed to use on anterior teeth. The Gracey 5/6 is used on anterior and premolar teeth. The Gracey 7/8 is designed for application on facial and linguals of posterior teeth. The Gracey 11/12 is designed for mesial surfaces of posterior teeth.

50.

C. The correct angulation between the instrument face and tooth surface is less than 90 degrees and greater than 45 degrees. A 70-degree angle is considered ideal.

11 Using Preventive Agents

D ental hygiene, as a science, studies and perfects the use of preventive agents in practice. In fact, dental hygienists use preventive agents in the routine practice of dental hygiene on a daily basis. Dental hygienists frequently provide consultative services regarding the use of fluoride, fluoridation, xylitol, and dental sealants.

In dental public health, dental hygienists develop programs using preventive agents to prevent and control diseases within certain populations. Preventive agents such as fluorides and dental sealants have been researched for decades and are among the top preventive measures in the field of public health.

chapter objectives

After completion of this chapter, the learner should be able to:

➤ Define and describe the different ways that fluorides are provided to patients and the advantages and disadvantages of fluoride

➤ Discuss the recommended optimal fluoride levels

➤ Discuss the fluoride supplements dosage schedule

➤ Discuss lethal and safe doses of fluoride

➤ Describe the mechanism of action of dental sealants

➤ Discuss sealant material

➤ Describe the application technique of dental sealants

➤ Discuss sealants in school programs

➤ Define xylitol and its use in prevention of dental caries

I. Fluoride

A. Fluoride is an essential nutrient in the formation of teeth and bones.

B. Fluoride is stored in the crystal lattice of fluorapatite.

C. Fluoride acquisition can be both topically and systemically.

1. Topical fluoride (post-eruptive fluoride) exposure inhibits demineralization and enhances remineralization. Laboratory and longitudinal studies suggest that fluoride prevents dental caries predominately after eruption of the tooth. The specific actions include inhibition of demineralization, enhancement of remineralization, and inhibition of bacterial activity in plaque.

2. Systemic fluoride (pre-eruptive fluoride) is taken in by drinking and eating food with fluoride and is made available to the developing teeth by way of the blood plasma to the tissues surrounding the tooth bud; after tooth mineralization, but before tooth eruption, fluoride deposition continues in the surface of the enamel after tooth eruption.

D. Toxicology of fluoride

1. Acute toxicity refers to the rapid intake of an excess dose over a short time, such as a child eating a large quantity of toothpaste. See Table 11-1■ for lethal and safe doses of fluoride. Symptoms of acute fluoride toxicity include nausea, vomiting, diarrhea, abdominal pain, and increased salivation and thirst. Treatment of acute toxicity includes:

   a. Call 911

   b. Induce vomiting

   c. Administer milk or lime water

2. Chronic toxicity can result in dental fluorosis. Patients with dental fluorosis generally have a low risk of dental caries. It is the form of enamel hypomineralization due to excessive ingestion of fluoride during the development of the teeth; may appear as a white spot or as severe browning of tooth and may include pitting of the surface; skeletal fluorosis may include isolated instance of osteosclerosis. The pediatric population are exhibiting more cases of mild fluorosis, possibly due to the ingestion of child-flavored toothpaste and the multiples types of fluoride available.

E. Defluoridation

1. The process of removing naturally occurring fluoride from water supplies; the Environmental Protection Agency (EPA) monitors this process

2. This is done when the fluoride content is well over 1 ppm

3. Some fluoride will be left in water for the prevention of dental caries

TABLE 11-1 LETHAL AND SAFE DOSES OF FLUORIDE

A. Lethal and safe dosages of fluoride for a 70-kg adult

Certainly Lethal Dose (CLD)

5–10 g NaF

or

32–64 mg F/kg

Safely Tolerated Dose (STD) = 1/4 CLD

1.25–2.5 g NaF

or

8–16 mg F/kg

B. CLDs and STDs of fluoride for selected ages

Age (years)	Weight (lbs)	CLD (mg)	STD (mg)
2	22	320	80
4	29	422	106
6	37	538	135
8	45	655	164
10	53	771	193
12	64	931	233
14	83	1,206	301
16	92	1,338	334
18	95	1,382	346

From Heifetz, S.B., & Horowitz, H.S. The Amounts of Fluoride in Current Fluoride Therapies: Safety Considerations for Children. *ASDC J. Dent. Child.*, 51, 257. July–August, 1984. Reprinted with permission.

F. Methods of administration

    1. Water fluoridation is the addition of fluoride in public water supplies, when it is not naturally occurring at a significant amount (Figures 11-1■, 11-2■, 11-3■). The Centers for Disease Control and Prevention (CDC) has a

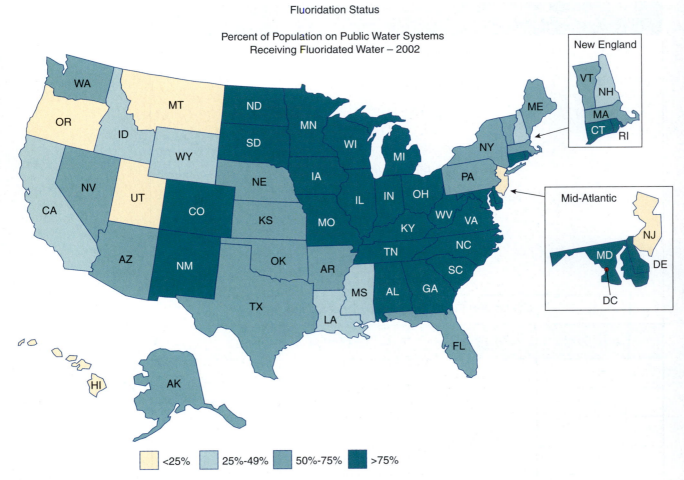

FIGURE 11-1 ■ Fluoridation of Public Water Systems in the United States.

Source: Centers for Disease Control and Prevention, Atlanta, Georgia, 2002.

website that can be used to identify individual community water supplies' fluoride content.

    a. Water fluoridation can result in as many as 20–40% fewer enamel caries in adults and 8–37% in adolescents

    b. Fluoride compounds added to water supplies include sodium silicofluoride, sodium fluoride, and hydrofluorosilicic acid

    c. Optimal recommended concentration in community drinking water can range from .7–1.2ppm, which prevents fluorosis; see Table 11-2■ for recommended fluoride levels

    d. The U.S. Environmental Protection Agency (EPA) monitors fluoridation

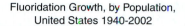

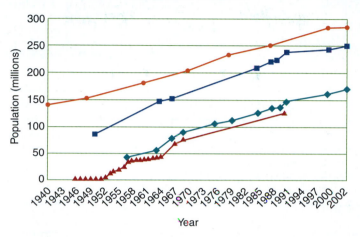

FIGURE 11-2 ■ Fluoridation Growth, by Population, in the United States, 1940–2002

Source: Centers for Disease Control and Prevention, Atlanta, Georgia, 2002.

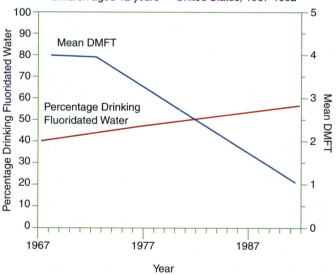

FIGURE 11-3 ■ Fluoridation and Dental Decay

Source: Achievements in Public Health, 1990–1999. Fluoridation of Drinking Water to Prevent Dental Caries. MMWR. Oct. 22 1999/48(41); 933–940.

TABLE 11-2 RECOMMENDED OPTIMAL FLUORIDE LEVELS

Annual Average of Maximum Daily Air Temperature (°F)	Optimal Fluoride Level (ppm)
40.0–53.7	1.2
53.8–58.3	1.1
58.4–63.8	1.0
63.9–70.6	0.9
70.7–79.2	0.8
79.3–90.5	0.7

Source: CDC, National Center for Prevention Services. Dental Disease Prevention Activity, 1991.

e. Water fluoridation is cost effective at $.31/person in communities larger than 50,000 persons and $2.12/person in communities less than 10,000. The CDC's 2001 recommendations for using fluoride to prevent dental caries reports that in 1991, the annual cost of water fluoridation in the United States was $0.72 per person.

f. One study estimated that prevention of dental caries, largely atrributed to fluoridation and fluoride-containing products, saved $39 billion (1990 dollars) in dental care expenditures in the United States during the years 1979–1989

g. Opponents of water fluoridation have claimed it increased the risk for cancer, Down syndrome, heart disease, osteoporosis, and bone fracture, AIDS, low intelligence, Alzheimer's disease, allergic reactions, and other health conditions. No credible evidence suggests an association between flouridation and any of these conditions. The safety of fluoride has been evaluated frequently and the CDC, ADHA, and ADA remain supportive of water fluoridation.

h. Water fluoridation is most effective for ages 6 mos.–14 yrs.

2. School fluoridation is the adding of fluoride at approximately 5 ppm to a school's water supply to decrease dental caries in the student population. Two studies on school water fluoridation revealed findings that indicated that children in a school system with fluoridation had a decrease in decay that ranged from 39–48% after 12 years in the school system. The increase of fluoride per ppm is due to the fact that children consume only part of their water consumption during school hours. School water fluoridation has been phased out in several states. Operations of small fluoridation systems were problematic in several instances.

3. Some foods naturally contain fluoride, whereas some food sources contain fluoride because of the inclusion of fluoridated waters

4. Fluoride can be ingested systemically through water, prescribed supplements, foods and beverages that contain fluoride, and swallowed dentifrices. The halo effect refers to the unintentional addition of fluoride to a concentrated beverage or food that is from a water supply containing fluoride in a city other than where it is consumed. See Table 11-3■ for fluoride supplement dosage recommendations.

5. Fluoridated salt has been used in some countries to deliver fluoride to populations for the purpose of decreasing dental caries.

6. Bottled water can introduce varying levels of fluoride and many times the amount of fluoride is not identified on the bottle. However, some bottled water has fluoride added and is actually marketed for the addition of fluoride.

G. Professionally administered fluoride

1. Fluoride foams, gels, and rinses are delivered by trays or the swabbing method and mouthrinses may be administered by the dental hygienist. Fluoride foams are the most widely used in dental practice today due to the pleasant taste. Fluoride gels are not as common, as patients favor the foams. In-office fluoride rinses are seldom used due to unpleasant taste, instability, tooth staining, and gingival sloughing (Tables 11-4■ and 11-5■).

TABLE 11-3 RECOMMENDED DIETARY FLUORIDE SUPPLEMENT* SCHEDULE

Age	Fluoride concentration in community drinking water[†]		
	<0.3 ppm	0.3–0.6 ppm	>0.6 ppm
0–6 months	None	None	None
6 months–3 years	0.25 mg/day	None	None
3–6 years	0.50 mg/day	0.25 mg/day	None
6–16 years	1.0 mg/day	0.50 mg/day	None

* Sodium fluoride (2.2 mg sodium fluoride contains 1 mg fluoride ion).

[†] 1.0 parts per million (ppm) = 1 mg/L.

Sources:

Meskin LH, ed. Caries diagnosis and risk assessment: a review of preventive strategies and management. *J Am Dent Assoc* 1995; 126(suppl):1S–24S.

American Academy of Pediatric Dentistry. Special issue: reference manual 1994–95. *Pediatr Dent* 1995; 16(special issue):1–96.

American Academy of Pediatrics Committee on Nutrition. Fluoride supplementation for children: interim policy recommendations. *Pediatrics* 1995;95:777.

Source: CDC MMWR Recommendations & Reports, August 17, 2001/50(RR14); 1–42.

TABLE 11-4 EVIDENCE-BASED CLINICAL RECOMMENDATIONS FOR PROFESSIONALLY APPLIED TOPICAL FLUORIDE			
Risk Category	**Recommendation**	**Grade of Evidence**	**Strength of Recommendation**
< 6 Years			
Low	May not receive additional benefit from professional topical fluoride application*	Ia	B
Moderate	Varnish application at 6-month intervals	Ia	A
High	Varnish application at 6-month intervals	Ia	A
	OR		
	Varnish application at 3-month intervals	Ia	D**
6 to 18 Years			
Low	May not receive additional benefit from professional topical fluoride application*	Ia	B
Moderate	Varnish application at 6-month intervals	Ia	A
	OR		
	Fluoride gel application at 6-month intervals	Ia	A
High	Varnish application at 6-month intervals	Ia	A
	OR		
	Varnish application at 3-month intervals	Ia	A**
	OR		
	Fluoride gel application at 6-month intervals	Ia	A
	OR		
	Fluoride gel application at 3-month intervals	IV	D***
18 + Years			
Low	May not receive additional benefit from professional topical fluoride application*	IV	D
Moderate	Varnish application at 6-month intervals	IV	D#
	OR		
	Fluoride gel application at 6-month intervals	IV	D***

TABLE 11-4 EVIDENCE-BASED CLINICAL RECOMMENDATIONS FOR PROFESSIONALLY APPLIED TOPICAL FLUORIDE

Risk Category	Recommendation	Grade of Evidence	Strength of Recommendation
High	Varnish application at 6-month intervals	IV	D#
	OR		
	Varnish application at 3-month intervals	IV	D#
	OR		
	Fluoride gel application at 6-month intervals	IV	D***
	OR		
	Fluoride gel application at 3-month intervals	IV	D***

* Fluoridated water and fluoride toothpastes may provide adequate caries prevention in this risk category. Whether or not to apply topical fluoride in such cases is a decision that should balance this consideration with the practitioner's professional judgment and the individual patient's preferences.

** Emerging evidence indicates that applications more frequent than twice per year may be more effective in preventing caries.

*** Although there are no clinical trials, there is reason to believe that fluoride gels would work similarly in this age group.

Although there are no clinical trials, there is reason to believe that fluoride varnish would work similarly in this age group.

Laboratory data demonstrate foam's equivalence to gels in terms of fluoride release; however, only two clinical trials have been published evaluating its effectiveness. Because of this, the recommendations for use of fluoride varnish and gel have not been extrapolated to foams.

Because there is insufficient evidence to address whether or not there is a difference in the efficacy of sodium fluoride versus acidulated phosphate fluoride gels, the clinical recommendations do not specify between these two formulations of fluoride gels. Application time for fluoride gel and foam should be four minutes. A one-minute fluoride application is not endorsed.

Definitions:

Levels of Evidence

Ia Evidence from systematic reviews of randomized controlled trials
Ib Evidence from at least one randomized controlled trial
IIa Evidence from at least one controlled study without randomization
IIb Evidence from at least one other type of quasi-experimental study
III Evidence from nonexperimental descriptive studies, such as comparative studies, correlation studies, cohort studies and case-control studies
IV Evidence from expert committee reports or opinions or clinical experience of respected authorities

* Amended with permission of the BMJ Publishing Group from Shekelle and colleagues. (Shekelle PG, Woolf SH, Eccles M, Grimshaw J. Clinical guidelines: developing guidelines. Brit Med J 1999;318(7183):593–6.

Grading of Recommendations

A Directly based on category I evidence
B Directly based on category II evidence or extrapolated recommendation from category I evidence
C Directly based on category III evidence or extrapolated recommendation from category I or II evidence
D Directly based on category IV evidence or extrapolated recommendation from category I, II or III evidence

TABLE 11-5 PROCEDURES TO REDUCE FLUORIDE INGESTION DURING TOPICAL GEL-TRAY APPLICATION	
Patient	Seat upright Instruct not to swallow Tilt head forward with trays; tilt away from side with cotton-roll holder
Trays	Custom-made or appropriate size with absorptive liners; post-dam; border rim Use minimum amount of gel: 2 mL per tray, less for small tray; no more than total of 5 mL for large trays
Isolation	Use saliva ejector with maximum efficiency suction Cotton-roll holder technique: position for security, stability; place saliva absorber in cheek
Attention	Do not leave patient unattended
Timing	Use a timer; do not estimate
Completion	Tilt head forward for removal of tray or cotton-roll holder Request patient to expectorate for several minutes; do not allow swallowing Wipe excess gel from teeth with gauze sponge Use high-power suction to draw out saliva and gel Instruct patient not to rinse, eat, drink, or brush teeth for at least 30 minutes

Recommendations based on *Oral Health Policies for Children: Protocol for Fluoride Therapy,* American Academy of Pediatric Dentistry, 211 E. Chicago Avenue, Chicago, IL 60611. Reprinted with permission.

2. Fluoride varnish can be used as a cavity varnish, to treat tooth sensitivity, or to prevent caries. Although the FDA has approved it for use as a cavity varnish or agent for tooth sensitivity, it is frequently used off label to remineralize demineralized areas of "white spots" on young children to help prevent early childhood decay (Tables 11-6■ and 11-7■).

3. Fluoride mouthrinses that are used weekly in school rinse programs in areas without water fluoridation contain 0.20% NaF (900 ppm). The rinse uses 5 mL (younger children) or 10 mL (older children), swished for 60 seconds and expectorated.

   a. Weekly rinse is the most common school-based program in the United States

   b. Requires little time (5 minutes/week), inexpensive, easy to learn, well accepted, and can be carried out by teachers with minimal dental hygiene supervision

4. Prophy pastes generally contain small amounts of fluorides; however, this fluoride should not replace a professionally applied fluoride treatment as a source of topical fluoride

TABLE 11-6 FLUORIDE VARNISH INDICATIONS AND CONTRAINDICATIONS

Indications/Risk Factors

Fluoride varnish application is indicated for infants and children with a moderate or high risk of developing cavities. A child is considered at risk if he or she:

Has had cavities in the past or has white spot lesions and stained fissures

Continues to use the bottle past 1 year of age or sleeps with a bottle containing liquids other than water

Breast-feeds on demand at night past the age of 1

Has a developmental disability

Chronically uses high sugar oral medications

Has frequent (three or more times per day) cariogenic snacks

Has visible plaque on the teeth

Has parents/caregivers who neglect brushing the child's teeth

Does not drink water with an optimal amount of fluoride or does not get proper fluoride supplementation

Has family members with a history of caries or untreated decay

Engages in prolonged or ad lib use throughout the day of a bottle or sippy cup containing liquids other than water

Contraindications

Fluoride varnish application is contraindicated for children with a low risk of cavity formation who consume optimally fluoridated water or children who receive routine fluoride treatments through a dental office

Ulcerative gingivitis and stomatitis

Known allergies or reactions to colophony (colophonium) (used in a variety of products for its ability to make things sticky) or similar agents

Avoid ingestion during application

Not to be used as a systemic treatment

---

    5. Glass ionomer cement restoratives and sealant materials have fluoride-releasing properties

  H. Home fluorides (self-administered fluorides) prescriptions

    1. Fluoride supplements are dietary supplements that can be administered as a pill, chewable tablet, lozenge, drop, or mouth rinse for swallowing after rinsing

    2. These are prescribed by a physician, nurse practitioner, dentist, or dental hygienist (depending on state law)

    3. Prescription fluoride gels can be used at home for patients at risk; patients either brush them on the teeth or place in a custom tray

TABLE 11-7 FLUORIDE VARNISH APPLICATION PROCEDURES

Pre-Application Instructions

Remind the parent to give the child something to eat and drink before coming to receive a fluoride application

Advise the parent that the child's teeth may become discolored temporarily as fluoride varnish has an orange-brown tinge (if using a colored varnish)

Tell the parent that the residual varnish can be brushed off the following day

Application

Gently remove excess saliva or plaque with a gauze sponge
Use your fingers and sponges to isolate the dry teeth and keep them dry

You will usually be able to isolate a quadrant of teeth at a time, but may have to work with fewer teeth in some children; infants are easiest because they have only anterior teeth

Apply a thin layer of the varnish to all surfaces of the teeth; avoid applying varnish on large open cavities

Once the varnish is applied, you need not worry about moisture (saliva) contamination; the varnish sets quickly

Post-Application Instructions

The child should wait 30 minutes to eat and should eat a soft, nonabrasive diet for the rest of the day; the child should also avoid eating crunchy or hard food for 4 hours or more

It is normal for the teeth to appear dull and yellow until they are brushed

Repeat the application once every 3 months regardless of risk factor

I. Home fluorides (self-administered fluorides; non-prescription)

    1. Over-the-counter (OTC) fluoride products include toothpastes, mouthrinses, and floss (Figure 11-4■)

        a. Fluoridated toothpastes generally contain sodium fluoride (NaF) 0.24% (1100 ppm), sodium monofluorophosphate (Na_2PO_3F) 0.76%, or an extra-strength at Na_3PO_3F contains 1500 ppm

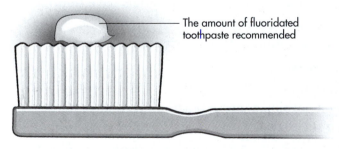

The amount of fluoridated toothpaste recommended

FIGURE 11-4 ■ Correct Amount of Fluoridated Toothpaste

b. The American Dental Association Seal of Acceptance program is a voluntary program and not regulated nor required by the federal or state governments

c. Mouthrinses that are sold OTC includes 0.05% NaF, 0.044% APF, or 0.63% SnF. A single container must contain no more than 120 mg of fluoride

d. Fluoride can be incorporated into unwaxed dental floss. Interproximal surfaces of teeth treated *in vitro* with fluoride-impregnated dental floss acquired significantly (approximately threefold) more enamel fluoride than those treated with plain dental floss. The number of *in vivo* interproximal areas harboring *Streptococcus mutans* was reduced significantly after treatment with fluoride-impregnated dental floss. Further studies should be done to establish the biological, physiochemical, manufacturing, and practical aspects of fluoride-impregnated dental floss.

II. Pit and Fissure Sealants

A. Mechanisms of action

1. Dental sealant is an organic polymer that bonds to the enamel surfaces of the pit and fissures by mechanical retention

2. Sealants are 100% effective in preventing pit and fissure caries when retained and remain retained in about 85% of the cases for up to 5–7 years

B. Goals of sealants

1. Seal off the pit and fissure surfaces

2. Fill the pit and fissure as deeply as possible

3. Prevent bacteria from collecting in the pit and fissures

C. Sealant material

1. Sealant material is a polymer resin (BisGMA) that may be:

a. Filled (glass or quartz particles)

b. Unfilled

c. Fluoride-releasing filled

d. Polymerization may occur with the use of an external light source (photopolymerized) or by the inclusion of a catalyst mixed with the sealant (self-curing or autopolymerization)

D. Bonding

1. Bonding is a hydrophilic agent utilized after the etching of the surface, which produces irregularities or micropores, sometimes referred to as tissue tags

2. Sealant material then bonds to the tooth surface areas via retention in these micropores

E. Techniques for application

    1. Assessment of tooth includes a tooth with no interproximal decay and deep pit and fissures

    2. It has been theorized that teeth should not be treated with fluoride prior to sealant application including teeth polished with prophy paste that contains fluoride; however, the application of fluoride prior to sealant placement is no longer a contraindication for sealant placement

F. Application procedure (Table 11-8■)

TABLE 11-8 APPLICATION PROCEDURE	
Polish	Clean occlusal surface with pumice, air polisher, or toothbrush
Rinse and dry	Rinse and dry tooth surface and isolate tooth by the use of cotton rolls, triangles, and/or gauze

Acid etch	Apply acid etch (phosphoric acid) to create micropores according to manufacturer's directions
	
	🔑 Acid etch may come in a variety of forms;
	    Liquid, use cotton pellets to apply
	    Gel
	    Semi-gel

Rinse and dry	Rinse and dry tooth; isolate tooth
Application of material	Apply sealant by covering pits and fissures but not overfilling the surface 🔑 Self-cured sealant will need to be applied after mixing sealant and catalyst; light-cured sealant will need to be applied and a light source will need to be placed on top of surface for the manufacturer's recommended time
Examine sealant	Check sealant adhesion and occlusion and adjust if necessary 🔑 If sealant is placed incorrectly in the interproximal area, acid etch can be used to remove it so flossing may be accomplished
Sealant failure	If sealant has not adhered to the tooth surface, rinse and dry tooth and repeat the etching and sealant placement procedures

G. Sealants in school programs. Many times programs are implemented in schools that provide dental sealants in the school setting. Dental hygienists and dental assistants screen children and then place dental sealants on first and second molars. In some states dentists must supervise sealant programs, which decreases their cost effectiveness. Despite the availability of highly effective measures for primary prevention, dental caries (tooth decay) remains one of the most common childhood chronic diseases. When properly placed, dental sealants are almost 100% effective in preventing caries on the chewing surfaces of first and second permanent molar teeth. However, sealants remain underused, particularly among children from low-income families and from racial/ethnic minority groups. Schools traditionally have been a setting for both dental disease prevention programs and for oral health status assessment (Figure 11-5■).

III. Other Preventive Agents

A. Fluoride custom trays are made by the dental hygienist to hold fluoride for patients at high risk of dental caries

    1. They are made of thermoplastic material

    2. Patients at high risk include those with medical conditions/diseases or taking medicines causing xerostomia, those with orthodontic or full-mouth restoratives with a high history of caries. In particular, patients undergoing radiation therapy for cancer experience severe xerostomia, making them excellent candidates for fluoride custom trays.

B. Chemotherapeutic agents to control or prevent dental caries will necessitate a more holistic understanding of the plaque microcommunity. Shotgun suppression of the entire flora without acknowledging the overall effect on ecology is unlikely to succeed. Chemotherapeutic approaches must be better targeted against specific microbes, with the goal of reestablishing an ecologically stable noncariogenic plaque. In addition, chemotherapy will need to be coupled with mechanical measures to reduce or eliminate reservoirs for recolonization.

C. Xylitol is a sugar substitute that has shown promising results in reducing dental caries and ear infections. Xylitol has been shown to provide a measure of resistance to drops in salivary or plaque pH after a carbohydrate challenge. The nonfermentability of xylitol by many oral bacteria and its interference with bacterial metabolism are probably responsible for these results. However, the characteristic that xylitol does not lower the pH of dental plaque below 5.7 *in vivo* is shared by most other polyols. *Streptococci mutans* can metabolize sorbitol and mannitol but not xylitol. One study of 14 days' duration also found

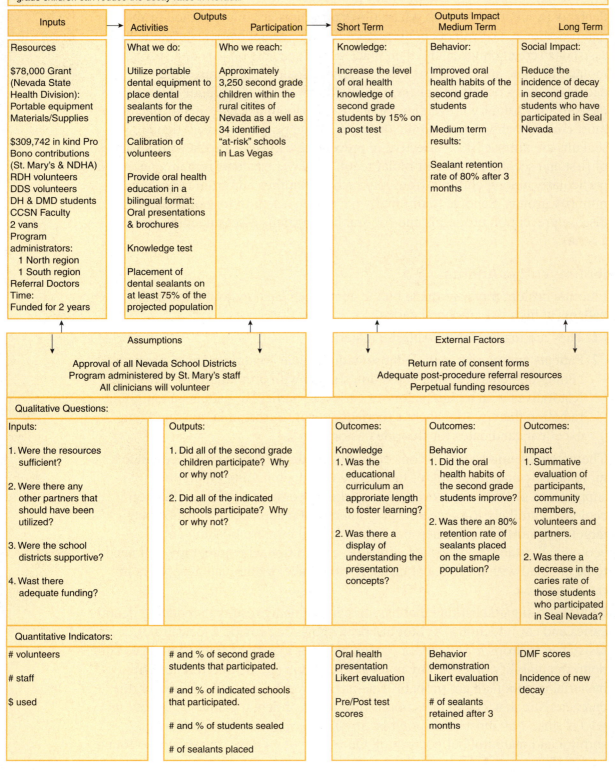

Situation: Nevada children experience some of the highest decay rates in the Nation. Evidence shows that dental sealants are an effective preventive protocol to reduce the incidence of decay. A portable expansion of the St. Mary's Sealant program that targets second grade children can reduce the decay rates in Nevada.

Inputs	Outputs		Outputs Impact		
	Activities	Participation	Short Term	Medium Term	Long Term

Inputs

Resources

$78,000 Grant (Nevada State Health Division):
Portable equipment
Materials/Supplies

$309,742 in kind Pro Bono contributions (St. Mary's & NDHA)
RDH volunteers
DDS volunteers
DH & DMD students
CCSN Faculty
2 vans
Program administrators:
   1 North region
   1 South region
Referral Doctors
Time:
Funded for 2 years

Activities — What we do:

Utilize portable dental equipment to place dental sealants for the prevention of decay

Calibration of volunteers

Provide oral health education in a bilingual format:
Oral presentations & brochures

Knowledge test

Placement of dental sealants on at least 75% of the projected population

Participation — Who we reach:

Approximately 3,250 second grade children within the rural cities of Nevada as a well as 34 identified "at-risk" schools in Las Vegas

Short Term — Knowledge:

Increase the level of oral health knowledge of second grade students by 15% on a post test

Medium Term — Behavior:

Improved oral health habits of the second grade students

Medium term results:

Sealant retention rate of 80% after 3 months

Long Term — Social Impact:

Reduce the incidence of decay in second grade students who have participated in Seal Nevada

Assumptions

Approval of all Nevada School Districts
Program administered by St. Mary's staff
All clinicians will volunteer

External Factors

Return rate of consent forms
Adequate post-procedure referral resources
Perpetual funding resources

Qualitative Questions:

Inputs:

1. Were the resources sufficient?

2. Were there any other partners that should have been utilized?

3. Were the school districts supportive?

4. Wast there adequate funding?

Outputs:

1. Did all of the second grade children participate? Why or why not?

2. Did all of the indicated schools participate? Why or why not?

Outcomes — Knowledge

1. Was the educational curriculum an appriorate length to foster learning?

2. Was there a display of understanding the presentation concepts?

Outcomes — Behavior

1. Did the oral health habits of the second grade students improve?

2. Was there an 80% retention rate of sealants placed on the smaple population?

Outcomes — Impact

1. Summative evaluation of participants, community members, volunteers and partners.

2. Was there a decrease in the caries rate of those students who participated in Seal Nevada?

Quantitative Indicators:

volunteers

staff

$ used

and % of second grade students that participated.

and % of indicated schools that participated.

and % of students sealed

of sealants placed

Oral health presentation
Likert evaluation

Pre/Post test scores

Behavior demonstration
Likert evaluation

# of sealants retained after 3 months

DMF scores

Incidence of new decay

FIGURE 11-5 ■ Logic Model

Source: Peterson, S. (2003). Dental Public Health Workshop, Albuquerque, NM.

that sorbitol produced a plaque pH response to sucrose challenge that was similar to that of xylitol.

1. Xylitol is found in berries, fruit, vegetables, mushrooms, and birch wood

2. Xylitol can be delivered in teeth via mints, gums, and lozenges to help reduce dental caries

3. After chewing food or products containing xylitol, bacteria do not absorb well on the surface of the tooth and the amount of plaque is decreased

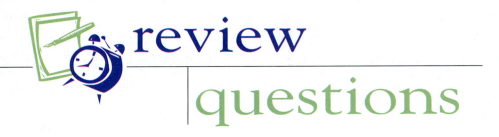
DIRECTIONS Each of the questions or incomplete statements below is followed by suggested answers or completions. Select the **one** answer that is best in each case.

1. Some loss of tooth structure occurs during polishing; therefore, which of the following MUST be applied in an attempt to replace the lost protection?
   A. Sealants
   B. Fluoride
   C. An amalgam
   D. A varnish

2. Which of the following is considered the MOST effective treatment for hypersensitive teeth?
   A. Acidulated phosphate fluoride
   B. Sodium fluoride
   C. Stannous fluoride
   D. A and B only
   E. B and C only

3. Repeated application of a topical fluoride will NOT cause enamel mottling because
   A. Topical fluoride is too weak to produce mottling
   B. The tooth is already calcified and cannot be altered
   C. The glycerin base of the polishing agent will protect the tooth from mottling
   D. Both A and C

4. Which of the following will decrease the retention and effectiveness of a pit and fissure sealant?
   A. Improper technique
   B. Abrasive dentifrice
   C. Saliva contamination of the etched enamel
   D. Consistent use of a hard-bristled toothbrush
   E. All of the above

5. Fluoride-induced enamel hypoplasia or hypocalcification is
   A. More caries-prone
   B. Caries-resistant
   C. Hypersensitive to temperature changes

6. MOST fluoride is excreted through the
   A. Small intestine
   B. Kidneys
   C. Liver
   D. Feces
   E. Sweat glands

7. MOST fluoride is absorbed in the
   A. Liver
   B. Small intestine
   C. Sweat glands
   D. Urine
   E. Kidneys

8. The pH of acidulated fluoride gels is in the range of
   A. 1–3
   B. 3–5
   C. 5–7
   D. 7–9
   E. 9–11

9. Fluorosis may result from excessive fluoride consumed during
   A. The mineralization stage of tooth development
   B. The maturation stage of tooth development
   C. Either the mineralization or the maturation stage of tooth development

10. Which of the following is an advantage of a school-based fluoride program?
    A. It is the most effective method of reducing dental caries.
    √B. It can be implemented by nondental personnel.
    C. It can achieve maximum effectiveness with monthly application.
    D. It is the least expensive method of administering fluoride.

11. In communities without fluoridated water supplies, the MOST cost-effective method of delivering fluoride to 6- to 12- year-old children is through
    A. Fluoride tablets
    B. School water fluoridation
    C. Brushing with a fluoride gel
    D. A fluoride mouthrinse program

12. Which of the following factors need not be considered in deciding whether pediatric fluoride supplements should be prescribed?
    A. Age of the patient
    B. Amount of fluoride in the drinking water
    C. Conscientiousness of the patient or parents
    D. Type of topical fluoride applied professionally

13. A 3-year-old child who lives in a nonfluoridated area has rampant decay. Which of the following home-care regimens, with parental supervision, is suitable for this child?
    A. Fluoride tablets
    B. Fluoride dentifrice
    C. Fluoride mouthrinse
    D. Brush-on gel
    E. Fluoride drops

14. Fluoride uptake in teeth depends on which of the following factors?
    A. Amount of fluoride delivered → ingested
    B. Type of fluoride delivered
    C. Form of fluoride delivered
    D. Length of time of exposure to fluoride delivered

15. Ideally, the optimum concentration of fluoride in community drinking water is in the range of
    A. 0.2–1.0 ppm
    B. 0.6–1.2 ppm
    C. 1.0–2.0 ppm
    D. 1.2–2.5 ppm

16. Which of the following types and concentrations of fluoride should be recommended to a head and neck cancer patient for home-care custom tray use?
    A. 0.4% stannous fluoride
    B. 1% neutral sodium fluoride
    C. 1.23% acidulated phosphate fluoride
    D. A and C only
    E. A and B only

17. Which of the following types of fluoride is reported to cause staining of demineralized enamel and porcelain?
    A. Stannous fluoride
    B. Acidulated phosphate fluoride
    C. Neutral sodium fluoride

18. Which of the following fluorides is recommended for a patient with bulimia nervosa?
    A. Stannous fluoride
    B. Neutral sodium fluoride
    C. Acidulated phosphate fluoride

19. The length of time of retention of sealants depends almost entirely on the
    A. Anatomy of the pit and fissure
    B. Precision of the technique
    C. Age of the material
    D. Amount of penetration
    E. Type of etchant utilized

20. Sealants should be applied
    A. As soon as possible following eruption
    B. At the age of 12
    C. At the age of 15
    D. After all permanent teeth have erupted
    E. To primary teeth only

21. Duraphat® (Colgate Oral Pharmaceuticals), 5% sodium fluoride varnish, is used for the treatment of
    A. Dentinal hypersensitivity
    B. Dental caries prevention
    C. Reducing demineralization and enhancing remineralization of incipient lesions
    D. A and B only
    E. A, B, and C

22. In sealant and composite placement, etching functions to which of the following?
    A. Increase the surface tension
    B. Expose the more porous dentin
    C. Produce a hard, lustrous surface
    D. Break down the calcium fluoride layer
    E. Produce micropores in the enamel surface

23. Penetration of sealant resins depends on each of the following properties EXCEPT one. Which one is the EXCEPTION?
    A. Viscosity of the sealant material
    B. Setting time
    C. Surface area
    D. Curing mechanism

24. The primary reasons for etching enamel before placing a sealant are to
    A. Increase the size of micropores
    B. Decrease surface irregularities to increase the area for retention
    C. Form a smooth surface to increase surface energy
    D. Create a chemical bond between enamel and sealant

25. Sealants prevent dental caries by creating a protective physical bond with the tooth. As long as the sealant remains intact, caries will not develop beneath it.
    A. Both statements are TRUE.
    B. Both statements are FALSE.
    C. The first statement is TRUE; the second is FALSE.
    D. The first statement is FALSE; the second is TRUE.

26. The MOST effective control or preventive measures for pit and fissure caries include
    A. Topical fluoride applications
    B. Pit and fissure sealants
    C. Prophylactic odontotomy
    D. Amalgam restorations
    E. All of the above

27. Which of the following materials are thermoplastic?
    A. Athletic mouthguard material
    B. Alginate impression material
    C. Dental amalgam material
    D. Zinc oxide–eugenol material

28. Mouthguards can be
    A. Custom-made
    B. Stock
    C. Mouth-formed
    D. All of the above

29. Wearing athletic mouthguards prevents concussions.
    A. True
    B. False

30. Professional athletes are more susceptible to oral–facial injuries than young children participating in sports.
    A. True
    B. False

31. Thermoplastic material will _____ upon heating and _____ upon cooling.
    A. Soften, reharden
    B. Harden, soften
    C. Harden, stay hard
    D. Soften, melt

32. Which method of systemic fluoride is MOST economical for caries prevention?
    A. Community water fluoridation
    B. Dietary fluoride supplements
    C. Naturally occurring in foods
    D. Professional fluoride treatment

33. What is the appropriate dietary fluoride supplement, in milligrams, for a 3-year-old patient who lives in an area with 0.4 ppm of fluoride in the water?
    A. None
    B. 0.25 ppm
    C. 0.5 ppm
    D. 1 ppm

34. All of the following indicate use of a professional topical fluoride EXCEPT one. Which one is the EXCEPTION?
    A. Wearing orthodontic appliances
    B. Compromised salivary flow
    C. Low community water fluoride level
    D. Primary teeth

35. For an adult patient, the maximum amount of fluoride recommended for a professionally applied topical treatment (tray technique), in milliliters, is
    A. 0.2
    B. 0.25
    C. 2.0
    D. 2.5

36. Which of the following professional topical fluorides has a recommended concentration of 1.23%?
    A. Acidulated phosphate fluoride
    B. Monofluorophosphate
    C. Sodium fluoride
    D. Stannous fluoride

37. What is the first sign of acute fluoride toxicity?
    A. Abdominal pain
    B. Diarrhea
    C. Nausea
    D. Vomiting

38. All of the following factors increase the severity of chronic fluoride toxicity EXCEPT one. Which one is the EXCEPTION?
    A. Increase in consumption of naturally fluoridated water
    B. Swallowing an excess amount of fluoride during a professional fluoride treatment
    C. Elevated intake of fluoride in food
    D. Low-calcium diet

review questions

39. Which of the following relates to auto-polymerization?
    A. Setting time cannot be controlled once catalyst is added
    B. Shorter polymerization time
    C. No mixing of materials
    D. Requires no special curing light

40. The goal(s) of sealants include
    A. Seal off the pit and fissure surfaces
    B. Fill the pit and fissure as deeply as possible
    C. Prevent bacteria from collecting in the pit and fissures
    D. All of the above

41. Polymerization may occur with the use of an external light source (autopolymerized) or by the inclusion of a catalyst mixed with the sealant (self-curing).
    A. Both statements are TRUE.
    B. Both statements are FALSE.
    C. The first statement is TRUE; the second statement is FALSE.
    D. The first statement is FALSE; the second statement is TRUE.

42. Fluoridation is the process of removing naturally occurring fluoride from water supplies and is done when the fluoride content is well over 1 ppm.
    A. Both statements are TRUE.
    B. Both statements are FALSE.
    C. The first statement is TRUE; the second statement is FALSE.
    D. The first statement is FALSE; the second statement is TRUE.

43. Prophy pastes generally contain small amounts of fluorides; however, this fluoride should not replace a professionally applied fluoride treatment as a source of topical fluoride.
    A. Both statements are TRUE.
    B. Both statements are FALSE.
    C. The first statement is TRUE; the second statement is FALSE.
    D. The first statement is FALSE; the second statement is TRUE.

44. Which patient would most benefit from a fluoride custom tray.
    A. 57-year-old undergoing radiation therapy for cancer
    B. 3-year-old child with a high caries risk factor
    C. 12-year-old patient with severe disabilities causing uncontrollable shaking
    D. 20-year-old with a history of no caries

45. Xylitol is a sugar substitute that has shown promising results in reducing dental caries and indigestion.
    A. Both statements are TRUE.
    B. Both statements are FALSE.
    C. The first statement is TRUE; the second statement is FALSE.

46. Enamel hypomineralization can be caused by
    A. Fluorosis
    B. Sodium bicarbonate
    C. Carbomide peroxide
    D. B and C only

47. When applying sealant material to a pit and fissure surface it is necessary to first apply what to the surface?
    A. A catalyst
    B. Acid etchant
    C. Fluoride
    D. Chlorohexidine gluconate

48. Which fluoride can cause scratching to a porcelain crown?
    A. Sodium fluoride
    B. Stannous fluoride
    C. Acidulated phosphate fluoride
    D. Monosodium fluoride

49. After chewing food or products containing xylitol, bacteria do not absorb well on the surface of the tooth and the amount of plaque decreases.
    A. Both statements are TRUE.
    B. Both statements are FALSE.
    C. The first statement is TRUE; the second statement is FALSE.
    D. The first statement is FALSE; the second statement is TRUE.

50. Water fluoridation is MOST effective for which age group?
    A. Prenatal
    B. 6 months–14 years
    C. 14 years–16 years
    D. 45 years–50 years

review questions

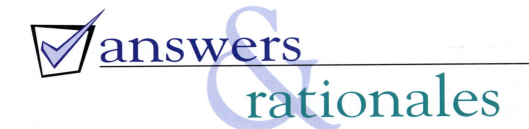

answers & rationales

1.

B. Some loss of the fluoride-rich tooth structure does occur during polishing. The rate of abrasion can be controlled through speed, pressure, and amount of abrasive used. Fluoride should be applied after tooth polishing.

2.

E. Fluoride applications are considered to be the most effective treatment for hypersensitive teeth. This includes self-applied fluoride by the patients. Sodium fluoride and stannous fluoride are commonly used to treat hypersensitive teeth. Acidulated phosphate fluoride is contraindicated for treatment of hypersensitivity due to the high acid pH.

3.

B. Repeated application of a topical fluoride will not cause enamel mottling because the tooth is already calcified and cannot be altered. The greatest amount of fluoride is taken up from topical preparations applied soon after eruption. Effectiveness of topical fluoride depends on its ability to deposit fluoride as fluorapatite in the tooth surface.

4.

E. Improper technique, abrasive dentifrices, water contamination of the etched enamel, and a hard-bristled toothbrush are all factors that will decrease the retention and effectiveness of a pit and fissure sealant. Precise technique must be used without contamination. Contaminants that will cause the sealant to fail are saliva and water.

5.

B. Ingestion of drinking water containing fluoride concentrations greater than 1 ppm during tooth development may result in enamel hypoplasia or fluorosis. The extent of the damage is dependent on the duration of ingestion, the timing of the ingestion (during development), and the intensity or concentration. Fluorosis ranges from white spots to mottled brown and white discolorations. There may also be pitting of the enamel. Enamel hypoplasia is caries resistant.

6.

B. Most fluoride is excreted through the kidneys, with a small amount excreted by the sweat glands.

7.

B. Most fluoride is rapidly absorbed by the small intestine and stomach. Maximum blood levels are reached within 30 minutes of intake. In young children, about one-half of the fluoride intake deposits in calcifying bones and teeth. Fluoride is stored in mineralized tissues (99% of the body fluoride). The teeth store small amounts, with the highest levels on the tooth surface.

8.

B. The pH of acidulated phosphate–fluoride gels is 3.0–3.5; sodium fluoride (2%) has a basic pH of 9.2. Stannous fluoride (8%) has a pH of 2.1–2.3.

9.

A. Fluoride is essential to the formation of sound teeth. It is deposited during the formation of the enamel. Sources of fluoride include drinking water and other ingested fluoride, such as tablets, drops, and foods. If there is an excess of fluoride during the mineralization stages, a defective enamel matrix can form. This can lead to dental fluorosis.

10.

B. The use of a weekly rinse is the most common school-based program in the United States. Advantages are that it requires little time (about 5 minutes once weekly for an entire class); is inexpensive; is easy to learn and well accepted by participants; and can be carried out by nondental personnel. Responsibility for providing the correctly mixed solution and safe storage can be taken by school officials and a supervising dental hygienist.

11.

B. School water fluoridation is a satisfactory method of bringing the benefits of fluoridation to children living in communities without fluoridated water supplies.

12.

D. When determining the need for pediatric fluoride supplements, you need to consider the age of the patient, the amount of fluoride in the patient's drinking water, and the conscientiousness and motivation level of the patient or parents. Supervision must also be provided. The type of topical fluoride applied professionally is not a factor that you need to consider.

13.

A. For a 3-year-old in a nonfluoridated area, tablets should be prescribed. For children from birth to 2 years of age, fluoride drops are primarily used. The tooth contact of the chewable tablet provides the enamel surface with protective fluoride.

14.

D. Uptake of fluoride depends on the amount of fluoride ingested (not delivered) and the length of time of exposure. Fluoride is a natural constituent of enamel. The surface has the highest concentration and the amount decreases rapidly toward the interior layers of the tooth.

15.

B. The optimum fluoride level for water in temperate climates is 1 ppm. For warmer climates and colder climates the amount can be adjusted from 0.6 ppm to 1.2 ppm.

16.

E. Stannous fluoride and neutral sodium fluoride are recommended for head and neck cancer patients to protect them from post-irradiation caries. Daily fluoride applications are recommended while the patient is receiving radiation therapy. Custom trays are made prior to the start of therapy and the patient places the fluoride gel from the tray in the mouth for 4 minutes a day.

17.

A. Stannous fluoride may discolor tooth-colored restorations and margins. There may also be staining of the teeth in demineralized areas, pits, fissures, and grooves.

18.

B. A multiple fluoride preventive program is recommended for a patient with bulimia in an attempt to counteract dental erosion. A fluoride dentifrice, neutral sodium fluoride 0.05% rinse preparation, and a daily gel tray application with neutral sodium is recommended.

19.

B. The length of time of retention of sealants depends almost entirely on the precision of the technique. Each step in the preparation of the tooth and the application of the sealant must be carefully performed. Improper technique is probably the major cause of early loss of a sealant from the tooth surface.

20.

A. Applications of sealants should be made as soon as possible following eruption. When application is delayed, caries may start, and the surface no longer can be considered for sealant. When possible, sealants can be applied before full eruption, provided there is no tissue flap to interfere with application.

21.

E. Sodium fluoride varnishes have been proven to be effective in reducing dentinal hypersensitivity, in preventing dental caries, and in reducing demineralization and enhancing remineralization of incipient lesions.

22.

E. Etching tooth surfaces creates a larger surface area that has micropores to help sealant retention.

23.

C. Sealants are retained in the tooth by bonding a sealant has with the tooth surface area. Etching the tooth increases the tooth's surface area for this bonding to occur.

24.

A. Etching increases the micropores, which increases the surface area. The more surface area, the better the sealant is retained.

25.

A. Sealants decrease caries activity in the pit and fissures of teeth where sealants remain intact. They do this by preventing bacterial plaque biofilm to form in the pit and fissures and demineralization to eventually occur. As long as sealants are retained in the pit and fissures, dental caries will not occur, because demineralization will not occur in these areas.

26.

B. The most effective method to prevent pit and fissure caries is dental sealants because if a sealant is retained, pit and fissure demineralization will not occur. Fluoride is most effective on the smooth surfaces of the tooth.

27.

A. Thermoplastic materials will soften upon heating and harden upon cooling. Athletic mouthguards are thermoplastic.

28.

D. Athletic mouthguards can be bought in a sporting goods store in various sizes as stock mouthguards, or bought to be boiled and then fit to the teeth. Dental offices can fabricate a custom mouthguard from a dental cast of the individual. This is a custom-made mouthguard.

29.

A. Wearing an athletic mouthguard helps prevent concussions by absorbing the force from a blow to the head. Usually when a blow occurs, a person will bite down with extreme force, thus causing or making worse a concussion.

30.

B. Young, inexperienced athletes are more likely to sustain injuries from traumas during athletic events than professional athletes.

31.

A. Thermoplastic materials will soften upon heating and harden upon cooling.

32.

A. Community fluoridation is the most economical systemic method for caries prevention. Dietary fluoride supplements and food that naturally contain fluoride are sources of systemic fluoride, but are not as economical as community fluoridation. Professional fluoride treatment is a topical form of fluoridation.

33.

B. A 3-year-old child would require a supplemental fluoride of 0.25 if the community water supply is <0.4 ppm of fluoride. However, a 3-year-old child may be prescribed 0.5 mg of fluoride if the concentration of fluoride in the water is less than 0.3 ppm. A supplement of 1 mg would never be prescribed to a 3-year-old.

34.

C. Low community water fluoridation level is not an indication for applying professional topical fluoride.

35.

D. An adult patient would receive 2.5 ml of fluoride during a professional fluoride treatment. A child fluoride treatment would contain 2.0 ml of fluoride. It is important to administer the correct amount to receive the full benefit of fluoride to reduce the chance of toxicity.

36.

A. Acidulated phosphate fluoride has a recommended concentration of 1.23%. This is obtained by combining 2.0% sodium fluoride and 0.34% hydrofluoric acid. Monofluorophosphate is found in dentifrices only. Professionally, sodium and stannous fluorides are available at 2% and 8%, respectively.

37.

C. The first sign of acute fluoride toxicity is nausea. Following nausea, the patient may also experience vomiting, abdominal pain, and diarrhea.

38.

B. Swallowing an excess amount of fluoride during a professional fluoride treatment is an example of acute, not chronic, fluoride toxicity. Factors that increase the severity of chronic fluoride toxicity include an increase in the consumption of fluoridated water, elevated intake of fluoride in food, and a low calcium diet.

39.

A. Autopolymerization or self-cured sealants require the mixing of a monomer and a catalyst. Once the catalyst is added, the setting time cannot be controlled. Light-cured or photopolymerization involves a shorter polymerization time, no mixing of materials, and a special curing light.

40.

D. Sealants prevent decay by sealing off the pit and fissure surfaces, filling the pit and fissure as deeply as possible, and preventing bacteria from collecting in the pit and fissures.

41.

A. Polymerization is when the monomers are cross-linked and become polymers. This is what happens when sealants "harden." This may occur with the use of an external light source (autopolymerized) or by the inclusion of a catalyst mixed with the sealant (self-curing).

42.

B. Defluoridation is removing naturally occurring fluoride from a water supply and is only done when the fluoride content is well over 1 ppm.

43.

A. Although most commercially available prophy pastes contain fluoride, they are not recommended to replace a professionally applied topical fluoride.

44.

A. Patients undergoing radiation therapy experience xerostomia, which subsequently increases the risk for dental caries. In addition, many older patients have gingival recession on some teeth, which increases the risk for root caries, thus making a fluoride custom tray an effective option for prevention of dental caries.

45.

C. Xylitol is a sugar substitute that has shown effectiveness in preventing dental caries and ear infections, but has not shown effectiveness in preventing indigestion.

46.

A. Enamel hypomineralization can be caused by ingesting too much fluoride.

47.

B. Applying acid etchant to the tooth surface before applying sealant material serves to create micropores in the tooth surface, thus increasing surface area, which helps bonding occur.

48.

C. Acidulated phosphate fluoride can cause scratching on ceramic and porcelain restorations.

49.

A. The theory of how xylitol prevents dental caries is that bacteria (especially those associated with tooth demineralization) tend to not adhere to tooth surfaces after ingesting xylitol.

50.

B. Water fluoridation is most effective when teeth are developing during the first 6 months to age 14.

12 Providing Supportive Treatment Services

Providing supportive treatment encompasses the science of dental materials. This science focuses on the study of materials used to restore or replace missing tooth structure, bone, and soft tissues. Dental hygienists study these materials in relation to the maintenance of health and prevention of further disease. In fact, preventing material failure is a focus of dental hygiene. Additionally, dental hygienists educate patients on specific materials and treatment modalities and provide detailed instruction on the daily maintenance of these materials.

chapter objectives

After completion of this chapter, the learner should be able to:

➤ Describe the properties and manipulation of materials
➤ Describe polishing natural and restored teeth
➤ Describe impressions and preparing study casts
➤ Define all other supportive structures

I. Properties and Manipulation of Materials

A. Characteristics of an ideal dental material

    1. Biocompatibility

    2. Adhere to tissues when necessary

    3. Easy to manipulate

    4. Cleanable

    5. Repairable

    6. Fiscally responsible

    7. Resistant to corrosion

    8. Dimensionally stable

    9. Minimal thermal and electrical conductivity

    10. Esthetically pleasing

    11. Tasteless

B. Regulation of dental materials

    1. Food and Drug Administration (FDA) regulates safety and efficacy of dental materials and devices

    2. Occupational Safety and Health Administration (OSHA) provides guidelines for safety and welfare of those in the workplace; OSHA enforces the completion of Material Safety Data Sheets (MSDS); MSDS are a document with a description of the chemicals in a product, and pertinent other data including such things as safe handling and emergency procedures; in accordance with OSHA regulations, it is the manufacturer's responsibility to produce an MSDS and the employer's responsibility to communicate its contents to employees

C. Dental restorations classifications

    1. Direct restoration is fabricated directly in the oral cavity

    2. Indirect restorations are fabricated using cast replica or oral structures involved

    3. Types of restorations include the following:

        a. Inlay replaces intracoronal tooth structure (Figure 12-1■)

        b. Onlay replaces intracoronal tooth structure including at least one cusp (Figure 12-2■)

        c. Veneer replaces the facial surface of anterior teeth (Figure 12-3■)

        d. Crown replaces extracoronal tooth structure and is cemented to tooth structure or implant (Figure 12-4■)

        e. Implant(s) replaces the missing tooth or teeth (Figure 12-5■)

        f. Fixed partial denture (bridge) replaces missing tooth or teeth and is cemented to adjacent teeth (Figure 12-6■)

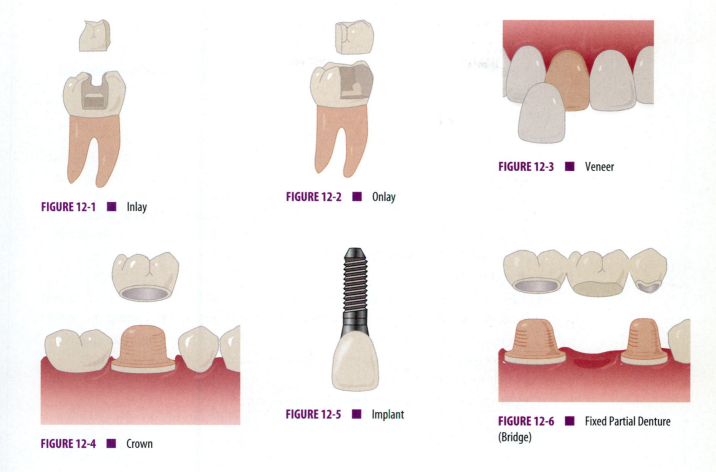

FIGURE 12-1 ■ Inlay

FIGURE 12-2 ■ Onlay

FIGURE 12-3 ■ Veneer

FIGURE 12-4 ■ Crown

FIGURE 12-5 ■ Implant

FIGURE 12-6 ■ Fixed Partial Denture (Bridge)

      g. Removable partial denture replaces missing teeth and is often retained with aid of clasps (Figure 12-7■)

      h. Complete denture replaces a fully endentulous arch (Figure 12-8■)

  D. Dimensional change

     1. Change occurring in dimension of material whether it be shrinkage or expansion

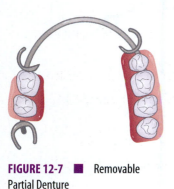

FIGURE 12-7 ■ Removable Partial Denture

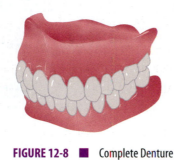

FIGURE 12-8 ■ Complete Denture

2. Oftentimes this change is caused by temperature

3. Sometimes referred to as microleakage or percolation

4. Microleakage is undesirable because of possible irritation of the pulp and recurrent decay

E. Thermal conductivity

1. Rate of heat flow of the material

2. Metals, such as amalgam or gold restoratives, have high heat flow, whereas plastic and ceramics (i.e., composites or porcelain) have a low rate of heat. Basically, materials with high thermal conductivity values are good conductors of heat and cold. So, when using a material that is a good thermal conductor, such as amalgam, it is appropriate to insulate the tooth first with a dental cement, which is a poor thermal conductor.

F. Electrical properties

1. Tarnish is a surface reaction in metals seen as the discoloration of surface and is reversible; tarnish can be removed with a finishing and polishing procedure

2. Corrosion is the dissolution of metal and is irreversible; when the material has corroded it is necessary to replace the material since finishing and polishing cannot restore

3. Galvanism is the generation of electrical currents between two dissimilar metal restoratives that the patient can feel; during a galvanic shock, saliva acts as an electrolyte conductor (Figure 12-9■)

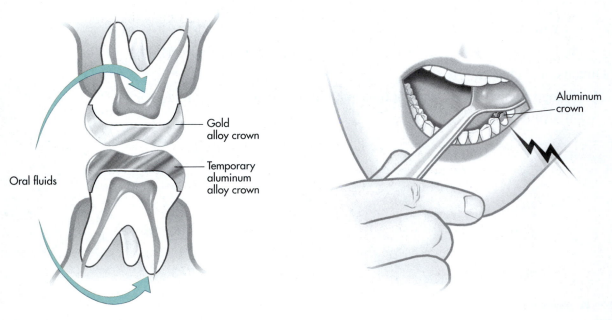

Oral fluids

Gold
alloy crown

Temporary
aluminum
alloy crown

Aluminum
crown

FIGURE 12-9 ■ Galvanism

G. Adhesion and cohesion

    1. Adhesion is the force of attraction between two different objects or surfaces that holds them together; one example would be a cemented orthodontic band that falls off once the patient is at home; the cement is still attached to the band; the problem was adhesion, probably due to saliva contamination.

    2. Cohesion is the force of attraction within an object that holds it together. Using the same scenario as above, the patient returns with cement on the band and the tooth; the problem was cohesion, probably due to the mixing of the cement.

H. Wettability

    1. A measure of the affinity of a liquid for a solid as indicated by the spreading of a drop of liquid sometimes referred to as the contact angle.

    2. A material that has good wettability would remain in close contact, such as sealant materials, fluoride, etc. (Figure 12-10■)

I. Stress and strain

    1. Restorations are subjected to stresses from mastication action. These forces act on teeth and/or material, producing different reactions that can lead to deformation and can ultimately compromise their durability over time. Stress is a materials' response to force (Figure 12-11■).

        a. Compressive: material is squeezed together

        b. Tensile: material is pulled apart

        c. Shear: material is forced to slide back and forth

    2. Strain is the change in length produced by stress. One example of strain is to bend a paper clip back and forth; the permanent change caused by the constant stress is called strain.

J. Elastic modulus, toughness, resilience, and strength

    1. Elastic modulus is the measure of stiffness of a material

    2. Toughness is the ability of a material to resist fracture or simply the energy necessary to fracture a material

    3. Resilience is the ability of a material to resist permanent deformation

    4. Strength is the greatest stress that can be withstood without rupture

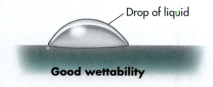

Good wettability

FIGURE 12-10 ■ Wettability

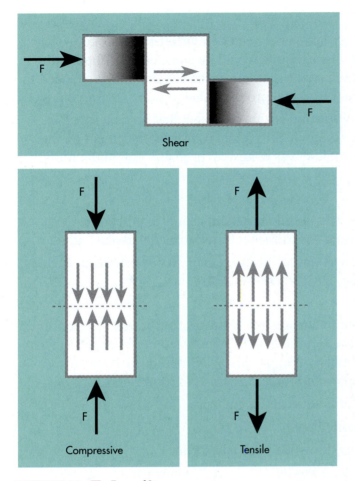

FIGURE 12-11 ■ Types of Stress

K. Ductility and malleability

1. Ductility is the ability of a material to withstand deformation under tension without fracturing; consequently, low ductility indicates brittleness of a material

2. Malleability is the ability of a material to withstand deformation under compression

L. Flow, creep, and fatigue

1. Flow is the continual permanent deformation under load of an amorphous or noncrystalline solid

2. Creep is the time-dependent deformation of an object subjected to constant stress or the flow of that material

3. Fatigue is the weakening of a material caused by repeated loading at a stress level below the fracture strength

M. Hardness

    1. Materials' resistance to indentation. A hardness property value is the result of a defined measurement procedure. Restorative materials with high hardness tend to resist abrasion.

    2. Surface hardness is a parameter frequently used to evaluate material surface resistance to plastic deformation by penetration.

    3. The usual method to achieve hardness value is to measure the depth or area of an indentation left by an indenter of a specific shape with a specific force applied for a specific time. There are four common standard test methods for expressing the hardness of a material: Brinell, Rockwell, Vickers, and Knoop. Each of these methods is divided into a range of scales, defined by a combination of applied load and indenter geometry.

        a. The Brinell hardness test method consists of indenting the material with a 10 mm diameter hardened steel or carbide ball subjected to a load; it is the oldest method to measure surface hardness and is applicable to test metal and alloys

        b. The Rockwell hardness test method consists of indenting the test material with a diamond cone or hardened steel ball indenter; this method is useful to evaluate surface hardness of plastic materials

        c. The Vickers hardness test method consists of indenting the test material with a diamond; it is suitable to be applied to determine the hardness of small areas and for very hard materials

        d. The Knoop hardness is more sensitive to surface characteristics of the material

        e. Moh's Hardness Scale provides a scale of material hardness rates, with diamond being the hardness

N. Imbibition

    1. The taking-up of fluid in the colloid system

    2. Referred to as "swelling" seen in alginate impression material

O. Syneresis

    1. The exudation of liquid film on the surface of a gel

    2. Referred to as "evaporation or condensation" seen in alginate impression material

P. Color

    1. Dimensions

        a. Hue is the dominant color of an object

        b. Value is the lightness of an object

        c. Chroma is the intensity or extent of saturation of a certain color

2. Definitions

    a. Metamerism means that colors look different under different light sources

    b. Fluorescence is the absorption of nonvisible light released by material as visible light

    c. Opacity is the degree to which passage of light is prevented

    d. Transulency is the dispersion of light through a material such that objects cannot be seen through it

    e. Transparency is the passage of minimally distorted light through a material such that objects may be clearly seen through it

Q. Dynamic properties

    1. The property witnessed at extremely high rates of loading, such as an impact

    2. The amount of energy the material is able to absorb

    3. Seen in the effects of the prevention of concussions and oral trauma due to wearing an athletic mouthguard

R. Manipulation of materials

    1. Stages of manipulation

        a. Mixing time is the time from the onset of the procedure to the completion of mixing

        b. Working time is the time from the onset of mixing until the onset of the initial setting time

        c. Initial setting time is the time at which the material is resistant to further manipulation

        d. Final setting time is the time at which the material is practically set as defined by its resistance to indentation

    2. Intervals of manipulation

        a. Three different stages occur during the manipulation

        b. Mixing is the length of time of the mixing stages

        c. Working is the length of time there is to work with a material before it sets

        d. Setting time is the length of time it takes for a material to set

    3. Material systems

        a. Systems by which dental materials commonly are dispensed:

            (1) Powder/liquid

            (2) Powder/water

            (3) Paste/paste

            (4) Paste/light

4. Reactions

    a. Physical is the reaction that occurs when a material solidifies by drying or cooling; an exothermic reaction, such as the heat felt on the base when a study model is setting

    b. Chemical is the reaction that solidifies by the bonding process; polymerization reaction, such as that seen when a sealant is being polymerized by a light source

II. Polishing Natural and Restored Teeth

A. Goals

    1. Reduces chance of decay

    2. Easier to keep clean

    3. Esthetics

    4. Less irritation to tissues

B. Principles

    1. Abrasion is the wearing-away or removal of material by the act of rubbing, cutting, or scraping

    2. Cutting is the removing of material by a shearing-off process

    3. Finishing is the process by which a restoration or appliance is contoured to remove excess material and produce a reasonably smooth surface

    4. Polishing refers to the final removal of material from restoration or appliance to result in a smooth surface; polishing always follows finishing

C. Factors that affect cutting, finishing, and polishing

    1. Hardness: The hardness of an abrasive as well as the hardness of the material to be abraded; Moh's scale refers to diamond as the hardest abrasive

    2. Shape: A spherical particle will be less abrasive than an irregularly cut particle (Figure 12-12■)

    3. Size: Larger particles abrade more rapidly than smaller particles; grit size of prophy paste refers to coarse, medium, fine, and extra fine grit

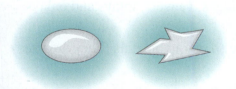

FIGURE 12-12 ■ The shape of particles affects their abrasiveness.

4. Pressure: The more pressure applied, the more abrasion will be accomplished

5. Speed: The faster the abrasive is applied, the more abrasion will be accomplished

6. Lubrication: Adding lubricators such as water will decrease the abrasive effect

7. Instruments with cutting edges and abrasive particles impregnated will result in abrasion

D. Polishing

1. Pumice is a natural glass that is rich in silica; produced from volcanoes

2. Polishing paste may contain pumice, silicon dioxide, or zirconium silicate and usually contains fluoride

3. Selective polishing refers to polishing the teeth only when stain cannot be removed with hand or ultrasonic instrumentation; Evidence-based practice dictates the use of selective polishing

E. Polishing restored teeth

1. There are various agents used when polishing restorations dependent upon the type of restoration to be polished.

2. Polishing paste sizes of fine, medium, coarse, and extra course are not regulated nor set by standards; therefore, the label identity is not necessarily indicative of the grit

3. See Table 12-1■ for a list of commonly used abrasives

F. Dental restorative materials

1. Amalgam is a metal alloy with one of its elements consisting of mercury; used to fill cavity preparations. Amalgams generally are used to fill restorations in the posterior regions.

2. Composite is esthetic restorative cement composed of polymers (resin) and glass particles (fillers). Composites can be used for anterior restorations, bonding, veneers, and inlays.

3. Glass ionomer cement used for Class V cavity preparations and sealants; newer glass ionomer restorations release fluoride.

4. Porcelain is an esthetic restoration that can be used for jacket crowns, porcelain fused to metal crowns and bridges, veneers, inlays and onlays, and very rarely, denture teeth.

5. Gold is an alloy of gold and other noble (precious) metals. They are used for gold foils, crowns, and bridges.

6. Acrylic plastics may be soft and flexible or rigid and brittle and can be used for dentures and denture teeth, denture liners, and oral appliances.

TABLE 12-1 POLISHING AGENTS	
Aluminum oxide	Used to *smooth* enamel (after a slight fracture or chip) or finish metal alloys and ceramic materials
Carbides	Used to cut cavity preparations or finish composite restorations: • Silicon carbide • Boron carbide • Tungsten carbide
Chalk	Used to polish teeth, gold and amalgam restorations, and plastic materials; sometimes it is referred to as whiting or calcium carbonate
Cuttle	A fine grade of quartz, although it was historically derived from fish bones; it is used to finish gold alloys, acrylics, and composites
Diamond	Used to finish and polish composite restorations, and to cut crown and bridge preparations
Emery	Used to grind off rough areas and contour acrylic appliances and custom trays
Garnet	Used for grinding plastics and metal alloys
Pumice	A silicate that is used to polish enamel, gold foil, and dental amalgam and to finish acrylic denture bases
Rouge	Is red in color and is used on a rag wheel to polish gold alloys
Sand	Used to grind metals and plastics
Tin oxide	Used as a final polishing paste for enamel and metallic restorations
Tripoli	Used to polish gold alloys
Zirconium silicate	Used to polish enamel

G. Instruments and materials used to polish restorations

    1. Burs are attached to a handpiece and can either be instruments with cutting edges or impregnated with abrasive particles

    2. Disks are attached to a handpiece and impregnated with abrasive particles

    3. Powders are used during the polishing sequence in conjunction with a rag wheel

    4. Rag wheels are a cloth rag that is attached to the dental lathe and spin so they are able to polish teeth

    5. Rubber cups, brushes, and points are attached to a prophy angle or contra angle for the purpose of polishing

6. Stones can be used to impregnate burs, disks, and strips and as an ingredient in paste

7. Strips are impregnated with abrasives and are utilized in the interproximal area to polish teeth; the process used when polishing with a strip is similar to flossing

H. Bleaching of teeth

    1. Composition

        a. In-office systems—30–35% hydrogen peroxide

        b. In-home systems—10–15% carbamide peroxide

        c. Over-the-counter systems

    2. Technique

        a. In office systems are applied and activated by heat, light, or laser

        b. Home systems—Custom-made application tray holds bleach and is placed by patient

        c. Over-the-counter systems—Can be gel sold with boil-n-bite mouthguards, strips, or gel used when brushing

III. Making Impressions and Preparing Study Casts

A. Impressions are negative replications of the oral cavity, whether dentition or edentulous; impressions accurately record the oral cavity (Figure 12-13■)

    1. Used for study models, patient education, baseline data, appliance fabrication, and restoration fabrication

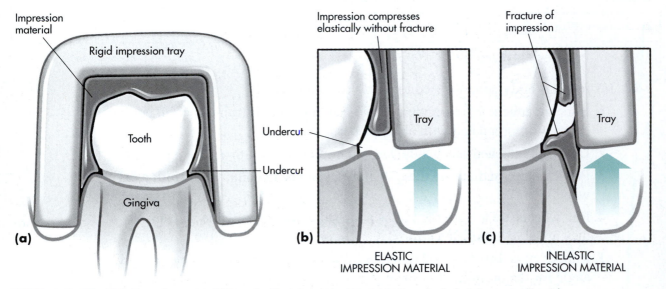

FIGURE 12-13 ■ (a) Making an Impression; (b) Removing Elastic Impression Material; (c) Removing Inelastic Impression Material

B. Requirements of an impression material

    1. Fluid enough to flow into or around area

    2. Must harden once positioned in the mouth

    3. Biocompatible

    4. Dimensionally stable

    5. Easy to handle

    6. Able to disinfect material

C. Inelastic (rigid) impression material

    1. Exhibits little or now spring-like quality when deformed

    2. Basically, any significant deformation produces a permanent change in the shape; cannot be used in undercut areas

    3. Can be used for edentulous procedures

    4. Includes plaster, compound, and zinc-oxide eugenol

        a. Plaster is used most frequently as a study model material; no longer used as an impression material

        b. Impression compound is a thermoplastic material that is supplied as plates or sticks

        c. Zinc-oxide eugenol is a phenol that is derived from oil of cloves

        d. An undercut is an area that has enough of a curve (e.g., a tooth) to make it difficult for a more rigid material to not tear upon removal

D. Elastic (flexible) impression material

    1. Can be removed from undercuts without undergoing any permanent distortion in shape; can be used for both dentulous and edentulous procedures

    2. Flexible hydrocolloids

        a. Hydrocolloids contain large amounts of water and have limited stability once they are removed from the mouth

        b. Agar-Agar—Reversible and transforms from a fluid paste to a rubber-like solid by a physical process that can be reversed simply by altering its temperature; made with seaweed.

        c. Alginate—Irreversible and supplied as a powder/water system; not as dimensionally accurate as agar, but easier to use

            (1) Major components include potassium alginate and calcium sulfate

            (2) Type I is fast setting and Type II is normal setting

            (3) Pour study models soon after taking impressions as it is not dimensionally stable for long periods of time

            (4) Syneresis, which results in shrinkage due to exuding or evaporating of fluids, will result; if waiting to pour, wrap in wet paper towel and place in plastic bag

(5) Imbibition is the swelling when water is absorbed in an alginate impression

(6) Instruct patients about the procedure prior to beginning; have them breath through their noses in an upright position to minimize gagging

3. Flexible, elastomeric, or rubber

a. Polysulfide rubber has high flexibility and tear strength but is long working and has high shrinkage on setting and stains

b. Silicone rubber sometimes referred to as condensation silicone; less dimensionally stable

c. Polyether rubber has a short working time and excellent dimensional stability and good wettability by gypsum, but has low flexibility and poor tear resistance

d. Polyvinyl siloxane referred to as addition silicone; this is most dimensionally stable

E. Model and die material

1. Models, casts, and dies are positive replications of the oral cavity

2. Model is used for observation

3. Cast is used for fabrication of restoration

4. Die is a cast used for a single tooth or a few teeth

5. Types of model material

a. Gypsum is calcium sulfate dehydrate, a rock that is ground to a powder and then mixed with water

b. Gypsum can be ground into irregularly shaped fluffy plaster or denser, regular-shaped particles for stone; the denser the particles, the stronger the stone

c. Gypsum is mined then it is heated and water is driven off; method of driving off water determines gypsum type

d. Plaster

e. Laboratory or model stone

f. Stone is stronger than plaster and model stone

g. Die stone is the strongest

h. High-strength die stone

6. Improper amount of water will adversely affect strength and setting expansion.

7. Lower-water/powder ratios within limits gives increased physical properties.

8. Electroplating are casts that are plated with metal to make them harder and stable.

9. Epoxy dies are resins that are toxic and not regularly used.

IV. Other Supportive Services

A. Temporary restorations may be in the form of a tooth filling or crown

1. Temporary restoratives are used to provide protection to the pulp, provide a palliative effect on the pulp, to be obtudant to the pulp, maintain tooth position, and provide esthetic properties

2. Materials used include zinc-oxide eugenol because it has a palliative effect on the pulp, MMA/PMMA filling materials, and bisacrylic filling materials

B. Rubber dams and matrices

1. Rubber dams provide an isolated working area for restorative procedures

2. See Table 12-2■ for the materials used in rubber dam placement

C. Margination is the process by which restorations are made flush with the enamel or cement surface (Figure 12-14■)

1. When a gap exists between these surfaces, plaque, food debris, and saliva can pass in and out of the gap; this is referred to as percolation or microleakage (Figure 12-15■)

D. Overhang removal is performed when the restoration is overhanging in the interproximal area

1. Contraindications include tooth sensitivity, recurrent decay, and defective restoration

2. Performing margination or overhang removal on a restoration will decrease tarnish, decrease corrosion, increase integrity of the junction of the tooth,

TABLE 12-2 MATERIALS	
Rubber dam	Rubber sheets provide isolation; holes are cut to allow for tooth position above the rubber dam field
Clamps	Used to provide stability and further isolation of materials
Lubricant	Allows easier work with the rubber dam isolation
Napkins	Used occasionally for the comfort of the patient's face
Rubber dam holders	Used for stabilization of the rubber dam and to stretch the rubber material
Matrix band	Utilized during a filling procedure to provide effective margination of the restoration

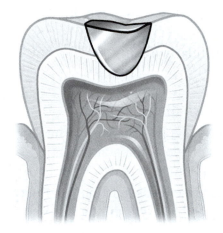

FIGURE 12-14 ■ Margination

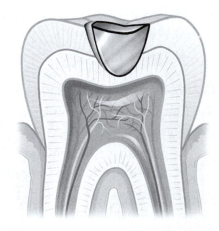

FIGURE 12-15 ■ Gap between Tooth and Restoration

decrease recurrent decay, improve gingival health, improve maintenance by the patient, increase patient comfort, improve appearance of restoration, and maintain tooth health and function

3. Procedure

(1) A bur may be used when the restoration is grossly overhanging

(2) A gold knife instrument may be used

(3) A prophen or EVA system is a handpiece that rotates and is impregnated with diamond chips that help reduce an overhang

(4) Polishing should then be accomplished to further smooth the restorative material; pumice and tin oxide are generally used to polish

E. Debonding is the removal of cements or any luting agent such as composite

1. Removal may be accomplished by mechanical instrumentation and polishing to smooth the area

2. The application of phosphoric acid can be used to remove the material

3. Dental hygienists often remove excess cement from orthodontic bands upon removal

F. Athletic mouthguards are utilized to prevent oral–facial trauma and concussions during athletics

1. Athletic mouthguards are made of thermoplastic material

2. They can be fabricated by the dental hygienist or purchased in the sporting goods section of a store as stock guard (small, medium, and large) or boil-n-bite guard (which the patient bites while softened to indent with his or her dentition).

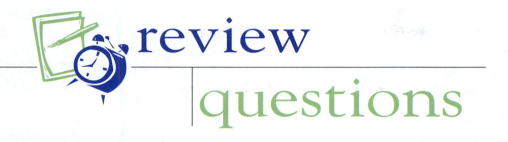

review questions

DIRECTIONS Each of the questions or incomplete statements below is followed by suggested answers or completions. Select the **one** answer that is best in each case.

1. In the United States, which of the following organizations must provide approval before a material can be marketed for dental use?
   A. International Standards Organization
   B. American Dental Association
   C. Occupational Safety and Health Administration
   D. Food and Drug Administration

2. For an adhesive to work on a given adherend, it must wet the surface well. All of the following aid wetting EXCEPT one. Which one is the EXCEPTION?
   A. A clean surface
   B. Fluoride
   C. High surface energy
   D. A smooth surface

3. Which of the following properties can be determined if an applied stress is proportional to a resulting strain for a given material?
   A. Modulus of elasticity
   B. Toughness
   C. Ductility
   D. Ultimate strength

4. All of the following increase the rate of abrasion EXCEPT one. Which one is the EXCEPTION?
   A. Increased pressure
   B. Abrasive harder than the surface being abraded
   C. Decreased speed of abrasive application
   D. Larger abrasive particle

5. Which physical property of an amalgam restoration is LIKELY to cause hot and cold sensitivity following its placement?
   A. Thermal conductivity
   B. Modulus of elasticity
   C. Toughness
   D. Creep

6. All of the following are dimensions of color EXCEPT one. Which one is the EXCEPTION?
   A. Hue
   B. Value
   C. Shade
   D. Chroma

7. Increased water/powder ratios (more water) will affect gypsum by
   A. Increasing its strength
   B. Decreasing its strength
   C. Increasing its abrasion resistance
   D. Decreasing its setting time

8. Alginate (irreversible hydrocolloid) impressions are used to fabricate all of the following EXCEPT one. Which one is the EXCEPTION?
   A. Bleach tray
   B. Three-unit fixed bridge
   C. Custom mouthguard
   D. Study cast

9. All of the following methods supply energy to a monomer (resulting in polymerization) EXCEPT one. Which one is the EXCEPTION?
   A. Heat activation
   B. Chemical activation
   C. Light activation
   D. Copolymerization

10. Which of the following materials is used to prepare the enamel for sealant and bonded orthodontic bracket applications?
    A. 10% hydrofluoric acid
    B. 10% citric acid
    C. 30–50% phosphoric acid
    D. EDTA

11. Which of the following cements provides chemical adhesion to tooth structure?
    A. Glass ionomer
    B. Zinc phosphate
    C. Zinc-oxide eugenol
    D. Resin

12. The combination of metals, which are mutually soluble in the molten state, is referred to as a(n)
    A. Composite resin
    B. Polymer
    C. Cement
    D. Alloy

13. Metals can be protected from corrosion in the oral environment by all of the following EXCEPT one. Which one is the EXCEPTION?
    A. Polishing the surface
    B. Including a noble metal in the alloy
    C. Including a metal that passivates in the alloy
    D. Placing the metal in contact with a dissimilar metal

14. Which form of mercury is of MOST concern for the dental professional?
    A. Vapor
    B. Droplets
    C. Combined with a dental amalgam alloy
    D. Metallic mercury

15. Materials used to protect the pulp from thermal stimulation, often experienced with metallic restorations, are classified as
    A. Varnishes
    B. Low-strength bases
    C. High-strength bases
    D. Liners

16. During an amalgam polishing procedure, which of the following factors can produce the largest biological effect?
    A. Odor
    B. Heat
    C. Debris
    D. Tin oxide

17. For a material to be considered a posterior restorative, all of the following criteria must be included EXCEPT one. Which one is the EXCEPTION?
    A. Ability to withstand high stresses
    B. Ability to withstand large temperature changes with no detrimental effects
    C. Minimal toxic or allergenic potential
    D. Ability to replicate the color of the tooth structure

18. Which of the following is an advantage of indirect restoration?
    A. Allows for optimum development of the form of a restoration
    B. Minimizes patient visits
    C. Less costly than direct restorations
    D. Requires fewer materials

19. A composite resin material that fails to release absorbed light lacks
    A. Metamerism
    B. Opacity
    C. Translucency
    D. Fluorescence

20. Which of the following is NOT an inelastic impression material?
    A. Impression compound
    B. ZOE impression paste
    C. Alginate
    D. Impression plaster

21. What can be done to increase working time when using a mix of reversible hydrocolloid (alginate) impression material?
    A. Increase the water/powder ratio
    B. Decrease the water/powder ratio
    C. Use cooler water
    D. Use warmer water

22. Which of the following is an acceptable method of disinfecting alginate impressions?
    A. Immerse in sodium hypochlorite for 30 minutes
    B. Immerse in alcohol for 30 minutes
    C. Spray with a glutaraldehyde or an iodophor and place in a sealed plastic bag for 10 minutes
    D. Immerse in sodium hypochlorite for 10 minutes

23. Which of the following is NOT a common component of a dental composite resin matrix?
    A. Silane
    B. BIS-GMA
    C. UDMA (urethane dimethacrylate)
    D. TEGDMA

24. Which of the following restorative materials releases significant amounts of fluoride?
    A. Dental amalgam
    B. Glass ionomer cement
    C. Gold alloys
    D. Dental porcelain

25. Which of the following materials has the greatest ultimate tensile strength?
    A. Composite resin
    B. Zinc phosphate cement
    C. Gold alloy
    D. Dental amalgam

26. Which of the following is the primary monomer used in fabricating denture bases?
    A. Methyl methacrylate
    B. TEGDMA
    C. BIS-GMA
    D. UDMA

27. Diagnostic casts made from alginate impressions are routinely used for all of the following EXCEPT
   A. To determine occlusion
   B. As the cast to fabricate a fixed partial denture
   C. To present a treatment plan to the patient
   D. To compare with subsequent models

28. The two principal methods of forming metallic objects used in dentistry are
   A. Cast and wrought
   B. Stamped and forged
   C. Distilled and cast
   D. Wrought and synthetic

29. The three methods of inducing a polymerization reaction in dentistry include all of the following EXCEPT
   A. Light curing
   B. Radioactive curing
   C. Heat curing
   D. Self-curing

30. Pit and fissure sealants represent a trade-off with composite resins in terms of physical and mechanical properties. In order to get the viscosity low enough to flow into the pits and fissures of teeth, what characteristic must be sacrificed?
   A. Color stability
   B. Strength
   C. The ability to use a light gun to cure it
   D. The ability to use it on primary teeth

31. The resistance to flowing demonstrated by a fluid is known as
   A. Thickness ration
   B. Viscosity
   C. Polymerization
   D. Liquid density

32. What do pit and fissure sealants, composites resins, acrylic appliances, and elastomeric impression materials have in common?
   A. They are all polymers.
   B. They all have to be heated before using.
   C. They can all be used as anterior filling materials.
   D. They are all products of secondary reactions.

33. Placing a base in the "bottom" of a cavity preparation serves what purpose?
   A. It helps hold the restoration in place.
   B. It helps insulate the pulpal tissue from the external environment.
   C. It kills any residual bacteria.
   D. It serves to add bulk to the cavity preparation.

34. Which of the following acts as an electrolyte in conjunction with a metal restoration to make up an electrical cell and cause galvanism?
   A. Bone
   B. Enamel
   C. Dentin
   D. Saliva

35. The brief but sharp electrical sensation one can receive when two dissimilar metals come into contact in the mouth is called
   A. Galvanic shock
   B. Alternating current corrosion
   C. Electrolyte explosion
   D. Electromagnetic pulse

36. Which of the following dental materials is a poor thermal conductor?
   A. Gold crowns
   B. Amalgam
   C. Composite resins
   D. Gold foil resins

37. All of the following are primary factors when considering the ideal restorative material EXCEPT
   A. Sustaining biting forces
   B. Resistance to abrasion
   C. Adaptability to the walls of the cavity
   D. Indestructibility to the fluids of the mouth
   E. Color

38. One should approach the subject of dental materials from the standpoint of
   A. What the material is chemically
   B. What happens to the material physically
   C. How the material is manipulated technically
   D. All of the above

39. The perfect method for altering the gelation period of an alginate impression material is to change the
   A. Water–powder ratio
   B. Temperature of the water
   C. Spatulation time of a mix
   D. Quantity of the reactor in the powder
   E. Quantity of the retarder in the powder

40. A complex set of chemical reactions that can weaken and eventually destroy a metal is called
   A. Tarnish
   B. Rust
   C. Hydrogen depletion
   D. Corrosion

41. The delayed expansion or secondary expansion that some zinc-containing amalgams exhibit for many months after their placement is thought to result from
   A. Poor quality control at the factory
   B. Moisture contamination during placement
   C. Overtrituration
   D. Mercury allergy in the patient

42. An increase in the temperature of the water used in mixing irreversible hydrocolloids will
   A. Prevent setting
   B. Shorten time to set
   C. Lengthen time to set
   D. Not affect time to set

43. What component of many cements has a definite soothing property on pulpal tissue?
   A. Zinc oxide
   B. Methyl methacrylate
   C. BIS-GMA
   D. Eugenol

44. The chief difference between model plaster powder and dental stone powder is
   A. Shelf life
   B. Chemical formula
   C. Solubility in water
   D. Particle size and shape

45. On a percentage basis, the main ingredient of a reversible hydrocolloid is
   A. Water
   B. Agar-agar
   C. Calcium alginate
   D. Potassium sulfate

46. The safety of the interaction of dental materials and tissue in the oral cavity (as well as the rest of the body) is assessed in studies grouped under the heading of
   A. Radioactivity studies
   B. Biocompatibility
   C. Carcinogenic potential
   D. Antigenic potential

review questions

47. There are several disadvantages associated with use of base metal dental casting alloys. Which of the following is an advantage that base metal alloys have over noble metal alloys?
    A. Base metal is easier to cast and finish.
    B. Base metal has a stronger porcelain bond.
    C. Base metal is much heavier (denser) than noble metal alloys.
    D. Base metal is stronger and thus more suited to long-span fixed bridges.

48. Which of the following would not be a likely test used to assay a material's biocompatibility?
    A. Toxicity test using bacterial cultures
    B. Pulp responses using extracted human teeth
    C. Carcinogenic potential using mice
    D. Antigenic potential using rabbits

49. Which of the following is not true concerning dental porcelain?
    A. Dental porcelains are ground glass with small amounts of tooth-colored paints added.
    B. Many porcelains rust at a temperature of over 2000°F.
    C. The glaze firing is the last firing and it produces a smooth, translucent surface.
    D. Dental porcelain has good biocompatibility but is very brittle.

50. If an alginate impression cannot be poured immediately, what must be done?
    A. The impression must be heated to body temperature for 15 minutes.
    B. The impression must be placed in a bowl of very cold water.
    C. The impression must be immersed in a solution of 15% calcium sulfate for 10 minutes.
    D. The impression must be kept in an environment of 100% relative humidity, such as in damp paper towels or a humidor.

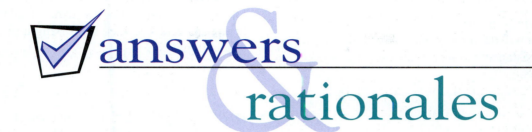

answers & rationales

1.

D. Since May 1976, the FDA has had regulatory jurisdiction over the safety and efficacy of medical and dental materials and devices. The ISO provides guidelines for international standards. The ADA provides a certification program for materials, which meet minimum standards. A certification is not required for a material to be marketed. OSHA is responsible for the safety and welfare of people in the workplace.

2.

B. The addition of a halogen atom, such as fluorine, reduces the surface energy and makes it more difficult to wet. A Teflon pan is an example of this. A clean or smooth surface is easier to wet than a dirty one. Also, a surface with a high surface energy wets easier than a surface with a low surface energy.

3.

A. Stress divided by strain below the proportional limit is equal to the modulus of elasticity for the material. Toughness is the energy required to cause fracture of a material. Ductility is the ability of a material to resist deformation under tension. Ultimate strength is the greatest stress that can be withstood without fracture.

4.

C. The rate of abrasion is decreased when the speed of application is decreased. Increased pressure, an abrasive harder than the surface being abraded, and larger particle sizes increase the rate of abrasion.

5.

A. Thermal conductivity describes the ability of a material to transmit heat. Metals, such as dental amalgam, typically have a high thermal conductivity and increase the likelihood of postoperative temperature sensitivity. The modulus of elasticity describes the stiffness of a material. Toughness is the energy required to cause fracture of a material. Creep is the gradual flow of a material under an applied stress, usually at temperatures approaching the melting point.

6.

C. Shade is commonly used to communicate and describe a color through the use of a shade guide. It includes all the dimensions: hue, value, and chroma. Hue describes the predominant wavelength of a color. Value describes the brightness or darkness of a color. Chroma describes the strength of the hue or how much of a wavelength is being seen.

7.

B. Increasing the water/powder ratio of a gypsum product will decrease its strength, hardness, and abrasion resistance, but increase its setting time.

8.

B. Alginate does not reproduce the detail needed for the fabrication of fixed prostheses such as a three-unit bridge. Alginate is often used in the fabrication of bleach trays, custom mouthguards, and study casts.

9.

D. Copolymerization is the process of combining two or more monomers when creating a polymer. Methods of polymerization induction in dentistry include the use of heat, chemical, light, and/or microwave activation or a combination of these.

10.

C. Enamel acid etching is effectively accomplished with 30–50% phosphoric acid. Hydrofluoric acid is a strong acid that has been used to etch porcelain. Ten percent citric acid is a weak acid and does not predictably etch enamel. EDTA effectively removes the dentin smear layer, but does not effectively etch dentin.

11.

A. Materials based on polyacrylic or polycarboxylic acids create chemical adhesion to tooth structure. These include glass ionomer, zinc polycarboxylate, and resin-modified glass ionomer cements. Zinc phosphate and zinc-oxide eugenol cements provide mechanical retention. Resin cements also provide mechanical retention.

12.

D. An alloy is a combination of metals that are mutually soluble in the molten stage. Dental composite resins are composed of a polymer matrix with glass or ceramic fillers. Polymers are high-molecular-weight compounds resulting from the linking of low-molecular-weight compounds. Cements are generally hard, brittle materials formed by mixing a powder oxide with a liquid.

13.

D. Placing dissimilar metals in contact with another metal can increase corrosion. This combination can also cause a galvanic reaction and tooth sensitivity. Polishing reduces metal corrosion. Noble metals and metals that passivate reduce corrosion activity.

14.

A. Mercury vapor is available for inhalation, the most effective portal of entry to the human bloodstream. Therefore, precautions should be taken to prevent the vaporization of mercury. Droplets of mercury are less of a risk than mercury vapor. Mercury bound in dental amalgam presents a very low risk. Mercury is an occupational hazard and requires proper handling.

15.

C. A high-strength base with a minimum thickness of 0.5 mm is capable of providing thermal insulation for pulp tissue. Varnishes are used to decrease initial marginal leakage with dental amalgam and to diminish the movement of corrosion products through the dentin. Low-strength bases function as a barrier to irritating chemicals and provide a therapeutic benefit to the pulp. They are not thick enough to provide thermal protection. A suspension of calcium hydroxide is used to neutralize acids.

16.

B. The heat generated during polishing can cause pulp damage and release mercury vapor. Efforts should be taken to minimize these effects. An odor may be produced during polishing, but is not a significant biological threat. Debris produced during polishing should not cause any long-term biological effects. Tin oxide is often used to produce a polish layer when polishing dental amalgams.

17.

D. Although creating tooth-colored restorations is often desirable, it is not a requirement for a functioning restoration. Molar regions may experience stresses of 28,000 psi. Large temperature changes are common when eating. Restorative materials must be biologically compatible.

18.

A. An indirect restorative technique replicates a patient's oral structures. This allows for improved access in creating optimum contour and occlusal form of dental restorations. Indirect restorative techniques usually require more materials and multiple visits and are typically more costly than direct procedures.

19.

D. Fluorescence describes the ability of a material to absorb a nonvisible energy and then release visible light with longer wavelengths. This property adds to the vital appearance of esthetic restorations. Metamerism causes a material to have a different color under different light sources. Opacity describes the degree to which the passage of light through a material is inhibited. Translucency describes the dispersion of light through a material such that objects cannot be seen through it.

20.

C. Alginate is an elastic material and therefore is useful in making impressions of structures that contain undercuts. Impression compound and plaster and ZOE impression paste are inelastic.

21.

C. Cooler water will prolong gelation of alginate and provide more working time. The water/powder ratio of the material should not be changed. Increasing the water/powder ratio should not be used to increase working time. Decreasing the water/powder ratio does not increase working time. However, using warmer water does decrease working time.

22.

C. Immersion of alginate materials can cause imbibition (swelling) and significant dimensional change. They should be sprayed with a glutaraldehyde or an iodophor and sealed in a plastic bag for 10 minutes.

23.

A. Silane is used as a coupling agent between the matrix and the filler particles of a dental composite resin. BIS-GMA, UDMA, and TEGDMA are all common components of the matrix.

24.

B. Glass ionomer cements release fluoride over time. They contain fluoroaluminosilicate glasses. Dental amalgam, gold alloys, and dental porcelain do not release fluoride.

25.

C. The casting alloys are among the strongest materials used in dentistry. Of the materials given, the gold alloy would be expected to have the highest ultimate tensile strength. Composite resin and dental amalgam have intermediate strength values. Zinc phosphate cement has low strength values.

26.

A. Methyl methacrylate is the primary monomer in denture bases and forms poly(methyl methacrylate) on polymerization. TEGDMA, BIS-GMA, and UDMA are components in composite resins.

27.

B. Diagnostic casts can be made of the patient's mouth to study the dentition and to educate the patient. At the time the casts are made the patient will be interested in seeing the arrangement of the teeth. Tooth form and arrangement of the dentition can be observed. These casts are not of sufficient precision to allow fabrication of fixed dental prostheses.

28.

A. Casting involves heating a metal until molten and pouring or forcing it into a mold for it to harden. Some metals that are not brittle can be formed into useful shapes by the use of mechanical forces, such as rolling or wire drawing. Inlays, crowns, bridges, and particle denture frame works are usually cast, while wires and most orthodontic appliances are wrought.

29.

B. No polymers in dentistry use radioactive materials to effect the polymerization reaction. Heat curing is most commonly used for denture base resins, while light-cured and self-curing resins have many dental applications.

30.

B. The strength of a sealant is sacrificed in order to make it flow into the pits and fissures. Sealants are completely unfilled, making them weak as compared to composites. This is the primary reason that sealants that are left high on the occlusion usually come out quickly.

31.

B. Viscosity is a term describing how well a liquid flows under pressure. With water being given a value of 1.0, most dental liquids have a viscosity reading in the tens of thousands. The manufacturers of cements and cavity liners strive for low viscosity in their products, as long as they maintain their physical properties.

32.

A. All of the items listed are polymers. They all have long chains of identical repeating units known as "mers."

33.

B. A base is used to provide thermal insulation to protect the pulp. This is especially important in metallic restorations on the posterior teeth, as they conduct temperature well.

34.

D. A cause for sensitivity is the small currents created whenever two metals are present in the oral cavity. Because both restorations are wet with saliva, a small battery exists between the two metallic restorations. When the two restorations touch during mastication, the current produced by the battery may irritate the pulp and produce a sharp pain. These currents are referred to as galvanic currents.

35.

A. Galvanic shock is a type of electrical short circuit that can occur in the mouth. It usually involves two different metallic restorations that are not normally in contact. The amount of electricity involved in galvanic shock can range up to 1.0 microamperes and 500 millivolts.

36.

C. Composite resins, as a group, are poor thermal conducts. Metals, as a group, are excellent thermal conducts.

37.

E. The properties of restorative materials that are of primary importance are: (1) indestructibility in the fluids of the mouth, (2) adaptability to the walls of the cavity, (3) freedoms from shrinkage or expansion following placement in the cavity form, (4) resistance to attrition, (5) sustaining power against the force of mastication, (6) color or appearance, (7) low thermal conductivity, (8) convenience of manipulation, and (9) resistance to tarnish and corrosion.

38.

D. One should approach the subject of dental materials from the point of view of determining what the material is chemically, why it behaves as it does physically and mechanically, and how it is manipulated technically to develop the most satisfactory properties.

39.

B. The setting times of alginate impression material can be altered by changing the water–powder ratio or the mixing time. Neither of these methods is recommended, however, because slight deviations in proportion or mixing time can diminish certain properties of the gel. If gelation time is too altered, the best method is to vary the temperature of the after used in making the mix. The higher the water temperature, the shorter the gelation times.

40.

D. Tarnish is a very mild form of corrosion that usually involves a loss of luster on the surface of a metal and is often associated with some surface deposit. Rust is a type of corrosion most often involving the oxidation of iron. Corrosion is a very complex phenomenon involving not only the metal structure, but also the environment in which the metal is placed.

41.

B. Moisture contamination is to be avoided in all amalgam placements, but zinc-containing amalgams are especially sensitive to moisture. The actual chemical reaction is not fully understood but apparently the offending element is zinc. This delayed expansion takes place over several months and can result in expansion of up to 4%.

42.

B. If gelation time of the alginate is to be altered, the best method is to vary the temperature of the water used in making the mix. The higher the water temperature, the shorter the gelation times.

43.

D. Eugenol, a natural plant oil, is an important component of the zinc oxide–eugenol cements that are used to cement the temporary restorations on the teeth during the period between tooth preparation and final restoration seating.

44.

D. Plaster, stone, and improved stone are made up of hemihydrate particles whose size, shape, and porosity differ for each material. These physical differences in the hemihydrate particles are the basic facts that determine the manipulative conditions for mixing the particle and properties and usage of the hardened gypsum product.

45.

A. While the basic constituent of reversible hydrocolloid impression materials is agar-agar, present in a concentration of 8–15%, the principal ingredient by weight (@ 80–85%) is water.

46.

B. Biocompatibility is a broad term used to describe how safe a material is. The potential for cancer or allergy are just two types of tests performed.

47.

D. While base metal dental casting alloys are very sensitive in terms of the techniques used to cast, finish, and apply porcelain, they are quite strong. Many noble metal alloys are not suited for a long-span fixed bridge due to a tendency to flex under loading, which could pop the porcelain off. Base metal alloy advantages are principally found only in their strength and low density.

48.

B. While pulpal response is an important aspect of the biocompatibility of dental materials, the testing must be on intact teeth in a living subject. If the safety of the product has been established, human subjects are often used; if not, monkeys are appropriate. Because it uses living teeth, pulpal response is usually one of the last tests performed; all toxicity tests must have been performed prior to this.

49.

A. Dental porcelain is a mixture of feldspar and quartz. These two materials have extremely high (over 2000°F) fusing temperatures—much higher than that of glass. Metallic oxides are used to impart the proper shade to the porcelain. Paint would decompose at such temperatures.

50.

D. Alginate impressions are very susceptible to loss of water, which has a drastic effect on the accuracy of the resulting cast. While it is best to point an alginate impression immediately, it may be held for approximately 30 minutes in a humid atmosphere such as inside damp paper towels or in a humidor.

13 Professional Responsibility

Dental hygiene as a practice assumes the inherent responsibility of the individual provided when delivering dental care to a population. Ethical decision making is a cornerstone of a scientific discipline. In fact, dental hygiene, as a profession, develops ethical standards of care mandated for use by all dental hygienists. It is imperative that dental hygiene continually use ethical standards when providing patient care, conducting research, and informing and educating society on dental health issues.

chapter objectives

After completion of this chapter, the learner should be able to:

➤ Define and describe the ethical principles, including informed consent

➤ Define and discuss the regulatory process

➤ Describe patient and professional communication

I. Ethical Principles

A. Moral theories: Ethics consists of thoughts, concepts, values, and ideas regarding morality. Basically, ethics is concerned with studying human behaviors and the relationships between humans.

B. Moral development has been shown to occur in progressive steps or stages. Some theories focus on development related to age and cognitive development, whereas others see a relationship between education and moral development.

    1. Male justice orientation includes categorized stages in the moral development of male children. Piaget and Kohleber's models suggest that moral development is sequential and dependent on an individual's level of cognitive development.

    2. Female ethic of care by Gilligan suggests that women tend to see morality in the context of a relationship. Feminine moral reasoning is different from masculine moral reasoning. To survive, females have had to develop a sense of responsibility based on the universal principle of caring.

    3. Cognitive development theory suggests that individuals act on their experiences in order to make sense of them, and that these experiences are the basis for which people construct meanings. Simply, this theory suggests that dental hygiene students are in a formative period of ethical development and that dental hygiene school is a powerful catalyst to ethical development.

C. Character can be defined as those qualities that are practiced consistently. The Character Counts Coalition defines character using the following core ethical values:

    1. Trustworthiness can be defined as the trait of deserving trust and confidence

    2. Respect can be defined as being honored and held in esteem

    3. Responsibility can be defined as the trait of being answerable to someone for something or being responsible for one's conduct

    4. Fairness can be defined as the ability to make judgments free from discrimination or dishonesty

    5. Caring can be defined as exhibiting concern and empathy for others

    6. Citizenship can be defined as membership in a community that involves rights, duties, and privileges

D. Ethical theories lay a foundation of decision making, whereas moral reasoning provides a frame of reference that assists the dental hygienist. Normative ethics describes a group of theories that provide, define, and describe a system of principles and rules that determine which actions are deemed right or wrong.

    1. Consequentilist or utilitarian ethics postulates that action or rules are right or good as they relate to producing good consequences

    2. Deontology or nonconsequentialism (Kantian) theorizes that an action is right when it conforms to a judgment or rule of conduct that meets some preestablished requirement or rule.

3. Virtue ethics places emphasis on the character traits of an individual. The virtue, character, and goodness of the person in living a good life is the cause of the action.

E. Ethical principles

    1. Nonmaleficence means that a healthcare provider's first obligation to the patient is to do not harm

        a. Provider ought not to inflict harm

        b. Provider ought to prevent harm

        c. Provider ought to remove harm

        d. Provider ought to do or promote good

    2. Beneficence actually requires that existing harm be removed. The premise of beneficence is to provide quality health care, which is a benefit to the patient.

    3. Autonomy is the ability to govern one's profession and to basically be self-determined and directed as a profession. Additionally, autonomy is based on respect for others and the belief that patients have the power to make decisions about issues that may affect their health.

    4. Justice refers to providing individuals or groups with what is owed, due, or deserved.

    5. Paternalism involves the dental hygienist doing what he or she thinks is best for the patient according to his or her ability and judgment.

    6. Veracity can be defined simply as being honest.

    7. Informed consent requires that the dental hygienist provides the patient with all relevant information needed to make a decision and it allows the patient to make the decision based on valid, understandable information provided by the provider.

    8. Confidentiality has to do with the power of trust that all information about the patient's health and status is kept in confidence and that it is respected by all dental providers.

    9. *Prima facie* duties can be described as duties that must be done at all times. *Prima facie* means "at first glance."

        a. Always do the act that is in accord with the stronger *prima facie* duty

        b. Always do the act that has the greatest of *prima facie* rightness over *pima facie* wrongness

F. Codes of ethics are the standards developed by dental hygienists for dental hygienists. See Figure 13-1■ for the complete set of ADHA Code of Ethics. Five fundamental principles and seven core values are included in the code.

    1. Principles

        a. Universality

        b. Complementarity

(text continues on p. 899)

1. **Preamble**

   As dental hygienists, we are a community of professionals devoted to the prevention of disease and the promotion and improvement of the public's health. We are preventive oral health professionals who provide educational, clinical, and therapeutic services to the public. We strive to live meaningful, productive, satisfying lives that simultaneously serve us, our profession, our society, and the world. Our actions, behaviors, and attitudes are consistent with our commitment to public service. We endorse and incorporate the Code into our daily lives.

2. **Purpose**

   The purpose of a professional code of ethics is to achieve high levels of ethical consciousness, decision making, and practice by the members of the profession. Specific objectives of the Dental Hygiene Code of Ethics are:

   - to increase our professional and ethical consciousness and sense of ethical responsibility.
   - to lead us to recognize ethical issues and choices and to guide us in making more informed ethical decisions.
   - to establish a standard for professional judgment and conduct.
   - to provide a statement of the ethical behavior the public can expect from us.

   The Dental Hygiene Code of Ethics is meant to influence us throughout our careers. It stimulates our continuing study of ethical issues and challenges us to explore our ethical responsibilities. The Code establishes concise standards of behavior to guide the public's expectations of our profession and supports existing dental hygiene practice, laws, and regulations. By holding ourselves accountable to meeting the standards stated in the Code, we enhance the public's trust on which our professional privilege and status are founded.

3. **Key Concepts**

   Our beliefs, principles, values, and ethics are concepts reflected in the Code. They are the essential elements of our comprehensive and definitive code of ethics, and are interrelated and mutually dependent.

4. **Basic Beliefs**

   We recognize the importance of the following beliefs that guide our practice and provide context for our ethics:

   - The services we provide contribute to the health and well being of society.
   - Our education and licensure qualify us to serve the public by preventing and treating oral disease and helping individuals achieve and maintain optimal health.
   - Individuals have intrinsic worth, are responsible for their own health, and are entitled to make choices regarding their health.
   - Dental hygiene care is an essential component of overall healthcare and we function interdependently with other healthcare providers.
   - All people should have access to healthcare, including oral healthcare.
   - We are individually responsible for our actions and the quality of care we provide.

FIGURE 13-1 ■ Code of Ethics for Dental Hygienists

Used with permission of American Dental Hygienists' Association, www.adha.org.

5. **Fundamental Principles**

These fundamental principles, universal concepts, and general laws of conduct provide the foundation for our ethics.

Universality: The principle of universality assumes that, if one individual judges an action to be right or wrong in a given situation, other people considering the same action in the same situation would make the same judgment.

Complementarity: The principle of complementarity assumes the existence of an obligation to justice and basic human rights. It requires us to act toward others in the same way they would act toward us if roles were reversed. In all relationships, it means considering the values and perspective of others before making decisions or taking actions affecting them.

Ethics: Ethics are the general standards of right and wrong that guide behavior within society. As generally accepted actions, they can be judged by determining the extent to which they promote good and minimize harm. Ethics compel us to engage in health promotion/disease prevention activities.

Community: This principle expresses our concern for the bond between individuals, the community, and society in general. It leads us to preserve natural resources and inspires us to show concern for the global environment.

Responsibility: Responsibility is central to our ethics. We recognize that there are guidelines for making ethical choices and accept responsibility for knowing and applying them. We accept the consequences of our actions or the failure to act and are willing to make ethical choices and publicly affirm them.

6. **Core Values**

We acknowledge these values as general guides for our choices and actions.

Individual autonomy and respect for human beings: People have the right to be treated with respect. They have the right to informed consent prior to treatment, and they have the right to full disclosure of all relevant information so that they can make informed choices about their care.

Confidentiality: We respect the confidentiality of client information and relationships as a demonstration of the value we place on individual autonomy. We acknowledge our obligation to justify any violation of a confidence.

Societal Trust: We value client trust and understand that public trust in our profession is based on our actions and behavior.

Nonmaleficence: We accept our fundamental obligation to provide services in a manner that protects all clients and minimizes harm to them and others involved in their treatment.

Beneficence: We have a primary role in promoting the well being of individuals and the public by engaging in health promotion/disease prevention activities.

FIGURE 13-1 ■ Code of Ethics for Dental Hygienists (cont.) *(continued)*

Justice and Fairness: We value justice and support the fair and equitable distribution of healthcare resources. We believe all people should have access to high-quality, affordable oral healthcare.

Veracity: We accept our obligation to tell the truth and assume that others will do the same. We value self-knowledge and seek truth and honesty in all relationships.

7. **Standards of Professional Responsibility**
We are obligated to practice our profession in a manner that supports our purpose, beliefs, and values in accordance with the fundamental principles that support our ethics. We acknowledge the following responsibilities:

To Ourselves as Individuals . . .
• Avoid self-deception, and continually strive for knowledge and personal growth.
• Establish and maintain a lifestyle that supports optimal health.
• Create a safe work environment.
• Assert our own interests in ways that are fair and equitable.
• Seek the advice and counsel of others when challenged with ethical dilemmas.
• Have realistic expectations of ourselves and recognize our limitations.

To Ourselves as Professionals . . .
• Enhance professional competencies through continuous learning in order to practice according to high standards of care.
• Support dental hygiene peer-review systems and quality-assurance measures.
• Develop collaborative professional relationships and exchange knowledge to enhance our own life-long professional development.

To Family and Friends . . .
• Support the efforts of others to establish and maintain healthy lifestyles and respect the rights of friends and family.

To Clients . . .
• Provide oral healthcare utilizing high levels of professional knowledge, judgment, and skill.
• Maintain a work environment that minimizes the risk of harm.
• Serve all clients without discrimination and avoid action toward any individual or group that may be interpreted as discriminatory.
• Hold professional client relationships confidential.
• Communicate with clients in a respectful manner.
• Promote ethical behavior and high standards of care by all dental hygienists.
• Serve as an advocate for the welfare of clients.
• Provide clients with the information necessary to make informed decisions about their oral health and encourage their full participation in treatment decisions and goals.
• Refer clients to other healthcare providers when their needs are beyond our ability or scope of practice.
• Educate clients about high-quality oral healthcare.

FIGURE 13-1 ■ Code of Ethics for Dental Hygienists (cont.)

To Colleagues . . .

- Conduct professional activities and programs, and develop relationships in ways that are honest, responsible, and appropriately open and candid.
- Encourage a work environment that promotes individual professional growth and development.
- Collaborate with others to create a work environment that minimizes risk to the personal health and safety of our colleagues.
- Manage conflicts constructively.
- Support the efforts of other dental hygienists to communicate the dental hygiene philosophy of preventive oral care.
- Inform other healthcare professionals about the relationship between general and oral health.
- Promote human relationships that are mutually beneficial, including those with other healthcare professionals.

To Employees and Employers . . .

- Conduct professional activities and programs, and develop relationships in ways that are honest, responsible, open, and candid.
- Manage conflicts constructively.
- Support the right of our employees and employers to work in an environment that promotes wellness.
- Respect the employment rights of our employers and employees.

To the Dental Hygiene Profession . . .

- Participate in the development and advancement of our profession.
- Avoid conflicts of interest and declare them when they occur.
- Seek opportunities to increase public awareness and understanding of oral health practices.
- Act in ways that bring credit to our profession while demonstrating appropriate respect for colleagues in other professions.
- Contribute time, talent, and financial resources to support and promote our profession.
- Promote a positive image for our profession.
- Promote a framework for professional education that develops dental hygiene competencies to meet the oral and overall health needs of the public.

To the Community and Society . . .

- Recognize and uphold the laws and regulations governing our profession.
- Document and report inappropriate, inadequate, or substandard care and/or illegal activities by any healthcare provider, to the responsible authorities.
- Use peer review as a mechanism for identifying inappropriate, inadequate, or substandard care and for modifying and improving the care provided by dental hygienists.
- Comply with local, state, and federal statutes that promote public health and safety.
- Develop support systems and quality-assurance programs in the workplace to assist dental hygienists in providing the appropriate standard of care.

FIGURE 13-1 ■ Code of Ethics for Dental Hygienists (cont.) *(continued)*

- Promote access to dental hygiene services for all, supporting justice and fairness in the distribution of healthcare resources.
- Act consistently with the ethics of the global scientific community of which our profession is a part.
- Create a healthful workplace ecosystem to support a healthy environment.
- Recognize and uphold our obligation to provide pro bono service.

To Scientific Investigation . . .

We accept responsibility for conducting research according to the fundamental principles underlying our ethical beliefs in compliance with universal codes, governmental standards, and professional guidelines for the care and management of experimental subjects. We acknowledge our ethical obligations to the scientific community:

- Conduct research that contributes knowledge that is valid and useful to our clients and society.
- Use research methods that meet accepted scientific standards.
- Use research resources appropriately.
- Systematically review and justify research in progress to insure the most favorable benefit-to-risk ratio to research subjects.
- Submit all proposals involving human subjects to an appropriate human subject review committee.
- Secure appropriate institutional committee approval for the conduct of research involving animals.
- Obtain informed consent from human subjects participating in research that is based on specifications published in Title 21 Code of Federal Regulations Part 46.
- Respect the confidentiality and privacy of data.
- Seek opportunities to advance dental hygiene knowledge through research by providing financial, human, and technical resources whenever possible.
- Report research results in a timely manner.
- Report research findings completely and honestly, drawing only those conclusions that are supported by the data presented.
- Report the names of investigators fairly and accurately.
- Interpret the research and the research of others accurately and objectively, drawing conclusions that are supported by the data presented and seeking clarity when uncertain.
- Critically evaluate research methods and results before applying new theory and technology in practice.
- Be knowledgeable concerning currently accepted preventive and therapeutic methods, products, and technology and their application to our practice.

Approved and ratified by the 1995 ADHA House of Delegates.

FIGURE 13-1 ■ Code of Ethics for Dental Hygienists (cont.)

    c. Ethics

    d. Community

    e. Responsiblity

  2. Values

    a. Autonomy

    b. Confidentiality

    c. Trust

    d. Nonmaleficence

    e. Beneficence

    f. Justice

    g. Veracity

II. Regulatory Process

A. The laws that affect dental hygiene practice are enacted and enforced by individual states. State government has three branches including the legislative, executive, and judicial branch. Each branch of government has a specific function and limited areas of authority, which is exclusive to that branch, as indicated in Table 13-1■.

  1. Legislative branch makes laws for the state, which would include laws affecting the licensing and practice of the dental hygienist.

  2. Executive branch carries out the laws passed by the legislature. This branch has the power to enforce laws made by the state legislators. An example of this branch is a police officer.

  3. Judicial branch interprets the laws the legislature passes. Judges do not make laws, they simply interpret existing laws.

B. The major bodies of law include common law, statutory law, constitutional law, and administrative law, which are listed in Table 13-2■.

  1. Common law is created by the courts via judicial decision and can be changed by the courts. It contains notions of common sense and precedent.

  2. Statutory law is written law, which is enacted by the legislature, helps promote justice, and can be changed by the legislature. Dental hygiene practice acts are statutory law.

TABLE 13-1 BRANCHES OF STATE GOVERNMENT

Branch of Government	Function
Legislative	Create laws
Executive	Enforce laws
Judicial	Interpret laws

TABLE 13-2 MAJOR BODIES OF LAW	
Type of Law	**Definition**
Common	Created and changed only by courts
Statutory	Created and changed by legislature
Constitutional	Created and changed by people
Administrative	Delegation of legislative power to an administrative agency

3. Constitutional law was developed after common law and statutory law. The people created it and the people have the power to change the law. It is the most powerful law; in fact, it takes precedence over both common law and statutory law.

4. Administrative law is the result of the legislative branch voluntarily delegating some of its lawmaking authority to the executive branch. Administrative agencies such as state dental boards fall within this law. The legislature has the authority to say when and if they can develop rules and regulations.

C. Generally, state legislative process includes two legislative bodies, the Senate and the House of Representatives, sometimes referred to as the Assembly or House of Delegates. Generally, the legislature meets for up to 6 months once a year.

D. Laws pertaining to dental hygiene are generally found in the state dental hygiene practice act. For the most part, laws pertaining to dental hygiene practice are found in state laws, sometimes referred to as the state "practice act." These statutory laws describe the allowable scope of practice, necessary dental supervision requirements, requirements necessary to obtain a dental hygiene license, and suspension and revocation of licensure procedures. Many states have rules and regulations developed by the state dental board to aid in interpreting the laws of the practice act.

1. State dental boards generally govern dental hygienists, although a few states have dental hygiene committees or advisory boards that work with the board to effectively govern dental hygienists.

2. Not all states have state dental boards.

3. State dental boards generally consist of several dentists, one or two dental hygienists, and one or two public members. Because of the fact that no state dental boards have an equal number of dentists and dental hygienists on the board, the dentists on the board are basically governing dental hygienists in the state with no chance for true governance for dental hygienists by dental hygienists.

4. The board is usually responsible for developing rules and regulations to interpret or further define the practice act, as well as granting and suspending or revoking licenses. This can become very limiting for dental hygienists, because the majority board members are dentists who can literally interpret the law to limit the practice of dental hygiene while increasing the functions that other on-the-job trained dental personnel can provide. Unfortunately, in many instances, the profession of dental hygiene has no power to affect their own practice, whereas dentists, who have limited education in dental hygiene science, make decisions regarding the practice of this science. Figure 13-2■ lists the state board representation of dental hygienists in each state. Figure 13-3■ includes states with individual dental hygiene committees.

5. Self-regulation of dental hygienists means that state governments turn to members of the dental hygiene profession for advice and assistance in carrying out the practice act. The basic guides for regulation for each profession are found in its practice act.

E. A rule is a statement of general applicability that implements, interprets law, or defines the practice and procedure requirements of an agency of a state government.

1. Thus, a rule establishes a requirement, sets a standard, establishes a fee or rate, provides a set procedure, and sets forth how a law will be implemented, gives guidance for compliance with law, describes the structure of an organization, or instructs members of the public on how they must deal with or practice before any agency.

2. Furthermore, mandatory rules are those required by statute to promulgate. The rule-making process is ongoing, and state dental boards may promulgate rules at any time provided that they follow the provision of the law regulating that process found in the state's administrative procedures. A rule can be changed by the board initiating the rule-making process or by a person petitioning the board to promulgate, amend, or repeal a rule.

F. All states have supervision requirements, meaning that dentists supervise dental hygienists (Figure 13-4■).

1. In 14 states, dental hygienists may provide services in certain settings under various forms of unsupervised practice.

2. Table 13-3■ defines the different types of supervisions of dental hygienists. Supervision is a major problem with respect to the utilization of dental hygienists. Supervision restricts the practice of dental hygiene usually to dental offices, and decreases the effectiveness of public health efforts. Furthermore, it sets a perception that dentists actually are educated in dental hygiene to a further extent than a dental hygienist.

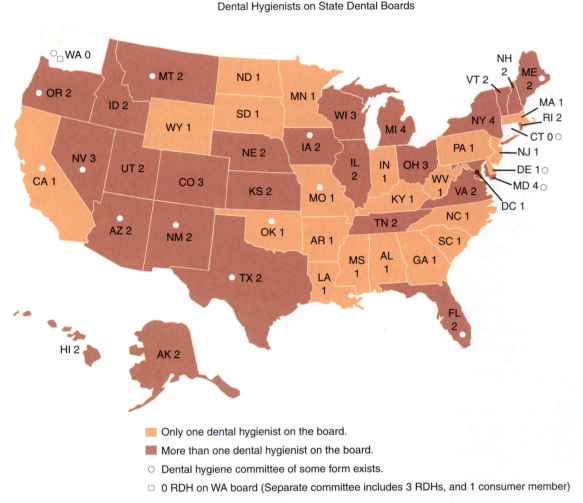

Dental Hygienists on State Dental Boards

■	Only one dental hygienist on the board.
■	More than one dental hygienist on the board.
○	Dental hygiene committee of some form exists.
□	0 RDH on WA board (Separate committee includes 3 RDHs, and 1 consumer member)

FIGURE 13-2 ■ State Board Representation of Dental Hygienists

Used with permission of American Dental Hygienists' Association, www.adha.org.

III. Professional and Patient Communication

A. Dental hygienists communicate with the entire dental workforce and other health care providers. Many times dental hygienists have dental assistants under their supervision. All members of the dental workforce should be treated with respect, dignity, and professionalism at all times.

B. Dental hygienists often assume a dentist–employer relationship with dentists who frequently employ dental hygienists. In some states, dental hygienists may employ dentists and this will probably increase as more states try to develop innovative dental care delivery systems.

Dental Hygiene Participation in Regulation

The following states have dental hygiene advisory committees or varying degrees of self-regulation for dental hygienists.

1. **Arizona:** The Arizona advisory committee consists of one dentist and one dental hygienist from the board, plus four additional dental hygienists and one public member. The committee serves as a forum for discussion of dental hygiene issues and advises the board on rules and proposed statute changes concerning dental hygiene education, regulation and practice. In addition the committee evaluates CE classes for expanded functions and monitors dental hygienists' compliance with CE requirements.

2. **California:** The Committee on Dental Auxiliary (COMDA) of the dental board consists of the public member of the board, two dentists (only one of whom can be a board member), three dental hygienists and three registered dental assistants. Duties include evaluating dental hygiene and dental assisting education programs, advising the board on discipline and recommending regulations concerning dental hygiene and dental assisting.

3. **Connecticut:** Connecticut is unique. Dental hygiene is directly under the health department, and although there is no standing dental hygiene committee, if there is a need to address rules or disciplinary matters, the department director has the ability to appoint an ad hoc committee of dental hygienists.

4. **Delaware:** Delaware's advisory committee is appointed by the governor and consists of three dental hygienists. During a recent sunset review of the board the committee was granted enhanced authority and now writes the examination for dental hygiene licensure (in conjunction with the dental board). Committee members also vote with the board on issues of dental hygiene licensure by credentials, disciplinary decisions and continuing education requirements for dental hygiene licensure.

5. **Florida:** Florida has both dental hygiene and dental assisting councils. The dental hygiene council is composed of four dental hygienists, one of whom sits on the board, and one dentist member of the board. The council is expected to develop all dental hygiene rules to submit to the board for its approval.

6. **Iowa:** Beginning in 1999, both dental hygienists on the dental board and one of the dentists became a dental hygiene committee of the board. This committee has the power to make all rules pertaining to dental hygiene. The board will be required to adopt those rules and enforce the committee rules.

7. **Maine:** Maine has a subcommittee on dental hygiene. The subcommittee consists of five members: one dental hygienist who is a member of the board; two dental hygienists appointed by the governor; two dentists who are members of the board and appointed by the president of the board. The duties of the subcommittee are to perform an initial review of all applications for licensure as a dental hygienist, submissions relating to continuing education of dental hygienists, and all submissions relating to public health supervision status of dental hygienists.

8. **Maryland:** Maryland's committee consists of three dental hygienists, one dentist, and one public member, all of whom are full voting members of the dental board. The committee was created during sunset review as a compromise to the creation of a separate dental hygiene regulatory board. According to statute, all matters pertaining to dental hygiene must first be brought to the committee for its review and recommendation.

FIGURE 13-3 ■ State Dental Hygiene Committees (*continued*)

Used with permission of American Dental Hygienists' Association, www.adha.org.

9. **Missouri:** A five member advisory commission, composed of the dental hygienists on the board and four dental hygienists appointed by the governor was created by the state legislature in 2001. The commission will make recommendations to the board concerning dental hygiene practice, licensure, examinations, discipline and educational requirements.

10. **Montana:** In 2002 the board assigned both dental hygienist members and one dentist member to be a standing committee to consider and address dental hygiene issues in a timely fashion. The committee will formulate specific recommendations to bring to the entire board for action.

11. **Nevada:** Legislation in 2003 added a third dental hygienist to the board, who together with a dentist appointed by the board, will constitute a dental hygiene committee that may formulate recommendations on dental hygiene rules for the board and be assigned additional duties by the board.

12. **New Mexico:** New Mexico has a board of dental health care comprised of five dentists, two dental hygienists and two public members. There is a dental hygiene committee comprised of five dental hygienists, two public members and two dentists. The committee selects two of its dental hygiene members to serve as the dental hygienists on the board. The board's public members and two of its dentist members are the dentist and public members of the committee. The committee adopts all the rules pertaining to dental hygiene and is also responsible for the discipline of dental hygienists. The board enforces the dental hygiene committee's rules.

13. **Oklahoma:** The dental hygiene advisory committee is comprised of the dental hygiene board and four additional dental hygienists appointed by the board.

14. **Oregon:** Under its authority to create standing committees, the Oregon dental board has appointed a committee comprised of three dentists, three dental hygienists, and one non-dental healthcare provider to advise the board concerning dental hygiene issues.

15. **Texas:** In 1995 a dental hygiene advisory committee comprised of three dental hygienists and two public members appointed by the governor and one dentist appointed by the board was established. All rules relating to the practice of dental hygiene must be submitted to the committee for review 30 days prior to board adoption. The committee has been responsible for researching and developing recent rules for licensure by credentials and the application of tetracycline fibers. Legislation in 2003 gave the committee the authority to propose specific rules for board action.

16. **Washington:** The state of Washington has a uniform disciplinary code which applies to all health professions and creates the regulatory bodies to implement each practice act. Dentistry and dental hygiene have separate practice acts. Dentists are regulated by the Dental Quality Assurance Commission (an independent dental board with no dental hygiene members). Dental hygienists are regulated by the Dental Hygiene Advisory Committee (comprised of three dental hygienists and one public member appointed by the department). Created in the early eighties, its original charge was to develop rules for dental hygiene education and licensure. Now, the committee has authority to originate all dental hygiene rules. Although nominally advisory, it meets and deliberates like a board. The department of health has consistently implemented rules as proposed by the committee.

Revised August 14, 2006

FIGURE 13-3 ■ State Dental Hygiene Committees

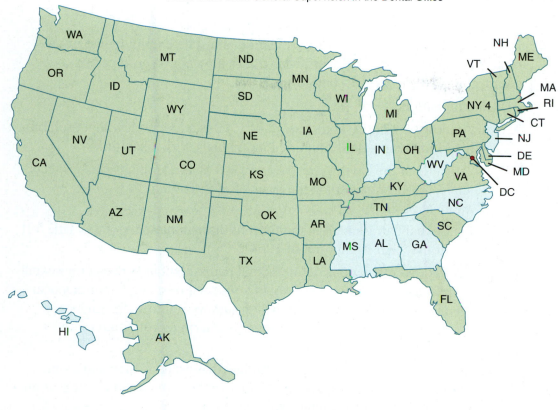

States that Permit General Supervision in the Dental Office

☐ States that permit General Supervision in private office.

☐ States that do not permit General Supervision in the private dental office.

Direct Supervision means that a dentist must be present in the facility when a dental hygienist performs prodcedures.

General Supervision means that a dentist has authorized a dental hygienist to perform procedures but need not be present in the treatment facility during the performance of those procedures.

FIGURE 13-4 ■ State Supervision Requirements

Used with permission of American Dental Hygienists' Association, www.adha.org.

TABLE 13-3 SUPERVISION OF DENTAL HYGIENISTS DEFINITIONS

Types of Supervision	Generally Accepted Definitions
Unsupervised, independent, collaborative practice	Dental hygiene practice without any supervision required from a dentist
General supervision	The practice of dental hygiene without the physical presence of a dentist; the dentist is still deemed to be "supervising"
Indirect/direct supervision	The dentist is in the facility while supervising

C. Employment laws: There are various federal and state employment laws to protect employees and employers. Many laws may not be enforced in companies with less than 15 employees.

    1. Discrimination

        a. Americans with Disabilities Act of 1990 is a federal law that prohibits discrimination against qualified individuals with disabilities

        b. Title VII of the Civil Rights Act of 1964 is a federal law that protects against discrimination on the basis of race, color, religion, sex, or national origin

            (1) Sexual harrassment in the form of discrimination violates Title VII of the Civil Rights Act of 1964

            (2) Federal regulations define sexual harassment as unwelcome sexual advances, requests for sexual favors, and other verbal or physical conduct of a sexual nature when submission to such conduct is made either explicitly or implicitly a term or condition of an indivual's employment

        c. Equal Pay Act of 1962 is a federal law that protects men and women who perform substantially equal work in the same establishment from sex-based wage discrimination

        d. Age Discrimination in Employment Act of 1967 is a federal law that prohibits discrimination based on age against any employee or applicant for employment who is at least 40 years of age; it applies to employers with 20 or more employees

        e. Equal Employment Opportunity Commission enforces federal laws against discimination in employment settings

    2. Family Medical Leave Act of 1993 is a federal law that makes available medically necessary leave to qualified employers with 50 or more employees

    3. Occupational Safety and Health Act of 1970 is a federal law intended to ensure safe and healthful working conditions for employees

D. Patient relationships: Dental hygienists have the inherent responsibility to maintain a professional relationship with each patient that includes communication and ensuring quality care. Jurisprudence is the philosophy and science of law and includes the establishment, regulation, and enforcement of legislation. Dental hygienists must complete jurisprudence exams and/or readings regarding state laws during the licensure process.

    1. Criminal law is a violation of a law or wrongful act against society. See Table 13-4■ for a comparison of criminal and civil law

TABLE 13-4 COMPARISON OF CRIMINAL LAW AND CIVIL LAW		
Item	**Criminal Law**	**Civil Law**
Initiator of legal action	Government (state, county, etc.)	Individual
Crime is against	Society	Individual
Agreement of jurors	Unanimous (all jurors)	51% (majority of jurors)
Payment of damages	Life, liberty, fine	Nominal, compensatory, punitive
Guilty of crimes	Beyond a reasonable doubt	Responsible for the crime

Source: Kimbrough, V.J., & Lautar, C.J. *Ethics, Jurisprudence and Practice Management in Dental Hygiene.* Upper Saddle River, NJ: Prentice Hall, 2003, p. 69.

2. Civil law is a violation of a law or wrongful act against an individual

    a. Tort law encompasses intentional or unintentional wrongs and can be acts of omission or commission

        (1) Negilence is an example of an unintentional tort

            (a) Malpractice actually is professional negligence; the patient was harmed due to lack of standard care

            (b) Three conditions must be met:

                i) There was an act of ommission or commission

                ii) There was failure to satisfy a standard of care

                iii) There was harm or injury to the patient

        (2) Assault and battery are examples of intentional torts

            (a) Assault is threatening to do harm to an individual; technical assult may occur even in the absence of the intention to harm, if there is no permission to touch

            (b) Battery is touching an individual with intent to harm the individual; technical battery may occur even in the absence of the intention to harm, if there is no permission to touch

        (3) Defamation is making false statements that harm an individual's reputation

            (a) Libel is written or published defamation

            (b) Slander is verbal defamation

    b. Contract law handles agreements and obligations; there are two types of contracts, implied and expressed:

        (1) Implied are assumed contracts such as patient presenting in the dental office is assuming the dental hygienist will be providing dental hygiene care

        (2) Expressed contracts are verbally stated or written agreements by the involved parties; treatment plans are examples of expressed contracts

    c. Abandonment is the termination of a patient, unless certain criteria are met

        (1) Care is no longer needed

        (2) The patient withdraws from the relationship

        (3) The care is transferred to another health care provider

        (4) Ample motive of withdrawal is given

        (5) The provider is unable to provide care

3. Risk management is used to prevent patient harm or neglect, financial loss, or possible legal gains.

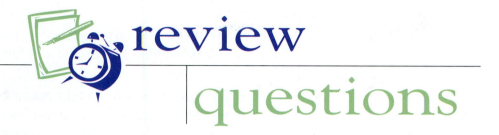

review questions

DIRECTIONS Each of the questions or incomplete statements below is followed by suggested answers or completions. Select the **one** answer that is best in each case.

1. Trustworthiness can be defined as the trait of
   A. Deserving trust and confidence
   B. Being honored and held in esteem
   C. Being answerable to a hiring calling
   D. Exhibiting concern for others

2. An individual who is honored and held in esteem is often called
   A. Trustworthy
   B. Fair
   C. Respected
   D. Responsible

3. A responsible person has a trait that is answerable to someone and is responsible for
   A. His or her conduct
   B. Being fair
   C. Exhibiting concern for others
   D. Citizenship of others

4. The ability to make judgments free from discrimination or dishonesty is termed
   A. Respect
   B. Trustworthiness
   C. Fairness
   D. Responsibility

5. Exhibiting concern and empathy for others is called
   A. Caring
   B. Citizenship
   C. Fairness
   D. Responsibility

6. This type of ethical theory describes a group of theories that provide, define, and describe a system of principles and rules that determine which actions are deemed right or wrong.
   A. Normative ethics
   B. Moral reasoning
   C. Virtue ethics
   D. Utilitarian ethics

7. Which type of ethics places emphasis on the character traits of an individual?
   A. Normative ethics
   B. Moral reasoning
   C. Virtue ethics
   D. Utilitarian ethics

review questions

8. A healthcare provider's first obligation to the patient is to do no harm, which is termed
   A. Nonmaleficence
   B. Beneficence
   C. Autonomy
   D. Veracity

9. Which of the following terms means that a dental hygienist should provide quality health care, which is a benefit to the patient?
   A. Nonmaleficence
   B. Beneficence
   C. Autonomy
   D. Veracity

10. Providing individuals or a group with what is owed, due, and/or deserved is called
    A. Autonomy
    B. Beneficence
    C. Justice
    D. Paternalism

11. Which ethical principle states that a provider should prevent harm, remove harm, and not inflict harm?
    A. Autonomy
    B. Beneficence
    C. Justice
    D. Nonmaleficence

12. The ability to govern's one's own profession and to basically be self-determined and directed as a profession is called
    A. Autonomy
    B. Beneficence
    C. Justice
    D. Nonmaleficence

13. Which principle is based on respect for others and the belief that patients have the power to make decisions about things that may affect their health?
    A. Autonomy
    B. Beneficence
    C. Justice
    D. Nonmaleficence

14. Being honest is called
    A. Justice
    B. Fairness
    C. Paternalism
    D. Veracity

15. Which principle states that the dental hygienist does what he thinks is best for the patient according to his ability and judgment?
    A. Justice
    B. Fairness
    C. Paternalism
    D. Veracity

16. Which of the following terms requires that the dental hygienist provides the patient with all the relevant information needed to make a decision and it allows the patient to make the decision based on valid, understandable information provided by the practitioner?
    A. Nonmaleficence
    B. Informed consent
    C. Paternalism
    D. Veracity

17. Which term has to do with the power of trust that all information about the patient's health and status is kept in confidence and is related to the respect of all patients and dental providers?
    A. Nonmaleficence
    B. Beneficence
    C. Trustworthiness
    D. Confidentiality

18. *Prima facie* duties can be described as duties that must be done at all times and the dental hygienist should always do the act that is in accord with the stronger *prima facie* duty.
    A. The first statement is TRUE; the second statement is FALSE.
    B. The first statement is FALSE; the second statement is TRUE.
    C. Both statements are TRUE.
    D. Both statements are FALSE.

19. Which of the following are principles contained in the ADHA Code of Ethics for dental hygienists?
A. Universality
B. Community
C. Responsibility
D. All of the above

20. Which of the following is NOT a value contained in the ADHA Code of Ethics for dental hygienists?
A. Autonomy
B. Justice
C. Beneficence
D. Virtue

21. This branch of government makes laws for the state.
A. Legislative branch
B. Executive branch
C. Administrative branch
D. Judicial branch

22. This branch of government enforces the laws passed by the legislature.
A. Legislative branch
B. Executive branch
C. Administrative branch
D. Judicial branch

23. This branch of government interprets the laws the legislature passes.
A. Legislative branch
B. Executive branch
C. Administrative branch
D. Judicial branch

24. Judges do not make laws, they simply interpret existing laws.
A. The first statement is TRUE, and the second statement is FALSE.
B. The first statement is FALSE, and the second statement is TRUE.
C. Both statements are TRUE.
D. Both statements are FALSE.

25. This body of law is created by the courts via judicial decision and can be changed by the courts. It contains notions of common sense and precedent.
A. Common law
B. Statutory law
C. Constitutional law
D. Administrative law

26. This body of law is the result of the legislative branch voluntarily delegating some of its lawmaking authority to the Executive branch.
A. Common law
B. Statutory law
C. Constitutional law
D. Administrative law

27. This body of law is written law, which is enacted by the legislature, helps promote justice, and can be changed by the legislature.
A. Common law
B. Statutory law
C. Constitutional law
D. Administrative law

28. Citizens have created this body of law and only citizens have the power to change this law. It is the most powerful law and takes precedent over other laws.
A. Common law
B. Statutory law
C. Constitutional law
D. Administrative law

29. Administrative agencies such as state dental boards fall within this law.
A. Common law
B. Statutory law
C. Constitutional law
D. Administrative law

30. Dental hygiene practice acts are actually which type of law?
    A. Common law
    B. Statutory law
    C. Constitutional law
    D. Administrative law

31. State dental boards govern dental hygiene practice and all states have dental boards.
    A. The first statement is TRUE; second statement is FALSE.
    B. The first statement is FALSE; second statement is TRUE.
    C. Both statements are TRUE.
    D. Both statements are FALSE.

32. The state dental board is usually responsible for developing rules and regulations to interpret or further define the practice act and also has the responsibility for granting and suspending or revoking licenses.
    A. The first statement is TRUE; second statement is FALSE.
    B. The first statement is FALSE; second statement is TRUE.
    C. Both statements are TRUE.
    D. Both statements are FALSE.

33. Self-regulation of dental hygienists means that state governments turn to members of the dental hygiene profession for advice and assistance in carrying out the practice act, and most states have implemented self-regulation for dental hygienists.
    A. The first statement is TRUE; the second statement is FALSE.
    B. The first statement is FALSE; the second statement is TRUE.
    C. Both statements are TRUE.
    D. Both statements are FALSE.

34. Which of the following is the term for the statement of general applicability that implements, interprets law, or defines the practice and procedure requirements of an agency of a state government?
    A. Regulation
    B. Rule
    C. Statute
    D. Practice act

35. Which type of supervision is defined by allowing a "supervised" dental hygienist to practice without a dentist on site?
    A. General supervision
    B. Direct supervision
    C. Indirect supervision
    D. Independent supervision

36. This is the federal law that states that older adults should have the same chance at gaining employment as all individuals.
    A. Family Medical Leave Act
    B. Civil Rights Act
    C. Equal Pay Act
    D. Age Discrimination in Employment Act

37. Criminal law is a violation of law or a wrongful act against an individual, whereas civil law is a violation of law or wrongful act against society.
    A. The first statement is TRUE; the second statement is FALSE.
    B. The first statement is FALSE; the second statement is TRUE.
    C. Both statements are TRUE.
    D. Both statements are FALSE.

38. Which of the following laws encompass intentional or unintentional wrongs and can be acts of omission or commission?
    A. Criminal law
    B. Tort law
    C. Unintentional law
    D. Both B and C

39. Which term best reflects professional negligence?
    A. Ommission
    B. Commission
    C. Tort ✓
    D. Malpractice

40. Negilence is an example of an unintentional tort and professional negligence is when the patient was harmed due to law of standard of care.
    A. The first statement is TRUE; the second statement is FALSE.
    B. The first statement is FALSE; the second statement is TRUE.
    C. Both statements are TRUE.
    D. Both statements are FALSE.

41. Which of the following conditions must be met in a malpractice case?
    A. There was an act of ommission or commission
    B. There was failure to satisfy standards of care
    C. There was harm or injury to the patient
    D. All of the above

42. Assault and battery are examples of intentional torts and assault is touching an individual with intent to harm the individual.
    A. The first statement is TRUE; the second statement is FALSE.
    B. The first statement is FALSE; the second statement is TRUE.
    C. Both statements are TRUE.
    D. Both statements are FALSE.

43. Technical battery may occur even in the absence of the intention of harm, if there is no permission to touch, whereas technical assault may occur even in the absence of the intention to harm, if there is no permission to touch.
    A. The first statement is TRUE; the second statement is FALSE.
    B. The first statement is FALSE; the second statement is TRUE.
    C. Both statements are TRUE.
    D. Both statements are FALSE.

44. Which of the following is the best term for writing or publishing statements that harm an individual reputation?
    A. Defamation
    ✓B. Libel
    C. Slander
    D. Both A and C

45. Which of the following would be a patient presenting in a dental office for a dental prophylaxis?
    A. Civil contract
    B. Implied contract
    C. Expressed contract
    D. Informed consent

46. Signing a health history is a form of which contract or consent?
    A. Civil contract
    B. Implied contract
    C. Expressed contract
    D. Informed consent

47. Abandonment is the termination of a patient and can be done after one no-show appointment.
    A. The first statement is TRUE; the second statement is FALSE.
    B. The first statement is FALSE; the second statement is TRUE.
    C. Both statements are TRUE.
    D. Both statements are FALSE.

48. Which of the following is used to prevent patient harm or neglect, financial loss, or possible legal gains?
    A. Expressed consent
    B. Civil contract
    C. Implied consent
    D. Risk management

49. Planning treatment options for a patient regardless of patient finances is an example of which character trait?
    A. Responsibility
    B. Fairness
    C. Virtue
    D. Veracity

50. Changing progress notes to reflect what should have happened during an appointment would be breaking which character trait?
    A. Responsibility
    B. Fairness
    C. Virtue
    D. Veracity

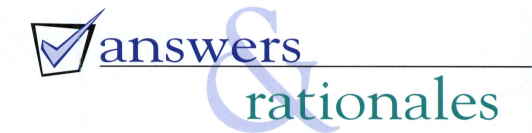

1.

A. Trustworthiness can be defined as the trait of deserving trust and confidence. An individual who is trustworthy would be a healthcare provider whom you would feel comfortable discussing signs and symptoms of possible diseases/conditions.

2.

C. An individual who is honored and held in esteem is often called respected. Healthcare providers are usually respected for their ability to treat patients in need and to help prevent diseases. Healthcare providers should show respect to their patients, which in turn will yield respect from their patients.

3.

A. A responsible person has a trait that is answerable to someone and is responsible for his or her conduct. A healthcare provider must be responsible to his or her patient and always conduct him- or herself in a professional manner.

4.

C. The ability to make judgments free from discrimination or dishonesty is termed fairness. A healthcare provider must always develop plans and treat patients with fairness that is based on treatment need.

5.

A. Exhibiting concern and empathy for others is called caring. Healthcare providers should always exhibit care for their patients and must always treat patients as they themselves would want to be treated.

6.

A. Normative ethics describes a group of theories that provide, define, and describe a system of principles and rules that determine which actions are deemed right or wrong. They include Consequentialist or Utilitarian, Deontology or Nonconsequentialism (Kantian), and Virtue ethics.

7.

C. Virtue ethics places emphasis on the character traits of an individual.

8.

A. Nonmaleficence means that a healthcare provider's first obligation to the patient is to do no harm. Basically, a healthcare provider ought not to inflict harm, ought to prevent harm, ought to remove harm, and ought to do or promote good.

9.

B. Beneficence means that a dental hygienist should provide quality health care, which is a benefit to the patient.

10.

C. Justice is when a dental hygienist is providing individuals or a group with what is owed, due, and/or deserved.

11.

D. Nonmaleficence means that a dental hygienist should prevent harm, remove harm, and not inflict harm. Dental hygienists should prevent diseases/conditions, treat and/or refer diseases/conditions appropriately, and practice current, safe treatment modalities.

12.

A. Autonomy is the ability to govern's one's own profession and to basically be self-determined and directed as a profession. Although organized dental hygiene has assumed a direction for the profession, legally dental hygiene is still governed by dentistry.

13.

A. Autonomy is a principle that is based on respect for others and the belief that patients have the power to make decisions about things that may affect their health. Dental hygienists must strive for patient/provider autonomy.

14.

D. Veracity is another term for honesty. Obviously, as in all aspects of life, honesty is mandatory for a dental hygiene provider.

15.

C. Paternalism is the principle that implies that the dental hygienist does what he or she thinks is best for the patient according to his or her ability and judgment.

16.

B. Informed consent requires that the dental hygienist provide the patient with all the relevant information needed to make a decision and it allows the patient to make the decision based on valid, understandable information provided by the pracitioner. It was instituted after failure to provide such information to patients resulted in death and illness.

17.

D. Confidentiality has to do with the power of trust that all information about the patient's health and status is kept in confidence and is related to respect of all patients and dental providers. In the United States, HIPAA enforces this principle.

18.

C. *Prima facie* duties can be described as duties that must be done at all times and the dental hygienist should always do the act that is in accord with the stronger *prima facie* duty.

19.

D. Universality, community, responsibility, and complementarity and ethics are principles contained in the ADHA Code of Ethics for dental hygienists.

20.

D. Individual autonomy and respect for human beings, societal trusts, nonmaleficence, beneficence, justice, fairness, and veracity are values contained in the ADHA Code of Ethics for dental hygienists.

21.

A. The Legislative branch of government makes laws for the state. State senators and representatives, sometimes called congressmen, are usually these lawmakers.

22.

B. The Executive branch of government enforces the laws passed by the legislature.

23.

D. The Judicial branch of government interprets the laws the legislature passes.

24.

C. Judges do not make laws; they simply interpret existing laws.

25.

A. Common law is created by the courts via judicial decision and can be changed by the courts. It contains notions of common sense and precedent.

26.

D. Adminstrative law is the result of the Legislative branch voluntarily delegating some of its lawmaking authority to the Executive branch. The state dental board has this authority.

27.

B. Statutory law is written law, which is enacted by the legislature, helps promote justice and can be changed by the legislature. Dental practice acts are examples of this type of law.

28.

C. Constitutional law was created by citizens. They have created this body of law and only citizens have the power to change this law. It is the most powerful law and takes precedent over other laws.

29.

D. Administrative agencies such as state dental boards fall within administrative law.

30.

B. Dental hygiene practice acts are actually examples of statutory law.

31.

A. State dental boards govern dental hygiene practice and most states have dental boards.

32.

C. The state dental board is usually responsible for developing rules and regulations to interpret or further define the practice act and also has the responsibility for granting and suspending or revoking licenses.

33.

A. Self-regulation of dental hygienists means that state governments turn to members of the dental hygiene profession for advice and assistance in carrying out the practice act; most states do not have self-regulation for dental hygienists.

34.

B. A rule is a statement of general applicability that implements, interprets law, or defines the practice and procedure requirements of an agency of a state government.

35.

A. General supervision is defined by allowing a "supervised" dental hygienist to practice without a dentist on site.

36.

D. The Age Discrimination in Employment Act is the federal law that states that older adults should have the same chance at gaining employment as all individuals.

37.

D. Criminal law is a violation of law or wrongful act against society, whereas civil law is a violation of law or wrongful act against an individual.

answers & rationales

38.

D. Tort laws encompass intentional or unintentional wrongs and can be acts of omission or commission.

39.

D. Malpractice is basically professional negligence by a healthcare provider.

40.

C. Negilence is an example of an unintentional tort and professional negligence is when the patient was harmed due to law of standard of care.

41.

D. The following conditions must be met in a malpractice case: (1) There was an act of ommission or commission, (2) there was failure to satisfy standard of care, and (3) there was harm or injury to the patient.

42.

A. Assault and battery are examples of intentional torts; battery is touching an individual with intent to harm the individual.

43.

C. Technical battery may occur even in the absence of the intention of harm, if there is no permission to touch, whereas technical assault may occur even in the absence of the intention to harm, if there is no permission to touch.

44.

B. Libel is the term for writing or publishing statements that harm an individual's reputation.

45.

B. Implied contract would be when a patient is presenting in a dental office for a dental prophylaxis.

46.

C. Signing a health history is a form of expressed contract.

47.

C. Abandonment is the termination of a patient and can be done after one no-show appointment.

48.

D. Risk management is used to prevent patient harm or neglect, financial loss, or possible legal gains.

49.

B. Planning treatment options for a patient regardless of patient finances is an example of fairness.

50.

D. Changing progress notes to reflect what should have happened during an appointment would be breaking veracity. It is of upmost importance to be honest as a dental hygiene provider.

Community Health and Research Principles

14 Promoting Health and Preventing Disease within Groups

Dental public health defined is the science and art of preventing and controlling dental disease and promoting dental health through organized community efforts. Basically, it is the delivery of oral health care, research, and education, with an emphasis on the utilization of the dental hygiene sciences, delivered to a target population.

Dental hygienists increasingly are becoming important health care providers in the dental public health arena. Dental hygienists play a crucial role in dental public health by bringing dental services to groups of people, developing health care policy, conducting research, and providing clinical care. With an increased emphasis on improving public access to oral health care, the opportunities for dental hygienists to promote oral health in the community are numerous. Dental hygiene practitioners who will be practicing in this new century need skills on how to effectively position and practice dental hygiene in the dental public health setting.

chapter objectives

After completion of this chapter, the learner should be able to:

➤ Define target populations

➤ Discuss teaching strategies

➤ Describe health promotion

➤ Discuss health education theories, learning, and teaching principles

➤ Describe education materials for target populations

➤ Describe programs that work to prevent disease within groups

I. Target Populations

   A. Definition: A group of people with similar characteristics

   B. In order to ensure program effectiveness, it is helpful to have contact with your target population

   C. Dental hygienists must concentrate on teaching caregivers, those individuals that provide care to patients

   D. These groups may include teachers, family or home health caregivers, nurse's assistants, aides, etc.

   E. When working with programs targeted at any population, it is helpful to have community leaders supporting your program

   F. Second- and sixth-grade classes are targeted for a dental sealants program because of the eruption dates of the first and second molars

   G. School fluoridation and school fluoride mouthrinse programs are targeted for children in nonfluoridated communities

   H. Socioeconomic status (SES) includes education, income, occupation, and culture; SES frequently is used as it relates to dental health issues, for example, a low SES yields an increased risk for caries

   I. Some populations face obstacles when trying to access dental hygiene and dental care; these are often termed barriers to care (Box 14-1■)

BOX 14-1

Barriers to Dental Hygiene and Dental Care

Age	Language	Habit
Culture	Limited finances	Lack of faith in treatment
Education	Misunderstanding	Fear
Transportation	Values	Safety of treatment
Illiteracy	Attitudes	Denial of disease
No dental providers	Belief in invulnerability	Convenience
Social issues	Education levels	Provider conflicts

Source: Nathe, C. *Dental Public Health* (2nd ed). Upper Saddle River, NJ: Prentice Hall, 2005.

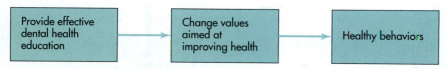

FIGURE 14-1 ■ Goals of Dental Health Education

II. Teaching Strategies

A. Health education is the education of health behaviors that brings an individual to a state of health awareness (Figure 14-1■); an example of a health education activity would be to provide an interactive lesson on the benefits and types of athletic mouthguards to a group of coaches at an annual state coaches' meeting

B. Health promotion is the informing and motivating of people on health behaviors; an example of a health promotion activity would be to sponsor a day that dental hygienists from the community make boil-n-bite mouthguards for school athletes during a tournament

C. Behavior change is when a target population adopts positive health behaviors.

    1. When teaching a target population to adopt positive health behaviors, it is necessary to change the opinions and subsequent values they may have about oral health

    2. Behavior change will not commence until value adoption is complete

    3. Value adoption and a change in a behavior must take place; merely providing dental health education or promotional activity to a target population does not ensure that behavior will change

    4. Without motivation, no learning can take place

III. Health Education Theories

A. The Health Belief model suggests that for an individual to display readiness to take action to avoid disease or to act in a preventive manner, he or she would need to believe he or she was susceptible and that the disease has serious consequences and that it is important

B. Stages of learning depict an individual's natural progression from knowledge absorption to value adoption

C. Classical conditioning suggests that individuals become conditioned to specific stimuli to act in a specific way

D. Operant conditioning is based on the concepts of reward and punishment

E. Modeling behavior can facilitate learning through imitation

IV. Learning Principles

A. Involvement of the group is necessary for learning to take place

B. School teachers should serve as role models during the year on positive dental health values and behaviors

BOX 14-2

Lesson Plan Development

Assessment
- Assess target population's needs, interests, and abilities
- Assess resources

Dental Hygiene Diagnosis
- Formulate findings from assessment
- Prioritize goals

Planning
- Broad goal formulation
- Specific objectives
- Select teaching method(s)

Implementation
- Be prepared
- Effective teacher characteristics

Evaluation
- Qualitative measurement
- Quantitative measurement
- Information provided to appropriate parties

Source: Nathe, C. *Dental Public Health* (2nd ed.). Upper Saddle River, NJ: Prentice Hall, 2005.

V. Teaching Principles

   A. Utilize the dental hygiene process of care when planning a lesson (Box 14-2■)

   B. There are various methods of teaching to utilize when presenting information to a population (Box 14-3■)

VI. Educational Materials

   A. Develop materials that can be utilized for the intended target population

BOX 14-3

Teaching Methods

Lecture	Self-study
Discussion	Inquiry
Presentation	Simulation
Interaction	Demonstration
Activities	

Source: Nathe, C. *Dental Public Health.* Upper Saddle River, NJ: Prentice Hall, 2000.

B. Types of materials

1. Slide series

2. Overhead transparencies

3. Flip chart

4. Actual models of interventions (i.e., toothbrushes, floss, instruments, etc.)

5. Books

6. Pamphlets

7. CD-ROMs, DVDs, and videotapes

8. Worksheets, puzzles, word finds, etc.

C. Professionally produced materials

1. Materials are developed by dental hygiene and dental organizations

2. Materials may be developed by dental industry

3. When distributing educational materials, be careful to scrutinize your materials so that you are not blatantly promoting dental care products and most importantly, that the information is factual

VII. Community Preventive Programs

A. Dental hygiene treatment including the oral examination, radiographs, periodontal debridement, selective polishing, application of fluoride and sealants, and education

B. Fluoridation

1. Water fluoridation has proven to be cost effective

2. The only claim made by opponents that cannot be discredited is that fluoridation of public water supplies may violate human rights (Box 14-4■)

3. Advocates of water fluoridation may find it beneficial to develop long-term strategies for adoption

4. See section on Preventive Agents for more information on fluoridation

---

BOX 14-4

Water Fluoridation Oppositions

- Violation of personal freedom
- Cause of disease(s) and/or medical conditions: cancer, AIDS, fatigue, etc.
- Forced medication
- Communist plot
- An abuse of police power

Source: Nathe, C. *Dental Public Health* (2nd ed.). Upper Saddle River, NJ: Prentice Hall, 2005.

    5. Methods utilized to implement water fluoridation

        a. Administrative decision by elected officials; for example, mayor and/or city council decision, etc.

        b. Initiative petition and/or referendum may be employed

        c. State legislative action may be taken

C. Other fluoride modalities

    1. School water fluoridation

    2. School fluoride mouthrinse programs

    3. Dietary fluoride supplements

    4. Professional fluoride applications

        a. Gels

        b. Foams

        c. Rinses

        d. Varnishes

    5. OTC (over-the-counter) fluoride dentifrices, mouthrinses, impregnated floss, and strips

D. Dental sealants

    1. In collaboration with fluoride, dental sealants are proven to be 85% effective in preventing pit and fissure caries

    2. Recommended for children and young adults and those at an increased risk for pit and fissure caries; recommended for all ages

    3. For example, the average cost of applying one dental sealant is less than half the cost of one amalgam restoration

E. Oral cancer examination

    1. Dental hygienist or dentist provides examination to screen for oral cancer

    2. Education targeted at signs and symptoms of oral cancer and lifestyle choices to decrease the chance of oral cancer

    3. The implementation of tobacco cessation programs

        a. Ask

        b. Advise

        c. Refer

    4. Early detection has a tremendous effect on mortality rates

F. Athletic mouthguards

    1. Can be made by the dental hygienist or bought at a store that sells sporting supplies

    2. Use of athletic mouthguards prevents oral trauma and concussions (Table 14-1■)

TABLE 14-1 TYPES OF MOUTHGUARDS	
Type of Mouthguard	**Description**
Stock	Not custom-made Can be purchased in athletic stores or discount department stores Not preferred due to poor fit and excess bulk
Mouth-formed	Referred to as "boil-n-bite" Comes in stock sizes, but can be heated in water and then placed in the mouth for a more exact fit Can become distorted Not definitive to dentition
Custom-made	Made in the dental office Fabricated from the patient's study model Reduces injuries because it fits better

Source: Nathe, C. Oral Appliances. In M. Gladwin & B. Bagby, *Clinical Applications of Dental Materials.* Philadelphia: Lippincott Williams and Wilkins, 1999.

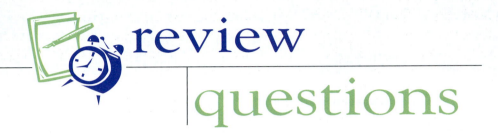
DIRECTIONS Each of the questions or incomplete statements below is followed by suggested answers or completions. Select the **one** answer that is best in each case.

Testlet 1: Questions 1–10

The nursing supervisor at the tenth district health department contacted the Boulder County Dental Hygiene Component (BCDHC) with dental concerns for students in the district. During routine checkups, the supervisor had noticed a high incidence of dental neglect within the Jackson Senior High School (JSHS) student population, as evidenced by severe decay, poor dietary habits, and inadequate home care. The BCDHC then sent surveys to the parents in the school district regarding dietary conditions in the home, socioeconomic status of the household, dental home care procedures, and access to routine dental care. Oral hygiene and caries status of the JSHS students were assessed in the classrooms with the use of the plaque index (PI) and DMF index. The group PI average was 2.5 and the group DMFT was as follows: D = 250, M = 5, and F = 25.

1. The use of surveys and classroom examination are integral components of
   A. Conducting a needs assessment
   B. Prioritizing needs
   C. Setting program goals
   D. Developing implementation strategies

2. The BCDHC analyzed data gathered from questionnaires and surveys. They voted unanimously "to increase access to dental care for low-income families." This is an example of a(n)
   A. Program objective
   B. Process evaluation
   C. Implementation strategy
   D. Program goal

3. A task force appointed by the BCDHC to obtain approval for a school-wide dental screening and treatment day contacts the district school superintendent. This is an example of a(n)
   A. Needs assessment
   B. Program objective
   C. Implementation strategy
   D. Program planning

4. A special committee is appointed by the BCDHC to review program objectives and evaluate if they are being met. This is part of an ongoing process known as
   A. Resource identification
   B. Program evaluation
   C. Community profiling
   D. Definition of needs

5. The BCDHC agrees to sponsor a "Jackson Senior High School Day of Smiles" event where area dentists, assistants, and hygienists donate their time to treat 100% of the JSHS stridence requiring care. This is an example of a(n)
   A. Program objective
   B. Process evaluation
   C. Implementation strategy
   D. Program goal

6. The BEST way to address this population's needs during this 1-day event is by
   A. Placing sealants on permanent molars
   B. Performing thorough teeth cleaning on the students
   C. Having a volunteer dentist restore or extract the carious teeth
   D. Providing fluoride treatments

7. A PI average of 2.5 indicates that this population
   A. Has severe periodontitis
   B. Has poor plaque control skills
   C. Needs dietary counseling
   D. Has generalized fluorosis

8. When analyzing the DMFT data, the high group D value and relatively low group M and F values probably indicates that this population
   A. Does not have regular access to dental care
   B. Has demonstrated an ability to control plaque
   C. Needs periodontal therapy
   D. Demonstrates the most calculus on the lingual surfaces

9. Obtaining DMFTs on the students before the "Day of Smiles" is an example of
   A. Establishing program objectives
   B. Obtaining baseline data
   C. Identifying a chief complaint
   D. Investigating surveys

10. Comparing the group DMFT data obtained before the "JSHS Day of Smiles" to the group DMFT data obtained on the participants 90 days after the Day of Smiles is an example of
    A. Process evaluation
    B. Product evaluation
    C. Program revision
    D. Identifying constraints

Testlet 2: Questions 11–15

A state board of health has just hired a veteran dental hygienist with 25 years of experience who must now begin to think on the group level rather than the individual patient level. She has been asked to assess the dental status of all second graders in a nonfluoridated school district. Dental hygiene students are available to help with screenings and gain experience with gathering data through various indices.

11. In a private practice setting, the dental status of a client is determined by an examination. In the public health setting, the examination would MOST closely parallel
    A. A survey
    B. Program planning
    C. Goal setting
    D. Program operation

12. After information is collected, the next step is to
    A. Establish goals
    B. Develop a strategic plan
    C. Conduct program appraisal
    D. Establish program funding

13. Water testing has been completed. Due to a minimal amount of fluoride in the water, approval has been obtained from the school board for a school water fluoridation program. What is the recommended concentration of fluoride for school water supplies?
    A. 1 ppm
    B. 2 ppm
    C. 3.5 ppm
    D. 4.5 ppm

14. The socioeconomic status of the second graders receiving the MOST benefit from classroom dental health presentations would be which one of the following?
    A. High
    B. Middle
    C. Low
    D. All

15. Which of the following approaches would be BEST to ensure that the entire school community of children are taught dental health?
    A. Have dental hygiene students teach oral health as part of their public health practicum
    B. Have volunteer dental hygienists from the local dental hygiene component teach oral health to the school community
    C. Teach the school nurse methods of oral hygiene
    D. Train the teachers in methods of oral hygiene

16. Fluoridation is the adjustment of the fluoride ion content in a(n)
    A. Gel solution
    B. Water supply
    C. Aerosol spray
    D. Ingestible tablet

17. Fluorides are stored in skeletal tissues. Even when concentrations reach 8 ppm, no impairment in general health can be detected.
    A. Both statements are TRUE.
    B. Both statements are FALSE.
    C. The first statement is TRUE; the second statement is FALSE.
    D. The first statement is FALSE; the second statement is TRUE.

18. Water fluoridation ranks as a very successful primary oral health measure because
    A. It demonstrates to the public that caries and tooth loss are not inevitable
    B. Its greatest benefit is to halt dental caries in the earliest possible stage
    C. Its clinical efficacy and effectiveness are well established in the dental literature
    D. All of the above

19. Based on results of recent fluoride studies, prenatal fluoride supplements are recommended in communities where water supplies are fluoridated. The results demonstrated a reduction of caries in primary teeth by 20%.
    A. Both statements are TRUE.
    B. Both statements are FALSE.
    C. The first statement is TRUE; the second statement is FALSE.
    D. The first statement is FALSE; the second statement is TRUE.

20. Controversy surrounding fluoridation of the drinking water has once again resurfaced. Opponents feel that fluoridated drinking water is a
    A. Violation of individual rights
    B. Risk factor for bone cancer
    C. Risk factor for Down's syndrome
    D. All of the above

21. The human body possesses a prompt and efficient excretory mechanism for fluorides; however, this does not minimize the danger of long-term accumulation of fluorides, which can be toxic.
    A. Both statements are TRUE.
    B. Both statements are FALSE.
    C. The first statement is TRUE; the second statement is FALSE.
    D. The first statement is FALSE; the second statement is TRUE.

22. If the dental hygienist is asked to present a community dental health presentation for a deaf audience, the dental hygienist should
    A. Switch the lights on and off to attract the group's attention, give written information for reinforcement, and immediately begin the program
    B. Enlist the support of an interpreter, review the program with him or her, and ask the interpreter to make comments or corrections when necessary
    C. Present using sign language with written material to augment the presentation
    D. Switch the lights on and off to attract the group's attention, allow the audience to read handouts before initiating the program, and use sign language with an interpreter

23. Which of the following age groups are most subject to rampant dental caries?
    A. Young children with poor oral hygiene, adults with gingival recession
    B. Young children with poor oral hygiene
    C. Adults with gingival recession
    D. Rampant caries are not age-related

24. Dental fluorosis is defined as
    A. Hypermineralization of the enamel caused by overingestion of fluoride immediately after tooth eruption
    B. Hypermineralization of the enamel caused by overingestion of fluoride during tooth development
    C. Hypomineralization of the enamel caused by overingestion of fluoride immediately after tooth eruption
    D. Hypomineralization of the enamel caused by overingestion of fluoride during tooth development

25. What percentage of U.S. children exhibit some form of fluorosis?
    A. 7–15%
    B. 20–25%
    C. 25–33%
    D. 40–50%

26. Fluoridation has several mechanisms for caries inhibition. Included are enhancement of remineralization enamel, inhibition of glycolysis, incorporation of fluoride into the enamel hydroxyapatite crystal, and bactericidal action.
    A. Both statements are TRUE.
    B. Both statements are FALSE.
    C. The first statement is TRUE; the second statement is FALSE.
    D. The first statement is FALSE; the second statement is TRUE.

27. In 1989, fluoridation of the public water supply was estimated to cost on the average
    A. 20 cents per person per year
    B. 51 cents per person per year
    C. $20 per person per year
    D. $51 per person per year

28. Prevention is the major objective of public health programs because it entails
    A. Ethics
    B. Teamwork
    C. Cost efficiency
    D. All of the above

29. Primary prevention covers those measures taken before any disease appears. Secondary prevention is synonymous with early disease control.
    A. Both statements are TRUE.
    B. Both statements are FALSE.
    C. The first statement is TRUE; the second statement is FALSE.
    D. The first statement is FALSE; the second statement is TRUE.

30. Education plays an important role in public health because
    A. Preventive measures are taught and learned
    B. It decreases the need for government intervention
    C. The programs allow for cost-efficiency
    D. A teamwork approach is necessary

31. Many factors such as climate, familial and genetic patterns, and socioeconomic status have been studied to determine their relationship to dental caries. Since the advent of fluoridation of public water supplies, socioeconomic status has been proven to be a powerful determinant of caries status in the community.
    A. Both statements are TRUE.
    B. Both statements are FALSE.
    C. The first statement is TRUE; the second statement is FALSE.
    D. The first statement is FALSE; the second statement is TRUE.

32. Nutritional status does directly influence prevalence of dental caries. Dietary factors do not.
    A. Both statements are TRUE.
    B. Both statements are FALSE.
    C. The first statement is TRUE; the second statement is FALSE.
    D. The first statement is FALSE; the second statement is TRUE.

33. Adults ingest approximately how many milligrams of fluoride daily?
    A. 1–3
    B. 10–30
    C. 100–200
    D. 250–500

34. Efforts to exclude highly sugared snacks from school vending machines is an example of which of the following?
    A. Health prevention
    B. Disease progression
    C. Health promotion
    D. Health services

35. _____ are most effective in reducing pit and fissure decay when remaining in the tooth surface.
    A. Water fluoridation
    B. Dental sealants
    C. Scaling gel
    D. Fluoride varnishes

36. Which of the children would MOST likely benefit from a sealant program?
    A. Kindergartners and first graders
    B. Second and sixth graders
    C. Third and fourth graders
    D. Fifth graders

37. Which of the following preventive measures affect both periodontal diseases and caries?
    A. Plaque control measures
    B. Fluoride supplements
    C. Chlorhexidine gluconate
    D. Sealants

38. Which of the following arguments advanced by anti-fluoridationists is the most difficult to dispute?
    A. Fluoride is a poison.
    B. Fluoridation may have injurious consequences.
    C. Fluoridation violates human rights.
    D. The benefits of fluoride are not proven.

39. In conducting a community fluoridation campaign, which of the following are most likely to result in adoption of fluoridation?
    A. Public debates
    B. Public endorsements by local leaders
    C. Spot announcements on radio and television
    D. Public endorsements by local dental and dental hygiene associations

40. The teaching of dental health behaviors that help patients become aware of dental health theories is termed
    A. Assessment
    B. Education
    C. Instruction
    D. Promotion

41. In communities without fluoridated water supplies, the most *frequently* used method of delivering systemic fluoride to 6- to 12-year-old children is through
    A. Fluoride tablets
    B. Fluoride vitamins
    C. School water fluoridation
    D. A fluoride mouthrinse program

42. Which of the following is an advantage of a school-based fluoride rinse program?
    A. It is effective in reducing dental caries.
    B. It cannot be implemented by nondental personnel.
    C. It can achieve maximum effectiveness with application twice daily.
    D. It is the most expensive method for administration of fluoride.

43. When dental health is neglected, it is largely because of
    A. Minimal inherent value to oral health
    B. The threatening nature of dental disease
    C. Insufficient health care delivery personnel
    D. Insufficient evidence of the effectiveness of preventive measures

44. In conducting a local campaign to reduce the availability of vending machines filled with soft drinks in public schools, which of the following are most likely to result in adoption of fluoridation?
    A. Teachers advocating support
    B. Endorsements by local leaders
    C. Advertisements on radio and television
    D. Public endorsements by local dental and dental hygiene associations

45. The adjustment of fluoride content in a community water supply is the most effective method of preventing dental caries in the population because fluoridation
    A. Serves more people than other methods
    B. Is the most economical method
    C. May have some beneficial topical effect
    D. Serves all segments of the population that drink water, without creating oral health disparities

46. In a nonfluoridated community, which preventive dental health program would have the maximum cost benefit for the control of caries in elementary school children?
    A. Dental health education program
    B. Fluoride mouthrinse program
    C. Restorative care program
    D. Parent–teacher education program

47. The scale that depicts a continuum leading from complete healthy function to death is termed the
    A. Assessment scale
    B. Healthy living measurement
    C. Quality scale
    D. Wellness scale

48. Selection of audiovisual and other teaching material should be based on
    A. Availability of free educational materials
    B. Appropriateness of health slogans
    C. Eye appeal
    D. Scientifically authenticated information

49. The fundamental requirement for all health information given to the layman is that it be
    A. Accurate in content
    B. Repeated frequently
    C. Presented in lay terms
    D. Attractive in design and color

50. What would be the best resources for dental health education materials?
    A. Dental employer's office
    B. Local nurses' society
    C. State educational departments
    D. American Dental Hygienists' Association

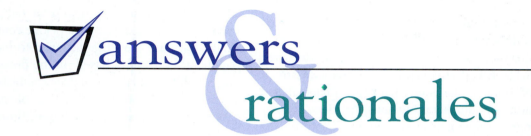

1.

A. A needs assessment, the first step in community planning, is used to obtain a profile of the community to ascertain the causes of the problem and helps in developing appropriate program goals and objectives in problem solving. A needs assessment identifies such things as community health status, population demographics, availability of manpower and facilities, and current ongoing programs and projects. Only after the needs assessment has been completed for the community are priorities for dealing with the identified problem(s) considered. Program goals can be established only after conduction of a needs assessment identifies areas of greatest concern. After a program plan based on analysis of the survey data, priorities and alternatives, community attitudes, and available resources has been developed, it must be approved by the community. Then, the program implementation begins.

2.

D. A program goal is a general statement about the overall purpose of a program to meet a defined problem. Program objectives are more specific than goals and describe the desired end result in a measurable way. Evaluation of a program is ongoing and occurs during program planning and implementation. Revisions to the program are based on evaluation results.

3.

C. Implementation strategies involve obtaining approval from appropriate personnel within the agency to determine rules, regulations, and possible limitations. Implementation strategies also include acquainting dental and dental hygiene professionals with the planned program, organizing the project, gathering necessary supplies, and identifying dental health education as it relates to the program. The needs assessment identifies the target group and defines programming needs. The assessment may utilize a variety of data collection methods such as surveys, dental indices, direct observations, questionnaires, interviews, and records from federal and state agencies. Program objectives are specific, measurable statements of what will be accomplished. Program planning within the community is much like developing a treatment plan to meet the dental needs of a patient in the private practice setting.

4.

B. Program evaluation is an ongoing process based on objectives serving as the standard of comparison to determine success or failure of the program. Resource identification is done during the needs assessment phase of program planning. Manpower, financial, and transportation considerations must be identified before program implementation. Community profiling is done during the needs assessment phase of program planning. The community profile of a population may include such characteristics as ethnic makeup, diet, socioeconomics status, education, and age. Defining the need of a population occurs during the needs assessment phase of program planning.

5.

A. A program objective is a specific, measurable statement of what will be accomplished. In this case, 100% of the students needing dental care (the percentage is specific and measurable) will receive it. Evaluation of a program is ongoing and occurs during program planning and implementation. Revisions to the program are based on evaluation results. Implementation strategies are developed during the planning stage of program development. A program goal is a broad general statement on the overall purpose of a program to meet a defined problem toward which program efforts are then directed.

6.

C. Because caries incidence is a nonreversible problem, preventive measures would not be effective in eliminating the existing caries. Restorative treatment is needed to optimize the dental health of the students. Placing sealants, performing cleanings, and providing fluoride treatments are preventive measures.

7.

B. The PI (plaque index) is designed to measure plaque removal based on the amount of plaque present at the time of evaluation. The possible range of scores is 0 to 3. An average PI of 2.5 indicates that there is a moderate to heavy accumulation of soft deposits within the gingival pocket and/or on the gingival margin that can be seen with the naked eye. The amount of debris indicates that plaque control is inadequate. Because the PI is designed to measure oral hygiene effectiveness based on the presence or absence of plaque and debris, it does not measure disease conditions of supporting structures of the teeth, dietary habits, or presence or extent of fluorosis.

8.

A. The high group D value represents a large percentage of carious lesions within the population. Because the group M and F values represent dental care rendered, their low values in this population suggest that dental care was not sought or obtained on a regular basis. The DMFT measures an individual's or group's caries experience and does not measure the amount of plaque, periodontal status, or presence or absence of calculus in a population.

9.

B. Baseline data are collected before program implementation. It is used to evaluate the success or failure of a given program by comparing baseline findings to program results. Program objectives are specific, measurable statements of what a program will accomplish. A survey is often initiated in response to a community's chief complaint. Investigation of surveys previously conducted by other researchers may help planners design new programs.

10.

B. Also known as "outcome evaluation," this process takes place at the end of the project and measures the impact of the program based on whether the program objectives were met. Process evaluation occurs during the project to evaluate procedures used to obtain data. Revisions to the program are based on the process evaluation. Program revisions are made during the course of the program and are based on evaluation results. Constraints may include such things as lack of manpower, inadequate financing, poor equipment, and anything else that impairs program operation.

11.

A. A needs assessment, which should occur first in an examination, most closely parallels a survey. Program planning parallels treatment planning. Goal setting does not come first and program operation parallels treatment.

12.

A. Develop a goal to meet each need. Goals must be developed before strategic planning can occur. Program appraisal is the evaluation stage, and program funding cannot be established until the program is determined.

13.

D. 4.5 ppm is the amount that has been shown to reduce caries up to 40%. Levels are at this concentration since ingestion is only taking place during the school hours. 1 ppm is the optimum level for community drinking water; 2 ppm and 3.5 ppm are not recommended for school water supplies.

14.

C. The low socioeconomic group has seen the least decline in caries according to the Surgeon General's Report, Healthy People 2000, and NHANES III. The high socioeconomic group has seen the sharpest decline in caries, so the lower the SES, the more they benefit from classroom presentations on dental health.

15.

D. Training the teachers is the best method of ensuring that the entire school community has been reached with dental health. They are present with the children every day to reinforce health habits and incorporate dental units in health and in science. Dental hygiene students and volunteer hygienists will do a great job presenting, but are only there once. The school nurse is not one-on-one with the second-grade classes daily.

16. B

C. Fluoridation is the controlled adjustment of the fluoride ion content of a domestic water supply to the optimum concentration that will provide maximum protection against dental caries.

17.

C. Fluoride is taken up at the tooth surface from both fluoridated drinking water and topical application. Some is deposited harmlessly within the skeletal system, even at 8 ppm.

18.

A. Increased public awareness resulting from caries prevention activites of water fluoridation has had a major impact as to how the public views tooth loss. Public acceptance of water fluoridation was essential for initiation and continuation of this public health program.

19.

B. Results of many studies have shown no benefit of use of prenatal flouride supplements.

20.

D. The fluoride controversy reemerged with arguments launched concerning water fluoridation's relationship to cancer.

21.

A. The human body possesses an efficient excretory mechanism for flourides. No damage to the human body has been reported from fluoridation of domestic water supplies.

22.

D. For a community presentation for deaf audiences, flashing lights on and off is necessary to attract the group's attention. Interpreters are used to interpret only and probably have little knowledge concerning a dental hygiene–related topic. Allow ample time for the audience to review handouts prior to the beginning of the presentation because deaf individuals depend on reading for communication, and also must rely on their sight to follow the presenter and/or interpreter.

23.

A. Rampant caries may be seen in children with poor oral hygiene or adults with xerostomia and gingival recession.

24.

D. Fluorosis occurs when excessive amounts of fluoride are ingested during tooth development.

25.

B. Fluorosis now seen in 22–25% of children.

26.

A. It was thought for many years that the mechanisms of fluoride was limited to incorporation of fluoride in the enamel hydroxyapatite crystal. The mechanism for the effectiveness of fluoride in the prevention of dental caries is multifactorial.

27.

B. The estimated cost in 1989 per person per year was 51 cents. However, costs have been shown to vary from 12 cents to $5.41 per person per year.

28.

D. It is more ethical to prevent disease than to cure disease. Teamwork is necessary to handle large groups efficiently, and delegation of responsibilities to aux-iliary personnel is utilized. Cost-efficiency plays a major role because prevention is cheaper than the cure.

29.

C. Primary prevention deals with the prepathogenic state of disease and involves health promotion and specific protection. Secondary prevention occurs in early pathogenesis. This involves early diagnosis and prompt treatment.

30.

B. Prevention, cost-efficiency, and teamwork are fundamental principles of public health. However, in a democratic society where government regulation is small, it is important for the public to understand why they must undertake proper health measure by their own volition. The individual must learn why such regulations are of value in order to increase compliance.

31.

A. After assessment and evaluation of many global studies to determine predictive and risk factors for dental caries, socioeconomic status was determined to be a powerful determinant factor of caries status in any community.

32.

B. Recent studies indicate that nutritional factors, defined as absorption of nutrients, have no bearing on caries development. However, dietary factors, relating to how patients select the food that they eat, have a clear influence on caries development.

33.

C. Adults ingest 100–200 mg of fluoride daily and have for many years. Acute fluoride poisoning occurs in adults when 250–500 mg are ingested over a 24-hour period.

34.

C. Health promotion is the activity that promotes healthy ideas and concepts to motivate individuals to adopt healthy behaviors.

35.

B. Dental sealants are the most effective modality to prevent pit and fissure decay. Fluoride therapies are most effective on smooth surfaces of teeth.

36.

B. Sealants are most effective when placed shortly after eruption so that decay has not started. Children that have recently had their first and second molars erupt are in second and sixth grade.

37.

A. Controlling plaque accumulation significantly affects both dental caries and periodontal diseases.

38.

C. Antifluoridationists frequently argue that adding fluoride to public water supplies is a violation of their rights.

39.

B. Endorsements by local leaders are very effective at promoting ideas and concepts as defined in the social cognitive theory.

40.

B. Health education is defined as the education of health behaviors that bring an individual to a state of health awareness.

41. C

D. School mouthrinse programs are most frequently employed in areas with fluoridated water. They are generally easier for schools to adopt and can be operated with minimal help from a dental professional.

42.

A. School fluoride mouthrinse programs are very effective at reducing dental decay.

43.

A. In order to maintain optimal oral health, an individual must value oral health. Values must be in place for healthy behaviors to commence.

44.

B. Social cognitive theory states that individuals make choices based on knowledge, behavior, and environment. Having a leader promote the idea will lend support from others.

45.

D. The adjustment of fluoride content in a community water supply is the most effective method of preventing dental caries in the population because fluoridation serves all segments of the population that drink water, without creating oral health disparities.

46.

B. When targeting dental caries in children, a school fluoride mouthrinse program would be most effective in an area without fluoride in the local water supply.

47.

D. The wellness scale defines a state of illness and death, leading from complete healthy function of individuals with areas in between for quality of life indicators.

48.

D. All materials provided for dental health education must be scientifically accurate.

49.

A. The fundamental requirement for patient education material must be that the information provided is correct.

50.

D. The organization that would have patient education materials available to the public would be the American Dental Hygienists' Association and federal agencies such as CDC and NIDCR.

15 Participating in Community Programs

Dental hygienists frequently provide dental health presentations to target populations, as discussed in the preceding chapters. Actually planning a dental health program entails more than just providing dental health education to a group. It generally consists of providing dental hygiene and dental treatment geared toward a population's needs.

Program planning is much more than just planning a program; it encompasses the assessment, diagnosis, implementation, and evaluation of programs in addition to the "planning" stage. Increasingly, dental hygienists are playing a vital role in developing oral health programs for communities.

chapter objectives

After completion of this chapter, the learner should be able to:

➤ Develop and plan community programs

➤ Discuss government programs at various levels

➤ Discuss how to evaluate community programs

➤ Describe dental indexes

➤ Participate in community programs

➤ Describe dental public health

TABLE 15-1 A COMPARISON OF THE PROVISION OF DENTAL HYGIENE CARE FOR A PRIVATE PATIENT AND FOR A COMMUNITY	
What the Dental Hygienist Does in Private Practice	**What the Dental Hygienist Does in Public Health**
Assessment	**Assessment**
Conducts initial health assessment by reviewing health and dental history with patient	Conducts a needs assessment of the target populations
Conducts a comprehensive oral examination	Analyzes needs of the community
Dental Hygiene Diagnosis	**Dental Hygiene Diagnosis**
Provides dental hygiene diagnosis of the patients	Provides dental hygiene diagnosis of the community
Planning	**Planning**
Develops a treatment plan based on diagnosis, patient interaction, and the priorities and method of payment; utilizes assessment mechanisms that are measurable	Develops a program based on analysis of needs assessment data, priorities and alternatives, community interaction, and the resources available; utilizes assessment mechanisms that are measurable
Selects appropriate healthcare workers to provide comprehensive care	Selects appropriate labor to implement program
Implementation	**Implementation**
Implements self-generated treatment plan effectively, changing plan when necessary	Implements self-generated program plan effectively, changing the plan when necessary
Evaluation	**Evaluation**
Evaluation of treatment via dental, gingival, and periodontal evaluations	Evaluates program via index and community evaluations

Source: Nathe, C. *Dental Public Health* (2nd ed.). Upper Saddle River, NJ: Prentice Hall, 2005.

I. Community Programs

    A. Comparing dental public health programs with private practice will aid in the understanding of hygienists' roles (Table 15-1■).

    B. When initiating a dental public health program, it is necessary to first contact the head administrator for approval and support

    C. *Collaborative* efforts between administration, dental hygienists, populations, caregivers, and communities are needed to ensure effectiveness of programs

    D. When operating a dental public health program it must have a significant number of individuals involved

II. Government Programs at Various Levels

A. International—The World Health Organization (WHO) is the United Nations' specialized agency for health, established in 1948. WHO's objective is the attainment by all peoples of the highest possible level of health. Health is defined in WHO's Constitution as a state of complete physical, mental, and social well-being and not merely the absence of disease or infirmity.

    1. WHO is governed by 192 Member States through the World Health Assembly; the Health Assembly is composed of representatives from WHO's Member States

    2. The main tasks of the World Health Assembly are to approve the WHO program and the budget for the following biennium and to decide major policy questions

    3. WHO coordinates programs for developing countries and gathers epidemiological data for comparison across nations. WHO establishes principles of primary healthcare to maintain health

    4. WHO develops means to summarize treatment needs of international populations utilizing minimal equipment (e.g., Community Periodontal Index of Treatment Needs [CPITN])

B. Federal: United States Government

    1. Primarily within the jurisdiction of the Department of Health and Human Services (DHHS), including U.S. Public Health Service, Centers for Disease Control and Prevention, National Institutes of Dental and Craniofacial Research, Centers for Medicare and Medicaid

    2. Examples of federally funded dental activities

        a. Biological research

        b. Disease prevention and control

        c. Planning and development programs in dental labor

        d. Education and services research

        e. Regulation and compliance functions (quality assessment)

        f. Programs concerned with provision of dental services

C. State level—Departments of Health and Human Services

    1. Provides consultation services to local health departments

    2. Directly administers some programs (especially those in rural areas)

    3. Allocates prevention block grant funds and Medicaid dental funding

    4. Example: many states report spending a portion of their Maternal and Child Health Services funds on dental-related services

D. Local level

    1. People-to-people level of public health that provides direct services

    2. Directly administers county and city programs

3. Initiates dental health legislative measures (such as fluoridation)

4. Although the division of responsibilities in delivering oral health programs to the community is delineated, it is clear that budget constraints are hampering program development and implementation at all levels

5. Evidence suggests that dental health care programs that are part of neighborhood, rural, migrant, and homeless health centers—founded largely through federal dollars—have experienced extreme difficulties in recent years owing to budget constraints

III. Process of Program Development

A. Assessment, which includes problem identification

B. Dental hygiene diagnosis, which identifies priority need determinations

C. Planning, which includes the following:

    1. Identification of goals and objectives. Goals are defined as broad statements that reflect the final outcome that is expected from the target population. Objectives are developed to provide detailed information that includes specific, observable actions/behaviors that should be completed during the program.

    2. Identification of resources and constraints

    3. Consideration of alternative implementation strategies

D. Evaluation, which occurs during all development stages (called formative evaluation) and at the end of a particular project or the end of the program (called the summative evaluation). Evaluation can be both qualitative, which answers the why and how of a dental program, and quantitative, which provides numerical evaluation of a program.

IV. Assessment

A. Needs assessment is an organized, systemic approach to identify the target group in order to define programming needs

B. Assessing the dental needs of the population via dental indexes and/or surveys

C. Focus on community organization of power (local politics), leadership, facility, resources, median age, SES, etc.

D. Assessing resources, which include facilities, funding, personnel, supplies, and equipment

E. Needs assessment evaluates population by identifying its

    1. Health status

    2. Community profile

    3. Demographics

    4. Income

       5. Funding availability

       6. Community and financial leaders

       7. Facilities

       8. Manpower

       9. Current and ongoing programs and projects

  F. Needs assessment is a vital part of planning a community dental health program

       1. Defines problems and determines severity

       2. Identifies target groups for programming

       3. Collects necessary data for planning

       4. Collects baseline data for program evaluation

V. Dental Hygiene Diagnosis

  A. Formulated after completing a comprehensive assessment

  B. Professional dental needs developed

VI. Program Planning

  A. Prioritization of dental needs from dental hygiene diagnosis during the planning stage of program development

  B. Goals and objectives

       1. When planning a program it is necessary to develop measurable goals and objectives so that the program can be effectively evaluated

  C. Labor force planning

       1. Need is defined as a normative, professional judgment as to the amount and kind of health care services required to attain or maintain health. Types of need may be conditions or diseases that need to be treated or prevented or the need for a particular healthcare provider

       2. Demand is the particular frequency or desired frequency of dental care from a population. Demand may be the public demanding a particular service, treatment, or preventive therapy or may be the demand for a particular type of healthcare provider

          a. A great example of the difference between need and demand can be seen when looking at the fact that although the state health department projects that 50% of the population needs dental hygiene treatment, the state dental hygienists' association's report suggests that 30% of a dental hygienist's schedule remains unfilled

          b. These two statements emphasize the difference between need and demand

       3. Supply is the quantity of dental care services available, which can be defined in terms of procedures/services/treatment options available or the number of dental providers or clinical facilities available to the public

4. Utilization is the number of dental care services actually consumed, not just desired; this can be of importance when speculating on the available supply of personnel to meet the demand and/or need

VII. Implementation

A. Implementation of the activities, timetables, costs, and possible alternatives

B. Modification of plan as necessary

C. Changing plans as needed to ensure program effectiveness

D. Important to have management for effective coordination, thus smooth operation

VIII. Evaluation

A. Utilize effective dental indexes and surveys to evaluate program (Box 15-1■)

B. Qualitative evaluation is evaluation utilizing personal interviews, short items, and fill-in-the-blank items on surveys; some see this as unscientific, but definitely helpful in evaluation and making useful revisions to a program

C. Quantitative evaluation is evaluating the program utilizing dental indexes and items with numerical value on surveys

D. Formative evaluation is evaluating the program during operation to ensure an effective program; helps in making necessary changes during program operation

E. Summative evaluation is completed at the end of the program to evaluate program effectiveness

IX. Dental Indexes (Table 15-2■)

A. A dental index is a method used to measure a disease or condition

B. Characteristics of a dental index

    1. Clarity: criteria are understandable

    2. Simplicity: easily memorized

    3. Objectivity: not subject to individual interpretation

    4. Validity: measures what is intended

    5. Reliability: reproducible examiner consistency and calibration

    6. Sensitivity: ability to detect small degrees of difference

    7. Acceptability: no pain or suffering caused to subjects and that the index is fiscally responsible

X. Dental Public Health Defined

A. The science and art of preventing and controlling dental disease and promoting dental health through organized community efforts

B. It is a form of dental practice that serves the community as a patient rather than as an individual

BOX 15-1

Dental Hygiene Program Planning Paradigm

ASSESSMENT

Assessment via surveys, existing data, or dental screenings:
Populations' dental needs
Demographics
Facility
Personnel (workforce)
Existing resources
Funding

↓

DENTAL HYGIENE DIAGNOSIS

Prioritization of needs

Formulation of diagnosis to provide goals and objectives for blueprint

↓

PLANNING

Identify methods to measure goals
Develop blueprint
Address constraints and possible alternatives described

↓

IMPLEMENTATION

Program will begin operation
Revision and changes identified and employed

↓

EVALUATION

Measuring of goals via surveys and dental indices
Qualitative and quantitative evaluation
Ongoing revisions employed

↵

Source: Nathe, C. *Dental Public Health* (2nd ed.). Upper Saddle River, NJ: Prentice Hall, 2005.

C. It is concerned with the dental health education of the public, with research and the application of the findings of research with the administration of programs of dental care for groups and with the prevention and control of disease through a community approach (from the American Board of Dental Public Health)

TABLE 15-2 COMMON DENTAL INDEXES

Index	Definition	Scoring
Plaque, Debris, and/or Calculus Indexes		
PHP: Patient Hygiene Performance	Assesses the extent of plaque and debris over a tooth surface; this index is particularly helpful when measuring different surfaces of a tooth; it actually divides the tooth into five surfaces.	Scores range from 0 to 5, with 0 being excellent and 5 being poor
PHP-M: Patient Hygiene Performance—Modified	A modification of the PHP index so that less teeth are evaluated and generalizations are made; Ramfjord teeth are generally chosen	Scores range from 0 to 5, with 0 being excellent and 5 being poor
Plaque control record	Records the presence of bacterial plaque on individual tooth surfaces; four to six surfaces are recorded depending on the purpose of the research	Score is either 0 or 1 depending on if plaque is present or not present
Plaque-free score	Determines the location, number, and percent of plaque-free surfaces of individual motivation and instruction; four surfaces are recorded; interproximal bleeding can also be documented	Score is either 0 or 1 depending on if plaque and/or bleeding is present or not present
PL1: Plaque index	Assesses the thickness of plaque at the gingival area	Scores range from 0 to 3 depending on amount of plaque
OHI: Oral hygiene index	Measures existing plaque and calculus as an indication of oral cleanliness; the OHI has two components, the debris index and the calculus index; the practitioner can evaluate both or just one	Scores range from 0 to 3 depending on the severity of plaque and/or calculus accumulation
OHI-S: Simplified oral hygiene index	The same as the OHI, but only used on six specific teeth; generally the Ramjford teeth are selected	Scores range from 0 to 3 depending on the severity of plaque and/or calculus accumulation
VMI: Volpe-Manhold index	Assesses the supragingival calculus after a dental cleaning	Measures three planes of calculus on six anterior teeth by bisecting the center of the lingual surface, using the diagonal measurement through the mesio-incisal angle of the tooth through the greatest areas of calculus and using a diagonal measurement through the disto-incisal angle of the tooth

TABLE 15-2 COMMON DENTAL INDEXES (*CONTINUED*)

Index	Definition	Scoring
Bleeding Indexes		
GBI: Gingival bleeding index	Records the presence or absence of gingival inflammation as determined by bleeding from interproximal gingival sulci; floss is used to determine bleeding	Score is either 0 or 1 depending on bleeding
SBI: Sulcus bleeding index	Locates areas of the gingival sulcus bleeding upon gentle probing; four areas are scored and a probe is used to determine bleeding	Scores range from 0 to 5 depending on bleeding and appearance of papillary and marginal gingiva
Eastman interdental bleeding index	Measures papillary bleeding; a wooden interdental cleaner is used	Score is either 0 or 1 depending on presence of bleeding
GI: Gingival index	Assesses the severity of gingivitis based on color, consistency, and bleeding; developed by Loe and Silness; probe is used in four gingival areas	Scores range from 0 to 3 depending on type of bleeding
MGI: Modified gingival index	A modified GI can omit the distal area	Scores range from 0 to 3 depending on type of bleeding
P-M-A: Papillary marginal attached index	Assesses the extent of gingival changes including papillary, gingival margin, and attached gingiva in large studies	Scores range from 0 to 3 depending on severity of gingival inflammation
Periodontal Diseases Index		
PI: Russell periodontal index	Assesses and scores the periodontal disease status of populations in large studies	Scores range from 0 to 8 depending on severity of disease
PDI: Periodontal disease index	Assesses the prevalence and severity of gingivitis and periodontitis to show the periodontal status of an individual or a group; used for longitudinal studies in the assessment of etiological factors and therapeutic procedures	Scores range from 0 to 3 depending on severity of disease
CPITN: Community periodontal index of treatment needs	Screens and monitors individual or group periodontal treatment needs; uses a specially designed probe	Scores range from 0 to III depending on periodontal treatment need

(*continued*)

TABLE 15-2 COMMON DENTAL INDEXES (*CONTINUED*)

Index	Definition	Scoring Methods
PSR: Periodontal screening and recording	A modified version of the CPITN to screen and monitor individuals or group periodontal needs using a specialized probe	Scores range from 0 to III depending on periodontal treatment need
LPA: Loss of periodontal attachment	Assesses the loss of periodontal attachment	Scores are taken from loss of attachment readings per surface area in millimeters
ESI: Extent and severity index	Measures the extent and severity of loss of alveolar bone utilizing radiographs	Scores are take from loss of alveolor bone readings in millimeters
GPI: Gingival periodontal index	Assesses the gingivitis and pocket depth in the dentition	Scores range from 0 to 3 depending on severity of disease
Dental Caries Indexes		
DEFT or DEFS: Decayed, extracted, filled primary teeth or tooth surfaces	Calculates the status of decayed, extractions, and filled primary teeth or tooth surfaces as indicated by the T or S at the end of the acronym; when measuring tooth surfaces, which is more sensitive, radiographs are used	Score is either 0 or 1 depending on decay, filled, or missing status of tooth or tooth surface
DMFT or DMFS: Decayed, missing, filled permanent teeth or tooth surfaces	Calculates the status of decayed, missing, and filled teeth or surfaces within the dentition, an indicator of dental caries activity as indicated by the T or S at the end of the acronym; when measuring tooth surfaces, which is more sensitive, radiographs are used	Score is either 0 or 1 depending on decay, filled, or missing status of tooth or tooth surface
RI: Root caries index	Calculates the status of root caries, usually recommended for adult surveys	The ratio of the number of teeth with carious lesions of the root and restorations of the root to the number of teeth with exposed root surfaces
Malocclusion Indexes		
Index of orthodontic treatment need	Defines specific, distinct categories of treatment need, while including a measure of function; it has been shown to be easy to use for epidemiological studies, acceptable to the profession and public and amenable to statistical analysis	Scores range from 0 to 5 depending on need for orthodontics
HLD: Handicapping Labiolingual Deviation index	Assesses orthodontic treatment needs based on HLD when recorded in Angle's classification	The angle classification for each patient is also recorded with the HLD variables; the mean and the percentage of the total score for each variable are calculated

TABLE 15-2 COMMON DENTAL INDEXES (*CONTINUED*)

Index	Definition	Scoring Methods
Occlusal index	Assesses the various characteristics of occlusion including dental age, molar relation, overbite, overjet, posterior crossbite, posterior open bite, tooth displacement, midline relations, and missing permanent maxillary incisors	Utilizes a variety of measurement scores for each of the nine characteristics assessed
Dental aesthetic index	Assesses esthetics of occlusion based on the impact it has on the social and psychological well-being of the individual	Consists of 10 occlusal traits related to dentofacial anomalies according to the three components of dentition, spacing–crowding, and occlusion
Dental Fluorosis Indexes		
Developmental defects of dental enamel	Scores enamel opacities, regardless of origin to avoid any bias	This index recognizes three types of defects, namely, opacities (white/cream, yellow/brown), hypoplasias (pits, horizontal grooves, vertical grooves, missing enamel), and discolored enamel; the defects can occur on a tooth surface as single or multiple well-demarcated areas or as poorly demarcated diffuse patches or fine lines; defects localization was assessed on three anatomical surfaces (buccal, lingual, and occlusal) and specified segments of a tooth crown
Fluorosis index	Rate of fluorosis within a population, sensitive to very mild through severe cases; developed by Dean	Scored with a 6-point scale
Fluorosis risk index	Assesses fluorosis, particularly the specific time of enamel formation	Developed for use in analytical epidemiological studies; designed to permit a more accurate identification of associations between age-specific exposures to fluoride sources and the development of enamel fluorosis; the FRI divides the enamel surfaces of the permanent dentition into two developmentally related groups of surface zones, designated either as having begun formation during the first year of life (classification I) or during the third through sixth years of life (classification II); data from the first use of this index in a population-based case-control study are given to illustrate the high reliability of the index, its validity, and its unique utility for the identification of risk factors of enamel fluorosis

(continued)

Index	Definition	Scoring Methods
Tooth surface index of fluorosis	Rate of fluorosis within a population; more sensitive than the Fluorosis Index	Scoring ranges from 0 to 7 depending on severity of fluorosis
Other Indexes		
Cleft lip/palate	Calculated as the terms of rate in the number of births in a population	Rates
Oral cancer	Calculated as the terms of rate in a population, sometimes broken down into strata	Rates

review questions

DIRECTIONS
Each of the questions or incomplete statements below is followed by suggested answers or completions. Select the **one** answer that is best in each case.

Testlet 1: Questions 1–10

A high school health class has 40 students, 14 to 16 years of age. Two public health dental hygienists are asked to assess the oral health of the students. Before gathering any data, the hygienists meet to select examination procedures and review indexes to be used. Both agree to use the DMFT examination. The hygienists then conduct DMFT examinations on 10 volunteer patients at the public health facility and compare and calibrate their results. When their clinical techniques produce the same clinical findings within the volunteer patient pool, the public health hygienists conduct DMFT evaluations on the health class students. The total DMFT of the class is 160.

1. The DMFT examinations conducted by the public health dental hygienists on the volunteers before examining the health class students will increase
   A. Sampling error
   B. Interexaminer reliability
   C. Sensitivity
   D. Predicative value

2. What is the group DMFT?
   A. 1.6
   B. 8.0
   C. 4.0
   D. 16

3. If D = 40, M = 44, and F = 76, what percent of the teeth have untreated caries?
   A. 40%
   B. 25%
   C. 16%
   D. 4%

4. The relatively high F value (76) would indicate that this population
   A. Has no access to dental care
   B. Has a high incidence of tooth extractions
   C. Is in need of aggressive periodontal therapy
   D. Has access to restorative dental care

5. The amount of untreated caries in this population at the time of the examination is known as the
   A. Caries incidence
   B. Caries prevalence
   C. Hidden caries
   D. Primary caries

6. The public health hygienists agree to conduct annual DMFTs on these 40 students for 10 years. This type of study is
   A. Retrospective
   B. Cross-sectional
   C. Longitudinal
   D. Experimental

7. The M component of the group DMFT in this population assumes that missing teeth have been lost as a result of
   A. Caries
   B. Periodontal involvement
   C. Congenital defects
   D. Poor oral hygiene

8. What percentage of the examined teeth has received dental treatment?
   A. 76%
   B. 75%
   C. 40%
   D. 44%

9. When considering DMFTs 5 years after the initial examinations, the test population consists of 21 former students. This is an example of
   A. Sampling error
   B. A probability sample
   C. Quantifiability
   D. Sample attrition

10. The DMFTs for the 21 test subjects are D = 20, M = 5, and F = 25. How does the data of unmet dental needs compare with the initial findings?
    A. There is a much greater need for dental treatment within the test population 5 years after the first examination.
    B. The sample population has maintained the same decay rate over the last 5 years.
    C. The need for dental treatment in the test population is much lower 5 years after the initial examination.
    D. Decay rates and extractions have markedly decreased since the first DMFT was conducted 5 years ago.

Testlet 2: Questions 11–15

A new dental hygiene graduate accepts a position in a migrant worker camp as part of a loan-forgiveness program. There are 56 adults and 92 children who need to be screened and be on a prevention program. Over half of the adults smoke.

11. The first thing to be done is
    A. Test the water for fluoride content
    B. Teach dental health education in group settings
    C. Assess the needs of the group
    D. Begin oral prophylaxis as soon as possible

12. Which of the following indices will be MOST helpful for the hygienist to use in assessing the periodontal treatment needs of the adults?
    A. CPITN
    B. FRI
    C. EIB
    D. PII

13. Which of the following indices is MOST appropriate to determine the caries experience of the preschool children in the camp?
    A. DMFT
    B. DMF
    C. deft
    D. DMFS

14. The "e" in the deft index stands for
    A. Erupted
    B. Exfoliated
    C. Primary teeth indicated for extraction
    D. Extracted

15. Which of the following would be an example of a risk factor in the migrant camp group?
    A. Age
    B. Gender
    C. Race
    D. Smoking

16. The Ramfjord teeth commonly used to simplify dental indexes include
    A. Maxillary right first molar, left central incisor, and left first premolar; mandibular left first molar, right central incisor, and right first premolar
    B. Maxillary right first molar, left central incisor, and left first molar; mandibular left first molar, left central incisor, and right first molar
    C. The division of the mouth into sextants: maxillary molars and mandibular incisors
    D. Only the premolars, both maxillary and mandibular

17. If the major purpose of an epidemiologist's research is to determine caries susceptibility as opposed to immediate treatment needs, the best caries index to use is
    A. DMFT
    B. DMFS
    C. CPITN
    D. TSIF

18. Dental health surveys overestimate dental needs more so than private practitioners because
    A. They are conducted under ideal conditions
    B. They utilize standardized examiners
    C. They result in congruencies between need and demand for care
    D. The statement is FALSE; dental needs are underestimated

19. A special characteristic of the Root Caries Index (RCI) as compared to other dental indexes is
    A. A carious lesion is only included in the count when it appears below the CEJ
    B. A carious lesion is included in the count when it appears above or below the gingival margin
    C. It is unique in that it includes the concept of teeth at risk
    D. It is based on 28 permanent teeth, excluding third molars

20. For epidemiological studies, the best available index for the measurement of periodontitis is the
    A. Sulcus Bleeding Index
    B. Periodontal Index
    C. Community Periodontal Index of Treatment Needs
    D. Indirect method of scoring loss of periodontal attachment

21. The Klien and Palmer Index can be recorded as DMFT or DMFS. The DMFS would be the recommended choice in which of the following situations?
    A. Radiographs are not available
    B. Time is a limiting factor in the screening process
    C. The examiner is not highly skilled in the detection of caries
    D. There is a need to detect sensitive changes in caries incidence
    E. All of the above

22. Females have been found to have higher DMF scores than males. One could also conclude from these findings that females are more caries susceptible than their male counterparts.
    A. Both statements are TRUE.
    B. Both statements are FALSE.
    C. The first statement is TRUE, the second statement is FALSE.
    D. The first statement is FALSE, the second statement is TRUE.

23. The OHI-S measures which of the following?
    A. Dental care
    B. Debris
    C. Gingival bleeding
    D. Both B and C

review questions

24. A treatment category of I on the community Periodontal Index of Treatment Needs (CPITN) indicates that
    A. Bleeding was observed upon probing or pressure
    B. Calculus was felt during probing and 3.5–5.5 mm pockets were recorded
    C. Improved oral hygiene and scaling are necessary
    D. This index does not include treatment categories

25. The effectiveness of a dental health program can be measured by
    A. The degree to which it meets program objectives
    B. The number of participants involved
    C. The cost of the program
    D. The length of the program
    E. All of the above

26. Which of the following indices is used to measure oral debris?
    A. Plaque Index
    B. Gingival Index
    C. Decayed, Missing, and Filled Surfaces
    D. Decayed, Missing, and Filled Teeth

27. Sensitivity, a characteristic of a diagnostic test, should determine if a high proportion of individuals who are tested for a disease and found positive
    A. Will not subsequently develop the disease
    B. Will subsequently develop the disease
    C. Has little place in oral epidemiology even though a positive test was determined
    D. Will seek treatment once notified of the results

28. When a patient comes to a dental office, the first procedure is an examination. The first step in a public health program is
    A. Analysis
    B. Survey
    C. Diagnosis
    D. Treatment

29. The most important determinants of dental utilization are
    A. Socioeconomic status, dentate status, and gender
    B. Socioeconomic status and gender
    C. Dentate status and gender
    D. Undetermined at this time

30. Which of the following caries indexes applies to primary dentition?
    A. DMF
    B. DEF
    C. DMFS
    D. Def
    E. OHI-S

31. Which of the following indexes should be used to estimate most severe periodontal disease?
    A. OHI
    B. OHI-S
    C. PI
    D. GI

32. Medicare, Title XVIII of the Social Security Act, pays for dental as well as medical care for patients age 65 and over. All types of dental care are included in this coverage.
    A. Both statements are TRUE.
    B. Both statements are FALSE.
    C. The first statement is TRUE, second statement is FALSE.
    D. The first statement is FALSE, second statement is TRUE.

33. Medicaid, Title XIX of the Social Security Act, approaches public-supported dental care providing
    A. Dental care for mothers and children receiving Aid to Families with Dependent children benefits
    B. Emergency dental treatment for everyone regardless of ability to pay
    C. Dental care (screening, diagnosis, treatment) to needy children up to at least 20 years of age

34. The most important concept of Winslow's definition of public health is
    A. The art and science of preventing disease
    B. Promoting mental and physical efficiency
    C. Promotion through organization community effort
    D. Health is not merely the absence of disease or infirmity

35. The minimum population level that is necessary to support a public health department is
    A. 4,000–5,000
    B. 7,500–10,000
    C. 10,000–15,000
    D. 35,000–50,000

36. Which level of the health department offers direct services to the individual?
    A. Local
    B. State
    C. National
    D. International

37. Education plays an important role in public health because
    A. Preventive measures are taught and learned
    B. It decreases the need the government intervention
    C. The programs allow for cost-efficiency
    D. A teamwork approach is necessary

38. Milestones in dental public health in the early twentieth century were characterized by all of the following EXCEPT
    A. The Dental Department of the U.S. Public Health Service was founded in 1919
    B. G.V. Black led discussion on fluoride at the Colorado State Dental Association in 1908
    C. Fones opened a training school for dental nurses in New Zealand

39. Health Maintenance Organizations (HMOs) are similar to preferred provider organizations (PPOs) in that they both are nontraditional methods for delivering and financing dental care. PPOs, however, are more of a financing arrangement than a structure.
    A. Both statements are TRUE.
    B. Both statements are FALSE.
    C. The first statement is TRUE; second statement is FALSE.
    D. The first statement is FALSE; second statement is TRUE.

40. Currently, a public health problem is defined as a health issue that
    A. Results in public demand for immediate intervention by the government
    B. Causes or potentially causes widespread morbidity and/or mortality
    C. Has caused widespread morbidity and/or mortality
    D. Involves a perception on the part of the public, public health authorities, and the government that a public health problem is occurring
    E. Both B and D

41. Severe caries is operationally defined in groups of children as a DMFT of 7.0. Five percent of children in the United States today will fall into this category.
    A. Ask, advise, assist and arrange for all patients to stop using tobacco
    B. Not personally use any form of tobacco
    C. Conduct diligent oral exams on both patients who report and those who do not report tobacco use
    D. All of the above

42. DMF surfaces have an advantage over DMF tooth counts because they are
    A. More economical
    B. Concerned with permanent dentition
    C. A simple, expedient index
    D. A more sensitive measurement

review questions

43. When organizing and providing dental care services, need may be defined as
    A. The particular frequency or desired frequency of dental care from a population
    B. A normative, professional judgment as to the amount and kind of services
    C. The quantity of dental care services
    D. The number of dental care services actually consumed by a given population

44. Dental public health or community dental health is best defined as
    A. Health care provided to maintain the health of the poor
    B. Rendering health care services and deducing the nature of health problems
    C. Protecting people's health through privately funding agencies
    D. Activity directed toward the improvement and protection of the health of a population group

45. Evaluation of a community-based dental care program is
    A. An ongoing process
    B. Important to provide qualitative and quantitative documentation of the program
    C. Not an important consideration during the planning phase
    D. Both A and B
    E. A, B, and C

46. Prevention is the major objective of a public health program because it entails
    A. Ethics
    B. Teamwork
    C. Cost efficiency
    D. All of the above

47. Which of the following demonstrates the most effective and efficient use of a dental public health hygienist's time?
    A. Conducting regular oral health screenings
    B. Rendering oral prophylaxes and topical fluoride treatments
    C. Delivering dental health instruction to elementary and secondary school children
    D. Organizing teachers to implement a school-based program involving self-application of topical fluoride

48. Dental public health is the science of providing oral health care and education to the public and emphasizes the science of
    A. Restorative dental care
    B. Prosthodontics
    C. Dental hygiene
    D. Emergency dental care

49. Demand for dental care is strongly influenced by
    A. Supply of dental manpower
    B. Needs of the population
    C. The level of dental knowledge
    D. Oral health expectations
    E. Social values

50. In a press release, a state health commission stated that 90% of the population had untreated cavities. The state dental hygiene association conducted a survey that showed that 50% of practicing dental hygienists had two or more unfilled appointment hours per day. What is the best explanation for the difference in data?
    A. The dental association survey was conducted poorly.
    B. The health commission projection was incorrect.
    C. The health commission based its figure on need for care, the dental hygiene association on current demand for care.
    D. The health commission based its figure on current demand for care, the dental hygiene association on need for care.

☑ answers & rationales

1.

B. Reaching agreement between two or more examiners is termed interexaminer reliability. It requires initial agreement on interpretation of diagnostic criteria followed by a period of training with repeated patient examinations to ensure that examiners are comparable. Sampling error results from the research sample not perfectly representing the base population. Sensitivity describes the ability of a measuring instrument to detect clinically relevant changes in the condition being measured. Predictive value refers to the ability of a diagnostic test to predict the probability that a person who tests positive will have the disease or condition (positive predictive value) or who tests negative will not have the disease or condition (negative predictive value).

2.

C. The total DMFT is divided by the number of individuals examined to calculate the group DMFT. The calculation is as follows: $160 \div 40 = 4.0$ (group DMFT). Based on the calculation used to determine the group DMFT of a study population, 1.6, 8.0, and 16 are incorrect values.

3.

B. To determine the percentage of untreated caries, divide the "D" component total by the total DMFT. The calculation is:

Total DMFT $= D + M + F = 40 + 44 + 76 = 160$

$D \div$ total DMFT $= 40 \div 160 = 0.25$

$0.25 \times 100\% = 25\%$ (of teeth examined have untreated caries)

Based on the calculations used to determine the percent of the group DMFT needing restorative care, 40%, 16%, and 4% are incorrect values.

4.

D. The "F" value in a DMFT examination refers to those teeth that have been filled. Filled teeth are assumed to have decayed before restoration. Because teeth must be diagnosed as carious and restored in the dental setting, access to care must be in place.

5.

B. The prevalence of a disease in a population is the proportion of existing cases of the disease in the population at one point in time or during a specified period of time. Incidence is the proportion of a new condition or disease within a population during a specified period of time. Hidden caries is the term used to describe dentinal caries found radiographically beneath an apparently sound occlusal surface, and primary caries are those carious lesions occurring on unrestored teeth.

6.

C. Longitudinal studies require at least two series of measurements among the same population at different times to determine the progress of the condition over a specified time period. A retrospective study is descriptive in nature and investigates previously collected data. In cross-sectional study, the health conditions in a representative cross section of a population are assessed at one time. An experimental study is designed to test the efficacy or effectiveness of a therapeutic drug, preventive material, or a treatment protocol by manipulating conditions.

7.

A. Only those teeth that are missing as a result of unrestorable caries are considered in the "M" category. Teeth extracted for orthodontic reasons are not considered in the "M" category. The DMFT is an index that measures caries experience, is not used to evaluate periodontal health, and does not include congenitally missing teeth or poor oral hygiene.

8.

B. To calculate what percentage of the examined teeth have received dental treatment, the "M" and "F" values are totaled and divided by the group DMFT. A percentage is calculated as follows:

$M + F = 120$

$120 \div 160 = 0.75$

$0.75 \times 100\% = 75\%$ (the percentage of teeth that have received dental treatment)

Based on the calculations used to determine the percentage of teeth that have received dental treatment from this group's DMFT score, 76%, 40%, and 44% are incorrect answers.

9.

D. Sample attrition refers to the decrease in number of subjects over the course of the study owing to such things as relocation, health issues, or loss of interest. Efforts to minimize sample attrition help to increase the validity of a study. Sampling error refers to the error that results from the sample not representing the base population. A probability sample is one in which the chance of each person being chosen in the sample is known. Quantifiability refers to the ability of an index to be analyzed statistically so that the status of a group can be expressed by a distribution, mean, median, or other statistical measure.

10.

A. To calculate the percentage of unmet dental needs in a DMFT score, the "D" value is divided by the total DMFT and converted to a percentage. The unmet dental needs of the sample population, examined 5 years after the initial DMFT examinations were performed, can be calculated as follows:

$D = 20$

Total DMFT $= D + M + F = 20 + 5 + 25 = 50$

$D \div$ Total DMFT $= 20 \div 50 = 0.4$

$0.4 \times 100\% = 40\%$ (unmet dental needs of the sample population 5 years after the initial DMFT examinations were performed)

The initial DMFT examination findings conducted on the 40 high school students can be used to calculate the unmet dental needs of the sample population in a like manner. The calculations in this case are as follows:

$D = 40$

Total DMFT $= D + M + F = 40 + 44 + 76 = 160$

$D \div$ Total DMFT $= 40 \div 160 = 0.25$

$0.25 \times 100\% = 25\%$ (unmet dental needs of the sample population at the initial DMFT examination)

Therefore, 40% of the sample population demonstrates unmet dental needs 5 years after the initial examinations compared with 25% needing restorative care initially.

11.

C. Assessment of needs and program planning come first. Teaching brushing and flossing are part of program implementation. Oral prophylaxis is part of program operation, and testing the water for fluoride content would take place after needs assessment.

12.

A. CPITN will assess periodontal treatment needs of a large group. FRI index is designed to identify risk factors for fluorosis. FIB index measures bleeding with an interdental stimulator. The PII will give us plaque scores; however, treatment information is needed first.

13.

C. deft will count decayed and filled primary teeth, as well as primary teeth indicated for extraction. DMFT counts permanent decayed, missing, and filled teeth. DMFS is decayed, missing, and filled permanent surfaces. For mixed dentitions, two indices must be used, one for the deciduous dentition and one for the permanent dentition.

14.

C. The "e" in deft stands for primary teeth indicated for extraction; deft does not measure erupted, exfoliated, or extracted teeth.

15.

D. Smoking is the risk factor that can be modified. Age, race, and gender cannot be modified, but it is possible to stop smoking.

16.

A. The Ramjford teeth, by definition, are those included in answer A.

17.

A. The results of the DMFT index yields a group's caries susceptibility without use of radiographs. However, the DMFS measures carious, missing, or filled surfaces and often incorporates use of radiographs. The CPITNM and the TSIF are not used for measurement of caries. Use of radiographs in diagnosis of DMF surfaces is of far greater importance for determining immediate treatment need, whereas visual exams without radiographs can estimate caries susceptibility.

18.

D. Dental health surveys often underestimate dental treatment due to complicating factors. Criteria used to diagnose caries may vary; incongruence occurs between patients' perceived needs and the practitioner's idea of need; surveys look at short-term findings whereas practitioners must be concerned with long-term outcomes for patients; treatment philosophies change rapidly.

19.

C. The Root Caries Index (RCI) is unique as compared to DMF and other indexes because it takes into account "teeth at risk." A tooth is considered to be at risk of dental root caries if enough gingival recession has occurred to expose the cementum to the oral environment.

20.

D. The indirect method of scoring loss of periodontal attachment (LPA) utilizes a fixed point, the CEJ, in partial calculation of the index. The first step is a traditional measure of pocket depth, the second measure is the measurement from gingival crest to the CEJ, and the final calculation is step one minus step two. Other indexes that utilize the first step only may give inaccurate readings because the level of the gingival is not always static.

21.

D. The Klein and Palmer Index can be recorded as "S" for surface and "T" for tooth. Surface counts are more sensitive than tooth counts. DMFS requires the use of radiographs, is more time-consuming, and requires that the examiner be highly skilled in the use of the index.

22.

C. While the first statement is true and may be explained by earlier tooth eruption patterns in females and utilization of dental care, current research demonstrates that it is erroneous at this time to assume from these findings that females are more caries-susceptible than males.

23.

B. The OHI-S measures plaque and calculus on six surfaces of six teeth. Caries and gingival bleeding are not determined by this index.

24.

C. The CPITN is an index of treatment needs rather than an index for determining periodontal status.

25.

A. The results of a program are measured against the objectives developed during planning. Effectiveness deals with the attainment of objectives. Efficiency deals with cost-effectiveness.

26.

A. The Plaque Index is used to determine accumulation of plaque and oral debris. The Gingival Index is used to determine, as the name indicates, bleeding and gingival health. DMFS and DMFT are caries indices.

27.

B. By definition, sensitivity is a proportion of positive tests with subsequent disease. It should not be confused with the term specificity, which by definition is the proportion of negative tests without subsequent disease.

28.

B. When a patient comes to the dental office or clinic, the dental provider first performs a careful examination. The first step in modern public health procedures is identical to that used by the dental clinic, only here it is the community that must be examined. It is called survey instead of examination.

29.

A. The future use of dental services will most likely be linked to the patient's gender, high socioeconomic status, and presence of most or all natural teeth.

30.

D. Lowercase letters are used for measuring caries susceptibility in primary dentition. OHI-S is a debris index, and a primary dentition counterpart is not reported in the dental literature.

31.

C. The OHI and OHI-S are debris indexes and do not measure severity of periodontal disease. The GI index is confined to measurements within the gingival. The PI is used to measure presence and severity of periodontal disease.

32.

B. Medicare does cover medical care for this population. Dental benefits are limited to those dental problems such as fractures and oral cancer that require hospitalization.

33.

C. The Medicaid program instituted in 1968 required states to provide dental screening, diagnosis, and treatment for needy children up to at least age 20 years.

34.

C. Winslow's definition utilizes the concept of organized community efforts of all individuals within a population.

35.

D. To be well supported by available tax funds, the 35,000–50,000 population is targeted. The essence of public health is dealing with large groups. Due to this fact, public health officials are educated with this orientation. Often it is more cost-efficient for two small counties to combine to form the target population.

36.

A. The local health department provides such direct functions as home visits, dental clinics, and supervision of local water supplies. The state and national levels perform supervisory and administrative functions. The international level often works with worldwide health promotion and prevention.

37.

B. Prevention, cost-efficiency, and teamwork are fundamental principles of public health. However, in a democratic society where government regulation is small, it is important for the public to understand why they must undertake proper health measures by their own volition. The individual must learn why such regulations are of value in order to increase compliance.

38.

C. Alfred Fones trained Irene Newman to be the first dental hygienist in the world.

39.

A. These two forms for delivery and financing of dental care became a more accepted part of health care in the 1980s. Often discussed together, they do differ because PPOs typically involve contracts between insurers and a number of practitioners. Patients are allowed to select from whom they will receive dental care depending on whether or not the practitioner participates in the PPO arrangement. Participants are much more limited in selection of practitioners.

40.

E. Dental public health originally was defined as a condition or situation that caused widespread death and/or disease, whereas a body of knowledge existed that could review the situation but was not being applied. Today, the definition has been expanded to include public health governmental perception of such a problem.

41.

C. By definition, severe caries is now classified by a DMFT score of 7.0 or above. Twenty percent of U.S. children still suffer from severe caries today.

42.

D. A more sensitive measure for dental caries is DMFS. It reaches its greatest usefulness when dental radiographs are incorporated. In cases of high caries attack rates where almost no unaffected teeth remained, the DMFS demonstrates well a more accurate caries count than DMFT because only a whole tooth is taken into account in the other index.

43.

B. Need can be defined as a normative, professional judgment as to the amount and kind of services required to attain and maintain health. Demand is the particular frequency or desired frequency of dental care of a population. Supply is defined as the quantity of dental care services available. Utilization is the number of dental care services actually consumed by a given population.

44.

D. Dental public health is defined as concern for and activity directed toward the improvement and protection of the health of a population group. It is not limited to the health of the poor, to rendering health services, or to deducing the nature of health problems. Also, it is not defined by the method of payment for health services or by the agency supplying those services.

45.

D. Evaluation is an ongoing process and actually is thought about in the planning phase when objectives and goals are being developed. It is also important that you are able to provide qualitative and qualifiable documentation of the program to the target population, administrators, funding agency, and public on an ongoing basis.

46.

D. It is more ethical to prevent disease than to cure disease. Teamwork is necessary to handle large groups efficiently, and delegation of responsibilities to dental hygienists is efficient. Cost-efficiency plays a major role because prevention is cheaper than the cure.

47.

D. Organizing teachers to implement a fluoride mouthrinse program and acting as a consultant to the program is the most effective way to work as a public health dental hygienist. It is an excellent way to integrate dental health into the school curriculum and an effective method to reach the most individuals.

48.

C. Dental public health focuses on first preventing disease, which is the essence of dental hygiene.

49.

E. Social values define demand of dental hygiene services. If individuals value oral health, they will seek and demand dental care.

50.

C. The state health commission based its figures on need for services, which is defined as a professional judgment of the amount and kind of health care services required whereas the state dental hygienists' association based its figures on demand for services, which is defined as the particular frequency or desired frequency of dental care from a population.

16 Analyzing Scientific Literature, Understanding Statistical Concepts, and Applying Research Results

The practice of dental hygiene is based on evidence-based published research that documents evidence that the science is effective. Dental providers make decisions that are derived from documented evidence rather than anecdotal tradition. This is commonly referred to as *evidence-based* practice.

It is important for the practitioner to be able to fully understand basic research principles so that he or she may make decisions based on evidence. Moreover, dental hygienists must be able to critically evaluate scientific literature and dental care products and modalities. Dental hygienists must continually make decisions when planning and implementing treatment, educating patients, and evaluating products and modalities. Science and technology are forever changing and when assuming the professional responsibility inherent in patient treatment, dental hygienists must employ state-of-the-art practice.

chapter objectives

After completion of this chapter, the learner should be able to:

➤ Analyze scientific literature

➤ Describe and apply statistical concepts

➤ Apply research results

BOX 16-1

Criteria for Judging a Research Report

- When was the work published?
- Where was it published?
- Are the qualifications of the authors appropriate?
- Is the purpose clearly stated?
- Is the experimental design clearly described?
- Have the possible influences on the findings been identified and controls instituted?
- Has the sample been appropriately selected?
- Has the reliability of the scoring been assessed?
- Is the experimental therapy compared appropriately to the control therapy?
- Is the investigation of sufficient duration?
- Is the statistical analysis appropriate to answer the research questions or hypotheses?
- Have the research questions or hypotheses been answered?

I. Critiquing Research (Box 16-1■)

A. Purpose of study should explain what is to be studied

B. Research problem and goal clearly identified

C. Review of literature included, which is thorough and reviews current literature and research and landmark (benchmark) studies published in peer-reviewed journals

D. Methods should be described including research designs, statistical tests, and materials to be used in study

E. Discussion of results clearly described and conclusions justifiable

F. Recommendations for further research included

G. Study is published in peer-reviewed journal, ensuring effective critique of research

   1. Peer-reviewed is usually blind review and frequently termed refereed

   2. Primary sources should come from original research studies

II. Descriptive Statistics Are Used to Describe Datasets

A. Measures of central tendency

   1. Mean is the arithmetic average ($x = \Sigma\, x/n$). A dental hygienist has just probed the facial mesial area of the 6 Ramfjord teeth. The measurements were 5,3,3,4,5,5. What is the mean? Answer = 4.2

   2. Median is the middle item of the dataset (the midpoint). A dental hygienist has just probed the facial mesial area of the 6 Ramfjord teeth. The measurements were 5,3,3,4,5,5. What is the median? Answer = 4.5

   3. Mode is the most frequently occurring number in the dataset; there can be two modes (bimodal) or three modes (trimodal), etc. A dental hygienist has just probed the facial mesial area of the 6 Ramfjord teeth. The measurements were 5,3,3,4,5,5. What is the mode? Answer = 5

B. Measures of dispersion or spread

    1. Range is the measurement of the highest score minus the lowest score (highest score − lowest score = range). A dental hygienist has just probed the facial mesial area of the 6 Ramfjord teeth. The measurements were 5,3,3,4,5,5. What is the range? Answer = 2

    2. Variance is the sum of the square deviations of the sample mean divided by one less than the total numbers of items; the larger the variance, the more data items are spread about the means. A dental hygienist has just probed the facial mesial areas of the 6 Ramfjord teeth. The measurements were 5,3,3,4,5,5. What is the variance? Answer = .66

    3. Standard deviation is the square root of the variance. A dental hygienist has just probed the mesial area of the 6 Ramfjord teeth. The measurements were 5,3,3,4,5,5. What is the standard deviation? Answer = .81.

III. Inferential Statistics Are Used to Test Hypothesis

  A. Parametric statistics

    1. Data must meet certain criteria (such as large enough sample and interval or ratio scale data)

    2. *t*-test—Used to test the difference between two mean scores

      a. t-*test for independent samples*—Tests the difference between means of two groups of subjects

      b. *t*-test for correlated samples

        (1) Tests difference between two means in the same group

        (2) Example—Pretest/post-test

  B. Nonparametric statistics

    1. Used when data do not meet assumptions of parametric statistics

    2. χ^2 (chi square)—Used to test the difference between frequency distributions

      a. Determines whether significant difference exists between observed number of cases within designated categories and expected number predicted in null hypothesis

      b. Tests independence of categorical variables to compare two or more distributions, especially useful for analyzing nominal data

    3. Mann-Whitney U-test

      a. Nonparametric counterpart to *t*-test for independent samples—Used with ordinal data

    4. Sign test

      a. Nonparametric counterpart to *t*-test for correlated samples—Used with ordinal data

IV. Graphing Data

   A. Data can be depicted on histogram or bar graph, frequency polygon, scattergram, or pie chart (Figure 16-1■)

V. Distribution

   A. Normal distribution is sometimes called the bell curve; it is a frequency distribution of scores that when graphed yields a bell-shaped curve; it implies that most scores fall around the measures of central tendency (Figure 16-2■)

   B. Skew means that extreme scores affect the distibution. In fact, a skew refers to the tail of the distribution with the fewest scores. A negatively skewed distribution occurs when a few extreme scores are to the left; this is when the

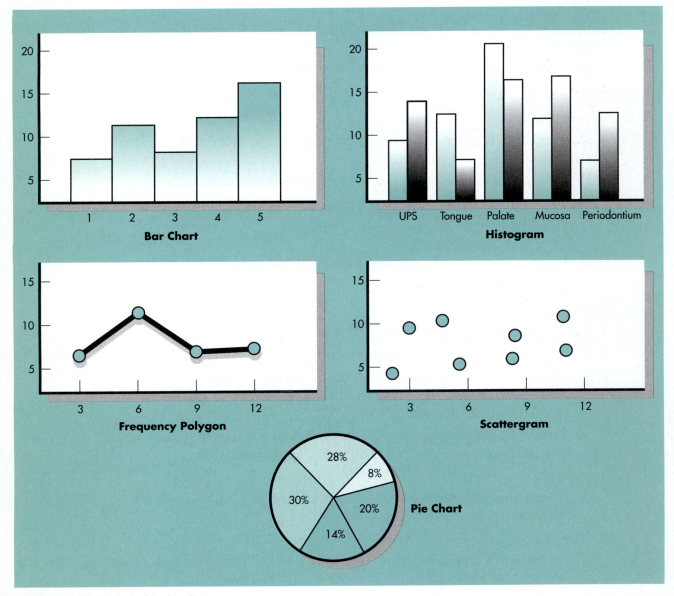

FIGURE 16-1 ■ Methods of Graphing Data

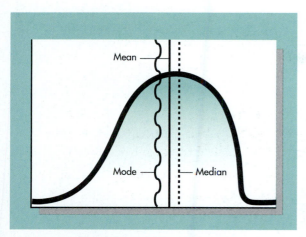

FIGURE 16-2 ■ Normal Distribution (Bell Curve)

mean is usually smaller than the median because it is pulled in the direction of the extremely low scores. A positively skewed distribution indicates a few extreme scores in the right half of the curve. In a positively skewed distribution, the mean is always greater than the median since it is pulled in the direction of the extremely high scores (Figure 16-3■).

VI. Correlation

A. Correlation measures the extent of the linear relationship between two variables.

B. In a positive linear relationship, the scores being correlated vary together—when one score is high, the other score is high; an example could be an increase in sugar, which may yield an increase in dental caries

C. In a negative relationship, the scores are inverse—when one score is high, the other score is low; an example could be an increase in fluoride application, which may yield a decrease in dental caries

D. A perfect correlation relationship would be close to +1 or −1.

E. Cooefficients close to 0 would yield little relation, and a 0 would yield no relation.

VII. Statistical Signficance

A. Significant *p*-values indicate that the association between the dependent and independent variables was not due to random chance, thus they are statistically significant

B. Basically, small *p*-values indicate rare chance occurrences and a statistically significant result (< .05), whereas large *p*-values indicate that chance occurrences were likely to have accounted for the occurences, thus this demonstrates that the data is biased and not statistically significant

C. Basically, small *p*-values indicate rare chance occurrences and statistically significant results

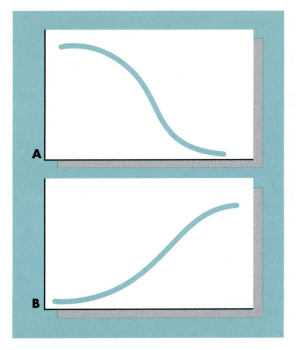

FIGURE 16-3 ■ Skewed Distribution

VIII. Errors
  A. Type I error is concluding that the null hypothesis is false when it is actually true
  B. Type II error is concluding that the null hypothesis is true when it is actually false

IX. Hypothesis
  A. Research (positive) hypothesis
      1. Stated in terms that express the prediction of the investigator
      2. Brand Y does significantly reduce supragingival calculus formation
  B. Null hypothesis
      1. The researcher is attemptng to discover a difference by disproving the null
      2. There is no statistically significant difference between brand Y and a placebo when comparing the formation of supragingival calculus

X. Sampling
  A. Sampling is done to generalize research; it is necessary to use a small sample of the population due to time and feasability
  B. Random sampling
      1. Every possible subject is selected independently and has an equal chance of being selected
      2. Random sampling is the preferred method

    3. This can be done by lottery for a small sample or by computer selection for a larger sample

C. Systematic sampling

    1. Systematic technique samples every *n*th subject

    2. This method may be accomplished by choosing every 9th number in a telephone book

D. Convenience sample

    1. Sampling subjects that are readily available

    2. Using a sample of patients from Dr. Fones's dental practice

E. Stratified sampling

    1. Research has the ability to further stratify the sample during the study by defining information such as age, gender, income level, or educational levels of subjects; the investigator can further generalize results to these strata

XI. Applying Research Results: Definitions of Terms

A. Mortality is the ratio of the number of deaths from a given disease or condition to the total number of cases reported

B. Morbidity is the ratio of sick (affected) individuals to well individuals in a community

C. Prevalence is the number of all existing cases of a disease or condition in a population at a given time

D. Incidence is the number of new cases of a disease or condition in a population over a given time

E. Epidemic is a disease or condition occurring among many individuals in a community or region at the same time, usually spreading rapidly and often referred to as an outbreak

F. Pandemic is a widespread outbreak of disease or condition across a region or continent

G. Endemic is a relatively low but constant level of occurrence of a disease or condition in a population; the common cold may be an endemic, although during some months it may become an epidemic in a particular locality or region

H. Risk factors are characteristics of an individual or population that may increase the likelihood of experience of a given health problem; examples include tobacco habits, age, gender, SES, etc.

I. Surveillance is the method of systems used to monitor disease in a population periodically or on an ongoing basis

J. Etiology is the theory of causation of disease

K. Placebo is the controlled variable

XII. Research Methods: The Different Types of Approaches to Conducting Research (Box 16-2■)

A. Descriptive studies

1. Examine data collected without specific hypotheses to be tested and are designed to describe disease or condition within a population and relationships between it and other variables without establishing causality

2. Classified as either incidence or prevalence studies

a. Incidence study—Describes the number of new cases of a disease within a specified time period

BOX 16-2

Study Types

Blind	When the subject does not know whether or not he or she is receiving actual treatment
	🔑 Double blind ensures that both the researcher and the subject do not know whether or not the subject is receiving actual treatment
Cross-over	When the subject is tested on two different treatments at different times
Split-mouth	Half of the mouth is used for one treatment and the other half as a control or a different treatment
Longitudinal study	An investigation over a long period of time
Prospective study (experimental)	Clinical trials
	🔑 Investigation of tooth-desensitizing agents on hypersensitive root surfaces
Retrospective (*ex post facto*)	Looks at a group of people with the disease in the past
	🔑 Utilizing past medical records to describe a mother's fluoride uptake during gestation compared to child's current dental health
Epidemiological research	Study of those factors that influence the occurrence and distribution of health, disease, defect, disability, and death in populations
	🔑 Useful in determining the needs of populations
Descriptive research	Involves description, documentation, analysis, and interpretation of current conditions
Health researcher	An individual who conducts research germane to the study of health and disease
Health evaluator	An individual whose responsibility it is to select relevant data on health issues and form an evaluative judgment
Case study	Intensive investigation of a person, a family, a group, a social institution, or an entire community in a natural setting

    b. Prevalence study—Describes total number of cases of disease at a point in time (termed "point prevalence") or during a period of time (known as "period prevalence")

  3. Increase understanding of multifactorial causes of disease by

    a. Describing normal biological processes

    b. Observing natural history of diseases

    c. Providing distribution statistics of disease in the population

    d. Identifying determinants of disease

    e. Testing hypotheses for disease prevention and control

    f. Planning and evaluating health care services

B. Experimental studies

  1. Longitudinal and prospective and test hypotheses designed to answer a particular question to establish causality

  2. Characteristics of an experimental study include

    a. Manipulation of one or more independent variables (IV)

C. Independent variable is the condition of the experiment that is manipulated or controlled or the "experimental" variable. In this scenario, Arm & Hammer Dental Care PM® toothpaste is the independent variable. What are the effects of Arm & Hammer Dental Care PM® toothpaste on halitosis?

D. Measurement of one or more dependent variables (DV), the measure thought to change as a result of the manipulation of the independent variable. In this scenario, halitosis is the dependent variable. What are the effects of Arm & Hammer Dental Care PM® toothpaste on halitosis?

  1. Occurrence of IV before measurement of DV

  2. Concept of control group

  3. Example of an experimental study—Clinical trial tests the efficacy of an agent or procedure

    a. Controlled experimental study of group comparison based on epidemiological principles and designed to test hypothesis that a particular agent or procedure favorably alters the natural history of the disease

    b. Overall aim is to ensure the only difference between the groups is that the test group receives the agent under study and the control group does not

    c. Extraneous variables that are not related to the purpose of the study but may influence the outcome; for example, if you are studying the outcome of dental health education during Children's Dental Health Month in February, the results may be affected by the additional promotion of dental health in that month

    d. Clinical trials require specific considerations such as

      (1) Choice of study population (should be determined by the purpose of the trial)

      (2) Adequate numbers of test subjects

      (3) Comparability of study and control groups

      (4) Placebo use in control group; placebo is the common "sugar pill," a nontreatment

      (5) Control of operational procedure

      (6) Reliability in diagnosis

      (7) Duration of the trial

      (8) Statistical analysis

      (9) Ethical considerations

    e. Pilot study is the small study that is done prior to a large study to help ensure validity and reliability

E. Other types of studies used frequently in epidemiological endeavors

  1. Analytical study

    a. Descriptive study analyzing the occurrence of a disease or condition relative to characteristics within the population or environment

    b. Seeks to analyze relationships between and among variables

  2. Longitudinal study—Study approach used in either descriptive or experimental protocols in which repeated measures are used while observing a sample over time

  3. Prospective study—Longitudinal study that can be either descriptive or experimental in which subjects are observed and data collected over time to determine if a disease or condition develops

  4. Retrospective study—A descriptive study that investigates previously collected data

  5. Developmental study—Descriptive study that examines progression or development of disease, condition, or program over a period of time using a longitudinal or cross-sectional approach

    a. Cohort study—One group (cohort) of subjects is followed over a period of time to observe development of disease (prospective)

    b. Case history—Group with disease or condition is compared to a group without the disease or condition to determine variables or factors that relate to its occurrence (retrospective); also known as *ex post facto* study

    c. Cross-sectional—Representative cross section of a population is observed at one point in time to determine occurrence of disease or condition and relate its occurrence to other variables or factors within the population

F. Considerations when designing an epidemiological study

  1. Validity of the measure is the degree to which the research measured what it was supposed to measure

    a. Internal validity (IV)

      (1) Degree to which change in IV actually brought about the change in DV

      (2) Influenced by control of extraneous variables and group equivalency

    b. External validity

      (1) Degree to which the results of the study can be generalized from sample to population

      (2) Influenced by type and size of sample

    c. Components of validity

      (1) Sensitivity—Measure is sensitive if it will test positive when the disease or condition is present

      (2) Specificity—Measure is specific if it will test negative when the disease or condition is absent

      (3) Predictive value—Ability of a measure to identify presence and absence of a disease or condition

    d. Increasing validity

      (1) Correct theoretical assumption relative to the hypothesis

      (2) Bias elimination

      (3) Extraneous variable control

      (4) Representative sample

      (5) Equivalent groups

      (6) Reliable measurement instruments, methods, and examiners

      (7) Length of study must produce meaningful results

  2. Reliability

    a. Measure reliability, which is the ability of a study to be reproduced and still yield the same results

      (1) Instrument reliability

        (a) Consistent

        (b) Reproducible

      (2) Examiner reliability

        (a) Intraexaminer reliability—Within one examiner

        (b) Interexaminer reliability—Between two or more examiners

    b. Increasing reliability

      (1) Standardization of study conditions

      (2) Examiner calibration

(3) Use of established reliable measures

(4) Conduction of pretest questionnaires and interviews designed for the study

(5) Careful administration of study

XIII. Epidemiology

A. Multifactorial study of health and disease in populations

B. Seeks to examine effects of host factors, biology, physical environment, and lifestyle on health

C. Epidemiological studies require that disease be measured quantitatively

D. Host factors

1. Age

2. Gender

3. Race

4. Immunity

E. Biological causes

1. Bacteria

2. Virus

3. Protozoa

F. Physical environmental factors

1. Sun

2. Industrial pollutants

3. Radiation

G. Lifestyle considerations

1. Education

2. Socioeconomic status

3. Drug and alcohol consumption

4. Diet

XIV. Methods of Measuring Oral Diseases

A. Counts

1. Simplest form of measuring any disease

2. Involves counting the number of cases of particular disease state

3. Most useful with unusual conditions of low prevalence

B. Proportions

1. Count can be turned into a proportion by adding a denominator

2. Determines prevalence

      3. Proportions *do not* include time dimension

      4. Example: The count of caries-free children age 3–5 years can be divided by the population of the group to give the prevalence:

         a. Total sample size = 400

         b. Number of caries-free children in sample population = 20

         c. Prevalence = number of caries-free children ÷ total sample size

         d. Prevalence = 20 ÷ 400

         e. Prevalence of caries-free children = 0.05 or 5% of the total sample population

C. Rates

      1. Proportion that uses standardized denominator and a time dimension

      2. Not often used in oral disease measures

XV. **Distribution of Oral Diseases and Conditions—An understanding of the distribution and determinants of oral diseases within populations is necessary for dental practitioners to provide expert guidance to the community on public health matters related to oral health; the following epidemiological findings provide the basis for that understanding:**

A. Prevalence of dental caries

      1. Ancient humans

         a. Low caries

         b. High attrition rate

         c. Coarse diet

      2. Modern humans

         a. High caries prevalence rate in United States

         b. Current decrease in caries prevalence due to

            (1) Water fluoridation

            (2) Fluorides

            (3) Fluoride toothpaste

            (4) Dental sealant placement

            (5) Emphasis on caries prevention

      3. Underdeveloped countries—Low prevalence associated with dietary patterns (less processed foods, refined carbohydrates, and sugar)

B. Factors associated with dental caries

      1. Susceptibility of teeth

         a. Molars are attacked before premolars

         b. Mandibular molars are attacked before maxillary molars

         c. Higher incidence in pits and fissures than on smooth surface caries

2. Age

   a. Two specific types of caries are associated with age

   (1) Early childhood caries (rampant caries in 1- to 3-year-olds)—More prevalent in lower socioeconomic status (SES) and Hispanic populations

   (2) Root caries (caries of the cemental root surfaces)

   (a) Higher prevalence in developed countries, in elderly, and in lower SES groups

   (b) Xerostomia is a risk factor

3. Gender

   a. Males have lower DMF scores than females

   b. Females seek out dental care more often than males

   c. Females have earlier eruption patterns than males

4. Race and ethnicity

   a. Higher caries prevalence in African Americans

   b. More untreated caries in Hispanics and African Americans owing to lower SES rather than inherent tendency to develop caries

5. Diet (total oral intake of substances that provides nourishment and/or calories)—Frequency of sugar intake increases caries risk in susceptible individuals

6. Nutrition (absorption of nutrients)—No association between nutritional deficiency in infancy and caries development

7. Familial influence

   a. Genetics have limited influence

   b. Family environment is strong factor

   c. Intrafamilial transmission of cariogenic flora can occur

8. SES status (income, education, occupation, attitudes, and values)—Most powerful determinant of dental caries in United States

C. Prevention of dental caries

1. Host factors

   a. Easiest to address with public health measures

   b. Examples

   (1) Fluorides

   (2) Pit and fissure sealants

2. Oral hygiene

   a. Difficult to control in public health programs

   b. Not well correlated to caries incidence

   c. Control of dietary sugar is difficult

3. Prevalence of periodontal diseases

    a. 70% of adults in all countries are affected by some type, form, and level of periodontal disease

    b. Low rate of severe periodontal disease in U.S. population

    c. Higher rate of mild to moderate periodontal disease

    d. Higher rate of mild gingivitis versus moderate to severe cases

4. Factors associated with periodontal disease

    a. Plaque

        (1) Etiological factor

        (2) Risk depends on type of bacteria and host response

    b. Age

        (1) Greater prevalence and severity of periodontal diseases in elderly

            (a) Not a natural consequence of aging

            (b) Due to accumulation and progression of disease

        (2) Greater prevalence of gingivitis in children

            (a) Due in part to inflammatory response associated with eruption

            (b) Oral hygiene may be inadequate in children

    c. Caries—Extraction of teeth and subsequent drifting is associated with periodontal breakdown

D. Prevention of periodontal disease

    1. Oral hygiene

    2. Regular periodontal maintenance

    3. Adjunctive aids (antimicrobial administration)

E. Oral cancer frequency of occurrence by location

    1. Pharynx

    2. Tongue

    3. Floor of the mouth

    4. Lip

    5. Buccal mucosa

F. Percentages

    1. 3.1% of new cases of cancer are oral

    2. Oral cancer accounts for 1.8% of cancer deaths

G. Associated risk factors with oral cancer

    1. Gender

        a. Twice as prevalent in males

        b. Twice as many deaths in males

    2. Age—Higher prevalence in elderly

    3. Tobacco use—Greatest risk factor for oral cancer

   4. Alcohol consumption

   5. Sun exposure—Dramatically increases risk of lip cancer

   6. Poorly fitted dentures

H. Cleft lip and palate occurrence

   1. 6,000 children born with clefts annually

   2. Associated risk factors

      a. Heredity

      b. Maternal drug consumption during first trimester

      c. Influenza and fever in first trimester

I. Malocclusion—Associated risk factors

   1. Oral habits such as thumb sucking

   2. Early extraction of teeth

   3. Heredity

J. Edentulism

   1. Prevalence

      a. Higher prevalence in elderly

      b. Prevalence is decreasing

   2. Associated risk factors

      a. Fluoride use has decreased incidence

      b. Prevention and control of periodontal diseases have increased retention of teeth

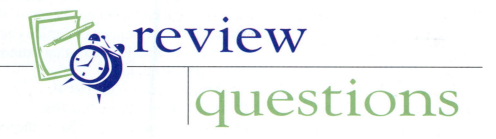

review questions

DIRECTIONS Each of the questions or incomplete statements below is followed by suggested answers or completions. Select the **one** answer that is best in each case.

Testlet 1: Questions 1–10

There are 10 million patients living with HIV in the global community. In many areas of the world HIV has become endemic within the community. In other communities, infection with HIV has been increasing rapidly. A dental hygiene researcher with the World Health Organization (WHO) is conducting a few studies in several countries. She is studying the oral manifestations of HIV infection and the oral manifestations associated with treatment modalities provided to individuals with HIV infection.

1. There are 10 million HIV-positive patients worldwide. A new case occurs every 15–20 seconds.
   A. First statement is prevalence of HIV; second statement is incidence.
   B. First statement is incidence of HIV; second statement is prevalence.
   C. The above statements describe an endemic.
   D. The above statements describe mortality rates related to HIV.

2. Some individuals are able to live with HIV, if they receive the appropriate medical care. The term *morbidity*, used in epidemiology, refers to
   A. Death
   B. Disease and disability
   C. Reasons as to why disease and death occur in a population
   D. Loss of subjects

3. Various ways in which epidemiological studies can be conducted by the researcher include
   A. Collecting data to describe normal oral anatomy and physiology
   B. Measuring distribution of disease in populations
   C. Conducting and evaluating clinical trials
   D. All of the above

4. Endemic refers to the
   A. Cause of the disease
   B. Occurrence of disease beyond normal expectancy
   C. Expected level of disease found within a particular locality
   D. Sudden outbreak of disease

review questions

5. Dietary histories of all patients entering the hospital with HIV infection are compared to the dietary histories of patients whose DMF scores are low and also to patients whose DMF scores are high to determine the relationship between diet and caries. This is an example of what type of study?
   A. Cohort
   B. Prospective
   C. Retrospective
   D. Both A and B

6. The epidemiology of HIV-associated periodontal disease is much more difficult to study than dental caries because of
   A. Involvement of more than one structure, greater accumulation later in life, problems with quantitative assessment, and inability to correctly assess impairment in tooth function
   B. Greater accumulation later in life, problems with quantifiable assessment, and inability to correctly assess impairment in tooth function
   C. Involvement of more than one structure, greater accumulation later in life, and problems with quantitative assessment
   D. Reversible shifts in gingivitis, problems with quantitative assessment, and inability to correctly assess impairment in tooth function

7. Older patients with HIV who suffered increased coronal caries are at greater risk for root caries. It was estimated in a 1985–1986 U.S. survey that over half of the dentate employed adult population and senior studies exhibited at least one carious root surface lesion.
   A. Both statements are TRUE.
   B. Both statements are FALSE.
   C. The first statement is TRUE; the second statement is FALSE.
   D. The first statement is FALSE; the second statement is TRUE.

8. Susceptibility to periodontitis increases with HIV infection, but not as part of the disease process. Dentate or partially edentulous patients with HIV are at an extreme risk of total tooth loss.
   A. Both statements are TRUE.
   B. Both statements are FALSE.
   C. The first statement is TRUE; the second statement is FALSE.
   D. The first statement is FALSE; the second statement is TRUE.

9. HIV-associated gingivitis precedes periodontitis. Areas of the mouth affected by gingivitis will most likely become affected in later years by periodontitis.
   A. Both statements are TRUE.
   B. Both statements are FALSE.
   C. The first statement is TRUE; the second statement is FALSE.
   D. The first statement is FALSE; the second statement is TRUE.

10. Prevalence is used to measure dental caries in the HIV population when
   A. Radiographs are available
   B. Animal studies are performed to determine progression of lesion
   C. Caries rates and tooth loss are expected to be high
   D. Caries rates are expected to be low

Testlet 2: Questions 11–20

A study was conducted by the State Dental Hygienists' Association on dental hygiene clinical practice. Half of all dental hygienists work more than 38 hours per week. On the average it takes 60 minutes to complete an oral exam, radiographs, and standard prophylaxis. More dental hygienists practice with one operatory and no dental assistants than any other staffing pattern. The State Dental Hygienists' Association has been trying to create a dental care delivery pattern after dentists' typical practice, which includes the use of two operatories and a dental assistant. This decreases the amount of time to complete an oral exam, radiographs, and standard oral prophylaxis, while increasing productivity.

11. After the initial study, a subsequent study was conducted on this new concept in dental hygiene care delivery. The extent to which the objectives are achieved in this new practice endeavor are measured is by comparing continuing program data to
    A. Program paradigm
    B. Government standards
    C. Baseline program data
    D. Professionally established criteria

12. Distortion of intraoral data gathered by several hygienists could be caused by
    A. Inconsistency between examiners
    B. Bias of the dentist
    C. Students' desire to please
    D. Influence of other students in the school

13. The study actually found a normal distribution of data, which is sometimes referred to as the
    A. Skewed data graph
    B. Bell curve
    C. Histograph
    D. Bar curve

14. What measures the extent of the linear relationship between two variables?
    A. Bell curve
    B. Correlation
    C. Linear curve
    D. Both A and B

15. The scores being correlated vary together in which linear relationship?
    A. Positive
    B. Inverted
    C. Negative
    D. Both B and C

16. Which is closest to a perfect correlation?
    A. +98
    B. 0
    C. +1.5
    D. −1

17. Small p-values indicate rare chance occurrences and statistically significant results ($<.05$), whereas large p-values indicate that the chance occurrences were likely to have accounted for the occurrences.
    A. Both statements are TRUE.
    B. Both statements are FALSE.
    C. The first statement is TRUE; the second statement is FALSE.
    D. The first statement is FALSE; the second statement is TRUE.

18. Which error is concluding that the null hypothesis is false when it is actually true?
    A. Type I
    B. Type II
    C. Type III
    D. Type IV

review questions

19. The two operatory/dental assistant practice modality does significantly increase practice productivity is which type of hypothesis?
    A. Null
    B. Positive
    C. Neutral
    D. None of the above

20. In this investigation, only some practices were studied. Which type of sampling is done so every possible subject is selected independently and has an equal chance of being selected?
    A. Random
    B. Systematic
    C. Convenience
    D. Stratified

Testlet 3: Questions 21–30

A dental hygiene professor is involved in an interdisciplinary study of obstructive sleep apnea (OSA). The medical researcher is investigating the effectiveness of two oral appliances for the treatment of OSA, while the dental hygiene professor is investigating the effects on periodontal health and occlusion from both oral appliances.

21. A convenience sample is chosen for every *n*th subject with OSA at the local sleep study clinic and can be further stratified during the study to define information such as age, gender, or income level.
    A. Both statements are TRUE.
    B. Both statements are FALSE.
    C. The first statement is TRUE; the second statement is FALSE.
    D. The first statement is FALSE; the second statement is TRUE.

22. The ratio of the number of deaths from OSA is termed
    A. Prevalence
    B. Incidence
    C. Morbidity
    D. Mortality

23. The number of new cases of OSA is referred to as
    A. Prevalence
    B. Incidence
    C. Morbidity
    D. Mortality

24. A newspaper article that defines the cases of OSA in a population of overweight individuals is defining its
    A. Prevalence
    B. Incidence
    C. Morbidity
    D. Mortality

25. When OSA occurrs among many individuals in a community or region at the same time it is termed
    A. Epidemic
    B. Endemic
    C. Pandemic
    D. Outbreak

26. The "occasional bad night's rest" generally is endemic within a population; however, the OSA can become an epidemic if enough risk factors are present.
    A. Both statements are TRUE.
    B. Both statements are FALSE.
    C. The first statement is TRUE; the second statement is FALSE.
    D. The first statement is FALSE; the second statement is TRUE.

27. Characteristics of an individual or population that may increase the likelihood of OSA of a given population is termed
    A. Endemic
    B. Risk factors
    C. Surveillance
    D. Etiology

28. Which type of study examines data collected without specific hypothesis to be tested and is designed to describe diseases or conditions within a population without establishing causality?
    A. Descriptive
    B. Experimental
    C. Clinical
    D. Correlational

29. The oral appliances in this study are the
    A. Dependent variable
    B. Independent variable
    C. Extraneous variable
    D. Placebo

30. The measure thought to change as a result of the oral appliance is termed the
    A. Dependent variable
    B. Independent variable
    C. Extraneous variable
    D. Placebo

Testlet 4: Questions 31–40

A dental hygienist is studying the effects of several mouthwashes in her clinical practice. Before she began the study she did a review of all previous studies on the mouthwashes she was planning on investigating. She was actually investigating the ability to reduce halitosis on a group of patients.

31. The study of halitosis is looking at the etiology, which is the theory of the cause of a
    A. Discipline
    B. Field
    C. Disease/condition
    D. Natural phenominaa

32. This investigation studies a new brand of mouthwash that claims to reduce bad breath. What is bad breath?
    A. Dependent variable
    B. Independent variable
    C. Extraneous variable
    D. Placebo

33. If you are studying the outcome of the mouthwashes on halitosis during Dental Hygiene Month in October, you have introduced what to the study?
    A. Dependent variable
    B. Placebo
    C. Controlled atmosphere
    D. Extraneous variable

34. A control group generally experiments with the
    A. Independent variable
    B. Placebo
    C. Extraneous variable
    D. Both B and C

35. A small study that is done prior to a large study to ensure validity and reliability is termed a
    A. Placebo
    B. Pilot
    C. Autorun
    D. Cross-over

36. The degree to which change in the independent variable actually brought about the change in the dependent variable is
    A. Internal validity
    B. External validity
    C. Reliability
    D. Extraneous control

37. The degree to which the results of the study can be generalized from the sample to the general population is
    A. Internal validity
    B. External validity
    C. Reliability
    D. Extraneous control

38. The ability of a study to be reproduced and still yield the same results is
    A. Internal validity
    B. External validity
    C. Reliability
    D. Extraneous control

39. When more than one examiner is serving in a study, which reliability is essential?
    A. Intraexaminer reliability
    B. Interexaminer reliability
    C. Consistency reliability
    D. Both A and B

40. Which value is the ability of a measure to identify presence and absence of a disease or condition?
    A. Sensitivity
    B. Specificity
    C. Predictive
    D. Both A and C

Testlet 5: Questions 41–50

When studying periodontal disease in a population, a dental hygiene researcher first reviewed risk factors of periodontal disease. She then designed a study that measured periodontal diseases in a large population, risk factors, and disease progression.

41. Host factors of periodontal diseases may include which of the following?
    A. Age
    B. Gender
    C. Race
    D. All of the above

42. The simplest form of measuring periodontal diseases are (is)
    A. Proportions
    B. Rates
    C. Counts
    D. Surveillance

43. The count of gingivitis-free teenagers age 13–16 years can be divided by the population of the group is termed
    A. Proportions
    B. Rates
    C. Counts
    D. Surveillance

44. Females generally have a lower plaque score than males and plaque score refers to a dental index measuring periodontal disease.
    A. Both statements are TRUE.
    B. Both statements are FALSE.
    C. First statement is TRUE; the second statement is FALSE.
    D. First statement is FALSE; the second statement is TRUE.

45. Periodontal diseases are more prevalent in which population?
    A. Infants
    B. 1- to 3-year-olds
    C. Pregnant women
    D. Adolescent boys

46. When half of the mouth is used for one treatment and the other half as a control group it is referred to as
    A. Blind study
    B. Cross-over
    C. Split-mouth
    D. *Ex post facto*

47. Utilizing past medical records to describe a mother's dietary intake during gestation compared to a child's gingival health is an example of which type of study?
    A. Blind study
    B. Cross-over
    C. Split-mouth
    D. *Ex post facto*

48. An intensive study of a person's, families', group's, or community's periodontal status is termed
    A. Blind study
    B. Case study
    C. Teaching case
    E. *Ex post facto*

49. A term used when the subject does not know whether he or she is receiving actual treatment is
   A. Blind study
   B. Double-blind study
   C. Refereed study
   D. Case study

50. An investigation of the effects of gel to soft calculus before debridement would likely be
   A. Longitudinal
   B. Descriptive
   C. Experimental
   D. Case study

review questions

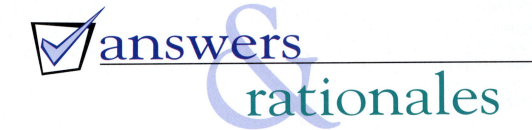

answers & rationales

1.

A. Prevalence is the number of existing cases at a certain point in time. Incidence refers to the number of new cases over a specific period of time.

2.

B. Morbidity refers to the amount of disease or disability in a population. Death rates are synonymous with mortality. Epidemiology has been termed the diagnostic procedure in mass disease.

3.

D. Collecting data to describe normal body processes such as temperature, measuring distribution of disease in populations, and conducting and evaluating clinical trials are appropriate uses of epidemiological studies.

4.

C. Endemic refers to the expected level of disease that occurs within a particular locality.

5.

C. Retrospective studies look at events or experiences in patients' pasts to determine if inferences can be drawn concerning etiological factors of a disease under study. Cohort studies, also known as prospective studies, look at a group of patients free of disease and follow them to a given point in the future to determine causes of disease.

6.

A. Due to involvement of both gingival and bone, periodontal disease is more difficult to study. The increased accumulation with age contributes to the difficulty. Problems with establishing a reliable and valid quantitative instrument for measuring periodontal disease and assessing tooth function impairment also increases the difficulty of studying periodontal disease.

7.

A. It has now been determined that patients with gingival recession who experienced high coronal caries rates will most likely experience high root surface caries rates.

8.

B. Post-1980 studies have indicated that elderly dental or partially dentate patients are actually less susceptible to periodontitis. Highly susceptible individuals exhibit signs/symptoms of disease when they are young.

9.

C. Basic, clinical, and epidemiological research from the 1970s on have revealed that while gingivitis precedes periodontitis, only a fraction of the sites affected by gingivitis will ultimately suffer periodontitis.

10.

D. Prevalence is useful when caries counts are low. It is useful in ancient skull studies where many teeth are lost due to reasons other than caries. It is best utilized when one or two carious teeth are the criterion for differences in affected individuals from unaffected individuals.

11.

C. Program objectives should always be measured from baseline data collected before implementation of a program or modality.

12.

A. All examiners must be calibrated to ensure valid data.

13.

B. Normal distribution is sometimes called the bell curve; it is a frequency distribution of scores that when graphed yields a bell-shaped curve. IT implies that most scores fall around the measures of central tendency.

14.

B. Correlation measures the extent of the linear relationship between two variables.

15.

A. In a positive linear relationship the scores vary together; if one score is high, the other score is high, if one score is low, the other score is low. The opposite is true of a negative or inverted relationship, if one score is high, the other score is low.

16.

D. A perfect correlational relationship is +1 or –1. The signs (+/–) indicate the nature of the relationship, the number 1 indicates the strength.

17.

A. In order to ensure that the independent variable actually manipulated or did not manipulate, a small p value is necessary. This ensures that it is likely that the independent variable did or did not affect the dependent variable and provides the ability that the results are statistically significant.

18.

A. Type I error concludes that the null hypothesis is false when it is actually true. Type II error concludes that the null hypothesis is true when it is actually false.

19.

B. A positive hypothesis is stated in terms that express the predication of the investigator.

20.

A. Random sampling is done so every possible subject is selected independently and has an equal chance of being selected.

21.

D. A convenience sample is chosen because subjects are readily available and a systematic sample is chosen for every nth subject. Stratified sampling is when the sample is stratified to gather defined, specific information on the population.

22.

D. Mortality is the ratio of the number of deaths from a given disease or condition.

23.

B. Incidence is the number of new cases of a disease or condition in population over a given time.

24.

B. Morbidity is the ratio of sick (affected) individuals in a community.

25.

A. Epidemic is a disease or condition occurring among many individuals in a community or region at the same time.

26.

A. The common cold is a perfect example of an endemic that at times can become an epidemic.

27.

B. Risk factors are characteristics of an individual or population that may increase the likelihood of experience of a given population.

28.

A. Descriptive studies examines data collected without specific hypotheses to be tested and is designed to describe diseases or conditions within a population without establishing causality.

29.

B. Independent variable is the condition of the experiment that is manipulated or controlled.

30.

A. Dependent variable is the measurement of the manipulated independent variable.

31.

C. Etiology is the study of the causation of a disease.

32.

A. Bad breath is the dependent variable and the new brand of mouthwash is the independent variable.

33.

D. Because the month of October is celebrated by many hygienists who promote dental hygiene during that time, you may introduce the segment during a time period that individuals hear more about dental health and this would be an extraneous variable.

34.

B. A placebo is used by the control group instead of the independent variable.

35.

B. A pilot study is a smaller version of a larger study to be conducted. This helps control the larger study.

36.

A. Internal validity is the degree to which change in the independent variable actually brought about the change in the dependent variable.

37.

B. External validity is the degree to which the results of the study can be generalized from the sample to the general population.

38.

C. Reliability is the ability of a study to be reproduced and still yield the same results.

39.

C. Both reliabilities are essential. Each examiner needs to be consistent and they both have to be calibrated together as well.

40.

C. Predictive value is the ability of a measure to identify presence and absence of a disease or condition.

41.

D. Host factors include age, race, gender, and immunity.

42.

C. Counts are the simplest form of measuring any disease.

43.

A. Proportion is the count with the addition of a denominator.

44.

D. The DMF is a dental index that measures caries activity within a population; however, males generally have a lower DMF score than females.

45.

B. During pregnancy women generally have more gingival inflammation and infection.

46.

C. Split-mouth design is when half of the mouth is used for one treatment and the other half as a control or a different treatment.

47.

D. *Ex post facto* or retrospective design looks at a group's prior disease, condition, or risk factors.

48.

B. Case study is an intensive study of a person, family, group, or community in a natural study.

49.

A. A blind study is when the subject does not know whether he or she is receiving actual treatment.

50.

C. An experimental study would be a clinical study with an independent variable, control, and dependent variable.

appendix a

simulated national board dental hygiene examination 1

DIRECTIONS Each of the questions or incomplete statements below is followed by suggested answers or completions. Select the **one** answer that is best in each case.

1. All of the following cranial nerves assist in the movement of the eyeball EXCEPT:
   A. Optic nerve
   B. Oculomotor nerve
   C. Trochlear nerve
   D. Abducens nerve

2. The sense of taste from the posterior third of the tongue is carried by fibers of the:
   A. Trigeminal nerve
   B. Hypoglossal nerve
   C. Facial nerve
   D. Glossopharyngeal nerve

3. Muscles of mastication are innervated by:
   A. Efferent fibers of the trigeminal nerve
   B. Efferent fibers of the facial nerve
   C. The glossopharyngeal motor nerves
   D. Afferent fibers of the facial nerve

4. The cerebrospinal fluid is produced by the
   A. Choroid plexus
   B. Subarachnoid granulations
   C. Pia mater
   D. Falx cerebri

5. The nerve that innervates the mucous membranes of the pharynx and is the sensory component of the gag reflex is the
   A. Facial nerve
   B. Glossopharyngeal nerve
   C. Hypoglossal nerve
   D. Trigeminal nerve

6. Which of the following supplies blood to the temporomandibular joint?
   A. Facial artery
   B. Pterygoid arteries from the maxillary artery
   C. Lingual artery
   D. Superficial temporal and maxillary branches
   E. Masseteric artery

7. In normal occlusion, the buccal cusps of maxillary teeth occlude
   A. With the lingual surface of mandibular teeth
   B. With the buccal surface of mandibular teeth
   C. In the central sulci of mandibular teeth
   D. Cusp tip to cusp tip

8. The mandibular permanent second molar differs from the mandibular permanent first molar in the number of
   A. Cusps
   B. Roots
   C. Lingual grooves
   D. Marginal ridges

9. The permanent tooth that has the longest crown is the
   A. Maxillary lateral incisor
   B. Maxillary central incisor
   C. Mandibular canine
   D. Maxillary first molar

10. The anterior tooth MOST likely to have a bifurcated root is the permanent
    A. Maxillary canine
    B. Mandibular canine
    C. Maxillary central incisor
    D. Mandibular lateral incisor
    E. Mandibular central incisor

11. A tooth occasionally exhibits a lingual groove that extends from the enamel onto the cemental area of the root. This is MOST likely to be the permanent
    A. Maxillary canine
    B. Maxillary third molar
    C. Maxillary central incisor
    D. Maxillary lateral incisor
    E. Mandibular second premolar

12. Which one of the following types of oral mucosa is not keratinized under normal conditions?
    A. Buccal mucosa
    B. Vermillion border on the lips
    C. Incisive papillae
    D. Hard palate
    E. Gingiva

13. The anterior two-thirds of the tongue develops from the
    A. Third arch mesenchyme
    B. Copula
    C. Hypobranchial eminence
    D. Tuberculum impar and adjacent tissue

14. The premaxilla contains tooth buds of the
    A. Incisors and cuspids
    B. Incisors, cuspids, and bicuspids
    C. Incisors
    D. Incisors, cuspids, bicuspids, and molars

15. The salivary glands arise from
    A. The ectodermal germ layer
    B. The endodermal germ layer
    C. Ectodermal and endodermal germ layers
    D. Oral mesenchyme

16. Active transport differs from facilitated diffusion in that active transport
    A. Moves a substance against a concentration gradient
    B. Requires a carrier
    C. Requires energy from magnesius adenosine triphosphate (Mg ATP)
    D. Is exemplified by the movement of sodium and potassium across cell membranes
    E. All of the above

17. Which of the following is (are) NOT associated with a skeletal muscle?
    A. Sarcolemma
    B. Myofibrils
    C. Intercalated disc
    D. Mitochondria
    E. Actin and myosin

18. A single motor neuron and the muscle cells supplied by its axon branches is termed
    A. An efferent neuron
    B. A motor unit
    C. A motor end plate
    D. A sarcoplasmic reticulum
    E. An annulospiral ending

19. Depolarization occurs with a
    A. Transfer of sodium ions to the inside of a neuron
    B. Transfer of potassium ions to the outside of a neuron
    C. Reversal of charge across the nerve cell membrane making the outside of the fiber positive with respect to the inside

20. Of the following substances, the ones that are generally most readily usable as a source of energy for heterotrophic bacteria are
    A. Proteins
    B. Vitamins
    C. Carbohydrates
    D. Ammonium salts

21. Formation of glucose from noncarbohydrate substances is called
    ✓ A. Gluconeogenesis
    B. Glycogenesis
    C. Glucogenesis
    D. Glycolysis

22. Pernicious anemia is associated with
    A. Iron deficiency
    B. Aminopyrine therapy
    C. Vitamin K deficiency
    D. Vitamin B_{12} deficiency

23. An adequate intake of vitamin C is necessary for good repair of a wound because it promotes
    A. Growth of epithelium
    B. Production of collagens
    C. Budding of capillaries
    D. Phagocytosis of cell fragments

24. The pH of foodstuffs is a very important consideration in predicting the cariogenicity of food. The safe pH area is considered to be
    A. Above 6.5
    B. About 7
    C. Above 6
    D. 5.5 to 6.0

25. The average American diet is lower in calcium than the recommended dietary allowance because calcium readily forms insoluble compounds.
    A. Both statement and reason are correct and related
    B. Both statement and reason are correct but not related
    C. The statement is correct but the reason is not
    D. The statement is not correct but the reason is an accurate statement
    E. Neither statement nor reason is correct

26. Certain amino acids need not be present in the diet of an animal because of its ability to synthesize them. An important source of the carbon of these amino acids is
    A. The metabolism of carbohydrates
    B. The metabolism of fatty acids
    C. Carbon dioxide
    D. Nucleic acid

27. Cells that phagocytize microorganisms are of which type?
    A. Neutrophils
    B. Macrophages
    C. Lymphocytes
    D. All of the above
    E. A and B only

28. The cell wall of Gram-positive microorganisms may include all of the following EXCEPT
    A. Lipopolysaccharides
    B. Lipoteichoic acids
    C. Peptidoglycans
    D. Penicillin binding proteins
    E. Teichoic acids

29. Serious complications of untreated group A streptococcal pharyngitis include
    A. Acute glomerulonephritis
    B. Rheumatic fever
    C. Moniliasis
    D. All of the above
    E. A and B only

30. Microbiological safety equipment for protection of health care workers recommended in OSHA standards include
    A. Gloves
    B. Face mask or shield
    C. Eye goggles
    D. Gowns and aprons
    E. All of the above

31. *Prevotella (Bacteroides) melaninogenicus* is best characterized as
    A. An aerobic Gram-negative rod
    B. An anaerobic Gram-positive rod
    C. A virulent oropharyngeal pathogen
    D. A common agent of caseous necrosis
    E. An anaerobe that produces pigmented colonies

32. The only "cold sterilizer" solution capable of destroying bacterial spores, viruses, and vegetative bacteria is
    A. 90% isoprophyl alcohol
    B. 2% glutaraldehyde
    C. Chlorhexidine
    D. Iodophors
    E. Quaternary ammonium

33. Autoclave efficiency should be checked regularly by using
    A. Heat-activated autoclave tapes that change colors
    B. Plastic strips designed to melt at 121°C
    C. Culture plates of viable bacteria
    D. Vials of culture media containing a pH indicator and a thermophilic spore-forming bacteria
    E. Vials with different acid and base chemical indicators

34. The best method for sterilizing cutting instruments is
    A. Autoclave for 15 minutes at 15 pounds of pressure at 121°C
    B. Benzalkonium chloride
    C. Boiling water
    D. 10% hypochlorite
    E. 70% ethyl alcohol

35. A Gram-negative anaerobic organism normally found in the upper respiratory tract and in mixed anaerobic infections is
    A. *Clostridium perfringens*
    B. *Enterococcus faecalis*
    C. *Provotella (Bacteroides) melaninogenicus*
    D. *Streptococcus pneumoniae*
    E. *Bordetella pertussis*

36. Animal experimentation has contributed much to our knowledge of caries, particularly experimentation of the gnotobiotic rat. The best definition of this term would be
    A. A completely germ-free rat
    B. Any rat being fed a cariogenic diet
    C. A previously germ-free rat that has been inoculated by a known organism
    D. A germ-free rat that has been inoculated by an unknown organism

37. Which one of the following is a Gram-negative anaerobic rod?
    A. *Fusobacterium nucleatum*
    B. *Clostridium prefringens*
    C. *Peptostreptococcus*
    D. *Candida albicans*
    E. *Neisseria meningitidis*

38. The difference between a benign and a malignant tumor is
    A. The speed with which a patient dies from the tumor
    B. The response to chemotherapy or radiation therapy
    C. The rate of growth
    D. The ability of the tumor to metastasize

39. Addison's disease is characterized by which one of the following?
    A. Stomach ulcers
    B. Decreased adrenal function
    C. Increased skin pigmentation
    D. Decreased pituitary function
    E. Polyps of the gastrointestinal tract

40. Vitiligo describes which of the following conditions?
    A. Acquired depigmentation of areas of the skin
    B. Benign pigmented nevi
    C. Albinism
    D. Ochronosis

41. The normal continuous breakdown of red blood cells in the reticuloendothelial system results in deposition of what in the liver and spleen?
    A. White blood cells
    B. Hematoidin
    C. Hematin
    D. Porphyrins
    E. Hemosiderin

42. An inflammatory reaction characterized by an outpouring of abundant fluids is known as which type of inflammation?
    A. Catarrhal
    B. Hemorrhagic
    C. Serous
    D. Acute
    E. Fibrinous

43. Radiographically, a periapical cyst and a periapical granuloma
    A. Show different peripheral remodeling characteristics
    B. Are distinguished by the presence of lamina dura
    C. Are indistinguishable
    D. Contain foci of calcification
    E. More than one of the above

44. A 50-year-old woman is examined in a dental office. She smokes, is sensitive to sunlight, and has had basal cell carcinoma of the lower lip. She has a medical history of intestinal polyps and has had a hysterectomy. Upon dental clinical examination, she is found to have yellow elevated areas on the mucosa of her lower lip and on her buccal mucosa, bilaterally. She is not aware of the presence of these yellow elevated areas. This patient most likely has, from a dental point of view, which of the following?
    A. Stomatitis nicotina
    B. Fordyce granules
    C. Peutz-Jeghers syndrome
    D. Multiple lipomas
    E. Lupus erythematosis

45. Which of the following is not an oral manifestation of AIDS?
    A. Kaposi's sarcoma
    B. Desquamative gingivitis
    C. Candidiasis
    D. Major aphthous ulcers
    E. Oral hairy leukoplakia

46. The state of teeth joined together only by cementum is diagnosed as
    A. Fusion
    B. Concrescence
    C. Budding
    D. Gemination

47. Two tooth buds are joined together during development and may appear clinically as a macrodont. The probable diagnosis is
    A. Budding
    B. Fusion
    C. Gemination
    D. Concrescence
    E. Dilaceration

48. A radiograph shows that the roots of a lower molar are severely curved to almost 90 degrees. This is diagnosed as
    A. Turner's tooth
    B. Hypoplasia
    C. Teratology
    D. Hutchinson's tooth
    E. Dilaceration

49. Which of the following are two types of amelogenesis imperfecta?
    A. Formative; mature
    B. Autosomal dominant; autosomal recessive
    C. Enamel hypoplasia; enamel hypocalcification
    D. Yellow; dark brown

50. A healthcare worker develops a positive reaction to a tuberculin skin test. After proper medical evaluation, the worker may be placed on long-term dosage of
    A. Insulin
    B. Rifampin
    C. Isoniazid (INH)
    D. Vancomycin

51. In using nitrous oxide–oxygen analgesia, one must keep in mind that
    A. The patient is put to sleep during the analgesia
    B. Local anesthetic most often is used to supplement the analgesia
    C. At most, a concentration of 10% nitrous oxide and 90% oxygen is sufficient for most analgesia
    D. In no way does nitrous oxide analgesia relax the patient

52. In considering the pharmacological properties of nitrous oxide, one can see that the gas is
    A. An irritant
    B. Lighter than air
    C. Colorless
    D. An organic solvent

53. Which one of the following conditions would not require the patient to have antibiotic prophylaxis prior to gingival therapy?
    A. History of endocarditis
    B. Cardiac pacemaker
    C. Heart-valve replacement
    D. Prosthetic joint replacements

54. A drug that is used for the treatment of epilepsy and that may produce excessive gingival enlargement is
    A. Phenobarbital
    B. Lincomycin
    C. Dilantin (phenytoin)
    D. Nystatin

55. A synonym for penicillin V is
    A. Phenoxymethyl penicillin
    B. Oxacillin
    C. Phenoxyethyl penicillin
    D. Methicillin

56. The most important advantage of penicillin V over penicillin G is that penicillin V
    A. Costs less per 100 tablets
    B. Is easier to remember than G
    C. Can be given to patients who are allergic to penicillin G
    D. Is stable at low gastric pH

57. Codeine, a widely used analgesic in dentistry,
    A. Is a natural constituent of opium
    B. May be given only by injection
    C. Has a calming effect on gastric mucosa
    D. Is contraindicated for use in cough

58. When the following drugs are given parenterally, which one is most effective for pain?
    A. Codeine
    B. Oxycodone
    C. Meperidine
    D. Morphine

59. The Drug Enforcement Administration (DEA) number is required for all of the following drugs except
    A. Dolophine (methadone)
    B. Meperidine
    C. Tetracycline
    D. Alphaprodine

60. Which of the following factors influence body temperature?
    A. Time of day, hemorrhage, pathology, application of external heat
    B. Heart rate, pathology, hemorrhage
    C. Respiration, time of day, application of external heat
    D. Hemorrhage, respiration, heart rate, time of day

61. If a radial pulse cannot be found or taken, which of the following alternative areas can be used?
    A. Femoral artery or jugular artery
    B. Brachial artery or facial artery
    C. Facial artery or temporal artery
    D. Jugular artery or temporal artery

62. Diastolic pressure represents which of the following?
    A. Aortic pressure
    B. Ventricular relaxation
    C. Heart rate
    D. Ventricular contraction

63. A mesognathic profile is usually associated with which of the following classifications of malocclusion?
    A. Class I
    B. Class II
    C. Class III

64. How many basic measurements are made on each tooth in periodontal charting?
    A. Two
    B. Four
    C. Six
    D. Eight
    E. Ten

65. When measuring the depth of a periodontal pocket, the measurement is made from the base of the pocket or the attached periodontal tissue to
    A. The cementoenamel junction
    B. The height of the gingival margin
    C. A fixed point
    D. The unattached periodontal tissue

66. Which of the following conditions can possibly affect the accuracy of periodontal charting?
    A. Bleeding, bone loss, and gingival enlargement
    B. Gingival enlargement and gingival recession
    C. Gingival recession, bone loss, and bleeding
    D. Bone loss and bleeding
    E. Ulcerated interdental papillae and bleeding

67. Most periodontal pocket depths up to what depth are usually related to a normal, healthy gingival sulcus?
    A. 3 mm
    B. 4 mm
    C. 5 mm
    D. 6 mm
    E. 7 mm

68. Which statement BEST describes what periodontal disease and dental caries have in common?
    A. The etiology of both can always be directly attributed to poor oral hygiene
    B. They are the most common chronic dental diseases
    C. Both diseases are infections
    D. Both diseases cause inflammation
    E. All of the above

69. A patient who manifests a peculiar inflammation of the marginal and attached gingiva and demonstrates ulcerated and necrotic epithelium that sloughs (or peels off) with air blasts probably has
    A. Red mouth syndrome
    B. Chronic desquamative gingivitis
    C. Periodontitis
    D. Necrotizing ulcerative gingivitis
    E. Hyperplastic gingiva

70. A mesial cavity in a mandibular right second premolar is classified as a
    A. Class I
    B. Class II
    C. Class III
    D. Class IV
    E. Class V

71. Which of the following types of dental stains can become embedded in decalcified surface enamel?
    A. Orange stain
    B. Black line stain
    C. Brown stain
    D. Green stain

72. A retrognathic profile is usually associated with which of the following classifications of malocclusion?
    A. Class I
    B. Class II
    C. Class III

73. A tooth in supraversion is
    A. In a position labial to normal
    B. In a position lingual to normal
    C. Elongated above the line of occlusion
    D. In a position buccal to normal

√74. The source of minerals for subgingival calculus is
    A. Saliva
    B. Blood
    C. Gingival sulcular fluid
    D. Food

75. Which of the following terms is used to describe a flat, nonraised lesion?
    A. Vesicle
    B. Macule
    C. Bulla
    D. Ulcer

76. Dental x-ray machines that use more than 70 kVp are required to have a total filtration of at least
    A. 0.5 mm of aluminum
    B. 1.5 mm of aluminum
    C. 2.0 mm of aluminum
    D. 2.5 mm of aluminum

77. A radiograph that is too light in density may be caused by
    A. Overdeveloping the film
    B. Using an exhausted developer
    C. Using high kilovoltage
    D. Too much radiation exposure time

78. Periapical or bitewing radiographs that exhibit the error of overlapping proximal structures are a result of
    A. Incorrect vertical positioning
    B. Incorrect vertical positioning of the cone
    C. Incorrect horizontal positioning of the cone
    D. Incorrect vertical angulation, but correct horizontal angulation

79. Radiographic examinations should be made on patients
    A. At least every 2 years
    B. At various intervals depending on their dental history
    C. At least every 3 years
    D. Whenever professional judgment dictates

80. On intraoral radiographs, dark areas around the necks of teeth are sometimes misinterpreted as carious lesions. These areas result from
    A. Attrition
    B. Abrasion
    C. The mach band effect
    D. Cervical burnout
    E. All of the above

81. Oral structures of greater density may require increased penetration by x-ray photons. This may be accomplished by
    A. Increasing the mA
    B. Increasing the exposure time
    C. Increasing the kVp
    D. Decreasing the exposure time

82. A processed film that is clear and has no image may be a result of which of the following errors?
    A. Placing the film in the fixer prior to its development
    B. A saliva leak into the film packet
    C. Reversing the film packet in the mouth
    D. Exposing the film to white light prior to processing

83. In processing radiographs, which of the following is a function of the fixing solution chemicals?
    A. Softens the emulsion
    B. Causes silver deposits at the sites of exposed crystals
    C. Develops the exposed silver halide salts
    D. Removes the undeveloped silver halide salts
    E. All of the above

84. Which of the following cells are LEAST sensitive to radiation (radioresistant)?
    A. Epithelial cells of the gastrointestinal tract
    B. Lymphocytes
    C. Erythrocytes
    D. Nerve cells
    E. Fibroblasts

85. Black lines on a film may be produced by
    A. Fixer spills onto the film prior to processing
    B. High temperature
    C. Static electricity
    D. Air bubbles

86. Panoramic radiographs are very useful for many reasons, but they may NOT accurately depict which of the following?
    A. Interproximal caries
    B. Presence of foreign bodies
    C. The relationship of one intraoral structure to another
    D. Fractures of the mandible

87. Intensifying screens used when extraoral radiographs are made
    A. Aid in decreasing radiation exposure to the patient
    B. Contain silver bromide crystals
    C. Increase radiographic sharpness
    D. Reduce film fog

88. The function of the raised dot on a dental film is to identify the
    A. Side of the film that should be next to the tongue
    B. Side of the film that should be toward the line of occlusion
    C. Side of the film that should be facing the x-ray beam
    D. Maxillary or mandibular teeth, depending on how the film is placed in the mouth

89. Cone cutting (partial image) on a radiograph is caused by
    A. Pointed plastic cone of radiation
    B. Underexposure
    C. Improper coverage of the film with the primary beam of radiation
    D. Placing the film in reverse to the beam of radiation
    E. All of the above

90. A hypochlorite solution for cleaning dentures contains which of the following ingredients?
    A. Calgon™, chlorine bleach, and water
    B. Acetic acid, water, and chlorine bleach
    C. Chlorine bleach, water, and vinegar
    D. Water, Calgon™, and sodium chloride

91. Which of the following is (are) contraindicated when polishing, due to the production of increased frictional heat?
    A. Rapid abrasion
    B. Coarse abrasive polish
    C. Dry agents
    D. Heavy pressure
    E. All of the above

92. A material composed of particles of sufficient hardness and sharpness to cut or scratch a softer material when drawn across its surface is called
    A. An abrasive
    B. A cleanser
    C. A polish
    D. A dentifrice

93. The process by which all forms of life, including bacterial spores and viruses, are destroyed describes the process of
    A. Sterilization
    B. Cleaning
    C. Disinfecting
    D. Decontamination

94. When is a tooth MOST susceptible to a dental caries attack?
    A. A year after eruption
    B. Soon after eruption
    C. The tooth is consistently susceptible

95. Prolonged use of hydrogen peroxide is most likely to produce which of the following conditions?
    A. Black hairy tongue
    B. Gingival hypersensitivity
    C. Decalcification
    D. Geographic tongue
    E. Candidiasis

96. Instruments receive the MOST wear from
    A. Autoclaving
    B. Scaling
    C. Gas sterilization
    D. Sharpening
    E. Ultrasonic cleaning

97. A patient taking diphenylhydantoin sodium probably has
    A. Rheumatic fever
    B. Tuberculosis
    C. Rheumatism
    D. Diabetes
    ✓E. Epilepsy

98. The MOST frequent error in the use of alginates for impressions is
    A. Having too much water in the mix
    B. Delaying the pouring of the cast
    C. Having too much powder in the mix
    D. Water added to the powder is too hot
    E. Wax is not added to the tray

99. Oral irrigators (water irrigation devices) are NOT useful for
    A. Removing bacterial plaque
    B. Stimulating the gingiva
    C. Dislodging debris from orthodontic appliances
    D. All of the above

100. Which of the following will decrease the retention and effectiveness of a pit and fissure sealant?
    A. Improper technique
    B. Abrasive dentifrice
    C. Water contamination of the etched enamel
    D. Consistent use of a hard-bristle tooth-brush
    E. All of the above

101. During mouth-to-mouth resuscitation or rescue breathing, the emergency operator should breathe into the victim's mouth and release at a rate of
    A. 6–7 times per minute
    B. 10 times per minute
    C. 12–20 times per minute
    D. 30 times per minute
    E. 60 times per minute

102. When performing cardiopulmonary resuscitation, the ratio of compressions to breaths is
    A. 10 compressions, then 1 breath
    B. 15 compressions, then 2 breaths
    C. 12 compressions, then 2 breaths
    D. 8 compressions, then 1 breath

103. When performing the Heimlich maneuver or abdominal thrusts, where do you place your fist and how are the thrusts given?
    A. At the lower tip of the breastbone and with an upward thrust
    B. On the navel and with a straight back thrust
    C. Just above the navel and well below the lower tip of the breastbone with a quick upward thrust

104. Which of the following is the MOST effective chemotherapeutic agent against bacterial plaque biofilm?
    A. Listerine™
    B. Zinc chloride
    C. Chlorhexidine
    D. Hydrogen peroxide
    E. Sodium perborate

105. Chemical agents that are EPA registered for surface disinfection include
    A. Quaternary ammonia compounds, iodophors, alcohol
    B. Alcohol, sodium hypochlorite, glutaraldehydes
    C. Sodium hypochlorite, iodophors, synthetic phenols
    D. Glutaraldehydes, quaternary ammonia compounds, sodium hypochlorite

106. Which of the following will contribute to the prevention of disease transmission and lessen the chance of cross-contamination?
    A. Utilization of barriers
    B. High-volume aspiration
    C. Antiretraction valves
    D. Flushing water lines
    E. All of the above

107. When performing gingival curettage, the face of the curette blade forms which angle with the soft-tissue pocket wall?
    A. 45°
    B. 60°
    C. 70°
    D. 90°

108. Airabrasive polishing is contraindicated in patients with
    A. Respiratory conditions
    B. Exposed cementum or dentin
    C. Soft, spongy gingiva
    D. Composite restorations
    E. A sodium-restricted diet
    F. All of the above

109. Overheating during amalgam polishing may cause injury to
    A. Osteoclasts
    B. Ameloblasts
    C. Osteoblasts
    D. Odontoblasts

110. Ending instrument sharpening strokes on a downward strike will assist in
    A. Rounding of the edge
    B. Preserving the contour of the blade
    C. Preventing dullness of the blade
    D. Preventing formation of a wire edge

111. When using an ultrasonic scaler, the patient may experience sensitivity. Which of the following alterations in technique can be made to lessen sensitivity?
    A. Lighten the pressure of the instrument against the tooth or deposit
    B. Lower the power setting
    C. Increase the water flow
    D. Maintain constant motion
    E. All of the above

112. MOST fluoride is excreted through the
    A. Small intestine
    B. Kidneys
    C. Liver
    D. Feces
    E. Sweat glands

113. The pH of acidulated fluoride gels is in the range of
    A. 1–3
    B. 3–5
    C. 5–7
    D. 7–9
    E. 9–11

114. Fluorosis may result from excessive fluoride consumed during
    A. The mineralization stage of tooth development
    B. The maturation stage of tooth development
    C. Either the mineralization or the maturation stage of tooth development

115. Which of the following is an advantage of a school-based fluoride program?
    A. It is the most effective method of reducing dental caries
    B. It can be implemented by nondental personnel
    C. It can achieve maximum effectiveness with monthly application
    D. It is the least expensive method of administering fluoride

116. Which of the following factors need NOT be considered in deciding whether pediatric fluoride supplements should be prescribed?
    A. Age of the patient
    B. Amount of fluoride in the drinking water
    C. Conscientiousness of the patient or parents
    D. Type of topical fluoride applied professionally

117. A 3-year-old child who lives in a non-fluoridated area has rampant decay. Which of the following home-care regimens, with parental supervision, is suitable for this child?
    A. Fluoride tablets
    B. Fluoride dentifrice
    C. Fluoride mouthrinse
    D. Brush-on gel
    E. Fluoride drops

118. Which of the following have been demonstrated to be the MOST effective in inhibiting microbial plaque?
    A. Fluoride
    B. Antibiotics
    C. Chlorhexidine
    D. Water irrigation devices

119. Toothbrush selection for a patient should be primarily and most importantly based on which of the following?
    A. Whether the toothbrush is ADA-approved
    B. Type of bristles
    C. State of health of the periodontium
    D. Anatomic configuration of the teeth and gingiva
    E. Individual patient's needs

120. In order to clean properly and most efficiently, in general, patients should be advised to floss
    A. Before bedtime
    B. As often as possible
    C. Before brushing
    D. After brushing

121. Fluoride uptake in teeth depends on which of the following factors?
    A. Amount of fluoride delivered
    B. Type of fluoride delivered
    C. Form of fluoride delivered
    D. Length of time of exposure to fluoride delivered

122. Ideally, the optimum concentration of fluoride in community drinking water is in the range of
    A. 0.2–1.0 parts per million (ppm)
    B. 0.6–1.2 ppm
    C. 1.0–2.0 ppm
    D. 1.2–2.5 ppm

123. Which of the following types and concentrations of fluoride should be recommended to a head and neck cancer patient for home-care custom tray use?
    A. 0.4% stannous fluoride
    B. 1% neutral sodium fluoride
    C. 1.23% acidulated phosphate fluoride
    D. A and C only
    E. A and B only
    F. A, B, and C

124. Which of the following types of fluoride is reported to cause staining of demineralized enamel and porcelain?
    A. Stannous fluoride
    B. Acidulated phosphate fluoride
    C. Neutral sodium fluoride

125. A symptom is referred to as any departure from the normal that may be indicative of disease. Which of the following are symptoms observed by the patient?
    A. Objective symptoms
    B. Subjective symptoms
    C. Cardinal symptoms
    D. Signal symptoms

126. Which of the following fluorides is recommended for a patient with bulimia nervosa?
    A. Stannous fluoride
    B. Neutral sodium fluoride
    C. Acidulated phosphate fluoride

127. Sealants should be applied
    A. As soon as possible following eruption
    B. At the age of 12
    C. At the age of 15
    D. After all permanent teeth have erupted
    E. To primary teeth only

128. Calculus can attach to the tooth by way of
    A. Attachment by means of an acquired pellicle
    B. Direct contact between calcified intercellular matrix and tooth surface
    C. Attachment to minute irregularities and undercuts in the tooth surface
    D. A and B only
    E. B and C only
    F. A, B, and C

129. Which of the following crystalline salts is most prevalent in dental calculus?
    A. Octocalcium phosphate
    B. Hydroxyapatite
    C. Brushite
    D. Whitlockite

130. Which of the following stains is composed of chromogenic bacteria and fungi?
    A. Metallic stain
    B. Green stain
    C. Black line stain
    D. Yellow stain

131. Changes in the types of organisms occur within plaque as it matures. At which time do vibrios and spirochetes appear?
    A. 1–7 days
    B. 7–14 days
    C. 14–21 days
    D. 21–28 days

132. Which of the following are indicated for use on titanium implants?
    A. Carbon steel instruments
    B. Ultrasonic scaling instruments
    C. Stainless steel instruments
    D. Gold instruments
    E. Plastic instruments

133. If a patient exhibits shortness of breath, dizziness, palpitation, or cold sweats following the administration of a local anesthetic, the patient
    A. Is allergic to the anesthetic
    B. Is probably apprehensive about dental treatment and reacting to the injection
    C. Is possibly abusing illicit drugs
    D. Has been given too much anesthesia

134. A patient's record
    A. Begins with the initial examination and continues as long as the patient is under care
    B. Should be reviewed and updated at each appointment
    C. Must be legible
    D. Is confidential
    E. All of the above

135. When establishing the recall frequency for patients, it should be based on which of the following?
    A. The patients' desire
    B. The maintenance of their oral health
    C. The effectiveness of their oral hygiene
    D. B and C only
    E. A, B, and C

136. Your patient begins to complain of fatigue, nausea, and tachycardia, and you notice a fruity, acetone odor to his or her breath. The patient is probably suffering from
    A. Hypoglycemia
    B. Alcohol overdose
    C. Hyperglycemia
    D. Epilepsy
    E. Halitosis

137. Which of the following BEST describes the objective of root planing?
    A. Removal of factors that promote gingival inflammation
    B. Removal of diseased epithelial attachment
    C. Removal of diseased attached gingiva
    D. Removal of diseased sulcular epithelium
    E. All of the above

138. Which of the following instruments is the most versatile for periodontal instrumentation?
    A. Contra-angled sickle scaler
    B. Curette
    C. Chisel
    D. Hoe
    E. File

139. Exposed cementum and dentin predispose the patient to
    A. Acute dental caries
    B. Hypersensitive teeth
    C. Periodontal pockets
    D. Gingival enlargement

140. Gingival curettage includes the removal of
    A. Diseased sulcular epithelial lining
    B. Necrotic cementum
    C. Inflamed connective tissue
    D. A and B only
    E. A and C only

141. Which of the following local factors is (are) implicated in the etiology of periodontal disease?
    A. Calculus
    B. Mouth breathing
    C. Smoking and/or drug use
    D. Tooth malposition
    E. Faulty restorations
    F. All of the above

142. When bacteria invade through some break in the gingival tissue, the result can be a
    A. Periapical abscess
    B. Periodontal abscess
    C. Gingival abscess
    D. Radicular cyst

143. The gingival cyst occurs as a painless, bluish-gray nodule in the gingiva and has the appearance and consistency of a mucocele. On a dental radiograph it
    A. Cannot be detected
    B. Appears radiopaque and well circumscribed
    C. Appears radiolucent and well circumscribed

144. Calculus is harmful to gingival and periodontal tissues for all of the following reasons EXCEPT
    A. It provides a haven for plaque and is irritating
    B. It provides a permeable surface that can store toxic irritants
    C. Calculus is covered by plaque
    D. It is a mechanical irritant

145. The severity of periodontal disease is determined by the
    A. Probing depths
    B. Degree of mobility
    C. Amount of bleeding
    D. Shape of the gingiva

146. Furcation involvement is BEST detected by which of the following methods?
    A. Use of an explorer
    B. Use of a Nabers probe
    C. Use of radiographs
    D. Use of a curette
    E. All of the above

147. Which of the following factors would influence instrument selection?
    A. Tissue state
    B. Length of the clinical crown
    C. Sulcular or pocket depth
    D. Amount of calculus
    E. Accessibility of the areas involved
    F. All of the above

148. Phase I of periodontal therapy includes
    A. Treatment of dental emergencies
    B. Removal of overhangs
    C. Patient education
    D. Extraction of hopeless teeth
    E. All of the above

149. The term peri-implantitis BEST describes which of the following clinical conditions?
    A. Inflammatory response in the peri-implant tissues
    B. Bone loss around an osseointegrated implant
    C. Gingivitis associated with an osseointegrated implant
    D. Suppuration around an osseointegrated implant

150. The organism(s) MOST commonly associated with the etiology of juvenile periodontitis include
    A. *Actinobacillus actinomycetemcomitans*
    B. *Capnocytophaga sputigena*
    C. *Actinomyces viscosus*
    D. A and B only
    E. A and C only
    F. A, B, and C

151. The Perio Chip®, a gelatin chip, contains 2.5 mg of which of the following antimicrobials used in adjunctive periodontal maintenance?
    A. Triclosan
    B. Chlorhexidine gluconate
    C. Tetracycline
    D. Doxycycline hyclate

152. Diagnostic casts made from alginate impressions are used routinely for all of the following reasons EXCEPT
    A. To determine occlusion
    B. As the cast used to fabricate a fixed partial denture
    C. To present a treatment plan to the patient
    D. To compare with subsequent models

153. The two principal methods of forming metallic objects used in dentistry are
    A. Cast and wrought
    B. Stamped and forged
    C. Distilled and cast
    D. Wrought and synthetic

154. The three methods of inducing a polymerization reaction in dentistry include all of the following EXCEPT
    A. Light curing
    B. Radioactive curing
    C. Heat curing
    D. Self-curing

155. Exhibiting concern and empathy for others is called
    A. Caring
    B. Citizenship
    C. Fairness
    D. Responsibility

156. Which type of ethical theory describes a group of theories that provide, define, and describe a system of principles and rules that determine which actions are deemed right or wrong?
    A. Normative ethics
    B. Moral reasoning
    C. Virtue ethics
    D. Utilitarian ethics

157. Which type of ethics places emphasis on character traits of an individual?
    A. Normative ethics
    B. Moral reasoning
    C. Virtue ethics
    D. Utilitarian ethics

158. A healthcare provider's first obligation to the patient is to do no harm, which is termed
    A. Nonmaleficence
    B. Beneficence
    C. Autonomy
    D. Veracity

159. Which of the following terms describes a dental hygienist's responsibility to provide quality health care that benefits the patient?
    A. Nonmaleficence
    B. Beneficence
    C. Autonomy
    D. Veracity

160. Providing individuals or a group with what is owed, due, and/or deserved is called
    A. Autonomy
    B. Beneficence
    C. Justice
    D. Paternalism

161. Which ethical principle states that a provider should prevent harm, remove harm, and not inflict harm?
    A. Autonomy
    B. Beneficence
    C. Justice
    D. Nonmaleficence

162. The ability to govern one's own profession and to be self-determined and directed as a profession is called
    A. Autonomy
    B. Beneficence
    C. Justice
    D. Nonmaleficence

163. Which principle is based on respect for others and the belief that patients have the power to make decisions about things that may affect their health?
    A. Autonomy
    B. Beneficence
    C. Justice
    D. Nonmaleficence

164. Being honest is called
    A. Justice
    B. Fairness
    C. Paternalism
    D. Veracity

165. The Ramfjord teeth commonly used to simplify dental indexes include
    A. The maxillary right first molar, left central incisor, left first bicuspid, and the mandibular left first molar, right central incisor, and right first bicuspid
    B. The maxillary right first molar, left central incisor, left first molar, and the mandibular left first molar, left central incisor, and right first molar
    C. The division of the mouth into sextants from the upper right third molar to the first bicuspid, cuspid to cuspid, left first bicuspid to third molar and the lower right third molar to the first bicuspid, cuspid to cuspid, and left first bicuspid to third molar
    D. The use of any six surfaces of any six teeth as long as operationally defined by the examiner

166. Fluoridation is the adjustment of the fluoride ion content in a(n)
    A. Gel solution
    B. Water supply
    C. Aerosol spray
    D. Ingestible tablet

167. If the major purpose of an epidemiologist's research is to determine caries susceptibility as opposed to immediate treatment needs, the BEST caries index to use is
    A. DMFT
    B. DMFS
    C. CPITN
    D. TSIF

168. Fluorides are stored in skeletal tissues. Even when concentrations reach 8 ppm, no impairment in general health can be detected.
    A. The first statement is TRUE; second statement is FALSE.
    B. The first statement is FALSE; second statement is TRUE.
    C. Both statements are TRUE.
    D. Both statements are FALSE.

169. Water fluoridation ranks as a very successful primary oral health measure because
    A. It demonstrates to the public that caries and tooth loss are not inevitable
    B. Its greatest benefit is to halt dental caries in the earliest possible stage
    C. Its clinical efficacy and effectiveness are well established in the dental literature
    D. All of the above

170. Based on results of recent fluoride studies, prenatal fluoride supplements are recommended by both the ADA and AMA in communities where water supplies are fluoridated. The results demonstrated a reduction of caries in primary teeth by 20 percent.
    A. Both statements are TRUE.
    B. Both statements are FALSE.
    C. The first statement is TRUE; second statement is FALSE.
    D. The first statement is FALSE; second statement is TRUE.

171. Controversy surrounding fluoridation of the drinking water has once again resurfaced. Opponents feel that fluoridated drinking water is a
    A. Violation of individual rights
    B. Risk factor for bone cancer
    C. Risk factor for Down syndrome
    D. All of the above

172. The human body possesses a prompt and efficient excretory mechanism for fluorides; however, this does not minimize the danger of long-term accumulation of fluorides which can be toxic.
    A. The first statement is TRUE; second statement is FALSE.
    B. The first statement is FALSE; second statement is TRUE.
    C. Both statements are TRUE.
    D. Both statements are FALSE.

173. Dental health surveys overestimate dental needs more so than private practitioners because
    A. They are conducted under ideal conditions
    B. They utilize standardized examiners
    C. They reflect a congruence between need and demand for care
    D. The statement is false; dental needs are underestimated in dental health surveys

174. A special characteristic of the Root Caries Index (RCI) as compared to other dental indexes is
    A. A carious lesion is only included in the count when it appears below the cementoenamel junction
    B. A carious lesion is included in the count when it appears above or below the gingival margin
    C. It is unique in that it includes the concept of teeth at risk
    D. It is based on 28 permanent teeth, excluding third molars

175. For epidemiological studies, the BEST available index for the measurement of periodontitis is the
    A. Sulcus Bleeding Index
    B. Periodontal Index
    C. Community Periodontal Index of Treatment Needs
    D. Indirect method of scoring loss of periodontal attachment (LPA)

176. If the dental hygienist is asked to present a community dental health presentation for a deaf audience, the dental hygienist should
    A. Switch the lights on and off to attract the group's attention, give written information for reinforcement, and immediately begin the program
    B. Enlist the support of an interpreter, review the program with him or her, and ask the interpreter to interject appropriate comments when necessary
    C. Present using sign language with written materials to augment the presentation
    D. Switch the lights on and off to attract the group's attention, allow the audience to read handouts before initiating the program, and use sign language or an interpreter

177. The Klein and Palmer Index can be recorded as DMFT or DMFS. The DMFS would be the recommended choice in which of the following situations?
    A. When radiographs are not available
    B. When time is a limiting factor in the screening process
    C. When the examiner is not highly skilled in the detection of caries
    D. When there is a need to detect sensitive changes in caries incidence
    E. All of the above

178. Females have been found to have higher DMF scores than males. One could also conclude from these findings that females are more caries susceptible than their male counterparts.
    A. Both statements are TRUE.
    B. Both statements are FALSE.
    C. The first statement is TRUE; second statement is FALSE.
    D. The first statement is FALSE; second statement is TRUE.

179. The OHI-S measures which of the following?
    A. Dental caries
    B. Debris
    C. Gingival bleeding
    D. B and C only

180. A treatment category of II on the Community Periodontal Index of Treatment Needs (CPITN) indicates that
    A. Bleeding was observed upon probing or pressure
    B. Calculus was felt during probing and 3.5–5.5 mm pockets were recorded
    C. Improved oral hygiene and scaling are necessary
    D. This index does not include treatment categories

181. The MOST common cause of tooth loss in adult life prior to age 60 is
    A. Dental caries
    B. Periodontal disease
    C. Accidents
    D. Acquired immunodeficiency syndrome

182. The effectiveness of a dental health program can be measured by
    A. The degree to which it meets program objectives
    B. The number of participants involved
    C. The cost of the program
    D. The length of the program
    E. All of the above

183. Which of the following age groups is (are) MOST subject to rampant dental caries?
    A. Young children with poor oral hygiene, adults with gingival recession
    B. Young children with poor oral hygiene
    C. Adults with gingival recession
    D. Rampant caries are not age-related

184. Which of the following indices is used to measure oral debris?
    A. Plaque Index
    B. Gingival Index
    C. Decayed, Missing, and Filled Surfaces of Teeth (DMFS)
    D. Decayed, Missing, and Filled Teeth (DMFT)

185. Edentulism is closely related to oral hygiene practices of the patient. Partial edentulism is more closely related to the dentist's/patient's attitude toward extraction of the patient's teeth as the primary method of dental care.
    A. Both statements are true
    B. Both statements are false
    C. The first statement is true; second statement is false
    D. The first statement is false; second statement is true

186. Dental fluorosis is defined as
    A. Hypermineralization of the enamel caused by overingestion of fluoride immediately after tooth eruption
    B. Hypermineralization of the enamel caused by overingestion of fluoride during tooth development
    C. Hypomineralization of the enamel caused by overingestion of fluoride immediately after tooth eruption
    D. Hypomineralization of the enamel caused by overingestion of fluoride during tooth development

187. Sensitivity, a characteristic of a diagnostic test, should determine if a high proportion of individuals who are tested for a disease and found positive
    A. Will not subsequently develop the disease
    B. Will subsequently develop the disease
    C. Has little place in oral epidemiology even though a positive test was determined
    D. Will seek treatment once notified of the results

188. When a patient comes to a dental office, the first procedure is an examination. The first step in a public health procedure is
    A. Analysis
    B. Survey
    C. Diagnosis
    D. Treatment

189. The MOST important determinants of dental utilization are
    A. Socioeconomic status, dentate status, and gender
    B. Socioeconomic status and gender
    C. Dentate status and gender
    D. Undetermined at this time

190. What percentage of U.S. children exhibit some form of fluorosis today?
    A. 7–15%
    B. 20–25%
    C. 25–33%
    D. 40–50%

Testlet 1: Questions 191–195

A school dental hygienist works for all three elementary schools in the district. The dental hygienist has dental hygiene operatories in each school where she provides comprehensive dental care. Importantly, she carefully examines each student, which includes the use of dental indexes for use in evaluation of the program. She conducts in-service workshops for parents and teachers. She also teaches all classes on the importance of oral hygiene care and the development of dental diseases.

191. The scenario best describes which type of community-based program being conducted in the elementary schools by the dental hygienist?
    A. Fluoride
    B. Preventive
    C. Therapeutic
    D. Sealants

192. The dental hygienists are going to discuss the importance of good oral hygiene habits and the prevention of dental disease. Which of the following is the BEST technique(s) for teaching this material?
    A. Demonstration
    B. Distribution of brochures and class activities
    C. Lecture only
    D. Lecture with slides, posters, and class activities

193. Select the BEST combination method of dental indexes to determine the dental needs and formation of debris on the teeth.
    A. DMFT/deft and GI
    B. DMFS/defs and CPITN
    C. DMFT/deft and OHI-S
    D. DMFT/defs and DI-S

194. The FIRST step the dental hygienist needs to complete before starting clinical procedures such as exams and sealant placement is
    A. Identifying dental insurance reimbursement
    B. Determining the students' daily schedule
    C. Identifying the students that do not need dental treatment
    D. Gathering informed consent from the parents

195. What critical area of a preventive program has not been discussed regarding this program?
    A. Educational
    B. Prevention
    C. Referral
    D. Evaluation

Testlet 2: Questions 196–200

A high school class of 12 physically challenged students, 14 to 19 years of age, show a need for improved oral hygiene. The district dental hygienist has been asked by the high school nurse to assess their needs and to work with the nurse to implement a dental public health program to this class. The dental hygienist plans to set up a portable dental unit to orally screen the students and to implement an evaluative tool to understand the dental health knowledge of the group. In addition, he plans to provide oral hygiene instruction each month during the remainder of the school year, and the nurse will follow up with the instructions each Tuesday. The Patient Hygiene Performance (PHP) scores during the initial assessment of the class were 2.5, 2.75, 1.5, 3.0, 2.5, 2.0, 2.5, 2.75, 2.5, 2.5, 2.0, and 3.0. The mean OHI-S score of the 12 individuals was 4.8.

196. A complete dental assessment of the class should include all of the following EXCEPT one. Which one is the EXCEPTION?
  A. Plaque and gingival scores
  B. Dental hygiene treatment needs
  C. Individual dexterity skills
  D. Familial income and education level
  E. Level of physical disabilities

197. Based on the severity of the physical disabilities, the dental hygienist may need to make accommodations for all of the following EXCEPT one. Which one is the EXCEPTION?
  A. Oral hygiene instruction
  B. Transportation to area dentists if needed
  C. Utilization of the portable dental chair
  D. Selection of dental indices

198. Which of the following represents the mean PHP score?
  A. 2.45
  B. 2.0
  C. 2.75
  D. 2.25
  E. 2.95

199. Which of the following PHP scores represents the mode?
  A. 1.5
  B. 2.0
  C. 2.5
  D. 2.75
  E. 3.0

200. When performing a correlation test between the debris and calculus scores of this class, the correlation coefficient was +.94. The relationship between gingival disease and plaque accumulation according to this test is statistically
  A. Strong
  B. Moderate
  C. Weak
  D. No correlation

answers & rationales

1.

A. The optic nerve serves a sensory function to the eye and functions in vision. The oculomotor nerve, trochlear nerve, and abducens nerve all have a motor function and assist in the movement of the eyeball.

2.

D. The sense of taste from the posterior third of the tongue is carried by the glossopharyngeal nerve. The facial nerve carries taste sensation from the anterior two-thirds on the tongue; the glossopharyngeal nerve is motor to muscles that move the tongue.

3.

A. Muscles of mastication are classified as muscles of branchiomeric origin; this means that they are derived from embryonic branchial arches. For this reason, they are placed in the "special" category of functional components. Efferent implies motor nerves. Muscles of mastication are supplied by fibers from the trigeminal nerve.

4.

A. Cerebrospinal fluid is produced by the choroid plexus. The choroid plexus is a membranous partition extending into the cavity of each of the ventricles. It forms a semipermeable partition that filters cerebrospinal fluid from blood.

5.

B. The mucous membranes of the pharynx and the associated gag reflex receive sensory innervation from the glossopharyngeal nerve.

6.

D. The superficial temporal and deep auricles supply arterial blood to the temporomandibular joint. The deep auricular artery is a branch of the maxillary artery. Both the superficial temporal artery and the maxillary artery are terminal branches of the external carotid artery.

7.

B. The buccal cusps of the maxillary teeth occlude with the buccal surfaces of the mandibular teeth in normal occlusion. The maxillary posterior teeth are slightly buccal to the mandibular posterior teeth. The tip of the mesiobuccal cusp of the maxillary first molar is aligned directly over the mesiobuccal groove on the mandibular first molar. The distal buccal surface is more lingual than the mesiobuccal, allowing the distobuccal cusp to occlude properly with the lower first molar.

8.

A. The permanent mandibular second molar has four cusps. The permanent mandibular first molar has five cusps. The mandibular molars are larger than any other mandibular teeth.

9.

C. The mandibular canine has the longest crown, approximately 11 mm in length. The maxillary canine has a crown length of approximately 10 mm. The mandibular canine crown is narrower mesiodistally than the maxillary canine.

10.

B. The anterior tooth most likely to have a bifurcated root is the permanent mandibular canine. This variation is not rare.

11.

D. From a lingual aspect of the maxillary lateral incisor, it is not uncommon to find a deep developmental groove at the side of the cingulum. This is usually found on the distal side, which may extend up on the root for part or all of its length. The linguoincisal ridge is well developed and the lingual fossa more concave than the central incisor.

12.

A. Normal keratinized areas of the oral mucosa include the vermillion border of the lips, the hard palate, and the gingiva. The buccal mucosa, floor of the mouth, inferior surface of the tongue, and soft palate are nonkeratinized oral mucosa under normal conditions. All oral mucosa, whether keratinized, parakeratinized, or nonkeratinized, is of the stratified squamous type of epithelium.

13.

D. The anterior two-thirds of the tongue develop from the tuberculum impar and adjacent tissue. The first indication of tongue development appears around the fourth week *in utero*. Two fused distal tongue buds also help develop into the anterior two-thirds of the tongue.

14.

C. The premaxilla contains the tooth buds of incisors. It forms the anterior portion of the hard palate and the rim of the piriform aperture. The maxilla is the other bone that forms the premaxilla.

15.

D. The salivary glands arise from oral mesenchyme. During fetal life each salivary gland is formed in a specific location in the oral cavity. The primordia of the parotid and submandibular salivary glands appear 7–8 weeks *in utero*.

16.

E. Active transport moves a substance against a concentration gradient; facilitated diffusion, down a concentration gradient. Active transport requires a carrier and energy. Diffusion and osmosis, on the other hand, are referred to as passive transport because the driving force is the concentration gradient. The continual movement of sodium and potassium across the cell membrane is an example of substances that move by active transport.

17.

C. Sarcolemma, myofibrils, mitochondria, actin, and myosin are all associated with skeletal muscle. Skeletal muscle is striated and voluntary. Intercalated discs, representing specialized cell junctions, are present in cardiac muscle only.

18.

C. A single motor neuron and the muscle cells supplied by its axon branches are termed a motor end plate. Neurons have two types of processes: axons and dendrites. The axon of the motor nerve divides into several branches, which distribute to different muscle fibers.

19.

A. Depolarization is the first stage of conduction. It occurs when the permeability of the cell membrane to sodium increases. In the resting state, the interior of the nerve fiber is negative to the exterior by approximately 70 to 90 millivolts.

20.

C. A low-carbohydrate diet will reduce the number of lactobacilli, *Streptococcus salivaris*, iodophilic polysaccharide-storing streptococci, and *Streptococcus mutans*.

21.

A. When body metabolism requires glucose which is not available from recently digested carbohydrates, it calls on the liver to convert its stored glycogen into glucose through the process of glycolysis. When the store is depleted, the liver begins to make new glycogen from amino acids. This partial conversion of protein to glycogen in the liver is known as gluconeogenesis.

22.

D. Pernicious anemia is usually due to a lack of intrinsic factor, which prevents the absorption of physiological amounts of vitamin B_{12}.

23.

B. Ascorbic acid is absolutely essential for the fibroblast to produce its fibrous protein, collagen. An ascorbic acid deficiency will bring about a reversal of the differentiated cells to the more immature cell types. However, if ascorbic acid is administered the defect is promptly corrected.

24.

C. One must consider the pH of food as well as the sugar content; one cannot predict the cariogenicity of food by the sugar content alone. A pH above 6 = safe area; 6.0–5.5 = doubtful; below 5.5 = danger area for solubility of the tooth.

25.

B. Under ordinary conditions about 20–30% of the calcium is absorbed; the remaining amount is excreted in the feces, urine, and perspiration. The recommended dietary allowance of calcium for the average adult in the United States is 0.8 g per day. According to calcium-balance experiments, a mean intake of 500 mg daily for an adult of average weight is the minimum required to offset the usual 400 mg loss.

26.

A. Carbohydrates contain carbon, hydrogen, and oxygen, with hydrogen and oxygen occurring in a 2:1 ratio as in water. We now know that carbohydrates are not hydrates of carbon but are polyhydroxy-aldehydes, ketones, and their condensation products (these being combinations between aldehyde and ketone polyhydric alcohols with the elimination of water).

27.

E. Two cell types are involved in phagocytosis: the polymorphonuclear neutrophil and macrophage. Neutrophils are present in the bloodstream and are short-lived cells. Macrophages, on the other hand, are long-lived cells present throughout the connective tissue and around the basement membrane of small blood vessels. Both cell types migrate to sites of inflammation to engulf bacteria and discharge granules consisting of microbicidal substances.

28.

A. Lipopolysaccharide (or endotoxin) is the most significant structure in the cell wall of Gram-negative bacteria. It accounts for a variety of immunological reactions.

29.

E. Rheumatic fever and acute glomerulonephritis are nonsuppurative complications of group A streptococcal disease. In rheumatic fever, inflammatory changes in the heart, joints, blood vessels, and subcutaneous tissue are evident. Acute inflammation of the glomerulus with edema, hypertension, hematuria, and proteinuria are seen in glomerulonephritis caused by nephrogenetic strains of group A streptococci.

30.

E. All body fluids from patients should be considered potentially infectious. The healthcare worker should exercise precautions as mandated by OSHA by using personal protective equipment, which includes gloves, goggles, face shields, gowns or lab coats, and aprons.

31.

E. *Prevotella (Bacteroides) melaninogenicus* is one of the members of anaerobic Gram-negative bacteria that produces a dark pigment after several days' growth in blood agar plates.

32.

B. 2% glutaraldehyde is an alkalyzing agent highly lethal to essentially all microorganisms if sufficient contact time is provided and there is absence of extraneous organic material. It is effective for sterilizing apparatuses that cannot be heated. Other products such as alcohols, iodophors, chlorhexidine, and quaternary ammonium compounds are disinfectants.

33.

D. Autoclaves should be quality controlled to ensure that the temperature, pressure, packing, and timing are correct. A thermophilic microorganism, usually *Bacillus stearothermophilus,* is used as a biological indicator. These organisms are supplied with vials of culture medium containing a pH indicator. The vial is placed in the autoclave with the load and the autoclave is run under normal conditions. The vial is removed and the culture medium is released to mix with the thermophilic microoganisms. The vial is placed in an incubator for a specified period of time and then checked for growth of the organism. If no organisms grow, the autoclave was effective. If the organisms grow in the culture media, the autoclave did not render the contents of that load sterile.

34.

A. Autoclaves are usually operated at 121°C, which is achieved at a pressure of 15 psi for 15 minutes. Under these conditions spores are killed. The velocity of the killing increases logarithmically with a steam temperature of 121°C and is more effective than 100°C or boiling.

35.

C. *Prevotella (Bacteroides) melaninogenicus* is normal flora of the mouth and oropharynx. It may be found in anaerobic infections, which are frequently polymicrobic.

36.

C. The term gnotobiotic has been used to designate an animal bearing a known microbial flora. Gnotobiotic may also be used to include the germ-free animal, but common usage has restricted this term to animals bearing one or more known and no unknown microorganisms. For animals born and reared in the usual animal quarters, the term conventional has been used.

37.

A. *Fusobacterium nucleatum* is a Gram-negative non-spore-forming anaerobic rod. *Clostridium prefringens* is a Gram-positive spore-forming rod. *Candida albicans* is a yeast. *Neisseria meningitidis* is a member of the aerobic Gram-negative cocci. *Peptostreptococcus* is a Gram-positive cocci.

38.

D. The major distinguishing feature between benign and malignant tumor is the ability of the latter to metastasize to distant sites.

39.

C. Addison's disease is a clinical condition resulting from chronic adrenocortical insufficiency. It is characterized by skin pigmentation, extreme weakness, and low blood pressure. A hormone is responsible for the increase in skin pigmentation.

40.

A. Acquired depigmentation of areas of the skin is known as vitiligo. The size and distribution of areas of vitiligo can vary. This is not to be confused with partial albinism.

41.

E. Hemosiderin is deposited in the liver and spleen during the normal continuous breakdown of red blood cells in the reticuloendothelial system. Hemosiderin may be formed locally or systemically where there is an excessive destruction of erythrocytes in the circulation.

42.

C. Serous inflammation is an inflammatory reaction characterized by an outpouring of abundant fluids. Serous inflammation occurs particularly in acute inflammations of serous cavities.

43.

C. A periapical cyst and a periapical granuloma are indistinguishable radiographically.

44.

B. Fordyce granules are ectopic sebaceous glands, entrapped embryonically in oral soft tissues. The most common sites are the buccal mucosa and the lips. They are described clinically as yellow spots, only slightly elevated on oral mucosa.

45.

B. Desquamative gingivitis is an oral manifestation of a number of mucocutaneous diseases such as lichen planus, pemphigus, or pemphigoid. It is not a manifestation of AIDS, as are the other choices.

46.

B. The condition of teeth joined together only by cementum is termed concrescence. It is thought to arise as a result of traumatic injury. Concrescence may occur before or after the teeth have erupted.

47.

B. Fusion of teeth is a condition produced when two tooth buds are joined together during development and appear as a macrodont. This is not to be confused with true macrodontia, in which all teeth are larger than normal.

48.

E. The condition in which the roots of mandibular molars are severely curved to almost 90 degrees is termed dilaceration. This is thought to be caused by trauma during tooth development. Dilacerated teeth can present problems at the time of extraction.

49.

C. Enamel hypoplasia and enamel hypocalcification are two types of amelogenesis imperfecta. Amelogenesis imperfecta represents a group of hereditary defects of enamel unassociated with any other generalized defects. It is entirely an ectodermal disturbance.

50.

C. Healthcare workers or anyone who develops a positive tuberculin skin test may, after proper chest radiography and medical consultation, be placed on prophylactic long-term, generally one year, Isoniazid therapy.

51.

B. Relative analgesia primarily employs the use of nitrous oxide–oxygen, but pain control must be given concomitantly with local anesthetic. Nitrous oxide offers comfort to the dental patient and an increased patient acceptance of dental procedures. Because of increased patient acceptance, the treatment administration is more relaxed.

52.

C. Nitrous oxide is a nonirritating, colorless gas. It has little or no odor. It is stored in a blue cylinder at 750 psi.

53.

B. Because they do not involve the endocardium per se, cardiac pacemakers will not necessitate antibiotic prophylaxis. Cardiac pacemakers may be affected by electronic devices such as ultrasonic scaling devices, pulp testers, and electrosurgical equipment.

54.

C. Phenytoin (Dilantin) produces excessive gingival enlargement in some patients who are treated with this drug. It is a highly effective anticonvulsant drug. The severity of the gingival enlargement differs. It is not seen in every patient taking this drug.

55.

A. A synonym for phenoxymethyl penicillin is penicillin V. The usual adult dose of penicillin V is 250–500 mg every 6 hours. Trade names for penicillin V include PenVeeK and Penicillin V K.

56.

D. Penicillin V is more resistant than penicillin G to acid inactivation in gastric secretions. Therefore, it has a measurably improved intestinal absorption because of its conversion into a soluble alkaline salt at the pH of the duodenal contents. Oral penicillin V gives higher and better sustained levels of penicillin activity than does oral buffered penicillin G at various dosage levels.

57.

A. Next to morphine, codeine is the most important alkaloid of opium. Codeine is only one-sixth as potent as morphine. It is less narcotic and less addictive and produces less constipation and less nausea.

58.

D. Morphine is the standard to which all other strong analgesics are compared. Morphine promotes drowsiness, depresses reasoning, stimulates imagination, and produces euphoria. It depresses the respiratory and cough centers, contracts pupils, and elicits vomiting.

59.

C. Tetracycline is an antibiotic, and antibiotics are not controlled by the Drug Enforcement Administration. Methadone, meperidine, and alphaprodine require DEA numbers for prescription. The DEA is an arm of the Department of Justice.

60.

A. Time of day, hemorrhage, pathology, and application of external heat are all factors that influence body temperature. Other factors include starvation and physiologic shock. Normal human temperature is 37°C or 98.6°F.

61.

C. If a radial pulse cannot be found or taken, the temporal or facial arteries can be used as alternative sites for taking pulse rate. Exercise, stimulants, eating, strong emotions, and heart disease can increase pulse rates. Sleep, depressants, low vitality from prolonged illness, and fasting can decrease pulse rates.

62.

B. Diastolic pressure represents ventricular relaxation. Systolic pressure represents ventricular contraction. Normal adult blood pressure is 120/80.

63.

A. A mesognathic profile is usually associated with Class I occlusion. Class II occlusion is associated with a retrognathic profile. Class III occlusion is associated with a prognathic profile.

64.

C. Six basic measurements are made in periodontal charting on each tooth: mesial, broad surface, and distal on buccal or facial aspect; and mesial, broad surface, and distal on lingual aspect. In addition to charting pocket depths, other periodontal problems should also be charted. These include recession, furcation involvement, mucogingival involvement, and width of the attached gingiva.

65.

B. Pocket depths measure the depth of the sulcus from the base of the pocket to the height of the gingival margin. Probed attachment level refers to the measurement of the position of the attached periodontal tissue at the base of the sulcus to a fixed point. Pocket depth and attachment level are important in the evaluation of the patient's periodontal status.

66.

B. Gingival enlargement and gingival recession can affect the accuracy of periodontal charting. Gingival enlargement may represent a pseudopocket or gingival pocket, in which there may be no bone loss or involvement of the deeper periodontal structures. On the other hand, in the presence of gingival recession, the operator may get a very low reading upon probing (1–2 mm), which in ordinary circumstances would represent healthy conditions. However, in the case of recession, the gingiva could be in very poor condition. This point should emphasize the necessity of determining bone level and the height of the gingiva and charting them both on the periodontal chart.

67.

A. Most periodontal pocket depths up to 3 mm are usually related to a normal, healthy gingival sulcus. Periodontal pockets are divided into gingival and periodontal types. They are further categorized by their position in relation to alveolar bone. Healthy sulci are shallow and may be only 0.5 mm. The average depth of the healthy sulcus is about 1.8 mm.

68.

B. Periodontal disease and dental caries are the two most common chronic dental diseases. Both are caused primarily by the presence of dental plaque. Preventive measures can eliminate both of these oral diseases extensively.

69.

B. A patient who manifests a peculiar inflammation of the gingiva and demonstrates ulcerated and necrotic epithelium that sloughs off with air blasts probably has chronic desquamative gingivitis. Chronic desquamative gingivitis has no known etiology. It occurs most frequently in women.

70.

B. A mesial cavity in a mandibular right second premolar is classified as a Class II. Class II cavities are found in proximal surfaces of premolars and molars.

71.

D. Dark green stain occasionally becomes embedded in surface enamel. Often the enamel under the stain is decalcified. Green stain results from oral uncleanliness and originates from chromogenic bacteria and fungi.

72.

B. A retrognathic profile is usually associated with Class II occlusion. Class I occlusion is associated with a mesognathic profile. Class III occlusion is associated with a prognathic profile.

73.

C. A tooth in supraversion is elongated above the line of occlusion. A tooth in labioversion is in a position labial to normal. A tooth in lingoversion is in a position lingual to normal.

74.

C. The source of minerals for subgingival calculus is the gingival sulcular fluid. The source of minerals for supragingival calculus is the saliva. The mode of attachment for calculus is the acquired pellicle.

75.

B. A macule is a circumscribed area not elevated above the surrounding skin or mucosa. It may be identified by its color, which contrasts with the surrounding tissue. Vesicles and bullae are classified as elevated blisterform lesions. Ulcers are classified as depressed lesions.

76.

D. The peak voltage of an x-ray machine determines the total amount of filtration required. Below 70 kVp, the total filtration should be 1.5 mm of aluminum. When the kilovoltage is above 70 kVp, the recommended amount is 2.5 mm of aluminum.

77.

B. A weakened developer will not fully develop the latent image in the usual time, and the density of the radiograph will be too light. A rough indication of an exhausted developer solution can be obtained by matching a good density radiograph with one taken at a later time. Less density in the more recent radiograph indicates an exhausted developer. A film positioned backward in the patient's mouth will also result in a lack of density due to the attenuation of the primary beam by the lead backing of the film. Additionally, a kVp, mA, or exposure time that is too low or a target film distance (TFD) that is too great results in a film that is too light.

78.

C. Incorrect horizontal angulation produces the same result in the bisecting, paralleling, or bitewing techniques. The radiograph will show overlapping of the proximal images of adjacent teeth. To correct this error, the central ray of the x-ray beam should be directed horizontally through the contact points of the proximal surfaces of the teeth. This direction for posterior teeth is usually somewhat anterior-posterior.

79.

D. Currently there are no specified lengths of time between which radiographs should be made on various types of patients in various age groups. The old description of "routine radiographs" has no place in today's practice of radiation reduction. The decision for radiographic examinations is therefore based on professional judgment as far as dental radiography is concerned.

80.

D. The area of the tooth between the enamel-covered crown and the portion of the root superimposed upon by alveolar bone attenuates fewer photons than the areas superior and inferior to it. As a result, a dark area referred to as cervical burnout is seen on the radiograph.

81.

C. Photons move through space in a straight line and have a wave pattern. The greater the energy a photon has, the shorter the photon's wavelength. In the x-ray region of the electromagnetic spectrum, the shorter the wavelength of the photon (a high kVp), the easier it is for the photon to pass through matter. Long wavelength, low-energy (a low kVp) photons are called "soft x-rays." Oral structures of greater density require increased penetration or a high kVp.

82.

A. Film will become clear if it is placed in the fixer prior to its development. This type of clear film is identical to an unexposed (to radiation) film that is processed.

83.

D. The function of the fixing solution is to remove the undeveloped silver halide salts. If the crystals (salts) are not removed, the image will be obscured. A second function of the fixing solution is to harden the emulsion which was softened by agents in the developing solution.

84.

D. The cells that are the most sensitive to the biologic effects of radiation have been found to be those that are least differentiated, immature, and are experiencing or will experience mitotic activity. Conversely, cells of nervous tissue and mature bone, which are well differentiated, are the least sensitive.

85.

C. A film packet should never be opened forcefully, especially when the darkroom air is dry. This could produce static electricity, which appears characteristically as dark streaks on the processed radiographs. The film should be held by the edges to prevent crimping or fingernail pressure, which appears as a crescent-shaped dark area. Bending a film can also produce a black line because the emulsion is sensitized to energy.

86.

A. Despite their many advantages (broad coverage, anatomical relationships, the speed and ease with which they are made, and the exposure reduction when compared to a complete mouth survey), panoramic radiographs, as a result of magnification, distortion, and interproximal overlap, frequently are not usable for determining the existence and/or extent of interproximal caries.

87.

A. Intensifying screens consist of tiny calcium tungstate crystals bonded in a uniform layer on a firm x-ray penetrable base material. These screens are generally used in pairs with a double-emulsion base. This method of recording the image of an object requires much less radiation to the patient compared with when the x-ray film alone is used.

88.

C. Every radiograph has an embossed or raised dot to help indicate the film orientation. When the film packet is placed in the mouth, the raised portion of the dot faces the x-ray machine. This assists in aligning films for proper placement into film mounts.

89.

C. If the central ray is not directed at the center of the film, cone cutting will result. The unexposed or white part of the film will not be in the path of radiation. *Cone cut* is the term commonly used to describe a radiograph made when the primary beam of an x-ray does not completely cover the film.

90.

A. A hypochlorite solution for cleaning dentures contains 2 teaspoons Calgon™, 1 tablespoon chlorine bleach, and 4 ounces water. Accumulations of stains and deposits on dentures vary between individuals in a manner similar to natural teeth. Denture pellicle forms readily after a denture is cleaned.

91.

E. Rapid abrasion, coarse abrasive polish, dry agents, and heavy pressure are all contraindicated when polishing. All of these factors increase frictional heat. Some loss of tooth structure occurs during polishing.

92.

A. A material composed of particles of sufficient hardness and sharpness to cut or scratch a softer material when drawn across its surface is an abrasive. Silex and flour of pumice are most often used in tooth polishing agents. Tin oxide is used for polishing amalgams. Jeweler's rouge is used to polish gold.

93.

A. The process by which all forms of life, including bacterial spores and viruses, are destroyed describes the process of sterilization. Sterilization can be achieved effectively through dry heat or autoclaving. Chemical vapor sterilization is used, but has more limitations.

94.

B. A tooth is most susceptible to a dental caries attack soon after eruption. A tooth is also the most susceptible to fluoride soon after eruption. Soon after eruption is often an excellent time to apply pit and fissure sealants.

95.

A. Prolonged use of hydrogen peroxide for the treatment of necrotizing ulcerative gingivitis may produce a black hairy tongue. Hairy tongue may also be attributed to the use of antibiotics and systemic corticosteroids. With this condition, there is an elongation of the filiform papillae, which become matted and entrap bacteria, fungi, cellular debris, and foreign material. Discontinued use of the causative agent and careful daily brushing of the tongue should be of some benefit. Hydrogen peroxide is often recommended for acute gingival conditions. Salt water rinses can be used in place of hydrogen peroxide rinses. Geographic tongue is a condition of unknown cause. Clinically, the tongue will have small, round to irregular areas of dekeratinization and desquamation of the filiform papillae. The desquamated areas appear red with white to yellow elevated margins. Over time the patterns will change and appear to move across the tongue. Geographic tongue is also referred to as benign migratory glossitis.

96.

D. Instruments receive the most wear from sharpening. A sharpening stone should be available at all times during scaling and root planing. The sharpening device must then be kept sterilized.

97.

E. A patient taking diphenylhydantoin sodium probably has epilepsy. Diphenylhydantoin sodium is used for controlling seizures. Often these patients have Dilantin-induced gingival fibromatosis. The condition is also called Dilantin hyperplasia or phenytoin-induced hyperplasia.

98.

B. The most frequent error in the use of alginates for impressions is delaying the pouring of the cast. Undue dehydration or water loss from the alginate will distort the impression. Thus, the final cast will be inaccurate.

99.

A. Oral irrigators (water spray devices) are useful for loosening debris from the gingival sulcus and dislodging debris from orthodontic appliances. Oral irrigators will disrupt bacterial plaque, but will not remove it. Use of oral irrigation is sometimes referred to as hydrotherapy.

100.

E. Improper technique, abrasive dentifrices, water contamination of the etched enamel, and a hard-bristle toothbrush are all factors that will decrease the retention and effectiveness of a pit and fissure sealant. Precise technique must be used without contamination. Contaminants that will cause the sealant to fail are saliva and water.

101.

C. During mouth-to-mouth resuscitation or rescue breathing, repeat 12 times per minute for an adult, 20 times per minute for a child, and 20 times per minute for an infant. Maintain a hold under the patient's neck. At all times the airway must remain unobstructed.

102.

B. Cardiopulmonary resuscitation is administered when breathing and heart action have stopped. Without both of these, oxygen cannot be carried to the cells and a deficiency occurs quickly. Within 4 to 6 minutes, there may be irreversible brain damage. CPR includes cardiac compressions and breaths. When CPR is being performed by one person, 15 compressions are delivered followed by two ventilations. When CPR is performed by two persons, the same ratio applies.

103.

C. The Heimlich maneuver is performed in the event of an airway obstruction from a foreign body. The thrusts are given to provide pressure against the diaphragm that compresses the lungs, increasing pressure to the lungs, forcing air through the trachea and forcing the obstruction out. If the patient is sitting or standing, wrap the arms around the waist and make a fist. Hold the fist, thumb side down, above the navel and below the breastbone or xiphoid. Press the fist into the abdomen with quick upward thrusts.

104.

C. To date, chlorhexidine is the most effective chemical antiplaque and antigingivitis agent available. Listerine™, a phenolic compound, can be somewhat effective as an antiplaque, antigingivitis agent, but does not have the substantivity or the same bactericidal activity that chlorhexidine does. Hydrogen peroxide is an oxygenating agent and is effective in debridement, but does not have the bactericidal activity that chlorhexidine does. Zinc chloride is an astringent.

105.

C. Chemical germicides manufactured for disinfection are regulated and registered by the Environmental Protection Agency. Sodium hypochlorite, iodophors, and synthetic phenols are EPA registered and ADA accepted as surface disinfectants. Alcohol has been shown to be ineffective as a disinfectant; therefore, it is not EPA registered. Quaternary ammonium compounds have been shown to be ineffective as disinfectants, but have been shown to be effective cleaning agents.

106.

E. Utilization of barriers, high-volume suction, and antiretraction valves have all been shown to lessen the chance of cross-contamination. The water lines to the handpiece and the air/water syringe tip should also be flushed before each patient to lessen the chance of contamination

107.

C. In gingival curettage, the face of the blade should be positioned at a 70-degree angle with the soft tissue pocket wall or sulcular epithelium. The curette should be positioned at the bottom of the pocket, pressure applied with the finger on the outside of the pocket, with smooth even vertical strokes. The area should be flushed to remove debris and pressure applied to achieve close adaptation of the tissue to the tooth.

108.

F. The airabrasive polisher uses air and water pressure to propel fine particles of sodium bicarbonate in a warm spray. The spray must be kept in constant motion about 4–5 mm away from the tooth surface, angled away from the gingival margin. Precautions must be followed to minimize the contamination from aerosol production. The airabrasive is contraindicated in patients with respiratory conditions; a restricted sodium diet; a communicable disease; exposed cementum or dentin; soft, spongy gingiva; and nonmetallic restorations.

109.

D. The odontoblasts are cells of the pulp and the dentin. They form the organic matrix of the dentin and provide nutrition to the dentin and possibly play a role in the pain sensation of a tooth. They are also responsible for the formative, nutritive, and defensive functions of the pulp. The cells of the dentin should not be insulted by bacterial toxins, strong drugs, undue operative trauma (such as amalgam polishing), unnecessary thermal changes, or irritating restorative materials.

110.

D. Ending your series of sharpening strokes with a downward strike will prevent the formation of minute metal projections (wire edge) on the cutting edge.

111.

E. If sensitivity is experienced while using the ultrasonic scaler, you should evaluate the following: your pressure against the tooth, the water flow, the power setting, and your motion. Ultrasonic strokes should be applied lightly to the deposit; too much pressure will remove tooth structure. The handpiece and working end are cooled by the constant flow of water. Sensitivity and damage to the tooth may occur if there is an inadequate amount of water flowing through the handpiece. Constant motion of the instrument and the correct angulation of the tip to the tooth are also essential for correct operation of the ultrasonic scaler.

112.

B. Most fluoride is excreted through the kidneys, with a small amount excreted by the sweat glands.

113.

B. The pH of acidulated phosphate-fluoride gels is 3.0–3.5. Sodium fluoride (2%) has a basic pH of 9.2. Stannous fluoride (8%) has a pH of 2.1–2.3.

114.

A. Fluoride is essential to the formation of sound teeth. It is deposited during the formation of the enamel. Sources of fluoride include drinking water and other ingested fluoride, such as tablets, drops, and foods. If there is an excess of fluoride during the mineralization stage, a defective enamel matrix can form. This can lead to dental fluorosis.

115.

B. The use of the weekly rinse is the most common school-based program in the United States. Advantages are that it requires little time (about 5 minutes once weekly for an entire class); is inexpensive; is easy to learn and well accepted by participants; and can be carried out by nondental personnel. Responsibility for providing the correctly mixed solution and safe storage can be taken by school officials and a supervising dental hygienist.

116.

D. When determining the need for pediatric fluoride supplements, you need to consider the age of the patient, the amount of fluoride in the patient's drinking water, and the conscientiousness and motivation level of the patient or parents. Supervision must also be provided. The type of topical fluoride applied professionally is not a factor that you need to consider.

117.

A. For a three-year-old in a nonfluoridated area, tablets should be prescribed. For children from birth to two years of age, fluoride drops are primarily used. The tooth contact of the chewable tablet provides the enamel surface with protective fluoride.

118.

C. Chlorhexidine has been tested extensively and has been shown to be the most effective antiplaque and antigingivitis chemotherapeutic agent available. Chlorhexidine is active against a wide range of Gram-positive and Gram-negative organisms and fungi. It is rapidly adsorbed to teeth and pellicle and released slowly, thus prolonging the bactericidal effect.

119.

E. In selecting a toothbrush for a patient, the patient's manual dexterity, motivation and willingness, status of periodontal health, and the position of the patient's teeth should all be considered. All of these factors relate to the needs of the individual patient

120.

C. For most patients, dental floss is best used before brushing to assure that caries-susceptible proximal surfaces will be as free as possible from plaque and that the fluoride from the dentifrice used during brushing will be able to reach the proximal surfaces for caries prevention.

121.

D. Uptake of fluoride depends on the amount of fluoride ingested (not delivered) and the length of time of exposure. Fluoride is a natural constituent of enamel. The surface has the highest concentration and the amount decreases rapidly toward the interior layers of the tooth.

122.

B. The optimum fluoride level for water in temperate climates is 1 part per million (ppm). For warmer and colder climates, the amount can be adjusted from 0.6 to 1.2 ppm.

123.

E. Stannous fluoride and neutral sodium fluoride are recommended for head and neck cancer patients to protect them from post-irradiation caries. Daily fluoride applications are recommended while the patient is receiving radiation therapy. Custom trays are made prior to the start of therapy and the patient places the fluoride gel from the tray in the mouth for four minutes a day.

124.

A. Stannous fluoride may discolor tooth-colored restorations and margins. There may also be staining of the teeth in demineralized areas, pits, fissures, and grooves.

125.

B. Subjective symptoms such as pain, tenderness, and itching are symptoms observed by the patient. Objective symptoms are frequently called signs. A sign is any abnormality that may indicate a deviation from normal or disease that is discovered by a professional while examining a patient. Examples of signs are changes in color, shape, or consistency of a tissue not observable by the patient.

126.

B. A multiple fluoride preventive program is recommended for a patient with bulimia in an attempt to counteract dental erosion. A fluoride dentifrice, neutral sodium fluoride 0.05 percent rinse preparation,

and a daily gel tray application with neutral sodium is recommended.

127.

A. Applications of sealants should be made as soon as possible following eruption. When application is delayed, caries may start, and the surface no longer can be considered for sealant. When possible, sealants can be applied before full eruption, provided there is no tissue flap to interfere with application.

128.

F. Calculus is more readily removed from some tooth surfaces than others. The ease of removal is related to the mode of attachment of the calculus to the tooth surface. Calculus can attach by means of the acquired pellicle, by mechanical locking into undercuts or minute irregularities in the tooth, or by direct contact between the intercellular matrix and the tooth surface.

129.

B. At least two-thirds of the inorganic matter of calculus is crystalline, principally apatite. Predominating is hydroxyapatite, which is the same crystal present in enamel, dentin, cementum, and bone. Calculus also contains octocalcium phosphate, brushite, and whitlockite.

130.

B. Green stain is composed of chromogenic bacteria and fungi. Black line stain is similar to calculus in that it is composed of microorganisms. Yellow stains are usually caused by food pigments.

131.

B. Plaque consists of a complex mixture of microorganisms that occur primarily as microcolonies. The population density is very high and increases as plaque ages. Changes in the types of organisms occur within plaque as it matures. Vibrios and spirochetes appear from day 7 to day 14. More Gram-negative and anaerobic organisms appear. Also during this time, signs of inflammation are beginning to be observable. Early plaque consists of cocci, filaments, and slender rods.

132.

E. Plastic instruments are indicated for use on titanium implants, as metal instruments scratch the titanium surface. Scratching a titanium implant surface with an unlike metal can create a battery or the production of ferric chloride (a caustic chemical) that can lead to implant failure.

133.

B. The most frequently observed adverse reactions are those associated with the administration of local anesthetics. The majority of these reactions are stress-related (psychogenic). Injection of local anesthetics with the patient in an upright position is most likely to produce a psychogenic reaction. Palpitations, headache, sweating, mild shaking, dizziness, and breathing difficulty are usually of psychogenic origin or are related to the administration of large doses of vasoconstrictors and are not allergic in nature. Allergic reactions normally involve itching or a rash on the skin, diarrhea or nausea, runny nose or watery eyes, wheezing or laryngeal edema, or tachycardia or hypotension.

134.

E. A patient's record is a legal document that begins with the initial appointment the patient has in your office. These records must be reviewed and updated at each appointment and are maintained as long as the patient is under your care. Patient records are confidential and must be legible.

135.

D. The recall frequency depends on the needs of each patient. The primary objectives are the prevention of

new disease as well as the recurrence of disease. The appointment frequency depends on the patient's ability to control plaque, the rate of calculus formation, extent of previous treatment, restorative considerations, and systemic factors. Appointment intervals vary from 2 to 6 months.

136.

A. Hypoglycemia results when a patient has too much insulin or too little food in his or her system. The cause is lowered blood glucose with an excess of insulin. The symptoms may occur suddenly and include the following: fatigue, nausea, tachycardia, dizziness, sweating, headache, and the patient's breath may have a fruity, acetone odor. The treatment involves the administration of sugar or glucagon, depending on the patient's consciousness.

137.

A. The objective for successful root planing involves removal of factors that promote gingival inflammation (plaque, calculus, altered cementum) and irregular, roughened root surfaces. The technique for root planing is basically the same as for scaling. The difference between scaling and root planing should be the degree of resulting smoothness.

138.

B. Curettes are the most widely used and most effective and versatile of the periodontal instruments. The design of the curette allows it to be inserted subgingivally with less chance of trauma to the tissue. The curve of the blade of the curette adapts to the curved surfaces of the teeth. Most curettes are smaller and thinner than other scaling instruments, allowing for increased tactile sensitivity and ease in insertion. The universal curette can be adapted to all surfaces of the teeth. The Gracey curettes are the most commonly used area-specific curettes. Their design features permit maximum access to certain areas of the oral cavity. They are particularly useful in planing deep periodontal pockets.

139.

B. Exposed cementum and dentin predispose the patient to hypersensitive teeth. Hypersensitive teeth can be treated with fluoride or iontophoresis. The patient can help control it with plaque control, diet, nonabrasive dentifrices, and self-applied fluorides.

140.

E. Gingival curettage includes the removal of diseased sulcular epithelium and inflamed connective tissue. Scaling removes calculus. Root planing removes residual calculus and altered cementum.

141.

F. Local factors implicated in the etiology of periodontal disease are: calculus, mouth breathing, smoking and/or drug use, tooth malposition, and faulty restorations. The American Academy of Periodontology has classified periodontal disease into four types. Type I is gingivitis, Type II is early periodontitis, Type III is moderate periodontitis, and Type IV is advanced periodontitis.

142.

C. Gingival abscesses occur when bacteria invade through some break in the gingival tissue. They can occur as a result of mastication, oral hygiene procedures, or dental treatment. The gingival sulcus is rarely involved at the onset.

143.

A. The origin of the gingival cyst is probably from remnants of the dental lamina or as a result of traumatic implantation of surface epithelium into gingival connective tissue. The overlying epithelium is intact and smooth. The lesion may appear white to blue.

144.

D. Calculus is mineralized plaque; therefore, it causes irritation to the tissue. Submarginal calculus is always covered by active plaque, which is in direct contact with the sulcular epithelium. Its permeable surface serves as an excellent storage place for bacteria.

145.

A. Pocket formation and probing depths represent the severity of periodontal disease. Mobility and bleeding are also associated with periodontal disease, but the depth of periodontal pockets determines the severity of the condition.

146.

B. The presence of furcation involvement is best detected by use of special curved probes such as a Nabers-1 or a Nabers-2 probe.

147.

F. When selecting the appropriate instrument, you must consider the length of the clinical crown, pocket depth, amount of calculus, accessibility of the area to be scaled, and the tissue state. Longer shanks with more acute bends are necessary to scale or plane posterior areas with deeper pocket depths. Curettes with fine flexible shanks would not be indicated for a patient with tenacious calculus. Large, bulky blades are inappropriate in patients with firm, nonretractable tissue.

148.

E. A dental treatment plan involves various phases. Phase I therapy is also called initial therapy. It may involve any or all of the following: patient education and establishment of therapist-patient alliance, treatment of dental emergencies, oral hygiene instructions, scaling and root planing, caries control, removal of overhangs and other inadequate restorations, endodontics, extraction of hopeless teeth, temporary stabilization, occlusal adjustment, and reevaluation. Reevaluation is done throughout all phases of treatment. Phase II therapy is called surgical and restorative therapy. It includes periodontal surgery and/or final restorative treatment. Phase III is the maintenance phase. In this phase, long-term follow-up care is provided.

149.

A. Peri-implantitis is similar to chronic adult periodontitis and is preceded by gingivitis characterized by gingiva that is edematous, enlarged, red, and/or hyperplastic. If peri-implantitis is untreated, the inflammation will increase in severity, resulting in bleeding upon probing, increased probing depths, mobility, fistulas, osteitis, and radiographic signs of bone loss.

150.

D. Juvenile periodontitis is a periodontal condition usually affecting permanent first molars and incisors of adolescents. The most prevalent organisms associated with this condition are *Actinobacillus actinomycetemcomitans* and *Capnocytophaga sputigena*. The periodontal breakdown progresses rapidly and often appears to become arrested.

151.

B. The active ingredient in PerioChip® is 2.5 mg of chlorhexidine gluconate.

152.

B. Diagnostic casts can be made of the patient's mouth to study the dentition and to educate the patient. At the time the casts are made, the patient will be interested in seeing the arrangement of the teeth. Tooth form and arrangement of the dentition can be observed. These casts are not of sufficient precision to allow fabrication of fixed dental prostheses.

153.

A. Casting involves heating a metal until molten and pouring or forcing it into a mold for it to harden. Some metals that are not brittle can be formed into useful shapes by the use of mechanical forces, such as rolling or wire drawing. Inlays, crowns, bridges, and partial denture frameworks are usually cast, while wires and most orthodontic appliances are wrought.

154.

B. No polymers in dentistry use radioactive materials to effect the polymerization reaction. Heat curing is most commonly used for denture base resins, while light-cured and self-curing resins have many dental applications.

155.

A. Exhibiting concern and empathy for others is called caring. Healthcare providers should always exhibit care for their patients and must always treat patients as they themselves would want to be treated.

156.

A. Normative ethics describes a group of theories that provide, define, and describe a system of principles and rules that determine which actions are deemed right or wrong. They include Consequentilist or Utilitarian, Deontology or Nonconsequentionalism (Kantian), and Virtue ethics.

157.

C. Virtue ethics places emphasis on the character traits of an individual.

158.

A. Nonmaleficence means that a health care provider's first obligation to the patient is to do no harm. Basically, a health care provider ought not to inflict harm, and ought to prevent harm, ought to remove harm, and ought to do or promote good.

159.

B. Beneficence means that a dental hygienist should provide quality health care that is a benefit to the patient.

160.

C. Justice is when a dental hygienist is providing individuals or a group with what is owed, due, and/or deserved.

161.

D. Nonmaleficence means that a dental hygienist should prevent harm, remove harm, and not inflict harm. Dental hygienists should prevent diseases/conditions, treat and/or refer diseases/conditions appropriately, and practice current, safe treatment modalities.

162.

A. Autonomy is the ability to govern one's own profession and to basically be self-determined and directed as a profession. Although organized dental hygiene has assumed a direction for the profession, legally, dental hygiene is stilled governed by dentistry.

163.

A. Autonomy is a principle that is based on respect for others and the belief that patients have the power to make decisions about things that may affect their health. Dental hygienists must strive for patient/provider autonomy.

164.

D. Veracity is another term for honesty. Obviously, as in all aspects of life, honesty is mandatory for a dental hygiene provider.

165.

A. The Ramfjord teeth, by definition, are those included in answer A.

166.

B. Fluoridation is the controlled adjustment of the fluoride ion content of a domestic water supply to the optimum concentration that will provide maximum protection against dental caries.

167.

A. The results of the DMFT index yields a group's caries susceptibility without use of radiographs. However, the DMFS measures carious, missing, or filled surfaces and often incorporates use of radiographs. The CPITN and the TSIF are not used for measurement of caries. Use of radiographs in diagnosis of DMF surfaces is of far greater importance for determining immediate treatment need, whereas visual exams without radiographs can estimate caries susceptibility.

168.

C. Fluoride is taken up at the tooth surface from both fluoridated drinking water and topical application. Some is deposited harmlessly within the skeletal system, even at 8 ppm.

169.

A. According to Burt, increased public awareness resulting from caries prevention activities of water fluoridation has had a major impact as to how the public views tooth loss. Public acceptance of water fluoridation was essential for initiation and continuation of this public health program.

170.

B. According to Burt, results of many studies have shown no benefit of use of prenatal fluoride supplements.

171.

D. In the January 1990 issue of *Science*, the fluoride controversy reemerged with arguments launched concerning water fluoridation's relationship to cancer. Burt disputes charges that fluoridation is unsafe.

172.

A. The human body possesses an efficient excretory mechanism for fluorides. No damage to the human body has been reported from fluoridation of domestic water supplies.

173.

D. Dental health surveys often underestimate dental treatment due to complicating factors. Criteria used to diagnose caries may vary; incongruencies occur between patients' perceived needs and practitioners' ideas of need; surveys look at short-term findings while practitioners must be concerned with long-term outcomes for patients; and treatment philosophies change rapidly.

174.

C. The Root Caries Index (RCI) is unique as compared to DMF and other indexes because it takes into account "teeth at risk." A tooth is considered to be at risk of dental root caries if enough gingival recession has occurred to expose the cementum to the oral environment.

175.

D. The indirect method of scoring loss of periodontal attachment (LPA) utilizes a fixed point, the cementoenamel junction (CEJ), in partial calculation of the index. The first step is a traditional measure of pocket depth, the second measure is the measurement from gingival crest to the CEJ, and the final calculation is step one minus step two. Other indexes utilizing the first step only may give inaccurate readings because the level of the gingiva is not always static.

176.

D. For a community presentation for deaf audiences, flashing lights on and off is necessary to attract the group's attention. Interpreters are used to interpret only and probably have little knowledge concerning a dental hygiene-related topic. Allow ample time for the audience to review handouts prior to the beginning of the presentation because deaf individuals depend on reading for communication, and also must rely on their sight to follow the presenter and/or interpreter.

177.

D. The Klein and Palmer Index can be recorded as "S" for surface and "T" for tooth. Surface counts are more sensitive than tooth counts. DMFS requires the use of radiographs, is more time-consuming, and requires that the examiner be highly skilled in the use of the index.

178.

C. While the first statement is true and may be explained by earlier tooth eruption patterns in females and utilization of dental care, current research demonstrates that it is erroneous at this time to assume from these findings that females are more caries-susceptible than males.

179.

B. The OHI-S measures plaque and calculus on six surfaces of six teeth. Caries and gingival bleeding are not determined by this index.

180.

C. The Community Periodontal Index of Treatment Needs (CPITN) is an index of treatment needs rather than an index for determining periodontal status. These are the four treatment categories: 0 = no treatment necessary; I = improved oral hygiene needed; II = improved oral hygiene and scaling needed; and III = improved oral hygiene, scaling, and complex treatment needed.

181.

A. Periodontal disease, for many years, was thought to be the major cause of tooth loss. Recently, research has revealed that dental caries is the primary cause of tooth loss at almost all ages, with the exception of the very old.

182.

A. The results of a program are measured against the objectives developed during planning. Effectiveness deals with the attainment of objectives. Efficiency deals with cost-effectiveness.

183.

A. Rampant caries may be seen in children with poor oral hygiene or adults with xerostomia and gingival recession.

184.

A. The Plaque Index is used to determine accumulation of plaque and oral debris. The Gingival Index is used to determine, as the name indicates, bleeding and gingival health. DMFS and DMFT are caries indices.

185.

B. Just the opposite is true. While edentulism reflects attitude toward treatment by both patient and dentist, partial edentulism seems to be more closely related to oral hygiene.

186.

D. Fluorosis occurs when excessive amounts of fluoride are ingested during tooth development.

187.

B. By definition, sensitivity is a proportion of positive tests with subsequent disease. It should not be confused with the term *specificity*, which, by definition, is the proportion of negative tests without subsequent disease.

188.

B. When a patient comes to the dental office or clinic, the dentist first performs a careful examination. The first step in modern public health procedures is identical to that used by the dental clinician, only here it is the community that must be examined. It is called a survey instead of an examination.

189.

A. The future use of dental services will most likely be linked to the patient's gender (female), high socioeconomic status, and presence of most all natural teeth.

190.

B. Dean, in his early work with fluoridation, reported that 7–16% of children exhibited some form of fluorosis. However, this figure has increased in children today, with various studies reporting from 22 to 25%.

191.

B. This school-based dental clinic focuses on all aspects of prevention including assessment, education, and therapy.

192.

D. These methods utilize many aspects to help all learners comprehend the material and remain interactive between the teacher and the learner. Most important, learner participation is necessary for comprehensive understanding of the material.

193.

C. DMFT/deft will reveal dental caries status and will allow for mixed dentition, without the time devoted to taking radiographs, which is needed in the DMFS/defs. OHI-S will reveal plaque and calculus status.

194.

D. Consent is always necessary before any process is started.

195.

C. A strong referral program is always necessary to ensure comprehensive patient care.

196.

D. When assessing a program for students, familial income and education are the least important factors to analyze.

197.

D. Selection of dental index has nothing to do with a physical disability. The use of a dental index is done to ascertain the desired information about dental disease, status, or need.

198.

C. The means is the arithmetic average of the data.

199.

C. The mode is the most frequently occurring number in a set of data.

200.

A. Any score close to +1 or −1 is a strong correlation.

patient history
synopsis

CASE 1
Age 36
Sex F
Height 5′ 4″
Weight 180lbs/81.8kg

VITAL SIGNS
Blood pressure 130/90
Pulse rate 77
Respiration rate 18

1. Under the care of a physician
☐ Yes ☒ No

2. Hospitalized within the last 5 years
☐ Yes ☒ No

3. Has or had the following conditions:
None

4. Current medication(s)
Patient is taking the contraceptive Ortho-Novum 1/50.

5. Smokes or uses tobacco products
☐ Yes ☒ No

6. Is pregnant
☐ Yes ☒ No ☐ N/A

Medical History: A year ago, the patient lost 75 lbs. while taking Redux (dexfenfluramine hydrochloride) for a period of 6 months. The patient reports she is allergic to penicillin.

Dental History: Five years ago, the patient received periodontal treatment and since, maintenance therapy. The patient reports brushing and flossing her teeth at least twice daily. She also clenches her teeth occasionally. Her last dental visit was 6 months ago for a recall appointment.

Social History: The patient reports a history of weight problems throughout adulthood and a family history of hypertension.

Chief Complaint: Periodontal maintenance therapy; sensitivity to cold

---

ADULT CLINICAL EXAMINATION

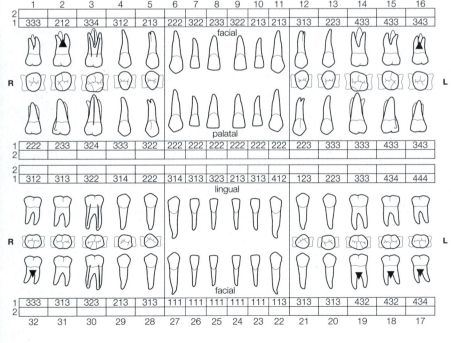

	1	2	3	4	5	6	7	8	9	10	11	12	13	14	15	16
2																
1	333	212	334	312	213	222	322	233	322	213	213	313	223	433	433	343

facial (R … L)
palatal

1	222	233	324	333	322	222	222	222	222	222	222	223	333	333	433	343
2																

2																
1	312	313	322	314	222	314	313	323	213	313	412	123	223	333	434	444

lingual (R … L)
facial

1	333	313	323	213	313	111	111	111	111	111	113	313	313	432	432	434
2																
	32	31	30	29	28	27	26	25	24	23	22	21	20	19	18	17

Current Oral Hygiene Status
1. Good oral hygiene
2. Slight calculus

Supplemental Oral Examination Findings
1. .5 mobility #23, 25, 26
2. Class I mobility #24
3. Root canal therapy #30

Ⓜ Clinically visible carious lesion
✖ Clinically missing tooth
△ Furcation
▲ "Through and through" furcation

Probe 1: initial probing depth
Probe 2: probing depth 1 month after scaling and root planing

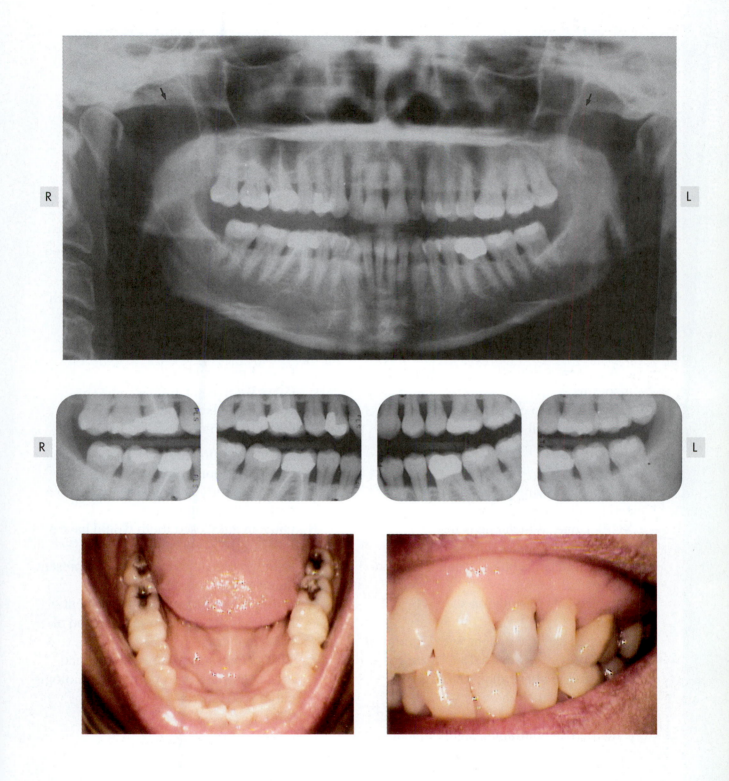

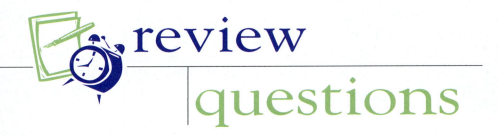

review
questions

DIRECTIONS Each of the questions or incomplete statements below is followed by suggested answers or completions. Select the **one** answer that is best in each case.

---

1. What is the clinical significance of the reported past use of the weight reduction medication, Redux™?
   A. There is no clinical significance
   B. A common side effect is esophageal spasms
   C. It is known to cause valvular spasms
   D. It causes renal damage
   E. It produces a painless enlargement of the liver

2. All of the following procedures are indicated for this client before treatment EXCEPT one. Which one is the EXCEPTION?
   A. The clinician should consult a pharmacological reference
   B. A medical consultation should be obtained
   C. Premedicate the patient with 2 grams of Cephalexin® 1 hour before treatment
   D. Inform the client about the diastolic blood pressure reading
   E. Conclude there is no health condition that would contraindicate treatment

3. On examining the intraoral images, which of the following classifications BEST describes the client's occlusion?
   A. Class I ideal occlusion
   B. Class I malocclusion
   C. Class II, division 1
   D. Class II, division 2
   E. Class III occlusion

4. Which of the following is NOT an accurate description of tooth mobility?
   A. Tooth mobility is typically graded on a scale of 0 through 3
   B. Only an ankylosed tooth would have a score of 0 tooth mobility
   C. Radiographs do not accurately represent the degree of tooth mobility
   D. Bidigital evaluation with instrument handles is the conventional method of measurement
   E. This patient has tooth mobility readings consistent with normal physiological movement

case study 1 questions

5. Examine the panoramic radiograph and intraoral camera image of the mandibular arch. What, MOST likely, is the identity of the mass located in the right and left premolar regions of the mandible?
   A. Condensing osteitis
   B. Primary molar root tips
   C. Bilateral mandibular tori
   D. Salivary stones at the duct orifices
   E. Chronic focal sclerosing osteomyelitis

6. Considering the clinical and radiographic information, which of the following Case Types BEST classifies this client's disease progression?
   A. I
   B. II
   C. III
   D. IV
   E. V

7. Of the following, which one MOST likely accounts for the client's reported sensitivity to cold?
   A. Exposed cementum
   B. Teeth clenching
   C. Recurrent caries
   D. Tooth mobility

8. Which of the following descriptions is NOT accurate regarding furcation involvement?
   A. A Shepherd's hook explorer and Nabors probe are instruments used to determine the degree of involvement
   B. Furcation occurs when the loss of attachment extends into the bifurcation or trifurcation of multirooted teeth
   C. Class I involvement indicates an early lesion in which the concavity of the furcation is detected
   D. The interradicular bone is resorbed, exposing a through-and-through tunnel in Class II involvement
   E. Class III involvement is indicated when the radiographs demonstrate an obvious radiolucency within the furcation

9. Examine the molar bitewings. What correction is necessary to minimize the overlapping of the interproximal surfaces of the molar teeth?
   A. Decrease the positive vertical angulation
   B. Direct the central ray to the center of the film
   C. Move the horizontal angulation more forward
   D. Align the PID in a negative vertical angulation
   E. Direct the horizontal angulation more posterior

10. Which of the following observations is NOT demonstrated on the bitewing radiographs?
   A. Root caries on 5, 11, 13, 19
   B. Generalized mild to moderate horizontal bone loss
   C. Class II amalgam restorations on 2, 5, and 14
   D. 3 and 30 have been endodontically treated with gutta percha
   E. Occlusal amalgams on 1, 2, 15, 16, 17, 18, 31, 32

case study 1 questions

11. In many clients, oral contraceptives may cause a condition mimicking pregnancy gingivitis. What bacteria would predominate in this condition?
    A. *Mutans streptococcus*
    B. *Streptococcus salivarius*
    C. *Prevotella intermedia*
    D. *Porphymonas gingivalis*

12. What is the correct description of the structure identified by the arrows on the panoramic photo?
    A. Fracture of the zygomatic process of the temporal bone
    B. Space between the maxilla and the lateral pterygoid plate
    C. Suture between the processes that form the zygoma
    D. Fine posterior boundary of the infraorbital canal
    E. Posterior wall of the maxillary sinus cavity

13. Which of the following reevaluation intervals is most appropriate for this patient?
    A. 1 month
    B. 2 months
    C. 3 months
    D. 6 months

14. Should antibiotics be necessary to treat this patient, what would be the drug of choice?
    A. Amoxicillin
    B. Clindamycin
    C. Cephalexin
    D. Erythromycin

15. What would you recommend to this client regarding her clenching of teeth?
    A. A full acrylic mouth guard
    B. Composite restorations on worn surfaces
    C. Repositioning splint
    D. No treatment needed

✓answers & rationales

1.

C. This diet drug causes valvular damage, increasing the risk of bacteria during oral procedures. The diet drugs Pondimin® and Redux™ were removed from the market because of potential cardiac and pulmonary side effects including valvular damage and pulmonary hypertension. Clients who have taken these drugs must be assumed to have a valvular damage until proven otherwise and precautions must be taken before undertaking procedures that are likely to induce a bacteremia. Any client who has taken these drugs in the past requires a medical consultation from his/her physician to determine any cardiac damage and the necessity of antibiotic prophylaxis before dental procedures to prevent endocarditis.

2.

E. Conclude that the client has had no health conditions that would contraindicate treatment. This client is at high risk for developing endocarditis from scaling and polishing procedures. It is best to err on the side of caution than to proceed without proper investigation, consultation, or precautions.

3.

B. The mesiobuccal cusp of the maxillary molar occludes in the buccal groove of the mandibular molar and the maxillary canine occludes between the mandibular canine and first premolar on the right and left sides. These observations are consistent with Class I occlusion, although the anterior teeth are crowded. The best classification of this dentition would be Class I malocclusion or Class I occlusion with anterior crowding.

4.

E. This client has tooth mobility readings consistent with normal physiological movement. Typically, normal physiological movement is not graded. This client has scores ranging from .5 mm to 1 mm, which indicates that the involved teeth have slightly greater mobility than normal and up to 1 mm of movement buccolingually.

5.

C. On the panoramic radiograph, areas of increased bone density are evident just inferior to the mandibular canine and premolar teeth. This is common radiographic presentation of mandibular tori. In the mandibular arch intraoral camera view, the mandibular tori appear on the lingual surface of the mandible adjacent to the canine and premolar teeth. Condensing osteitis, root tips, salivary stones, and chronic focal sclerosing osteomyelitis are not evident on the intraoral camera image.

6.

B. The client presents with mild periodontitis with probing depths measuring from 3 to 4 mm from the cementoenamel junction (CEJ). Recession is present in all sextants and furcation involvement was noted on several maxillary and mandibular molars. There is radiographic evidence of furcation involvement on teeth #s 19 and 30 and clinical evidence of .5–1 mm mobility of the mandibular anterior teeth. Although the client is predominantly a Case Type II, the clinical evidence of furcation involvement and tooth mobility places her into the Case Type III classification.

7.

A. The cementum is exposed as a result of gingival recession and bone loss. The exposed root surfaces tend to be more sensitive to cold air and fluids. There is no clinical evidence of recurrent caries or enough tooth mobility to warrant cold sensitivity. The client assessment does not denote tooth clenching.

8.

D. Interradicular bone is resorbed, exposing a through-and-through tunnel in Class II involvement. In Class II furcation involvement, the explorer or probe can enter the furcation but not extend through to the other side. The description in the correct answer is consistent with Class III furcation involvement rather than Class II.

9.

C. To correct horizontal overlap, the horizontal angulation needs to be directed in a more forward direction. The horizontal angle was aligned too far posterior resulting in interproximal overlap. To correct this error, move the horizontal angle forward until the horizontal angle directs the x-rays through the contacts of the molar teeth. Adjusting vertical angulation does not correct overlapping. Directing the central ray corrects conecutting, not overlapping. Redirecting the horizontal angulation more posterior would maximize rather than minimize the overlapping.

10.

A. The radiolucent areas on the interproximal root surfaces are consistent with cervical burnout but not root caries. Cervical burnout is a phenomenon of x-ray penetration of cervical tooth anatomy. The cervical tooth anatomy is thinner and thus more radiolucent than the enamel above it and alveolar crest below it.

11.

B. *Provotella intermedia* predominates in all types of hormonal gingivitis. *S. Salivarius* is not linked to development of gingivitis; it is a common inhabitant of saliva. *Porphymonas gingivalis* is common in all types of periodontal disease, but is not considered the primary etiologic agent in pregnancy gingivitis. *Mutans streptococcus* is implicated as the primary etiologic agent in human caries.

12.

C. This structure is the zygomaticotemporal suture. It is the radiolucent diagonal junction between the zygomatic process of the temporal bone and the temporal process of the zygomatic bone. Together these processes form the zygoma.

13.

C. This patient is periodontally maintained, and a 3-month recall is appropriate for maintenance of this patient.

14.

B. Clindamycin is the drug of choice for patients allergic to penicillin. Amoxicillin and cephalexin both should not be given to patients allergic to penicillin.

15.

A. A full acrylic mouth guard is the first choice for the treatment of bruxism. A repositioning splint is used for severe bruxism and looks like the traditional night guard but has certain functions built into it. This device protects your teeth when you do grind but, in addition, it reduces your urge to grind.

patient history
synopsis

CASE 2	VITAL SIGNS
Age 16	Blood pressure 140/85
Sex F	Pulse rate 80
Height 5'4"	Respiration rate 20
Weight 165lbs/75kg	

1. Under the care of a physician

☐ Yes   ☒ No

2. Hospitalized within the last 5 years

☐ Yes   ☒ No

3. Has or had the following conditions:

None

4. Current medication(s)

She has been advised to take 400–1,000 mg of folate and 30 mg of ferrous sulfate tid, but often forgets to take her medications. The client has vitamin B_{12} injections monthly.

5. Smokes or uses tobacco products

☐ Yes   ☒ No

6. Is pregnant

☐ Yes   ☒ No   ☐ N/A

Medical History: This client has a history of morbid obesity. Two years ago she weighed 200 lbs. Repeated weight loss attempts with fad diets have failed. The client has multiple chronic nutrient deficiencies, including folate and vitamin B_{12}.

Dental History: The client's radiographs indicate extensive interproximal caries, with one tooth requiring endodontic therapy. She brushes twice a day and flosses once a day.

Social History: This client is a sophomore in high school and lives at home.

Chief Complaint: "My teeth hurt."

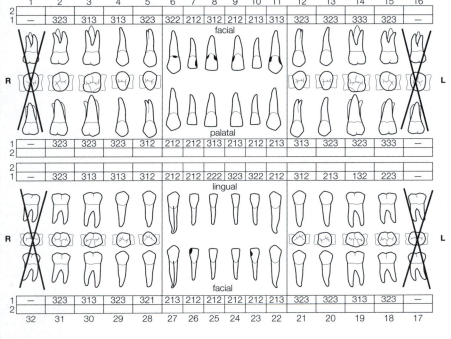

ADULT CLINICAL EXAMINATION

Current Oral Hygiene Status
1. Plaque scores are below 20%

Supplemental Oral Examination Findings
1. Periodontal data reveal all pocket depths are 3mm or less

 Clinically visible carious lesion

 Clinically missing tooth

△ Furcation

▲ "Through and through" furcation

Probe 1: initial probing depth

Probe 2: probing depth 1 month after scaling and root planing

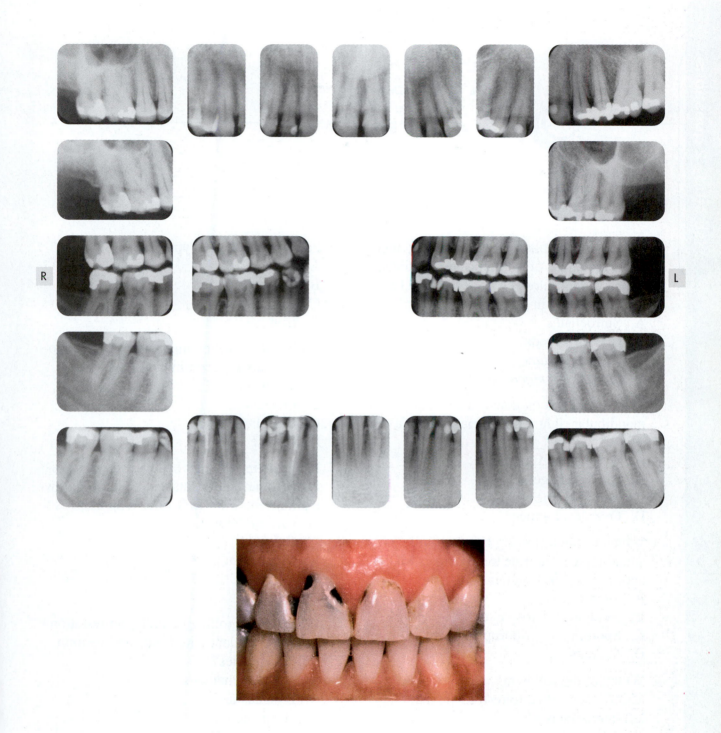

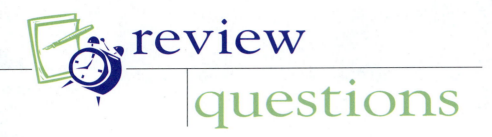

review questions

1. Since this client has no bleeding on probing and a few areas of 3-mm pocket readings, which of the following bacteria would be more prevalent in her plaque?
   A. Spirochetes
   B. Cocci and rods
   C. *Fusobacterium*
   D. *Mutans streptococcus*

2. The radiolucent diagonal lines on the mandibular right molar periapical are a result of:
   A. Overlapped films
   B. Light leakage
   C. Film bending
   D. Overdevelopment

3. Which of the following types of professional topical fluoride treatments is MOST appropriate for this client?
   A. Stannous
   B. Acidulated phosphate
   C. Sodium monofluorophosphate
   D. Sodium

4. Which of the following materials was MOST likely used to restore the maxillary left lateral incisor?
   A. Dental amalgam
   B. Composite resin
   C. Gold alloy
   D. Glass ionomer cement

5. Ferrous sulfate is a type of
   A. Vitamin B
   B. Calcium
   C. Hormone
   D. Iron

6. Which of the following is a good anticariogenic snack to recommend to this client?
   A. Crackers
   B. Pretzels
   C. Carrots
   D. Cheese

7. In evaluating the diet history, this client is likely to have poor intakes of all the following nutrients EXCEPT one. Which one is the EXCEPTION?
   A. Calcium
   B. Vitamin D
   C. Vitamin C
   D. Thiamin

8. Which of the following oral manifestations would be evident with folate and vitamin B_{12} deficiencies?
   A. Angular cheilosis
   B. Dysgeusia
   C. Dysphagia
   D. Oral candidiasis

case study 2 questions

9. The clinician determined that the density of the bitewing radiographs was lower than desired. Of the following, which one would NOT have caused the problem?
   A. Underestimation of the client's size and stature
   B. Exposure time was at too high of a setting
   C. Weak or exhausted developer chemicals
   D. Processing temperature was too low
   E. Exposure button was released too soon

10. Ferrous sulfate is being taken
    A. As needed
    B. Before meals
    C. Twice a day
    D. Three times a day

11. Folate and vitamin B_{12} are important for the integrity of the oral mucosa because they are involved in DNA synthesis, cell growth, and maintenance.
    A. Both statement and reason are correct and related
    B. Both statement and reason are correct, but not related
    C. The statement is correct, but the reason is not
    D. The statement is not correct, but the reason is
    E. Neither the statement nor the reason is correct

12. The MOST appropriate recommendation for this client is to see a(n)
    A. High school counselor
    B. School psychologist
    C. Oral surgeon
    D. Dietitian

13. According to the principles, of dietary counseling, how should the dental hygienist assess the patient's eating habits?
    A. Ask patient to keep a record of all food and beverage intake for a specified length of time, usually 3–5 days
    B. Ask patient to tell you what she normally eats during the day
    C. Ask the patient what type of exercise program she is on
    D. Determine the patient's motivation based on how much she weighs

14. During the restorative treatment this client will be anesthetized with Lidocaine 2%, 1:100,000 epinephrine. What is the maximum permissible dose this client can have in milligrams?
    A. 370 mg
    B. 300 mg
    C. 400 mg
    D. 250 mg

15. During the restorative phase of this client's treatment the dentist asks the dental hygienist to administer the anesthetic. Minutes following your initial injection, the client seems nervous and complains of dizziness, lightheadedness, and a racing heart. Her color is ashen and her extremities feel cold and clammy. Which of the following BEST labels the clinical symptom described?
    a. Systemic toxic overdose
    b. Urticaria
    c. Allergic reaction
    d. Syncope

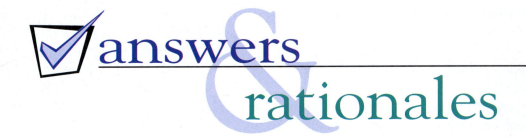

answers & rationales

1.

B. The client has small amounts of plaque owing to her good home care measures. Gram-positive cocci and few rods predominate at this stage. Spirochetes and vibrios are common in mature plaque. *Fusobacterium* are more common in the middle stages of plaque development.

2.

C. Film bending causes radiolucent diagonal lines on a radiograph. Films that stick together during processing will usually have the outline border of the other film and will have dark and white areas, not lines. Since x-rays are sensitive to light, the exposed areas will appear black. The entire density of the film will appear radiolucent with overdevelopment.

3.

D. The appropriate professional topical fluoride for this client is sodium because she has composite restorations. Sodium fluoride does not etch the glass particles in composite restorations. Stannous fluoride has a strong metallic taste, which should be considered when treating a patient. It also causes brown staining in carious tooth structures. Acidulated phosphate fluoride has the disadvantage of possibly etching ceramic or porcelain restorations and should be used with caution. Sodium monofluorophosphate fluoride is recognized as effective and safe for over-the-counter toothpaste use.

4.

B. Composite resin is often used as a direct esthetic material, especially in an area where significant strength of the material is required. Dental amalgam and gold alloy are not recommended for anterior restorations for esthetic reasons. Glass ionomer cement is a brittle material and not recommended for restorations that are subjected to high stress or wear.

5.

D. Ferrous pertains to iron. Ferrous sulfate is prescribed to treat iron deficiency. It does not refer to vitamin B, calcium, or hormones.

6.

D. Cheese has been found to be anticariogenic, possibly because of its high calcium and phosphate concentrations. However, crackers and pretzels are retentive polysaccharides that could promote tooth decay. Carrots are an excellent source of fiber.

7.

D. Thiamin is found in abundance in enriched crackers, breads, and pastas that this client consumes. However, she would be deficient in calcium and vitamins D and C.

8.

A. Angular cheilosis is a common oral manifestation of B-vitamin deficiencies. Dysgeusia refers to a distortion in taste. Dysphagia refers to difficulty in swallowing. Neither is an oral manifestation of B-vitamin deficiencies. Oral candidiasis is not an oral manifestation of folate and vitamin B_{12} deficiencies.

9.

B. This selection would produce a high density or dark radiograph rather than a low density radiograph. Underestimation of the client's size and stature, weak or exhausted developer chemicals, low processing temperature, and releasing the exposure button would result in a low density image.

10.

D. As stated in the client's medication listing, she is taking ferrous sulfate tid (three times a day). The abbreviations for a needed, before meals, and twice a day are PRN, AC, and bid, respectively.

11.

A. Both the statement and reason are related and correct regarding folate and vitamin B_{12}.

12.

D. Since this client has a history of morbid obesity, nutritional deficiencies, and a high decay rate, it would be highly recommended she see a dietitian for proper nutritional counseling. A school counselor or psychologist would not be qualified in the area of nutrition. It is hoped her dentition will be restored and will not require oral surgery for the removal of any teeth.

13.

A. Asking the patient to keep a record of all food and beverage intake will allow the dental hygienist to code each food item according to the food groups of the food guide pyramid, estimate the number of servings of each food according to food group, and code foods that contain sugar and/or cooked starches.

14.

B. The client can receive 300 mg. The absolute maximum dose of Lidocaine is 300 mg, even if the patient's weight is higher, and the calculation based on weight indicates that this patient can receive more than 300 mg.

15.

D. Syncopy is the sudden transient loss of consciousness that usually occurs secondary to a period of cerebral ischemia. Symptoms include anxiety, pallor, diaphoresis, tachycardia followed by bradycardia, decreased blood pressure (transient increase in blood pressure followed by rapid decrease), loss of consciousness, dilatation of pupils, nausea.

patient history
synopsis

CASE 3	VITAL SIGNS
Age 32	Blood pressure 145/90
Sex F	Pulse rate 90
Height 5'7"	Respiration rate 18
Weight 145lbs/65.9kg	

1. Under the care of a physician

☐ Yes   ☒ No

2. Hospitalized within the last 5 years

☐ Yes   ☒ No

3. Has or had the following conditions:

None

4. Current medication(s)

She reports taking Prozac and oral contraceptives at bedtime and Proventil 3–4 times/day.

5. Smokes or uses tobacco products

☐ Yes   ☒ No

6. Is pregnant

☐ Yes   ☒ No   ☐ N/A

Medical History: The client has been diagnosed with asthma and clinical depression. She states her mother was a diabetic and her father died of a heart attack at age 45.

Dental History: She has had routine dental treatment throughout her life and received a dental prophylaxis 9 months ago. She reports that she brushes her teeth twice a day and flosses once a day.

Social History: The client has earned a Master's degree in computer science, manages the computer networks of a major regional bank, and is the wife of an insurance executive.

Chief Complaint: "I am unhappy with the way my front teeth look."

ADULT CLINICAL EXAMINATION

	1	2	3	4	5	6	7	8	9	10	11	12	13	14	15	16
2/1	—	323	333	324	433	323	323	323	323	323	323	323	323	323	424	—

facial

R   L

palatal

| 1/2 | — | 323 | 333 | 324 | 533 | 323 | 322 | 332 | 323 | 323 | 323 | 323 | 323 | 434 | 423 | — |

| 2/1 | — | 434 | 333 | 323 | 323 | 332 | 223 | 323 | 323 | 323 | 323 | 324 | 434 | 434 | 423 | — |

lingual

R   L

facial

| 1/2 | — | 434 | 434 | 323 | 233 | 232 | 222 | 323 | 323 | 323 | 323 | 324 | 434 | 434 | 423 | — |

| | 32 | 31 | 30 | 29 | 28 | 27 | 26 | 25 | 24 | 23 | 22 | 21 | 20 | 19 | 18 | 17 |

Current Oral Hygiene Status
1. Brushes twice per day.
2. Flosses once per day.
3. Slight calculus

Supplemental Oral Examination Findings
1. Evidence of slight gingivitis

⊓ Clinically visible carious lesion

⊠ Clinically missing tooth

△ Furcation

▲ "Through and through" furcation

Probe 1: initial probing depth

Probe 2: probing depth 1 month after scaling and root planing

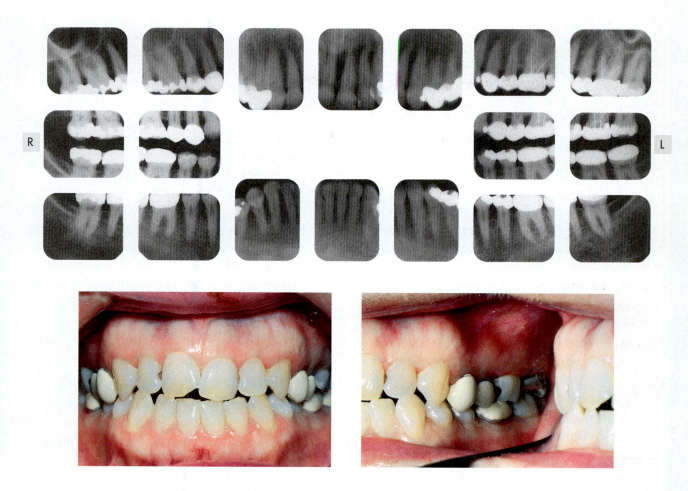

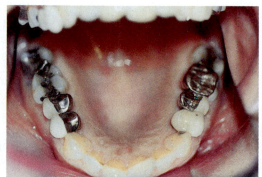

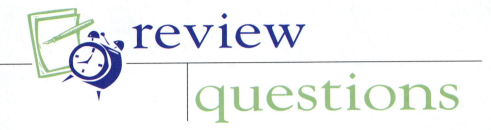

review questions

1. During treatment, the client starts experiencing dyspnea and wheezing on exhalation—characteristic of an acute asthmatic attack. The first step to be taken after seating the client in the most comfortable position is to
   A. Administer oxygen
   B. Prepare a cortocosteroid injection for the dentist to administer
   C. Assist the client in use of her own bronchodilator
   D. Administer sedation

2. All of the following are side effects of Proventil EXCEPT one. Which one is the EXCEPTION?
   A. Taste changes
   B. Xerostomia
   C. Ecchymoses
   D. Tooth discoloration

3. The radiographic survey demonstrates that the maxillary left first molar has undergone endodontic therapy. Close examination reveals a difference in radiodensity between the two buccal and palatal canals. Why is that difference observed?
   A. The canals were likely obstructed at different times
   B. Gold posts are present in the buccal canals
   C. Gutta percha is present in the buccal canals and a silver point in the palatal canal
   D. Gutta percha is present in the palatal canal and silver points in the buccal canals

4. By using the photographic and radiographic surveys, it can be determined that the mandibular first molar has been restored. Which of the following types of restoration is present?
   A. All-ceramic
   B. Porcelain fused to metal (metal ceramic)
   C. Indirect composite full coverage crown
   D. 3/4-gold crown

5. In evaluating the client's blood pressure, which of the following considerations would be MOST appropriate before treatment is rendered?
   A. Dental treatment can be rendered with no further consideration
   B. A medical referral is recommended before treatment is provided
   C. A medical referral is required before treatment is provided
   D. Blood pressure measurement should be retaken before treatment is provided

6. The restoration on the maxillary left first molar was fabricated using an indirect technique. Which of the following restorations is identified on this tooth?
   A. Full coverage crown
   B. 3/4-coverage crown
   C. Mesial-occlusal-distal onlay
   D. Mesial-occlusal-distal inlay

7. The restoration on tooth #7 shows discoloration along its edges. Which of the following is the MOST likely cause?
   A. Marginal leakage (percolation)
   B. Overpolymerization of the restorative material
   C. Improper flossing technique
   D. Improper brushing technique

8. The drugs, which she takes at bedtime, require which of the following abbreviations?
   A. qid
   B. bid
   C. PRN
   D. HS

9. The maxillary right central incisor has a Class II fracture of the mesial incisal angle. Which of the following materials would NOT be an appropriate choice for restoring this fracture?
   A. Glass ionomer cement
   B. Composite restoration
   C. Aluminous porcelain
   D. Gold alloy

10. Since there is a history of dental caries activity, presence of secondary decay, and multiple restorations, which of the following topical fluoride applications would be MOST appropriate for this client?
    A. Stannous fluoride
    B. Neutral sodium fluoride
    C. APF gel
    D. Sodium monofluorophosphate

11. Oral contraceptives may cause a condition mimicking pregnancy gingivitis. Which of the following bacteria would predominate in this condition?
    A. *Mutans streptococcus*
    B. *Streptococcus salivarius*
    ✓C. *Provotella intermedia*
    D. *Porphyromonas gingivalis*

12. The clinical examination reveals that tooth #3 requires a full-cast crown. To anesthetize the mesial buccal root, which of the following alveolar nerves must be innervated?
    A. Anterior superior
    B. Middle superior
    C. Posterior superior
    D. Inferior

13. What is the drug of choice to treat a severe asthmatic attack when the client's bronchodilator does not treat the condition?
    A. Benedryl
    B. Wyamine Sulfate
    C. Epinephrine
    D. Solucortef

14. When choosing a local anesthetic to administer to this client, which of the following local anesthetics should be avoided?
    A. Lidocaine
    B. Prilocaine
    C. Mepivacaine
    D. Articaine

15. This client has a family history of diabetes. Which of the following medical history questions may be a symptom of diabetes?
    A. Excessive thirst and urination
    B. Swollen ankles
    C. Difficulty laying in a supine position
    D. Chest pain following exertion

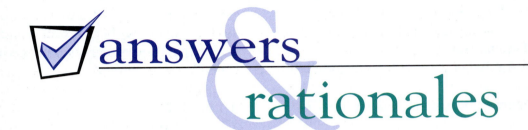

answers & rationales

1.

C. After the client has been placed in a comfortable position, she should use her own bronchodilator to manage an acute stage. If the episode continues after use of the bronchodilator, oxygen should be administered. The team member should then seek medical assistance. The injection of a corticosteroid may be necessary at this time. Administration of nitrous oxide would be used during the appointment if the client is fearful.

2.

C. Ecchymoses—discoloration of the mucous membranes—is not a common side effect of Proventil. However, it is not uncommon for the client to experience taste changes, xerostomia, and tooth discoloration while taking Proventil.

3.

D. Silver points were once the standard care in the obturation of canals undergoing endodontic treatment. They appear radiopaque within the canals. Timing of obturation is not significant. Gold posts are not used to obturate canals.

4.

B. The opacity on the radiograph and the metal along the lingual margin in the photograph indicate this is a porcelain fused-to-metal crown. All-ceramic and indirect composite restorations have no metal present. Three-quarter gold crowns have no tooth-colored components.

5.

D. The blood pressure should be verified before dental treatment. The client is borderline hypertensive and should be encouraged to be evaluated for hypertension by a physician. However, a consultation is not required for dental treatment.

6.

B. The restoration covers all of the lingual, interproximal, and occlusal surfaces. It extends slightly onto the facial surface and is therefore considered a 3/4-coverage crown. A full coverage crown covers all surfaces of the tooth. The palatal surface is covered and could not be an MOD inlay or onlay.

7.

A. The marginal staining is due to the ingress of fluid and its contents between the restoration and the tooth surface. This has been called microleakage or percolation. Complete, not overpolymerization, is desired. Proper brushing and flossing will not stop marginal leakage.

8.

D. HS means take at bedtime. Qid means to take four times a day. Bid and PRN means to take twice a day and "as needed," respectively.

9.

A. The only material given that would not be expected to function properly is the glass ionomer. The composite resin and aluminous porcelain are common choices for this situation. The gold alloy could be used if aesthetic desires dictate its use.

10.

C. The application of neutral sodium fluoride would be the best choice for this client. Stannous fluoride can stain pre-carious lesions. Acid-based fluoride products, such as acidulated phosphate, are contraindicated in the presence of existing composite and porcelain restorations. Sodium monofluorophosphate is used in over-the-counter dentifrices.

11.

C. *Provotella intermedia* is a common pathogen involved in hormonal gingivitis. *S. mutans* is implicated in human caries. *S. salivarius* is commonly found in saliva. *P. gingivalis* is not the primary etiological agent implicated in hormonal gingivitis.

12.

B. The middle superior alveolar nerve serves the maxillary premolar and maxillary first molars. The anterior alveolar nerve serves the maxillary central and lateral incisors, as well as maxillary canines. The posterior superior alveolar nerve serves the distobuccal and lingual roots of the maxillary first molars and the second and third molars. The inferior alveolar nerve innervates the mandibular teeth.

13.

C. Epinephrine is the drug of choice for a severe asthmatic attack. Epinephrine acts on all beta-adrenergic receptors.

14.

B. Prilocaine is the only amide local anesthetic that is metabolized predominantly in the lungs. This anesthetic should be avoided with patients who have asthma.

15.

A. The classic triad of diabetes symptoms is *polyuria* (frequent urination), *polydipsia* (increased thirst and consequent increased fluid intake), *polyphagia* (increased appetite).

patient history
synopsis

CASE 4	VITAL SIGNS
Age 50	Blood pressure 140/85
Sex M	Pulse rate 74
Height 5'10"	Respiration rate 20
Weight 185lbs/84kg	

1. Under the care of a physician
☐ Yes   ☒ No

2. Hospitalized within the last 5 years
☐ Yes   ☒ No

3. Has or had the following conditions:
None

4. Current medication(s)
The client takes Catapres.

5. Smokes or uses tobacco products
☒ Yes   ☐ No

6. Is pregnant
☐ Yes   ☐ No   ☒ N/A

Medical History: The client has recently developed a sore throat that seems to "hang on." He presents with a hacking cough that he relates to his pipe-smoking habit of 20 years. He enjoys hot, spicy Asian cuisine. After meals, he likes to suck on candy breath mints, which he holds in the buccal vestibule.

Dental History: Minor decay exists in facial areas of gingival recession. The client states he hasn't brushed today due to his recent sore throat. The client's last dental appointment was 2 years ago.

The client has a nervous facial tic and several moles that he states have been present since childhood without change.

Social History: The client is married and works as a car salesman.

Chief Complaint: None

ADULT CLINICAL EXAMINATION

	1	2	3	4	5	6	7	8	9	10	11	12	13	14	15	16
2 1	—	—	—	—	—	—	—	—	—	—	—	—	—	—	—	—

facial

R L

palatal

| 1 2 | — | — | — | — | — | — | — | — | — | — | — | — | — | — | — | — |

| 2 1 | — | — | — | 444 | 444 | 447 | 746 | 646 | 645 | 546 | 544 | 444 | 444 | 444 | — | — |

lingual

R L

facial

| 1 2 | — | — | — | 444 | 444 | 447 | 646 | 646 | 646 | 647 | 644 | 444 | 444 | 445 | — | — |
| | 32 | 31 | 30 | 29 | 28 | 27 | 26 | 25 | 24 | 23 | 22 | 21 | 20 | 19 | 18 | 17 |

Current Oral Hygiene Status
1. Heavy plaque
2. Client states he did not brush today due to recent sore throat

Supplemental Oral Examination Findings
1. Has white patches on his palate
2. Class I furcation on #19
3. A fixed, firm, nontender, left anterior node was palpable
4. Heavy stain

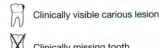

⌇ Clinically visible carious lesion

☒ Clinically missing tooth

△ Furcation

▲ "Through and through" furcation

Probe 1: initial probing depth

Probe 2: probing depth 1 month after scaling and root planing

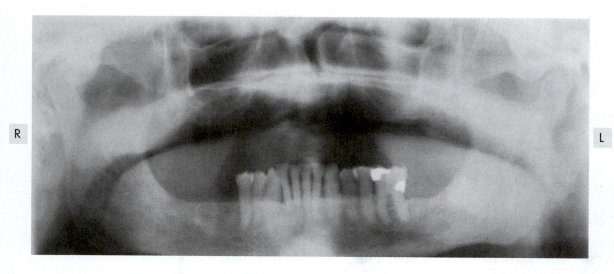

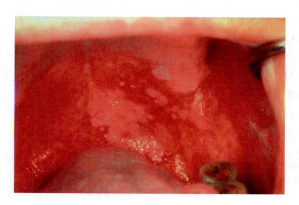

R   L

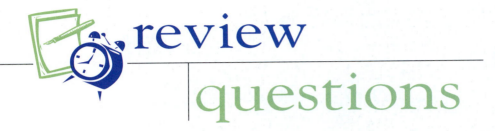

review questions

1. During the appointment, the client complains of an intense headache at the right temple and then leans over to vomit. In a slurred manner, he states the left side of his body has gone numb, then loses consciousness. Which of the following medical emergencies has occurred?
   A. Myxedema coma
   B. Acute adrenal insufficiency
   C. Hemorrhagic CVA
   D. Thyroid storm

2. Which of the following nerves primarily innervates muscles of facial expression?
   A. V
   B. III
   C. VII
   D. IX

3. Since the client has not brushed his teeth today, which of the following bacteria would be first to aggregate on his teeth?
   A. *Mutans streptococcus*
   B. *Streptococcus sanguis*
   C. *Streptococcus salivarius*
   D. *Provotella intermedia*

4. The drug class of Catapres is
   A. Antihyperlipidemic
   B. Antihypertensive
   C. Nonsteriodal ovulatory stimulant
   D. Urinary tract antibacterial

5. Which of the following terminology describes the lesion in the photograph?
   A. Diffuse leukoplakia
   B. Nodular leukoplakia
   C. Diffuse erythema
   D. Nodular erythema
   E. Speckled leukoplakia

6. Which of the following would be considered high-risk factors for this lesion?
   A. Tobacco use
   B. Spicy food consumption
   C. Breath mint abuse
   D. Alcohol consumption
   E. Oral tongue habits

7. Which of the following dictates the next course of treatment?
   A. Observation for 1 year
   B. Incisional biopsy
   C. Excisional biopsy
   D. Antibiotics
   E. Antifungal medication

8. Histological examination reveals top to bottom dysplastic epithelium with invasion of the basement membrane. Which of the following is the MOST likely diagnosis?
   A. Mild dysplasia
   B. Moderate dysplasia
   C. Severe dysplasia
   D. Carcinoma in situ
   E. Invasive carcinoma

9. Which of the following is the MOST likely explanation for the palpable cervical node?
   A. Drainage of an infection
   B. Drainage of the gingival inflammation
   C. Inflammation from spicy food consumption
   D. Metastasis of the oropharyngeal lesion

10. The MOST likely etiology for the minor carious lesions in the facial areas of gingival recession is
   A. Tobacco use
   B. Chronic sugar exposure
   C. Mouth breathing
   D. Toothpick habit

11. Which of the following periodontal case types best describes this patient?
   A. Type I
   B. Type II
   C. Type III
   D. Type IV
   E. Type V

12. What would be the most efficient way to remove this patient's stain?
   A. Air polishing
   B. Manual scaling
   C. Ultrasonic scaling
   D. Rubber-cup polishing

13. Each of the following clinical signs could be used as a motivating factor to advise this client to quit smoking EXCEPT one. Which one is the EXCEPTION?
   A. Extrinsic stains
   B. Lip hyperkeratosis
   C. Increased probe depth
   D. Gingival erythema

14. This client has heavy plaque around the gingival margin. Which oral hygiene device would be helpful for him to remove the plaque?
   A. Perio aid
   B. Proxy brush
   C. Dental floss
   D. Gauze strips

15. What type of recall should be advised for this patient?
   A. 1 month
   B. 12 months
   C. 3 months
   D. 6 months

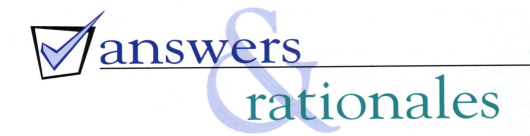

answers & rationales

1.

C. Symptoms of hemorrhagic CVA include a sudden onset of a headache, dizziness and vertigo, sweating and chills, nausea, and vomiting. Myxedema coma is a severe complication associated with hypothyroidism. Its symptoms include hypothermia, bradycardia, hypotension, and loss of consciousness. Clients with acute adrenal insufficiency (adrenal crisis) most generally exhibit lethargy, fatigue, and weakness. Thyroid storm is a result of untreated hyperthyroidism. Symptoms include an elevated body temperature, excessive sweating, vomiting, and abdominal pain.

2.

C. The trigeminal nerve is sensory via V_1 and V_2 and sensory and motor via V_3 to muscles of mastication. The oculomotor provides motor innervation to muscles of the eyeball. The glossopharyngeal provides sensory innervation to the posterior one-third of the tongue and motor to selected soft palate and pharynx muscles.

3.

B. *S. sanguis* is the first "colonizer" of tooth structures. *S. mutans* competes with *S. sanguis*, but is not the first colonizer. *S. salivarius* is found in saliva. *P. intermedia* is a periodontal pathogen found in mature plaque.

4.

B. Catapres is an antihypertensive medication.

5.

E. Areas of erythema and leukoplakia are referred to as "speckled leukoplakia" owing to interspersed areas of red and white appearances. Diffuse leukoplakia is not completely white in appearance. Nodular leukoplakia and erythema are not nodular in appearance. Diffuse erythema is not completely red in appearance.

6.

A. Tobacco usage frequently results in premalignant lesions. Use of breath mints, alcohol and spicy food consumption, and oral tongue habits are not considered high-risk factors.

7.

B. Unexplained lesions imply immediate investigation and would not be observed for an extended period of time. The lesion is too large for successful, complete excision with an excisional biopsy. Antibioties and antifungal medications are not indicated because there is no bacterial or fungal disease implicated.

8.

E. The top-to-bottom atypical proliferation of epithelium, with violation of the basement membrane, is by definition invasive carcinoma. Mild, moderate, and severe dysplasias are not defined as top-to-bottom dysplasias. Carcinoma in situ implies a top-to-bottom dysplasia, but without violation of the basement membrane.

9.

D. When the nodes are hard, fixed, and not tender, metastasis is suspicious. When the nodes are draining from an infection, they are tender and movable. Lymphadenopathy is unusual with mild gingivitis and, if present, would be tender and movable. Metastasis of the oropharyngeal lesion is not an etiology for lymphadenopathy.

10.

B. The client has a habit of sucking on breath mints, which have a high sucrose content. Smoking, mouth breathing, and a toothpick habit are not cariogenic.

11.

E. Radiographs exhibit excessive bone loss. Periodontal probing depths indicate advanced periodontitis.

12.

D. The use of sodium bicarbonate with high air pressure is an effective and efficient way to remove heavy stains.

13.

D. Gingival erythema is usually caused by inflammation. Patients who smoke usually have chronic rather than acute inflammation.

14.

A. The perio aid is effective in assisting patients to remove plaque along the gingival margin.

15.

C. A 3-month recall is important for a patient with advanced periodontitis.

case study 4 answers

patient history
synopsis

CASE 5	VITAL SIGNS
Age 43	Blood pressure 128/108
Sex F	Pulse rate 80
Height 5′1″	Respiration rate 16
Weight 175lbs/80kg	

1. Under the care of a physician

☒ Yes   ☐ No

Condition: Adult-onset diabetes and hypertension.

2. Hospitalized within the last 5 years

☐ Yes   ☒ No

3. Has or had the following conditions:

Diabetes, hypertension

4. Current medication(s)

The client takes Glucophage 500 mg daily.

5. Smokes or uses tobacco products

☐ Yes   ☒ No

6. Is pregnant

☐ Yes   ☒ No   ☐ N/A

Medical History: The client has adult-onset diabetes and hypertension. She is currently under the care of a physician for her diabetes, which was diagnosed 5 months ago. The initial attempt to manage the diabetes with diet modification was unsuccessful. The patient had knee surgery for a sports injury when she was in high school with no complications.

Dental History: The client had her premolars and third molars removed. When she was in high school, she wore braces for 2½; years. However, her dental care has been limited the past 10 years. She bruxes at night and has a habit of biting her nails. She brushes twice a day using a soft toothbrush, but does not floss. She exhibits evidence of periodontal disease, but has not been informed of her condition.

Social History: The client is divorced and currently holds a receptionist position.

Additional Findings: While taking the radiographs, the hygienist notes the client is having difficulty positioning her head.

Chief Complaint: "My gums bleed." In addition, she complains of bad breath, dry mouth, and that some of her teeth ache.

ADULT CLINICAL EXAMINATION

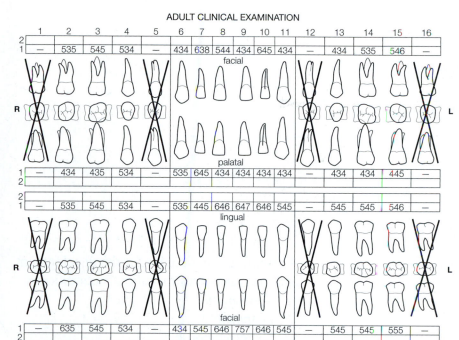

	1	2	3	4	5	6	7	8	9	10	11	12	13	14	15	16
2																
1	—	535	545	534	—	434	638	544	434	645	434	—	434	535	546	—

facial

R / L

palatal

1	—	434	435	534	—	535	645	434	434	434	434	—	434	434	445	—
2																

2																
1	—	535	545	534	—	535	445	646	647	646	545	—	545	545	546	—

lingual

R / L

facial

1	—	635	545	534	—	434	545	646	757	646	545	—	545	545	555	—
2																

| 32 | 31 | 30 | 29 | 28 | 27 | 26 | 25 | 24 | 23 | 22 | 21 | 20 | 19 | 18 | 17 |

Current Oral Hygiene Status
1. Heavy plaque
2. Heavy calculus

Supplemental Oral Examination Findings
1. General bleeding upon probing
2. Purulence at facial #24
3. Gingival red, rolled margins, blunted papilla
4. Grade I mobility #7, 23, 24, 25
5. Clefts at facial #8, 24
6. Root canal #10

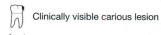

Clinically visible carious lesion

Clinically missing tooth

△ Furcation

▲ "Through and through" furcation

Probe 1: initial probing depth

Probe 2: probing depth 1 month after scaling and root planing

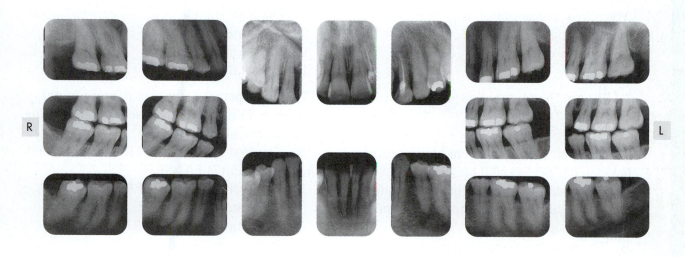

R / L

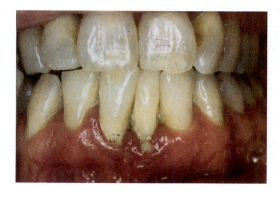

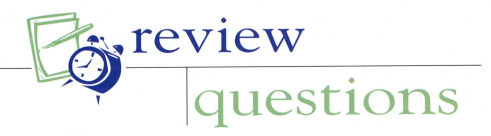

review questions

1. The status of this client's periodontal health would be described as
   A. Healthy
   B. Acute gingivitis
   C. Active periodontitis
   D. Healthy, with a past history of periodontitis

2. According to G.V. Black's classification, what class of restoration is present on teeth #s 2, 3, 13, and 14?
   A. A
   B. I
   C. II
   D. C
   E. V

3. What impact does this client's restorations have on her periodontal condition?
   A. The overhanging margins are plaque retentive and contribute to the inflammatory disease
   B. The restorative material is known to contribute to periodontal disease
   C. The restorations are of little concern; they do not contribute to the periodontal disease
   D. The restorations are the cause of the periodontal disease

4. A significant risk factor for the development and progression of this client's condition is
   A. Tobacco use
   B. Diabetes
   C. Hypertension
   D. Past history of orthodontic care

5. There is purulence present on the facial of #24. Its cause is
   A. Occlusal trauma
   B. Pulp infection
   C. Periodontal infection
   D. Physical injury

6. Diabetes increases the risk of periodontal disease. Periodontal disease complicates the management of diabetes.
   A. The first statement is TRUE; the second statement is FALSE.
   B. The first statement is FALSE; the second statement is TRUE.
   C. Both statements are TRUE.
   D. Both statements are FALSE.

7. Referring to the clinical and radiographic findings, the client's AAP Case Type is MOST likely
   A. I
   B. II
   C. III
   D. IV
   E. V

8. Compare the radiographic appearance of the bone at the mesial of #7 with the mesial of #19. Which of the following suggests active periodontal disease at #7?
   A. There is more bone loss at #7 than #19
   B. There is calculus present at #7 and not at #19
   C. There is a deeper pocket at #7 than #19
   D. The lamina dura does not appear at #7, but does at #19

9. Tooth #7 has been recommended for extraction. The MOST appropriate referral for this client is to a(n)
   A. Oral surgeon
   B. Dietitian
   C. Physician
   D. Periodontist

10. The masseter muscle plays an active role during bruxism. Which of the following structures represent the origin and insertion of the masseter muscle?
    A. Temporal fossa; coronoid process
    B. Greater wing of the sphenoid; anterior surface of the temperomandibular joint (TMJ) disc
    C. Zygomatic arch; angle of mandible, lateral surface
    D. Lateral surface of pterygoid plate; neck of the condyle

11. Which of the following would MOST likely correct the distortion that appears on the maxillary left molar radiograph?
    A. Increase vertical angulation
    B. Decrease vertical angulation
    C. Redirect the PID more posteriorly
    D. Place the film more inferior to the occlusal surfaces

12. Which of the following muscles is primarily responsible for the client's difficulty in tilting and rotating her head?
    A. Digastric
    B. Sternohyoid
    C. Mylohyoid
    D. Sternocleidomastoid

13. What type of diabetes does this patient probably exhibit?
    A. Type I
    B. Type II
    C. Gestational diabetes
    D. Pre-diabetes

14. During your treatment of this patient, she suddenly has trembling in the hands and arms, decreased muscle coordination, and confusion. What symptoms is she exhibiting?
    A. Hypoglycemia
    B. Hyperglycemia
    C. Diabetic coma
    D. Hypothyroidism

15. What emergency procedures should be taken for the above situation?
    A. Have client take an insulin injection
    B. Have the client eat food high in protein
    C. Have client eat or drink something sweet
    D. None of the above

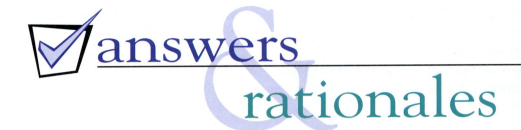

answers & rationales

1.

C. Generalized bleeding on probing indicates active inflammatory disease. Both the clinical examination and radiographs show evidence of periodontal destruction and furcation involvement. The client's condition would not be considered healthy since there is presence of bleeding on probing. This indicates active disease. Evidence of bone loss indicates the disease has progressed from gingivitis to periodontitis.

2.

B. Class I restorations are found on the occlusal surfaces of posterior teeth. Classes A and C are not part of G.V. Black's classifications. Class II is a two-surface posterior restoration. Class V describes restorations found at the cervical one third.

3.

C. Both the clinical and radiographic appearance of these Class I amalgams suggest that they are intact, sound restorations. They do not have overhanging margins and therefore have little impact on the development or progression of periodontal disease. An intact, smooth, non-plaque-retentive amalgam restoration does not contribute to periodontal disease. Restorations do not cause periodontal disease. If the margins of a restoration are adjacent to the gingival tissue and are plaque retentive, the restoration may contribute to periodontal disease.

4.

B. Diabetes increases the incidence of periodontal disease. There may be poor wound healing, increased incidence of periodontal abscesses, xerostomia, and burning mouth. The history does not include tobacco use. Hypertension is not considered a significant risk factor for the development and progression of periodontal disease. The presence of orthodontic bands or brackets may make plaque removal more difficult; however, past history of orthodontic care is not a risk factor.

5.

C. Radiographic and clinical findings identify pocket formation, bone loss, and supragingival calculus. These factors suggest a periodontal disease state. Purulence is related to the presence of microorganisms, not occlusal trauma. The radiographs do not show evidence of pulp pathology. There is no history of physical injury, and x-ray studies do not reveal evidence.

6.

C. Uncontrolled diabetes is a risk factor for the development and progression of periodontal disease. The bacterial infections found in periodontal disease may make it more difficult to manage the diabetes. The periodontal infections place additional burden on the host's defense mechanisms.

7.

C. Case Type III, moderate periodontitis, shows evidence of increased destruction of the periodontal structure and noticeable loss of bone support, possibly accompanied by an increase in tooth mobility. There may be furcation involvement in multirooted teeth.

8.

D. An indicator of active disease in bone is the loss of the crestal lamina dura. The lamina dura can be clearly identified at the mesial of #19 on the bitewings. The lamina dura is not defined on the periapical x-ray at #7. Although there may be more loss of bone support at #7 than at #19, bone level itself is not an indicator of active disease. The presence of calculus is not an indicator of active disease. Radiographs are valuable to assess calcified structures, but they have little value in assessing the status of soft tissue.

9.

C. Oral surgery procedures, associated with restricted food intake, require a medical consultation and temporary cessation of the medication. Referral to the oral surgeon is appropriate after a medical consultation. A referral to a dietitian is appropriate because the client is diabetic. The client could be referred to the periodontist after the tooth is extracted.

10.

C. The origin and insertion of the temporalis muscle are the temporal bone and coronoid process, respectively. The origin and insertion for the lateral pterygoid muscle are the greater wing of the sphenoid and anterior surface of the temperomandibular joint (TMJ), respectively. The origin and insertion of the medial pterygoid muscle are the lateral surface of the pterygoid plate and the neck of the condyle, respectively.

11.

A. To decrease the distortion evident on the maxillary left molar periapical, it would be necessary to increase the vertical angulation. Decreasing the vertical angulation would cause elongation. Redirecting the PID more posteriorly would cause a cone cut to occur. Placing the film more inferior to the occlusal surfaces would cut off the apices.

12.

D. The sternocleidomastoid is a large strap muscle in the neck that rotates and tilts the head. The digastric muscle is a minor muscle of mastication that depresses the mandible. The sternohyoid muscle helps to stabilize the hyoid bone. The mylohyoid muscle forms the floor of the mouth.

13.

B. Type 2 diabetes results from insulin resistance (a condition in which the body fails to properly use insulin), combined with relative insulin deficiency. Most Americans who are diagnosed with diabetes have type 2 diabetes. Type 1 diabetes results from the body's failure to produce insulin, the hormone that "unlocks" the cells of the body, allowing glucose to enter and fuel them. Gestational diabetes affects about 4% of all pregnant women. Pre-diabetes is a condition that occurs when a person's blood glucose levels are higher than normal but not high enough for a diagnosis of type 2 diabetes.

14.

A. The most common emergency facing victims of diabetes is hypoglycemia (low blood sugar). Hypoglycemia happens when the victim has taken too much medication, or took the right amount of medication but did not eat. Hypoglycemia can also happen as a result of infection or increased exertion.

15.

C. If the victim is conscious and able to follow your commands, have the victim eat or drink something sweet; juices work best. Victims can even eat frozen juice concentrate right out of the can.

patient history
synopsis

CASE 6
Age 37
Sex M
Height 6′
Weight 160lbs/73kg

VITAL SIGNS
Blood pressure 145/90
Pulse rate 80
Respiration rate 17

1. Under the care of a physician

☒ Yes ☐ No

Condition: Adult-onset diabetes and hypertension.

2. Hospitalized within the last 5 years

☐ Yes ☒ No

3. Has or had the following conditions:

Diabetes and hypertension

4. Current medication(s)

None

5. Smokes or uses tobacco products

☒ Yes ☐ No

Two packs a day

6. Is pregnant

☐ Yes ☐ No ☒ N/A

Medical History: The client has had significant weight loss and complains of being tired. He does have a physician of record.

Dental History: The reason for this visit is to have his teeth cleaned. The client's last visit to the dentist was 3 years ago. He routinely brushes once a day, but sometimes twice daily. He does not floss.

Social History: The client owns his own business and works many hours. He notes he has a stressful job and has three children who keep him busy with their outside activities.

Chief Complaint: "White patches in my mouth bleed when I try to scrape them off." His teeth are also cold-sensitive.

ADULT CLINICAL EXAMINATION

	1	2	3	4	5	6	7	8	9	10	11	12	13	14	15	16
2 1	—	425	323	423	323	423	545	545	544	434	323	324	323	523	526	—

facial

palatal

	1	2	3	4	5	6	7	8	9	10	11	12	13	14	15	16
1 2	—	324	323	323	323	423	434	435	545	545	323	323	323	523	425	—

2 1	526	626	635	524	323	323	565	666	656	545	424	434	323	434	535	644

lingual

facial

1 2	425	525	523	423	323	323	556	757	757	656	434	323	323	424	526	644

| 32 | 31 | 30 | 29 | 28 | 27 | 26 | 25 | 24 | 23 | 22 | 21 | 20 | 19 | 18 | 17 |

Current Oral Hygiene Status
1. Moderate plaque
2. Moderate calculus

Supplemental Oral Examination Findings
1. Pronounced bad breath
2. Moderate gingival inflammation, as well as color and texture change.
3. Gingiva bleeds easily
4. Palpable cervical lymph nodes

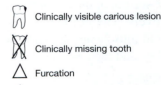

Clinically visible carious lesion

Clinically missing tooth

Furcation

"Through and through" furcation

Probe 1: initial probing depth

Probe 2: probing depth 1 month after scaling and root planing

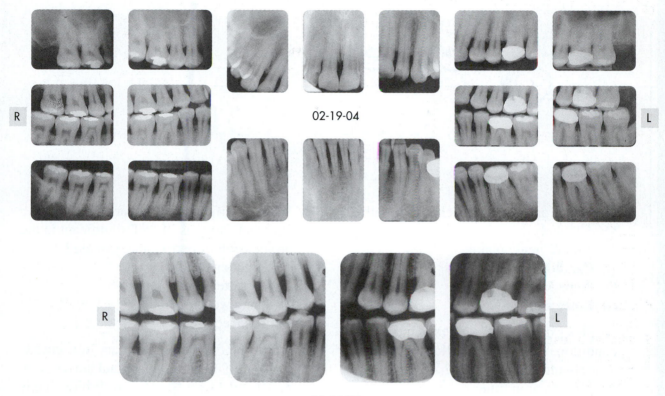

02-19-04

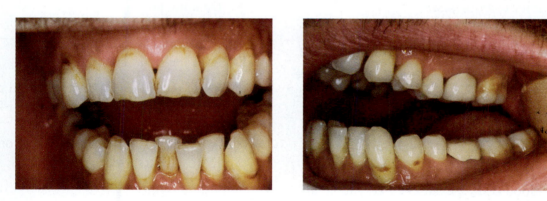

11-14-07

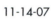

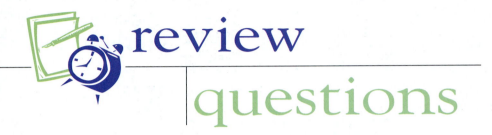

review
questions

1. The white patches in this client's mouth are MOST likely
   A. "Snuff" leukoplakia
   B. Candidiasis
   C. Hyperkeratosis
   D. Linea alba

2. To BEST diagnose this client's medical condition, which of the following medical tests should be performed?
   A. Prothrombin time
   B. Antibody assay test
   C. Liver enzyme test
   D. Partial prothrombin time

3. The symptoms displayed by this client are MOST likely due to which of the following conditions?
   A. Tuberculosis
   B. Hepatitis B
   C. HIV
   D. Hepatitis C

4. The blood cell type MOST likely to be affected by this client's disease is
   A. Thrombocytes
   B. B lymphocytes
   C. CD4 lymphocytes
   D. Neutrophils

5. What modifiable risk factor, noted in this client's history, is MOST significant in the progression of periodontal disease?
   A. High-stress job
   B. Hypertension
   C. Long working hours
   D. Tobacco use

6. All of the following auxiliary aids could be used to clean the proximal surfaces of #s 10 and 11 EXCEPT one. Which one is the EXCEPTION?
   A. Dental tape
   B. Interdental brush
   C. Interdental wood stimulator
   D. Bass method of toothbrushing

7. Which of the following factors could contribute to plaque retention at tooth #14?
   A. Porcelain-fused-to-metal crown
   B. A large MOD amalgam restoration
   C. Exposed furcation
   D. Extrinsic stain

8. Which of the following Gracey curets could be utilized on the distolinguals of teeth #s 30 and 31?
   A. 11
   B. 12
   C. 13
   D. 14

9. Referral to his physician is indicated for this client to
   A. Identify the cause of his tooth sensitivity
   B. Provide antibiotics for treatment of his periodontal disease
   C. Identify the cause of his breath odor
   D. Evaluate his significant weight loss

10. What AAP Case Type would classify this client?
    A. I
    B. II
    C. III
    D. IV

11. Which of the following techniques was MOST likely used to palpate the cervical lymph nodes?
    A. Bimanual
    B. Bilateral
    C. Digital
    D. Inspection

12. To prepare for treatment of this client, the dental hygienist should
    A. Double glove
    B. Use barriers as appropriate
    C. Sterilize all instruments twice
    D. Use a special "isolation" room

13. What tumor that is associated with the herpes virus may develop from this client's systemic illness?
    A. Candidiasis
    B. Leukoplakia
    C. Erythroplakia
    D. Kaposi's sarcoma

14. Which of the following is an effective treatment of oral candidiasis?
    A. Nystatin (Mycostatin)
    B. Monostat
    C. Glucosamine
    D. Prilosec

15. Utilizing the client's radiographs and dental charting, which area has the poorest prognosis?
    A. Maxillary anterior teeth
    B. Maxillary posterior teeth
    C. Mandibular anterior teeth
    D. Mandibular posterior teeth

case study 6 questions

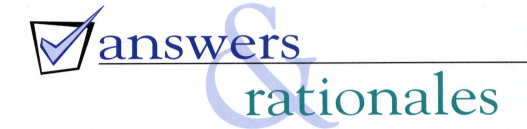

answers & rationales

1.

B. Candidiasis classically presents as white patches that leave a bloody area when rubbed off. The client had other risk factors that made candidiasis a likely diagnosis. The client gave no history of snuff use. Hyperkeratosis is a term for extra layers of keratinization in response to trauma. This was not the most likely diagnosis because of other risk factors.

2.

B. Antibody assays are tests used to determine what disease entity is present. Prothrombin time is a blood-clotting test. A liver enzyme test would be indicated if liver damage were suspected. Partial prothrombin time is a test of blood clotting ability.

3.

C. This client is most likely suffering from HIV. He displays lymphadenopathy, oral candidiasis, weight loss, fatigue, and bleeding gingiva. These are classic symptoms of this syndrome. Weight loss and fatigue are symptoms of tuberculosis and hepatitis B and C. However, candidiasis and bleeding tissues are not associated with TB, and there are no oral manifestations associated with hepatitis B and C.

4.

C. HIV destroys the CD4 T lymphocytes, weakening the immune system. Thrombocytes, or platelets, are cells that cause blood clotting, and B lymphocytes are the cells that produce antibodies; both are not affected by HIV. The HIV virus affects neutrophils, but the cells most harmed are the CD4 T lymphocytes.

5.

D. Tobacco use, especially smoking, has been identified as a significant factor in the development and progression of periodontal disease. The client, through smoking cessation, can alter this risk factor. Stress has been identified as a possible contributor to the progression of periodontal disease. Its significance is less well defined than the changeable risk factor of tobacco use. Hypertension and working long hours have not been identified as significant risk factors in the progression of periodontal disease.

6.

D. The Bass method of toothbrushing is used to clean the facials and linguals of teeth with pocketing. The bristles of the toothbrush are placed in the sulcus for cleaning. Because of the diastema between teeth #s 10 and 11, it is acceptable to use dental tape or interdental wood stimulators.

7.

A. Because of the overhanging or defective margin of the crown on tooth #14, more plaque is likely to accumulate. A large MOD amalgam with a defective proximal margin could contribute to plaque accumulation; however, this client does not have an amalgam on tooth #14. The clinical and radiographic evidence does not identify a furcation involvement. If one existed, it could contribute to plaque accumulation. There is no extrinsic stain noted on tooth #14.

8.

C. The Gracey curet 13 is designed for application on the distolinguals of teeth #s 30 and 31. The Gracey curet 11 and 12 are designed for use on the mesial surfaces of posterior teeth. The Gracey curet 14 would be applied on the distofacials of teeth #s 30 and 31.

9.

D. Referral to this client's physician would be indicated for his severe weight loss. The dentist would most likely be able to identify the cause for his tooth sensitivity and breath odor, as well as provide antibiotics to treat his periodontal condition.

10.

D. Advanced periodontitis is identified by its major loss of bone support, increase in tooth mobility, and probable furcation involvement. This client's condition is more severe than Case I gingival disease. Early periodontitis describes the progression of gingival inflammation with slight bone and connective tissue attachment loss. Moderate periodontitis is a more advanced disease with noticeable loss of bone support, increase in tooth mobility, and probable furcation involvement.

11.

B. Using both hands at the same time to examine corresponding structures on opposite sides of the body is called the bilateral palpation technique. Use of finger(s) and thumb from each hand, applied simultaneously, is the bimanual palpation technique. Digital palpation involves using a single finger. Inspection is not a valid tool to use to evaluate the client's TMJ.

12.

B. All clients should be treated with "universal precautions" as mandated by the Americans with Disability Act. Double gloving, sterilizing instruments twice, and use of a special isolation room violates universal precautions.

13.

D. Kaposi's sarcoma (KS) is a tumor caused by Kaposi's sarcoma-associated herpes virus (KSHV), also known as human herpes virus 8.

14.

A. Topical treatment (active only on the area where applied) is generally the first choice for oral candidiasis and usually works for mild-to-moderate cases. Topical treatments for oral candidiasis include lozenges (also called troches) and mouth rinses. One or two lozenges are taken for oral symptoms three to five times a day. They should be sucked slowly and not chewed or swallowed whole. Common brands are clotrimazole (Mycelex) and nystatin (Mycostatin).

15.

C. The mandibular anterior teeth have the most advanced periodontal status. With 7 mm pocket depths and 70% alveolar bone loss, the prognosis is not favorable for these teeth.

patient history
synopsis

CASE 7
Age 71
Sex M
Height 6′
Weight 190lbs/86kg

VITAL SIGNS
Blood pressure 130/80
Pulse rate 64
Respiration rate 18

1. Under the care of a physician
☐ Yes ☒ No
Condition: Type I diabetes

2. Hospitalized within the last 5 years
☐ Yes ☒ No

3. Has or had the following conditions:
Type I diabetes

4. Current medication(s)
Insulin

5. Smokes or uses tobacco products
☐ Yes ☒ No

6. Is pregnant
☐ Yes ☐ No ☒ N/A

Medical History: His last complete physical examination was 2 years ago at a Family Health Center. The client has no past history of surgeries except for skin grafts on his neck and chest due to a scalding burn when he was a toddler.

Dental History: A year ago the client came to the dental office for a routine prophylaxis appointment. It had been years since his last visit. His chief complaint at that time was "bleeding gums." There is evidence of existing restorations and missing teeth.

Social History: The client is the oldest of five brothers and is the only member of his family living in the state. He is on a fixed income and cannot afford extensive dental treatment. He is currently working part time.

Chief Complaint: "Food gets stuck in my cheeks. I'm also in a hurry to get to work, so I hope this doesn't take too long. I do want to keep my teeth."

ADULT CLINICAL EXAMINATION

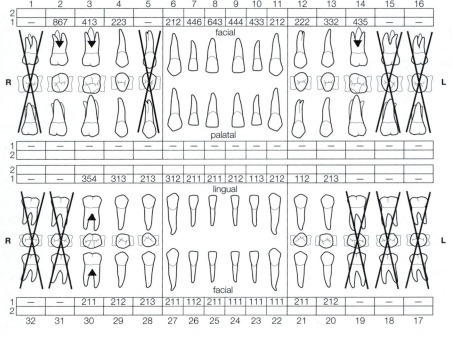

Current Oral Hygiene Status
1. Moderate calculus
2. Client does not floss regularly

Supplemental Oral Examination Findings
1. Class I mobility #28, 30
2. Class II mobility #29
3. #2 is in supraversion
4. Exudate #30

Clinically visible carious lesion

Clinically missing tooth

Furcation

"Through and through" furcation

Probe 1: initial probing depth

Probe 2: probing depth 1 month after scaling and root planing

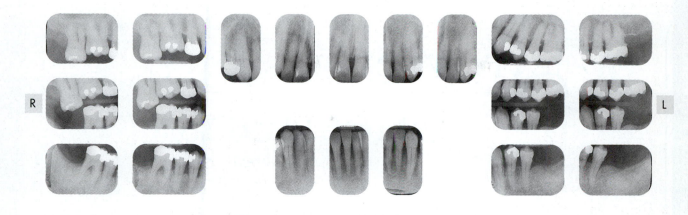

R   L

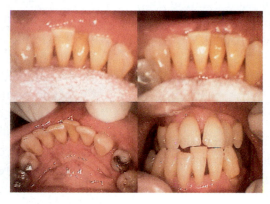

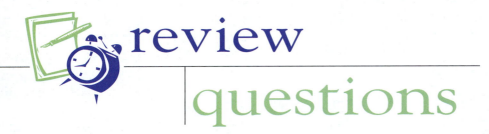

review questions

1. The client's complaint of accumulating food in the vestibule might suggest a malfunction of which of the following muscles?
   A. Risorius
   B. Buccinator
   C. Orbicularis oris
   D. Medial pterygoid

2. Since extensive scaling and pocket debridement are to be performed on the maxillary incisors, which of the following nerves would require anesthesia?
   A. Inferior alveolar and long buccal
   B. Mental and inferior alveolar
   C. Posterior superior alveolar and greater anterior palatine
   D. Anterior superior alveolar and nasopalatine

3. Local anesthesia was administered using 2% lidocaine plus epinephrine 1:50,000. About 5 minutes after the injection, the client experiences the following symptoms: sweating, pallor, headache, dizziness, and weakness. The pulse rate is 100 and the blood pressure is 140/90. The client's symptoms are MOST likely due to
   A. Drug reaction
   B. Anaphylactic allergic reaction
   C. Myocardial infarction
   D. Insulin shock

4. To have prevented this medical emergency, the clinician should have
   A. Taken the client's blood pressure reading first
   B. Maintained the client in a supine position
   C. Made certain the client was not allergic to any of the components of the local anesthesia
   D. Determined if the client had eaten and administered his medication before his appointment

5. The initial treatment for the emergency would be to administer
   A. Sugar in some form
   B. Oxygen and 15 units of insulin subcutaneously
   C. Oxygen and any available antihistamine
   D. Oxygen only

6. What is the BEST oral hygiene aid to recommend to this client to help remove plaque from the proximal areas of the mandibular anterior teeth?
   A. Toothpick
   B. Oral irrigation
   C. Interdental brush
   D. Child-size toothbrush

7. Radiopaque spurs, visible interproximally on the posterior films of all quadrants, are evidence of
   A. Bone
   B. Calculus
   C. Fixer spots
   D. Overhanging margins

8. Which of the following teeth clearly has a furcation involvement evident on the radiograph?
   A. Maxillary right first molar
   B. Maxillary left first premolar
   C. Maxillary left first molar
   D. Mandibular right first molar

9. What classification of restoration would be used to restore the facial fracture on tooth #9?
   A. III
   B. IV
   C. V
   D. VI

10. The mandibular left first premolar exhibits iatrogenic dentistry in the form of a(n)
    A. Open contact
    B. Overhang
    C. Fracture
    D. Leaky margin

11. The radiopaque areas on the distal of #8 and the mesial of #11 are a result of which of the following?
    A. Calcium hydroxide base
    B. Amalgam restorations
    C. Composite restorations
    D. Splashes of fixer

12. Based on the client's social, medical, and dental histories, what type of dental treatment would be MOST appropriate for him?
    A. Regular six-month prophylaxis appointments
    B. Referral to a periodontist for extensive treatment
    C. Referral to prosthodontist for complete dentures
    D. Three-month intervals for scaling and periodontal debridement

13. Why is tooth #2 in supraversion?
    A. Because of the class III furcations
    B. Because #31 is missing
    C. Because #32 is missing
    D. Because of extensive periodontal disease

14. What treatment is indicated for this patient to treat the supraversion?
    A. Implants to replace missing teeth
    B. Extraction of #2
    C. Bone grafting
    D. None of the above

15. Why is there exudate around tooth #30?
    A. There is an infection causing the accumulation of pus
    B. There is significant amount of bone loss
    C. The tooth needs to be extracted
    D. There is calculus present

case study 7 questions

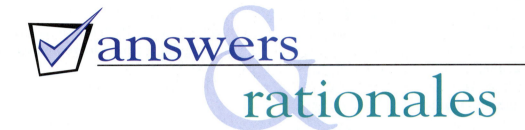

answers & rationales

1.

B. The buccinator muscle flattens the cheek, which pushes food out of the vestibule both vertically and horizontally. The risorius muscle is responsible for widening the mouth—as when a person smiles. The orbicularis oris muscle encircles the mouth and acts to close the lips. The medial pterygoid muscle has the function of elevating the mandible.

2.

D. The anterior superior branch supplies the maxillary centrals, laterals, and canines, whereas the nasopalatine branch innervates the soft tissue of the anterior one-third of the hard palate. The inferior alveolar innervation for the mandibular teeth and the long buccal nerve serve as afferent nerves for the mandibular teeth and skin of cheek, buccal mucous membranes, and buccal gingiva of the mandibular posterior teeth, respectively. The mental nerve (afferent) serves the chin, lower lip, and labial mucosa near the mandibular anterior teeth. The posterior superior nerve serves most portions of the maxillary molar teeth and the greater anterior palatine nerve serves the posterior hard palate.

3.

D. Symptoms of insulin shock include sweating, pallor, hunger, trembling, headaches, dizziness, and weakness. The client may also experience an increase in blood pressure and pulse rate. However, the respiration rate will remain normal or depressed. An allergic response to lidocaine is extremely rare. The client would most likely experience psychogenic responses, such as hyperventilation and vasodepressor syncope. The most common symptoms of anaphylactic shock include smooth muscle spasms, cardiovascular and acute respiratory distress, and skin reactions—a generalized rash. With myocardial infarction (heart attack), the client will experience severe pain in the sternum, difficulty in breathing, profuse sweating and nausea, with possible vomiting.

4.

D. With an insulin-dependent diabetic client, it is important to determine when insulin was last administered, as well as when the last meal was consumed. Checking the client's blood pressure, keeping him in a supine position, and determining his allergic status with the local anesthetic would not have prevented insulin shock.

5.

A. When a diabetic client goes into insulin shock, the first mode of action is to administer some form of sugar such as orange juice, candy, or a sugared soft drink. It is also vital to determine when insulin was administered. The administration of oxygen and an antihistamine would not assist the client in this situation.

6.

C. Because of bone loss and missing interdental papillae, an interdental brush is recommended to assist in removing plaque. The toothpick is used to clean along the marginal gingiva. Oral irrigation does not remove plaque. A child-size toothbrush would not provide access to the proximal areas as would the proximal brush.

7.

B. Interproximal calculus is projected as radiopaque spurs on radiographs. Bone, fixer spots, and overhangs are radiopaque, but not shaped as spurs at the interproximals of the posterior teeth.

8.

D. A radiolucent area is evident in the furcation of tooth #30, Teeth #s 3, 12, and 14 do not show evidence of furcation involvement.

9.

B. A Class IV involves the proximal and incisal angles of anterior teeth. A Class III involves proximal surfaces of incisors and canines. A Class V involves the cervical one third of facial or lingual surfaces. A Class VI involves the incisal edge of anterior teeth or the cups tips of posterior teeth.

10.

B. Improper use of the matrix band and wood wedge allowed excess amalgam to leak through onto the distal of #21. There is no evidence of an open contact, fracture, or leaky margin on tooth #21.

11.

A. Calcium hydroxide base material is more radiopaque than composite material used on anterior teeth. An amalgam restoration is even more radiopaque than calcium hydroxide and composite material. Fixer spots are not as configured as anterior restoration materials.

12.

D. Since the client is retired and on a fixed income, maintenance appointments every 3 months would be best. Because of his periodontal status, it would be more appropriate to have him on a 3-month rather than 6-month recall. Referral to a periodontist would not be feasible because of the client's limited income, and since he wants to keep his teeth, referral for complete dentures should not be recommended.

13.

B. If a tooth does not have another tooth to occlude with, the tooth will begin to descend out of the pocket.

14.

B. With this patient's financial situation, extraction would be the best option.

15.

A. The presence of exudate is an indication of an infection in the area.

patient history
synopsis

CASE 8
Age 68
Sex F
Height 5′7″
Weight 180lbs/82kg

VITAL SIGNS
Blood pressure 142/86
Pulse rate 84
Respiration rate 16

1. Under the care of a physician
☒ Yes ☐ No
Condition: Heart problems

2. Hospitalized within the last 5 years
☐ Yes ☒ No

3. Has or had the following conditions:
A fast heartbeat

4. Current medication(s)
Diltiazem, Estratest, Atenolol, and Medroxyprophyl

5. Smokes or uses tobacco products
☐ Yes ☒ No

6. Is pregnant
☐ Yes ☒ No ☐ N/A

Medical History: The client notes that she has heart problems (a fast heartbeat). She complains of shortness of breath and states she has been treated for ulcers.

Dental History: The client has a full upper denture that was placed at age 40. Her lower removable partial was placed at age 53. She cleans her teeth with baking soda three times a week, but does not use an auxiliary aid to clean under the mandibular bar since it is too time-consuming. She realizes the importance of removing plaque and states she does clean her denture and partial every night.

Social History: The client currently works part time as a secretary for a law firm.

Chief Complaint: At the initial appointment, the patient wants to have her lower partial adjusted. "Food also gets trapped under my partial."

ADULT CLINICAL EXAMINATION

Current Oral Hygiene Status
1. Heavy calculus
2. States that she relies on the hygenist to maintain the health of her oral cavity

Supplemental Oral Examination Findings
1. Crepitance on left TMJ
2. 1 month evaluation after prophylaxis, the tissue around #'s 22, 27 and 28 were inflamed with rolled margins.

Clinically visible carious lesion

Clinically missing tooth

Furcation

"Through and through" furcation

Probe 1: initial probing depth

Probe 2: probing depth 1 month after scaling and root planing

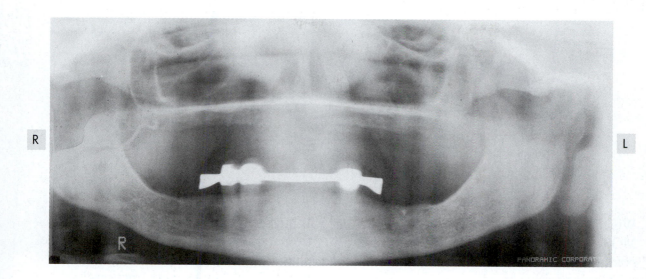

R   L

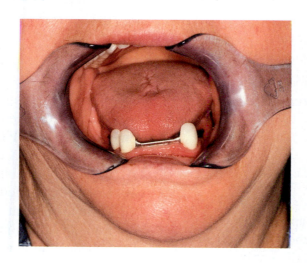

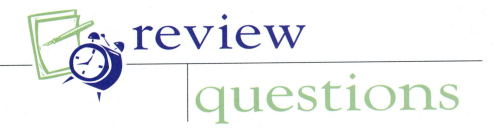

review questions

1. Which of the following bacteria would be MOST predominant at the evaluation appointment?
   A. Gram-positive cocci
   B. Gram-negative cocci
   C. Gram-positive spirochetes
   D. Gram-negative spirochetes

2. Which of the following toothbrush techniques is MOST appropriate to recommend to this client?
   A. Fones
   B. Bass
   C. Roll
   D. Charters

3. All of the following are appropriate physiotherapy aids to recommend for this client to help clean under the mandibular bar EXCEPT one. Which one is the EXCEPTION?
   A. Interdental brush
   B. Oral irrigating device
   C. Wooden interdental cleaner
   D. Super Floss®

4. The MOST appropriate referral for this client is to a(n)
   A. Occupational therapist
   B. Psychologist
   C. Dietitian
   D. Physical therapist

5. Which of the following numbers, taken from the client's vital signs, represents the phase of the cardiac cycle in which the heart relaxes between contractions?
   A. 142
   B. 86
   C. 84
   D. 16

6. All of the following protocol should be used to help reduce the risk of a medical emergency EXCEPT one. Which one is the EXCEPTION?
   A. Call the physician
   B. Use stress reduction
   C. Have the patient sit in a supine position for at least 2 minutes before releasing
   D. Schedule longer appointment times

7. When using a periodontal probe to determine the clinical attachment level of tooth #27, what is the reference point on the tooth to begin measurement readings?
   A. Marginal ridge
   B. CEJ
   C. Apical margin of the crown
   D. Mandibular bar

8. What is the MOST likely cause of bleeding at probing the mesial of #28?
   A. Heavy plaque
   B. Heavy pressure while exploring
   C. Poorly contoured crown margin
   D. Diseased gingival tissue

case study 8 questions

9. At which stage of the learning ladder is this client regarding plaque removal?
   A. Unawareness
   B. Awareness
   C. Self-interest
   D. Involvement

10. All of the following factors could lower the client's blood pressure EXCEPT one. Which one is the EXCEPTION?
   A. Exercise
   B. Ulcers
   C. Use of Atenolol
   D. Use of Diltiazem

11. What is the proper cleaning technique to clean this client's full denture without a soft liner?
   A. Place in water with mouthwash for 1 minute
   B. Scrub with a denture brush
   C. Immerse in solution of one part 5% sodium hypochlorite (Clorox) and three parts water
   D. Use a cotton swab and water and clean with a soft brush

12. What is the client taking Estratest for?
   A. To control high blood pressure
   B. To control her fast heartbeat
   C. To treat her ulcers
   D. To treat her menopausal symptoms

13. During the oral examination the dental hygienist asks the client to remove her upper denture. The client states, "I don't have any teeth up there—why should I remove my denture?" How should the dental hygienist proceed?
   A. Explain to the client that she needs to examine the tissue under the denture to ensure that the denture is fitting properly, and that there are no lesions under the denture
   B. The dental hygienist needs to understand that the patient may be self-conscious without her denture, so she should not push the issue
   C. Ask the dentist for assistance
   D. Dismiss the patient and hope that she will allow you to remove the denture next time

14. What is papillary hyperplasia of the palate?
   A. A condition caused by excessive smoking
   B. A response caused by irritants such as heavy plaque and calculus
   C. A form of denture stomatitis
   D. Benign tumor of the palate

15. All of the following is a cause of papillary hyperplasia of the palate EXCEPT for one. Which is the EXCEPTION?
   A. Ill-fitting denture
   B. Poor denture hygiene
   C. Excessive pressure of an ill-fitting denture
   D. Increased estrogen levels

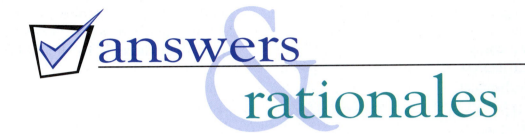

answers & rationales

1.

D. Gram-negative spirochetes, associated with inflammation, would be most predominant at the evaluation appointment since gingivitis is present. Gram-positive microorganisms are associated with healthy tissues and early plaque development.

2.

B. The Bass toothbrushing technique is most appropriate because it stimulates and cleans the gingival tissues along the tooth structure and adapts to the margins of the fixed partial denture. The toothbrush bristles are directed in the gingival sulcus for thorough plaque removal. Since it is easy to learn, the Fones technique could be recommended to use because the patient does not brush on a daily basis. However, it would not be a toothbrushing method of choice. The roll technique should not be considered since it does not provide gingival stimulation. The Charters technique could be considered, but it is more difficult to comprehend and apply than the Bass method.

3.

B. The oral irrigating device does not remove plaque. The interdental brush, wooden interdental cleaner, and Super Floss® would all be appropriate for use under the mandibular bar since they are capable of removing debris without causing trauma.

4.

C. Referral to a dietitian would be the most appropriate because the client is overweight. Weight reduction could benefit the client's elevated blood pressure. Referral to an occupational therapist, psychologist, or physical therapist is not appropriate for this client.

5.

B. The diastolic reading of the blood pressure represents the phase of the cardiac cycle in which the heart relaxes between contractions. This client's diastolic reading is 86. The systolic reading of the blood pressure represents the phase of the cardiac cycle in which the left ventricle of the heart contracts and blood is forced through the aorta and pulmonary artery. This client's systolic reading is 142. The client's pulse is 84, which is the intermittent throbbing sensation felt when finger(s) are pressed against an artery. The respiration rate, 16, indicates how well the body is providing oxygen to the tissues.

6.

D. Shorter appointments would be indicated to assist with stress reduction protocol and help reduce anxiety. It is appropriate to contact the physician if the clinician has questions or concerns regarding the treatment of this client. To decrease the risk of a medical emergency, it is important to use stress reduction protocol and have the client sit up at least 2 minutes before releasing.

7.

C. To determine the clinical attachment level, a fixed point on the tooth must be selected first. In this case, the fixed point is the apical margin of the crown. Although the marginal ridge is a fixed point on the occlusal surface of the tooth, it would not be a good reference point to use to determine attachment loss, since the distance would be greater than the probe readings. The cementoenamel joint (CEJ) is the point used when obtaining the clinical attachment level. In this case, the CEJ is not visible since the crown covers it. The mandibular bar is not an appropriate reference point since it is not attached to the tooth in question.

8.

D. The cause of bleeding on probing indicates diseased gingival tissues. The tissue has lacerated pocket walls, which bleed on gentle probing. Heavy plaque and a poorly contoured crown margin are causative factors of diseased gingival tissues; however, neither is the direct cause of bleeding on probing. Heavy pressure while exploring involves use of a different assessment instrument.

9.

B. The client does not use an auxiliary aid to remove plaque from under the mandibular bar because it is too "time-consuming." This indicates she is at the awareness level of the learning ladder—she has the correct information, but it does not offer any personal meaning. The patient is aware of the importance of plaque removal, establishing her at a higher level than unawareness. However, she does not have an interest to act, which demonstrates a lack of self-interest or involvement in the stages of the learning ladder.

10.

B. The client's blood pressure is slightly elevated. The client's past history of having ulcers would not affect her blood pressure. Exercise would help with weight reduction and, in turn, assist with decreasing her blood pressure. Atenolol is an antihypertensive drug. Diltiazem is a calcium channel blocker, which is also prescribed to reduce high blood pressure.

11.

C. Dentures without soft liners should be immersed in Clorox and water.

12.

D. Estratest is used to treat menopausal women who suffer from hot flashes but do not get relief from estrogen-only therapy.

13.

A. It is important to examine the tissue under the denture for improper wearing of the denture, and any oral lesions that are precancerous.

14.

C. Papillary hyperplasia is a form of denture stomatitis.

15.

D. Papillary hyperplasia is caused by the denture alone. Hormones do not play a role in the cause of papillary hyperplasia.

patient history
synopsis

CASE 9
Age 42
Sex F
Height 5′7″
Weight 135lbs/61kg

VITAL SIGNS
Blood pressure 122/78
Pulse rate 80
Respiration rate 16

1. Under the care of a physician

☐ Yes   ☒ No

2. Hopitalized within the last 5 years

☒ Yes   ☐ No

Reason: Multiple childbirths

3. Has or had the following conditions:

Rheumatic fever and numbness on her extremities

4. Current medication(s)

Calen

5. Smokes or uses tobacco products

☐ Yes   ☒ No

6. Is pregnant

☐ Yes   ☒ No   ☐ N/A

Medical History: The client has a history of rheumatic fever and numbness on her extremities. She denies having been told of the presence of a heart murmur and has never taken antibiotics before dental treatment. She is allergic to Bactrim.

Dental History: The client reports receiving regular dental care throughout her life. She has multiple restorations. She has had no problem with her previous treatment. Her last visit was 6 months ago.

Social History: The client is a mother of 5 children.

Chief Complaint: Her teeth look yellow.

ADULT CLINICAL EXAMINATION

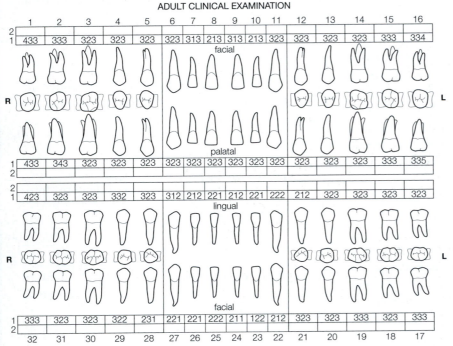

Current Oral Hygiene Status
1. Good oral hygiene

Supplemental Oral Examination Findings
1. None

		Clinically visible carious lesion
		Clinically missing tooth
		Furcation
		"Through and through" furcation

Probe 1: initial probing depth

Probe 2: probing depth 1 month
after scaling and root planing

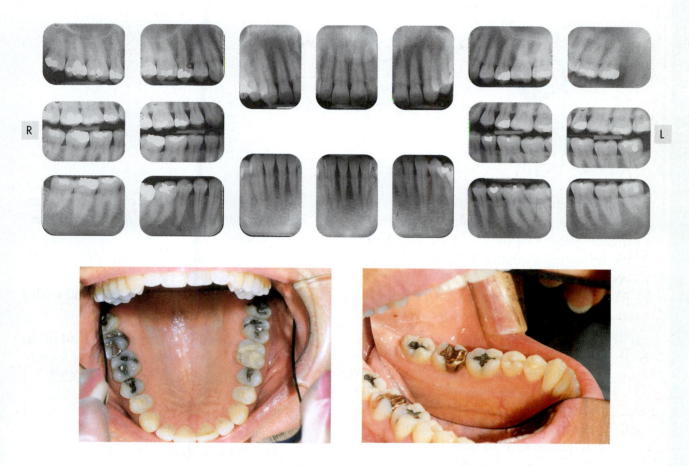

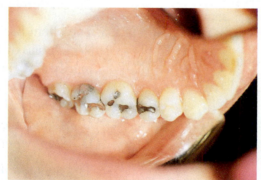

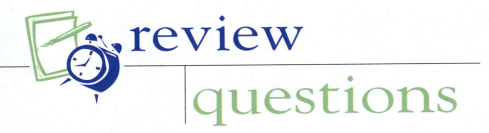

review questions

1. A gingivectomy is indicated for the mandibular right third molar. After reviewing the client's medical history, which of the following assessments should be made prior to treatment?
   A. A history of rheumatic fever requires antibiotic prophylactic therapy for all dental treatment.
   B. A history of rheumatic fever requires antibiotic prophylactic therapy for some dental treatment, but not for minor surgical procedures.
   C. The client has never been premedicated with antibiotics for dental treatment and therefore does not need it.
   D. A medical consultation is required to determine the cardiac status of this client.

2. The classification of restoration on the maxillary right second premolar is
   A. I
   B. II
   C. III
   D. IV

3. Which of the following materials was MOST likely used to restore the maxillary right second premolar?
   A. Dental amalgam
   B. Composite resin
   C. Gold alloy
   D. Glass ionomer cement

4. The probable cause of the overhang on the maxillary left second premolar may be due to improper
   A. Condensation of the amalgam
   B. Polishing of the restoration
   C. Placement of the matrix band and wedge
   D. Burnishing of the restoration

5. Since this client has healthy tissue, all of the following microorganisms would be found EXCEPT one. Which one is the EXCEPTION?
   A. Predominately Gram-positive
   B. Aerobic cocci
   C. Anaerobic spirochetes
   D. Predominately Gram-negative

6. The client has several occlusal restorations. Which one of the following bacteria is primarily associated with coronal caries?
   A. *Mutans streptococcus*
   B. *Lactobacillus*
   C. *Actinomyces*
   D. *Staphylococcus*

7. The dental amalgam on the mandibular right first molar is to be polished. Which of the following is NOT a reason for minimizing heat during this procedure?
   A. Pulp damage
   B. Weakened marginal areas by adversely affecting mercury concentration
   C. Release of mercury vapor
   D. Discoloration of the tooth

8. The mandibular right second molar has an existing restoration fabricated by an indirect technique. What material was MOST likely used to restore this tooth?
   A. Dental amalgam
   B. Composite resin
   C. Gold alloy
   D. Glass ionomer

9. What is the radiolucent band visible on the radiograph at the neck of tooth #9?
   A. An artifact
   B. Caries
   C. Cervical burnout
   D. Incisive foramen

10. Side effects of antihypersensitive drugs are MOST likely to include all of the following EXCEPT one. Which one is the EXCEPTION?
    A. Postural hypotension
    B. Gingival hyperplasia
    C. Xerostomia
    D. Increased gag reflex

11. Tooth # 31 is classified as a
    A. Gold onlay
    B. Gold inlay
    C. Gold crown
    D. None of the above

12. What should the dental hygienist recommend for the patient's yellow teeth?
    A. Brush and floss more frequently.
    B. Put patient on a 3-month recall to have her teeth polished more often.
    C. Suggest an at-home bleaching system.
    D. Inform the patient that not much can be done for her yellow teeth.

13. What is the structure of home bleaching systems?
    A. 10% carbamide peroxide applied in a custom-fitted tray
    B. 5.3% carbamide peroxide applied in a custom-fitted tray
    C. 30% hydrogen peroxide gel or paste applied in a custom-fitted tray
    D. 20% hydrogen peroxide gel or paste applied in a custom-fitted tray

14. Which of the following types of stains bleach the quickest?
    A. Tetracycline stains
    B. Gray stains
    C. Yellow stains
    D. Orange stains

15. All of the following are common side effects of bleaching EXCEPT for one. Which is the EXCEPTION?
    A. Tooth sensitivity
    B. TMJ pain due to wearing the tray
    C. Gingival irritation
    D. Over whitening

case study 9 questions

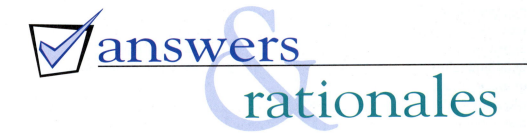

answers & rationales

1.

D. The presence or absence of a heart murmur should be verified. A history of rheumatic fever with no valvular replacement does not require antibiotic prophylaxis. Although the client has not been premedicated for past care, her cardiac status should be determined.

2.

B. Class II restorations involve the proximal surfaces of posterior teeth. Class I restorations involve the pits and fissures of teeth. Class III and IV restorations involve the proximal surfaces and incisal edges of anterior teeth, respectively.

3.

A. The material in tooth #4 is dental amalgam. Composite resins and glass ionomers are tooth-colored restorations. Gold alloys do not typically present with evidence of corrosion.

4.

C. Improper placement of the matrix and wedge can cause overhanging restorations. The amalgam in tooth #13 appears well condensed. Polishing techniques could be used to remove the overhang. Burnishing is used to smooth the surface of an amalgam.

5.

C. Anaerobic bacteria are found predominately in diseased tissues. All the remaining bacteria can be found in healthy tissue.

6.

A. The primary bacteria associated with the initiation of coronal caries is *Mutans streptococcus*. *Lactobacillus* is involved with advanced smooth surface caries. *Actinomyces* has been associated with root surface caries. *Staphylococcus* is not associated with dental caries.

7.

D. Heat generated by polishing should not discolor tooth structure. Heat generation can cause pulp damage and mercury to vaporize. It can also increase the mercury concentration, decreasing the strength of the amalgam in thin marginal areas.

8.

C. Gold alloy is a metallic material used for indirect restorations. Dental amalgam and glass ionomers are used as direct restorative materials. The restoration present is too radiopaque to be a composite restoration.

9.

C. Cervical burnout appears radiolucent because of the concavities between the facial and lingual root surfaces. An artifact is a manmade error, which can be radiolucent or radiopaque. Root surface caries have a "ditched out" appearance with some degree of bone loss. Incisive foramen is an opening in the midline in the hard palate.

10.

D. Increased gag reflex is not a side effect associated with antihypertensive drugs. Gingival hyperplasia is associated with most of the calcium channel blockers used as antihypersensitives. Postural hypotension and xerostomia are associated with antihypersensitive medications.

11.

A. Since the gold restoration includes the lingual mesial cusp, the restoration is classified as a gold onlay.

12.

C. At-home bleaching systems are effective for the treatment of yellow stain.

13.

A. 10% carbamide peroxide is typically used for at-home bleaching in a custom-fitted tray. 5.3% carbamide peroxide is used in the thin polyethylene strips, and 30% hydrogen peroxide gel or paste is used for in-office light or heat-activated bleaching systems.

14.

C. Yellow stains bleach faster than gray stains. Tetracycline-stained teeth bleach very slowly or not at all.

15.

B. There is no evidence that states bleaching trays cause TMJ disorders.

case study 9 answers

1. Under the care of a physician

☐ Yes   ☒ No

2. Hospitalized within the last 5 years

☐ Yes   ☒ No

3. Has or had the following conditions:

Abdominal discomfort, nausea, and vomiting

4. Current medication(s)

None

5. Smokes or uses tobacco products

☐ Yes   ☒ No

6. Is pregnant

☐ Yes   ☐ No   ☒ N/A

Medical History: The client has not been under the care of a physician for the past 5 years, but reports recent symptoms of abdominal discomfort, nausea, and vomiting. He is allergic to penicillin.

Dental History: The client's last dental treatment was 1 year ago. A full-mouth series was taken at that time and nonsurgical periodontal therapy was completed by the dental hygienist. The client states he was diagnosed with periodontal disease over 11 years ago, but has not been able to afford treatment. He has received annual cleaning and emergency extractions #s 14 and 30.

Social History: The client's occupation is construction work. He is married and has six children. He reports experiencing financial difficulties.

Chief Complaint: "My gums bleed when I brush."

ADULT CLINICAL EXAMINATION

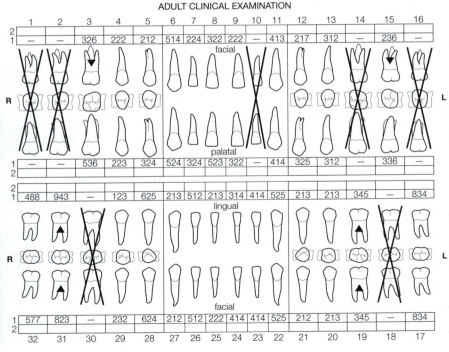

	1	2	3	4	5	6	7	8	9	10	11	12	13	14	15	16
2 1 (facial)	—	—	326	222	212	514	224	322	222	—	413	217	312	—	236	—
1 2 (palatal)	—	—	536	223	324	524	324	523	322	—	414	325	312	—	336	—

	32	31	30	29	28	27	26	25	24	23	22	21	20	19	18	17
2 1 (lingual)	488	943	—	123	625	213	512	213	314	414	525	213	213	345	—	834
1 2 (facial)	577	823	—	232	624	212	512	222	414	414	525	212	213	345	—	834

Current Oral Hygiene Status

1. Moderate plaque, calculus, and stain
2. Brushes twice a day, but does not floss

Supplemental Oral Examination Findings

1. Class I mobility #31
2. Class II mobility #12, 15
3. Generalized attrition and cervical abrasion
4. Localized areas of dentinal hypersensitivity
5. Gingiva exhibits generalized marginal redness, edema, and bleeding on probing

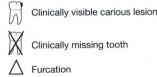

☐ Clinically visible carious lesion

☒ Clinically missing tooth

△ Furcation

▲ "Through and through" furcation

Probe 1: initial probing depth

Probe 2: probing depth 1 month after scaling and root planing

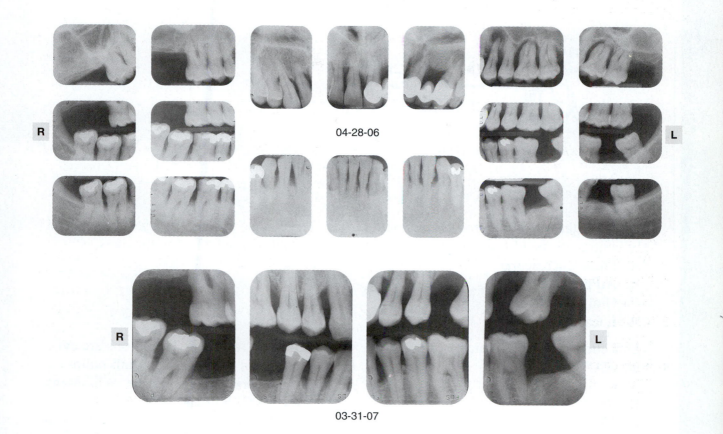

04-28-06

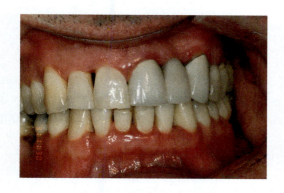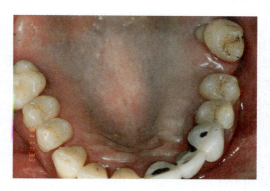

03-31-07

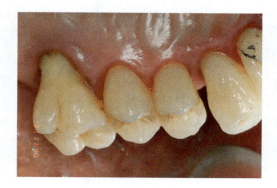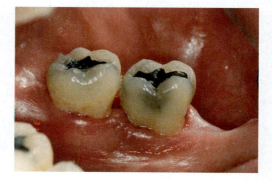

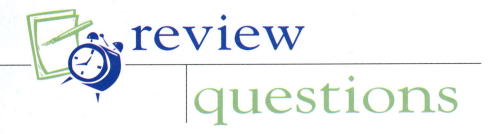

review questions

1. Which of the following procedures would be contraindicated for this client?
   A. Phase microscope
   B. Air polishing
   C. Oral irrigation
   D. Local anesthesia

2. This client represents which of the following AAP Case Types?
   A. I
   B. II
   C. III
   D. IV
   E. V

3. Which of the following ultrasonic instrument tips would be BEST to use for debridement on the lingual aspect of tooth #31?
   A. Modified (thin) straight ultrasonic
   B. Modified (thin) curved right
   C. Modified (thin) curved left
   D. Standard rigid

4. All of the following antimicrobial/antibiotic adjuncts can be considered for use with this client EXCEPT one. Which one is the EXCEPTION?
   A. Tetracycline fiber placement
   B. Chlorhexidine gluconate in ultrasonic unit
   C. Daily stannous fluoride home irrigation
   D. Oral penicillin
   E. Daily phenolic compound rinses

5. The clinical attachment level on the direct lingual of tooth #3, in millimeters, is
   A. 5
   B. 6
   C. 8
   D. 10

6. All of the following conditions are evident in this client's full mouth radiographic series EXCEPT one. Which one is the EXCEPTION?
   A. Calculus
   B. Amalgam overhang
   C. Furcation involvement
   D. Vertical bone loss
   E. Periapical pathology

7. All of the following home care recommendations are appropriate and address the client's chief complaint EXCEPT one. Which one is the EXCEPTION?
   A. Interdental brush
   B. Desensitizing dentifrice
   C. Sulcular flossing
   D. Antimicrobial mouth rinse
   E. Perio-Aid (toothpick in holder)

8. Based on the data provided, what is the MOST appropriate continued care regimen for this client?
   A. 3 months
   B. 4 months
   C. 6 months
   D. 12 months

9. Which of the following terms BEST describes the lingual tissue between teeth #s 31 and 32?
   A. Bulbous
   B. Blunted
   C. Cratered
   D. Festooned
   E. Flattened

10. Because of the client's periodontal condition relative to his age and length of time since a physician last examined him, a referral for medical examination may be indicated. Which of the following undiagnosed medical conditions is MOST likely suspected as a contributing factor to this client's physical symptoms?
    A. Thyroid disease
    B. Diabetes
    C. Tuberculosis
    D. Hepatitis C

11. All of the following instruments may be appropriate to debride the mesial surface of tooth #3 EXCEPT one. Which one is the EXCEPTION?
    A. Columbia 4R/4L
    B. Gracey 15/16
    C. Gracey 5/6
    D. Modified (thin) curved right ultrasonic tip
    E. Modified (thin) curved left ultrasonic tip

12. Which of the following Gracey curets is LEAST appropriate to use to debride the facial surface and furcation on tooth #15?
    A. 3/4
    B. 7/8
    C. 11/12
    D. 13/14

13. Which of the following probes is the instrument of choice for the detection and classification of furcation involvements?
    A. William's probe
    B. PSR probe
    C. Nabers probe
    D. UNC15 probe

14. The client will need to be anesthetized for the scaling procedures. Considering his medical history, which of the following should be taken into consideration?
    A. Limit the amount of vasoconstrictor used
    B. Limit the amount of amide anesthetic used
    C. Limit the amount of ester topical anesthetic used
    D. None of the above; there is no problem with the administration of a local anesthetic for this client

15. Which injections are needed to anesthetize the mandibular right quadrant for deep cleaning?
    A. Right IA, lingual, buccal
    B. Right IA, lingual, buccal, mental
    C. Right incisive, buccal, lingual
    D. Right IA, lingual, incisive

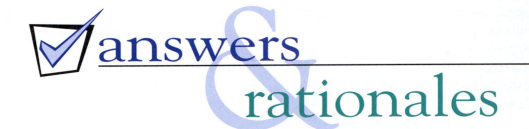

answers & rationales

1.

B. The use of airpolishing is contraindicated for a patient with an anterior porcelain-fused-to-metal bridge, generalized recession, and exposed cementum and dentin. Air polishing has demonstrated pitting and wear to porcelain, erosion of dental cements, and damage to margins of dental castings. Ultrasonic scaling is indicated for calculus removal and debridement in deep pockets, furcations, and root concavities. Antimicrobial oral irrigation may be helpful in controlling the client's periodontal disease. The phase contrast microscope may help to motivate the client into more stringent homecare and treatment recommendations. Periodontal debridement may be more efficient and comfortable for the patient if local anesthesia is used.

2.

D. This client presents with AAP Case Type IV—advanced periodontitis. There is evidence of advanced loss of alveolar bone, furcations, and increased mobility, all indicators of AAP Case Type IV. This client's periodontal condition is beyond AAP Case Types I, II, and III. Owing to the client's lack of finances, he has never received the recommended periodontal surgery and therefore could not be classified as AAP Case Type V, refractory periodontitis.

3.

C. The lingual of tooth #31 has 2-mm recession, a 5-mm pocket, Class II furcation involvement, with light to moderate plaque and calculus. The modified (thin) curved left is designed for use on the mandibular right lingual. Its design is specified for removal of light to moderate calculus, plaque, and endotoxins and provides access into furcations and pockets greater than 4 mm. The modified (thin) straight tip is designed primarily for patients with AAP Case Type I, exhibiting 3 to 4 mm pockets and minimal to no bone loss. The modified (thin) right is designed for application on the mandibular facial of #31. The standard rigid tip is designed to remove heavy or tenacious calculus.

4.

D. The client is allergic to penicillin; therefore another antibiotic would need to be selected if antibiotic therapy is deemed necessary. The new paradigm in periodontal therapy includes use of antimicrobial adjuncts such as tetracycline, chlorhexidine, and daily phenolic compound rinses.

5.

D. When the gingival margin has receded apically to the CEJ, the clinical attachment level is determined by measuring the distance from the base of the pocket to the CEJ. The pocket depth of 5 mm is added to the recession measurement of 5 mm, giving the clinical attachment a measurement of 10 mm.

6.

B. Class II restorations are only evident on teeth #s 29 and 30. Neither restoration exhibits an overhang on the radiographs. Vertical bone loss, periapical pathology (#12), and furcation involvement (on most molars) are evident on the radiographs.

7.

B. While a desensitizing dentifrice is an appropriate recommendation for the client's dentinal hypersensitivity, it does not address the client's chief complaint of bleeding gingiva. Regular use of the proxy brush, sulcular flossing, antimicrobial mouth rinses, and perio aid (toothpick) would improve plaque control and reduce gingival inflammation and bleeding.

8.

A. The client has advanced periodontitis and is unable to afford definitive periodontal treatment—periodontal surgery. In addition, the client's home care is noncompliant. Therefore, a 3-month continued care interval is most appropriate for this client to debride the periodontal pockets and monitor his periodontal condition.

9.

D. The term *festooned* refers to enlargement of the marginal gingiva with the formation of a lifesaver-like gingival prominence.

10.

D. With hepatitis C, the symptoms include abdominal discomfort, nausea, and vomiting. The symptoms of thyroid disease, diabetes, and tuberculosis do not include those stated above.

11.

C. The Gracey curet 5/6 is designed for use on anterior and premolar teeth. The Columbia 4R/4L is a universal instrument that can be used on the entire dentition. The Gracey curet 15/16 is designed to provide access to the mesials of posterior teeth. The modified curved right ultrasonic tip can access the lingual aspect of #3 and the modified curved left tip can access the facial of #3.

12.

A. The Gracey curet 3/4 is designed for use on the anterior teeth and not appropriate for use on #15. The Gracey curet 7/8 and 9/10 are designed for use on the facial and lingual surfaces of posterior teeth. The Gracey curet 11/12 and 13/14 are designed for use on the mesial and distal surfaces of posterior teeth, respectively.

13.

C. The Nabers probe is curved and has a blunted tip and is used to detect bone loss in the furcation areas of bifurcated and trifurcated teeth.

14.

B. Amide local anesthetic are metabolized in the liver. Should the client have hepatitis C he will metabolize the anesthetic at a slower rate.

15.

A. The inferior alveolar, lingual, and buccal injections will anesthetize the entire mandibular right quadrant. The mental and incisive nerves are branches of the IA nerve and will be anesthetized with the IA injection.

appendix b

simulated national board dental hygiene examination 2

1. The major artery that extends through the pterygopalatine fossa is the
   A. Facial artery
   B. Maxillary artery
   C. Superficial temporal artery
   D. Internal carotid artery

2. The infratemporal fossa is important in dentistry because it contains the
   A. Origin of the mandibular nerve
   B. Facial artery
   C. Buccinator muscle
   D. Salivary glands
   E. Muscles of mastication and many of the nerves and vessels supplying the mouth

3. The maxillary sinuses develop
   A. During the third month of fetal life
   B. At birth
   C. After the permanent teeth have erupted
   D. During the sixth to eighth years
   E. At about 12 years

4. The line of demarcation between the loose alveolar mucosa and the more dense alveolar mucosa adjacent to teeth is the
   A. Retromolar papilla
   B. Palatoglossal fold
   C. Mucogingival junction
   D. Sulcus terminalis
   E. Pterygopalatine junction

5. A fold of mucous membrane that helps anchor the tongue to the mouth floor in the midline is the
   A. Fauces
   B. Philtrum
   C. Frenulum
   D. Nasolabial fold
   E. Anterior median fold

6. The superior and inferior ganglia are associated with which cranial nerve?
   A. Trigeminal
   B. Facial
   C. Glossopharyngeal
   D. Vagus
   E. Hypoglossal

7. Which of the following permanent molars frequently exhibits a small fifth cusp attached to the lingual surface of the mesiolingual cusp?
   A. Maxillary second molar
   B. Maxillary first molar
   C. Mandibular first molar
   D. Mandibular second molar

8. A comparison of primary and permanent teeth will show which of the following differences in form?
   A. The crowns of primary anterior teeth are wider mesiodistally in comparison with their crown length than are the permanent teeth.
   B. The roots of primary anterior teeth are narrower and longer than those of permanent teeth
   C. Cervical ridges positioned buccally on the primary molars are more pronounced than on permanent teeth
   D. All of the above

9. The first evidence of calcification of the primary lateral incisor is seen at approximately which of the following ages?
   A. 2 months in utero
   B. 4 months
   C. 6 months
   D. 4 1/2 months in utero
   E. 1 1/2 years

10. The roots of the permanent third molars are completely formed at which of the following ages?
    A. 10–12 years
    B. 13–14 years
    C. 14–16 years
    D. 18–25 years

11. Deciduous teeth are exfoliated by which of the following processes?
    A. Pressure from the permanent tooth pushes the primary tooth out.
    B. The primary tooth undergoes resorption from the crown apically to the root.
    C. The primary tooth undergoes resorption from the apical portion of the root upward

12. Bitter and sour taste sensations of the tongue are mediated by the intermediofacial nerve by the chorda tympani. Sweet and salty tastes of the tongue are mediated by the glossopharyngeal nerve.
    A. First statement TRUE; second statement FALSE
    B. First statement FALSE; second statement TRUE
    C. Both statements TRUE
    D. Both statements FALSE

13. Hertwig's epithelial sheath is derived from the
    A. Inner dental epithelium and stratum intermedium
    B. Inner dental epithelium and stellate reticulum
    C. Outer dental epithelium and stellate reticulum
    D. Outer dental epithelium and stratum intermedium
    E. Inner dental epithelium and outer dental epithelium

14. After the tooth is formed, the dental papilla becomes
    A. The dental sac
    B. Dentin
    C. The dental pulp
    D. bone

15. Hunger-Schreger bands are best demonstrated by
    A. Transmitted light
    B. Diffracted light
    C. Reflected light
    D. Polarized light

16. Hormones
    A. Catalyze intracellular biochemical reactions
    B. Enter into chemical reactions without being degraded or depleted
    C. Are chemical substances that (1) are produced by endocrine glands, (2) travel through the circulatory system, and (3) exert their influence on specific structures
    D. All of the above

17. Calcitonin
    A. Potentiates the effect of parathyroid hormone
    B. Is secreted by the thyroid gland
    C. Is released in response to excess serum calcium
    D. All of the above
    E. B and C only

18. Cortisol
    A. Increases the flux of amino acids in the body
    B. Mobilizes stored fat
    C. Promotes gluconeogenesis
    D. All of the above
    E. A and C only

19. Oxygen is carried in the blood
    A. As oxyhemoglobin
    B. Dissolved in plasma
    C. As carbaminohemoglobin
    D. Both A and B
    E. Both A and C

20. A disease caused by interference with the intrinsic–extrinsic factor mechanism is called
    A. Aplastic anemia
    B. Sickle-cell anemia
    C. Iron-deficiency anemia
    D. Pernicious anemia

21. Beriberi is prevalent in the Orient because a diet made up primarily of polished rice is deficient in
    A. Thiamin
    B. Vitamin A
    C. Vitamin C
    D. Riboflavin

22. The daily NRC/RDA (1989) requirement for iron by a normal adult female during childbearing years approximates
    A. 15 mg
    B. 18 mg
    C. 100 mg
    D. 1 g
    E. 10 g

23. The dominant factor in controlling the absorption of iron from the gastrointestinal tract is the
    A. Excretion of iron in the urine
    B. Excretion of iron in the stools
    C. Presence of reducing substances in the gut
    D. Physiological saturation of the mucosal cells with iron
    E. Concentration of the ferrous iron in bone marrow, spleen, and liver

24. Although rare, toxicity to vitamin excess by eating naturally occurring foodstuffs has been reported for vitamins
    A. A and D
    B. D and K
    C. B_1 and C
    D. B_2 and K
    E. B_2 and B_6

25. Which of the following nutrient deficiencies is frequently found in the diet of children in developed countries and has been associated with increased caries susceptibility in laboratory animals?
    A. Iron
    B. Zinc
    C. Vitamin E
    D. Protein
    E. Calcium

26. Amino acids are building blocks for
    A. Vitamins
    B. Minerals
    C. Proteins
    D. All of the above

27. Herpes zoster is thought to be the adult counterpart of which of the following diseases?
    A. Chickenpox
    B. Measles
    C. Mumps
    D. Smallpox
    E. Rubeola

28. An anaerobic *Streptococcus* is classified as a member of genus
    A. *Neisseria*
    B. *Peptostreptococcus*
    C. *Hemophilus*
    D. *Lactobacillus*
    E. *Enterococcus*

29. For optimal growth, microaerophilic bacteria grow best with
    A. Free access to air
    B. The presence of molecular oxygen only
    C. A complete absence of oxygen
    D. An atmosphere of low oxygen tension
    E. A mixture of nitrogen and hydrogen

30. MacConkey's agar is a medium best suited for selective growth of microorganisms such as
    A. *Streptococcus pyogenes*
    B. *Staphylococcus aureus*
    C. *Lactobacillus species*
    D. *Escherichia coli*
    E. *Hemophilus influenzae*

31. *Lactobacillus acidophilus* is a
    A. Gram-positive coccus
    B. Gram-positive rod
    C. Gram-negative coccus
    D. Gram-negative rod
    E. gram-variable spiral bacteria

32. Viruses that infect bacteria are known as
    A. Saprophytes
    B. Commensals
    C. Protoplasts
    D. Bacteriophages
    E. Spheroplasts

33. A substance that helps prepare bacteria for phagocytosis is a(n)
    A. Bacteriolysin
    B. Interferon
    C. Antitoxin
    D. Opsonin
    E. Hemolysin

34. Which characteristic is the most outstanding feature of genus Mycoplasma?
    A. Slow-replicating viruses
    B. Temperate bacteriophages
    C. Extracellular rickettsia
    D. Spiral bacteria
    E. Cell wall–deficient organisms

35. Chemotaxis is a function of which of the following cells?
    A. Erythrocytes
    B. Leukocytes
    C. Epithelial
    D. Endothelial
    E. All of the above

36. Diseases of lower animals that are transmissible to humans are known as
    A. Zoonoses
    B. Phycomycoses
    C. Geophilic
    D. Anthrophilic
    E. Dermatophytes

37. Ethylene oxide has which of the following action on bacteria?
    A. Bacteriostatic
    B. Antiseptic
    C. Disinfects
    D. Sterilizes
    E. Sanitizes

38. The first step in the sequence of steps in the vascular reaction associated with the inflammatory process is
    A. Increased vascular permeability
    B. Vasodilation
    C. Transient vasoconstriction
    D. Margination of leukocytes
    E. Slowing of blood flow and stagnation

39. Chemical products released into the blood during the inflammatory process can produce which one of the following?
    A. Lymphadenopathy
    B. Fever
    C. Bacteremia
    D. Pyemia
    E. Leukopenia

40. AIDS is characterized by a depletion of which type of cells?
    A. Polymorphonuclear leukocytes
    B. B Lymphocytes
    C. Helper T lymphocytes
    D. Suppressor T lymphocytes

41. A purulent inflammation is characterized by the production of mucin. It is a creamy opaque substance containing liquefied necrotic material and many red blood cells.
    A. First statement TRUE; second statement FALSE
    B. First statement FALSE; second statement TRUE
    C. Both statements TRUE
    D. Both statements FALSE

42. Granulomatous inflammation is present in which of the following diseases?
    A. Tuberculosis
    B. Fungal infections
    C. Sarcoidosis ✓
    D. All of the above

43. The most common benign soft-tissue lesion occurring in the oral cavity is the
    A. Papilloma
    B. Fibroma ✓
    C. Amalgam tattoo
    D. Verrucus vulgaris
    E. Pyogenic granuloma

44. Peripheral giant-cell granulomas always occur
    A. In the mandible
    B. In the maxilla
    C. In edentulous patients
    D. On the gingiva or alveolar process

45. The central giant-cell granuloma is not a destructive lesion. Radiographically, it appears radiopaque.
    A. First statement TRUE; second statement FALSE
    B. First statement FALSE; second statement TRUE
    C. Both statements TRUE
    D. Both statements FALSE

46. Which of the following is the most common site for a pleomorphic adenoma?
    A. Submaxillary salivary gland
    B. Lip
    C. Tongue
    D. Parotid gland
    E. Buccal mucosa

47. A dentigerous cyst originates through alteration of the reduced enamel epithelium
    A. After the crown and root are completely formed
    B. Before the crown is completely formed
    C. After the crown is completely formed
    D. After the crown is formed, but before the root is completely formed

48. A 50-year-old man who smokes a pipe is found to have lesions on his palate, underneath his denture. He says he removes the denture only to clean it. The lesions on his palate are erythematous, papillary projections. His chief complaint is an ill-fitting set of dentures that is 10 years old. This patient most probably has
    A. Stomatitis nicotina
    B. Traumatic ulcers
    C. Papillary hyperplasia
    D. Denture stomatitis
    E. Epulis

49. A white patch on the oral mucosa that cannot be rubbed off and cannot be ascribed to any other disease is most probably
    A. Lichen planus
    B. Leukoplakia
    C. Erythroplasia
    D. Squamous-cell carcinoma
    E. Candidiasis

50. The topical cortisone most commonly used in treating oral ulceration is
    A. Triamcinolone acetonide (Kenalog)
    B. Orabase
    C. Promethazine hydrochloride
    D. Oxycodone hydrochloride

51. In prescribing amoxicillin for prevention of bacterial endocarditis, one should give how much amoxicillin 1 hour prior to the oral prophylaxis appointment?
    A. 500 mg
    B. 1,000 mg
    C. 3,000 mg
    D. 2,000 mg

52. A patient with a mild to moderately severe oral infection who gives a history of allergy to penicillin should be given
    A. Cloxacillin
    B. Erythromycin
    C. Streptomycin
    D. Chloramphenicol
    E. Cephalexin

53. Pentazocine is sold under the trademark
    A. Ponstel
    B. Talwin
    C. Darvon
    D. Dilaudid

54. Which one of the following is a Schedule II controlled substance?
    A. Demerol
    B. Phenaphen
    C. Empirin with codeine 1/2 gr
    D. Tylenol with codeine

55. In discussing meperidine (Demerol), one finds that
    A. It is commonly used alone as a pre-anesthetic medication for anxiety
    B. It has a usual adult dose of 25 mg
    C. It is a good substitute drug for morphine
    D. Its ability to be combined with other drugs (e.g., aspirin) is quite limited

56. In general, barbiturates have the ability to
    A. Produce long-term cortical depression
    B. Provide sedation but no analgesia
    C. Provide sedation and analgesia
    D. Be sedative but not hypnotic

57. Promethazine (Phenergan) has all of the following properties except
    A. Anti-inflammatory
    B. Sedative
    C. Local anesthetic
    D. Antihistaminic

58. If a patient is allergic to salicylates (aspirin), you may prescribe
    A. Demerol
    B. Darvon compound
    C. Tylenol
    D. Codeine

59. If a patient gives a history of having been on a drug regimen of long-term chlorothiazide, one should be alert to
    A. Hypertension and diuresis
    B. Diabetes and poor healing
    C. Psychosis and mood elevation
    D. Heart disease and anticoagulation

60. Which of the following blood pressures is considered normal?
    A. 100/80 mm Hg
    B. 120/80 mm Hg
    C. 130/120 mm Hg
    D. 140/60 mm Hg
    E. 150/100 mm Hg

61. Nitroglycerine (glyceryl trinitrate) is used for the treatment of
    A. Diabetes
    B. Epilepsy
    C. Convulsions
    D. Angina pectoris
    E. Hypertension

62. If a patient has recently suffered a myocardial infarction, elective dental and dental hygiene appointments should be postponed for
    A. 6 weeks
    B. 1 month
    C. 3 month or longer
    D. More than 1 year

63. The best way to examine the dorsum of the tongue is to
    A. Ask the patient to say "ah" and depress the tongue with the mouth mirror
    B. Use a dental mirror for indirect vision
    C. Extend the tongue fully by grasping with a dry gauze square and use direct vision
    D. Palpate between the thumb and index finger

64. Subgingival calculus differs from supragingival calculus in
    A. Location
    B. Density
    C. Color
    D. A and C only
    E. A, B, and C

65. An enlargement of the marginal gingiva with the formation of a lifesaver-like gingival prominence describes
    A. Stillman's cleft
    B. Gingival cyst
    C. Gingival abscess
    D. Fistula
    E. McCall's festoon

66. A patient who evidences the typical signs of traumatic occlusion is likely to have radiographs that demonstrate which of the following?
    A. Widening of the periodontal space
    B. Angular bone destruction
    C. Thickening of the lamina dura
    D. All of the above

67. Which of the following periodontal factors cannot be determined through a radiographic evaluation alone?
    A. Height or contour of bone located on the facial or lingual surfaces of the teeth
    B. Presence or absence of periodontal pockets
    C. Presence or absence of occlusal trauma
    D. A and C only
    E. All of the above

68. Which of the following is the LEAST important diagnostic aid in recognizing the early stage of gingival disease?
    A. Gingival color
    B. Depth of the gingival crevice
    C. Stippling of the gingival tissue
    D. Hemorrhaging of the gingival tissue

69. Bleeding upon probing in the presence of periodontal disease is caused by which of the following histologic changes?
    A. Fibrosis associated with chronic inflammation
    B. Edema

70. Which of the following stains of the teeth will show up brilliant yellow under ultraviolet light?
    A. Chromogenic stain
    B. Erythroblastosis fetalis
    C. Fluorosis
    D. Tetracycline

71. A pathologic wearing away of the teeth through some abnormal mechanical process is called
    A. Erosion
    B. Attrition
    C. Abrasion
    D. Intrusion

72. A prognathic profile is usually associated with which of the following classifications of malocclusion?
    A. Class I
    B. Class II
    C. Class III

73. Acquired pellicle is initially derived from
    A. Saliva
    B. Tooth structure
    C. Bacterial products
    D. Dietary components

74. The standard regimen for antibiotic premedication is
    A. 2 grams of clindamycin 1 hour before the appointment
    B. 2 grams of amoxicillin 1 hour before the appointment
    C. 2 grams of amoxicillin 1 hour before the appointment and 1 gram 6 hours later
    D. 2 grams of clindamycin 1 hour before the appointment and 1 gram 6 hours later

75. MOST fluoride is absorbed in the
    A. Liver
    B. Small intestine
    C. Sweat glands
    D. Urine
    E. Kidneys

76. To reduce radiation exposure when taking radiographs, the operator should
    A. Stand behind a suitable barrier
    B. Stand at least 4 feet away from the patient and 125 degrees away from the central beam
    C. Use speed D film
    D. Stand behind the head of the x-ray unit

77. Of all the periapical views included in a paralleling technique full-mouth series of radiographs, which region is closest to satisfying all the principles of shadow casting and parallel placement of the film?
    A. The maxillary molar view
    B. The maxillary premolar view
    C. The mandibular molar view
    D. The mandibular premolar view

78. All of the following landmarks occur in the anterior region of the maxilla EXCEPT the
    A. Nasal fossae
    B. Hamular process
    C. Median palatal suture
    D. Nasal septum
    E. Incisive foramen

79. Which of the following is a radiolucent restorative material?
    A. Amalgam
    B. Acrylic
    C. Silver points
    D. Gold

80. Which of the following combinations of structures appear radiolucent in a radiograph?
    A. Nasal fossae, mental foramen, periodontal ligament space
    B. Nasal fossae, incisive canal, genial tubercle
    C. Hamular process, nutrient canal, nasal septum
    D. Maxillary sinus, internal oblique ridge, mental foramen

81. Which of the following extraoral projections is most useful in the diagnosis of maxillary sinus conditions?
    A. Lateral skull projection
    B. Water's view
    C. Posteroanterior projection
    D. Lateral oblique projection

82. A lateral oblique of the mandible (Lateral Jaw) radiograph is most frequently used for observing structures in
    A. Both the maxilla and mandible for early periodontal disease detection
    B. The posterior teeth for periapical disease
    C. Areas such as the symphysis of the mandible for possible fractures
    D. Posterior areas of the mandible and/or maxillae that are too large to be depicted on a periapical film

83. If an exposure time of 30 impulses produces the proper density for an intraoral film at a focal spot film distance of 8 inches, what exposure time would be required to produce the same density at a 16-inch distance?
    A. 60 impulses
    B. 90 impulses
    C. 120 impulses
    D. 150 impulses

84. In panoramic radiography, the focal trough is the
    A. Slit where excess radiation is filtered
    B. Area that is in focus when the mA and kVp are adjusted
    C. Zone of sharpness
    D. Area that is collimated

85. In the rare event someone who works in a dental office has no shielding available and cannot leave the room, he or she should stand at least how many feet from the x-ray machine?
    A. 3
    B. 4
    C. 5
    D. 6
    E. 7

86. Which of the following is the BEST attenuator of an x-ray beam?
    A. Aluminum
    B. Zinc
    C. Lead
    D. Tin
    E. Tungsten

87. An anatomical landmark located in the mandibular bicuspid area when superimposed on or adjacent to the apex of a tooth could easily be mistaken for periapical pathology. That landmark is the
    A. Submandibular fossa
    B. Mental foramen
    C. Mental fossa
    D. Mandibular canal

88. Which of the following is the periapical lesion that is LEAST likely to be seen on radiographs?
    A. An acute alveolar abscess
    B. A chronic alveolar abscess
    C. A cyst
    D. A granuloma

89. Digital imaging systems used in dentistry replace film with an alternative sensor known as a (an)
    A. PID (position indicating device)
    B. CCD (charged-couple device)
    C. TLD (thermoluminescent dosimeter)
    D. MRI (magnetic resonance imaging)

90. Which of the following types of mouthwashes are prepared to relieve pain?
    A. Astringents
    B. Anodynes
    C. Buffering agents
    D. Oxygenating agents

91. A toxic reaction to a local anesthetic (due to intravascular injection) is treated with
    A. Oxygen and supportive therapy
    B. Mouth-to-mouth resuscitation
    C. Barbiturates for convulsions and supportive therapy
    D. Administration of an antihistamine and supportive therapy

92. Which of the following surface disinfectants has residual biocidal action?
    A. Chlorines
    B. Iodophors
    C. Quaternary ammonium compounds
    D. Phenols

93. The incubation period for hepatitis B virus is
    A. 2–6 days
    B. 2–6 weeks
    C. 2–6 months

94. The first step in the prevention of disease transmission is
    A. Washing of the operator's hands
    B. Placing gloves on the operator's hands
    C. Taking the patient's medical history
    D. Being sure the dental operatory is disinfected and instruments are sterilized

95. Which of the following methods of sterilization kills bacterial spores in the shortest time?
    A. Dry heat oven
    B. Chemical vapor
    C. Steam autoclave
    D. Ethylene oxide

96. A scientifically effective face mask will
    A. Prevent passage of microorganisms
    B. Have minimal marginal leakage
    C. Filter particles
    D. All of the above

97. The most widely used local anesthetics are
    A. Amides
    B. Esters
    C. Ethyls
    D. Amines

98. Of all the topical anesthetics, which of the following types is the LEAST desirable?
    A. Ointment
    B. Gel
    C. Liquid
    D. Spray

99. The most widely used method of conscious sedation is
    A. Hypnosis
    B. Nitrous oxide-oxygen
    C. Tranquilizers
    D. Intravenous administration of sedatives

100. When using topical anesthetics to alleviate tissue discomfort and to relieve patient anxiety, it is important to limit
    A. The amount applied
    B. The concentration used
    C. The area of application
    D. A and B only
    E. A, B, and C

101. Which of the following is added to local anesthetics to decrease absorption into the blood, thus increasing duration of the anesthetic and decreasing toxicity of the anesthetic?
    A. Epinephrine
    B. Paraben
    C. Sodium metabisulfite
    D. Sodium chloride

102. Which of the following design characteristics is NOT useful in a curette used to reach heavy, tenacious calculus in a deep pocket on a molar?
    A. A long shank
    B. A multiangled shank
    C. A fine, flexible shank

103. A patient experiencing tachycardia has a pulse rate
    A. Less than 140 bpm
    B. Greater than 70 bpm
    C. Less than 50 bpm
    D. Greater than 150 bpm

104. Fluoride-induced enamel hypoplasia or hypocalcification is
    A. More caries-prone
    B. Caries-resistant
    C. Hypersensitive to temperature changes

105. In order to open the angulation of a curette blade in relation to the tooth surface, the shank must be moved
    A. Toward the tooth
    B. Away from the tooth
    C. Parallel to the tooth
    D. Perpendicular to the tooth

106. The initial instruction in patient education is best given at the beginning of the appointment because
    A. The patient will see the importance of home care because the hygienist has placed emphasis on its importance
    B. At the end of the appointment, time may be limited, the patient may be tired, and the gingiva may be sensitive
    C. After the plaque and calculus are removed, the opportunity to show the patient what is to be accomplished is lost
    D. A and B only
    E. B and C only
    F. A, B, and C

107. In communities without fluoridated water supplies, the most cost-effective method of delivering fluoride to 6- to 12-year-old children is through
    A. Fluoride tablets
    B. School water fluoridation
    C. Brushing with a fluoride gel
    D. A fluoride mouthrinse program

108. Bruxism can cause
    A. Acute pulpitis
    B. Wear facets
    C. Occlusal trauma
    D. Muscle fatigue and limited opening
    E. B, C, and D only
    F. A, B, C, and D

109. Generalized gingival bleeding may be associated with which of the following conditions?
    A. Infectious mononucleosis
    B. Leukemia
    C. Agranulocytosis
    D. Cyclic neutropenia
    E. B and C only
    F. B and D only
    G. A, B, C, and D

110. Which of the following conditions may be seen in a patient with cerebral palsy?
    A. Attrition and/or fractured teeth
    B. Periodontal disease
    C. Difficulty with mastication and swallowing
    D. A and B only
    E. B and C only
    F. A, B, and C

111. The first step in patient education is
    A. Disclosing the patient
    B. Developing rapport with the patient
    C. Demonstrating brushing and flossing

112. Which of the following conditions may be associated with improper flossing?
    A. Cuts of the papillae
    B. Destruction of the attachment fibers
    C. Abrasion
    D. All of the above

113. Two weeks after treatment, the success of your root planing and oral hygiene instructions may be determined by
    A. Smooth roots
    B. No bleeding upon probing
    C. No plaque upon disclosing
    D. No calculus

114. When treating a patient suffering from hypertension, which of the following should be considered?
    A. Stress management
    B. Treatment planning
    C. Chair position
    D. Monitoring vital signs
    E. Drug side effects
    F. A, B, and D only
    G. A, D, and E only
    H. A, B, C, D, and E

115. Your patient has an increase in pulse and blood pressure, appears cold and clammy, and has chest pains radiating to the arm and neck. This attack lasts approximately 3 to 5 minutes. Which of the following conditions is related to these symptoms?
    A. Myocardial infarction
    B. Angina pectoris
    C. Cardiac arrest
    D. Congestive heart failure

116. A patient suffering from which of the following may exhibit symptoms such as weakness, dyspnea, rapid heart rate, difficulty breathing, or nocturia.
    A. Right heart failure
    B. Coronary thrombosis
    C. Left heart failure
    D. Angina pectoris

117. If your patient begins to experience a seizure, your response should be to
    A. Discontinue treatment
    B. Stay calm
    C. Place the patient in a supine position
    D. Monitor the patient's vital signs
    E. A and C only
    F. A, B, C, and D

118. Headache, confusion, impaired speech, respiratory difficulty, and unequal pupils are all symptoms of
    A. An allergic reaction
    B. A drug overdose
    C. A cerebrovascular accident
    D. Hypertension

119. When treating a patient with Alzheimer's disease, which of the following should be considered?
    A. Disorientation and mood swings
    B. The length of the appointment
    C. Communication difficulty
    D. Motor problems
    E. A and C only
    F. A, B, C, and D

120. When treating a patient suffering from congestive heart failure, which of the following should be considered?
    A. Stress management
    B. Appointment length
    C. Chair position
    D. Supplemental oxygen
    E. A, B, and C
    F. A, B, C, and D

121. Which of the following drugs can be associated with gingival hyperplasia?
    A. Cyclosporine
    B. Nifedipine
    C. Diltiazem
    D. A and C only
    E. A, B, and C

122. A pocket formed by gingival enlargement without apical migration of the junctional epithelium is which of the following?
    A. Absolute pocket
    B. Pseudopocket
    C. Periodontal pocket
    D. True pocket

123. Which of the following does NOT occur in the periodontal ligament as a result of aging?
    A. Hypercalcification
    B. Decrease in vascularity
    C. Decrease in fibroplasia
    D. Increase in elastic fibers
    E. Decrease in mitotic activity

124. Periodontal dressings
    A. Maintain patient comfort
    B. Control surgical bleeding
    C. Provide some splinting of mobile teeth
    D. All of the above

125. Which attachment apparatus of the periodontium is LEAST affected by occlusal trauma?
    A. Gingival attachment
    B. Periodontal ligament
    C. Alveolar bone
    D. Cementum

126. Which of the following oral hygiene aids is appropriate for cleaning a Class II furcation?
    A. Toothpick in a holder
    B. End tuft brush
    C. Interdental brush
    D. Oral irrigator

127. Which of the following terms is currently used, replacing the term "Early-Onset Periodonitis"?
    A. Juvenile periodontitis
    B. Aggressive periodontitis
    C. Prepubertal periodontitis
    D. None of the above

128. Periodontitis is preceded by gingivitis. All untreated gingivitis does not necessarily proceed to periodontitis.
    A. The first statement is TRUE; second statement is FALSE
    B. The first statement is FALSE; second statement is TRUE
    C. Both statements are TRUE
    D. Both statements are FALSE

129. Progression of periodontal disease appears to be a cyclic process with periods of exacerbation and quiescence. This explains why chronic periodontitis may exist for many years without rapid bone loss and without certain loss of teeth.
    A. The first statement is TRUE; second statement is FALSE
    B. The first statement is FALSE; second statement is TRUE
    C. Both statements are TRUE
    D. Both statements are FALSE

130. In the presence of periodontal disease, the spread of inflammation into the deeper structures of the periodontium follows which of the following pathways?
    A. Bony
    B. Perivascular
    C. Intraepithelial

131. Which of the following antibiotics has been used in the treatment of *A. actinomycetemcomitans* infections in localized aggressive periodontitis (formerly known as localized juvenile periodontitis)?
    A. Doxycycline
    B. Minocycline
    C. Penicillin VK
    D. A only
    E. A and B

132. Which of the following controlled-release delivery systems for site-specific antimicrobial therapy is nonresorbable and requires later removal by the clinician?
    A. Actisite®
    B. Perio Chip®
    C. Atridox®
    D. None of the above

133. Atridox® is composed of 10% doxycycline hyclate in what type of formulation?
    A. Liquid
    B. Powder
    C. Paste
    D. Gel

134. Which of the following products utilizes a subantimicrobial-dose doxycycline as its active ingredient to inhibit collagenase activity in the treatment of periodontal disease?
    A. Periogard™
    B. Peridex™
    C. Periostat®
    D. Periocline®

135. Pit and fissure sealants represent a trade-off with composite resins in terms of physical and mechanical properties. In order to get the viscosity low enough to flow into the pits and fissures of teeth, what characteristic must be sacrificed?
    A. Color stability
    B. Strength
    C. The ability to use a light gun to cure it
    D. The ability to use it on primary teeth

136. What do pit and fissure sealants, composite resins, acrylic appliances, and elastomeric impression materials have in common?
    A. They are all polymers
    B. They all have to be heated before using
    C. They can all be used as anterior filling materials
    D. They are all products of secondary reactions

137. An increase in the temperature of the water used in mixing irreversible hydrocolloids will
    A. Prevent setting
    B. Shorten time to set
    C. Lengthen time to set
    D. Not affect time to set

138. What appearance does a properly acid-etched surface have?
    A. Slightly pink with a definite shine
    B. Dull white and chalky
    C. Somewhat gray in color
    D. Identical to natural dentition

139. The process of mixing an amalgam is known as
    A. Amalgamation
    B. Condensation
    C. Trituration
    D. Carving

140. The powder used in mixing acrylic resin is referred to as the
    A. Monomer
    B. Dimer
    C. Polymer
    D. Initiator

141. Direct placement resins harden by two methods. What are these?
    A. Autopolymerization and self-curing
    B. Cold-curing and self-curing
    C. Autopolymerization and light-initiated polymerization
    D. Heat cure and cold cure

142. Zinc phosphate cement, upon setting, will
    A. Shrink slightly
    B. Expand slightly
    C. Neither shrink nor expand

143. There are four types of gypsum products approved for use in dentistry. Which of the following types is NOT used today?
    A. Type I impression plaster
    B. Type II model plaster
    C. Type III dental stone
    D. Type IV die stone

144. Why is dental stone vibrated after mixing?
    A. The mixing is not uniform and vibration completes the mixing
    B. The vibration shakes up any remaining particles
    C. The vibration makes the mixture more dense by removing any trapped air pockets
    D. The vibration halts the reaction and allows extended pouring times

145. Which of the following metals contributes to the corrosion resistance of a dental casting gold alloy?
    A. Zinc
    B. Gold
    C. Nickel
    D. Copper

146. If a topical fluoride is to be used in conjunction with a pit and fissure sealant, which sequence is used?
    A. Fluoride before sealant
    B. Fluoride should not be used
    C. Fluoride after sealant
    D. It doesn't make any difference

147. Inhibitors are added to the monomer of the denture base resins to
    A. Activate the monomer
    B. Increase shelf life
    C. Speed up the reaction
    D. Produce a softer polymer

148. Which of the following properties contributes greatly to the strength of a polymer?
    A. Covalent addition
    B. Biochemical adhesion
    C. Cross-linking

149. The cast chromium-cobalt alloy used for removable partial dentures has many advantages. Which of the following properties is NOT an advantage of this alloy system?
    A. Low specific gravity
    B. High flexibility
    C. Corrosion resistance
    D. High strength

150. The denture base resins should have which of the following physical properties?
    A. Adequate strength
    B. Satisfactory thermal properties
    C. Low specific gravity
    D. All of the above

151. Proper monitoring of oral hygiene around implants is absolutely imperative. Which of the following reasons BEST explains why?
    A. Plaque around the implant could cause corrosion, leading to failure of the implant from metal fatigue
    B. Improper brushing techniques could lead to calculus buildup on the implant
    C. Because there is no direct connective tissue attachment, the potential for infection is high
    D. There are no special precautions used to clean implants because they are not real teeth

152. In casting a restoration for a patient, the proper sequence of events is
    A. Cast, wax, polish, invest, burn out
    B. Polish, wax, invest, burn out, cast
    C. Wax, invest, burn out, cast, polish
    D. Invest, wax, cast, burn out, polish

153. After an alloy is cast for a dental restoration, a surface oxide must often be removed prior to polishing the restoration. This process is known as
   A. Investing
   B. Pickling
   C. Flux addition
   D. Passivation

154. One disadvantage of dental porcelain restorations is
   A. Brittleness
   B. Matching tooth color
   C. Expansion
   D. Radioactivity

155. Which of the following is not a value contained in the ADHA Code of Ethics for dental hygienists?
   A. Autonomy
   B. Justice
   C. Beneficence
   D. Virtue

156. This branch of government makes laws for the state.
   A. Legislative branch
   B. Executive branch
   C. Administrative branch
   D. Judicial branch

157. This branch of government enforces the laws passed by the legislature.
   A. Legislative branch
   B. Executive branch
   C. Administrative branch
   D. Judicial branch

158. This branch of government interprets the laws the legislature passes.
   A. Legislative branch
   B. Executive branch
   C. Administrative branch
   D. Judicial branch

159. Judges do not make laws, they simply interpret existing laws
   A. The first statement is TRUE, and the second statement is FALSE
   B. The first statement is FALSE, and the second statement is TRUE
   C. Both statements are TRUE
   D. Both statements are FALSE

160. This body of law is created by the courts via judicial decision and can be changed by the courts. It contains notions of common sense and precedent.
   A. Common law
   B. Statutory law
   C. Constitutional law
   D. Administrative law

161. This body of law is the result of the legislative branches voluntarily delegating some of its lawmaking authority to the Executive branch.
   A. Common law
   B. Statutory law
   C. Constitutional law
   D. Administrative law

162. This body of law is written law, which is enacted by the legislature, helps promote justice and can be changed by the legislature.
   A. Common law
   B. Statutory law
   C. Constitutional law
   D. Administrative law

163. Citizens have created this body of law and only citizens have the power to change this law. It is the most powerful law and takes precedent over other laws.
   A. Common law
   B. Statutory law
   C. Constitutional law
   D. Administrative law

164. Administrative agencies such as state dental boards fall within this law.
    A. Common law
    B. Statutory law
    C. Constitutional law
    D. Administrative law

165. Fluoridation has several mechanisms for caries inhibition. Included are enhancement of remineralization of enamel, inhibition of glycolysis, incorporation of fluoride into the enamel hydroxyapatite crystal, and bacteriocidal action.
    A. Both statements are TRUE
    B. Both statements are FALSE
    C. The first statement is TRUE; second statement is FALSE
    D. The first statement is FALSE; second statement is TRUE

166. Which of the following caries indexes applies to primary dentition?
    A. DMF
    B. DEF
    C. DMFS
    D. Def
    E. OHI-S

167. Which of the following indexes should be used to estimate MOST severe periodontal disease?
    A. OHI
    B. OHI-S
    C. PI
    D. GI

168. In 1989, fluoridation of the public water supply was estimated to cost on the average
    A. 20 cents per person per year
    B. 51 cents per person per year
    C. $20 per person per year
    D. $51 per person per year

169. Medicare, Title XVIII of the Social Security Act, pays for dental as well as medical care for patients aged 65 and over. All types of dental care are included in this coverage.
    A. Both statements are TRUE
    B. Both statements are FALSE
    C. The first statement is TRUE; second statement is FALSE
    D. The first statement is FALSE; second statement is TRUE

170. Medicaid, Title XIX of the Social Security Act, approaches public-supported dental care by providing
    A. Dental care for mothers and children receiving Aid to Families with Dependent Children benefits
    B. Emergency dental treatment for everyone regardless of ability to pay
    C. Dental care (screening, diagnosis, treatment) to needy children up to at least 20 years of age
    D. Emergency dental care to needy children up to at least 20 years of age

171. The most important concept of Winslow's definition of public health is
    A. The art and science of preventing disease
    B. Promoting mental and physical efficiency
    C. Promotion through organized community effort
    D. Health is not merely the absence of disease or infirmity

172. Prevention is the major objective of public health programs because it entails
    A. Ethics
    B. Teamwork
    C. Cost efficiency
    D. All of the above

173. Primary prevention covers those measures taken before any disease appears. Secondary prevention is synonymous with early disease control.
    A. The first statement is TRUE; second statement is FALSE
    B. The first statement is FALSE; second statement is TRUE
    C. Both statements are TRUE
    D. Both statements are FALSE

174. The minimum population level that is necessary to support a public health department is
    A. 4,000–5,000
    B. 7,500–10,000
    C. 10,000–15,000
    D. 35,000–50,000

175. Which level of the health department offers direct services to the individual?
    A. Local
    B. State
    C. National
    D. International

176. Education plays an important role in public health because
    A. Preventive measures are taught and learned
    B. It decreases the need for government intervention
    C. The programs allow for cost-efficiency
    D. A teamwork approach is necessary

177. Milestones in dental public health in the early twentieth century were characterized by all of the following EXCEPT which?
    A. The Dental Department of the U.S. Public Health Service was founded in 1919
    B. G.V. Black led discussion on fluoride at the Colorado State Dental Association in 1908
    C. Fones opened a training school for dental nurses in New Zealand
    D. Irene Newman became the first dental hygienist in 1906

178. Health Maintenance Organizations (HMOs) are similar to preferred provider organizations (PPOs) in that they both are nontraditional methods for delivering and financing dental care. PPOs, however, are more of a financing arrangement than a structure.
    A. Both statements are TRUE
    B. Both statements are FALSE
    C. The first statement is TRUE; second statement is FALSE
    D. The first statement is FALSE; second statement is TRUE

179. Currently, a public health problem is defined as a health issue that
    A. Results in public demand for immediate intervention by the government
    B. Causes or potentially causes widespread morbidity and/or mortality
    C. Has caused widespread morbidity and/or mortality
    D. Involves a perception on the part of the public, public health authorities, and the government that a public health problem is occurring
    E. B and D only

180. Many factors such as climate, familial and genetic patterns, and socioeconomic status have been studied to determine their relationship to dental caries. Since the advent of fluoridation of public water supplies, socioeconomic status has been proven to be a powerful determinant of caries status in the community.
   A. Both statements are TRUE
   B. Both statements are FALSE
   C. The first statement is TRUE; second statement is FALSE
   D. The first statement is FALSE; second statement is TRUE

181. Nutritional status does directly influence prevalence of caries. Dietary factors do not.
   A. Both statements are TRUE
   B. Both statements are FALSE
   C. The first statement is TRUE; second statement is FALSE
   D. The first statement is FALSE; second statement is TRUE

182. Severe caries is operationally defined in groups of children as a DMFT of 7.0. Five percent of children in the United States today will fall into this category.
   A. Both statements are TRUE
   B. Both statements are FALSE
   C. The first statement is TRUE; second statement is FALSE
   D. The first statement is FALSE; second statement is TRUE

183. Gingivitis precedes periodontitis. Areas of the mouth affected by gingivitis will most likely become affected in later years by periodontitis.
   A. Both statements are TRUE
   B. Both statements are FALSE
   C. The first statement is TRUE; second statement is FALSE
   D. The first statement is FALSE; second statement is TRUE

184. DMF surfaces have an advantage over DMF tooth counts because they are
   A. More economical
   B. Concerned with permanent dentition
   C. A simple, expedient index
   D. A more sensitive measurement

185. Prevalence is used to measure dental caries when
   A. Radiographs are available
   B. Animal studies are performed to determine progression of lesion
   C. Caries rates and tooth loss are expected to be high
   D. Caries rates are expected to be low

186. As a dental hygienist, your role in the community concerning tobacco use should be to
   A. Ask, advise, assist, and arrange for all patients to stop using tobacco
   B. Not personally use any form of tobacco
   C. Conduct diligent oral exams on both patients who report and those who do not report tobacco use
   D. All of the above

187. Adults ingest approximately how many milligrams of fluoride daily?
   A. 1–3
   B. 10–30
   C. 100–200
   D. 250–500

188. When organizing and providing dental care services, *need* may be defined as
    A. The particular frequency or desired frequency of dental care from a population
    B. A normative, professional judgment as to the amount and kind of services required to attain and maintain health
    C. The quantity of dental care services available
    D. The number of dental care services actually consumed by a given population

189. Dental public health, or community dental health, is BEST defined as
    A. Health care provided to maintain the health of the poor
    B. Rendering health care services and deducing the nature of health problems
    C. Protecting people's health through privately funded agencies
    D. Activity directed toward the improvement and protection of the health of a population group

190. Evaluation of a community-based dental care program is
    A. An ongoing process
    B. Important to provide qualitative and quantitative documentation of the program
    C. Not an important consideration during the planning phase
    D. A and B only
    E. A, B, and C

Testlet 1: Questions 191–195

A school dental hygienist was approached by the board of education to establish a dental health education curriculum for the students enrolled in the public school system. The board was concerned that the only dental health education students received was during Children's Dental Health month. The school system consists of 6,000 students, grades K–12. Health care facilities are available at each school, including a nurse, who was available twice a week.

191. Possible negative reactions and conflict could be avoided by obtaining support from which of the following?
    A. The board of dentistry
    B. The State Department of Education
    C. The school nurse and teachers
    D. The local dental hygiene association

192. To determine the oral hygiene knowledge of the target population the dental hygienists should
    A. Perform DMFS on all students
    B. Perform clinical examinations and radiographs
    C. Conduct a discussion group with the teachers
    D. Conduct a pretest dental questionnaire for the students

193. The best objective for this educational program would be which of the following? Following completion of the dental health curriculum,
    A. The students should have a 20% reduction in active, untreated dental caries
    B. The students should be able to describe dental disease etiology
    C. The students should be able to utilize dental services for their children
    D. The teachers should participate in dental school curriculum development

194. The best way to measure the effectiveness of the dental health curriculum is to compare
    A. Federal data banks with the local dental bank
    B. The NHANES for the last 5 years
    C. Posttest dental questionnaire with the pretest questionnaire
    D. Perform a DMFT or deft

195. After the program is developed, the most effective role for community dental hygienists would be as
    A. Teacher for classroom instruction
    B. Chairside instructor
    D. Evaluator of the success of the program
    E. Clinical hygienist

Testlet 2: Questions 196–200

The State Dental Division is involved in conducting a 5-year study on the use of sealants in conjunction with fluoride. The study involves all the public schools in the county, grades K–12. At the beginning of the study, none of the public schools had fluoridated water supplies, and fewer than 20% of the children attending these public schools had sealants. The total number of students in the county is 5,000. To decrease the number of subjects involved in the study, a random sample was taken from the 5,000 students; however, students who did not have their first molars could not participate. The sample size then consisted of 2,000 students, grades K–12. The sample was then further divided into two groups: Group 1 received sealants and fluoride, and Group 2 just received fluoride every 6 months for 5 years. Group 1 received sealants at the start of the study and professional fluoride treatments every 6 months for 5 years. Group 2 only received fluoride treatments every 6 months for 5 years. The State Dental Division then needed to gather information on the subjects' dental caries and plaque accumulation. A mean plaque index score of 2.6 (based on a 3.0 scale) was recorded for both Group 1 and Group 2 and at the end of the 5 years the plaque index for Group 1 was 2.0 and the plaque index for Group 2 was 2.3. There was high interrater reliability between the dental examiners.

196. What type of research study was conducted?
    A. Historical
    B. Experimental
    C. Cross-sectional
    D. Descriptive

197. The mean plaque index score for both groups at the beginning of the study revealed the students having
    A. No plaque
    B. Slight plaque
    C. Moderate plaque
    D. Severe plaque

198. Randomizing the sample suggests that the
    A. Subjects were total volunteers
    B. Every nth name on a list was selected
    C. Every student had equal chance to be included in the study
    D. A person in the experimental group will not be a member of the control group

199. What is the best choice to add fluoride to these public schools?
    A. Fluoride tablets; .25 mg sodium fluoride
    B. Fluoride tablets; .5 mg sodium fluoride
    C. Fluoride rinse; .5 mg sodium fluoride
    D. Fluorinated water; 2.0 ppm
    E. Fluorinated water; 7.0 ppm

200. When evaluating the study, what dental index would help compare the effectiveness of sealants and fluoride versus fluoride alone?
    A. DMFT
    B. Deft
    C. Gingival index
    D. Demineralization index

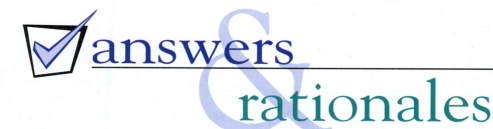

answers & rationales

1.

B. The major vessel that extends through the ptery-gopalatine fossa is the maxillary artery. The maxillary artery extends from a point anterior to the ear through the infratemporal fossa. It also extends into the pterygopalatine fossa where it divides its terminal branches.

2.

E. The infratemporal fossa is important in dentistry because it contains the muscles of mastication and many of the nerves and vessels supplying the mouth. The infratemporal fossa is the area extending inferiorly below the zygomatic arch. It extends medially, deep to the ramus of the mandible.

3.

C. The maxillary sinuses develop after the permanent teeth have erupted. The growth of the maxillary air sinus continues through adulthood. The maxillary air sinus sometimes infringes on the maxillary alveolar bone.

4.

C. The line of demarcation between the loose alveolar mucosa and the denser alveolar mucosa adjacent to the teeth is the mucogingival junction. The mucogingival junction is visible as the demarcation between the reddish loose mucosa and the pink alveolar mucosa adjacent to the teeth. The attached gingiva extends from the base of the gingival sulcus to the mucogingival junction.

5.

C. A fold of mucous membrane that helps anchor the tongue to the floor of the mouth is the frenulum. Sometimes the lingual frenulum is excessively tight, limiting movement of the tongue. The terms *frenum* and *frenulum* are used interchangeably.

6.

D. The superior and inferior ganglia are associated with the vagus nerve. The superior and inferior ganglia are located within the jugular foramen. The vagus nerve is the tenth cranial nerve.

7.

B. Frequently there is a small fifth cusp attached to the lingual surface of the mesiolingual cusp of the maxillary first molar. This fifth cusp is usually 2 mm cervical to the tip of the mesiolingual cusp. The fifth cusp varies greatly in shape and size. It may be a conspicuous, well-formed cusp or, at the other extreme, it may be barely discernible or absent, or there may even be a depression in this location.

exam 2 answers

8.

D. (1) The crowns of primary anterior teeth are wider mesiodistally in comparison with their crown length than are the permanent teeth (2) The roots of primary teeth are narrower and longer than those of permanent teeth (3) The cervical ridges positioned buccally on the primary molars are much more pronounced, especially on first molars, maxillary and mandibular.

9.

D. The first evidence of calcification of the primary lateral incisor is seen at approximately 4 1/2 months in utero. Hard tissue formation occurs in all primary teeth by the 18th week in utero. All primary teeth have usually erupted by 27 months of age.

10.

D. The roots of the permanent third molars are completely formed by 18 to 25 years of age. Third molars are the teeth most likely to be malformed. They are also commonly associated with dentigerous cysts.

11.

C. Before the permanent tooth can come into position, the primary tooth must be exfoliated; this is brought about by the phenomenon called resorption of the primary root. The permanent tooth in its follicle attempts to force its way into the position held by its predecessor. The pressure brought to bear against the primary root evidently causes resorption of the root, which continues until the primary crown has lost its anchorage, becomes loose, and is finally exfoliated.

12.

D. Bitter and sour taste sensations of the tongue are mediated by the glossopharyngeal nerve. Sweet and salty tastes of the tongue are mediated by the inter-mediofacial nerve. Taste occurs when a chemical substance contacts a receptor cell in the taste bud.

13.

E. Hertwig's epithelial root sheath is derived from the union of inner dental epithelium and outer dental epithelium. It does not contain a stratum intermedium or stellate reticulum. Hertwig's epithelial root sheath therefore develops from two layers of the enamel epithelium.

14.

C. After the tooth is formed, the dental papilla becomes confined within the dentin walls forming the primordium of the dental pulp. The dental papilla is derived from the inner enamel epithelium.

15.

C. Hunter-Schreger bands are best demonstrated by oblique reflected light as alternating dark and light strips of varying width. Hunter-Schreger bands are established by the change in direction of enamel rods. These bands originate at the dentinoenamel junction and pass outward, ending some distance from the outer enamel surface.

16.

C. Hormones regulate, increase, or decrease activity of particular systems. However, they are utilized or degraded in the process. Enzymes catalyze intracellular biochemical reactions without being degraded or depleted.

17.

E. Calcitonin is secreted by the thyroid gland. It is released in response to excess serum calcium. The effect of calcitonin, or thyrocalcitonin as it is sometimes called, is opposite that of parathyroid hormone.

18.

D. Cortisol increases the flux of amino acids in the body and mobilizes stored fat. It also promotes gluconeogenesis. Cortisol and other related corticosteriods are produced by the adrenal cortex.

19.

D. Each gram of hemoglobin can transport 1.34 mL of oxygen. Normally, 100 mL of blood contains 15 g of hemoglobin. Therefore, 100 mL of blood will contain 15×1.34 or 21.1 mL O_2 as oxyhemoglobin. A much lesser amount, approximately 0.3 mL, is dissolved in 100 mL of plasma.

20.

D. Pernicious anemia is usually due to lack of an intrinsic factor, which prevents the absorption of physiological amounts of vitamin B12.

21.

A. Beriberi is a thiamin deficiency disease. It is commonly found among those populations for whom polished rice is a dietary staple. Thiamin is found in the bran and germ layer of brown rice, but polished white rice has had the bran and germ layer removed, thus removing the source of thiamin. In the United States, thiamin is replaced during enriching processes for rice and other grains.

22.

A. The recommended daily allowance of iron for a woman of childbearing age is 15 mg per day, which will allow for accumulation of iron stores and will help take care of the increased needs for iron during menstruation and pregnancy. Previous editions of the National Research Council's Recommended Dietary Allowances (NRC/RDA) have recommended 18 mg per day for a woman of childbearing age.

23.

D. Humans have difficulty in absorbing iron efficiently. Absorption is improved in the presence of amino acids and ascorbic acid. The theory is not well understood but, according to the explanation of Granick's "Amucosal block theory," iron absorption is dependent upon the availability of apoferritin, a protein found in the intestinal mucosa, in order to complex the iron and form ferritin. When apoferritin becomes completely saturated with iron, no further absorption can take place.

24.

A. Toxicity can develop if 20–30 times the recommended allowance of vitamin A or carotene is ingested for long periods of time. It is best to avoid vitamin D intake in excess of 400 units per day. Huge amounts of vitamin D will induce a very intense calcification of the bone and even calcification of the arteries, as well as the formation of renal calculi.

25.

A. The mineral iron is often found to be deficient in the diet of children in both developed and third-world countries. There is suggestive animal experimental evidence of a relationship between an iron-deficient diet and increased caries susceptibility. The caries occur primarily on the smooth buccal surface because of reduced salivary volume and interference with the biosynthesis of salivary proteins, which are dependent on iron.

26.

C. Amino acids are ordinarily required for synthesis of tissue proteins, and the absence of any one of them could prevent the formation of proteins in the body.

27.

A. Reactivation of the varicella-zoster virus, the agent of chickenpox seen most commonly in children, is associated with herpes zoster. It increases in frequency with age and is seen most commonly in adults.

28.

B. An anaerobic streptococcus is classified as a member of genus *Peptostreptococcus*.

29.

D. Microaerophilic bacteria grows best at low oxygen concentration and cannot grow without oxygen.

30.

D. MacConkey's agar is a differential and selective medium that supports the growth of organisms such as *E. coli* and other members of the enteric bacilli. Gram-positive organisms like streptococci do not grow. *Hemophilus influenzae* is fastidious and requires a heme-containing medium for growth.

31.

B. *Lactobacillus acidophilus* is a gram-positive rod commonly found in the oropharyngeal flora. It has been believed to play some role in the pathogenesis of dental caries.

32.

D. Viruses are capable of reproduction only inside living cells. Those that grow inside bacteria are known as bacteriophages.

33.

D. Substances that prepare bacteria for phagocytosis are known as opsonins. They attach to the surface of the microbe and activate the complement pathway. The complement fragment C3b and a calcium-dependent mannose-binding protein are examples of opsonins.

34.

E. Mycoplasma are the smallest known free-living microorganisms, intermediate in size between bacteria and viruses. Although they evolved from Gram-positive ancestors, they lack a cell wall, which is their most distinguishing feature.

35.

B. Some bacteria produce chemical substances known as chemotaxins, which directionally attract leukocytes. The adherence of bacteria to the leukocyte activates the membrane and initiates engulfment.

36.

A. Many bacterial, rickettsial, and viral diseases are classified as zoonoses because they are acquired by humans either directly or indirectly from animals.

37.

D. Ethylene oxide is an alkylating agent, which is an effective sterilizing agent for heat-liable devices that cannot be treated at the temperatures achieved in the autoclave.

38.

C. The first step in the vascular reaction associated with the inflammatory process is transient vasoconstriction. This transient vasoconstriction produces a local anemia. It is replaced by hyperemia.

39.

B. Chemical products that are released into the blood during the inflammatory process can produce fever.

40.

C. AIDS is a disease characterized by a depletion of helper T lymphocytes.

41.

D. A purulent inflammation is characterized by the production of pus. It is a creamy opaque substance containing liquefied necrotic material and many white blood cells. A suppurative reaction usually results from a bacterial infection.

42.

D. Granulomatous inflammation is a form of chronic inflammation. It is characterized by a focal accumulation of mononuclear leukocytes, chiefly macrophages, and is present in important diseases such as TB, fungal infections, and sarcoidosis.

43.

B. The most common benign soft-tissue lesion occurring in the oral cavity is the fibroma, which probably represents fibrous hyperplasia. The fibroma appears as an elevated lesion of normal color with a smooth surface and a sessile or pedunculated base.

44.

D. Peripheral giant-cell granulomas always occur on the gingiva or alveolar process, outside of bone. They occur most frequently anterior to molars. These lesions are most often dark red, vascular or hemorrhagic, and commonly ulcerated.

45.

D. The central giant-cell granuloma is a destructive lesion, appearing radiolucent with a smooth or ragged border in radiographs. The central giant-cell granuloma occurs predominantly in children or young adults. The mandible is more often affected than the maxilla, and it is more commonly found in females than males.

46.

D. The most common site for the pleomorphic adenoma is the parotid gland, but it can occur in any major or minor salivary gland. It occurs in a 6:4 ratio of females to males. This tumor usually does not show fixation to deeper tissues.

47.

C. A dentigerous cyst, which is also an odontogenic cyst, originates through alteration of the reduced enamel epithelium after the crown is completely formed. The dentigerous cyst is always associated with the crown of an unerupted tooth.

48.

C. Papillary hyperplasia is most often associated with ill-fitting dentures. The lesions are red, edematous papillary projections of the palate.

49.

B. Any white patch on the oral mucosa that cannot be rubbed off and cannot be ascribed to any other disease is most probably leukoplakia.

50.

A. Triamcinolone acetonide (Kenalog) has been used to treat some acute and chronic lesions of the oral mucosa, such as recurrent ulcerative stomatitis. As with all corticosteroids, triamcinolone acetonide is entirely suppressive, but not curative. It does not prevent recurrence of any oral lesions.

51.

D. Two grams (2,000 mg) of Amoxicillin should be given 1 hour prior to the procedure for prophylaxis against bacterial endocarditis.

52.

B. The antibacterial spectrum of erythromycin closely resembles that of penicillin. It is a drug of choice for patients that are allergic to penicillin. If the patient is allergic to penicillin and erythromycin, clindamycin could be administered.

53.

B. Talwin is marketed as the proprietary compound of the generic pentazocine. Talwin is a narcotic antagonist that is an effective analgesic when given orally. It is capable of producing hallucinations.

54.

A. Meperidine hydrochloride (Demerol) is classified as a Schedule II drug by the Controlled Substances Act. Demerol is a narcotic-analgesic. It has one-tenth the analgesic activity of morphine.

55.

C. Meperidine hydrochloride (Demerol) has both morphine-like and atropine-like properties and can be used for patients showing intolerance to morphine. It is more unlikely to produce gastrointestinal disturbance than morphine. A tolerance may result from meperidine HCl therapy.

56.

B. In general, barbiturates do not produce analgesia unless they are given in extremely high doses, which are not generally acceptable. High concentrations of barbiturates can be lethal. Barbiturates in high concentrations depress liver and kidney functions, reduce gastrointestinal mobility, and lower body temperature.

57.

A. Promethazine (Phenergan) is primarily antihistaminic, but it has side effects of local anesthesia and sedation. Its production of excessive sedation may be accompanied by dizziness, dryness of the mouth, uncoordination, blurred vision, and fatigue.

58.

C. Tylenol (acetaminophen) may be substituted for aspirin when allergy is a problem. Acetaminophen has the same analgesic properties and antipyretic effects as aspirin. It does not, however, have the anti-inflammatory activity of aspirin.

59.

A. Chlorothiazide, a diuretic used in the treatment of hypertension, may be one of the more common drugs encountered in hypertensive dental patients. Other commonly encountered diuretics include Hydro-Diuril, Lasix, and Aldactone.

60.

B. A blood pressure of 120/80 is considered normal. The top figure represents the systolic pressure. The bottom figure represents the diastolic pressure. Exercise, eating, stimulants, emotional disturbance, and menopause may increase blood pressure. Factors that may decrease a patient's blood pressure include fasting, rest, depressants, quiet emotion, fainting, blood loss, and shock.

61.

D. Nitroglycerine (glyceryl trinitrate) in 0.3–0.6 mg tablets may be placed sublingually and administered several times to help prevent and ward off an attack of angina pectoris. The patient will usually give a history of the condition. Overdosage will cause a fall in blood pressure. Nitroglycerin normally reduces or eliminates discomfort dramatically within 2–4 minutes. Nitroglycerin is also available in a spray or patch

62.

C. Myocardial infarction results from a sudden reduction or arrest of coronary blood flow. The symptoms include chest pains, cold sweat, weakness, shortness of breath, nausea, and lowered blood pressure. Elective dental and dental hygiene appointments should be postponed 3 months or longer, until the patient's physician has given consent.

63.

C. To observe the dorsum of the tongue, hold the tongue with a gauze square, retract the cheek, and move the tongue out, first to one side and then the other.

64.

E. Subgingival calculus differs from supragingival calculus in location, density, and color. Subgingival calculus is harder and more dense than supragingival calculus. Subgingival calculus is usually heaviest on proximal surfaces and lightest on facial surfaces.

65.

E. A festoon ("McCall's festoon") is an enlargement of the marginal gingiva with the formation of a life-saver-like gingival prominence. Frequently, the associated total gingiva is very narrow. Also, apparent recession is usually present.

66.

D. In the absence of local irritants severe enough to produce periodontal pockets, trauma from occlusion may cause excessive loosening of teeth. Thus, the periodontal ligament may widen. Vertical alveolar defects may occur in the alveolar bone without pockets.

67.

E. The following are periodontal factors that cannot be determined through radiographic evaluation alone: presence or absence of periodontal pockets, height or contour of bone located on the facial or lingual surfaces of the teeth, and presence or absence of occlusal trauma.

68.

C. Inflammation, bleeding upon probing, and pocket depths are the most important diagnostic aids or signs of gingival or periodontal disease. Gingiva may or may not be stippled whether healthy or inflamed. The presence or absence of stippling is not diagnostic.

69.

C. Gingival bleeding in the presence of periodontal disease is due to the ulceration of the sulcular epithelium. Additionally, capillaries become engorged and extend near the gingival surface.

70.

D. Discoloration of either primary or permanent teeth may occur as a result of tetracycline. The deposition occurs during prophylactic or therapeutic regimens instituted either in the pregnant female or postpartum in the infant. Tetracycline staining is often clinically confused with fluorosis.

71.

C. Abrasion is the mechanical wearing away of tooth substance by forces other than mastication. Erosion is the loss of tooth substance by a chemical process that does not involve known bacterial action. Attrition is the wearing away of a tooth as a result of tooth-to-tooth contact. Causes of abrasion include an abrasive dentifrice applied with vigorous horizontal toothbrushing, opening bobby pins, or holding items such as tacks or pins between your teeth.

72.

C. A prognathic profile is usually associated with Class III occlusion. Persons with prognathic profiles have normal maxillas and protruded mandibles. The buccal groove of the mandibular first permanent molar is mesial to the mesiobuccal cusp of the maxillary first permanent molar by at least the width of a premolar.

73.

A. Acquired pellicle is an amorphous, organic, tenacious membranous layer that forms on exposed tooth surfaces, restorations, and calculus. It is composed of glycoproteins from the saliva.

74.

B. The recommended standard regimen for patients able to take amoxicillin or penicillin is 2 grams of amoxicillin 1 hour before the appointment. For patients allergic to amoxicillin or penicillin, clindamycin or cephalexin are indicated.

exam 2 answers

75.

B. Most fluoride is rapidly absorbed by the small intestine and stomach. Maximum blood levels are reached within 30 minutes of intake. In young children, about one-half of the fluoride intake deposits in calcifying bones and teeth. Fluoride is stored in mineralized tissues (99% of the body fluoride). The teeth store small amounts, with the highest levels on the tooth surface.

76.

A. Standing behind a suitably constructed barrier will reduce the radiation to the operator to zero. Common usage has resulted in the recommendation of lead barriers. There are other suitable materials, such as steel, concrete, bricks, tile, or plaster when adequate thickness is used.

77.

C. When using the paralleling technique, it is usually necessary to use a relatively long tooth-to-film distance because of anatomic considerations. However, this violates one of the rules of shadow casting, namely that the distance from the object to the recording surface should be as short as possible. In the mandibular molar view, however, low muscle attachment allows the film packet to be placed quite close to the teeth and parallel to their long axes. Therefore, this approaches the ideal.

78.

B. The maxillary midline area depicts several radiographic landmarks. The nasal fossae, median palatal suture, and incisive foramen are radiolucent. The nasal septum is radiopaque. The hamular process is also radiopaque but is a part of sphenoid bone and is never seen on maxillary anterior radiographs.

79.

B. The radiopacity of dental materials is contingent on atomic weight. Materials with low anatomic weight, such as acrylic, are radiolucent. Materials with high atomic weight, indicating a greater density, are radiopaque.

80.

A. Radiolucent structures appear on a radiograph as relatively dark areas. Cavities and spaces will form radiolucent images because of their lack of density. Structures of greater density such as teeth and bone will appear radiopaque.

81.

B. The Water's view is a projection that enlarges the middle third of the face and is useful in the diagnosis of maxillary sinus and other pathologic conditions involving this part of the face. The posteroanterior skull projection is not effective for studying the maxillary sinus because of the superimposition of other cranial structures. The lateral skull is not effective because it superimposes the right and left sides. The lateral oblique projection is used primarily to survey the mandible.

82.

D. Lateral Jaw or lateral oblique of the mandible radiography is the term used to describe extraoral lateral projections of the mandible and/or the maxilla. At best, this projection entails a certain degree of oblique angulation. Any region examined by this technique will have well-proportioned images and will depict a larger area than the periapical technique.

83.

C. The inverse square law indicates that the intensity of a beam is 1/4 as great at 16 inches as it would be at 8 inches. Thus, four times as much exposure would be required if all other exposure factors remained the same.

84.

C. The tomogram or panograph is a radiograph that shows a sharp image of a layer of tissue with the layers above and below it being blurred. The width or thickness of the sharp layer (zone of sharpness or focal trough) varies with the angle of movement of the x-ray beam. A large angle produces a narrow focal trough; a small angle results in a wide focal trough.

85.

D. In this unlikely event, it is recommended that the office worker stand at least 6 feet from the source of radiation. This takes advantage of the inverse square law regarding the intensity of the beam of radiation.

86.

C. The best attenuator (absorber) of x-radiation of the energies used in diagnostic radiology is the one with the most mass per unit volume. Of the materials listed here, lead is best and is the most frequently used shielding material.

87.

B. The mental foramen may be superimposed or adjacent to the apex of mandibular bicuspid teeth and look much like a periapical lesion. A comparison of its appearance on the contralateral side will frequently rule out the possibility of its being a lesion.

88.

A. For a periapical lesion to be seen radiographically, there must have been a certain amount of tissue destruction. In the cases of chronic lesions, this will have occurred; but in the case of an acute lesion, this will not have occurred.

89.

B. A charged-couple device (CCD) is a solid-state electronic plate used to transmit signals directly into a computer in digital imaging systems.

90.

B. Anodyne mouthwashes are prepared to relieve pain. Their essential ingredients consist of phenol derivatives and essential oils. Astringent mouth rinses are used for shrinking tissues. Buffering agents reduce oral acidity and dissolve mucinous films. Oxygenating agents are effective in debridement. Antimicrobial mouth rinses reduce the oral microbacterial count and inhibit bacterial activity.

91.

D. On occasion, the dental patient will give a history of being "allergic" to local anesthetics. In most instances, careful questioning will show that syncope occurred following injection of a local anesthetic, but that no other untoward effects developed. This suggests that syncope was due to apprehension. Should a toxic reaction (hives, itching, edema, or flushed skin) occur, an antihistamine (orally, intravenously, or intramuscularly) and other supportive therapy should be administered.

92.

B. Iodophors are EPA registered and ADA accepted, biocidal within 5–10 minutes, and economical. They have been shown to be broad spectrum antimicrobials and have a prolonged or residual biocidal activity after application. They must be prepared daily, they may discolor some surfaces, and they may be inactivated by hard water.

93.

C. The incubation period for hepatitis B is 2–6 months versus hepatitis A, which is 15–50 days. The period of communicability varies and the presence of serum hepatitis B surface antigen (HBsAg) indicates communicability.

94.

D. Before any clinical procedure is performed, all equipment must be disinfected and/or sterilized as appropriate for the prevention of disease transmission. Prevention of cross-contamination begins at the very start of the appointment. The health status of dental patients is determined primarily by using the medical history. History taking should elicit information on the presence or absence of disease and identify patients at risk. Then, universal precautions should be utilized throughout the appointment.

95.

C. The steam autoclave is an effective method of sterilization with a maximum sterilization period of 30 minutes. Advances in the equipment have allowed for the application of higher temperature and pressure for shorter cycle times (3–5 minutes, 10 minutes, or 15–20 minutes). The other methods of sterilization require sterilization cycles of 30 minutes, 1–2 hours, or 10–16 hours.

96.

D. An effective face mask will prevent passage of organisms, have minimal leakage, and filter particles. The shape, material, and degree of absorption of the mask will influence its efficiency.

97.

A. The amide-type local anesthetics were introduced in the 1940s. Their widespread usage is due to the decrease in the frequency of allergic reactions versus the ester local anesthetics.

98.

D. The least desirable topical anesthetic is the spray or aerosol type because it is more concentrated than other types of topical anesthetics, increasing the potential for toxic reactions. Because of the spray, it is difficult to control the amount given and the area covered by the mist. There is also the possibility of inhalation by the patient.

99.

B. Nitrous oxide–oxygen sedation produces a state in which the patient is conscious but relaxed. The advantages of this method of sedation include rapid effect due to the inhalation of these gases, easy regulation by altering the concentrations, and rapid reversal by having the patient breathe pure oxygen at the completion of the dental procedure.

100.

E. Because topical anesthetics must be absorbed through the mucosa, they must be formulated in greater concentrations. The higher concentrations increase the potential for toxic reactions. Therefore, it is important to limit the amount used, the concentration used, and the area of application.

101.

A. Epinephrine is a vasoconstrictor added to local anesthetics to decrease the absorption of the anesthetic by the bloodstream, increasing the duration of the effect of the anesthetic and decreasing the toxicity of the anesthetic.

102.

C. Fine, flexible shanks are not appropriate for the removal of tenacious calculus. A curette with a rigid shank would be more appropriate. To reach calculus in a deep pocket on a molar, the curette of choice would be one with a long, multiangled shank.

103.

D. An unusually fast heartbeat or pulse rate is called tachycardia. This increase may be caused by exercise, stimulants, eating, strong emotions, extreme heat or cold, and some forms of heart disease. An unusually slow heart rate is called bradycardia and may be caused by sleep, depressants, fasting, quiet emotions, and low vitality from prolonged illness. While there is no absolute normal, the adult range for normal pulse rates is 60–100 beats per minute. Women have slightly higher normal pulse rates than men.

104.

B. Ingestion of drinking water containing fluoride concentrations greater than 1 part per million during tooth development may result in enamel hypoplasia or fluorosis. The extent of the damage is dependent on the duration of ingestion, the timing of the ingestion (during development), and the intensity or concentration. Fluorosis ranges from white spots to mottled brown and white discolorations. There may also be pitting of the enamel. Enamel hypoplasia is caries resistant.

105.

B. In order to insert a curette subgingivally, the face of the blade of the instrument must be flush to the tooth or at a 0-degree angle to the surface to be scaled. To establish the correct working angle, the shank of the instrument must be moved away from the tooth in order to open the angle of the blade to the tooth surface. The working angle should be more than 45 degrees and less than 90 degrees.

106.

F. Patient education is more effective when given at the beginning of the appointment. If the instruction is delayed, the patient may be in a hurry to leave, the hygienist's time may also be limited, the gingiva and teeth may be sensitive, and there will be no calculus or plaque remaining on the teeth to show the patient what needs to be accomplished. Patients also place more importance on home care techniques when the hygienist is motivated and places great importance on home care.

107.

B. School water fluoridation is a satisfactory method of bringing the benefits of fluoridation to children living in communities without fluoridated water supplies.

108.

F. Bruxism is the clenching or grinding of the teeth when the patient is not chewing or swallowing. Bruxism may lead to acute pulpitis, wear facets, occlusal trauma, and muscle fatigue. Most people are not aware of the habit until it is brought to their attention. Opinions differ as to the primary cause, but occlusal prematurities, muscle tension, and emotional factors have been implicated. Bruxism can be treated through behavioral, emotional, and interceptive modalities.

109.

G. Spontaneous gingival hemorrhage can occur with patients suffering from infectious mononucleosis, leukemia, agranulocytosis, or cyclic neutropenia. This bleeding (from the gingiva and other areas) is an important clinical sign suggesting a hematologic disorder.

110.

F. Patients with cerebral palsy have difficulty swallowing and chewing due to musculature dysfunction. Orally, they may exhibit problems with attrition, fractured teeth, dental caries, and periodontal disease. Cerebral palsy can occur at any age as a result of brain injury from a variety of causes.

111.

B. Patient education must be tailored to the patient's needs and motivation. The first step must be to develop rapport with your patient and assess his or her needs. A preventive program involves a series of cooperative steps taken by the patient and the dental team. The information provided must be applicable to everyday living.

112.

D. Improper flossing may cause cuts or clefts of the papillae. Abrasion and destruction of the gingival attachment may occur when excess pressure is applied.

113.

B. After root planing and oral hygiene instruction, the number of pocket microorganisms decreases substantially and there is a shift to aerobic, Gram-positive organisms. The gingiva reflects these changes with a decrease in gingival inflammation. A lack of bleeding upon probing indicates removal of the irritants.

114.

H. Hypertension means an abnormal elevation of blood pressure. It is a risk factor in many vascular diseases. Evaluation of blood pressure is essential in patient evaluation and treatment. When outlining a treatment plan and providing patient care, you must follow a stress reduction protocol to eliminate adverse effects on the patient's blood pressure. Postural hypotension (fainting, nausea, or dizziness) results when a person sits up quickly from a supine position. The patient's vital signs must be evaluated and recorded at all visits, and the patient referred to his or her physician if a problem is noted. Various side effects may be associated with medications prescribed for hypertension, and these side effects may affect your treatment plan and your patient care. Depression, fatigue, gastrointestinal disturbances, and xerostomia are possible side effects.

115.

B. Angina pectoris involves discomfort in the chest, which results from transient and reversible myocardial oxygen deficiency. Approximately 90% of angina attacks are related to coronary artery atherosclerosis. An attack may be precipitated by exertion, emotion, or a heavy meal. The symptoms are a feeling of weight on the chest, faintness, sweating, difficulty breathing, or clamminess. The attacks may last for seconds or minutes.

116.

C. Left heart failure alters output and causes respiratory difficulty because of the backup of fluid and blood into the lungs. The symptoms include weakness, fatigue, dyspnea, nocturia, increased blood pressure, increased heart rate, and anxiety or fear. The symptoms are more prominent at night and are relieved when the patient is sitting or in a semi-sitting position.

117.

F. In the event your patient begins to experience a seizure, your first response is to discontinue treatment. You must also remain calm. Place your patient in a supine position, do not restrain the patient, clear away all equipment, loosen the patient's clothing, turn the patient's head to one side, and monitor the patient's vital signs.

118.

C. Cerebrovascular accident or stroke is a sudden loss of brain function resulting from interference with the blood supply to a part of the brain. Predisposing factors include atherosclerosis, hypertension, drug abuse, cardiovascular disease, diabetes, and oral contraceptive use.

119.

F. Alzheimer's disease is one of the nonreversible types of dementia. Dementia is severe impairment of the intellectual abilities (thinking, memory, and personality). There are four stages of impairment: early, middle, advanced, and terminal. Later symptoms include physical immobility, unawareness, and total helplessness.

120.

F. Heart failure involves the inability or failure of the heart to pump blood at a rate necessary to meet the needs of the body tissues. The result is the collection of fluid in various body organs. In the treatment of a patient with congestive heart failure, stress reduction, appointment length, supplemental oxygen, and chair position should be considered. A medical consultation is recommended. Appointments should be scheduled in the morning and the length of the appointment should not exceed the patient's tolerance. Due to the patient's possible difficulty in breathing, the chair should be in a more semi-upright position and supplemental oxygen may be needed.

121.

E. Cyclosporine (an immunosuppressive), nifedipine, and diltiazem (calcium-blocking drugs) can all produce gingival hyperplasia as side effects of the drugs. Additionally, phenytoin can also produce gingival hyperplasia.

122.

B. A pseudopocket is a pocket formed by gingival enlargement without apical migration of the junctional epithelium. It does not involve the loss of bone. Pseudopockets are also referred to as gingival pockets, false pockets, or relative pockets. All gingival pockets are suprabony (the base of the pocket is coronal to the crest of the alveolar bone).

123.

A. The results of aging on the periodontal ligament include increase in elastic fibers and decrease in vascularity. Mitotic activity also decreases and there is a decrease in fibroplasia. The periodontal ligament may or may not widen with age. Also, with age, the amount of mucopolysaccharides and collagen fibers in the periodontal ligament decreases.

124.

D. Periodontal dressings are placed over surgical wounds following periodontal surgery and gingival curettage. They serve a variety of purposes including providing protection, maintaining patient comfort, splinting of mobile teeth, controlling bleeding, and shaping or molding the flap.

125.

A. The gingival attachment is least affected by occlusal force. Occlusal trauma does not cause gingival changes or pocket formation. The periodontal ligament may be crushed, hemorrhage, and in the chronic phase, it becomes wider. The cementum tears and fractures in the acute phase. In the chronic phase, there may be cemental hyperplasia or dentinal resorp-

tion. With occlusal trauma, there is resorption of the alveolar bone.

126.

A. A toothpick in a holder is indicated for plaque removal at or just under the gingival margin for concave tooth surfaces and for exposed furcations. In a Class II furcation, the bone has been destroyed to an extent that the area between the roots has moderate involvement, but instruments or oral hygiene aids may not pass through the area between the roots.

127.

B. The term "Early-Onset Periodontitis" was used in the 1989 AAP to describe destructive periodontal diseases that affect young patients. The terminology has now been changed to "Aggressive Periodontitis."

128.

C. Periodontitis is preceded by gingivitis; however, not all untreated gingivitis will proceed to periodontitis.

129.

C. Progression of periodontitis appears to be a cyclic process with periods of exacerbation and quiescence. Attachment loss worsens during the periods of exacerbation; however, if attachment loss is not severe, the patient may have chronic periodontitis for years without suffering tooth loss.

130.

B. In the presence of periodontal disease, the spread of inflammation into the deeper structures follows a perivascular pathway because the vascular channels offer less resistance than the fibers of the periodontal ligament.

131.

E. Tetracyclines as a group are bacteriostatic, inhibiting growth and multiplication by inhibiting protein synthesis. Doxycycline and minocycline have been used to treat Aa infections in localized aggressive periodontitis (formerly known as localized juvenile periodontitis) and refractory periodontitis.

132.

A. Actisite® is an ethylene vinyl acetate flexible fiber impregnated with 12.7 mg of tetracycline HCl. It is placed subgingivally into the periodontal pocket, where the tetracycline is released slowly over 7–10 days. It is nonresorbable and must be removed at a follow-up appointment.

133.

D. Atridox® is a biodegradable gel delivered via a syringe system to the diseased pocket for use in the treatment of chronic periodontitis to promote attachment level gain, to reduce pocket depths, and to reduce bleeding on probing.

134.

C. Periostat® capsules (20 mg twice daily) have proven effective in the inhibition of collagenase activity in individuals with periodontal disease.

135.

B. The strength of a sealant is sacrificed in order to make it flow into the pits and fissures. Sealants are completely unfilled, making them weak as compared to composites. This is the primary reason that sealants that are left high in occlusion usually come out quickly.

136.

A. All of the items listed are polymers. They all have long chains of identical repeating units known as "mers."

137.

B. If gelation time of the alginate is to be altered, the best method is to vary the temperature of the water used in making the mix. The higher the water temperature, the shorter the gelation time.

138.

B. A properly acid-etched surface has a distinctive appearance of dull white and chalky. Any other appearance is an indication that the acid etching has been contaminated and must be reapplied.

139.

C. An alloy, known as the amalgam alloy, is made by the manufacturer and generally is cut into small particles or filings. The mixing of these particles with mercury is known as trituration.

140.

C. The methyl methacrylate system often comes as a powder and liquid. The powder is composed primarily of beads of prepolymerized methacrylate.

141.

C. Autopolymerizing resins begin to set shortly after the two components are mixed together. Light-cured resins are already mixed together but will not begin to set until a bright light is placed close to the resin to initiate the polymerization reaction. Auto-cure, cold-cure, and self-cure are synonyms.

142.

A. Zinc phosphate cements shrink slightly during setting. The cement shrinks much more when it is in contact with air than when it is under water. Thus, the cement should not be allowed to dry out.

143.

A. Type I dental impression plaster is not used at all today due to the tremendous improvement in other impression-making systems.

144.

C. As the stone is mixed, air bubbles are incorporated into the mix. Vibration forces the air bubbles (which are less dense) to the surface of the mixture, making the entire mix more dense.

145.

B. The chief contribution of gold is to increase the tarnish resistance of the alloy. The tarnish resistance is in almost direct proportion to the gold content where the gold is combined with base metals. It has been estimated that the gold content of a successful dental gold alloy should be at least 75% by weight in order to resist tarnish in the mouth.

146.

C. Sealants should be applied first. If fluoride is applied first, the efficiency of the acid etching is diminished.

147.

B. The liquid is methyl methacrylate. A small amount of an inhibitor such as hydroquinone is usually present to aid in preventing polymerization of the monomer during storage.

148.

C. Cross-linking, the chemical attachment of one polymer strand to another, greatly increases the physical and mechanical properties of a polymer.

149.

B. Chromium–cobalt alloys are quite inflexible. They have essentially no ductility or malleability after

they are cast. All of the other properties seen in the question are advantages of chromium–cobalt alloys.

150.

D. A number of authors have listed the optimum properties of a denture base resin. The following desirable qualities indicate the wide variety of requirements; the order in which these properties are listed does not represent their relative importance (1) adequate strength characteristics; (2) satisfactory thermal properties; (3) dimensional stability in or out of oral fluids; (4) low specific gravity; (5) good chemical stability; (6) insolubility in and low sorption of fluids present; (7) absence of taste, odor, and oral tissues; (8) natural appearance; (9) stability of color and translucency; (10) reasonable adhesion to other plastics; (11) ease and accuracy in fabrication and repair; and (12) moderate cost.

151.

C. Any infection resulting from improper cleaning in this area could migrate down the implant toward the bone. This infection could have results ranging from simple implant failure to a life-threatening infection for the patient. Assurance that the patient can and will keep the implant clean is one of the most important criteria in patient selection.

152.

C. The wax pattern is encased in a special gypsum product (invest), which is placed in a hot oven (burnout), and molten metal is forced into the space provided by the burning out process (casting). The restoration is then polished.

153.

B. The flux is used while the alloy is on the molten stage. With pickling, the casting is placed in an acidic solution which reduces the surface oxides.

154.

A. The compressive strength of ceramic bodies is greater than either their tensile or their shear strength. The tensile strength is low because of the unavoidable surface defects. The shear strength is low because of the lack of ductility or ability to shear, caused by the complex structure of the glass ceramic materials. The shear and tensile strengths of the fired porcelain are so low that the slightest imperfection in the preparation of the cavity in the tooth may cause the jacket crown to fracture in service.

155.

D. Individual autonomy and respect for human beings, societal trusts, nonmaleficence, beneficence, justice and fairness, and veracity are values contained in the ADHA Code of Ethics for dental hygienists.

156.

A. The Legislative branch of government makes laws for the state. State senators and representatives, sometimes called congressmen, are usually these lawmakers.

157.

B. The Executive branch of government enforces the laws passed by the legislature.

158.

D. The Judicial branch of government interprets the laws the legislature passes.

159.

A. Judges do not make laws, they simply interpret existing laws.

160.

A. Common law is created by the courts via judicial decision and can be changed by the courts. It contains notions of common sense and precedent.

161.

D. Adminstrative law is the result of the Legislative branches voluntarily delegating some of its lawmaking authority to the Executive branch. The state dental board has this authority.

162.

B. Statutory of law is written law, which is enacted by the legislature, helps promote justice, and can be changed by the legislature. Dental practice acts are examples of this type of law.

163.

C. Constitutional law was created by citizens. They have created this body of law and only citizens have the power to change this law. It is the most powerful law and takes precedent over other laws.

164.

D. Administrative agencies such as state dental boards fall within this administrative law.

165.

A. It was thought for many years that the mechanism of fluoride was limited to incorporation of fluoride into the enamel hydroxyapatite crystal. According to Burt, the mechanism for the effectiveness of fluoride in the prevention of dental caries is multifactorial.

166.

D. Lowercase letters are used for measuring caries susceptibility in primary dentition. OHI-S is a debris index, and a primary dentition counterpart is not reported in the dental literature.

167.

C. The OHI and OHI-S are debris indexes and do not measure severity of periodontal disease. The GI index is confined to measurements within the gingiva. The Periodontal Index (PI) is used to measure presence and severity of periodontal disease.

168.

B. The estimated cost in 1989 per person per year was 51 cents. However, costs have been shown to vary from 12 cents to $5.41 per person per year.

169.

C. Medicare does cover medical care for this population. Dental benefits are limited to those dental problems such as fractures and oral cancer that require hospitalization.

170.

C. The Medicaid program instituted in 1968 required states to provide dental screening, diagnosis, and treatment for needy children up to at least age 20 years.

171.

C. Winslow's definition utilizes the concept of organized community effort. All individuals within the population, whether fatally ill from the disease, susceptible, or disease-resistant, are encompassed. The entire community is taken into account.

172.

D. It is more ethical to prevent disease than to cure disease. Teamwork is necessary to handle large groups efficiently, and delegation of responsibilities to auxiliary personnel is utilized. Cost-efficiency plays a major role because prevention is cheaper than the cure.

173.

C. Primary prevention deals with the prepathogenic state of disease and involves health promotion and specific protection. Secondary prevention occurs in early pathogenesis. This involves early diagnosis and prompt treatment.

174.

D. To be well supported by available tax funds, the 35,000–50,000 population is targeted. The essence of public health is dealing with large groups. Due to this fact, public health officials are educated with this ori-

entation. Often it is more cost-efficient for two small counties to combine to form the target population.

175.

A. The local health department provides such direct functions as home visits, dental clinics, and supervision of local water supplies. The state and national levels perform supervisory and administrative functions. The international level often works with worldwide health promotion and prevention.

176.

B. Prevention, cost-efficiency, and teamwork are fundamental principles of public health. However, in a democratic society where government regulation is small, it is important for the public to understand why they must undertake proper health measures by their own volition. The individual must learn why such regulations are of value in order to increase compliance. (Wearing a seat belt is mandatory in some states, yet many people refuse to wear a seat belt. When one learns how many lives are saved yearly, then one is more inclined to comply.)

177.

C. T. A. Hunter urged the founding of the training schools for dental nurses in New Zealand. In 1905, Alfred Fones trained Ms. Irene Newman in dental prophylaxis procedures. At that time, Dr. Fones was Chairman of the Legislative Committee of the Connecticut Dental Association. He introduced a bill to allow assistants to perform prophylaxes under direct supervision.

178.

A. These two forms for delivery and financing of dental care became a more accepted part of health care in the 1980s. Often discussed together, they do differ because PPOs typically involve contracts between insurers and a number of practitioners. Patients are allowed to select from whom they will receive dental care depending on whether or not the practitioner participates in the PPO arrangement. Participants of HMOs are much more limited in selection of practitioners.

179.

E. Blackerby originally defined a public health problem as (1) a condition or situation that caused widespread death and/or disease, (2) where a body of knowledge existed that could relieve the situation, and (3) the body of knowledge was not being applied. Today, the definition has been expanded to include public and governmental perception of such a problem.

180.

A. After assessment and evaluation of many global studies to determine predictive and risk factors for dental caries, socioeconomic status was determined to be a powerful determinant factor of caries status in any community.

181.

B. Recent studies indicate that nutritional factors, defined as absorption of nutrients, have no bearing on caries development. However, dietary factors, relating to how patients select foods that they eat, have a clear influence on caries development.

182.

C. By definition, severe caries is now classified by a DMFT score of 7.0 or above. Twenty percent of U.S. children still suffer from severe caries today.

183.

C. Basic, clinical, and epidemiological research from the 1970s on have revealed that while gingivitis precedes periodontitis, only a fraction of the sites affected by gingivitis will later suffer periodontitis.

184.

D. A more sensitive measure for dental caries is DMFS. It reaches its greatest usefulness when dental radiographs are incorporated. In cases of high caries attack rates where almost no unaffected teeth remain, the DMFS well demonstrates a more accurate caries count than DMFT because only the whole tooth is taken into account in the later index.

185.

D. Prevalence is useful when caries counts are low. It is useful in ancient skull studies where many teeth are lost due to reasons other than caries. It is best utilized when one or two carious teeth are the criterion for differentiating affected individuals from unaffected individuals (those with no history of dental disease).

186.

D. As role models, as well as health professionals in the community, dental hygienists have a responsibility to support cessation of all forms of tobacco use as well as to be aware of tobacco-associated general and oral health problems.

187.

A. Adults ingest 1–3 mg of fluoride daily and have for many years. Acute fluoride poisoning occurs in adults when 250–500 mg are ingested over a 24-hour period.

188.

B. Need can be defined as a normative, professional judgment as to the amount and kind of services required to attain and maintain health. Demand is the particular frequency or desired frequency of dental care from a population. Supply is defined as the quantity of dental care services available. Utilization is the number of dental care services actually consumed by a given population.

189.

D. Dental public health is best defined as a concern for and activity directed toward the improvement and protection of the health of a population group. It is not limited to the health of the poor, to rendering health services, or to deducing the nature of health problems. Also, it is not defined by the method of payment for health services or by the agency supplying those services.

190.

D. Evaluation is an ongoing process and actually is thought about in the planning phase when objectives and goals are being developed. It is also important that you are able to provide qualitative and quantitative documentation of the program to the target population, administrators, funding agency, and public on an ongoing basis.

191.

C. To ensure program acceptance, the organizational leaders should always support dental public health programs and be an integral part of the assessment and planning process.

192.

D. Since the question asked about knowledge, it is necessary to assess the knowledge.

193.

B. Since the students were supposed to have effective dental health education, the best way to determine that would be for the students to describe dental disease etiology.

194.

C. Pretest/posttest would be the most effective way to measure the effectiveness of the new curriculum.

195.

D. The dental hygienist could best be utilized by evaluation and presentation of program effectiveness.

196.

B. The student conducted researched treatment modalities.

197.

D. 2.6 out of 3.0 signifies heavy plaque accumulation.

198.

C. Randomization ensures equal participation chance in a study.

199.

C. The easiest and most likely to be adopted method of fluoride is the fluoride mouthrinse program.

200.

A. When evaluating sealants and fluoride, you evaluate the rate of caries, which is easily assessed in age group with permanent molars present by the DMFT.

patient history
synopsis

CASE 1	VITAL SIGNS
Age 77	Blood pressure 66/58
Sex F	Pulse rate 80
Height 5′ 2″	Respiration rate 18
Weight 130lbs/59kg	

1. Under the care of a physician

☒ Yes   ☐ No

Condition: Arthritis

2. Hospitalized within the last 5 years

☐ Yes   ☒ No

3. Has or had the following conditions:

Arthritis

4. Current medication(s)

Motrin and multivitamins

5. Smokes or uses tobacco products

☐ Yes   ☒ No

6. Is pregnant

☐ Yes   ☒ No   ☐ N/A

Medical History: The client has arthritis in both hands, a functional heart murmur, and ptosis of the left eye.

Dental History: The client's frequency of visits to the dental clinic is based on discomfort — she had a tooth extracted 2 years ago. Her last prophylaxis was 3 years ago. When asked about the importance of maintaining oral health, she states she would like to keep her teeth for the rest of her life. She brushes once a day when her arthritis is not bothering her. She does not use an interdental cleaning aid since she cannot manipulate the dental floss.

Social History: The client is retired with a high school diploma.

Chief Complaint: "I want to have my front tooth replaced."

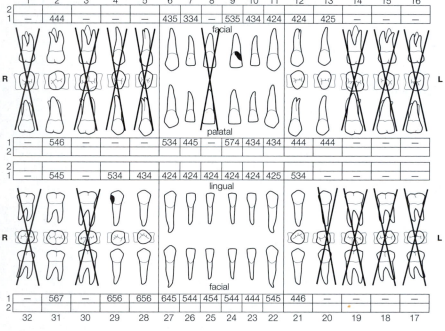

ADULT CLINICAL EXAMINATION

Current Oral Hygiene Status
1. Brushes once per day.

Supplemental Oral Examination Findings
1. Generalized moderate periodontitis and pigmentation
2. Bilateral mandibular and palatel tori
3. TMJ - difficulty opening
4. Class III mobility #9

⋔ Clinically visible carious lesion

⧓ Clinically missing tooth

△ Furcation

▲ "Through and through" furcation

Probe 1: initial probing depth

Probe 2: probing depth 1 month after scaling and root planing

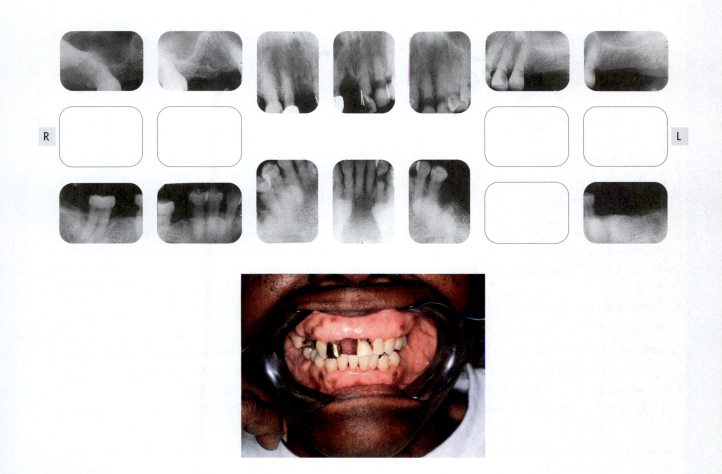

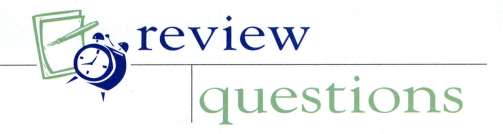

review questions

1. Using G. V. Black's classification, which one of the following would accurately classify the restoration on tooth #9?
   A. II
   B. III
   C. IV
   D. V

2. All of the following oral physiotherapy aids would be appropriate for this client EXCEPT one. Which one is the EXCEPTION?
   A. Automatic toothbrush
   B. Floss holder
   C. Oral irrigator
   D. Interdental brush

3. All of the following are appropriate practices for providing fluoride to the client's dentition EXCEPT one. Which one is the EXCEPTION?
   A. Dentifrice
   B. Dietary supplement
   C. Mouth rinse
   D. Professional fluoride treatment

4. What is the total (actual) recession, in millimeters, on tooth #21?
   A. 3
   B. 4
   C. 5
   D. 6

5. Which intraoral technique was used to determine the finding on the hard palate?
   A. Inspection
   B. Digital
   C. Bimanual
   D. Bilateral

6. Which of the following radiographs shows evidence of nutrient canals?
   A. Maxillary left molar
   B. Mandibular right molar
   C. Mandibular central incisor
   D. Mandibular right canine

7. The client has decided to have a removable partial made to replace tooth #8. All of the following materials are appropriate for obtaining an impression EXCEPT one. Which one is the EXCEPTION?
   A. Reversible hydrocolloid
   B. Addition silicone
   C. Irreversible hydrocolloid
   D. Polysulfide

8. All of the following vital signs are within normal/acceptable range EXCEPT one. Which one is the EXCEPTION?
   A. Blood pressure
   B. Pulse
   C. Respiration
   D. Temperature

9. Tooth mobility may be associated with all of the following EXCEPT one. Which one is the EXCEPTION?
   A. Alveolar bone loss
   B. Pregnancy
   C. NSAIDs
   D. Occlusal trauma

10. For this client, the MOST important reason to remove calculus from the root surface is because it
    A. Alters the dentin
    B. Irritates the junctional epithelium
    C. Harbors plaque organisms
    D. Is an irritant to the gingival sulcus

11. The client has difficulty opening her mouth. Which of the following muscles of mastication is MOST likely involved?
    A. Masseter
    B. Temporalis
    C. Internal (medial) ptyeroid
    D. External (lateral) pterygoid

12. Which of the following cranial nerves is involved with the client's ptosis of the left eye?
    A. Glossopharyngeal
    B. Facial
    C. Abducens
    D. Oculomotor

13. What is the pigmentation of the gingiva called?
    A. Amalgam tattoo
    B. Melanin pigmentation
    C. Fordyce granules
    D. Angular cheilitis

14. What is the pigmentation on the gingiva caused by?
    A. Amalgam particle embedded in the mucosa or gingiva
    B. Hereditary, or can occur following inflammation from injury
    C. Aberrant sebaceous glands
    D. Infection caused by *Candida albicans*

15. Following a prophylaxis, what is the next treatment indicated for this patient?
    A. Severe decay needs to be restored
    B. Fix the front tooth the patient is complaining about
    C. Periodontal surgery
    D. Extraction of #9

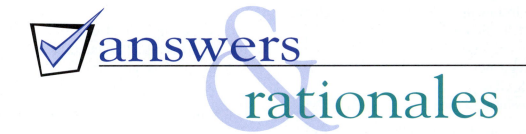

answers & rationales

1.

C. Tooth #9 exhibits a Class IV restoration involving the proximal surface and incisal edge. A Class II restoration involves the proximal surfaces of posterior teeth. A Class III restoration involves the proximal surfaces of anterior tooth. A Class V restoration involves the cervical one third of the facial or lingual surface.

2.

D. The interdental brush would be difficult to handle for this client because of her arthritis. Also, the contour of her gingival tissues does not allow for access to the proximal areas. Owing to the larger and/or longer handles, an automatic toothbrush, floss holder, and oral irrigator would be easier to grasp.

3.

B. A dietary fluoride supplement would not be beneficial for this client because she is over 16 years of age. Dietary fluoride supplements are indicated for those under 16 who use a private water supply without natural fluoride, whose water supply has less than optimum fluoride, and who live in a community where the water supply has not been fluoridated. A dentifrice and mouth rinse containing fluoride would be appropriate for this client because they both provide a low concentration of fluoride, which has a bacterio-static effect on the bacteria. A professional fluoride treatment would be indicated because there is evidence of dental caries.

4.

C. To get the total amount of attachment loss, the probing depth must be added to the amount of recession present. The amount of attachment loss is 5 mm because the probing depth is 3 mm and the amount of recession is 2 mm.

5.

B. The finding on the hard palate is tori. When palpating the hard palate, the digital method of examination is used that involves a single finger. Inspection, the visual examination of tissues, should be used in conjunction with the digital examination. Using only the inspection method may cause the examiner to overlook significant findings. Bimanual examination involves using the finger and thumb from each hand simultaneously. The bilateral examination method involves using both hands at the same time to examine corresponding structures on opposite sides of the body.

6.

C. The mandibular central incisor radiograph shows evidence of nutrient canals. These canals are radiolucent vertical lines located between the teeth.

7.

C. Irreversible hydrocolloid does not have adequate accuracy for predictable removable partials. Reversible hydrocolloid, addition silicone, and polysulfide are appropriate choices for impression materials.

8.

A. The client's blood pressure is slightly lower than the normal range for an elderly person—systolic, 90–140, and diastolic, 60–90. All other vital signs are within normal limits.

9.

C. NSAID is an anti-inflammatory drug that would not contribute to tooth mobility. Loss of bone support, occlusal trauma, and in some instances hormone alterations are associated with increased tooth mobility.

10.

C. Calculus is a major factor in gingival inflammation and is most damaging because its rough surface allows for plaque accumulation. Calculus can cause irritation to the tissue, but that is secondary to its ability to harbor plaque. Calculus does not alter dentin.

11.

D. The external (lateral) pterygoid pulls the head of the condyle down the posterior slope of the articular eminence. The masseter, temporalis, and internal (medial) pterygoid muscles assist in closing the mandible.

12.

D. The oculomotor is a motor nerve to the levator muscle that raises the upper eyelid. The glossopharyngeal is a motor nerve to the throat muscles. The abducens and facial nerves are motor nerves, which serve the lateral rectus and muscles of facial expression, respectively.

13.

B. Melanin pigmentation of the gingiva or mucosa.

14.

B. Melanin pigmentation is a hereditary condition; those with dark complexions are most commonly affected; can also occur following inflammation from injury.

15.

A. The client has several areas of dental decay, that need to be addressed prior to any other procedure.

case study 1 answers

patient history
synopsis

CASE 2
Age 41
Sex F
Height 5′ 3″
Weight 140lbs/64kg

VITAL SIGNS
Blood pressure 110/78
Pulse rate 72
Respiration rate 18

1. Under the care of a physician

☒ Yes ☐ No

Condition: Hypothyroidism

2. Hospitalized within the last 5 years

☐ Yes ☒ No

3. Has or had the following conditions:

Hypothyroidism and seasonal allergies

4. Current medication(s)

Synthroid 125 mg, Levoxyl 125 mg, meclizine, Naprosyn

5. Smokes or uses tobacco products

☒ Yes ☐ No
Occasionally

6. Is pregnant

☐ Yes ☒ No ☐ N/A

Medical History: The client has seasonal allergies and hypothyroidism. She is under the care of a physician for her hypothyroidism. Patient is concerned that the medication she is taking for her hypothyroidism is not working well.

Dental History: The client's past care has been limited to dental emergencies. She brushes her teeth twice a day, but does not floss or use any other cleaning aids.

Social History: The client cleans homes for a living. Owing to her recent move, she is worried about her two children not adjusting to their new school.

Chief Complaint: "My teeth hurt and sometimes my gums bleed when I brush."

ADULT CLINICAL EXAMINATION

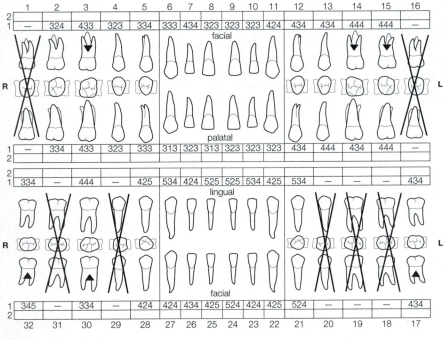

Current Oral Hygiene Status
1. Heavy Calculus
2. Brushes twice a day

Supplemental Oral Examination Findings
1. Generalized inflamation with bleeding on probing
2. Generalized recession
3. Class I mobility #7

⬆ Clinically visible carious lesion

✕ Clinically missing tooth

△ Furcation

▲ "Through and through" furcation

Probe 1: initial probing depth

Probe 2: probing depth 1 month after scaling and root planing

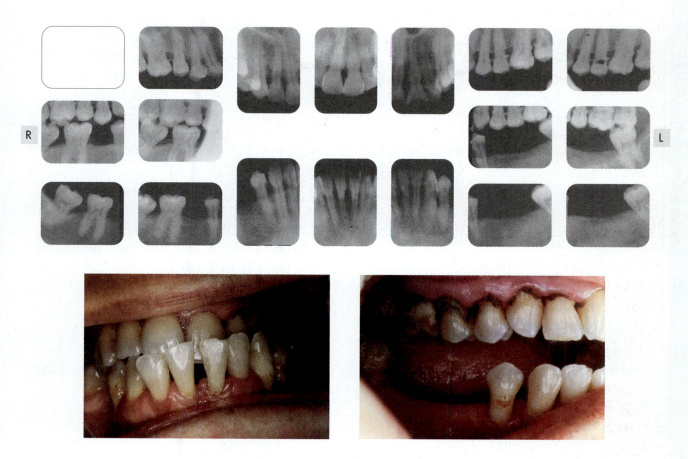

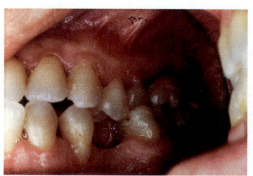

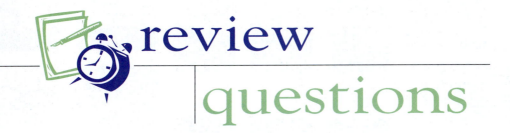

review questions

1. On the facial root surface of #28 there is evidence of
   A. Calculus
   B. Root caries
   C. Abrasion
   D. Tobacco stain

2. To accurately diagnose posterior bone level, which of the following radiographs would provide the MOST accurate diagnosis?
   A. Pantomogram
   B. Occlusal
   C. Vertical bitewings
   D. Horizontal bitewings

3. Teeth #s 6–10 and 22–27 show which of the following malrelationships?
   A. Overjet
   B. Edge-to-edge
   C. Overbite
   D. Crossbite

4. The MOST appropriate procedure for calculus removal on this client would be the use of
   A. Ultrasonic scaling
   B. Hoes
   C. Files
   D. Sonic scaling

5. All of the following are characteristics of hypothyroidism EXCEPT one. Which one is the EXCEPTION?
   A. Myxedema
   B. Cold intolerance
   C. Graves' disease
   D. Glossitis

6. All of the following medications are acceptable for clients with hypothyroidism EXCEPT one. Which one is the EXCEPTION?
   A. Synthroid
   B. Levoxyl
   C. Meclizine
   D. Naprosyn

7. The MOST appropriate referral for this client at this time is to a(n)
   A. School counselor
   B. Periodontist
   C. Oral surgeon
   D. Orthodontist

8. In addition to the heavy calculus deposits on the buccal surfaces of teeth #s 9–15, there is an accumulation of calculus on the occlusal surface of #14. This is probably due to
   A. The lack of opposing teeth, resulting in a reduction of mechanical plaque removal and therefore calculus formation
   B. Medications taken by the client
   C. The client not flossing
   D. The salivary flow delivered through Wharton's duct causing calculus formation

9. Which of the following BEST describes the pattern of bone loss in this client?
   A. Generalized horizontal
   B. Localized horizontal
   C. Generalized vertical
   D. Localized vertical

10. Calculus removal at the facial of the maxillary left first molar may result in tooth sensitivity owing to
    A. Occlusal caries
    B. Traumatized tissue
    C. Exposed dentinal tubules
    D. Altered occlusion

11. Nerve fibers associated with root hypersensitivity are
    A. A-delta fibers in the pulp
    B. Myelinated C fibers in the pulp
    C. Long neurons
    D. Cranial nerves III and VIII

12. Radiographs suggest the presence of root surface caries at the distal of #14. Which of the following microorganisms is implicated in the development of root caries?
    A. *Actinomyces viscosus*
    B. *Actinobacillus actinomycetemcomitans*
    C. *Fusobacterius nucleatum*
    D. *Prevotella intermedia*
    E. *Mutans streptococcus*

13. Which of the following periodontal maintenance appointments is most appropriate following definitive periodontal treatment for this patient?
    A. 4–6 weeks
    B. 7–9 weeks
    C. 10–12 weeks
    D. 13–15 weeks

14. Which of the following oral hygiene aids would be most effective for removing plaque in the furcation areas?
    A. Perio-Aid
    B. Floss with threader
    C. Interdental brush
    D. Rubber-tip stimulator

15. All of the following symptoms could indicate that the patient is receiving too much of her thyroid medication EXCEPT one. Which one is the EXCEPTION?
    A. Fatigue
    B. Nervousness
    C. Irritability
    D. Arrhythmia

case study 2 questions

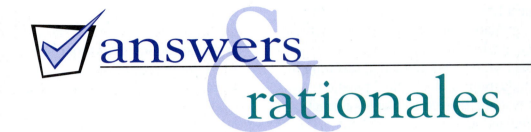

answers & rationales

1.

B. Root caries is the absence of tooth structure, but calculus and tobacco stain are deposits. Abrasion is the mechanical wearing away of tooth structure and appears smooth, shiny, and hard.

2.

C. Vertical placement of bitewings, instead of horizontal, gives the necessary view to show advanced bone loss. Occlusal film technique and the pantomogram are not useful in accurately diagnosing bone level.

3.

D. Overjet occurs when the maxillary incisors are facial to the mandibular incisors with a measurable horizontal distance. Edge-to-edge occurs when the maxillary and mandibular incisal surfaces meet. The vertical overlap of the maxillary over the mandibular teeth is overbite.

4.

A. Ultrasonic scaling is superior to sonic scaling owing to the increased frequency. Hoes and files would not be instruments of choice for this client's condition.

5.

C. Graves' disease is associated with hyperthyroidism, not hypothyroidism. Myxedema is the most severe form of hypothyroidism. The client may also experience cold intolerance and glossitis.

6.

C. Meclizine is an antihistimine. Synthroid, Levoxyl, and Naprosyn are used in treating hypothyroidism.

7.

A. Because the client is concerned about her children and has limited income, the first step should be to see the school counselor.

8.

A. Masticatory forces will help clean the occlusal surfaces of plaque. Because there are no opposing teeth, the cleansing action does not occur. Medications may contribute to calculus formation, but in this client, lack of opposing teeth is the cause. Flossing is beneficial for cleansing proximal, not occlusal, surfaces. Wharton's duct is located in the mandibular region. Salivary flow from the duct would have little impact on calculus formation in the maxillary molars.

9.

A. Horizontal bone loss is relatively constant throughout the mouth. Localized horizontal bone loss would suggest one or two isolated areas. Generalized vertical bone loss would suggest vertical or angular defects throughout the mouth. Localized vertical bone loss would suggest isolated areas of angular loss. None of the three apply.

10.

C. Calculus removal at #2 will expose dentinal tubules. These exposed tubules may cause tooth sensitivity, especially to cold and sweets. Traumatized tissue does not result in tissue sensitivity. There is no evidence of occlusal caries on #14. Calculus removal on the facial will not alter the tooth's occlusion.

11.

A. The myelinated A-delta fibers are irritated because of rapid fluid movement in the open dentinal tubules. Myelinated C fibers and long neurons are not associated with dentin hypersensitivity. Tooth innervation is from the trigeminal or 5th cranial nerve.

12.

A. *Actinomyces viscosis* is associated with root surface caries. *Actinobacillus actinomycemcomitans, Fusobacterium nucleatum,* and *Prevotella intermedia* are involved in the development of periodontal disease. *Streptococcus mutans* is an etiological agent in coronal caries.

13.

A. Patient has advanced periodontal condition and heavy calculus. Four to six weeks is an appropriate reevaluation interval.

14.

A. The Perio-Aid toothpick-in-holder is small enough to fit into a furcation area.

15.

A. Fatigue is not a symptom of too much thyroid medication. Increased doses often cause excitability reactions.

case study 2 answers

patient history
synopsis

CASE 3
Age 50
Sex F
Height 5' 7"
Weight 145lbs/66kg

VITAL SIGNS
Blood pressure 142/92
Pulse rate 74
Respiration rate 16

1. Under the care of a physician
☐ Yes　　☒ No

2. Hospitalized within the last 5 years
☐ Yes　　☒ No

3. Has or had the following conditions:
None

4. Current medication(s)
None

5. Smokes or uses tobacco products
☐ Yes　　☒ No

6. Is pregnant
☐ Yes　　☒ No　　☐ N/A

Medical History: The client had a complete hysterectomy seven years ago due to precancerous lesion in her uterus. She also had a wrist fracture 1 year ago.

Dental History: The patient visits the dentist every 6 months for a routine prophylaxis. She brushes at least twice a day with tartar-control toothpaste and flosses at least five times per week. She has not had any new carious lesions for five years.

Social History: The patient retired as a professor from a local university. She enjoys being involved in the community and is a member of several women's groups. She frequently eats fast food with her three young grandchildren.

Chief Complaint: "My tissues are tender when I brush. I'm also concerned about losing bone from my mouth."

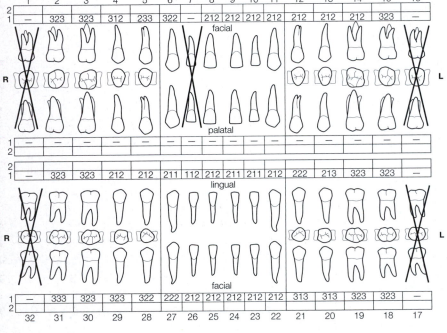

ADULT CLINICAL EXAMINATION

Current Oral Hygiene Status
1. Brushes twice daily
2. Flosses 5 times per week
3. Slight plaque

Supplemental Oral Examination Findings
1. Slightly fissured tongue

Clinically visible carious lesion

Clinically missing tooth

Furcation

"Through and through" furcation

Probe 1: initial probing depth

Probe 2: probing depth 1 month after scaling and root planing

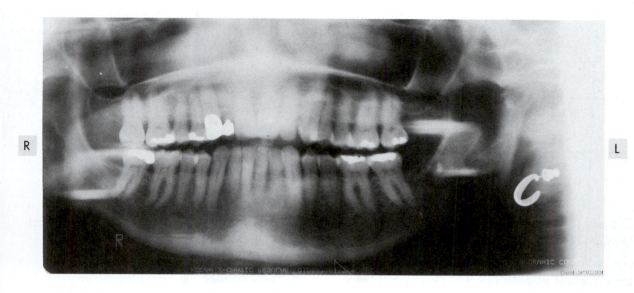

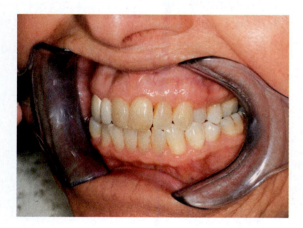 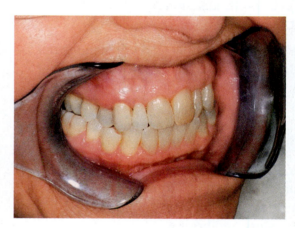

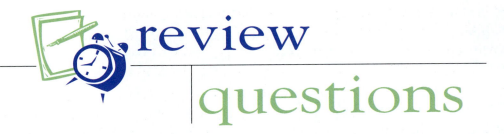

review questions

1. What is the Angle's classification for the molars on this client?
   A. Class I
   B. Class II, Division I
   C. Class II, Division II
   D. Class III

2. Which of the following teeth demonstrate a plaque-retentive factor?
   A. Maxillary right first premolar
   B. Maxillary right central incisor
   C. Mandibular left first molar
   D. Mandibular right second molar

3. What type of prosthesis is found in the maxillary right quadrant?
   A. Cantilever bridge
   B. Maryland bridge
   C. 3-unit fixed partial denture
   D. Laminate

4. Which of the following active ingredients is in the toothpaste this client uses?
   A. Potassium nitrate
   B. Triclosan
   C. Acidulated phosphate fluoride
   D. Pyrophosphate

5. Which of the following vital signs is NOT within normal limits?
   A. Blood pressure
   B. Pulse
   C. Respiration
   D. Temperature

6. Which of the following areas was palpated to obtain the pulse rate?
   A. Side of neck
   B. Side of face
   C. Bend in elbow
   D. Wrist

7. Using G. V. Black's classification, how would the restoration on tooth #19 be classified?
   A. I
   B. II
   C. V
   D. VI

8. When the dentition is occluded, which of the following is the correct term for the position of the molars?
   A. End-to-end
   B. Open-bite
   C. Crossbite
   D. Edge-to-edge

9. When reviewing the client's home care regimen, at which level is she positioned on the learning ladder?
   A. Awareness
   B. Self-interest
   C. Involvement
   D. Habit

10. If a sample of this client's plaque were examined with a phase microscope, which types of bacteria would MOST likely predominate?
    A. Gram-negative rods
    B. Gram-negative spirochetes
    C. Gram-positive cocci
    D. White blood cells

11. Given the medical and social histories, the client MOST likely suffers from which of the following conditions?
    A. Obesity
    B. Osteoporosis
    C. Depression
    D. Type 1 diabetes

12. On reviewing the client's history, total care should address all of the following EXCEPT one. Which one is the EXCEPTION?
    A. Exercise
    B. Caloric intake
    C. Calcium intake
    D. Hormone replacement therapy

13. Tooth #31 has which of the following overhanging restoration?
    A. Type I overhang
    B. Type II overhang
    C. Type III overhang

14. How would you treat the above condition?
    A. Treated with marginization procedure and repolishing of the restoration
    B. Replacement of restoration
    C. Treated with marginization procedure if predicted final result is good
    D. Repolishing of the restoration

15. Which of the following case types best describes this patients periodontal condition?
    A. Type I
    B. Type II
    C. Type III
    D. Type IV
    E. Type V

case study 3 questions

✓answers & rationales

1.

A. The Angle's classification is Class I. The mesial cusp of the maxillary first molar is aligned with the buccal groove of the mandibular first molar, and the cusp of the maxillary canine is positioned to the immediate distal of the mandibular canine. Classes II and III are not choices for this client's occlusion since she has a Class I occlusion for the reasons stated previously.

2.

D. Tooth #31 has a proximal restoration, which can be a plaque-retentive factor. Bacteria will more likely adhere to a restoration.

3.

A. Tooth #7 is the pontic of the cantilever bridge, which has only one abutment. A Maryland bridge would have metal fingers extending on the linguals of teeth #s 6 and 8. A three-unit fixed bridge would have #8 as an abutment with a crown. A laminate needs to have a tooth available to be attached and tooth #7 is missing. Also, it would not be durable enough to hold a pontic.

4.

D. The active ingredient in tartar-control toothpaste is pyrophosphate. Potassium nitrate and triclosan are active ingredients in antihypersensitivity and antigingivitis dentifrices, respectively. Acidulated phosphate fluoride is the only fluoride not added to dentifrices. It is used in in-office fluoride applications.

5.

A. The client's blood pressure, 144/92, is higher than the normal average, which is systolic 90–140, and diastolic, 60–90. The remaining vital sign readings are within the normal adult limits. Normal limits for the pulse are 60–100 and normal limits for the respiration rate are 12–20.

6.

D. To obtain the radial pulse, it is necessary to palpate the radial artery, which is located on the radial side of the wrist. The carotid artery is palpated on the side of the neck. The facial artery is palpated on the side of the face, near the angle of the mandible. The brachial artery is palpated at the antecubital fossa at the bend of the elbow.

7.

A. The alloy on tooth #19 is on the occlusal surface—a Class I restoration. A Class II restoration involves the proximal surface of posterior teeth. A Class V restoration involves the cervical one third of either the facial or lingual surfaces. A Class VI restoration involves the incisal edges of anterior teeth and cusps of posterior teeth.

8.

C. The first permanent molars are in crossbite. There is no evidence that the first molars are end-to-end, open-bite, or edge-to-edge.

9.

D. The client is at the habit level of the learning ladder. She demonstrates routine oral hygiene practices with her brushing and flossing. This client has surpassed the awareness, self-interest, and involvement stages of the learning ladder.

10.

C. The bacteria most likely found in a healthy mouth would be Gram-positive cocci. The remaining three, Gram-negative rods, spirochetes, and white blood cells, are present in diseased gingival tissues.

11.

B. For the client's height, her weight is within normal body weight range. Signs of depression include withdrawal from social contact and loss of appetite, which are not evidenced by this client. The symptoms of Type 1 diabetes are abrupt weight loss, weakness, and insulin dependency, none of which are evidenced by this client.

12.

B. Because the client's weight is within normal limits, her caloric intake appears to be fine. Exercise, calcium intake, and hormone replacement therapy are recommended for an individual suffering from osteoporosis.

13.

C. The overhang is more than one half of the interproximal space.

14.

B. A complete restoration replacement is needed.

15.

A. This patient is in great periodontal health. No pockets deeper than 3mm with no bone loss.

patient history
synopsis

CASE 4
Age 37
Sex F
Height 5′ 6″
Weight 185lbs/84kg

VITAL SIGNS
Blood pressure 142/92
Pulse rate 80
Respiration rate 16

1. Under the care of a physician

☒ Yes ☐ No

Condition: Multiple sclerosis

2. Hospitalized within the last 5 years

☐ Yes ☒ No

3. Has or had the following conditions:

Multiple sclerosis

4. Current medication(s)

Phentermine HCL (Fastin) and OTC medications for allergies

5. Smokes or uses tobacco products

☐ Yes ☒ No

6. Is pregnant

☐ Yes ☒ No ☐ N/A

Medical History: The patient has chronic allergies and sinus trouble and was recently diagnosed with multiple sclerosis. She is allergic to penicillin. She has a history of herpes labialis following sun exposure. The patient has a functional heart murmur.

Dental History: The patient's last dental visit was over 8 years ago. At that time she received a cleaning and examination. She brushes 2–3 times a day with a medium-hard toothbrush and experiences gingival bleeding. She never flosses and experiences chronic halitosis.

Social History: The patient works as a waitress. She is a single mother of two children. She reports being under stress due to financial problems.

Chief Complaint: "I need to have my teeth cleaned."

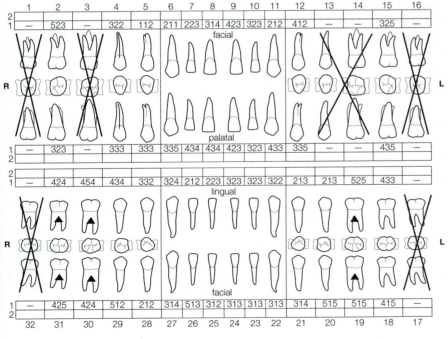

ADULT CLINICAL EXAMINATION

Current Oral Hygiene Status
1. Brushes 2-3 times per day
2. Never flosses
3. Heavy calculus

Supplemental Oral Examination Findings
1. Root canal #4
2. Generalized 4-5 mm pockets and 1-4 mm gingival recession
3. TMJ - pops
4. Grinds her teeth at night
5. Patient has xerostomia

Clinically visible carious lesion

Clinically missing tooth

Furcation

"Through and through" furcation

Probe 1: initial probing depth

Probe 2: probing depth 1 month after scaling and root planing

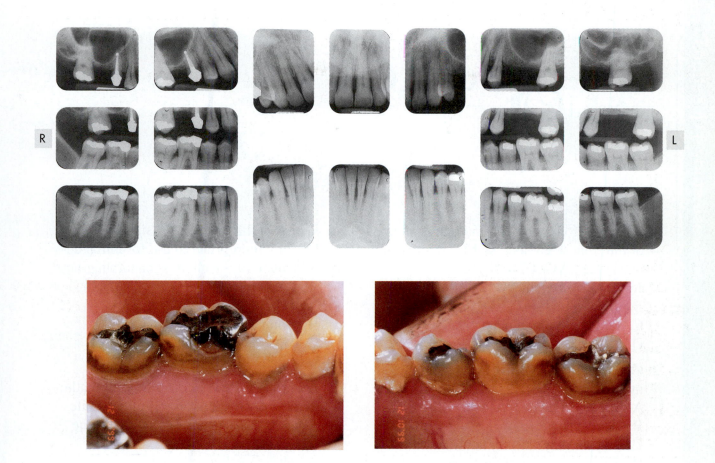

R   L

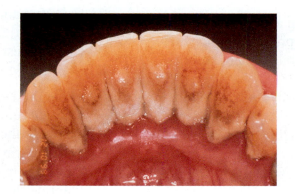

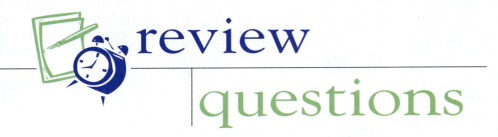
case study 4 questions

1. All of the following are oral manifestations of multiple sclerosis EXCEPT one. Which one is the EXCEPTION?
   A. TMJ dysfunction
   B. Xerostomia
   C. Gingival enlargement
   D. Recession

2. Which of the following is a symptom of multiple sclerosis?
   A. Lip and tongue tremor
   B. Lordosis
   C. Impaired eye-hand coordination
   D. Paralysis of facial muscles

3. Which of the following antibiotic premedication regimens is appropriate for this client?
   A. 2 g Amoxicillin orally 1 hour before procedure
   B. 600 mg Clindamycin orally 1 hour before procedure
   C. 2 g Cephalexin orally 1 hour before procedure
   D. No premedication needed

4. On the initial appointment, air polishing is contraindicated owing to all of the following EXCEPT one. Which one is the EXCEPTION?
   A. Gingival recession
   B. Hypertension
   C. Gingivitis
   D. Herpes labialis

5. Which of the following instruments is LEAST appropriate to use for initial debridement of the client's mandibular anterior lingual surfaces?
   A. Gracey curet
   B. Sonic scaler
   C. Hoe
   D. Sickle scaler

6. All of the following conditions are radiographically evident on this client's bitewings EXCEPT one. Which one is the EXCEPTION?
   A. Horizontal bone loss
   B. Early furcation involvement
   C. Calculus
   D. Class III restoration
   E. Caries

7. All of the following recommendations may be indicated for this client EXCEPT one. Which one is the EXCEPTION?
   A. Toothpick in a holder (Perio-Aid)
   B. Desensitizing dentifrice
   C. Fluoride rinse containing alcohol
   D. Use of a soft-bristled toothbrush

8. If the clinician chose to use an ultrasonic scaler, which of the following ultrasonic tips would be MOST effective in the initial debridement of this client's mandibular lingual surfaces?
   A. Modified (thin) straight
   B. Modified (thin) right
   C. Modified (thin) left
   D. Standard (traditional)

9. The clinical attachment level on the direct facial of tooth #6, in millimeters, is
   A. 2.
   B. 3.
   C. 4.
   D. 5.

10. All of the following procedures are indicated for this client EXCEPT one. Which one is the EXCEPTION?
    A. Finish and polish amalgam in #30
    B. Replace prosthesis of #s 3, 13, and 14
    C. Replace crown on #4
    D. Place sealants on #s 5, 12, 21, and 28

11. On this client, which of the following dental implants is contraindicated for replacement of teeth #s 13 and 14?
    A. Subperiosteal
    B. Transosteal
    C. endosseous
    D. An implant is not indicated

12. The client's prescription medication is contributing to all of the following conditions EXCEPT one. Which one is the EXCEPTION?
    A. Xerostomia
    B. Periodontal disease
    C. Hypertension
    D. Cervical abrasion

13. What is the cause of halitosis?
    A. Breakdown of carbohydrates
    B. Breakdown of fatty acids
    C. Anaerobic breakdown of proteins
    D. None of the above

14. How can a patient treat chronic halitosis?
    A. Gently cleaning the tongue surface twice daily with a tongue brush
    B. Maintaining proper oral hygiene
    C. Drinking several glasses of water a day
    D. All of the above
    E. None of the above

15. Which of the following are effective treatments for xerostomia?
    A. Chew sugarfree gum
    B. Use cold-temperature foods rather than hot-temperature foods
    C. Synthetic saliva
    D. All of the above
    E. None of the above

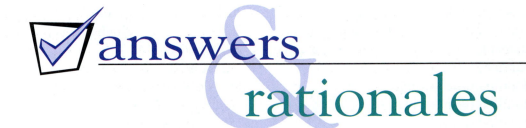

answers & rationales

1.

○ **B.** Recession is not associated with multiple sclerosis. However, TMJ dysfunction, xerostomia, and gingival enlargement are associated with multiple sclerosis.

2.

C. Lip and tongue tremor is associated with Parkinson's disease. Lordosis, an increased curvature of any part of the back, is associated with muscular dystrophy, and paralysis of facial muscles is associated with Bell's palsy.

3.

D. The client has a functional heart murmur that does NOT require antibiotic premedication.

4.

D. The client has a history of herpes labialis, which is a communicable disease and, thus, contraindicated for air polishing. However, no current herpes lesions were detected at this visit. Air polishing is contraindicated for clients with gingival recession, hypertension, and gingivitis.

5.

A. The Gracey curet is used for removal of light calculus deposits and root surface debridement. The hoe, file, and sickle scaler are used to remove heavy calculus and therefore are appropriate for initial debridement.

6.

D. A Class III restoration involves a proximal surface of an anterior tooth and does not involve the incisal angle. Horizontal bone loss and caries are evident on tooth #30, and calculus is evident on several posterior teeth.

7.

C. Because of the client's xerostomia, nonalcohol mouth rinses should be recommended. Alcohol will dry the oral mucosa. A toothpick holder (Perio-Aid) is effective for daily plaque removal in areas of early furcation. A daily desensitizing dentifrice is indicated for areas of dentinal hypersensitivity—noted on the facials of most of the client's teeth. Use of a soft-bristled toothbrush will help decrease gingival bleeding, often caused by using a medium-hard toothbrush.

8.

D. Because the client has medium to heavy calculus deposits on the mandibular anterior, a traditional ultrasonic tip, which is designed for removal of such deposits, would be most appropriate. Modified (thin) tips are used to deplaque and remove light to moderate calculus and endotoxins.

9.

D. When the gingival margin has receded apically to the CEJ, the clinical attachment level is determined by measuring the distance from the base of the pocket to the CEJ. In this client, the pocket depth of 2 mm on the direct facial of tooth #6 is added to the recession measurement of 3 mm, resulting in a clinical attachment level of 5 mm.

10.

A. The amalgam in tooth #30 is contraindicated for finishing and polishing, as the mesiolingual cusp is broken and secondary decay is present. Prosthetic replacement should be recommended for replacing teeth #s 3, 13, and 14. The lost crown on #4 should also be replaced. Sealants are recommended on clients when they are caries-active.

11.

B. A transosteal dental implant is placed completely through the bone and is designed strictly for use on the mandible. It cannot be placed in the maxilla. A subperiosteal dental implant may be placed in the mandible or maxilla when the width or depth of the bone is insufficient for an endosseous implant. An endosseous implant is placed within the maxillary or mandibular bone to support a fixed or removable prosthetic appliance.

12.

D. The client's cervical abrasion is most likely due to overbrushing with a medium to hard toothbrush and is not related to the drug Fastin. Side effects of Fastin include xerostomia, which has an indirect effect on caries, periodontal disease, and hypertension.

13.

C. The odors are produced mainly due to the anaerobic breakdown of proteins into individual amino acids, followed by the further breakdown of certain amino acids to produce detectable foul gases.

14.

D. Currently, chronic halitosis is not very well understood by most physicians and dentists, so effective treatment is not always easy to find. However, gently cleaning the tongue surface twice daily with a tongue brush, tongue scraper, or tongue cleaner to wipe off the bacterial biofilm, debris, and mucus; maintaining proper oral hygiene, including brushing, daily flossing, and periodic visits to dentists and hygienists may be effective in treating halitosis. Flossing is particularly important in removing rotting food debris and bacterial plaque from between the teeth, especially at the gumline; maintain water levels in the body by drinking several glasses of water a day.

15.

D. All of the above are effective treatments of xerostomia.

patient history
synopsis

CASE 5
Age 58
Sex F
Height 5′ 5″
Weight 165lbs/75kg

VITAL SIGNS
Blood pressure 120/82
Pulse rate 80
Respiration rate 22

1. Under the care of a physician
  ☒ Yes ☐ No
  Condition: Addison's disease; foot surgery

2. Hospitalized within the last 5 years
  ☐ Yes ☒ No

3. Has or had the following conditions:
  None

4. Current medication(s)
  Hydrochlorothiazide, Ranitidine, Hydrocordisone 20mg

5. Smokes or uses tobacco products
  ☐ Yes ☒ No

6. Is pregnant
  ☐ Yes ☒ No ☐ N/A

Medical History: The patient is allergic to penicillin and sulfa. Patient was diagnosed with Addison's disease 5 years ago.

Dental History: The patient's last dental visit was over 5 years ago. At that time she received a cleaning and examination. She brushes two times a day. She wears a full maxillary denture and never removes it to sleep at night. She cleans denture with a denture brush.

Social History: Patient did not comment on social history.

Chief Complaint: "I need to have my teeth cleaned."

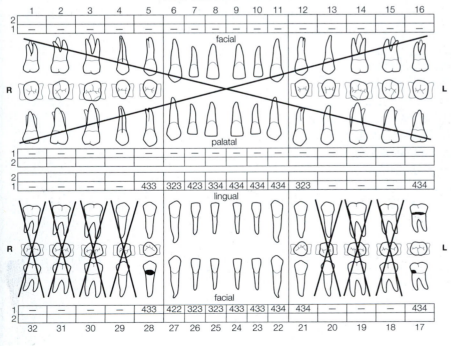

ADULT CLINICAL EXAMINATION

Current Oral Hygiene Status
1. Brushes 2 times per day
2. Heavy calculus

Supplemental Oral Examination Findings
1. Experiencing pain on #24, 25, 26
2. Generalized inflamation
3. Class II mobility #5, 22, 23, 27, 28
4. Class III mobility #24, 25, 26

Clinically visible carious lesion

Clinically missing tooth

Furcation

"Through and through" furcation

Probe 1: initial probing depth

Probe 2: probing depth 1 month
after scaling and root planing

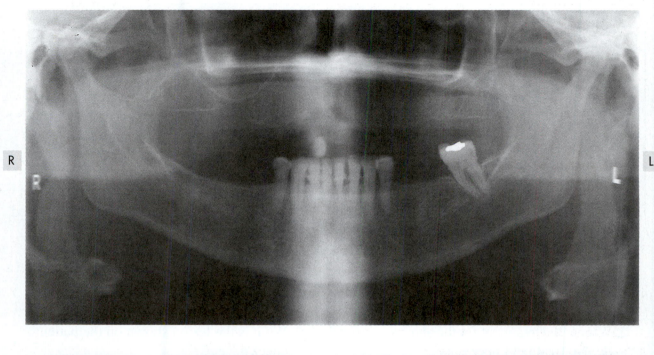

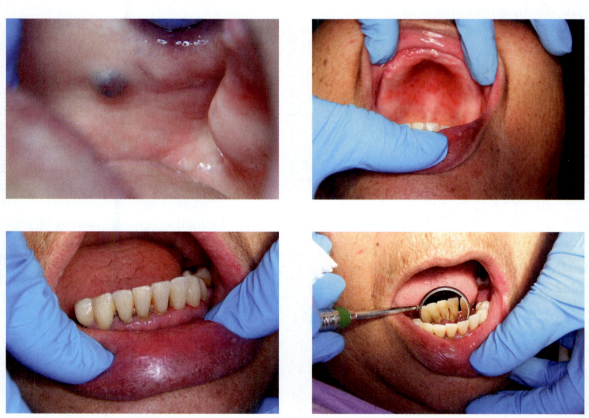

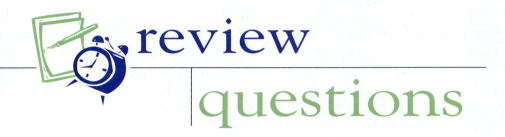

review questions

1. What is the condition on the palatal tissues called?
   A. Epulis fissuratum
   B. Papillary hyperplasia of the palate
   C. Pyogenic granuloma
   D. Lipoma

2. What is the treatment for the above condition?
   A. No treatment necessary
   B. Surgical removal and correction of denture flange
   C. Use of antibiotic ointment
   D. None of the above

3. Using G.V. Black's classification, which one of the following would accurately classify the decay on tooth #17?
   A. I
   B. II
   C. III
   D. IV
   E. V

4. This patient represents which of the following AAP Case Types?
   A. I
   B. II
   C. III
   D. IV
   E. V

5. What is the drug Hydrochlorothiazide used for?
   A. Treatment of Addison's disease
   B. Treatment of hypertension
   C. Treatment of cardiac arrthemias
   D. Treatment of hypothyrodism

6. What is the lesion shown on the patient's cheek?
   A. Lipoma
   B. Mucocele
   C. Hemangioma
   D. Fibroma

7. Which of the following describes Addison's disease?
   A. Endocrine disorder that produces chronic adrenal insufficiency, in which the body produces insufficient amounts of adrenal steroid hormones
   B. Endocrine disorder caused by high levels of cortisol in the blood
   C. Disorder caused by the administration of exogenous glucocorticosteroids to a patient with functional adrenal cortices
   D. None of the above

8. Which of the following best describes secondary adrenal insufficiency?
   A. Endocrine disorder that produces chronic adrenal insufficiency, in which the body produces insufficient amounts of adrenal steroid hormones
   B. Endocrine disorder caused by high levels of cortisol in the blood
   C. Disorder caused by the administration of exogenous glucocorticosteroids to a patient with functional adrenal cortices
   D. None of the above

9. Which of the following best describes Cushing syndrome?
   A. Endocrine disorder that produces chronic adrenal insufficiency, in which the body produces insufficient amounts of adrenal steroid hormones
   B. Endocrine disorder caused by high levels of cortisol in the blood
   C. Disorder caused by the administration of exogenous glucocorticosteroids to a patient with functional adrenal cortices
   D. None of the above

10. What is the pharmacological effect of hydrocortisone?
    A. Used to treat allergies and inflammation
    B. Used to treat yeast infections
    C. Used to treat hypertension
    D. Used to treat cardiac abnormalities

11. What would be the antibiotic of choice for this patient?
    A. Amoxicillin
    B. Penicillin V
    C. Carbenicillin
    D. Clindamycin

12. The dental hygienist will be administering a local anesthetic, Lidocaine 2% 1:100,000), for the deep scaling. What is the maximum permissible dose in carpules for this patient?
    A. 2.2 carpules
    B. 1.1 carpules
    C. 4.4 carpules
    D. 8 carpules

13. With an inferior alveolar nerve block, the solution should be deposited
    A. Into the mental foramen
    B. Medial to the condyle of the mandible
    C. Slightly superior to the mandibular foramen
    D. None of the above

14. When an injection damages a nerve trunk resulting in prolonged numbness, the condition is known as
    A. Neuralgia
    B. Parasthesia
    C. Trismus
    D. Neuritis

15. How can a clinician reduce muscle trismus?
    A. By avoiding repeated insertions of the needle
    B. By using a lower concentration of anesthetic solution
    C. By using more vasoconstrictor
    D. By warming the anesthetic solution before injection

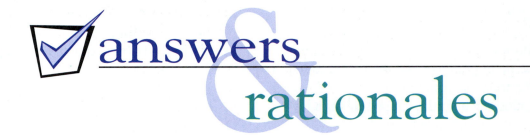

answers & rationales

1.

A. Epulis fissuratum is an irritation by improper fitting of dentures, and wearing the denture all night.

2.

B. Surgical removal of hyperplastic tissue is indicated, and correction of denture flange so that the condition will not reoccur.

3.

E. Tooth #17 exhibits a Class V carious lesion involving the cervical one-third of the facial or lingual surface.

4.

D. This patient presents with AAP Case Type IV, advanced periodontitis. There is evidence of advanced loss of alveolar bone and increased mobility, indicators of AAP Case Type IV.

5.

B. Hydrochlorothiazide is a popular diuretic drug that acts by inhibiting the kidney's ability to retain water. This reduces the volume of the blood, decreasing blood return to the heart and thus cardiac output and, by other mechanisms, is believed to lower peripheral vascular resistance. It is commonly used for the treatment of hypertension.

6.

C. Hemangioma is a neoplasm of blood. It is characterized by superficial lesions that are sessile-red or bluish-red; deeper lesions are of normal color and only palpable or slightly elevated on surface; vascular color not readily detectable in deeper lesions.

7.

A. Addison's disease is a cortisol deficiency and can lead to loss of consciousness and possible death. It can be corrected by the administration of physiological doses of exogenous cortisol.

8.

C. Secondary adrenal insufficiency is caused by the administration of exogenous glococorticosteroids to a patient with functional adrenal cortices. It can produce an adrenocortical hypofunction by producing a disuse atrophy of the adrenal cortex and thereby decreasing the ability of the adrenal cortex to increase corticosteroid levels in response to stressful situations.

9.

B. Cushing syndrome is the hypersecretion of cortisol, which causes elevated blood pressure, alters blood cell distribution, and causes a "buffalo hump" by increasing fat deposition in certain areas of the face and back.

10.

A. Cortisol is a corticosteroid hormone produced by the adrenal cortex that is involved in the response to stress; it increases blood pressure and blood sugar levels, may cause infertility in women, and suppresses the immune system. In pharmacology, cortisol is referred to as hydrocortisone, and is used to treat allergies and inflammation.

11.

D. Clindamycin is not a penicillin. Since the patient is allergic to penicillin, all other drugs would be contraindicated.

12.

A. Considering the patient's medical history, the patient is taking a beta blocker, which potentiates the action of epinephrine and other adrenergic amines by increasing the pressor potency two to six times. This drug must be given at the compromised dose of 2.2 carpules, or .04 mg.

13.

C. Anesthetic should be deposited slightly superior to the inferior alveolar foramen to allow gravity to assist the anesthetic into the foramen.

14.

B. Parathesia causes prolonged numbness and can be caused by irritation to the nerve following injection of contaminated solution.

15.

A. Muscle trismus is caused by continuous needle insertion.

case study 5 answers

patient history
synopsis

CASE 6
Age 59
Sex M
Height 5′ 10″
Weight 170lbs/77kg

VITAL SIGNS
Blood pressure 117/80
Pulse rate 76
Respiration rate 16

1. Under the care of a physician

☐ Yes ☒ No

2. Hospitalized within the last 5 years

☐ Yes ☒ No

3. Has or had the following conditions:

None

4. Current medication(s)

None

5. Smokes or uses tobacco products

☒ Yes ☐ No

Smoker for 30+ years

6. Is pregnant

☐ Yes ☐ No ☒ N/A

Medical History: No significant medical issues.

Dental History: The patient has never had a dental cleaning. Very nervous and embarrassed about his teeth due to lack of dental care.

Social History: His wife and daughter made the dental appointment for him.

Chief Complaint: Pain and swelling on left canine tooth.

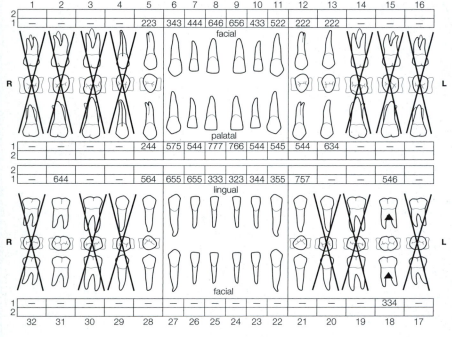

ADULT CLINICAL EXAMINATION

Current Oral Hygiene Status
1. Heavy calculus
2. Heavy staining

Supplemental Oral Examination Findings
1. Type I mobility # 24, 25, 8
2. Generalized recession
3. MGD 23-27
4. High frenum attachment

 Clinically visible carious lesion

Clinically missing tooth

Furcation

"Through and through" furcation

Probe 1: initial probing depth

Probe 2: probing depth 1 month
after scaling and root planing

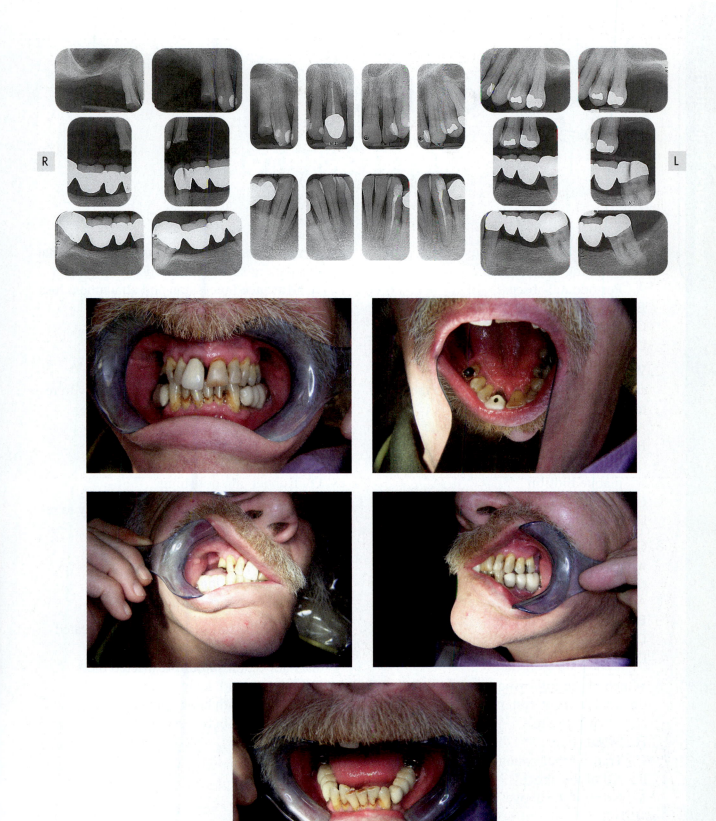

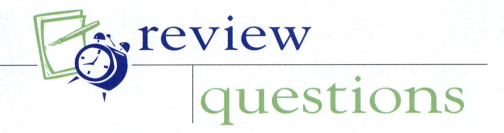

review questions

1. What is the most likely cause of the pain and swelling on tooth #22?
   A. Periodontal abscess
   B. Tooth fracture
   C. Large carious lesion
   D. Root sensitivity

2. Which of the following is important to discuss with this patient in regard to the heavy tobacco stains?
   A. Stains are primarily an esthetic problem
   B. Heavy tobacco stains cause a risk factor for the accumulation of bacterial plaque biofilm
   C. Tobacco stains cannot be removed
   D. None of the above

3. Considering this patient's smoking history, which of the following is the most important to evaluate?
   A. The degree of staining present
   B. The patient's breath
   C. Any benign and malignant changes
   D. None of the above

4. Which of the following are used as a nicotine replacement system?
   A. Chewing gum
   B. Nasal spray
   C. Transdermal system
   D. All of the above
   E. None of the above

5. Which of the following reasons indicate that this patient's prognosis is poor?
   A. Advanced recession and attachment loss
   B. Smoking
   C. Poor oral hygiene
   D. None of the above
   E. All of the above

6. What would be the most efficient way to remove the patient's heavy calculus?
   A. Air polishing
   B. Ultrasonic scaling
   C. Manual scaling
   D. Rubber cup polishing

7. What would be the most efficient way to remove the patient's heavy stain?
   A. Air polishing
   B. Ultrasonic scaling
   C. Manual scaling
   D. Rubber cup polishing

8. Which of the following is contraindicated for the use of the Prophy jet?
   A. Patients on sodium-restricted diets
   B. Patients with heavy stain
   C. Patients with heavy plaque
   D. Patients with recession

9. What is the cause of this patient's mucogingival involvements?
   A. Gingival recession resulting in inadequate attached gingiva
   B. Probing depths extending to or beyond the mucogingival junction into the alveolar mucosa
   C. High frenum attachment
   D. All of the above
   E. None of the above

10. Which of the following periodontal Case Types best describes this patient?
    A. Type I
    B. Type II
    C. Type III
    D. Type IV
    E. Type V

11. What radiographic periodontal conditions characterize the selection of the Case Type in question 10?
    A. Triangulation is widening of the periodontal ligament space and generalized slight horizontal bone loss of less than 20%
    B. Bone loss may be apparent in both horizontal and vertical planes with localized furcation involvement
    C. Advanced vertical and horizontal patterns of bone loss and furcation involvement
    D. None of the above

12. What is the most probable cause of the supraerupted tooth #8?
    A. The patient's occlusion
    B. Extensive bone loss
    C. The root canal
    D. The patient's crown

13. The dental hygienist begins treatment on the patient. During the treatment the patient suddenly has rapid, shallow breathing, confusion, vertigo (dizziness), paresthesia (numbness or tingling of extremities), carpopedal spasm (cramping of hands or feet), and chest tightness. What condition is the patient exhibiting?
    A. Syncopy
    B. Hyperventilation
    C. Postural hypotension
    D. Anaphylaxis

14. What is the proper first-response treatment for a patient who is hyperventilating?
    A. Breath into a paper bag
    B. Keep patient in supine position
    C. Inject patient with epinephrine
    D. Call EMS

15. Which of the following can help reduce the occurrence of this medical emergency?
    A. Complete medical history evaluation
    B. Physical evaluation
    C. Stress reduction protocol
    D. All of the above
    E. None of the above

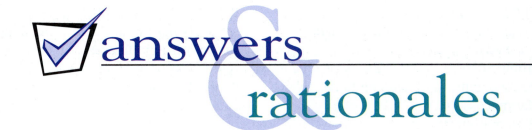

answers & rationales

1.

A. Periodontal abscess occurs where preexisting periodontitis is present. This infection occurs in the walls of the periodontal pocket as a result of bacterial invasion into the periodontal tissue, while abscesses usually spontaneously occur in patients with untreated periodontitis.

2.

B. Heavy tobacco stains cause a breeding ground for the rapid accumulation of bacterial plaque biofilm.

3.

C. It is extremely important to evaluate the oral cavity for any benign or malignant changes. Smoking increases the chance of oral cancer.

4.

D. All of the above are used as nicotine replacement systems.

5.

E. All of the above contribute to the patient's poor prognosis.

6.

B. Ultrasonic scalers involve a rapidly vibrating water-cooled tip that fractures and dislodges calculus deposits and flushes debris from pockets.

7.

A. Air polishing removes plaque and stain as effectively as rubber cup polishing and requires less time.

8.

A. The prophy jet should not be used on patients who are on sodium-restricted diets. Sodium bicarbonate is the main ingredient in the paste.

9.

E. A mucogingival defect is a discrepancy in the relationship between the free gingival margin and the mucogingival junction. All of the above are common conditions that cause mucogingival conditions.

10.

D. This patient has advanced periodontitis and is classified as Case Type IV.

11.

C. Severe chronic periodontitis is characterized by generalized extensive horizontal and vertical bone loss of more than 50% and numerous furcation involvements.

12.

B. Changes in tooth position in a patient with advanced periodontitis is related to the amount of bone loss in the area.

13.

B. The patient has expressed that he is nervous about dental treatment. Therefore, the most probable explaination of his symptoms is hyperventilation.

14.

A. Instruct patient to breathe into a paper bag to enrich carbon dioxide, or to hold breath for 10 seconds then breathe, then repeat. Patient should be placed in upright position. Call EMS should the symptoms continue.

15.

D. All of the above are important to consider for a patient who is apprehensive about dental care.

patient history
synopsis

CASE 7	VITAL SIGNS
Age 60	Blood pressure 130/95
Sex M	Pulse rate 80
Height 5′ 10″	Respiration rate 18
Weight 210lbs/95kg	

1. Under the care of a physician

☒ Yes ☐ No

Condition: Epilepsy

2. Hospitalized within the last 5 years

☒ Yes ☐ No

Reason: Knee replacement surgery

3. Has or had the following conditions:

Epilepsy

4. Current medication(s)

Dilantin, Depakote

5. Smokes or uses tobacco products

☐ Yes ☒ No

6. Is pregnant

☐ Yes ☐ No ☒ N/A

Medical History: Patient is an epileptic and is currently being treated for his condition. He also has indicated that he has been depressed a lot lately. Patient had his right knee replaced 1 year ago.

Dental History: The patient has not visited the dentist for many years.

Social History: Single and works as a parking attendant

Chief Complaint: Swollen, bleeding gums

ADULT CLINICAL EXAMINATION

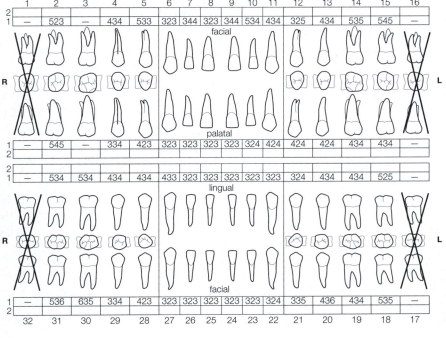

Current Oral Hygiene Status
1. Generalized gingival hyperplasia
2. Generalized bleeding
3. Moderate plaque & calculus

Supplemental Oral Examination Findings

Clinically visible carious lesion

Clinically missing tooth

Furcation

"Through and through" furcation

Probe 1: initial probing depth

Probe 2: probing depth 1 month after scaling and root planing

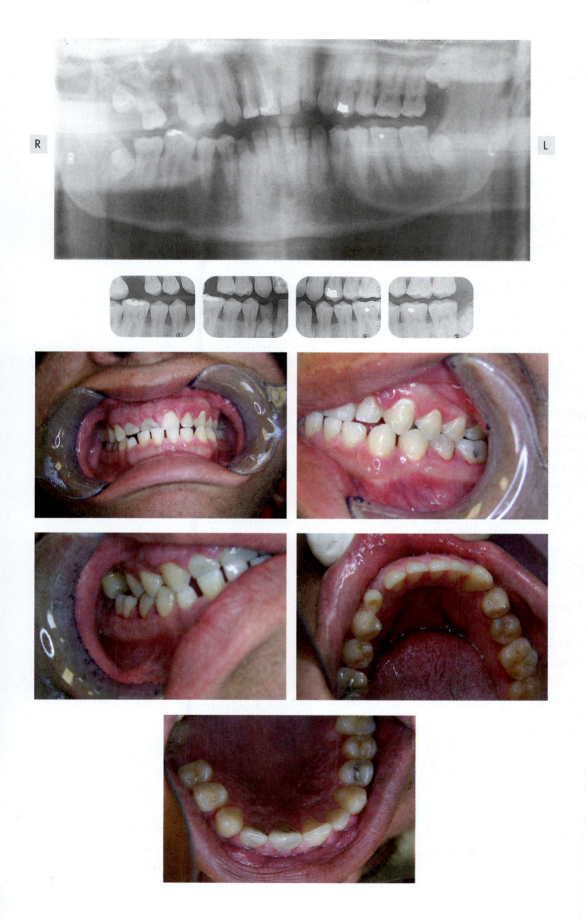

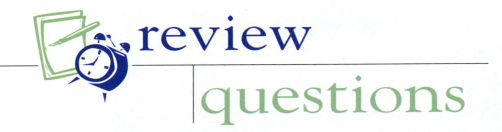

review
questions

1. What is this patient's generalized gingival hyperplasia most likely caused by?
   A. The use of phenytoin
   B. The use of Depakote
   C. Poor oral hygiene
   D. Moderate calculus

2. What is the patient taking Depakote for?
   A. For the treatment of epilepsy and depression
   B. For the treatment of chronic headaches
   C. For the treatment of gingival hyperplasia
   D. None of the above

3. The preferred oral antibiotic regimen for adult SBE premedication is:
   A. Clindamycin 2.0g orally, 1 hr prior to treatment
   B. Clindamycin 600 mg orally, 2 hr prior to treatment
   C. Amoxicillin 2.0g orally, 1 hr prior to treatment
   D. Amoxicillin 600 mg orally, 1 hr prior to treatment

4. What is the reason why antibiotic premedication is needed for this patient?
   A. For his epilepsy
   B. For his depression
   C. For his knee replacement
   D. None of the above
   E. All of the above

5. What is status epilepticus?
   A. A tonic-clonic seizure
   B. A petit mal seizure
   C. A grand mal seizure
   D. A seizure that persists for more than 1 hour

6. During the dental hygiene treatment, the patient goes into a seizure. What is the most common cause of the episode?
   A. Flickering of the dental light
   B. Taking the patient's vital signs
   C. Physical evaluation of patient before treatment
   D. None of the above

7. The patient's anterior occlusal bite is in:
   A. End to end
   B. Crossbite
   C. Overjet
   D. Overbite

8. Which of the following characterizes tooth #27?
   A. Retained primary tooth
   B. Microdont
   C. Supernumerary tooth
   D. Macrodont

9. Which of the following procedures should be conducted on teeth #s 7 and 8?
   A. Pulp vitality testing
   B. Toludine blue testing
   C. Exfloliative cytology
   D. None of the above

10. What is the following assessment of this patient's diastolic blood pressure?
   A. Within normal range
   B. Prehypertensive
   C. Stage 1 hypertension
   D. Stage 2 hypertension

11. Which of the following describes the diastolic pressure?
   A. The effect of ventricular relaxation
   B. The effect of ventricular contraction
   C. The difference between the systolic and diastolic pressures
   D. None of the above

12. This patient has an epileptic seizure during the dental procedure; what is the best treatment for this emergency?
   A. Remove patient from dental chair, and have him lie on the floor until the symptoms are gone
   B. Leave patient in dental chair (supine is ideal), remove sharp items, and wait until symptoms are gone
   C. Place a tongue depressor in his mouth to protect his tongue
   D. None of the above

13. What is the drug of choice for prolonged seizures?
   A. Epinephrine
   B. Diazepam (Valium)
   C. Dilantin
   D. Benedryl

14. Which of the following are effects of gingival hyperplasia?
   A. Poses dental biofilm control problems
   B. May alter tooth eruption
   C. May interfere with speech
   D. May affect mastication
   E. All of the above

15. Which of the following is a treatment for gingival hyperplasia?
   A. Change in drug prescription
   B. A program of prevention and control
   C. Gingivectomy
   D. All of the above
   E. None of the above

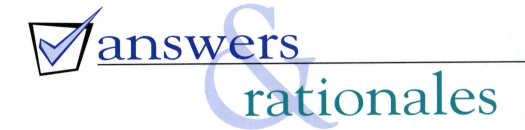

✓ answers & rationales

1.

A. Gingival enlargement or overgrowth in response to plaque accumulation can be exaggerated by medications such as phenytoin (used for seizures).

2.

A. Depakote has dual action. It is used for the treatment of depression and epilepsy. It is also used for migraine headaches, but the patient does not have a history of severe headaches.

3.

C. Amoxicillin 2.0g orally, 1 hour prior to treatment is the drug of choice for SBE premedication if the patient is not allergic to penicillin.

4.

C. SBE premedication is indicated within the first 2 years of joint replacement.

5.

D. A seizure that persists for more than 1 hour or repeated seizures that produce a fixed and enduring epileptic condition for more than 1 hour.

6.

A. An acute triggering disturbance, such as sleep, menstrual cycle, fatigue, flickering lights, or physical or psychological stress can cause an epileptic seizure.

7.

B. The mandibular teeth are facial rather than lingual to the maxillary teeth.

8.

A. This patient has a retained primary tooth. Tooth #27 is visible on radiographs.

9.

A. Pulp vitality test, which is the method used to test a suspected nonvital tooth. Teeth #s 7 and 8 are darker than the other teeth, so vitality testing is indicated.

10.

C. The patient's diastolic pressure is stage 1 hypertension, a reading between 90–99. Stage 2 hypertension is a reading >100. Prehypertension has a reading between 80 and 89, and normal is <80.

11.

A. The effect of ventricular relaxation. The systolic pressure is the effect of ventricular contraction, and the pulse pressure is the difference between the systolic and diastolic pressures.

12.

B. Leave patient in dental chair (supine is ideal), and protect patient from injury by removing sharp items and wait until symptoms are gone. If seizure is still occurring within 5 minutes activate emergency medical system.

13.

B. Diazepam IV if seizure progresses to status epilepticus.

14.

E. All of the above are effects of gingival hyperplasia

15.

D. All of the above are treatments for gingival hyperplasia. Change in drug prescription to a different drug with a lower chance of causing gingival enlargement; gingivectomy is indicated if a sufficient band of attached gingiva exists. A program of prevention and control should be started immediately.

case study 7   answers

patient history
synopsis

CASE 8
Age 69
Sex F
Height 5′ 5″
Weight 150lbs/68kg

VITAL SIGNS
Blood pressure 138/92
Pulse rate 79
Respiration rate 16

1. Under the care of a physician

☒ Yes　　☐ No

Condition: Diabetes, two previous heart attacks

2. Hospitalized within the last 5 years

☒ Yes　　☐ No

Reason: Two previous heart attacks

3. Has or had the following conditions:

Diabetes, heart problems

4. Current medication(s)

Insulin, Nitroglycerine, Coumadin

5. Smokes or uses tobacco products

☐ Yes　　☒ No

6. Is pregnant

☐ Yes　　☒ No　　☐ N/A

Medical History: Patient had two previous heart attacks and is an insulin-dependent diabetic.

Dental History: The patient has not visited the dentist for many years. The patient states she brushes her teeth whenever she gets around to it.

Social History: Widow whose only income is Social Security.

Chief Complaint: "Tooth hurts upper right."

Current Oral Hygiene Status

Supplemental Oral Examination Findings
1. Generalized recession

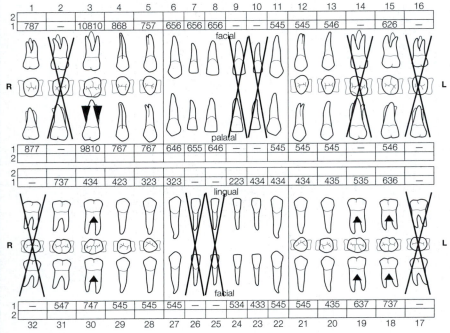

ADULT CLINICAL EXAMINATION

Clinically visible carious lesion

Clinically missing tooth

Furcation

"Through and through" furcation

Probe 1: initial probing depth

Probe 2: probing depth 1 month after scaling and root planing

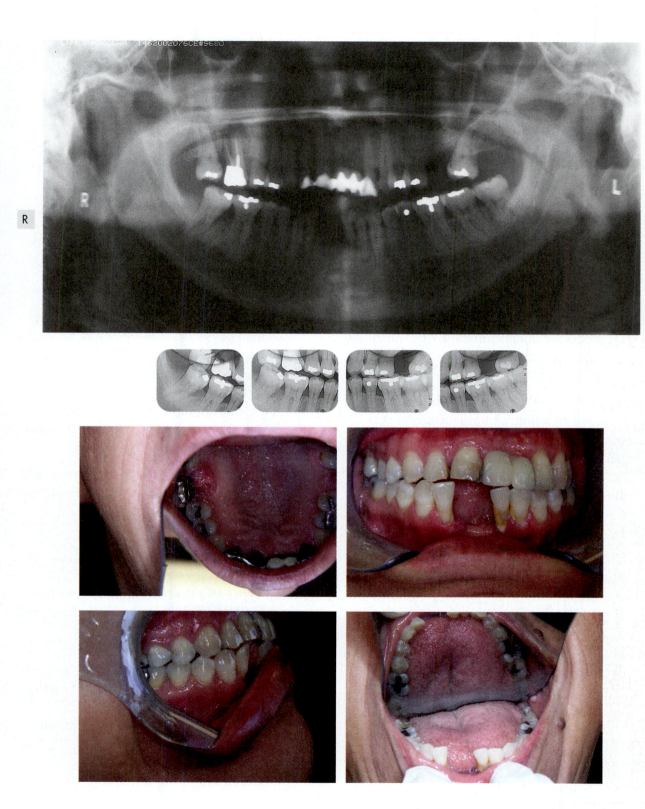

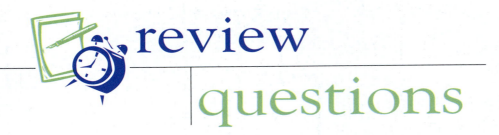

review questions

1. What is the appropriate course of periodontal therapy for this patient?
   A. General gross debridement
   B. Periodontal debridement by the quadrant
   C. Oral hygiene instruction only
   D. Periodontal debridment by the quadrant under anesthesia
   E. Hand instrumentation

2. According to this patient's clinical examination, radiographic examination, and periodontal assessment, what is the correct periodontal diagnosis?
   A. Case Type I—Gingivitis
   B. Case Type II—Early Periodontitis
   C. Case Type III—Moderate Periodontitis
   D. Case Type IV—Advanced Periodontitis

3. The best rinse for this patient's oral health needs is:
   A. Scope
   B. 0.12% chlorhexidine gluconate rinse
   C. Listerine
   D. 0.05% NaF rinse
   E. Warm saline rinse

4. If the patient had a heart attack 1 month before her scheduled periodontal debridements, what would be the appropriate course of action?
   A. Postpone appointments for 1 month and obtain physician consent before treatment
   B. Postpone appointments for 3 months or more and obtain physician consent before treatment
   C. Postpone appointments for 6 months and obtain physician consent before treatment
   D. Proceed with planned treatment

5. Which medication may cause xerostomia and exacerbate this patient's oral health condition?
   A. Hydrochlorothiazide (HCT)
   B. Coumadin
   C. Aspirin
   D. Insulin

6. What types of microorganisms would most likely be found in the pockets around teeth #s 3 and 4?
   A. Gram-positive cocci
   B. Rods and filamentous forms
   C. Vibrios, spirochetes, and other Gram-negative organisms
   D. Gram-negative motile spirochetes and rods

7. In what position would you place your patient in the event of syncope?
   A. Supine
   B. Semi-upright
   C. Trendelenburg
   D. Maxillary positioning (chin-up)
   E. Mandibular positioning (chin-down)

8. If this patient were to experience ketoacidosis (diabetic coma), what would be the appropriate course of action?
   A. Terminate oral procedure
   B. Activate 911
   C. Keep patient warm
   D. Administer oxygen by nasal cannula
   E. All of the above

9. What is the lesion on the patient's palate next to tooth #3?
   A. Fistula
   B. Abscess
   C. Fibroma
   D. Mucocele

10. What is the cause of this lesion?
    A. Abscess
    B. Cyst
    C. Pericoronitis
    D. Ulceration

11. Which of the following is the most appropriate treatment of the above lesion?
    A. Drainage
    B. Surgical excision
    C. Prescription for Pen VK 500 mg
    D. Nothing, the lesion will resolve on its own

12. Which of the following is a relative contraindication to the administration of anesthetic to this patient?
    A. Epinephrine
    B. Lidocaine
    C. Benzocaine
    D. None of the above

13. When mild toxic local anesthetic overdose reaction occurs, the proper treatment would be:
    A. Protect patient, monitor vital signs, and give oxygen
    B. Place tongue depressor between the teeth to prevent the patient from biting their tongue, monitor vital signs, and give oxygen
    C. Give Valium 10 mg IM
    D. Give epinephrine IM
    E. None of the above

14. When severe local anesthetic toxic overdose reaction occurs, the proper treatment would be:
    A. Immediate administration of valium IV
    B. Administration of valium if seizures have not abated after 15 minutes of seizures
    C. Give epinephrine IV
    D. Inhalation of amly nitrate
    E. None of the above

15. During the dental hygiene procedure the patient begins to have a crushing chest pain. What is the first response the dental hygienist should do?
    A. Call EMS
    B. Administer CPR
    C. Administer nitroglycerine
    D. Administer oxygen

1.

D. For diabetic patients, the clinician should limit the number of teeth treated at each visit. Allow short appointments for stress management. Debridement by the quadrant under anesthesia is appropriate for pain control, thorough deposit removal, and homeostasis.

2.

D. The American Academy of Periodontology's Case Type IV, by definition, is further progression of periodontitis with major loss of alveolar bone support, usually accompanied by increased tooth mobility. There is furcation involvement in multirooted teeth.

3.

B. Chlorhexidine gluconate has been shown to be the most effective antiplaque and antigingivitis chemotherapeutic agent available. Scope and Listerine are antimicrobial rinses, with Listerine having a therapeutic effect on gingivitis only. Sodium fluoride prevents dental caries. Warm saline rinses only serve to soothe tissues after instrumentation and promote tissue healing.

4.

B. Elective dental and dental hygiene appointments may need to be postponed 3 months or more until the patient's physician has given consent for treatment.

5.

A. Hydrochlorothiazide (HCT), a diuretic, is implicated in causing xerostomia. None of this patient's other medications specifically cause xerostomia.

6.

D. In a disease pocket, the microflora consists primarily of Gram-negative, motile spirochetes and rods.

7.

C. Trendelenburg position (supine with the heart higher than the head on a surface inclined downward about 45 degrees) is preferred for those patients experiencing syncope.

8.

E. All steps listed would be appropriate for the emergency management of ketoacidosis.

9.

A. Fistula is a pathological sinus or abnormal passage that leads from an abscess to the surface of the gingiva or mucosa.

10.

A. Abscess causes the development of a fistula, which drains the abscess.

11.

C. Pen VK is the drug of choice for an abscess if the patient is not allergic to penicillin.

12.

A. Epinephrine and other sympathomemic amines inhibit peripheral glucose uptake by the tissues and increase glucose release by the liver. Hyperglycemia can result. Epinephrine is, therefore, an antagonist to antidiabetic agents, and a relative contraindication.

13.

A. Protect patient and monitor vital signs during the mild convulsive period (consider 10 mg Valium IV if convulsive period is prolonged longer than 15 minutes)

14.

A. If convulsions from the overdose continue longer than 15 minutes or become more severe, immediate administration of Valium IV is indicated.

15.

C. Administer nitroglycerin 0.2–0.6 mg sublingually; may be repeated in 5 minutes, up to three times over 15 minutes if angina pain does not subside with nitroglycerin; treat as myocardial infarction and activate EMS immediately.

case study 8 answers

patient history
synopsis

CASE 9
Age 22
Sex F
Height 5′ 7″
Weight 145lbs/66kg

VITAL SIGNS
Blood pressure 110/69
Pulse rate 46
Respiration rate 22

1. Under the care of a physician
☐ Yes   ☒ No

2. Hospitalized within the last 5 years
☒ Yes   ☐ No
Reason: Appendectomy

3. Has or had the following conditions:
None

4. Current medication(s)
Ortho Cyclin

5. Smokes or uses tobacco products
☒ Yes   ☐ No

6. Is pregnant
☐ Yes   ☒ No   ☐ N/A

Medical History: Takes oral contraceptives and smokes twice daily.

Dental History: The patient is congenitally missing nine teeth, edentulous #523–26, and wears a partial. Patient has an intraoral piercing. The patient is currently undergoing dental implant treatment. She brushes two times daily and flosses three times per week. She states that there is generalized bleeding while flossing.

Social History: Single and currently a college student.

Chief Complaint: "Sensitivity to cold and crunchy food. I have pain on my upper molars."

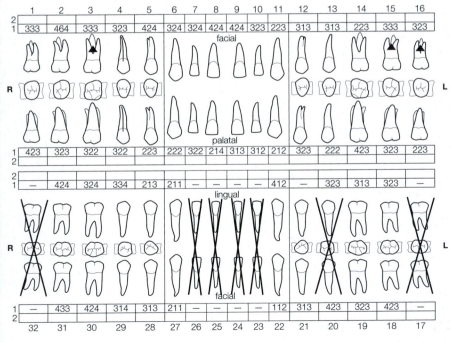

ADULT CLINICAL EXAMINATION

Current Oral Hygiene Status
1. Brushes 2 times per day
2. Flosses 3 times per week
3. Gingival slightly inflammed

Supplemental Oral Examination Findings
1. Sensitivity to cold
2. Oral tongue piercing
3. Retained primary teeth
4. Congenitally missing 9 teeth
5. Partial denture

 Clinically visible carious lesion

 Clinically missing tooth

 Furcation

 "Through and through" furcation

Probe 1: initial probing depth

Probe 2: probing depth 1 month
after scaling and root planing

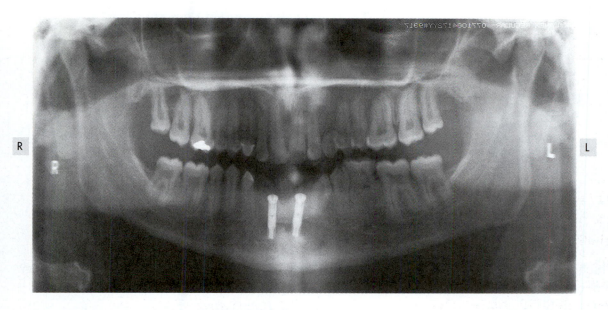

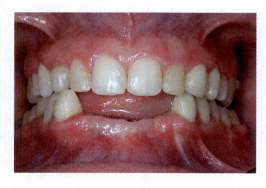

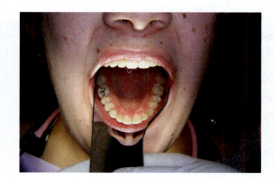

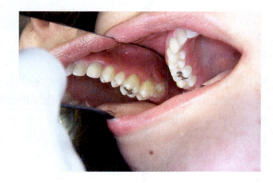

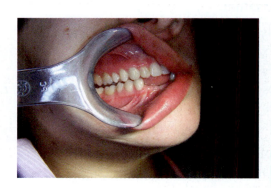

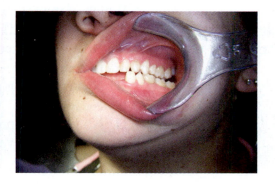

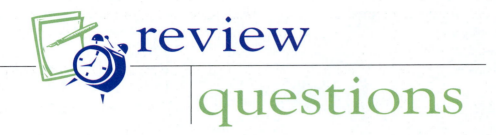

review questions

1. Which of the following primary teeth are retained?
   A. Q, M, G
   B. R, M, K
   C. R, N, K
   D. R, M, L

2. Which of the following is the term to identify the eruption of permanent teeth into the positions of exfoliated primary teeth?
   A. Mixed dentition
   B. Avulsion
   C. Succedaneous
   D. Exfoliation

3. Typically between what ages does a patient have mixed dentition?
   A. Ages 6–12
   B. Ages 4–12
   C. Ages 5–14
   D. Ages 4–14

4. Which of the following permanent teeth usually are the first to erupt?
   A. Maxillary central incisors
   B. Maxillary lateral incisors
   C. Mandibular central incisors
   D. Mandibular lateral incisors

5. What type of dental implants were used on this patient?
   A. Endosseous
   B. Subperiosteal
   C. Transosteal
   D. None of the above

6. During the patient selection phase of dental implants, which of the following is the most important factor to consider in assessing if a patient qualifies to receive dental implant?
   A. Adequate attached gingiva
   B. Radiographic evidence of adequate depth of alveolar bone
   C. No gingival inflammation
   D. All of the above
   E. None of the above

7. Which of the following systemic conditions is a contraindication to implant placement?
   A. Uncontrolled diabetes mellitus
   B. Hypertension
   C. Hypothyroidism
   D. Moderate alcohol consumption

8. Which of the following shows evidence that the implant is healthy?
   A. No pain or discomfort reported by the patient
   B. No bone loss or peri-implant radiolucency
   C. No mobility
   D. No increased probing depths
   E. All of the above

9. Which of the following instrumentation technique is acceptable for titanium implants?
   A. Plastic instruments
   B. Use of ultrasonic scaler
   C. Stain removal with rubber cup and polishing paste
   D. All of the above
   E. None of the above

10. Which of the following describes the gingiva on the buccal of tooth #2?
    A. Floss cleft
    B. McCall's festoon
    C. Stillman's cleft
    D. Bulbous papilla

11. Which of the following is the most common dental problem associated with tongue piercing?
    A. Trauma to the lingual anterior gingival
    B. Dental abrasion
    C. Chipping of teeth
    D. Salivary flow stimulating effect

12. Which of the following is a mechanism of naturally occurring desensitization over time?
    A. Sclerosis of dentin
    B. Neural activity
    C. Iontophoresis
    D. Physical blocking

13. Which of the following agents should be recommended to this patient for a self-applied treatment for desensitization?
    A. Fluoride varnish
    B. Stannous fluoride .4% utilizing tray delivery
    C. 5% Glutaraldehyde and 35% hydroxyethylmethacrylate
    D. .4% stannous fluoride gel

14. Which of the following toothbrushing method is indicated for this patient?
    A. Circular: the Fones method
    B. Scrub-brush
    C. Charters method
    D. Modified Stillman

15. Which of the following oral hygiene adjunct should be recommended to this patient?
    A. End tuft brush
    B. Perio aid
    C. Wooden interdental cleaner
    D. Gauze strips

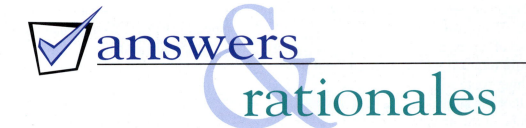

answers & rationales

1.

B. Utilizing the patient's radiographs, the following primary teeth are retained: R, M, K.

2.

C. Succedaneous is the eruption of permanent teeth into the positions of exfoliated primary teeth. Mixed dentition is the combination of primary and permanent teeth. Avulsion is the traumatic separation of teeth from the alveolus. Exfoliation is the loss of primary teeth following resorption of root structure.

3.

A. Typically a patient's mixed dentition begins at age 6 and ends at age 12.

4.

C. The mandibular central incisors are the first to erupt at approximately 6 years of age.

5.

A. Endosseous implants were placed in the mandibular anterior region. Endosseous implants are placed within the bone and are usually blade, screw, and cylinder types. Subperiosteal implants are placed over the bone, under the periosteum, and transosteal implants are placed through the bone.

6.

B. Radiographic evidence of adequate depth of alveolar bone is needed to place an implant into, through, or over the bone.

7.

A. Uncontrolled diabetes is a risk factor for the placement of dental implants due to the patient's inability to heal quickly and effectively.

8.

E. All of the above are important factors to assess the long-term success of a dental implant.

9.

A. Plastic instruments are indicated for titanium implants. Severe abrasion can result from the use of an ultrasonic scaler, and stain removal should not be routinely conducted. Stain removal is indicated only for esthetic purposes and the use of rubber cups with nonabrasive agents is required.

10.

C. Stillman's cleft is an area of localized recession in a V-shape. It may extend several millimeters toward or into the mucogingival junction. A floss cleft is created by incorrect flossing. It usually appears as a vertical linear line or V-shaped fissure in the marginal gingiva. McCall's festoon is an enlargement of the marginal gingiva with the formation of a lifesaver-like gingival prominence.

11.

C. Although all of the answers may occur from oral piercing, chipping of teeth is the most common.

12.

A. Sclerosis of dentin occurs naturally by the mineral deposition within the dentinal tubules as a result of traumatic stimuli. It creates a thicker, highly mineralized layer of peritubular dentin. Neural activity is when pain is registered by depolarization. Iontophoresis is the use of a low-voltage electric current to impregnate the tooth with fluoride ions. Physical blocking is when periodontal soft tissue grafts cover the sensitive dentinal surface.

13.

D. .4% stannous fluoride gel is a self-applied agent used as a desensitizing agent. All other agents are used for professional in-office use.

14.

D. Since this patient has sensitivity and gingival recession, the modified Stillman minimizes the possibility of gingival trauma. The circular Fones method and the scrub-brush method may be detrimental to adults by overbrushing.

15.

B. The perio-aid or toothpick in holder is used for the removal of biofilm at and just under the gingival margin. This is an effective way for this patient to clean biofilm from recessed areas. The single-tuft brush, gauze strips, and wooden interdental cleaner is appropriate when interdental gingiva are missing.

case study 9 answers

patient history
synopsis

CASE 10
Age 27
Sex M
Height 5' 11"
Weight 200lbs/91kg

VITAL SIGNS
Blood pressure 150/91
Pulse rate 66
Respiration rate 18

1. Under the care of a physician

☒ Yes   ☐ No

Condition: Hypertension, Hepatitis B

2. Hospitalized within the last 5 years

☒ Yes   ☐ No

Reason: Hepatitis B

3. Has or had the following conditions:

Hypertension, Hepatitis B

4. Current medication(s)

Diovan 10 mg daily, Zyrtec

5. Smokes or uses tobacco products

☒ Yes   ☐ No

Chews tobacco 2–3 times per day

6. Is pregnant

☐ Yes   ☐ No   ☒ N/A

Medical History: Patient has a history of hypertension and is currently taking Diovan. He was hospitalized for Hepatitis B. Patient claims that he has many allergies, to metals, food, pollen, etc.

Dental History: The patient's last cleaning was 2 years ago. He brushes two times daily and does not floss. The patient chews tobacco 2–3 times per day.

Social History: Single and works as an insurance agent.

Chief Complaint: Routine cleaning, occasional sensitivity to temperatures and concerned about changes on tooth #2.

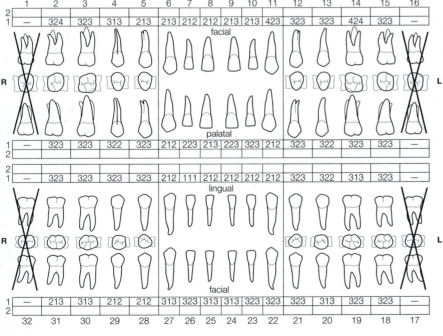

ADULT CLINICAL EXAMINATION

Current Oral Hygiene Status
1. Brushes 2 times per day
2. Doesn't floss
3. Localized recession
4. Slight calculus

Supplemental Oral Examination Findings
1. Bilateral linea alba
2. Bilateral fibrotic gingiva adjacent to #s 19 & 30
3. Leukoedema mandibular vestibule

⬱ Clinically visible carious lesion

⬲ Clinically missing tooth

△ Furcation

▲ "Through and through" furcation

Probe 1: initial probing depth

Probe 2: probing depth 1 month after scaling and root planing

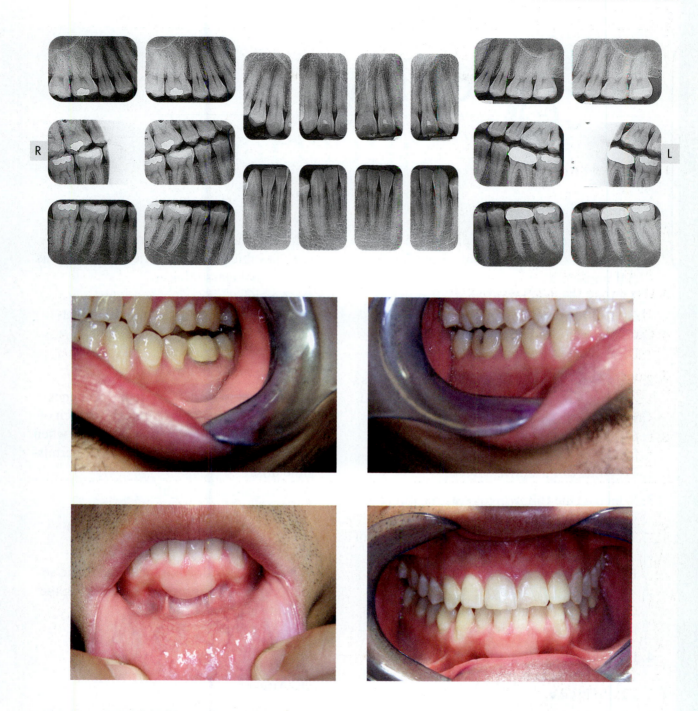

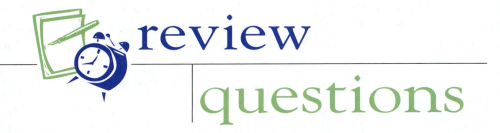

review questions

1. What type of periodontal procedure was conducted on the mandibular anterior facial gingival?
   - A. Free gingival graft
   - B. Double papilla flap
   - C. Laterally positioned flap
   - D. None of the above

2. What is the purpose of periodontal dressings?
   - A. Provide protection for a surgical wound
   - B. Assist in shaping newly formed tissue
   - C. Help prevent postreatment bleeding
   - D. All of the above
   - E. None of the above

3. Which of the following is true regarding a visible-light-cured dressing?
   - A. Setting does not begin until activation of light
   - B. Dressing becomes hard, brittle, and breaks easily
   - C. Commonly known as Coe-Pac
   - D. Main ingredient is zinc oxide

4. Leukodema is present in the right vestibule. What is most likely the cause of this condition?
   - A. A gingival infection
   - B. Smokeless tobacco
   - C. Toothbrush trauma
   - D. All of the above
   - E. None of the above

5. Which of the following periodontal problems has this patient experienced due to his use of smokeless tobacco?
   - A. ANUG
   - B. Localized recession and clinical attachment loss
   - C. Periodontal abscess
   - D. Inflamed gingiva

6. This patient is going to require local anesthesia for the dental prophylaxis. Which of the following is important to consider when determining the patient's maximum permissible dose?
   - A. The patient's weight
   - B. The patient's tobacco use
   - C. The patient's history of hepatitis B
   - D. The patient's history of allergies

7. Which of the following local anesthetic selection is most appropriate considering the patient's medical history?
   - A. Lidocaine
   - B. Prilocaine
   - C. Mepivacaine
   - D. Articaine

8. When administering the posterior superior alveolar injection, what should the needle depth be when using a short needle?
   - A. Three-fourths the depth
   - B. One-half the depth
   - C. Until bone is gently contacted
   - D. One-quarter the depth

Questions 9–11: Following the administration of the PSA injection you notice a faint bluish discoloration on her cheek. You check intraorally and find the same discoloration near the injection site along with swelling.

9. What is the most probable cause of this mark?
   A. The anesthetic cartridge was contaminated with alcohol
   B. The needle created a tear in the blood vessel
   C. The hygienist used a needle of too fine a gauge
   D. The hygienist injected too rapidly

10. What is this reaction called?
   A. Trismus
   B. Hematoma
   C. Needle breakage
   D. Paresthesia

11. What post-op care is most appropriate for this patient?
   A. Transporting her to the emergency room
   B. Applying cold packs for the next 3 days
   C. Applying cold packs for up to 12 hours using warm, moist packs the next day
   D. Applying heat for up to 12 hours using cold packs the next day

12. To perform a Simplified Oral Hygiene Index (OHI-S), which tooth surfaces are assessed?
   A. #3 L, #8 F, #14 L, #19 B, #24 F, #30 B
   B. #3 B, #8 F, #14 B, #19 L, #24 F, #30 L
   C. #3 B, #8 L, #14 B, #19 L, #24 L, #30 L
   D. #3 L, #8 L, #14 B, #19 L, #24 L, #30 B

13. If a molar tooth used in the OHI-S index is missing, which tooth would you use to replace it?
   A. The second molar
   B. The third molar
   C. The second premolar
   D. The first premolar
   E. Either A or B

14. When using the Patient Hygiene Performance (PHP) index, into how many subdivisions do you divide each tooth examined?
   A. 2
   B. 3
   C. 4
   D. 5
   E. 6

15. Which of the following best describes this patient's occlusion?
   A. Mesognathic
   B. Retrognathic
   C. Prognathic
   D. Crossbite

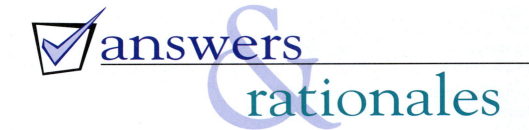

✓answers & rationales

1.

A. Free gingival graft was conducted to cover exposed roots by taking tissue from the patient's palate. A double papillae flap procedure uses the papillae from each side of the tooth and rotated over the midfacial aspect of the recipient tooth. A laterally positioned flap is used to move gingival from an adjacent tooth.

2.

D. All of the above are indications for the placement of periodontal dressings. They provide protection for a surgical wound from external irritation or trauma. They assist in shaping newly formed tissue to immobilize a graft and help prevent posttreatment bleeding by securing initial clot formation.

3.

A. The advantage of visible-light-cured dressings is that it does not begin to set until activation by the light-curing unit. Dressing becomes hard, brittle, and breaks easily, a disadvantage of a zinc oxide with eugenol dressing. Coe-Pac is a common name for chemical-cured dressing.

4.

B. Leukodema is an oral consequence of tobacco use.

5.

B. Localized recession and clinical attachment loss is a consequence of tobacco use. This patient required graft surgery to correct the attachment loss in the area of the smokeless tobacco use.

6.

C. In determining the patient's maximum permissible dose, the patient's history of hepatitis is important because most amide local anesthetics are metabolized in the liver. Therefore, the dose should not exceed 2.2 carpules.

7.

B. All amide local anesthetics are metabolized in the liver except for Prilocaine, which is metabolized primarily in the lungs. This is the drug of choice since there may be some liver dysfunction due to the hepatitis B.

8.

A. Three-fourths the depth of the short needle is indicated for the PSA injection. Going deeper than that, the clinician could enter the pterygoid venous plexus, causing a hematoma. Bone should never be contacted during a PSA injection.

9.

B. The needle created a tear in a vein or artery. The PSA injection is the most common injection that causes a hematoma.

10.

B. Hematoma is swelling and discoloration of the tissue resulting from effusion of blood into extravascular spaces.

11.

C. Applying cold packs for up to 12 hours; using warm, moist packs the next day is the treatment for hematoma. Swelling and discoloration will disappear after 7–14 days.

12.

B. The six surfaces used to assess oral cleanliness by the Simplified Oral Hygiene Index (OHI-S) are: #3 B, #8 F, #14 B, #19 L, #24 F, and #30 L.

13.

E. If a molar tooth used in the OHI-S is missing, you could use either the second molar or third molar directly behind the missing first molar. The only stipulation is that it be fully erupted.

14.

D. Each tooth is divided into five subdivisions: mesial third, middle third, and distal third, whereby the middle third is further subdivided into cervical middle and occlusal/incisal thirds.

15.

A. Mesognathic, having slightly protruded jaws and a relatively straight profile. Retrognathic: prominent maxilla and a mandible posterior to its normal relationship (convex profile). Prognathic: prominent, protruded mandible and normal maxilla (concave profile). Crossbite: Maxillary or mandibular posterior teeth are either facial or lingual to their normal position.

Glossary

Abandonment: the termination of a patient, unless certain set criteria are met.

Abduction: in functional anatomy, a movement which draws a limb away from the median (sagittal) plane of the body. It is thus opposed to adduction.

Abrasion: the wearing away or removal of material by the act of rubbing, cutting, or scraping.

Absorption: the movement of a drug into the bloodstream.

Acquired immunodeficiency syndrome (AIDS): a collection of symptoms and infections resulting from the specific damage to the immune system caused by the human immunodeficiency virus (HIV).

Acromegaly: a hormonal disorder that results when the pituitary gland produces excess growth hormone (hGH).

Acrylic plastics: soft and flexible or rigid and brittle materials used for dentures and denture teeth, denture liners, and oral appliances.

Active transport: substance is transported against gradient across a biological membrane by "carriers" that furnish energy for transportation of drug.

Acute adrenal insufficiency (adrenal crisis): a sudden lack of sufficient circulating adrenal hormones.

Acute herpetic gingivostomatitis: an acute, viral infection of the oral mucosa with a 7- to 10-day duration.

Added filtration: a metal filter, usually aluminum, installed by the manufacturer.

Addison's disease (also known as **chronic adrenal insufficiency**, or **hypocortisolism**): a rare endocrine disorder which results in the body not producing sufficient amounts of adrenal glucocorticoids and mineralocorticoids.

Adenoid cystic carcinoma: slow-growing malignancy most commonly found in minor salivary glands.

Adhesion (pavementing): white blood cells become sticky and adhere to walls of blood vessels.

Adhesion: the forces of attraction between two different objects or surfaces that hold them together.

Adrenal cortex: mediates the stress response through the production of mineralocorticoids and glucocorticoids, including aldosterone and cortisol respectively.

Adrenocorticotropic hormone (**ACTH** or **corticotropin**): a peptide hormone produced and secreted by the hypothalamus. It is an important player in the hypothalamic-pituitary-adrenal axis.

Aerosol: an artificially generated collection of particles (often pathogenic and capable of producing infection) suspended in air.

Affective domain: the learning domain that includes feelings, attitudes, and values; it is not easily measured.

Afferent neurons: otherwise known as sensory or receptor neurons; carry nerve impulses from receptors or sense organs *toward* the central nervous system.

Affinity: the tendency of a drug to bind to a receptor site.

Agent factors: biological or mechanical means for causing diseases or conditions.

Agonist: a molecule that selectively binds to a specific receptor and triggers a response in the cell.

Agranulocytosis: severe reduction in circulating granulocytes, especially neutrophils, resulting from either a defect in production or accelerated destruction.

Allergen: antigen that can exhibit allergic symptoms.

Allergy: hypersensitive response to an allergen.

Alveolar bone: see Alveolar process.

Alveolar mucosa: located below mucogingival junction.

Alveolar process: the thickened ridge of bone that contains the tooth sockets on bones that bear teeth. It is also referred to as the **alveolar bone**. In humans, the tooth-bearing bones are the maxilla and the mandible.

Alzheimer's disease (AD): a neurodegenerative disease characterized by progressive cognitive deterioration together with declining activities of daily living and neuropsychiatric symptoms or behavioral changes. It is the most common type of dementia.

Amalgam: a metal alloy with one of its elements consisting of mercury; used to fill cavity preparations.

Ameloblastic fibroma: a slow-growing, benign tumor made up of ameloblasts and fibroblasts.

Ameloblastoma: a slow-growing, benign, but locally invasive tumor of ameloblasts.

Amelogenesis imperfecta: abnormal enamel.

American Association of Public Health Dentistry (AAPHD): the organization that represents American public health dentists, dental hygienists, and the science of dental public health.

American Association of State and Territorial Dental Directors: the organization that represents state dental departments.

American Dental Association (ADA): the organization that represents American dentists and the science of dentistry.

American Dental Hygienists' Association (ADHA): the organization that represents American dental hygienists and the science of dental hygiene.

Amino acid: any molecule that contains both amine and carboxyl functional groups.

Anaphylactic: life-threatening, systemic allergic reaction; also called anaphylactic shock.

Anemia: disorder of oxygen-carrying capability either in RBCs or defect in hemoglobin molecule

Anergy: a diminished reactivity to a specific antigen because of immunosuppression. (e.g., a negative skin test in a TB-infected individual due to immunosuppression caused by HIV).

Angina pectoris: chest pain due to ischemia (a lack of blood and hence oxygen supply) of the heart muscle, generally due to obstruction or spasm of the coronary arteries (the heart's blood vessels).

Ankyloglossia: tongue-tied.

Anodontia: missing teeth.

Antagonism: clinical response is reduced by administration of second agent.

Anterior: situated before or toward the front.

Anterior superior alveolar branch: a branch off from the nerve just before its exit from the infraorbital foramen; it descends in a canal in the anterior wall of the maxillary sinus, and divides into branches which supply the incisor and canine teeth.

Anti-bacterial: acts against bacteria.

Antibiotic agents: produced by another microorganism to kill or inhibit the growth or multiplication of bacteria.

Antibiotic: a drug that kills or prevents the growth of bacteria.

Antibody: a soluble protein molecule produced and secreted by body cells in response to an antigen, capable of binding and inactivating that specific antigen.

Anticholinergic agent: a member of a class of pharmaceutical compounds which serve to reduce the effects mediated by acetylcholine in the central nervous system and peripheral nervous system.

Antigen: a substance capable of producing a specific immune response and reacting with an antibody, usually a large molecular weight protein.

Antigenic determinant: the specific molecular binding area on the surface of the cell that activates an immunological response.

Antihypertensives: a class of drugs that are used in medicine and pharmacology to treat hypertension (high blood pressure).

Anti-infective: a substance that acts against or destroys infections.

Antimicrobial: a substance that acts against microorganisms.

Antiseptics: antimicrobial substances that are applied to living tissue/skin to reduce the possibility of infection, sepsis, or putrefaction.

Antiviral: a substance that acts against viruses.

Aplastic anemia: a severe decrease of all circulating blood cells including RBCs, WBCs (leukopenia), and platelets (thrombocytopenia).

Aponeuroses: membranes separating muscles from each other.

Appendicular skeleton: the part of the skeleton that includes the pectoral girdle, the upper limbs, the pelvic girdle, and the lower limbs. The appendicular skeleton and the axial skeleton together form the complete skeleton.

Arachnoid mater: one of the three meninges, the membranes that cover the brain and spinal cord.

Asepsis: no living pathogens present; a sterile state.

Aseptic technique: a procedure that is performed under sterile conditions. This includes medical techniques and laboratory techniques, such as those used with microbiological cultures.

Assessment: the part of the dental hygiene process of care that carefully analyzes the program's target group and resources.

Atraumatic Restorative Treatment (ART): a dental sealant placed on a tooth surface with demineralization that has been removed by hand. This preventive/restorative dental method is utilized when a patient will have difficulty accessing restorative dental care.

Attached gingiva: gingiva that is continuous with the marginal gingiva. It is firm, resilient, and tightly bound to the underlying periosteum of alveolar bone. The facial aspect of the attached gingiva extends to the relatively loose and movable alveolar mucosa, from which it is demarcated by the mucogingival junction.

Autonomic drugs: drugs that exert stimulating or inhibiting effects on the two divisions of the autonomic nervous system (ANS), both parasympathetic (PANS) and sympathetic (SANS).

Autonomic nervous system (ANS): the part of the peripheral nervous system that controls homeostasis, that is the constancy of the content of tissues in gasses, ions and nutrients. It does so mostly by controlling cardiovascular, digestive, and respiratory functions, but also salivation, perspiration, diameter of the pupils, micturition (the discharge of urine), and erection.

Autonomy: based on respect for others and the belief that patients have the power to make decisions about issues that may affect their health.

Axial skeleton: the 80 bones in the head and trunk of the human body.

Axon or **nerve fiber:** a long, slender projection of a nerve cell, or neuron, that conducts electrical impulses away from the neuron's cell body or soma.

B cells: lymphocytes that play a large role in the humoral immune response as opposed to the cell-mediated immune response that is governed by T cells.

Bacteremia: presence of microbes in a normally sterile bloodstream.

Bactericidal: a substance that kills bacteria.

bacteriostatic: a substance that inhibits or retards growth of bacteria.

Barrier: something that prevents an individual or a group from receiving dental care.

Basal cell carcinoma (BCC): the most common skin cancer.

Bell's palsy: characterized by drooping muscles on the affected side of the face, due to malfunction of the facial nerve (VII cranial nerve).

Beneficence: a state that requires that existing harm be removed.

Benefits: the amount that the insurance entity will pay for covered dental services described in their policy.

Benign: the description of a growth that cannot metastasize (spread to other locations from point of origin); hence, it is not cancer.

Benzodiazepines: a class of psychoactive drugs considered as minor tranquilizers with varying hypnotic, sedative, anxiolytic, anticonvulsant, muscle relaxant, and amnesic properties, which are brought on by slowing down the central nervous system.

Bile (gall): a bitter, yellow or green alkaline fluid secreted by hepatocytes from the liver of most vertebrates. In many species, it is stored in the gallbladder between meals and upon eating is discharged into the duodenum where it excretes waste and aids the process of digestion of lipids.

Binary fission: the form of asexual reproduction in single-celled organisms by which one cell divides into two cells of the same size, used by most prokaryotes. This process results in the reproduction of a living cell by division into two equal or near-equal parts.

Blood level: concentration of anti-infective agent present in blood serum.

Blood plasma: the liquid component of blood, in which the blood cells are suspended.

Blood-brain barrier (BBB): endothelial cells packed tightly in brain capillaries that more greatly restrict passage of substances from the bloodstream than do endothelial cells in capillaries elsewhere in the body.

Bonding: a hydrophilic agent utilized after the etching of the surface of teeth, which produces irregularities or micropores, sometimes referred to as tissue tags.

Botulism: a rare, but serious paralytic illness caused by a nerve toxin, botulin, that is produced by the bacterium *Clostridium botulinum*.

Bradycardia: a slow heart rate.

Brain stem: the lower part of the brain, adjoining and structurally continuous with the spinal cord. Most sources consider the pons, medulla oblongata, and midbrain all to be part of the brainstem.

Bulla (plural, bullae): fluid-filled blister > 5 mm in diameter

Calcitonin: a 32 amino acid polypeptide hormone that is produced in humans primarily by the C cells of the thyroid, and in many other animals in the ultimobranchial body.

Calibration: ensuring consistency within and among examiner(s).

Candidiasis: commonly called yeast infection or thrush, this is a fungal infection of any of the *Candida* species, of which *Candida albicans* is the most common.

Capitation: a dental provider gets paid a specified dollar amount, for a given time period, to take care of the dental needs of a specified group of people.

Carbohydrates or saccharides: simple molecules that are straight-chain aldehydes or ketones with many hydroxyl groups added, usually one on each carbon atom that is not part of the aldehyde or ketone functional group.

Cardiac muscle: a type of involuntary mononucleated, or uninucleated, striated muscle found exclusively within the heart. Its function is to "pump" blood through the circulatory system by contracting.

Caring: exhibiting concern and empathy for others.

Carrier: a person harboring a specific infectious agent with no clinical manifestations and who serves as a source of potential infection; may be chronic or temporary.

Cast: a positive replica of teeth used for fabrication of restoration.

Catabolism: the metabolic process that breaks down molecules into smaller units. It is made up of degradative chemical reactions in the living cell.

Caudal: of, relating to, or being a tail.

Ceiling effect (plateau): a therapeutic effect that cannot be increased with a higher dose of the drug.

Cell membrane: a semipermeable lipid bilayer common to all living cells.

Cell-mediated (cellular) immunity: also known as delayed-type hypersensitivity (DTH) or Type IV hypersensitivity, this is an immune response that does not involve antibodies but rather involves the activation of macrophages, natural killer cells (NK), antigen-specific cytotoxic T-lymphocytes, and the release of various cytokines in response to an antigen.

Cementoblastoma: true neoplasm of cementum.

Cementogenesis: the formation of cementum, one of the three mineralized substances of a tooth. For cementogenesis to begin, Hertwig's epithelial root sheath must fragment. Once the root sheath fragments, the dentin that later forms the tooth's root comes in contact with the dental sac. This then stimulates the activation of cementoblasts to begin cementogenesis.

Cementoma (periapical cemental dysplasia): hyperplasia of the cementum.

Cementum: a specialized bony substance covering the root of a tooth.

Central papillary atrophy (median rhomboid glossitis): raised erythematous rhomboid-shaped area located in midline of tongue.

Centriole: in biology this is a barrel-shaped microtubule structure found in most animal cells and algae though not frequently in plants.

Cerebellum: a region of the brain that plays an important role in the integration of sensory perception and motor output.

Change agent: a person who lobbies to change laws, increasing access to care for the underserved populations.

Chemotaxis: moving of white blood cells toward the target area for the body's/defense against the injury.

Chlamydiae: a bacterial phylum whose members are obligate intracellular pathogens.

Chondroma: neoplasm of cartilage.

Chondrosarcoma: malignancy of cartilage resulting in bone lesions.

Chroma: the intensity or extent of saturation of a certain color.

Chronic adrenal insufficiency: see Addison's disease.

Cilium (plural cilia): an organelle found in eukaryotic cells. Cilia are thin, tail-like *projections* extending approximately 5–10 micrometers outwards from the cell body.

Circulatory system (scientifically known as the **cardiovascular system**): an organ system that moves substances to and from cells; it can also help stabilize body temperature and pH (part of homeostasis).

Circumduction: the circular (or, more precisely, conical) movement of a body part, such as a ball-and-socket joint or the eye. It consists of a combination of flexion, extension, adduction, and abduction. "Windmilling" the arms or rotating the hand from the wrist are examples of circumductive movement.

Cirrhosis: a consequence of chronic liver disease characterized by replacement of liver tissue by fibrotic scar tissue as well as regenerative nodules, leading to progressive loss of liver function.

Civil service employee: an employee of the federal government. A hygienist may work as a civil servant at various government entities.

Civilian Health and Medical Program of the Uniformed Services (CHAMPUS): health care services for military personnel and dependents.

Claims processing: the entire process of entering the procedures rendered until payment is collected or denial is determined.

Clindamycin: a lincosamide antibiotic used in the treatment of infections caused by susceptible microorganisms.

Clinical evaluation: any clinical method utilized to evaluate a dental public health program or research.

Clinician: a person who provides dental hygiene clinical care to the population.

Coccidioidomycosis (also known as **Valley fever, California valley fever**, and [incorrectly] **coccidiomycosis**): a fungal disease caused by *Coccidioides immitis* or *C. posadasii*.

Cognitive domain: the learning domain that consists of intellectual skills.

Cohesion: the forces of attraction within an object that hold it together.

Col: nonkeratinized tissue located between lingual and facial papilla.

Collaborative practice: the science of the prevention and treatment of oral disease through the provision of education, assessment, preventive, clinical, and other therapeutic services in a cooperative working relationship with a consulting dentist, but without general supervision as practiced in the state of New Mexico.

Collimation: restriction of size of x-ray beam.

Commercial insurance plans: an insurance plan that operates for a profit.

Communicable stage of a disease: the time during which the infectious agent may be transferred from an infected person to an uninfected one; the communicable period may include or overlap the incubation period.

Community dental health: see dental public health.

Complement: a step-by-step process (the complement cascade) by which more than 20 serum proteins mediate the antigen-antibody process.

Component organizations: the local components of the American Dental Hygienists' Association.

Composite: an esthetic restorative cement composed of polymers (resin) and glass particles (fillers).

Compressive stress: the stress that results from material being squeezed together.

Concrescence: the joining of adjacent teeth by cementum only.

Confidentiality: information about a patient is kept in confidence and is respected by all dental providers.

Congenital heart disease: anomalies of the structure of the heart following irregularities in development during the first 9 weeks in utero.

Congenital syphilis: syphilis present in utero and at birth; occurs when a child is born to a mother with secondary or tertiary syphilis.

Congestive heart failure (CHF): also called congestive cardiac failure (CCF) or just heart failure, this is a condition that can result from any structural or functional cardiac disorder that impairs the ability of the heart to fill with or pump a sufficient amount of blood throughout the body.

Conjunctivitis: commonly called "pinkeye" in the United States, this is an inflammation of the conjunctiva (the outermost layer of the eye and the inner surface of the eyelids), most commonly due to an allergic reaction or an infection (usually bacterial or viral).

Connective tissue: one of the four types of tissue in traditional classifications (the others being epithelial, muscle, and nervous tissue).

Consequentialist or **Utilitarian ethics:** the theory that postulates that actions or rules are right or good as they relate to producing good consequences.

Constant equilibrium: a balance of the drugs remaining between the unbound and bound form.

Constituent organizations: the state or regional components of the American Dental Hygienists' Association.

Consumer advocate: a person who provides dental health consultation to various target populations.

Contamination: an infectious agent on a body surface.

Continuous variable: a variable that can be expressed by a large and infinite number of measures along a continuum, can be expressed in a fraction, and is considered quantitative.

Contract: the agreement between the insurance entity and the group.

Contrast: the difference in densities among various regions on a radiograph.

Control: a group in a study that does not receive treatment or therapy.

Copayment: a portion of the costs of each service that is paid by the patient.

Coronal polishing: removal of stains and bacterial plaque (nonmineralized deposits) from surface of teeth with a hand or rotary instrument; frequently accomplished using a rubber cup with polishing agent on a slow speed handpiece.

Coronal suture: a dense, fibrous connective tissue joint that separates the frontal and parietal bones of the skull. At birth, the bones of the skull do not meet.

Correlation: the linear relationship between variables.

Corrosion: the dissolution of metal that is irreversible.

Corrugated: wavy elevations and depressions; also wrinkled.

Covalent: a description of chemical bonding that is characterized by the sharing of pairs of electrons between atoms.

Corticotropin: see Adrenocorticotropin.

Cranial: of or relating to the skull or cranium.

Creep: the time dependent deformation of an object subjected to constant stress, or the flow of that material.

Cretinism: a condition of severely stunted physical and mental growth due to untreated congenital deficiency of thyroid hormones (hypothyroidism). The term *cretin* refers to a person so affected.

Crown: a restoration that replaces extracoronal tooth structure and is cemented to tooth structure or implant.

Cultural diversity: the integration of an individual's or population's socioethnocultural background into dental hygiene care.

Culture and sensitivity: application of antimicrobial agent to culture to determine effective antibiotic. All infections not responding to antimicrobial therapy should be cultured and sensitivity tests performed. Also, cases of serious infections and infection in compromised patients.

Cushing's syndrome or **hypercortisolism** or **hyperadrenocorticism:** an endocrine disorder caused by high levels of cortisol in the blood.

Cyclic neutropenia: periodic cycles of neutrophils decrease with cycles of normal count, usually over 3 to 4 weeks.

Cytokine: a substance (e.g., lymphokines, interleukins, and interferons) produced by cells that affects other cells (e.g., lymphocytes and macrophages) and that mediate the immune response.

Cytolysis: the breaking apart (lysis) of bacteria or cells such as tumor or red blood cells, from the activation of complement.

Cytomegalovirus (CMV): a genus of herpesviruse.

Cytosol: the internal fluid of the cell; a portion of cell metabolism occurs here.

Cytotoxic T cell: a cell that belongs to a sub-group of T lymphocytes (a type of white blood cell) which are capable of inducing the death of infected somatic or tumor cells; they kill cells that are infected with viruses (or other pathogens), or are otherwise damaged or dysfunctional.

Data: the information that is collected by a researcher.

Debonding: the removal of cements or any luting agent, such as composite.

Deductible: the amount an individual enrolled in the insurance plan must pay toward covered services before the insurance entity begins paying.

Defamation: making false statements that harm an individual's reputation.

Defluoridation: the process of removing naturally occurring fluoride from water supplies.

Demand: the particular frequency or desired frequency of dental care from a population.

Dendrites: the branched projections of a neuron that act to conduct the electrical stimulation received from other neural cells to the cell body, or soma, of the neuron from which the dendrites project.

Dens in dente (dens invaginatus): a tooth within a tooth; enamel is deposited within the pulp chamber due to the invagination of the enamel organ.

Density: overall degree of blackness or darkness on the radiograph.

Dental assistant: the professional who assists the dental hygienist and/or dentist.

Dental claim form: the standard form utilized to file a claim or request authorization for a procedure.

Dental claim: a claim for payment made by the patient for a dental procedure that was rendered.

Dental fluorosis: chronic toxicity of fluoride taken systemically.

Dental hygiene: the art and science of preventive oral health.

Dental hygiene diagnosis: the formal diagnosis of a population's current dental hygiene status.

Dental hygiene process of care: The assessment, dental hygiene diagnosis, planning, implementation, and evaluation of dental hygiene care of a target population.

Dental hygiene treatment: periodontal debridement and oral hygiene instruction.

Dental hygienist: the professional who provides clinical and educational dental hygiene services to the public.

Dental indexes: the standardized methods used to describe the status of an individual or group with respect to an oral condition.

Dental lamina: a band of epithelial tissue seen in histologic sections of a developing tooth. The dental lamina is the first evidence of tooth development and begins at the sixth week in utero.

Dental necessity: a service provided by a dental provider that has been determined as a generally acceptable dental practice for the diagnosis and treatment of an individual.

Dental public health: the oral health care and education, with an emphasis on the utilization of the dental hygiene sciences, delivered to a target population.

Dental pulp: the part in the center of a tooth made up of living soft tissue and cells called odontoblasts. The odontoblasts are the sturctural cells of the tooth, however there are also other cells in the pulp. Those include: fibroblasts, granulocites, histiosites etc. It's commonly called "the nerve," although it contains many other structures which are not nerves.

Dental sealant: an organic polymer that bonds to the enamel surfaces of the pit and fissures, by mechanical retention, to prevent dental caries.

Dentin (dentine): the substance between enamel (substance in the crown) or cementum (substance in the root) of a tooth and the pulp chamber. Dentin is secreted by the odontoblasts of the dental pulp. The formation of dentin is known as dentinogenesis.

Dentinal dysplasia: abnormal dentin.

Dentinogenesis imperfecta: abnormal dentin.

Dentist: the professional who provides clinical and educational dental services to the public.

Dentistry: the art and science of restorative oral health.

Denture: a prosthetic device that replaces a fully endentulous arch.

Deontology or **nonconsequentialism (Kantian):** a theory that an action is right when it conforms to a judgment or rule of conduct that meets some preestablished requirement or rule.

Dependent variable: in a clinical study, the variable that is being tested.

Depression: the anatomical term of motion for movement in an inferior direction.

Descriptive statistics: procedures that are used to summarize, organize, and describe quantitative data.

Determinants of health: the factors that interact to create specific health conditions, including physical, biological, behavioral, social, cultural, and spiritual.

Developmental disability: a disability that occurs during uterine development.

DHCW: dental health care worker.

Diabetes insipidus (DI): a disease characterized by excretion of large amounts of severely diluted urine, which cannot be reduced when fluid intake is reduced.

Diabetes mellitus: a metabolic disorder characterized by hyperglycemia (high blood sugar) and other signs, as distinct from a single illness or condition.

Diastole: the period of time when the heart relaxes after contraction.

Die: a cast used for a single tooth or a few teeth.

Diencephalon: the region of the brain that includes the thalamus, hypothalamus, epithalamus, prethalamus, or subthalamus and pretectum.

Dietary fibers: the indigestible portion of plant foods that move food through the digestive system, absorbing water.

Diffuse: poorly identifiable margins that blend into normal tissue.

Diffusion: the net action of matter (particles or molecules), heat, momentum, or light whose end is to minimize a concentration gradient.

Dilaceration: abnormal root curvature caused by trauma during tooth formation.

Dimensional change: a change occurring in dimension of material whether it be shrinkage or expansion; it is sometimes referred to as microleakage or percolation.

Diphtheria: an upper respiratory tract illness characterized by sore throat, low-grade fever, and an adherent membrane (a pseudomembrane) on the tonsil(s), pharynx, and/or nose.

Direct restoration: a restoration fabricated directly in the oral cavity.

Disaccharide: a sugar (a carbohydrate) composed of two monosaccharides.

Discrete (categorical) variable: a variable that is made up of distinct and separate units or categories, also referred to as mutually exclusive, and is counted only in whole numbers.

Disease rates: the number of disease cases or deaths (expressed as a ratio) among a population or target group during a given time period.

Disinfectants: antimicrobial agents that are applied to non-living objects to destroy microorganisms, the process of which is known as disinfection.

Disinfection: the process of destroying pathogenic microorganisms by applying chemical or physical agents.

Distal: situated away from the point of attachment or origin or a central point, especially of the body.

Distribution: the movement of a drug throughout the body by plasma proteins in blood.

Dorsal: relating to, or situated near or on the back, especially of an animal or of one of its parts.

Droplet: a very small drop, such as a particle of moisture expelled during sneezing, coughing, or talking that may carry potentially infectious agents.

Drug allergy: reactions to drugs which may vary from a mild rash to anaphylaxis. They may be antigen–antibody reactions; not dose-related and not predictable; can be divided into four types of reactions depending on the type of antibody or cell-mediated reaction.

Ductility: the ability of a material to withstand deformation under tension without fracturing.

dura mater: the tough and inflexible outermost of the three layers of the meninges surrounding the brain and spinal cord.

Early and Periodic Screening, Diagnosis and Treatment (EPSDT): Persons under 21 years of age must be covered by Medicaid for medical, dental, and vision care.

Early childhood caries: dental caries that affects children; sometimes referred to as nursing bottle decay or baby bottle decay.

Early Head Start: the federal program that promotes the economic and social well-being of pregnant women and their children up to age three.

Ecchymosis: purple or purplish-red, nonelevated area of submucosal bleeding, larger than a petechiae.

Ectoderm: the start of a tissue that covers the body surfaces. It emerges first and forms from the outermost of the germ layers.

Edema: swelling of any organ or tissue due to accumulation of excess lymph fluid, without an increase of the number of cells in the affected tissue.

Educator: the person who educates and promotes dental health issues to various target populations.

Effect dose (ED50): a dose that produces a therapeutic response in 50% of the subjects given the drug.

Efferent nerves: otherwise known as motor or effector neurons, these are nerves that carry impulses *away* from the central nervous system to effectors such as muscles or glands.

Efficacy: the desired therapeutic response obtained when a sufficient amount of a drug is administered; not related to potency.

Elastic modulus: the measure of stiffness of a material.

Electromagnetic radiation: transmission of wave energy through space and matter as a combination of electric and magnetic fields.

Elevation: the anatomical term of motion for movement in a superior direction.

Embryology: the study of the development of an embryo.

Emigration: white blood cells leaving the blood vessels with plasma fluids and entering the injured tissue, due to chemotactic factors, following adhesion.

Emphysema: a type of chronic obstructive lung disease. It is often caused by exposure to toxic chemicals or long-term exposure to tobacco smoke.

Enamel hypocalcification: defect in enamel mineralization.

Enamel hypoplasia: defect in enamel organic matrix formation.

Enamel pearl: development of excess enamel on root due to misplaced ameloblasts.

Encephalitis: an acute inflammation of the brain, commonly caused by a viral infection.

Endemic: a relatively low, but constant level of occurrence of a disease or health condition in a population.

Endocarditis: an inflammation of the inner layer of the heart, the endocardium. The most common structures involved are the heart valves.

Endocrine system: a control system of ductless glands that secrete chemical messengers called hormones that circulate within the body via the bloodstream to affect distant cells within specific organs.

Endoderm: one of the germ layers formed during animal embryogenesis. Cells migrating inward along the archenteron form the inner layer of the gastrula, which develops into the endoderm.

Endodontic abscess: an infection of the tooth pulp; tooth will be nonvital.

Endogenous infection: an infection acquired as a result of self microflora.

Endoplasmic reticulum or ER: an organelle, found in all eukaryotic cells, that is an interconnected network of tubules, vesicles, and cisternae, that is responsible for several specialized functions: protein translation, folding, and transport of proteins to be used in the cell membrane (e.g., transmembrane receptors and other integral membrane proteins), or to be secreted (exocytosed) from the cell (e.g., digestive enzymes); sequestration of calcium; and production and storage of glycogen, steroids, and other macromolecules.

Enteral: by mouth (orally); many drugs in tablet, capsule, or drop form are taken this way.

Eosinophil granulocytes: commonly referred to as eosinophils (or less commonly as acidophils), these are white blood cells of the immune system that are responsible for combating infection by parasites in vertebrates.

Epidemic: widespread cases of disease in a region with greater than the expected number of cases for that population.

Epidemiology: see oral epidemiology.

Epididymis: a part of the human male reproductive system that is present in all male mammals.

Epidural space: the space outside the tough membrane called the dura mater (sometimes called the "dura"), and within the spinal canal, that is formed by the surrounding vertebrae.

Epilepsy: a common chronic neurological condition that is characterized by recurrent unprovoked epileptic seizures.

Epinephrine or adrenaline: a hormone; a catecholamine, a sympathomimetic monoamine derived from the amino acids phenylalanine and tyrosine.

Epistaxis: a spontaneous nose bleed.

Epithelial attachment: the place, located at the base of the sulcus, where epithelium attaches to the tooth.

Epithelium: a tissue composed of a layer of cells. In humans, it is one of four primary body tissues. Epithelium lines both the outside (skin) and the inside cavities and lumen of bodies.

Erythema multiforme: a disease affecting skin and mucous membranes.

Erythema: an abnormal redness of the skin caused by capillary congestion. It is one of the cardinal signs of inflammation.

Erythropenia: a decrease in circulating red blood cells (RBCs).

Essential nutrient: a nutrient required for normal body functioning that cannot be synthesized by the body.

Estrogens: a group of steroid compounds, named for their importance in the estrous cycle, and functioning as the primary female sex hormone.

Ethmoid: a light spongy cubical bone forming much of the walls of the nasal cavity and part of those of the orbits.

Ethnocentrism: the belief that one's culture is superior.

Etiology: the theory of causation for a disease or condition.

Eukaryotes: organisms with a complex cell or cells, where the genetic material is organized into a membrane-bound nucleus or nuclei.

Evaluation: the part of the dental hygiene process of care that encompasses the initial overview of a dental public health program.

Eversion: the movement of the sole of the foot away from the median plane.

Ewing's sarcoma: the common name for primitive neuroectodermal tumor.

Exclusive Provider Arrangement (EPA): a plan in which dental care providers contract with an employer (which eliminates the third party) and negotiate the fees for services offered to the employees.

Excretion: the process by which drugs and their metabolites are eliminated via urine, bile, sweat, saliva, lungs, tears, and milk. The kidney is the major organ of drug excretion.

Exostosis: hyperplasia of the bone.

Explanation of benefits: a form sent to the patient and provider explaining the payment for procedures, or denial of payment for procedures, rendered.

Exposure time: the length of time that film is exposed to produce x-rays.

Expressed contracts: verbally stated or written agreements.

Extension: a movement of a joint. For example, extension is produced by extending the flexed elbow. The arm is now straight; it has been extended. If the head is tilted all the way back, it is said to be extended.

Exudate: any fluid that filters from the circulatory system into lesions or areas of inflammation.

Facial nerve: the seventh (VII) of twelve paired cranial nerves. It emerges from the brainstem between the pons and the medulla, and controls the muscles of facial expression, and taste to the anterior two-thirds of the tongue. It also supplies preganglionic parasympathetic fibers to several head and neck ganglia.

Facilitated diffusion: the result of a drug being transported down the concentration gradient at a greater rate than passive diffusion; bound to specific carrier proteins.

Fairness: the ability to make judgments free from discrimination or dishonesty.

Fascia: specialized connective tissue layer which surrounds muscles, bones, and joints, providing support and protection, and giving structure to the body. It consists of three layers: the superficial fascia, the deep fascia, and the subserous fascia.

Fatigue: the weakening of a material caused by repeated loading at a stress level below the fracture strength.

Federation Dentaire Internationale (FDI): the organization that represents the international community of dentists.

Fee slip: form utilized by the dental provider that details the services rendered.

Fibromyalgia (FM or FMS): a chronic syndrome (constellation of signs and symptoms) characterized by diffuse or specific muscle, joint, or bone pain, fatigue, and a wide range of other symptoms.

Fibrous dysplasia (monostotic fibroosseous lesion of the jaws): unilateral asymptomatic enlargement of maxilla or mandible.

Filtration: the process of using a filter to mechanically separate a mixture of solids and fluids. Also, removes less penetrating x-rays, improving beam quality.

Finishing: the process by which a restoration or appliance is contoured to remove excess material and produce a reasonably smooth surface.

Fissured: deep grooves with no cracks or ulcerations.

Fixed partial denture (bridge): a prosthetic device that replaces a missing tooth or teeth and is cemented to adjacent teeth.

Flexion: a position that is made possible by the joint angle decreasing.

Flow: the continual permanent deformation under load of an amorphous or noncrystalline solid.

Fluorescence: the absorption of nonvisible light released by material as visible light.

Fluoridation: the addition of fluoride to drinking water.

Fluoride varnish: A varnish composed of fluoride that is applied to teeth to treat tooth sensitivity and prevent dental caries; particularly effective in the prevention of early childhood caries.

Fluoride: a salt of hydrofluoric acid.

Fluorosis: a form of enamel hypomineralization due to excessive ingestion of fluoride during the development of the teeth.

Foliate papillae: taste buds, the end-organs of the gustatory sense, are scattered over the mucous membrane of the mouth and tongue at irregular intervals and are localized at the side of the base of the tongue. They occur especially in the sides of the vallate papillae.

Fomite or fomes: an inanimate material or object on which pathogen agents may be carried.

Foramen ovale: one of the larger of the several holes (the foramina) at the base of the skull that transmits nerves through the skull. The foramen ovale is situated in the anterior part of the sphenoid bone, posteriolateral to the foramen rotundum.

Foramen rotundum: a circular hole in the sphenoid bone that connects the middle cranial fossa and the pterygopalatine fossa.

Fordyce granules: yellowish clusters of submucosal sebaceous glands.

Formative evaluation: an evaluation of the program during implementation; evaluating the process.

Free gingival groove: a depression located at the inferior border of free gingiva at a point opposite the alveolar crest.

Free gingiva: the outer boundary of the sulcus located at the crest of the alveolus; not attached.

Frontal bone: a bone in the human skull that resembles a cockle-shell in form.

Frontier: a geographic area that is even more sparsely populated than a rural area.

Fructose (or levulose): a simple sugar (monosaccharide) found in many foods and is one of the three most important blood sugars, along with glucose and sucrose.

Fusion: two teeth are fused into one, resulting in a macrodont; therefore, fewer than normal complement of teeth are present

Galactose (Gal; also called brain sugar): a type of sugar found in dairy products, in sugar beets, and other gums and mucilages.

Galvanism: the generation of electrical currents between two dissimilar metal restoratives that the patient can feel.

Ganglion: a tissue mass, which is composed mainly of somata and dendritic structures, that often interconnects with others to form a complex system of ganglia known as a plexus.

Giant cell tumor (giant cell granuloma): a neoplasm of multinucleated giant cells.

Gingiva (or gums): the mucosal tissue that lays over the jawbone.

Gingival curettage: removal of epithelial lining of periodontal pocket by scraping surface with an instrument, such as a curet.

Gingival sulcus: denotes space between gingiva and tooth.

Gingivitis: reversible inflammation of the gingival.

Glass ionomer: cement used for Class V cavity preparations and sealants; newer glass ionomer restorations release fluoride.

Glomerulonephritis (GN): a primary or secondary autoimmune renal disease characterized by inflammation of the glomeruli, the small blood vessels in the kidneys. It may be asymptomatic, or present with hematuria and/or proteinuria (blood protein in the urine).

Glomerulus: a capillary tuft surrounded by Bowman's capsule in nephrons of the vertebrate kidney.

Glossopharyngeal nerve: the ninth of twelve cranial nerves. It exits the brainstem from the sides of the upper medulla, just rostral (closer to the nose) to the vagus nerve.

Glucagon: a 29-amino acid polypeptide acting as an important hormone in carbohydrate metabolism.

Glucose (Glc): a monosaccharide (or simple sugar); it is the most important carbohydrate in biology.

Glycocalyx: a general term referring to extra cellular polymeric material produced by some bacteria, epithelia, and other cells.

Glycogen: (commonly known as **animal starch** although this name is inaccurate) a polysaccharide that is the principal storage form of glucose (Glc) in animal cells.

Gold: an alloy of gold and other noble (precious) metals. This is used for gold foils, crowns, and bridges.

Golgi apparatus: an organelle found in typical eukaryotic cells.

Gonorrhea: one of the most common sexually-transmitted diseases in the world; caused by gram-negative bacterium *Neisseria gonorrhoeae*.

Gout: also called metabolic arthritis, this is a disease caused by an inborn disorder of the uric acid metabolism. In this condition, monosodium urate crystals are deposited on the articular cartilage of joints and in the particular tissue like tendons.

Graves' disease: a thyroid disorder characterized by goiter, exophthalmos, "orange-peel" skin, and hyperthyroidism.

Group: see Target population.

Growth hormone: a 191-amino acid, single chain polypeptide hormone which is synthesized, stored, and secreted by the somatotroph cells within the lateral wings of the anterior pituitary gland, which stimulates growth and cell reproduction in humans and other animals.

Hairy tongue: proliferation of filiform papillae.

Hantaviruses: viruses belonging to the bunyaviridae family. There are five genera within the Bunyaviridae family: bunyavirus, phlebovirus, nairovirus, tospovirus, and hantavirus.

Hapten: a molecule that is not intrinsically immunological, but that may produce a response if combined with a specific antibody.

Hardness: a material's resistance to indentation.

HCW: health care worker.

Head Start: the federal program that promotes the economic and social well-being of families and children from three to five years of age.

Health behavior: an action that helps prevent illness and promote health.

Health education: the education of health behaviors that bring an individual to a state of health awareness.

Health promotion: the promotion of healthy ideas and concepts to motivate individuals to adopt healthy behaviors.

Healthy People 2010: the report released from the federal government which states the goals and objectives necessary to improve the health and quality of life for individuals and communities.

Hemangioma: neoplasm of blood vessels.

Hematoma: purple or purplish-red, elevated area of submucosal bleeding.

Hematuria: blood in urine.

Hemicellulose: any of several heteropolymers (matrix polysaccharides) present in almost all cell walls along with cellulose.

Hemolysis: rupture of erythrocytes with loss of hemoglobin.

Hemoptysis: coughing up blood.

Hemostasis: the physiologic process whereby bleeding is halted. Stopped bleeding is commonly referred to as coagulation, however, coagulation is only one type of hemostatic process.

Hepatitis A: formerly known as infectious hepatitis, this is an acute, infectious liver disease caused by the Hepatovirus hepatitis A virus

Hepatitis B: a disease of the liver that is caused by the Hepatitis B virus (HBV), a member of the Hepadnavirus family

Hepatitis C: a blood-borne, infectious, viral disease that is caused by a hepatotropic virus called Hepatitis C virus (HCV).

Hepatitis D: a disease caused by a small circular RNA virus (Hepatitis delta virus or hepatitis D virus, HDV). HDV is considered to be a subviral satellite because it can propagate only in the presence of another virus, the hepatitis B virus (HBV).

Hepatitis E: an acute viral hepatitis (liver inflammation) caused by infection with a virus called hepatitis E virus (HEV).

Hepatitis G and GB virus C (GBV-C): RNA viruses that were independently identified in 1995, and were subsequently found to be two isolates of the same virus.

Herpes simplex: a viral infection caused by one of two Herpes Simplex Viruses (HSV).

Herpes zoster: colloquially known as **shingles**, this is the reactivation of varicella zoster virus.

Hertwig's epithelial root sheath: a proliferation of epithelial cells located at the cervical loop of the enamel organ in a developing tooth. Hertwig's epithelial root sheath initates the formation of dentin in the root of a tooth by causing the differentiation of odontoblasts from the dental papilla.

Histamine: a biogenic amine chemical involved in local immune responses as well as regulating physiological function in the gut and acting as a neurotransmitter.

Histocompatible: transplant antigens are shared; unlikely to cause rejection response.

Histoplasmosis: also known as Darling's disease, this is a disease caused by the fungus Histoplasma capsulatum.

Hodgkin's lymphoma: also known as **Hodgkin's disease**, this is a type of lymphoma first described by Thomas Hodgkin in 1832. Hodgkin's lymphoma is characterized clinically by the orderly spread of disease from one lymph node group to another and by the development of systemic symptoms with advanced disease.

Homeostasis: the property of an open system, especially in living organisms, to regulate its internal environment to maintain a stable, constant condition, by means of multiple dynamic equilibrium adjustments, controlled by interrelated regulation mechanisms.

Honeycombed: containing several radiolucent compartments of the same size.

Hue: the dominant color of an object.

Humoral immunity: a condition in which a population of activated B lymphocytes become plasma cells, which produce specific antibodies in response to stimulus by a specific antigen; mediated by complement.

Hydrogen: is a chemical element that has the symbol **H** and an atomic number of 1.

Hyoid bone: is a bone in the human neck, not articulated to any other bone. It is supported by the muscles of the neck and in turn supports the root of the tongue.

Hyperpituitarism: the result of excess secretion of adenohypophyseal trophic hormones most commonly by a functional pituitary adenoma.

Hyperplasia: a general term for an increase in the number of the cells of an organ or tissue causing it to increase in size, usually as a response to stimuli or an irritant.

Hypersensitivity reactions: exaggerated or inappropriate response to an antigen; classified as Type I, Type II, Type III, or Type IV.

Hyperthyroidism (or "overactive thyroid gland"): the clinical syndrome caused by an excess of circulating free thyroxine (T_4) or free triiodothyronine (T_3), or both.

Hypertrophy: the increase in size of an organ or tissue resulting from an increase in size of individual cells; mimics neoplasia clinically and is usually a response to stimuli.

Hyperventilation (or overbreathing): the state of breathing faster and/or deeper than necessary, thereby reducing the carbon dioxide concentration of the blood below normal.

Hypocortisolism: See Addison's disease.

Hypoglycemia: a medical term referring to a pathologic state produced by a lower than normal amount of sugar (glucose) in the blood.

Hypothalamus: also known as the "master gland," this gland links the nervous system to the endocrine system via the pituitary gland.

Hypothyroidism: the disease state in humans and animals caused by insufficient production of thyroid hormone by the thyroid gland.

Idiosyncrasy: peculiar, or individual, reaction to drugs and/or food substances.

Idiosyncratic reaction: unexpected reaction to a drug, not predictable; most likely to affect the very young and old.

Imbibition: the taking up of fluid in the colloid system.

Immune response: the development of immunity or resistance to a foreign substance, which can be antibody mediated (humoral), cell-mediated (cellular), or both.

Immune system: a collection of mechanisms within an organism that protects against infection by identifying and killing pathogens.

Immunity: the resistance a person has against a disease.

Immunoglobin: a glycoprotein composed of L and H chains that functions as an antibody. The five subclasses based on the antigenic determinants are: IgA, IgD, IgG, IgM, IgE.

Implant: a titanium screw that is implanted in alveolar bone to replace a missing tooth or teeth.

Implementation: the part of the dental hygiene process of care that includes the actual operation of a program.

Implied contracts: assumed contracts.

Incidence: the number of new cases of a disease in a population over a given period of time.

Incisive foramen: a funnel-shaped opening seen in the middle line, immediately behind the incisor teeth. When the two maxillae are articulated.

Incubation period: the interval of time between the first contact with the infectious agent and the appearance of clinical symptoms and signs of the disease.

Independent contractor: a person who works for him- or herself in a governmental or private capacity.

Independent practice: the practice of dental hygiene without the supervision of a dentist, although the dental hygienist refers all dental needs to a dentist; sometimes called unsupervised practice or collaborative practice.

Independent variable: in a clinical study, the variable that is being manipulated.

Index: see dental indexes.

Indirect restoration: a restoration that is fabricated using cast replica or oral structures involved.

Infarct: death of tissue from lack of oxygen.

Infection: the state caused by the invasion, development, or multiplication of the infectious agent in the body; may be primary (original), latent (no clinical symptoms), recurrent (reactivation of primary infection), acute (rapid onset, abrupt resolution), chronic (slow onset, long duration), localized (confined to a particular area), or generalized or systemic (invades bloodstream and lymphatic system).

Infectious mononucleosis: a disease seen most commonly in adolescents and young adults, characterized by fever, sore throat, muscle soreness, and fatigue.

Infective endocarditis: disease caused by microbial infection of the heart valves.

Inferential statistics: used to make inferences or generalizations about a population based on data taken from a sample of that population.

Inferior: situated lower down.

Inferior alveolar nerve: a branch of the mandibular nerve, which is itself the third branch (V3) of the fifth cranial nerve, the trigeminal nerve (cranial nerve V).

Informed consent: providing the patient with relevant information needed to make a decision.

Infrahyoid muscles: a group of four pairs of muscles in the anterior part of the neck. (The term **infrahyoid** refers to the region below (inferior) to the hyoid bone in the neck.)

Infraorbital foramen: the opening located above the canine fossa, at the end of the infraorbital canal; it transmits the infraorbital artery, vein, and infraorbital nerve.

Inhalation (INH): into the lungs (gaseous, microcrystalline, volatile drugs, and bronchodilators)

Inherent filtration: unleaded glass window and oil bath through which the x-ray beam passes

Inlay: a restoration that replaces intracoronal tooth structure.

Integumentary system: the external covering of the body, comprised of the skin, hair, feathers, scales, nails, sweat glands, and their products (sweat and mucus).

Interdental gingiva: the oral mucosa that occupies the gingival embrasure, which is the interproximal space beneath the area of tooth contact. The interdental gingiva can be pyramidal or have a "col" shape.

Interdental papilla: tissue that occupies interdental space between two adjacent teeth.

Interferons (IFNs): are natural proteins produced by the cells of the immune system of most vertebrates in response to challenges by foreign agents such as viruses, bacteria, parasites, and tumor cells.

Interleukin: a cytokine that stimulates or affects the functions of lymphocytes and other cells.

International Federation of Dental Hygienists (IFDH): the organization representing the international community of dental hygienists.

Interval scale of measurement: the equal distance between any two adjacent units of measurement, but there is no meaningful zero point.

Intradermal: into the dermis; the site where usually small amounts of drugs (e.g., local anesthetic and tuberculin skin test) are injected.

Intramuscular injection: the injection of a substance directly into a muscle. It is one of several alternative methods for the administration of medications.

Intraperitoneal: into the peritoneal cavity.

Intrathecal: into the spinal subarachnoid space; used for treatment of certain forms of meningitis.

Intravenous therapy or **IV therapy:** the administration of liquid substances directly into a vein.

Inverse square law: the intensity of an x-ray beam varies inversely with the square of the source-film distance.

Ionic bonds: a type of chemical bond based on electrostatic forces between two oppositely-charged ions.

Ischemic heart disease: a heart condition resulting from oxygen deprivation to the myocardium as a result of coronary atherosclerosis.

Isoniazid: a first-line antituberculous medication used in the prevention and treatment of tuberculosis.

Jaundice (icterus): yellowish coloring of skin, mucous membranes, sclerae, and bodily excretions due to hyperbilirubinemia and deposition of bile pigments.

Kaposi's sarcoma: a fatal, metastasizing, malignant vascular cancer found in 90% of all patients with AIDS.

kVp: the adjustment that controls quality or penetrating power of x-rays; minor factor in controlling quantity of x-rays.

Kwashiorkor: a type of childhood malnutrition; there is some controversy over the possible causes, but it is commonly believed to be caused by insufficient protein intake.

Lacrimal bone: the smallest and most fragile bone of the face, it is situated at the front part of the medial wall of the orbit. It has two surfaces and four borders.

Lacto-ovovegetarian: a vegetarian who is willing to consume dairy products (i.e., milk and its derivatives, like cheese, butter, or yogurt) and eggs. Lacto means "milk" and ovo means "egg."

Lactose: a disaccharide that consists of β-D-galactose and β-D-glucose molecules bonded through a β1–4 glycosidic linkage. Lactose makes up around 2–8% of the solids in milk.

Lactose intolerance: the condition in which lactase, an enzyme needed for proper metabolization of lactose (a sugar that is a constituent of milk and other dairy products), is not produced in adulthood.

Lambdoid suture: a dense, fibrous connective tissue joint that separates the parietal and temporal bones of the skull from the occipital bone.

Lateral: of or relating to the side.

Law of Bergonié-Tribondeau: this describes the cells most sensitive to effects of radiation.

Learning domain: a way to differentiate the individual types of learning.

Leiomyoma: neoplasm of smooth (involuntary) muscle.

Lesson plan: a written document used in planning a presentation.

Lethal dose (LD50): the dose of a drug that produces death in 50% of the subjects given the drug.

Leukemia: a cancer of the blood or bone marrow that is characterized by an abnormal proliferation (production by multiplication) of blood cells, usually white blood cells (leukocytes).

Leukoedema: opalescent (milky) hue of the buccal mucosa resulting from increased intracellular edema.

Leukopenia: decrease in circulating white blood cells (WBCs).

Leukoplakia: a condition of the mouth that involves the formation of white leathery spots on the mucous membranes of the tongue and inside of the mouth. When not given as a diagnosis, it is a clinical description of a white lesion that does not rub off.

Libel: written or published defamation.

Lichen planus: white or gray thread-like papules in a linear or reticular arrangement.

Lignin: a chemical compound that is most commonly derived from wood and is an integral part of the cell walls of plants, especially in tracheids, xylem fibers and sclereids.

Lingual nerve: a branch of the mandibular nerve (CN V_3), itself a branch of the trigeminal nerve. The lingual nerve supplies sensory innervation to the mucous membrane of the anterior two-thirds of the tongue.

Lingual thyroid nodule: thyroid tissue remnant during developmental stages.

Lingual varices: enlarged tortuous veins on ventral surface of tongue.

lipids: fat substances used for energy storage, to serve as structural components of cell membranes, and that constitute important signaling molecules.

Lipoma: neoplasm of adipose (fat) tissue.

Long-term care facility: a facility that provides live-in care for patients with medical complications.

Lyme disease or **Lyme borreliosis:** the most common tick-borne disease in North America and Europe, and the fastest-growing infectious disease in the United States.

Lymphangioma: neoplasm of lymphatic vessels.

Lymphatic system: a complex network of lymphoid organs, lymph nodes, lymph ducts, lymph tissues, lymph capillaries, and lymph vessels that produce and transport lymph fluid from tissues to the circulatory system. The lymphatic system is a major component of the immune system.

Lysosomes: organelles that contain digestive enzymes (acid hydrolases).

Lysozyme: commonly referred to as the "body's own antibiotic" because it kills bacteria.

mA: controls quantity or number of x-rays.

Macrodont: denotes large tooth.

Macrolides: a group of drugs (typically antibiotics) whose activity stems from the presence of a macrolide ring, a large lactone ring to which one or more deoxy sugars, usually cladinose and desosamine, are attached.

Macronutrients: those nutrients that together provide the vast majority of metabolic energy to an organism.

Macule: a discolored spot on the skin that is flat and can only be seen and not felt.

Major histocompatibility complex (MHC): a cluster of genes that determines the histocompatibility of the species, determining what substances will be considered foreign or antigenic.

Malignant pleomorphic adenoma: malignancy arising from a preexisting, long-standing, benign pleomorphic adenoma.

Malignant: having the ability to metastasize; therefore, it is cancer.

Malleability: the ability of a material to withstand deformation under compression.

Malpractice: professional negligence.

Maltose: malt sugar, is a disaccharide formed from two units of glucose joined with an $\alpha(1 \rightarrow 4)$ linkage.

Managed care: the integration of health care delivery and financing.

Manager: the developer and coordinator of dental public health programs; sometimes referred to as an administrator.

Mandible: together with the maxilla, this is the largest and strongest bone of the face. It forms the lower jaw and holds the lower teeth in place.

Mandibular foramen: an opening on the internal surface of the ramus (posterior and perpendicularly oriented part of the mandible) for divisions of the mandibular vessels and nerve to pass.

Mandibular nerve: (V_3) is the largest of the three branches of the **trigeminal nerve**.

Marginal gingiva: the terminal edge of gingiva surrounding the teeth in collar-like fashion. In about 50% of cases, it is demarcated from the adjacent, attached gingiva by a shallow linear depression, the free gingival groove. Usually about 1 mm wide, it forms the soft tissue wall of the gingival sulcus. It may be separated from the tooth surface with a periodontal probe.

Margination: movement of white blood cells to the periphery of the venule; also the process by which restorations are made flush with the enamel or cement surface.

Maxilla: a fusion of two bones along the palatal fissure that form the upper jaw. This is similar to the **mandible**, which is also a fusion of two halves at the mental symphysis.

Maxillary: an artery that supplies deep structures of the face.

Maxillary nerve: is the second division of the trigeminal; it is a sensory nerve.

Mean: the average of scores.

Measurement: a particular method utilized to evaluate a dental public health program based upon the program objectives.

Median: the midpoint of scores.

Medicaid (Title XIX): money from federal, state, and local taxes pays bills for certain groups of people, including low-income, aged, blind, disabled, and members of families with dependent children.

Medicare (Title XVIII): a federal insurance program from a trust fund to pay medical bills of all people over age sixty-five.

Medulla oblongata: the lower portion of the brainstem.

Meiosis: the process by which one diploid eukaryotic cell divides to generate haploid cells called gametes.

Melanin pigmentations: focal brownish areas that may be racial in origin or indicative of a systemic disease.

Melanocyte-stimulating hormones (collectively referred to as **MSH**): a class of peptide hormones produced by cells in the intermediate lobe of the pituitary gland.

Meninges: the system of membranes that envelops the central nervous system.

Meningitis: the inflammation (infection) of the meninges which are the membranes that cover the brain and spine.

Mental foramen: one of two foramina located on the anterior surface of the mandible. It permits passage of the mental nerve and vessels. The mental foramen descends slightly in edentulous individuals.

Mental nerve: a general somatic afferent (sensory) nerve which provides sensation to the anterior aspects of the chin and lower lip as well as the buccal gingivae of the mandibular anterior teeth and the premolars. It is a branch of the posterior trunk of the inferior alveolar nerve, which is itself a branch of the mandibular division of the trigeminal nerve (CN V).

Mesoderm: the germ layer that forms in the embryos of animals. Mesoderm forms during gastrulation when some of the cells migrating inward to form the endoderm form an additional layer between the endoderm and the ectoderm.

Metabolism (biotransformation): the process of chemically converting a drug to a form that is usually more easily removed from the body.

Metamerism: a term that means that colors look different under different light sources.

Methotrexate: an antimetabolite drug used in treatment of cancer and autoimmune diseases.

Metropolitan: a large population nucleus, consisting of a city and surrounding suburban areas.

Microbiota: the living microscopic organisms of an area.

Microdont: a small tooth.

Micronutrients: essential elements needed for life in small quantities. They include microminerals and vitamins.

Microvilli (singular, **microvillus**): structures that increase the surface area of cells by approximately 600-fold (human), thus facilitating absorption and secretion.

Middle superior alveolar nerve: a nerve that drops from the infraorbital portion of the maxillary nerve to supply the sinus mucosa, the roots of the maxillary premolars, and the mesiobuccal root of the first molar.

Milliampere-seconds (mAs): combined density factor; product of milliamperage and time.

Minimum inhibiting concentrations (MIC): lowest concentration needed to inhibit visible growth of an organism on media after incubation for 18 to 24 hours.

Mitochondria: a membrane-enclosed organelle, found in most eukaryotic cells.

Mitosis: the process by which a cell duplicates its genetic information (DNA), in order to generate two, identical, daughter cells.

Modality: a clinical or educational dental hygiene treatment.

Mode: the score that occurs most often.

Model: a positive replica of the dentition used for observation.

Monocyte: a leukocyte, part of the human body's immune system that protects against blood-borne pathogens and moves quickly (aprox. 8–12 hours) to sites of infection in the tissues.

Monomorphic adenoma: glandular neoplasm.

Monosaccharide: the simplest form of carbohydrates.

Morbidity: the ratio of "sick" (affected) individuals to well individuals in a community.

Mortality: the ratio of the number of deaths from a given disease or health problem to the total number of cases reported.

Mucoepidermoid carcinoma: malignancy composed of epidermoid cells and mucin-secreting cells.

Mucogingival junction: the place where attached gingiva ends.

Multilocular: several radiolucent compartments with the same or varied sizes.

Multiple myeloma: malignancy of plasma cells affecting bone.

Multiple sclerosis: a chronic, inflammatory disease that affects the central nervous system (CNS).

Muscarinic receptors: those membrane-bound acetylcholine receptors that are more sensitive to muscarine than to nicotine.

Muscular dystrophy: a genetic condition that includes more than 30 genetic and hereditary muscle diseases.

Muscular system: the biological system of humans that allows them to move. The muscular system in vertebrates is controlled through the nervous system, although some muscles (such as the cardiac muscle) can be completely autonomous.

Myasthenia gravis: a neuromuscular disease leading to fluctuating muscle weakness and fatiguability.

Myelin: an electrically insulating phospholipid layer that surrounds the axons of many neurons.

Myocardial infarction (MI): commonly known as a heart attack, this is a disease state that occurs when the blood supply to a part of the heart is interrupted.

Myxedema: a skin and tissue disorder usually due to severe prolonged **hypothyroidism**.

Nasal bones: two small oblong bones, varying in size and form in different individuals; they are placed side by side at the middle and upper part of the face, and form, by their junction, "the bridge" of the nose.

Nasal septum: the wall that separates the left and right airways in the nose, dividing the two nostrils.

Natural killer (NK) cells: a form of cytotoxic lymphocyte which constitutes a major component of the innate immune system.

Necrotizing sialometaplasia: necrosis of salivary gland tissue with metaplasia of ducts.

Necrotizing ulcerative gingivitis: chronic or acute, punched-out papilla, very painful; treat with debridement, interoffice chlorhexidine irrigation, scale and root plane as able, consider systemic antibiotics and antifungal medication.

Need: A normative, professional judgment as to the amount and kind of health care services required to attain or maintain health.

Negilence: an example of an unintentional tort and occurs when the provider did not do necessary assessment or treatment.

Neoplasia ("new growth"): implies an uncontrolled growth.

Nephron: the basic structural and functional unit of the kidney. Its chief function is to regulate water and soluble substances by filtering the blood, reabsorbing what is needed, and excreting the rest as urine.

Nervous system: the system of an animal that coordinates the activity of the muscles, monitors the organs, constructs and also stops input from the senses, and initiates actions.

Nervous tissue: the fourth major class of vertebrate tissue. The function of the nervous tissue is communication between parts of the body. It is composed of neurons, which transmit impulses, and the neuroglia, which assist propagation of the nerve impulse as well as provide nutrients to the neuron.

Neurilemoma (schwannoma): neoplasm of Schwann's cells (produce myelin sheath).

Neuritis: the general inflammation of the peripheral nervous system. Symptoms depend on the nerves involved, but may include pain, paresthesias, paresis, or hypesthesia (numbness).

Neurofibroma: neoplasm of neural elements and fibrous connective tissue.

Neuroma: neoplasm of neural tissue.

Neurons: electrically excitable cells in the nervous system that function to process and transmit information. In vertebrate animals, neurons are the core components of the brain, spinal cord, and peripheral nerves.

Neurotransmitters: chemicals that are used to relay, amplify and modulate electrical signals between a neuron and another cell.

Neutrophil granulocytes: generally referred to as neutrophils, these are the most abundant type of white blood cells and form an integral part of the immune system.

Nitrous oxide: a chemical compound with chemical formula N_2O. Under room conditions, it is a colorless, non-flammable gas, with a pleasant, slightly sweet odor. It is used in surgery and dentistry for its anaesthetic and analgesic effects, where it is commonly known as laughing gas due to the euphoric effects of inhaling it.

Nodule: small, firm, palpable lesion above or below surrounding surface level.

Nominal scale of measurement: the organization of data into mutually exclusive categories, but the categories have no rank order or value.

Nonclinical evaluation: a method utilized when evaluating a dental public health program that does not measure clinical changes.

Non-Hodgkin lymphoma (NHL): describes a group of cancers arising from lymphocytes, a type of white blood cell.

Nonmaleficence: the term that means that a health care provider's first obligation to the patient is to do no harm.

Normal bell curve: a normal distribution of the mean, median, and mode.

Normative ethics: this describes a group of theories that provide, define, and describe a system of principles and rules that determine which actions are deemed right or wrong.

Nosocomial: infection acquired as a result of a hospital stay.

Nucleolus (plural - nucleoli): a "sub-organelle" of the cell nucleus, which itself is an organelle.

Nucleus: a membrane-enclosed organelle found in most eukaryotic cells.

Nursing home: see long-term care facility.

Nutrient: either a chemical element or compound used in an organism's metabolism or physiology.

Occipital bone: a saucer-shaped membrane bone situated at the back and lower part of the cranium that is trapezoid in shape and curved on itself. It is pierced by a large oval aperture, the foramen magnum, through which the cranial cavity communicates with the vertebral canal.

Odontogenic adenomatoid tumor (OAT): a slow-growing benign tumor.

Odontoma: benign tumor that forms enamel, dentin, and cementum.

Onlay: a restoration that replaces intracoronal tooth structure including at least one cusp.

Opacity: the degree to which passage of light is prevented.

Ophthalmic nerve: one of the three branches of the trigeminal nerve, the fifth cranial nerve. Like the maxillary branch of the trigeminal nerve, the ophthalmic branch carries sensory fibers only. The ophthalmic nerve passes through the cavernous sinus and exits the skull through the superior orbital fissure.

Opiate: describes any of the narcotic alkaloids found in opium.

Opportunist: bacteria that are normally benign that invade the host under favorable conditions.

Opsonization: the coating of an antigen or infectious agent by antibodies or complement that facilitates uptake of the foreign particle into the phagocytic cell.

Oral epidemiology: the study of the amount, distribution, determinant, and control of disease and health conditions among given populations.

Ordinal scale of measurement: the system organizes data into mutually exclusive categories which are rank ordered based on some criterion but the difference between ranks is not necessarily equal.

Osmosis: the net movement of a solvent across a semipermeable membrane from a region of high solvent potential to an area of low solvent potential.

Osteoarthritis: a condition in which low-grade inflammation results in pain in the joints, caused by wearing of the cartilage that covers and acts as a cushion inside joints.

Osteoblast: a mononucleate cell that is responsible for bone formation. Osteoblasts produce osteoid, which is composed mainly of Type I collagen. Osteoblasts are also responsible for mineralization of the osteoid matrix. Bone is a dynamic tissue that is constantly being reshaped by osteoblasts, which build bone, and osteoclasts, which resorb bone.

Osteocyte: a star-shaped cell that is the most abundant cell found in bone. Once osteoblasts become trapped in the matrix they secrete, they become osteocytes. Osteocytes are networked to each other via long processes that occupy tiny canals called canaliculi, which are used for exchange of nutrients and waste.

Osteoma: slow-growing neoplasm of bone.

Osteomyelitis: an infection of bone or bone marrow, usually caused by pyogenic bacteria or mycobacteria.

Osteoporosis: a disease of bone in which the bone mineral density (BMD) is reduced, bone microarchitecture is disrupted, and the amount and variety of non-collagenous proteins in bone is altered.

Osteosarcoma: malignant tumor of bone.

Overhang removal: a procedure performed when the restoration is over-hanging in the interproximal area.

Ovovegetarian: a person who does not eat meat or dairy products but does eat eggs.

P.A.N.D.A.: an acronym for Prevent Abuse and Neglect through Dental Awareness. An educational program aimed at helping dental providers recognize and report child abuse.

Palatine bone: a bone in the palate.

Pancreas: an organ in the digestive and endocrine system.

Pandemic: a widespread epidemic affecting the populations of extensive areas, perhaps the whole world.

Papillary: rough surface with small projections (cauliflower-like).

Papilloma: epithelial neoplasm induced by papilloma virus.

Papule: a small, solid and usually conical elevation of the skin.

Paradigm: a model used to explain a concept or theory.

Parameter: numerical characteristic of the population.

Paranasal sinuses: air-filled spaces, communicating with the nasal cavity, within the bones of the skull and face. Humans possess a number of paranasal sinuses, divided into subgroups that are named according to the bones within which the sinuses lie.

Parasympathetic nervous system: one of three divisions of the autonomic nervous system.

Parathyroid hormone (PTH) or **parathormone:** a substance secreted by the parathyroid glands as a polypeptide containing 84 amino acids. It acts to increase the concentration of calcium in the blood, whereas calcitonin (a hormone produced by the thyroid gland) acts to decrease calcium concentration.

Parenteral: infection by a route other than the alimentary tract, such as intramuscular, intravenous, or subcutaneous.

Parietal bones: bones in the human skull that form, by their union, the sides and roof of the cranium. Each bone is irregularly quadrilateral in form, and has two surfaces, four borders, and four angles.

Parkinson's disease: a degenerative disorder of the central nervous system that often impairs the sufferer's motor skills and speech.

Parotid gland: the gland found wrapped around the mandibular ramus, secretes saliva through Stensen's duct into the oral cavity to facilitate mastication and swallowing.

Parotiditis: inflammation of the parotid gland.

Particulate radiation: atomic nuclei or subatomic particles that travel at high velocity.

Passive immunity: the transfer of active humoral immunity in the form of ready-made antibodies, from one individual to another.

Paternalism: a health provider does what he or she thinks is best for the patient according to his or her ability and judgment.

Pathogen: a microorganism, or other substance that causes disease. An opportunistic pathogen causes disease when the immune system is compromised.

Pedunculated: narrow base that grows on a stalk.

Pellagra: a vitamin deficiency disease caused by dietary lack of niacin (vitamin B_3) and protein, especially proteins containing the essential amino acid tryptophan.

Pemphigoid: an autoimmune disease that affects the basal layer membrane area; antibodies are directed against hemidesmosomes, resulting in subepithelial separation.

Pemphigus: an autoimmune disorder that causes blistering and raw sores on skin and mucous membranes.

Penciclovir: an antiviral drug used for the treatment of various herpesvirus infections.

Penicillin (sometimes abbreviated **PCN**):   refers to a group of β-lactam antibiotics used in the treatment of bacterial infections caused by susceptible, usually gram-positive, organisms.

Percutaneous: through, or by way of, the skin.

Periodontal abscess: an abscess associated with periodontal structures primarily, not pulp; tooth may be vital.

Periodontal debridement: nonsurgical removal of tooth surface irritants.

Periodontal dressings: substance applied to cover gingival wounds during healing, which provides patient comfort by protecting the healing wound.

Periodontal ligament (PDL):   a specialized connective tissue that attaches a tooth to the jaw bone. This ligament helps the tooth withstand large compressive forces which occur during chewing, without destruction of the adjacent alveolar bone.

Periodontitis: inflammation of periodontal tissues and loss of connective tissue.

Peripheral nervous system or **PNS**:   part of the nervous system that consists of the nerves and neurons that reside or extend outside the central nervous system (the brain and spinal cord), to serve the limbs and organs, for example. Unlike the central nervous system, however, the PNS is not protected by bone or the blood-brain barrier, leaving it exposed to toxins and mechanical injuries. The peripheral nervous system is divided into the somatic nervous system and the autonomic nervous system.

Permeability: a measure of the ability of a material (typically, a rock or unconsolidated material) to transmit fluids.

Permucosal: through, or by way of, a mucous membrane.

Personal protective equipment (PPE):   those items mandated by OSHA, such as barrier gowns, masks, safety glasses, and face shields, that protect the HCW from transmission of disease.

Pertussis: also known as whooping cough, this is a highly contagious disease caused by the bacterium *Bordetella pertussis*; a similar, milder disease is caused by *B. parapertussis*.

Petechiae: small, pinpoint, nonelevated red spot of submucosal bleeding.

Phagocytosis: the process by which certain immunological cells ingest and destroy other cells.

Pharmacodynamic: the study of the biochemical and physiological effects of drugs on the body or on microorganisms or parasites within or on the body and the mechanisms of drug action and the relationship between drug concentration and effect.

Pharmacokinetics: the study of what happens to a drug once it enters, circulates, and leaves the body; what factors influence absorption, distribution, metabolism, and excretion (ADME).

Phenylketonuria: a human genetic disorder in which the body does not contain the enzyme phenylalanine hydroxylase, necessary to metabolize phenylalanine to tyrosine, and converts phenylalanine instead to phenylpyruvic acid.

Pia mater: the delicate innermost layer of the meninges—the membranes surrounding the brain and spinal cord.

Pineal gland (also called the **pineal body** or **epiphysis**):   a small endocrine gland in the brain.

Placebo: a preparation which is pharmacologically inert but which may have a medical effect based solely on the power of suggestion, a response is known as the placebo effect or placebo response.

Planning: the part of the dental hygiene process of care that includes the development of a program.

Pleomorphic adenoma (mixed tumor):   slow-growing, encapsulated, sessile neoplasm of glandular tissue.

Pleurisy: also known as **pleuritis**, this is an inflammation of the pleura, the lining of the pleural cavity surrounding the lungs, which can cause painful respiration and other symptoms. Pleurisy can be generated by a variety of infectious and non-infectious causes.

Pneumonia: an illness of the lungs and respiratory system in which the alveoli (microscopic air-filled sacs of the lung responsible for absorbing oxygen from the atmosphere) become inflamed and flooded with fluid.

Poliomyelitis: often called polio or infantile paralysis, this is an acute viral infectious disease which is spread from person-to-person via the fecal-oral route.

Polishing: the final removal of material from restoration or appliance to result in a smooth surface. Polishing always follows finishing.

Polycythemia: abnormal increase in RBC count; either absolute or relative.

Polymyositis: a type of inflammatory myopathy, related to dermatomyositis and inclusion body myositis. Polymyositis means "many muscle inflammation."

Polysaccharides: sometimes called glycans these are relatively complex carbohydrates.

Porcelain: an esthetic restoration that can be used for jacket crowns, porcelain fused to metal crowns and bridges, veneers, inlays and onlays, and very rarely, denture teeth.

Poster session: a method utilized to disseminate original research findings.

Posterior: situated behind.

Posterior superior alveolar branches: branches that arise from the trunk of the maxillary nerve just before it enters the infraorbital groove; they are generally two in number, but sometimes arise by a single trunk.

Potency: a measure of the activity of a drug in a biological system.

Potentiation: interaction of two or more drugs resulting in a greater-than-expected effect.

Practice act: a statute that defines the practice of dental hygiene or dentistry.

Preceptorship: the on-the-job training of dental hygienists, sometimes referred to as alternative education.

Preexisting condition: the condition of the mouth that exists prior to the patient being covered by an insurance entity.

Premium: the monthly amount due to the insurance entity by the group or the individual.

Prepaid group practice: a large group of dental providers that contract to groups of patients.

Prevalence: a numerical expression of the number of all existing cases of a disease in a population measured at a given point.

Prima facie duties: duties that must be done at all times.

Probenecid: a uricosuric drug primarily used in treating gout or hyperuricemia, that increases uric acid removal in the urine.

Procedure number: the number given to a specific procedure as designated in the *Codes on Dental Procedures and Nomenclature* published by the ADA.

Prodromal: early signs or warnings of impending disease.

Program planning: the process of developing a dental public health program.

Prokaryotes: organisms without a cell nucleus, or any other membrane-bound organelles. Most are unicellular, but some prokaryotes are multicellular.

Prolactin (PRL): a peptide hormone primarily associated with lactation.

Promulgate: to put a law into practice as done by state dental boards.

Pronation: a rotation of the forearm that moves the palm from an anterior-facing position to a posterior-facing position, or palm facing down.

Prophylaxis: involves mechanical plaque control procedures that can be performed by dental hygienist or dentist to prevent and control periodontal diseases, such as scaling, polishing, and flossing.

Protein binding: a drug is bound reversibly to plasma proteins, a storage site; a bound drug is not free to exert its action.

Proteins: relatively large organic compounds made of amino acids arranged in a linear chain and joined together by peptide bonds between the carboxyl and amino groups of adjacent amino acid residues.

Provider: a legally licensed dental hygienist or dentist that is operating within their scope of practice.

Proximal: next to or nearest the point of attachment or origin, a central point, or the point of view; especially located toward the center of the body.

Pruritus: severe itching.

Psychomotor domain: the learning domain that describes actions.

Pterygoid plexus: a muscle of considerable size that is situated between the temporalis and pterygoideus externus, and partly between the two pterygoidei.

Public health officer: see U.S. Public Health Service Officer.

Public health: see dental public health.

Pulmonary edema: swelling and/or fluid accumulation in the lungs.

Purpura: general term for submucosal, subcutaneous bleeding.

Pustule: vesicle or bulla filled with pus.

P-value: the probability that the findings from a study are due to chance.

Pyelonephritis: an ascending urinary tract infection that has reached the *pyelum* (pelvis) of the kidney (nephros in Greek). If the infection is severe, the term **"urosepsis"** is used interchangeably.

Qualitative evaluation: answering the why and how of a dental public health program or research project.

Quantitative evaluation: a numerical evaluation of a dental public health program or research project.

Quasi-experimental research design: a research design that does not include a control group.

Quinolones: a family of broad-spectrum antibiotics.

Rabies: a viral zoonotic disease that causes acute encephalitis (inflammation of the brain) in mammals.

Radiation absorbed dose: a measurement of quantity of any type of ionizing radiation received by a mass of any type of matter including patient's tissues.

Radiation biology: the study of the effects of ionizing radiation on biological or living systems.

Radiation dose equivalent: the measure used to compare biological effects or damage an exposed individual might expect to incur from (RBE, relative biological effectiveness) different types of radiation.

Radiation exposure dose: measure of radiation quantity or exposure that refers to the ability of x-rays to ionize air; measure is taken at the skin surface before radiation has penetrated patient's tissues.

Radiation: transmission of energy through space and matter in the form of waves or particles.

Range: the range is a measurement determined by subtracting the highest score from the lowest score.

Ratio scale of measurement: a measurement that contains all the characteristics of the preceding scales, but also has an absolute zero point determined by nature.

Receptor: a protein on the cell membrane or within the cytoplasm or cell nucleus that binds to a specific molecule (a ligand), such as a neurotransmitter, hormone, or other substance, and initiates the cellular response to the ligand.

Rectal: administered as suppositories, creams, enemas for local (hemorrhoids) or systemic (antiemetic) effects; slower onset of action.

Redistribution: drugs move from the site of action to other nonspecific sites.

Reduced enamel epithelium: sometimes called **reduced dental epithelium**, this overlies a developing tooth and is formed by two layers: a layer of ameloblast cells and the adjacent layer of cuboidal cells (outer enamel epithelium) from the dental lamina.

Reference Daily Intake (RDI): the daily dietary intake level of a nutrient considered sufficient to meet the requirements of nearly all (97–98%) healthy individuals in each life-stage and gender group.

Regional odontodysplasia (ghost teeth on x-ray): evidence of thin enamel and dentin with large pulp chambers.

Regulation: the state dental boards' procedure which further defines the law.

Reliability: the reproducibility of a research study.

Removable partial denture: a prosthetic device that replaces missing teeth and is often retained with the aid of clasps.

Reproductive system: the ensembles and interactions of organs and/or substances within an organism that strictly pertain to reproduction.

Research types: the way of categorizing research studies.

Researcher: a person who conducts research germane to the study of health and disease.

Resilience: the ability of a material to resist permanent deformation.

Resistance: the results that occur when microorganisms are unaffected by an antimicrobial agent; may be natural (always has been resistant) or acquired (develops resistance).

Resolution: ability of a radiograph to record and demonstrate separate structures that are close together.

Respiratory system: the system that generally includes tubes, such as the bronchi, used to carry air to the lungs, where gas exchange takes place.

Responsibility: the trait of being answerable to someone for something or controlling one's conduct according to accepted conventions.

Retrocuspid papilla: fibrous elevation lingual to mandibular canines.

Retrovirus: RNA is the core genetic material of this virus; the enzyme reverse transcriptase is required to convert RNA to proviral DNA.

Rhabdomyoma: neoplasm of striated (voluntary) muscle.

Rhabdomyosarcoma: malignancy of skeletal muscle; rapidly growing submucosal mass with induration.

Rheumatic fever: an inflammatory disease which may develop after a Group A streptococcal infection (such as strep throat or scarlet fever) and can involve the heart, joints, skin, and brain.

Rheumatoid arthritis (RA): traditionally considered a chronic, inflammatory autoimmune disorder that causes the immune system to attack the joints. It is a disabling and painful inflammatory condition, which can lead to substantial loss of mobility due to pain and joint destruction.

Ribosome: a small, dense organelle in cells that assembles proteins.

Rickets: a softening of the bones in children, potentially leading to fractures and deformity. The predominant cause is a vitamin D deficiency, but lack of adequate calcium in the diet may also lead to rickets.

Rickettsia: a genus of non-motile, gram-negative, non-spore-forming, highly pleomorphic bacteria that can present as cocci, or threadlike.

Rifampicin: a bactericidal antibiotic drug typically used to treat *Mycobacterium* infections, including tuberculosis and leprosy; and also has a role in the treatment of methicillin-resistant *Staphylococcus aureus* (MRSA) in combination with fusidic acid.

Risk factors: the characteristics of an individual or population that may increase the likelihood of experiencing a given health problem.

Risk management: a system used to prevent patient harm or neglect, financial loss or legal problems.

Root planing: smoothing of root surfaces, including removal of rough cementum or dentin that is impregnated with calculus and endotoxins.

Rotation: a motion that occurs when a part turns on its axis. The head rotates on the neck, as in shaking the head no.

Rules: the state dental boards' interpretation of a law.

Rural: a geographic area that is sparsely populated.

Sagittal suture: a dense, fibrous connective tissue joint between the two parietal bones of the skull.

Salt fluoridation: the addition of fluoride to salt, used in some countries to deliver fluoride to populations.

Scaling: removal of calculus and stain from surfaces of teeth with hand-activated instruments and/or sonic and ultrasonic scalers.

School fluoridation: the addition of fluoride at approximately 5 ppm to a school's water supply to decrease dental caries in the student population.

School mouthrinse programs: fluoride mouthrinses that are used weekly in school rinse programs in areas without water fluoridation; they contain 0.20% NaF (900ppm).

Sclerotic: appears more radiopaque than normal.

Selective polishing: polishing the teeth only when extrinsic stain and visible plaque cannot be removed with hand or ultrasonic instrumentation. Evidenced-based practice dictates the use of selective polishing.

Self-regulation: regulation of dental hygienists by dental hygienists.

Sequelae: long-term or permanent damage to organs or tissue as a result of disease.

Seroconversion: the presence of antibodies is changed from negative (seronegative) to positive (seropositive) after exposure to the etiological agents of the disease.

Serological marker or diagnosis: specific laboratory finding of an antibody or an antigen that identifies a disease.

Sessile: wide base without stalk.

Sharpey's fibers: a matrix of connective tissue consisting of bundles of strong collagenous fibers connecting periosteum to bone. They are part of the outer fibrous layer of periosteum, entering into the outer circumferential and interstitial lamellae of bone tissue.

Sharpness: ability of a radiograph to define an edge.

Shear stress: the stress when material is forced to slide back and forth.

Sialadenitis: inflammation of salivary gland tissue.

Sialodochitis: inflammation of salivary gland duct.

Sialolithiasis: stone formation.

Side effect: a dose-related reaction not part of the desired therapeutic outcome; occurs when the drug acts on a nontarget organ.

Sign: objective, observable, and measurable changes in the client's condition (e.g., fever).

Simple diffusion: substance moves from high concentration to low concentration.

Single procedure: a specific procedure designated by a specific code.

Sjögren's syndrome: lymphocytic infiltration of salivary glands resulting in loss of function.

Skeletal muscle: a type of striated muscle that is attached to the skeleton. Skeletal muscles are used to facilitate movement by applying force to bones and joints via contraction.

Skeletal system: the biological system providing physical support in living organisms.

Skew: the tail of a distribution formed by a few extreme scores.

Slander: verbal defamation.

Smooth muscle: a type of non-striated muscle, found within the "walls" of hollow organs and elsewhere like the bladder and abdominal cavity, the uterus, male and female reproductive tracts, the gastrointestinal tract, the respiratory tract, the vasculature, the skin, and the ciliary muscle and iris of the eye.

Social worker: a professional who works at helping individuals, or the community, enhance their capacity for social functioning.

Socioeconomic status (SES): an individual's comparative status in social and economic standing within a community.

Sound natural teeth: teeth that are either primary or permanent that have adequate hard and soft tissue support.

Spectrum: range of action of a drug.

Sphenoid bone: a bone situated at the base of the skull in front of the temporals and basilar part of the occipital.

Spinal cord: a thin, tubular structure that is an extension of the central nervous system from the brain and is enclosed in, and protected by, the bony vertebral column.

Spleen: an organ of the upper abdomen that functions in the destruction of old red blood cells and holds a reservoir of blood. It is regarded as one of the centers of activity of the reticuloendothelial system (part of the immune system).

Squamosal suture: arches backward from the pterion and connects the temporal squama with the lower border of the parietal: this suture is continuous behind with the short, nearly horizontal parietomastoid suture, which unites the mastoid process of the temporal with the region of the mastoid angle of the parietal.

Squamous cell carcinoma: a form of cancer of the carcinoma type that may occur in many different organs, including the skin, mouth, esophagus, prostate, lungs, and cervix.

Standard deviation: the measure of dispersion.

State Children Health Insurance Program (SCHIP): a program that was created by the federal government to cover individuals that have incomes too high to qualify for state medical assistance but cannot obtain private insurance. All states participate, but some do not cover dental.

STD: sexually transmitted disease.

Stella turcica: "turkish saddle," cavity within the sphenoid bone where the pituitary gland resides.

Sterilization: the elimination of all transmissible agents from a surface, a piece of equipment, food, or biological culture medium.

Stevens-Johnson syndrome: multisystem disease of erythema multiforme; usually involves ocular, oral, and genital regions.

Strain: the change in length produced by stress.

Strength: the greatest stress that can be withstood without rupture.

Streptococcus mutans: a Gram-positive, facultatively anaerobic bacteria commonly found in the human oral cavity and is a significant contributor to tooth decay.

Stress: a materials' response to force.

Stroke: a rapidly developing loss of part of brain function or loss of conciousness due to an interuption in the blood supply to all or part of the brain.

Subcutaneous injection: an injection administered into the subcutis, the layer of skin directly below the dermis and epidermis, collectively referred to as the cutis.

Sublingual glands: salivary glands in the mouth. They lie anterior to the submandibular gland under the tongue, beneath the mucous membrane of the floor of the mouth.

Submandibular glands: salivary glands located beneath the floor of the mouth. In humans, they account for 70% of the salivary volume.

Sucrose (common name: **table sugar**, also called **saccharose**): a disaccharide (glucose + fructose) with the molecular formula $C_{12}H_{22}O_{11}$.

Sugar alcohol: a hydrogenated form of carbohydrate, whose carbonyl group (aldehyde or ketone, reducing sugar) has been reduced to a primary or secondary hydroxyl group. They are commonly used for replacing sucrose in foodstuffs, often in combination with high intensity artificial sweeteners to counter the low sweetness.

Sulcular (crevicular) fluid: serum-like fluid that passes from gingival connective tissue through tissues into the sulcus; an inflammatory exudate.

Sulfonylurea derivatives: a class of antidiabetic drugs that are used in the management of diabetes mellitus type 2 ("adult-onset"). They act by increasing insulin release from the beta cells in the pancreas.

Summation: combined activities of two or more drugs that elicit identical or related pharmacological effects; effect is not greater.

Summative evaluation: an evaluation of all parts of an implemented program.

Superficial: relating to, or located near, a surface.

Superinfection, suprainfection: infection caused by the overgrowth of microbes different from the causative microorganism (e.g., *Candida* infection after antibiotic therapy).

Superior: situated higher up.

Supernumerary: extra teeth.

Supination: the rotation of the forearm so that the palm faces anteriorly, or palm facing up.

Supply: the quantity of dental care services available.

Suppressor T cells: a specialized subpopulation of T cells that act to suppress activation of the immune system and thereby maintain immune system homeostasis and tolerance to self.

Suprahyoid muscles: the muscles that include digastricus, stylohyoideus, geniohyoideus, and mylohyoideus.

Suprahyoid: a term that refers to the region above (superior to) the hyoid bone in the neck.

Surgeon general: the appointed administrator of the U.S. Public Health Service.

Surveillance: the methods or systems used to monitor disease and morbidity in a population periodically or on an ongoing basis.

Susceptible host: a person or organism not possessing resistance against an infectious agent.

Sympathetic nervous system: the system responsible for up- or down-regulating many homeostatic mechanisms in living organisms.

Symptom: subjective changes reported by the client (e.g., pain).

Synapses: specialized junctions through which cells of the nervous system signal to one another and to non-neuronal cells such as muscles or glands.

Syneresis: the exudation of liquid film on the surface of a gel.

Synergism: combination of two or more agonists producing an effect greater than can be achieved by the maximum dose of one of those drugs.

Syphilis: a sexually transmitted disease (STD) caused by *Spirochaeta* bacterium, *Treponema pallidum*.

Systemic fluoride (pre-eruptive fluoride): fluoride taken internally that is made available to the developing teeth by way of the blood plasma to the tissues surrounding the tooth bud; after tooth mineralization, but before tooth eruption.

Systemic lupus erythematosus (SLE or lupus): a chronic autoimmune disease that is potentially debilitating and sometimes fatal as the immune system attacks the body's cells and tissue, resulting in inflammation and tissue damage.

Systole: the contraction of the chambers of the heart, driving blood out of the chambers. The chamber most often discussed is the left ventricle.

T cells: cells belong to a group of white blood cells known as lymphocytes that play a central role in cell-mediated immunity. They can be distinguished from other lymphocyte types, such as B cells and NK cells by the presence of a special receptor on their cell surface that is called the T cell receptor (TCR).

Table clinic: a method utilized to disseminate past research studies and literature reviews of a specific topic.

Tachypnea: rapid respiration.

Talon cusp: accessory cusp found on the maxillary and mandibular anteriors.

Target population: a representation of a certain segment of the population.

Tarnish: a surface reaction in metals seen as the discoloration of surface and is reversible.

Taurodontism: elongated pulp chamber with short roots.

Temporal bone: a compound bone of the side of the skull of some mammals including humans.

Temporary restoratives: restorations used to provide temporary protection to the pulp, provide a palliative effect on the pulp, to be obtudant to the pulp, maintain tooth position, and provide esthetic properties.

Temporomandibular joint (TMJ): a diarthrodial joint that connects the condyle of the mandible (lower jaw) to the temporal bone at the side of a skull. As a modified hinge joint, not only does the TMJ enable the jaw to rotate open and closed, it also enables the jaw to translate forward and backward. The condyle can also move laterally and medially.

Tendon: a tough band of fibrous connective tissue that connects muscle to bone or muscle to muscle and is designed to withstand tension. Tendons are similar to ligaments except that ligaments join one bone to another. Tendons and muscles work together and can only exert a pulling force.

Tensile stress: the stress when material is pulled apart.

Teratogenic: adverse effect of a drug on the fetus, producing deformities.

Testosterone: a steroid hormone from the androgen group. Testosterone is primarily secreted in the testes of males and the ovaries of females although small amounts are secreted by the adrenal glands. It is the principal male sex hormone and an anabolic steroid. In both males and females, it plays key roles in health and well-being.

Tetracyclines: a group of broad-spectrum antibiotics whose general usefulness has been reduced with the onset of bacterial resistance.

Thalamus: a pair and symmetric part of the brain. It constitutes the main part of the diencephalon.

Therapeutic Index (TI): the ratio of the median lethal dose (LD50) to the median effective dose (ED50); express the safety of the drug; the greater the TI, the safer the drug.

Therapeutic services: the services the dental hygienist provides that benefit the patient. These may include periodontal debridement, polishing, fluoride application, local anesthesia, dental sealants, education, and behavior modification interventions.

Thermal conductivity: the rate of heat flow of the material.

Three-party system: the dental provider renders the service and a sponsor of the patient pays for the service: (e.g., the insurance company or employer pays the dental provider for the service).

Thrombocytes: the cell fragments circulating in the blood that are involved in the cellular mechanisms of primary hemostasis leading to the formation of blood clots.

Thrombocytopenia: a decrease in circulating platelets.

Thymus: an organ located in the upper anterior portion of the chest cavity. It is of central importance in the maturation of T cells.

Thyroid hormones: thyroxine (T_4) and triiodothyronine (T_3), are tyrosine-based hormones produced by the thyroid gland.

Thyroid-stimulating hormone (also known as **TSH** or **thyrotropin**): a hormone synthesized and secreted by thyrotrope cells in the anterior pituitary gland which regulates the endocrine function of the thyroid gland.

Tic douloureux: a painful condition in which the trigeminal nerve is affected by pressure or degeneration.

Tonsils: areas of lymphoid tissue on either side of the throat. An infection of the tonsils is called tonsillitis. Most commonly, the term "tonsils" refers to the palatine tonsils that can be seen in the back of the throat.

Tooth enamel: the hardest and most highly mineralized substance of the body and which, with dentin, cementum, and dental pulp, is one of the four major tissues which make up the tooth. It is the normally visible dental tissue of a tooth and must be supported by underlying dentin. Ninety-six percent of enamel consists of mineral, with water and organic material composing the rest.

Topical: local application to oral mucous membranes, skin, and other epithelial surfaces for local or systemic effects (e.g., anesthetic).

Topical fluoride (post-eruptive fluoride): fluoride application that inhibits demineralization and enhances remineralization.

Total filtration: the sum of inherent and added filtration.

Toughness: the ability of a material to resist fracture or simply the energy necessary to fracture a material.

Toxemia: presence of toxin in the bloodstream.

Toxic effect: the result that exceeds the amount of desired effect; dose-related, predictable.

Toxoplasmosis: a parasitic disease caused by the protozoan *Toxoplasma gondii.*

Transdermal: providing continuous controlled release of medication through semipermeable membrane after application to intact skin (e.g., estrogen/nicotine patches).

Transmission (horizontal): one individual passes an infectious agent to another.

Transmission (vertical): an infectious agent is passed from one generation to another, across the placenta, or through breast milk.

Transparency: the passage of minimally distorted light through a material such that objects may be clearly seen through it.

Transulency: the dispersion of light through a material such that objects cannot be seen through it.

Trigeminal nerve (the **fifth cranial nerve**, also called the **fifth nerve** or simply **V**): the nerve responsible for sensation in the face. Sensory information from the face and body is processed by parallel pathways in the central nervous system.

Tuberculosis (abbreviated as **TB** for **tubercle bacillus**): a common and deadly infectious disease caused by the mycobacterium *Mycobacterium tuberculosis* or *Mycobacterium bovis.*

Tumor: swelling; frequently used interchangeably with neoplasm.

Two-party system: the dental provider renders the service and the patient pays the dental provider for the service.

U.S. Public Health Service Officer: a dental hygienist or dentist that is a commissioned officer of the U.S. Public Health Services.

UCR (Usual, customary, and reasonable fee): the fee that reflects the average dentist fee per service in the immediate local region.

Unbound drug: a drug that can cross membranes to the site of action, bind to cell receptor, and cause an action.

Unilocular: only one radiolucent compartment.

Universal precautions (universal standards): the philosophy of infection control in which all human blood and some human bodily fluids are treated as if known to be infected with blood-borne pathogens (BBP).

Urban: a concentrated human settlement, usually consisting of at least 2,500 people.

Urinary system: the organ system that produces, stores, and eliminates urine. In humans it includes two kidneys, two ureters, the urinary bladder, two sphincter muscles, and the urethra.

Urticaria (also called **hives**): vascular reaction of skin, characterized by wheals or papules.

Utilization: the number of dental care services actually consumed.

Validity: the degree to which the research study measured what it was supposed to measure.

Value: the lightness of an object.

Variance: the squared deviation of each score from the mean's sum.

Vasoconstrictor (also **vasopressor** or simply **pressor**): any substance that acts to cause vasoconstriction (narrowing of the lumena of blood vessels) and usually results in an increase of the blood pressure.

Vasodilation: the process whereby blood vessels in the body become wider following the relaxation of the smooth muscle in the vessel wall.

Vector: the carrier that transfers an infectious microorganism from one host to another. Biological vectors may be arthropods, insects, or other living carriers in whose body the microorganism multiplies.

Vegan: one who practices veganism—does not consume or use animal products, notably meat, fish, poultry, eggs, and dairy products.

Vehicle: the object or substance serving as an intermediary in which the infectious organism is transported and introduced into a new susceptible host.

Veneer: a restoration that replaces the facial surface of anterior teeth.

Ventral: of, or relating to, the belly.

Ventricular diastole: the ventricles are relaxing, while **atrial diastole** is when the atria are relaxing.

Vesicle: fluid-filled blister < 5 mm in diameter.

Virion: the complete virus particle consisting of the nucleoid (genetic information) and the capsid (protective protein shell).

Virulence: the degree of pathogenicity; ability to invade host, toxin production, number of microorganisms present.

Virus: a subcellular entity that gains entrance to living cells and is capable of replication only within those cells; may contain DNA or RNA.

Vomer: one of the unpaired facial bones of the skull. It is located in the midsagittal line, and touches the sphenoid, the ethmoid, the left and right palatine bones, and the left and right maxillary bones.

Warfarin (also known under the brand names of Coumadin®, Jantoven®, Marevan®, and Waran®): an anticoagulant medication that is administered orally or, very rarely, by injection.

Warthin's tumor (papillary cystadenoma lymphomatosum): glandular neoplasm.

Water fluoridation: the addition of fluoride in public water supplies, when it is not naturally occurring at a significant amount.

Well-circumscribed: well-defined border with clearly defined margins.

Wettability: the measure of the affinity of a liquid for a solid as indicted by the spreading of a drop of liquid; sometimes referred to as the contact angle.

Window period: the time between exposure, resulting in infection and the serological antibody marker; the infectious agent is transmissible, but the antibody test is negative.

Xerostomia: dryness of mouth owing to reduced salivary flow.

Xylitol: a sugar substitute that has shown promising results in reducing dental caries and ear infections.

Zygomatic bone: a paired bone of the human skull. It articulates with the maxilla, the temporal bone, the sphenoid bone, and the frontal bone. It forms part of the orbit and is commonly referred to as the cheekbone. It is situated at the upper and lateral part of the face: it forms the prominence of the cheek, part of the lateral wall and floor of the orbit, and parts of the temporal and infratemporal fossae.

References

CHAPTER 1

Aquir, A. *Giant's Atlas of Anatomy* (10th ed.). Philadelphia: Lippincott Williams & Wilkins, 1999.

Brand, R. & Isselhard, D. *Anatomy of Orofacial Structures* (6th ed.). St. Louis: Mosby, 1998.

Brand, R. & Isselhard, D. *Study Guide to Accompany the Sixth Edition of Anatomy of Orofacial Structures.* St. Louis: Mosby, 1998.

Darby, M. *Comprehensive Review of Dental Hygiene* (6th ed.). St. Louis: Mosby, 2006.

Fremgen, B. & Frucht, S. *Medical Terminology: An Anatomy and Physiology Systems Approach* (2nd ed.). Upper Saddle River, NJ: Prentice Hall, 2002.

Gardner, M. *Basic Anatomy of the Head and Neck* (1st ed.). Philadelphia: Lea & Febiger, 1992.

Grant, J.C. *A Method of Anatomy* (2nd ed.). Baltimore: Williams & Wilkins, 1940.

Hiatt, J. & Gartner, L. *Texbook of Head and Neck Anatomy* (1st ed.). Baltimore: Williams & Wilkins, 1987.

Karst, N. & Smith, S. *Dental Anatomy: A Self-Instructional Program* (10th ed.). Stamford, CT: Appleton and Lange, 1998.

King, B. & Showers, M.J. *Human Anatomy and Physiology* (6th ed.). Philadelphia: W.B. Saunders Co., 1963.

Mader, S.S. *Understanding Human Anatomy and Physiology* (3rd ed.). Dubuque, IA: Wm. C. Brown Publishers, 1997.

Martinti, H. & Bartholomew, E. *Essentials of Anatomy and Physiology* (2nd ed.). Upper Saddle River, NJ: Prentice Hall, 1999.

Melphi, R. *Permar's Oral Embryology and Microscopic Anatomy* (9th ed.). Philadelphia: Lea & Febiger, 1994.

Moore, K. *The Developing Human* (1st ed.). Philadelphia: W.B. Saunders Co., 1973.

Moore, K.L. & Dalley, A.F. *Clinically Oriented Anatomy* (4th ed.). Philadelphia: Lippincott Williams & Wilkins, 1999.

Reed, G. & Sheppard, V. *Basic Structures of the Head and Neck* (1st ed.). Philadelphia: W.B. Saunders Co., 1976.

Rice, J. *Medical Terminology with Human Anatomy* (5th ed.). Upper Saddle River, NJ: Prentice Hall, 2005.

Rosse, C. & Gaddum-Rosse, P. *Hollinshead's Textbook of Anatomy* (5th ed.). Philadelphia: Lippincott-Raven, 1997.

Smith, S. & Karst, N. *Head and Neck Histology and Anatomy.* Stamford, CT: Appleton and Lange, 2000.

Thomas, C. *Taber's Cyclopedia Medical Dictionary* (16th ed.). Philadelphia: F.A. Davis Company, 1989.

Woefel, J.B. & Scheid, R.C. *Dental Anatomy: Its Relevance to Dentistry* (5th ed.). Baltimore: Williams & Wilkins, 1997.

CHAPTER 2

D'Amico, D. & Barbarito, C. *Health and Physical Assessment in Nursing.* Upper Saddle River, NJ: Prentice Hall, 2007.

Fremgen, B. & Frucht, S. *Medical Terminology: An Anatomy and Physiology Systems Approach* (2nd ed.). Upper Saddle River, NJ: Prentice Hall, 2002.

Martinti, H. & Bartholomew, E. *Essentials of Anatomy and Physiology* (2nd ed.). Upper Saddle River, NJ: Prentice Hall, 1999.

Netter, F. *Digestive System, Vols 1–3.* New York: Ciba, 1971.

Netter, F. *Endocrine System and Selected Metabolic Diseases.* New York: Ciba, 1970.

Netter, F. *Heart.* New York: Ciba, 1971.

Netter, F. *Kidneys, Ureters, and Urinary Bladder.* New York: Ciba, 1973.

Netter, F. *Nervous System.* New York: Ciba, 1968.

Netter, F. *Reproductive System.* Summit, NJ: Ciba, 1954.

Rice, J. *Medical Terminology with Human Anatomy* (5th ed.). Upper Saddle River, NJ: Prentice Hall, 2005.

CHAPTER 3

Davis, J.R. & Stegeman, C.A. *The Dental Hygienist's Guide to Nutritional Care* (1st ed.). Philadelphia: W.B. Saunders Co., 1998.

Dietary guidelines for Americans 2005 (6th ed.). Hyattsville: U.S. Departments of Agriculture and Health and Human Services. *Home and Garden Bulletin* 232-CP, 2005.

Food and Nutrition Board. *Dietary Reference Intakes: Calcium, Phosphorus, Magnesium, Vitamin D, and Fluoride.* Washington, D.C.: National Academy of Sciences, 1997.

Insel, P., Turner, E., & Ross, D. *Nutrition.* Jones and Bartlett, 2001.

Mahan, L.K. & Escott-Stump, S. *Krause's Food, Nutrition, and Diet Therapy* (9th ed.). W.B. Saunders Co., 1996.

Palmer, C. *Diet and Nutrition in Oral Health* (2nd ed.). Upper Saddle River, NJ: Prentice Hall, 2007.

Whitney, N. & Rolfes, S. *Understanding Nutrition.* Boulder, CO: Wadsworth, 1999.

Zeman, F. & Ney, D. *Applications in Medical Nutrition Therapy* (2nd ed.). Upper Saddle River, NJ: Prentice Hall, 1996.

CHAPTER 4

Alcamo, I.E. *Fundamental of Microbiology* (5th ed.). Menlo Park, CA: Addison Wesley Longman, 1997.

Black, J.G. *Microbiology Principles & Applications* (3rd ed.). Upper Saddle River, NJ: Prentice Hall, 1996.

Janusz, S. *Adventures in Learning.* Champaign, IL: Periodontology Board Review, 1999.

Jensen, M., Wright, D., & Robison, R. *Microbiology for the Health Sciences* (4th ed.). Upper Saddle River, NJ: Prentice Hall, 1997.

Madigan, M.T., Martinko, J.M., & Parker, J. *Brock Biology of Microorganisms* (8th ed.). Upper Saddle River, NJ: Prentice Hall, 1997.

Nester, E.W., Roberts, C.E., & Nester, M.T. *Microbiology: A Human Perspective.* Dubuque, IA: Wm. C. Brown Publishers, 1995.

Schaechter, M., Engleberg, N.C., Eisenstein, B.I., & Medoff, G. *Mechanisms of Microbial Disease* (3rd ed.). Baltimore: Williams & Wilkins, 1998.

Wilkins, E.M. *Clinical Practice of the Dental Hygienist* (10th ed.). Philadelphia: Lippincott Williams & Wilkins, 2009.

Willet, N.P., White, R.R., & Rosen, S. *Essential Dental Microbiology.* Norwalk, CT: Appleton & Lange, 1991.

CHAPTER 5

Ibsen, O. & Phelan J. *Oral Pathology for the Dental Hygienist* (3rd ed.). Philadelphia: W.B. Saunders, 2000.

Langlais, R.P. & Miller C.S. *Color Atlas of Common Oral Conditions.* Philadelphia: Williams & Wilkins, 1998.

Newland, R., Meiller, T., Wynn, R., & Crossley, H. *Oral Soft Tissue Diseases.* Hudson, OH: Lexi-Comp, 2001.

Neville, D. & Allen B. *Oral and Maxillofacial Pathology.* Philadelphia: W.B. Saunders, 1995.

Regezi, S. *Oral Pathology: Clinical-Pathologic Correlation,* (3rd ed.). Philadelphia: W.B. Saunders Co., 1999.

CHAPTER 6

Adams, M.P., Josephson, D.L., Holland, L.N., *Pharmacology for Nurses: A Pathophysiologic Approach* (2nd ed.). Upper Saddle River, NJ: Prentice Hall, 2007.

Christ, D. *High-Yield Pharmacology.* Philadelphia: Lippincott Williams & Wilkins, 1999.

D'Amico, D., & Barbarito, C., *Health and Physical Assessment in Nursing.* Upper Saddle River, NJ: Prentice Hall, 2005.

Gage, T. & Pickett, F. *Mosby's Dental Drug Reference* (4th ed.). St Louis: Mosby, 1999.

Haveles, E. *Pharmacology for Dental Hygiene Practice.* Cincinatti: Delmar, 1997.

Requa-Clark, B. *Applied Pharmacology for the Dental Hygienist* (4th ed.). St. Louis: Mosby, 2000.

Whynn, R., Meiller, T., & Crossley, H. *Drug Information Handbook for Dentistry* (5th ed.). Hudson, OH: Lexi-Comp, 1999.

Yagiela, J.A., Neidle, E.A., & Dowd, F.J. *Pharmacology and Therapeutics for Dentistry* (4th ed.). St Louis: Mosby, 1998.

CHAPTER 7

Annals of Periodontology: 1996 World Workshop in Periodontics, vol. 1. Chicago: American Academy of Periodontology, 1996.

Cooper, M.D. & Wiechmann, L. *Essentials of Dental Hygiene: Preclinical Skills.* Upper Saddle River, NJ: Prentice Hall, 2005.

Cooper, M.D. & Wiechmann, L., *Essentials of Dental Hygiene: Clinical Skills.* Upper Saddle River, NJ: Prentice Hall, 2005

Darby, M.L. & Walsh, M.M. *Dental Hygiene Theory and Practice.* Philadelphia: W.B. Saunders, 1995.

Weinberg, M.A., Westphal, C., Froum, S.J., & Palat, M., *Comprehensive Periodontics for the Dental Hygienists* (2nd ed.). Upper Saddle River, NJ: Prentice Hall, 2006.

Wilkins, E.M. *Clinical Practice of the Dental Hygienist* (10th ed.). Philadelphia: Lippincott Williams & Wilkins, 2009.

Woodall, I.R. *Comprehensive Dental Hygiene Care* (4th ed.). St. Louis: Mosby, 1993.

CHAPTER 8

Frommer, H. *Radiology for Dental Auxiliaries* (7th ed.). St. Louis: Mosby, 2001.

Goaz, P.W. & White S.C. *Oral Radiology: Principles and Interpretation* (3rd ed.). St Louis: Mosby-Yearbook, 1994.

Haring, J.I. & Lind, L. *Dental Radiography: Principles and Techniques.* Philadelphia: W.B. Saunders, 1996.

Hodges, K.O. *Concepts in Nonsurgical Periodontal Therapy.* Cincinnati: Delmar Publishers, 1997.

Holm-Pedersen, P. & Loe, H. *Textbook of Geriatric Dentistry* (2nd ed.). Copenhagen: Munksgaard, 1996.

Johnson, O., McNally, M., & Essay, C. *Essentials of Dental Radiography for Dental Assistants and Hygienists* (8th ed.). Upper Saddle River, NJ: Prentice Hall, 2007.

Papas, A.S., Niessen, L.C., & Chauncey, H.H. *Geriatric Dentistry, Aging and Oral Health.* St Louis: Mosby-Yearbook, 1991.

Physicians' Desk Reference (52nd ed.). Montvale, NJ: Medical Economics Company, 1998.

Razmus, T.F. & Williamson, G.F. *Current Oral and Maxillofacial Imaging.* Philadelphia: W.B. Saunders, 1996.

Thomson-Lakey, E. *Exercises in Oral Radiography Techniques: A Laboratory Manual.* Upper Saddle River, NJ: Prentice Hall, 2003.

White S. & Pharoah, M. *Oral Radiology Principles and Interpretation.* St. Louis: Mosby, 2000.

Woodall, I.R. *Comprehensive Dental Hygiene* (4th ed.). St Louis: Mosby-Yearbook, 1993.

CHAPTER 9

American Red Cross *First Aid – Responding to Emergencies.* St Louis: Mosby Lifeline, 2006.

Centers for Disease Control. *HIV/AIDS Surveillance report.* Online. http://www.cdc.gov/nchstp/hiv_aids/stats/hasr1001.pdf. 1998;1:3.37–40.

Cooper, M.D. & Wiechmann, L. *Essentials of Dental Hygiene: Preclinical Skills.* Upper Saddle River, NJ: Prentice Hall, 2005.

Cooper, M.D. & Wiechmann, L. *Essentials of Dental Hygiene: Clinical Skills.* Upper Saddle River, NJ: Prentice Hall, 2005

Darby, M.L. & Walsh, M.M. *Dental Hygiene Theory and Practice.* Philadelphia: W.B. Saunders, 1995.

Evans, D. *HIV Diagnostic Tests.* Online. http://www.projinf.org/fs/HIVDiagTest.htm1\#CommonLabTests. 1997:1–14.

Evans, D. *Project Inform Perspective: Number 21-March 1997.* Online. http://www.projinf.org/pub/21/ViralLoad.html. 1997;1–3.

Hughes, M., et al. CD4 cell count as a surrogate endpoint in HIV clinical trials: A metaanalysis of studies of the AIDS Clinical Trials Group. *AIDS* 1998;12:1823–32.

Hughes, M., et al. Monitoring plasma HIV-1 RNA levels in addition to CD4+ lymphocyte count improves assessment of antiretroviral therapeutic response. *Annals of Internal Medicine* 1997;126:929–38.

Little, J.W. & Falace, D. *Dental Management of the Medically Compromised Patient.* St. Louis: Mosby, 1997.

Malamed, S. *Handbook of Local Anesthesia* (5th ed.). St. Louis: Mosby, 2004.

Malamed, S. *Medical Emergencies in the Dental Office* (5th ed.). St. Louis: Mosby, 2003.

Mancano, M. Focus on selected meperidine and codeine drug interactions. *Pharmacy Times,* April 2000.

O'Toole, M. *Miller-Keane Encyclopedia and Dictionary of Medicine, Nursing, & Allied Health.* Philadelphia: W.B. Saunders, 1996.

Rhoades, R. & Pflanzer, R. *Human Physiology.* Philadelphia: W.B. Saunders, 1992.

Stein, D.S., Korcik, J.A., & Vermund, S.H. CD4+ lymphocyte cell enumeration for prediction of clinical courses of human immunodeficiency virus disease: A review. *J of Inf Diseases* 1992;165:352–63.

Treatment Strategy. *Project Inform Discussion Paper.* San Francisco: Treatment Strategy, 1996.

UNAIDS Press Release: AIDS moves up to fourth place among would-be killers. Online. http://www.unaids.org/highband/press/whr99.html 1999:1–2.

Weinberg, M.A., Westphal, C., Froum, S.J., & Palat, M. *Comprehensive Periodontics for the Dental Hygienists* (2nd ed.). Upper Saddle River, NJ: Prentice Hall, 2006.

Whitney, N. & Rolfes, S. *Understanding Nutrition.* Boulder, CO: Wadsworth, 1999.

Wilkins, E.M. *Clinical Practice of the Dental Hygienist* (10th ed.). Philadelphia: Lippincott Williams & Wilkins, 2009.

Woodall, I.R. *Comprehensive Dental Hygiene Care* (4th ed.). St. Louis: Mosby, 1993.

CHAPTER 10

Cooper, M.D. & Wiechmann, L. *Essentials of Dental Hygiene: Clinical Skills.* Upper Saddle River, NJ: Prentice Hall, 2005.

Cooper, M.D. & Wiechmann, L. *Essentials of Dental Hygiene: Preclinical Skills.* Upper Saddle River, NJ: Prentice Hall, 2005.

Darby, M. *Comprehensive Review of Dental Hygiene* (6th ed.). St Louis: Mosby, 2006.

Darby, M.L. & Walsh, M.M. *Dental Hygiene Theory and Practice.* Philadelphia: W.B. Saunders, 1995.

Fedi, P.F. & Vernino, A.R. *The Periodontal Syllabus* (3rd ed.). Baltimore: Williams & Wilkins, 1995.

Newman, M.G., Takei, H.H., Klokkevold, P.R., & Carranza, R.E. *Clinical Periodontology* (10th ed.). Philadelphia: W.B. Saunders, 2006.

Schwartz, M., Lamster, I.B., & Fine, J.B. *Clinical Guide to Periodontics* Philadelphia: W.B. Saunders, 1995.

Weinberg, M.A., Westphal, C., Froum, S.J., & Palat, M. *Comprehensive Periodontics for the Dental Hygienists* (2nd ed.). Upper Saddle River, NJ: Prentice Hall, 2006.

Wilkins, E.M. *Clinical Practice of the Dental Hygienist* (10th ed.). Philadelphia: Lippincott Williams & Wilkins, 2009.

Woodall, I. *Comprehensive Dental Hygiene Care* (4th ed.). St Louis: Mosby, 1993.

CHAPTER 11

Darby, M.L. & Walsh, M.M. *Dental Hygiene Theory and Practice* (2nd ed.). Philadelphia: W.B. Saunders, 2003.

Nathe, C. *Dental Public Health: Contemporary Practice for the Dental Hygienist.* (2nd ed.). Upper Saddle River, NJ: Prentice Hall, 2005.

Wilkins, E.M. *Clinical Practice of the Dental Hygienist* (10th ed.). Philadelphia: Lippincott Williams & Wilkins, 2009.

CHAPTER 12

Craig, R., O'Brien, W., & Powers, J. *Dental Materials: Properties and Manipulation* (5th ed.). St. Louis: Mosby, 1992.

Craig, R.G., O'Brien, W.J., & Powers, J.M. *Dental Materials: Properties and Manipulation* (6th ed.). St Louis: Mosby, 1996.

Darby, M.L. *Mosby's Comprehensive Review of Dental Hygiene* (6th ed.). St Louis: Mosby, 2006.

Ferrace, J. *Materials in Dentistry: Principles and Applications* (2nd ed.). Philadelphia: Lippincott Williams & Wilkins, 2000.

Gladwin, M. & Bagby, M. *Clinical Aspects of Dental Materials.* Philadelphia: Lippincott Williams & Wilkins, 2000.

Phillips, R.W. & Moore, B.K. *Elements of Dental Materials* (5th ed.). Philadelphia: W.B. Saunders, 1994.

CHAPTER 13

Beemsterboer, P.L. *Ethics and Law in Dental Hygiene.* Philadelphia: W.B. Saunders. 2002.

Flynn, E.P. *Issues in Health Care Ethics.* Upper Saddle River, NJ: Prentice Hall, 2000.

Kimbrough, V.J. & Lautar, C.J. *Ethics, Jurisprudence and Practice Management.* (2nd ed.). Upper Saddle River, NJ: Prentice Hall, 2007.

Morris, W.O. *The Dentist's Legal Advisor.* St. Louis: Mosby, 1995.

Ozar, D.T. & Sokol, D.J. *Dental Ethics at Chairside.* (2nd ed.). Washington, DC: Georgetown University Press, 2002.

CHAPTER 14

Nathe, C. *Dental Public Health: Contemporary Practice for the Dental Hygienist* (2nd ed.). Upper Saddle River, NJ: Prentice Hall, 2005.

U.S. Department of Health and Human Services. *Healthy People 2010.* Hyattsville, MD: U.S. Department of Health and Human Services, National Center for Health Statistics, 2001.

U.S. Department of Health and Human Services. *Oral Health in America: A Report of the Surgeon General.* Rockville, MD: U.S. Department of Health and Human Services, National

Institute of Dental and Craniofacial Research, National Institutes of Health, 2000.

CHAPTER 15

American Association of Public Health Dentistry and American Board of Public Health: Dental public health: The past, present, and future. *J Am Dent Assoc* 117:171–76, 1988.

Burt, B.A. & Eklund, S.A. *Dentistry, Dental Practice, and the Community,* Philadelphia: W.B. Saunders, 1999.

Corbin, S.B. & Martin, F.R. The future of dental public health report—preparing dental public health to meet the challenges: Opportunities of the 21st century. *J Public Health Dent* 54:80, 1994.

Dean, H.T. The investigation of physiological effects by the epidemiological method. In: Moulton, F.R., ed: *Fluorine and Dental Health.* Washington, DC, American Association for the Advancement of Science, 1942, pp. 23–71.

Ferjerskov, H.S., et al. A new method for assessing the prevalence of dental fluorosis—the Tooth Surface Index of Fluorosis. *J Am Dent Assoc* 109:37–41, 1984.

Fisher, F.J. A field survey of dental caries, periodontal disease and enamel defects in Tristan da Cunha. *Br Dent J* 125:447–53, 1968.

Gluck, G.M. & Morganstein, W.M. *Jong's Community Dental Health* (4th ed.). St Louis: Mosby, 1998.

Greenstein, G. The role of bleeding upon probing in the diagnosis of periodontal disease. *J Periodontol* 55:684–88, 1984.

Klein, H., Palmer, C., & Knutson, J.W. Studies of dental caries. I. Dental status and dental needs of elementary school children. *Public Health Rep* 53:751–65, 1938.

Locker, D. & Slade, G.D. Association between clinical and subjective indicators of oral health status in older adult populations. *Gerontology* 11:108–14, 1994.

Nathe, C. *Dental Public Health: Contemporary Practice for the Dental Hygienist* (2nd ed.). Upper Saddle River, NJ: Prentice Hall, 2005.

Ramfjord, S.P. Indices for prevalence and incidence of periodontal disease. *J Periodontol* 30:51–59, 1959.

Russell, A.L. A system of scoring for prevalence surveys of periodontal disease. *J Dent Res* 35:350–59, 1956.

Takeuchi, M. Epidemiological study on dental caries in Japanese children before, during, and after World War II. *Int Dent J* 11:443–57, 1961.

CHAPTER 16

Darby, M. & Bowen, D. *Research Methods for the Oral Health Professionls: An introduction.* Pocatello, ID: JT McCann, 1986.

DeBiase, C. *Dental Health Education Theory and Practice.* Philadelphia: Lea & Febiger, 1991.

Index

Page numbers followed by *f* indicate figure; those followed by *t* indicate table.